Redfern's NURSING OLDER PEOPLE

Redfern's
NURSING
OLDER PEOPLE

FIFTH EDITION

Fiona M. Ross, BSc, PhD, RN, CBE
Professor Emerita in Health and Social Care
Kingston University

Ruth Harris, BSc (Hons), MSc, PhD, RN
Professor of Health Care for Older Adults
Care for Long Term Conditions Research Division
Florence Nightingale Faculty of Nursing, Midwifery & Palliative Care
King's College London

Joanne M. Fitzpatrick, BSc (Hons), PhD, RN, PGCEA
Reader in Older People's Healthcare
Care for Long Term Conditions Research Division
Florence Nightingale Faculty of Nursing, Midwifery & Palliative Care
King's College London

Clare Abley, BSc (Hons), MSc, PhD, RN, PGDL, PGCert Dementia Studies
Nurse Consultant Vulnerable Older Adults
The Newcastle upon Tyne Hospitals NHS Foundation Trust
Honorary Clinical Senior Lecturer
Institute of Population and Health Sciences
Newcastle University, Newcastle upon Tyne

ELSEVIER

ELSEVIER

© 2024, Elsevier Limited. All rights reserved.

First edition 1986
Second edition 1991
Third edition 1999
Fourth edition 2006

REDFERN'S NURSING OLDER PEOPLE
ISBN: 978-0-7020-8246-7

Notices

Practitioners and researchers must always rely on their own experience and knowledge in evaluating and using any information, methods, compounds or experiments described herein. Because of rapid advances in the medical sciences, in particular, independent verification of diagnoses and drug dosages should be made. To the fullest extent of the law, no responsibility is assumed by Elsevier, authors, editors or contributors for any injury and/or damage to persons or property as a matter of products liability, negligence or otherwise, or from any use or operation of any methods, products, instructions or ideas contained in the material herein.

Executive Content Strategist: Robert Edwards
Content Project Manager: Ayan Dhar

Printed in Bell & Bain Limited, Glasgow

Last digit is the print number: 9 8 7 6 5 4 3 2 1

CONTENTS

SECTION 4 Postscript: New Directions and Reflections on Caring for Older People

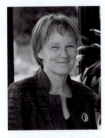

Fiona M. Ross is professor emerita in Health and Social Care at Kingston University, London. She has a background in community nursing and social policy and a longstanding interest in the care of older people. She was joint editor with Sally Redfern on the third and fourth editions of this book. Fiona has had senior roles at King's College London and St George's at the University of London and was dean at Kingston University and St George's. She has been director of research for the Leadership Foundation for Higher Education, director of education at the Academic Health Sciences Network, a non-executive on an NHS Trust board and chair of Princess Alice Hospice. Currently she is an independent governor on the Court of Westminster University.

Professor Fiona M. Ross, CBE, PhD, BSc, RN, DN

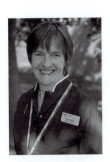

Clare Abley is a nurse consultant for vulnerable older adults at the Newcastle upon Tyne Hospitals NHS Foundation Trust and honorary clinical senior lecturer, Institute of Population and Health Sciences, Newcastle University. She has over 35 years of experience working with older people in both hospital and community settings in London, Cardiff and Newcastle and in 2000 was one of the first nurse consultants appointed in the UK. Most recently her work has focused on the care of people living with dementia. She is the Trust lead for dementia. In 2019 she completed an NIHR Clinical Lectureship to improve general hospital care for older people with cognitive impairment, which culminated in the Dementia Care Leaders' Toolkit. Link to Trust profile: https://www.newcastle-hospitals.nhs.uk/home/nmahps/our-strategy/improve-quality/dementia-care/clare-abley/

Dr Clare Abley PhD, MSc, BSc (Hons), RN, PGDL

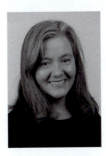

Ruth Harris is professor of Health Care for Older Adults at King's College London. She has a clinical background in acute medical nursing and the care of older people. She worked as a primary nurse in a King's Fund funded Nursing Development Unit and as the senior primary nurse/ward manager in a nursing-led intermediate care unit and acute care of older people ward. Her research focuses on understanding how complex nursing and interprofessional interventions contribute to healthcare delivery, patient outcome, and patient experience of care, particularly for older people and those with long-term conditions. Ruth is a member of the Editorial Board of the International Journal of Nursing Studies. For further information please see: https://www.kcl.ac.uk/people/ruth-harris

Professor Ruth Harris PhD, MSc, BSc (Hons), RN

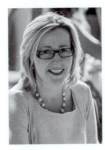

Joanne M. Fitzpatrick is a Reader in older people's health care at King's College London. Joanne graduated as a registered nurse (adult) with a BSc (Hons) from Ulster University before completing her PhD at King's College London and PGCEA at the University of Surrey. Joanne is an NMC registered nurse teacher. Joanne specialised in gerontological nursing. Her research focuses on health and social care of older people, particularly for those living in the care home sector, and workforce issues pertaining to nurses who care for older people. Joanne is a member of the editorial board for the *International Journal of Older People Nursing*. For further information, including her latest publications, visit: https://www.kcl.ac.uk/people/joanne-fitzpatrick

**Dr Joanne M. Fitzpatrick
BSc (Hons), PhD, RN, PGCEA**

Clare Abley, PhD, MSc, PGDL, BSc (Hons), RN
Nurse Consultant Vulnerable Older Adults
The Newcastle upon Tyne Hospitals NHS Foundation Trust
Newcastle upon Tyne
United Kingdom
Honorary Clinical Senior Lecturer
Institute of Population and Health Sciences
Newcastle University, Newcastle upon Tyne
United Kingdom

Richard Adams, PhD, RN
Chief Executive Officer
Sears Healthcare Ltd
Newbury, United Kingdom

Antony Arthur, BA (Hons), MSc, PhD
Professor Emeritus of Nursing Science
School of Health Sciences
University of East Anglia
Norwich, United Kingdom

Abigail Mary Barkham, PhD, BSc (Hons), RGN
Southern Health NHS Foundation Trust
Hampshire, United Kingdom
Visiting Fellow
Faculty of Health & Social Sciences
Bournemouth University
Dorset, United Kingdom

Jane Berg, RGN, DipDN, MSc, FHEA
Director of Skills Knowledge & Research
Education & Research
Princess Alice Hospice, Esher
Surrey, United Kingdom
Honourary Lecturer
Faculty of Health, Social Care and Education
Kingston University London
Surrey, United Kingdom

Christine Brown Wilson, PhD, BSc (Hons), PFHEA, RN
Professor Nursing (Education)
School of Nursing and Midwifery
Queen's University Belfast
Northern Ireland, United Kingdom

Caroline Chill, MBBS, DRCOG, DFSRH
Clinical Director for Healthy Ageing
Health Innovation Network
London, United Kingdom

Sarah Ann Cowley, DBE, BA, PhD, PGDE, RGN, RHV
Professor Emerita Dame
Faculty of Nursing and Midwifery
King's College London
London, United Kingdom

Jonathan Darley, MSci
Former Project Manager
Health Innovation Network
London, United Kingdom

Katie A. Davis, BN (Nursing), MSc, PhD, RN (Mental Health), FHEA
Lecturer in Mental Health Nursing
Nursing and Community Health
Glasgow Caledonian University
Glasgow, United Kingdom

Nisha Dhanda, BSc (Hons) Audiology, PG.Dip. Rehabilitative Audiology, MEd Learning and Teaching in Higher Education
Assistant Professor of Public Health
Institute of Applied Health Research
University of Birmingham
United Kingdom

Tommy Dickinson, PhD, RN, FEANS, ANEF, FAAN
Professor of Nursing Education & Head of Department of Mental Health Nursing
Florence Nightingale Faculty of Nursing, Midwifery and Palliative Care
King's College London
London, United Kingdom

Lindsay Dingwall, RN, BN Nursing & SQP (Adult Nursing), PG Cert THE, MRes
Clinical Care Quality Manager
Balhousie Care Group
Scotland, United Kingdom

Samantha Dorney-Smith, RN (Adult), BSc (Nursing), Specialist Practitioner (Practice Nursing), Nurse Prescriber
Nursing Fellow
Pathway
London, United Kingdom
Ad hoc Advisor
Homeless and Inclusion Health Programme
Queen's Nursing Institute
London, United Kingdom

Denis Duignan, BEng, MSc, PGCert, PGDip
Head of Digital Transformation and Technology
Health Innovation Network
London, United Kingdom

Margaret Dunham, PhD, MSc, BSc, RGN
Associate Professor in Nursing & Pain Management
School of Health & Social Care
Edinburgh Napier University
Edinburgh, United Kingdom

Heather M. Fillmore Elbourne, RN, PhD
Health Care Nurse Scientist
Independent Consultant
Halifax, Nova Scotia, Canada

Joanne M. Fitzpatrick, BSc (Hons), PhD, RN, PGCEA
Reader in Older People's Healthcare
Florence Nightingale Faculty of Nursing, Midwifery and Palliative Care
King's College London
London, United Kingdom

Brendan Garry, MSc, BSc, PgDip, PgCert, RN, DN, QN, RNT, MAcadMEd, SFHEA
Lecturer
Division of Nursing, Midwifery and Social Work
University of Manchester
Manchester, United Kingdom

Irene Gilsenan, MEd, BA (Hons), RGN, EN(G) Diploma in Education, Certificate in Education, ILM Level 3, D32/33, D34, ENB 998, 182, Post Grad Certificate in Clinical Audit
Practice Development Co-ordinator (Evidence Based Practice)
Learning, Education & Development
Sheffield Teaching Hospitals NHS Foundation Trust
Sheffield, United Kingdom

Dinah Gould, PhD, RN, RNT, FRCN
Independent Consultant
London, United Kingdom
Honorary Professor
City, University of London
United Kingdom

Laura Green, RN, PhD, MSc, BSc, Adv Dip (nursing), SFHEA
Lecturer in Adult Nursing
Division of Nursing, Midwifery and Social Work
University of Manchester
Manchester, United Kingdom

Sue M. Green, RN, PGCert, BSc, MedSci, PhD
Professor Nursing Science
Bournemouth University
Bournemouth, Dorset, United Kingdom

Nan Greenwood, BSc, MSc, PhD
Professor emerita
Faculty of Health, Social Care and Education
Kingston University and St George's University of London
London, United Kingdom

Jane Griffiths, PhD, BNurs, RN, DNCert
Senior Lecturer
Division of Nursing, Midwifery and Social Work
University of Manchester
Manchester, United Kingdom

Ruth Harris, RN, BSc (Hons), MSc, PhD
Professor of Health Care for Older Adults
Care for Long Term Conditions Research Division
Florence Nightingale Faculty of Nursing, Midwifery and Palliative Care
King's College London
London, United Kingdom

Rebecca Henry, MRPharmS, Dip Clin Pharm, Dip Psych Pharm, MCMHP, IP
School of Health Sciences
University of Southampton
Southampton, Hants, United Kingdom
Advanced Mental Health Pharmacist
Winchester Community Mental Health Team
Southern Health NHS Foundation Trust
Winchester, Hants, United Kingdom

Sharron Hinchliff, PhD, BSc (Hons)
Professor of Psychology and Health
Division of Nursing and Midwifery
University of Sheffield
Sheffield, United Kingdom

Maria Horne, PhD, MA (Health Research), BA (Hons), Dip Community Health Studies, SCPHN (HV), SCM, RGN, Queen's Nurse
Associate Professor in Community and Public Health (Queens Nurse)
School of Healthcare
University of Leeds
West Yorkshire, United Kingdom

Briony F. Hudson, PhD
Associate Director, Internal Research Development
Research and Policy Team
Marie Curie, London
United Kingdom
Honorary Research Fellow
Marie Curie Palliative Care Research Department
Division of Psychiatry
University College London
London, United Kingdom
Research Fellow
Pathway

Colin Hughes, BSc (Hons), Dip, MSc, RMN, SFHEA
Lecturer (Education) Mental Health
School of Nursing and Midwifery
Queens University
Belfast

Rebecca Jarvis, MA, BA, DGDip (Management)
Churchill Fellow
Former Director of Operations
Health Innovation Network
London, United Kingdom

Fenella Jolly, PgDip Women's Studies, RN
Clinical Nurse Manager
Health Inclusion Team – Homeless and HIU
Integrated Local Services
Guy's and St Thomas' NHS Foundation Trust
London, United Kingdom

Elizabeth Anne Keat, BSc (Hons) Specialist Community Public Health Nursing, RN, Queen's Nurse
Homeless Integration Lead
Leeds Community Healthcare NHS Trust
Leeds, United Kingdom

Rachel Kirby, MRCP, MBBS, BSc
Specialist Registrar
St Helens and Knowlsey Teaching hospitals, NHS Trust
Prescot, United Kingdom

Sue Latter, PhD, BSc (Hons), PGDipHV, RN
Professor of Health Services Research
School of Health Sciences
University of Southampton
Southampton, United Kingdom

Andree Christine le May, BSc (Hons), PhD, RGN, PGCE(A)
Professor emerita
School of Health Sciences
Univerisity of Southampton
Southampton, United Kingdom

Roy Litvin, BSc (Hons), MA, PGCE, RN, FHEA
Lecturer in Mental Health Nursing Education
Florence Nightingale Faculty of Nursing, Midwifery & Palliative Care
King's College London
London, United Kingdom

Daniel Marsden, RNLD, MSc, SCLD, FHEA
Senior Lecturer
School of Nursing
Canterbury Christ Church University, Chatham
Kent, United Kingdom
Honourary Senior Lecturer in Research
Kingston University
Surrey, United Kingdom

Caroline McGraw, RN, BSc (Hons), PGCert, PGDip, MSc, PhD
Honourary Research Fellow
School of Health and Psychological Sciences
City University, London
London, United Kingdom

Krishna Misra, MRCGP, MBBS, DRCOG, DFFP
Joint GP Clinical Lead, Asylum and Refugee Health Services
Health Inclusion Team
Guy's and St Thomas' NHS Foundation Trust
London, United Kingdom

Caroline Nicholson, PhD, Msc, BSc (Hons), RGN, FEHA
Professor of Palliative Care and Ageing
School of Health Sciences
University of Surrey, Guildford
Surrey, United Kingdom

Margaret Orange, Prof(Doc), MBA, MA (Mental Health), RMN
Associate Director (Addictions Governance)
Addiction Services
Cumbria, Northumberland, Tyne and Wear NHS
Foundation Trust, Newcastle Upon Tyne
United Kingdom

Joanne Paton, PhD, MSc, BSc
Associate Professor in Podiatry
School of Health Professions, Faculty of Health
University of Plymouth
Devon, United Kingdom

Gillian Elizabeth Pedley, PhD, MSc, BSc (Hons), PGCEA, RN, SFHEA
Associate Professor
Director for Workforce Development
School of Nursing
Faculty of Health, Social Care and Education
Kingston University and St George's University of London
London, United Kingdom

Bridget Penhale, BA, MSc
Reader Emerita in Mental Health of Older People
School of Health Sciences
University of East Anglia, Norwich
Norfolk, United Kingdom

Maria Teresa Ponto, PhD, MSc Health Psychology, BA Psychology, RN, RM
Associate Professor (Retired)
Faculty of Health, Social Care and Education
Kingston University, Kingston upon Thames
Surrey, United Kingdom

Rachel S. Price, RN (Mental Health), BSc, MSc, Specialist Practitioner, FHEA
Senior Lecturer
Manchester Metropolitan University
Manchester, United Kingdom

Helen Pryce, PD (Health), MSc, PGCert Hearing Therapy, BA(Hons)
Reader in Audiology
College of Health and Life Sciences
Aston University
Birmingham
United Kingdom

Edward Purssell, PhD, MSc (Microbiology), BSc, RN (Adult and Child)
Associate Professor
Faculty of Health, Education, Medicine and Social Care
Anglia Ruskin University
Chelmsford, United Kingdom

Raphael Rogans-Watson, MBBS, BSc, MRCP, DPMSA
Consultant Geriatrician and Physician
Royal Sussex County Hospital
Brighton
University Hospitals Sussex NHS Foundation Trust
West Sussex, United Kingdom
Clinical Research Fellow
Pathway
London, United Kingdom

Fiona M. Ross, CBE, BSc, PhD, RN
Professor emerita in Health and Social Care
Faculty of Health, Social Care and Education
Kingston University
London, United Kingdom

Patricia A. Schofield, PhD, RGN, PGDipEd
Professor of Clinical Nursing (Pain & Ageing)
School of Nursing and Midwifery (Faculty of Health)
University of Plymouth
Plymouth, United Kingdom

Caroline Shulman, MBBS, DCH, DRCOG, MRCGP, DTM&H, MSc, PhD
Clinical Lead
Homeless Health Programme
Healthy London Partnership
London, United Kingdom
Honorary Clinical Senior Lecturer
Marie Curie Palliative Care Research Department
Division of Psychiatry
University College London, London
United Kingdom
Senior Clinical Research Fellow
Pathway, London
United Kingdom

Fay Sibley, MSc, BSc
Former Head of Healthy Ageing
Health Innovation Network
London, United Kingdom

Tiago Manuel Horta Reis da Silva, BSc (Hons) (Nurs), BSc (Hons) (TCM), MBAcC, PGCertHE, PGDipHE, MSc, RN, FHEA
Lecturer in Nursing Education
Adult Nursing
Kings College London
London, United Kingdom
Lecturer
Traditional Chinese Medicine
Escuela Superior Medicina Tradicional China
Spain
Lecturer and Director of West Medicine Sciences
Traditional Chinese Medicine and West Medicine Sciences
Greece

Paul Simpson, PhD
Lecturer in Sociology, Arthur Lewis Building
University of Manchester, Oxford Road
Manchester, United Kingdom

Karen Spilsbury, PhD, RN
Professor
Chair in Nursing and Academic Director for Nurturing
Innovation in Care Home Excellence in Leeds
(NICHE-Leeds)
University of Leeds
Leeds, United Kingdom

Penelope Stanford, PhD, MSc, BSc (Hons), PGDE, RN, OND, RNT, SFHEA
Senior Lecturer
Division of Nursing, Midwifery and Social Work
University of Manchester
Manchester, United Kingdom

Emma Stanmore, PhD, MRes, BNurs (Hons), DN, RN
Reader
Division of Nursing, Midwifery and Social Work
University of Manchester
Manchester, United Kingdom

Vasiliki Tzouvara, BA, MSc, PhD, GMBPsS, FHEA
Lecturer in Mental Health
King's College London
Care for Long Term Conditions Research Division, FNMPC
57 Waterloo Road
London, United Kingdom

Emma Vardy, FRCP, PhD, PGDip, MBChB, BMedSci
Professor
Consultant Geriatrician
Northern Care Alliance NHS Foundation Trust
Salford, United Kingdom
Honorary Clinical Chair
Manchester Academic Health Science Centre
Faculty of Biology, Medicine and Health
University of Manchester
Manchester, United Kingdom

Christina Victor, BA, MPhil, PhD
Professor of Gerontology and Public Health
College of Health, Medical and Life Sciences
Brunel University London
Uxbridge, United Kingdom

Julie Whitney, PhD, MSc, BSc (Hons), MCSP
Lecturer in long term conditions and population health sciences
School of Life Course & Population Sciences
King's College London and Consultant
Practitioner in Gerontology
King's College Hospital
London, United Kingdom

Sue Woodward, RN, MSc, PGCEA, PhD, FRCN
Senior Lecturer
Florence Nightingale Faculty of Nursing, Midwifery and
Palliative Care
King's College London
London, United Kingdom

Janelle Yorke, PhD, MRES, RGN
Professor
School of Nursing, Midwifery and Social Work
University of Manchester
Manchester, United Kingdom;
Executive Chief Nurse
The Christie NHS Foundation Trust
Manchester, United Kingdom

PREFACE

I am honoured to be asked to write a preface to this new edition of *Nursing Older People*. A fifth edition is long overdue. The fourth was published in 2006, since when so much has changed in health and social care policy, practice and prevention of ill health. Now that I have joined the ranks of the book's client group, in age if not yet in poor health, I shall treasure the opportunity to acquire a copy of the fifth edition as a valuable reference to dip into when needed to help stave off future infirmities that creep up on me.

I am thrilled to see a new group of editors joining Fiona Ross for this new edition. I know them all as past students and colleagues and am delighted they have overtaken me in their growth and contribution to knowledge and practice in the care of older people. To be overtaken in your career by former students is, I believe, the highest reward a teacher can achieve.

This edition has been a huge undertaking for the editors and contributors in the amount of work required, needing to be rewritten and expanded. I am so pleased the emphasis on warm-bloodedness and person-centredness of previous editions continues. Nursing students and future practitioners will have a valuable resource to consult, for many years to come, before another edition is required as knowledge and policies change and evolve. The learning and practice outcomes derived from this book by nurses of the future will help them improve the quality of care for older people. In fact, many other practitioners who work in all areas of health and care for older people would also benefit from having access to a copy.

My best wishes to you all.
Sally Redfern
21 August 2022

Ageing and Old Age

Introduction

Fiona M. Ross, Ruth Harris, Joanne M. Fitzpatrick, Clare Abley

The fifth edition of *Nursing Older People* is a complete re-write. Our friend, colleague, inspiration and sometime teacher Sally Redfern has retired to Suffolk, so we are a new team. Sally Redfern was a pioneer and academic advocate for the highest quality of care for older people. She believed nurses should be both knowledgeable and understanding in their care, and her research was known internationally for its excellence and contribution to improving nursing practice.

Fiona Ross has assembled a strong new editorial team for the fifth edition: Ruth Harris, Joanne Fitzpatrick and Clare Abley. All are experts in gerontological nursing and currently active in the field as senior academics (Ruth and Joanne) and a nurse consultant with an academic appointment (Clare). We all worked with or were taught by Sally over the years at King's College London, and this book retains Sally's values and the warm-blooded, person-centred emphasis of the last edition. We are delighted to announce in honour of her enduring contribution, the book is now known as *Redfern's Nursing Older People.*

The approach and content of the book will be of interest and relevance to practitioners from all disciplines who work in a wide range of care settings for older people. Our aim is to convey the depth of knowledge needed to develop the complex and sometimes delicate skills required for nursing interventions and support of older people. Even though major advances have been made in health and social care and gerontological nursing, older people today continue to be among the least privileged of service users. We hope the accessible evidence-based information in this book will give practitioners the confidence to challenge the status quo and look for ways to improve the quality of care and thus seek to change that underprivileged status.

This introductory chapter outlines the scope and approach of the book and its focus on evidence-based care and the effectiveness of interventions that support independence in old age. The book takes a person-centred approach to understanding and meeting older people's needs and problems nurses and other practitioners deal with every day, such as to improve the difficulties faced by

problems of pain, immobility, breathlessness, eating and drinking and eliminating. This, therefore, is not a disease-centred book. Readers who expect to find information about treatments for common diseases in older people, such as mature-onset diabetes or hypertension, will be disappointed. For that kind of knowledge, we refer them to the many medical texts available.

Words are important and subject to changing fashion. In the preface to the third edition, we wrote about our reluctant decision to change the book's title from *Nursing Elderly People* to *Nursing Older People* to pre-empt criticism from readers who regard *elderly* as a pejorative word. That it has become so continues, in our view, to be cause for regret because of its pedigree and origins in the Anglo-Saxon word *eld*, which forms the root of words that convey wisdom on account of age and experience. An example is the term *alderman*, meaning an elected councillor in local government. We do not condone use of *the elderly* as a collective noun because of its erroneous and ageist assumption of homogeneity and denial of individual differences. It seems, though, that *elderly* has gone the way of *geriatrics*, another misused and banished word. Although we would prefer to use words in their original meaning, we have sustained this change by referring to senior citizens as older people. Older is not as specific as elderly because it is a relative term that applies to any age; a 5-year-old child is older than a 4-year-old. As underlined in the earlier editions, misuse of language is a serious issue because it creates stereotypes of identity and behaviour that have a powerful and often damaging effect on individuals so labelled. We are not suggesting words should never change; language naturally evolves over time. But when a collective term is needed—and some question whether one is ever needed—a return to the magnificent *elders* would be welcome and would help those of us who have not yet got there to recognise the wisdom of individuals who have and to learn from them.

The last edition was published in 2006. Much has changed in policy and nursing practice since then. We commissioned a new team of contributors for 15 chapters, and for most chapters the senior author is joined by other experts. Our writers are authorities in expert practice, have published in their field and are drawn from the disciplines of nursing, allied health professions, social sciences and medicine. There are new chapters on frailty, the use of alcohol as a growing problem in old age, digital technology and nursing older people with intellectual disabilities. We made the decision to embed core themes throughout rather than isolated in a separate chapter. For example, we encouraged contributors to cover diversity within their specialist areas. Similarly, assessment is embedded throughout and applied in a bespoke way in, for example, frailty, pressure ulcer prevention and medicine management. Again, it is part of our philosophy not to have a separate chapter on rehabilitation. Our view is rehabilitation is too huge a subject for any single chapter to do it justice. Instead, we see rehabilitation as a continuous thread that is more explicit in some chapters—on mobility, care of feet, hearing, sight, nutrition and elimination, for example. The book was written during the COVID-19 global pandemic. Therefore, we encouraged contributors to consider the impact in relation to their particular areas. In this way discussion of periods of acute infections, successive lockdowns and recovery are embedded throughout and illustrated, for example, in infection control, public health and the response of caregivers and experiences of care at the end of life.

This edition has other changes to make the material more accessible. We encouraged contributors to be selective and limit the number of references and where possible to cite review articles. Chapters mostly include, where appropriate, mini stories, case studies or fragments from the experience of ageing and nursing care to bring material to life. Chapters conclude with a summarised set of learning points.

Three sections and a postscript in this edition are arranged differently to the last edition. Section 1, on ageing and old age, contains four updated and rewritten chapters on what it means to be old, demographic and epidemiological trends in ageing, and the psychology and biology of human ageing. Chapter 2 explores the meaning of old age from biological, psychological, social and political perspectives. It draws on the sociological and gerontological literature to discuss influences of the life course on roles of older people in the family and society, integration and isolation, and intergenerational challenges. Chapter 3 updates information on demographic and epidemiological trends in ageing with particular emphasis on the four countries of the United Kingdom. Chapter 4 reviews psychological theories of ageing and discusses factors that influence successful ageing, adaptation and satisfaction in later life. It contains an additional section on the role of emotions in later life. Biological theories and mechanisms of ageing and the implications of physiological changes are covered

in Chapter 5. A new Chapter 6 on frailty and the important role nurses can play in its recognition, assessment and prevention is added to this edition.

Section 2 covers people, policy and the place of care in eight chapters. Chapter 7 reviews the major policy changes that have influenced health and social care service development and delivery for older people, including social care. The chapter also discusses citizenship and the role of older people in the policy-making process and policy response to meeting the needs of difference and diversity. Chapter 8, on healthy ageing and well-being, discusses public health as the context for prevention. It considers wider determinants of health and social care and inequalities in ageing, and it proposes models to guide nurses in practical action to improve health and well-being. The place of care is important for older people, and the next three chapters discuss community care, hospitals and independent living with options of extra care. Specifically, Chapter 9 reviews the organisation and use of community and primary care services by older people. Chapter 10 considers nursing care of older people in hospitals, including good practice in assessment and discharge processes as well as interventions to minimise the risk of adverse outcomes of hospitalisation, in particular deconditioning, falls and delirium. In Chapter 11 care homes are described as nurse-led units and the homes of people first that seek to support individuals to live full, meaningful and engaging lives while managing a range of physical, psychological, cognitive or mental health needs. The contribution of care home nurses as critical thinkers, autonomous practitioners and dynamic leaders is discussed. The final three chapters in this section review the evidence and experience of specific challenges for some older people and caregivers. Chapter 12 discusses the role of nursing in supporting better health care for older people who are homeless or marginalised from society, paying attention to questions of complex health conditions, inclusion, access to mainstream services and routes out of homelessness. In Chapter 13 the role and needs of informal unpaid carers looks at the emotional, psychological and financial costs and questions nurses should ask in assessment. The final chapter in this section discusses abuse and safeguarding and issues nurses should be alert to as well as the boundaries of accountability, confidentiality and when to raise concerns.

Section 3, on nursing care of older people, emphasises independence, autonomy and self-fulfilment. It contains 21 chapters, new ones on alcohol use, older people with intellectual disabilities and the role of technology and digital tools in the care and support of older people. The rest are substantially updated or completely rewritten by new authors. Chapter 15 focuses on the factors that shape and influence communication between older people and nurses, challenges older people face and strategies caregivers can use to improve their communication skills. Chapter 16 continues the discussion of communication with particular focus on the experiences of older people living with hearing impairment and disability. The chapter highlights the stigma of deafness, describes assessment of hearing loss in some detail and shows what can be done to help people manage their hearing loss by using personal and environmental aids and behavioural tactics to maximise communication and interaction. Chapter 17 addresses the concepts of ocular anatomy and physiology, common eye conditions, the impact of visual impartment and ultimately how to support the well-being of older people in whatever health care context. Promoting safe mobility is discussed in Chapter 18, which considers the effects of ageing on the musculoskeletal system, risks associated with mobility, long-term conditions, assessment and management with a focus on preventing falls and promoting safe mobility. Chapter 19 continues the theme of mobility by addressing caring for feet. Nurses have an important role in promoting and educating older people about preventive self-foot care. People with breathing problems have mobility difficulties, too, and Chapter 20 highlights the normal pathophysiological changes associated with breathing in older people and shows what can be done to assess and improve the quality of life for individuals with breathing difficulties, particularly due to chronic airway disease, pneumonia and COVID-19.

Chapter 21, on eating and drinking, covers the many factors that influence food and fluid intake in older people, malnutrition and good nutritional care, including assessment. As we see in Chapter 22, many older people are at risk of less-than-perfect control over their elimination. It is a nursing responsibility to assess each individual and then to plan care in collaboration with other members of the multidisciplinary team. That care should attempt to remedy any bladder or bowel problem and to maximise the individual's ability to cope with elimination in a continent manner. In this area nurses can make a significant contribution to the comfort, dignity and well-being of individuals who come into their care.

Infection prevention and control and thermoregulation in older people are the topic of Chapter 23, which incorporates the risks of infection, the principles of infection prevention applied to older people and how to manage thermoregulatory challenges. The COVID-19 pandemic highlighted the importance of prevention of infection, especially for high-risk groups such as older people. In Chapter 24 the care and maintenance of healthy skin in ageing is discussed from the perspective of the best evidence-based practice. It includes the assessment, management and prevention of pressure ulcers and wound care. Sleep and rest are of paramount importance to the restoration of health and maintenance of

well-being but can be disturbed by many factors in later life. This is often overlooked by nurses and other practitioners. Chapter 25 discusses the physiological, psychological and social components of sleep, evidence-based interventions for nursing and practical strategies that may make a difference to the comfort and rest of older people.

Sexuality and relationships in later life are the subject of Chapter 26, which highlights that relationships, sexual expression and intimacy remain important aspects of older people's lives. As we learn in this chapter, addressing these issues is a central tenet of nursing older people; crucial to this, it is imperative to foster a climate where permission to discuss sexuality and intimacy is implicit in care settings, care processes and practice. Pain, the subject of Chapter 27, is often assumed to be an inevitable consequence of old age because of the prevalence of chronic disease and multiple pathology, but this need not be so. Thorough individualised assessment and appropriate treatment with a range of pharmacological and non-pharmacological interventions can lead to a pain-free life or one where quality of life is enhanced.

Delirium and care of the older person living with dementia are addressed in Chapters 28 and 29, respectively. Delirium is a commonly occurring but poorly understood and underrecognised condition. Using clinical and biographic knowledge alongside assessment tools, nurses can play a central role in detecting, treating and preventing delirium to improve outcomes for older people. Dementia is more complex. It can affect memory, orientation, thinking, comprehension, language, learning capacity and judgement. Chapter 29 shows the experience of living with dementia can be challenging for individuals who live with the condition and those who provide care, but evidence suggest personalised dementia care can reduce these challenges and enhance quality of life. Likewise, nurses can do much to improve the quality of life of older people living with depression, the subject of Chapter 30. Though very common in older people, depression often goes undetected. Nurses have a major role in its identification, assessment, management and prevention. General nursing approaches and specific evidence-based therapies such as cognitive behavioural psychotherapy and interpersonal therapy are covered in this chapter.

Chapter 31, on medicine management, covers evidence and best knowledge of risks for older people in polypharmacy, drug interactions, medicine management errors and near misses and the nurse's role in safeguarding procedures. It emphasises the need to start low and go slow when prescribing new medications and the importance of reviewing medication regularly for indications, interactions, adverse drug reactions, adherence and appropriate dosage, including dose reduction. It includes the development in current thinking toward shared decision making with older people and the role of nurses in prescribing and medicine management. Chapter 32, on alcohol use, begins by outlining the history and policy context as well as the prevalence of alcohol problems in old age. The chapter then focuses on the effective management of alcohol use, providing in-depth information on both assessment and intervention. The notion alcohol use in the ageing population should be everybody's business and not dealt with solely by specialist mental health/drug and alcohol services, as has been the case in the past, is emphasised in this chapter. A new chapter in this section recognises the growing number of people with an intellectual disability who are living into older age. Drawing on contemporary debates and new research, Chapter 33 frames discussion of evolving needs, the importance of supporting independence and planning for the future. Chapter 34 considers end-of-life care, dying, bereavement and loss and shows how nurses can support dying people and their families, making this final phase of living a positive experience. Finally, this section has a new chapter on the role of technology and digital tools in the care and support of older people. This is an important and rapidly changing field nurses need to keep abreast of. Digital literacy accelerated at pace during the pandemic as final goodbyes to the dying were said using tablets and phones. Inevitably by the time this book is published, new devices and digital interventions will have come into the mainstream and may have overtaken some of the material here. But fundamental issues such as digital exclusion for some older people as a factor determining inequalities will not become dated and should remain on the agenda.

We conclude the book with our reflections in a post-script. This gives us an opportunity to draw together and reflect on themes that run throughout the book and provide pointers to future action. Throughout the narrative we intersperse photographs, extracts from literature and poetry and stories that highlight our themes. We set out to draw attention to important issues for older people: images of ageing, the importance of valuing personal relationships, balancing rights and risk-taking, rehabilitation, empowerment and involvement of older people. We discuss key issues for workers, including interprofessional working, specialist roles for nurses who work with older people, education and the importance of ensuring service-user perspectives in evaluating high-quality care.

We hope you enjoy this book as a useful and stimulating contribution to the development of services for older people and their families and friends that will improve both their experiences and clinical outcomes of care.

ACKNOWLEDGEMENTS

We are forever grateful to Sally Redfern for encouraging us to do a fifth edition and writing the preface. Our sincere thanks to all those who have written chapters, sharing their knowledge and expertise on a wide selection of topics important in the care of older people. We thank our families and friends for inspiration, support and keeping us going and those who have generously contributed photos. Finally thank you to the Elsevier team and in particular Veronica Watkins, who started us off, and more recently Ayan Dhar, who patiently worked with us on the production.

What Is Old Age?

Christina Victor

This chapter considers some of the background issues relevant to nursing older people. We first consider definitions of old age, followed by consideration of the stereotypes and attitudes that are commonly held about both old age and the ageing process. Finally, we consider some of the methodological approaches used to study ageing.

WHAT IS OLD AGE?

What is old age? When does it start? These apparently simple questions are, in reality, rather complex, and the answers not as straightforward as might be expected. In this section we look at the main approaches to the definition of old age. The term *OLD AGE*, sometimes referred to as *SENESCENCE*, is often used to describe the last stage of the normal lifespan. This definition is of limited utility as it does not define the attributes that identify old age or describe the criteria that make it distinct from other phases of life. Looking at research, policy and practice, we can identify three main approaches to the identification and definition of old age. Each of these is discussed briefly. This short review illustrates the very arbitrary way in which old age is defined and counsels us to be cautious about how such terms are used in research, policy and practice.

BIOLOGICAL AGEING

The study of the biological aspects of ageing is discussed in detail in Chapter 5. The main point to note here is there is no readily available, easy-to-operationalise measure or biological definition of old age. Hence all the definitions we tend to use in research, policy development and the provision of services are essentially indirect and largely socially constructed. As such they have only a very tenuous relationship to the biological ageing of both individuals and populations. It is therefore important that all those who work with older people or with specialist services for older people recognise the fundamentally arbitrary nature of the definitions used to identify and define their client group and the fluidity of such definitions culturally and historically.

Normal ageing is characterised by progressive and irreversible changes in both structure and function with time (Kirkwood, 2005). Age-related changes (termed *SENESCENCE*) are not observed in all biological populations because of the influence of disease or predatory action. Some populations do not live long enough to grow old. Within a given population, the chance (or probability) of death increases with age. Put another way, the percentage of survivors from a given population decreases with time; this form of analysis is known as survivorship analysis. In other words, there is an increasing chance or probability of death with age. This type of analysis illustrates two important concepts in ageing research: maximum lifespan and life expectancy.

Maximum lifespan is best defined as the greatest age a member of a population can attain under optimal conditions. It remains a matter of contention as to whether there is a maximum lifespan for humans and what this 'theoretical maximum' could be (Kirkwood, 2005). The longest verified lifespan is that of Jeanne Calment (1875–1997), a French woman who lived to 122. Life expectancy is the number of years an individual can expect to live from a given time point. Expectation of life is often calculated from birth but can be calculated from any age (e.g., expectation of life from, for example, age 60). Life expectancy varies between and within populations and over time. In the United Kingdom, life expectancy at birth has increased by approximately 31 years for men and 33 years for women, to 79 and 83 years, respectively, since 1900. This is largely due to increased infant survival resulting from improvements in public health such as the control of common infectious diseases. The continuation of such improvements is not inevitable. For example, early estimates for the United Kingdom and United States suggest the excess mortality from COVID-19 has reduced life expectancy at birth by a year (Marois et al., 2020).

CHRONOLOGICAL AGE

The most widely used marker of old age is chronological age, or the length of time from birth a person has lived, usually counted in years. Age is extensively used across societies as a social regulator. We use age to determine when children must start formal education, obtain a driver's licence, hold criminal responsibility, vote, marry or purchase alcohol. However, there is no unanimity across countries—although we may infer it over time—in the chronological ages used to define when people can or must undertake particular activities. Furthermore, we can use chronological age as a social differentiator only when there is a reliable and comprehensive system for recording and authenticating age, usually via universal birth and death registration systems. For example, in England and Wales the formal registration of births and deaths was introduced on July 1, 1837.

Most biological and physiological parameters show a gradual age-related decline rather than a clear break point at which we could identify old age. The chronological age used to define old age is largely arbitrary, with both cultural and temporal variations. It is rooted in the cultural values and norms of each society. One example is the definition of old age based around eligibility for health and social welfare benefits such as retirement pensions. This approach to the definition of old age relates it to participation in the formal labour market and formal retirement policies (Phillipson, 1998). Age of eligibility for pensions has become a prevalent proxy, albeit a rather arbitrary one, for the onset of old age. Consequently, in the United Kingdom, old age was often considered to start at 60 for women and 65 for men. However, the abolition of compulsory retirement brought a focus on extending working lives and equalisation of retirement policies. One interesting area of research is the relationship—or lack of—between chronological age and how old people perceive themselves, a concept known as subjective age identity. Individuals may not perceive themselves as being old despite having achieved a specified number of calendar years. For example, a woman in her mid-40s may be defined by others as 'middle-aged' (or by the medical profession as premenopausal), yet she may still consider herself 'young' and entirely reject this view. Disjunction between chronological and felt age may have its roots in our negative views of ageing and a reluctance of older people to accept a stigmatised and damaged identity (see Pickard, 2016). However, it does have implications for nurses, as it means 'the old lady' for whom they are caring may not accept this label and not respond positively to being addressed as such.

Given the diversity of the population in terms of race, class and gender, we cannot presume comparable health status and health care needs across people of the same chronological age. For example, Nazroo (2017) shows the least-affluent third of the population aged 50 or older experiences levels of frailty equivalent to those 10 or more years older in the most-affluent third. The issue of the diversity of the ageing experience and the heterogeneous nature of the older population is examined further in Chapter 3 (see also Gilleard & Higgs, 2020; Pickard & Robinson, 2019; Torres, 2020). The imprecise relationship between chronological age and biological ageing has implications for the development and provision of health services for older people (Chapter 7). Services for older people that use chronological age as an entry criterion use only a very crude proxy measure for biological ageing and health care needs. While such decisions are pragmatic, the limitations implicit in these approaches require acknowledgement.

OLD AGE AS A STAGE IN THE LIFE CYCLE

The idea that life is divided into a series of distinct stages or phases is not new or confined to the academic community. It was common in the Middle Ages to divide the lifespan into a series of phases and to allocate individuals to a phase according to their age. In *As You Like It*, Shakespeare describes the classic 'seven ages' of man, with old age as a distinct phase, while Erikson proposed eight phases (see Pickard, 2016). With this life-cycle approach, chronological age is loosely related to each of the phases; hence we can both classify the life course and divide the population into approximate age groups. This approach is pervasive and forms part of popular discourse about how individuals make sense of the pattern of their lives. Research has shown people have clear ideas as to how major role transitions, such as marriage, parenthood or retirement, relate to some 'ideal' chronological age and how their own life has followed or deviated from this ideal pattern, as evidenced by such common statements as 'I married early (or late)' or 'I had my children (child) late (or early)'.

However, again, problems persist with the life-cycle approach that are not just theoretical or conceptual. For example, it is difficult to operationalise this type of definition of old age. How do the stages relate to specific chronological ages? It is not always clear that the phases are sequential and that an individual should progress in a linear fashion through each segment; neither can we presume a homogeneous pattern across different subgroups within a population or across populations. One development in the life-cycle approach to the study and definition of ageing has been the identification of the third and fourth ages. (Neugarten 1974) was the first to draw the distinction between the 'young old' (up to about 75 years) and the 'old old' (over 75 years). This segmentation of later life, or old age, has reappeared as the third and fourth ages proposed by (Laslett 1991). The third age is seen as a time of opportunity and activity. People are typified as mature adults freed from child-care and labour-market responsibilities and who have sufficient resources to take advantage of this 'free' time. In contrast, the fourth age is seen as final dependence, decrepitude and death. Empirically it is clear the experience of old age is much more complex than the simple divisions into third and fourth ages (see Higgs & Gilleard, 2015).

Theoretical Perspectives on Old Age

The theoretical basis for social gerontology is limited. Much of the focus of gerontological research has been on the documentation of the 'facts' about ageing rather than theoretical development. However, a number of theoretical concepts and developments have influenced the nature and content of the study of ageing, and these have implications for the provision of nursing and other services for older people. These major theoretical perspectives are briefly outlined and the key assumptions underlying them presented. Identification of the values and assumptions that underpin research concerned with ageing and other areas is important because it highlights the limitations of the way research questions are posed and answered—or why they are asked in the first place. More discussion of theories of ageing is found in Chapter 4.

STRUCTURAL–FUNCTIONALIST THEORIES

Structural–functionalist theories operate at the macro, or societal, level. The basic unit of analysis is society, which is conceived as a set of interrelated parts, or social institutions or structures, that are integrated into a relatively stable structure. These parts are studied both as individual components and as elements for the maintenance of society. It is assumed each element of the system has functional consequences for society overall. From this perspective, it is the task of researchers to analyse the individual social elements, their relationship to other parts and the role they play in preserving society. The structural–functionalist perspective has been influential in the area of ageing research with two important theories, activity theory and disengagement theory, that are essentially functionalist in nature. Other theories from this tradition, but not considered for reasons of space, include modernization theory, role transition theory, continuity theory and social integration theory. A key element of the functionalist perspective is the emphasis on maintaining equilibrium, which neglects the important areas of social change and social conflict. Furthermore, this research perspective accords little power to individuals; rather, they are theorised as passive social actors.

THEORIES FOCUSED ON INDIVIDUAL ADAPTATION

(Havinghurst 1961) developed the activity theory of ageing, which, at its most reductionist, states that adjustment, or adaptation, is the key concern of individuals as they age and is best achieved by those who adapt to ageing by remaining as active as they were in midlife. Such activity could be achieved either by maintaining pre-existing roles or activities or by adopting new ones. The underlying premise of this perspective is a positive relationship between activity and life satisfaction. Social and health policies derived from the activity theory of ageing stress activity and interaction as the vehicles for 'successful ageing' (Rowe & Kahn, 1997).

(Cumming and Henry 1961) developed disengagement theory, which is diametrically opposed to the implicit assumptions of the activity theorists, who strongly believe activity, engagement and involvement are the keys to successful ageing. Disengagement theory proposes successful ageing, for both the society and the individual, is best achieved by the progressive reduction of social roles and relationships with age and the withdrawal of older individuals from society. This facilitates a smooth transfer of power to the young with a minimum of disruption to society as a whole. From this perspective, disengagement is seen as necessary because of the inevitability of death, the presumed decline in abilities with age, the value placed on youth and the need for society to continue to function efficiently. To age successfully, the individual is required to reduce activity and involvement and hand over responsibility to the next generation. At the same time the individual withdraws from society, society also withdraws from the individual.

The third theory, continuity theory, argues that as people grow older, they maintain, as far as possible, habits, behaviours and lifestyles adopted in earlier ages (Atchley, 1989). If activities are dropped, continuity theorists argue, it is because of personal limitations or external barriers rather than a direct choice of individuals to disengage.

There are problems with these approaches to the study of ageing. Activity theory makes the not-easily-empirically-verified assumption that old age is a time of psychological and social adjustment. It presumes people have the resources to reconstruct or maintain middle-aged lifestyles or to substitute new roles for older, lost roles in later life. This does not allow for individuals who cannot replace roles, either because of resource limitations or because they are not easily replaced (e.g., widowhood). It has been demonstrated that older people can demonstrate high satisfaction without maintaining high levels of activity or in the face of declining levels of activity (Victor, 2005). Disengagement—as indicated by variables such as widowhood or retirement—is not often voluntary, inevitable or universal. The term *disengagement* is not defined and can be subject to variability of interpretation; one person's disengagement may be another's engagement and activity. What is the reference point against which disengagement is measured?

Both activity and disengagement theory assume the solution to the social problem of ageing is successful ageing achieved by different routes. These two approaches assume a consensus as to what constitutes successful ageing that in reality does not exist, and both are highly prescriptive and value-laden and do not take into account the diversity of the experience of ageing. Furthermore, such approaches to ageing, and indeed the whole orientation of research aimed at identification and definition of successful ageing, can be used to blame older people for the often marginal condition they find themselves in. The logic of these approaches is that older people are in poor circumstances because they have not been successful in adapting to the challenge of ageing, conveniently unrelated to the provision of support and benefits for older people.

The activity and disengagement approaches to old age are concerned with adaptation at the individual level. Age stratification theory, although still an essentially functionalist approach concerned with social integration, operates at the collective level. This perspective views age as a universal criterion for the allocation of social roles (Riley et al., 1972). Age is conceptualised as the crucial factor in the allocation of social roles and the accompanying rights and privileges. The focus of attention is on relationships between and within different age strata. People are divided according to chronological age or life stage, such as middle aged or young, or in terms of cohort experiences, such as baby boomers. Each stratum can then be analysed in terms of the roles played and the value ascribed to such roles by society. Again this is a limited approach. Its key assumptions are that vertical stratification is inherent in all social systems, and the inequalities created as a result of this stratification are both inevitable and politically acceptable. Again the heterogeneous nature of this approach does not encapsulate the diversity of older people or explicitly recognise the importance of class, gender and ethnicity.

CONFLICT THEORY

Conflict theory operates at a macro, rather than an individual, level. Conflict theory is concerned with the ways social structures and social change affect ageing at both individual and collective levels. Researchers who study this theoretical perspective are of the view that conflict and instability are central to social life and are the prime factors in the organization of people into groups. As such, conflict theory places emphasis on what divides groups rather than the values they share.

Inequality theory argues the inequalities characteristic of other stages of life are maintained in later life. Those who were poor in midlife remain so in old age, while the wealthy maintain their privileged lifestyle. One exemple of this approach in the field of gerontology is the notion of structured dependency, which argues the dependency of older people so frequently documented is 'socially constructed' (Townsend, 1981). This theory is concerned with how and why society restricts the life chances of older people via institutions such as retirement and pensions. These are tools for the management of the economy but ones Townsend (1981) argues resulted in the marginalization and dependence of older people. He also argues we must recognise the potential conflicts of interest between older people and the not so old, especially over the allocation of scarce health and social welfare resources—for example, the so-called intergenerational conflict. Critiques of inequality theory have largely focused on the dominance of economic factors, give little credit to other influences, are highly deterministic and suggest older people are compelled or coerced into particular positions, all of which give the impression of a conspiracy theory applied to social policy.

INTERPRETATIVE THEORIES

Interpretative theories operate at the microsociological level and assume choice, or free will, is the most basic aspect of human behaviour. They focus on social interaction within specific settings and view communication—usually language—as key to the understanding and analysis of society. The focus is on understanding the way individuals perceive their world and others in it and the meaning they attribute to these experiences. For example, explanations for the care of older people by their families from this perspective would investigate the meaning of such terms as OBLIGATION, DUTY and RESPONSIBILITY and look at how caregiving is negotiated between the parties involved rather than as response to external social norms (a functionalist perspective). The main criticism of interpretative approaches is the level of analysis. Interpretative theories are often concerned with the minute details of daily life rather than dealing with the large-scale structures and processes of society. However, micro-level approaches can be very illuminating tools when studying the process of care and caregiving.

It is evident from what we have looked at so far that no single theoretical approach may be universally applied to the study of ageing. For all its limitations, biological work in ageing has been very influential in the development of ageing research. Within the fields of medicine and nursing, in particular, the biomedical approach has been enormously influential. This approach to the study of ageing has concentrated on determining physiological and biological explanations of ageing and the health of older people. However, the biomedical approach denies the importance of psychological or social factors in determining people's health experience or other aspects of ageing. No account is taken of factors such as class, gender and ethnicity in explaining the existence of disease and illness or in the utilization of health services. The pre-eminence of the biomedical approach has resulted in the relative neglect of issues such as health promotion and prevention in favour of an emphasis on illness, treatment and management. Furthermore, by denying the importance of social and psychological factors in understanding ageing, we portray the individual as a passive entity who has little influence on the events that happen to them.

The experience of ageing is not a fixed and inevitable consequence of chronological age. Rather, it is a multifaceted experience that results from the complex interrelationship between psychological, social and biological variables. Rowe and Kahn (1997) argue social factors may be more important than biological or genetic factors in influencing the quality of later life. This complexity needs to be recognised in the enterprise of ageing research, which is almost always multidisciplinary in nature.

Old Age: Attitudes, Myths and Stereotypes

A stereotype is a caricature-type summary of the attributes, positive or negative, of specific social groups, such as older people, adolescents or asylum-seekers, which can be descriptive or prescriptive (Centre for Ageing Better, 2020). Descriptive stereotypes focus on the characteristics of specific groups and can be negative—for example, old people are unable to learn new skills like using smartphones—or positive, such as older people are more polite. Prescriptive stereotypes focus on expectations about how specific groups should or should not behave. For example, older people shouldn't live in three-bedroom houses but should move into smaller houses to make way for families to occupy larger ones. Importantly, stereotypes influence how we respond to and interact with people, such as the infantilisation of older people and considering old age as a second childhood. Applying labels to older people, such as DEPENDENT, can stigmatise them and serves to marginalise them from wider society. This can influence how older adults behave if their behaviour is being monitored for signs of physical or mental decline and the challenge for the older person is to maintain independence and social competence. Negative images of older people may discourage nurses from entering gerontological nursing because of stigma by association.

One important manifestation of the negative stereotyping of older people has been the development of the notion of ageism. Like racism and sexism, ageism implies wholesale stereotyping and discrimination against a specific subgroup in society. Ageism describes discrimination against people simply on the basis of their chronological age, not just old age, and may be implicit or explicit. Explicit ageism is protected by law. Abrams et al. (2015) described societal attitudes toward older people as demonstrating 'benign indifference', meaning ageism is indirect rather than direct. In a range of forums, policy, practice and media, older people are often represented as a burden because of the largely deficit-focused representation of old age. Terms such as the GREY TSUNAMI, the DEMOGRAPHIC TIMEBOMB or the RISING TIDE OF DEMENTIA largely represent older people as a burden rather than as the triumph that population ageing represents. One consequence of the burden/deficit narrative is the creation of intergenerational conflict between younger and older people, as illustrated in some debates about the management of COVID-19 and discussion about how to raise money from taxes to support improvement in social care. However, older people are not simply defined by their age but also class, gender and ethnicity.

Sontag (1978) used the term DOUBLE STANDARD, or jeopardy of ageing, to describe the double disadvantages experienced by older women in terms of health and other resource outcomes such as behavioural norms and expectations. Other developments of this perspective include the triple jeopardy felt by older adults from minority communities who experience the disadvantages of age, racism and low socioeconomic status. These perspectives encompass ideas around intersectionality—in other words, ageing is shaped by intersecting characteristics like age, gender, ethnicity and socioeconomic status. To fully understand health and well-being outcomes in old age, we need to examine these characteristics in combination rather than individually.

Methodological Issues in the Study of Ageing

As well as being theoretically and conceptually challenging, the study of later life and ageing is methodologically challenging. In this section we examine some of the key methodological issues and approaches the student of ageing should be familiar with (see Luszczyńska, 2020). We focus identify the key challenges specific to ageing research and relevant methodological issues.

IDENTIFYING AGE DIFFERENCES

Observed differences between people of different age groups in, for example, cognitive function may arise either because of ageing (i.e., they are age effects) or other reasons, such as cohort or period effects—or, even more confusing, some combination of these. This serves to emphasise that practitioners need to be very cautious in inferring patients' problems are due to their age or because of ageing.

Age Effects

Strehler (1982) proposed four criteria for observed biological changes to be classed as part of age effects—in other words, part of normal ageing rather than pathological or disease process:

Universal: The change happens to everyone regardless of their ethnicity, social and physical environment.

Progressive: Onset is gradual rather than the result of an acute or catastrophic event.

Intrinsic: The change should be the result of natural processes rather than harmful environmental exposures.

Deleterious: The change reduces the ability of the person to cope.

Hence for dementia—or grey hair or wrinkles—to be a true age effect, it should happen to everyone. The requirement for universality in particular is an important way of distinguishing pathology from ageing. Most of the health problems and disease older people experience are often tritely attributed to ageing, which, given the test of universality, is palpably untrue. In the field of social gerontology,

universality, progressiveness and deleteriousness are important tests for the veracity of an observed age difference (in, for example, loneliness) to be accepted as a true age effect.

COHORT EFFECTS

Cohort effects reflect the influence of historical time and are attributes specific to a particular generation or cohort. As well as being defined by age, cohorts may be defined on the basis of social class, ethnicity or other variables. A good example of cohort effect was the very high number of never-married women that resulted from the high death rate in men in the United Kingdom during World War I. Will the baby boomer generation, who are the children of the post-war welfare state, present a similar profile when they reach old age? We cannot answer with any degree of certainty. We must always be aware that the patterns and problems seen among older people today may reflect cohort rather than age effects and, as such, may not be repeated by subsequent generations.

PERIOD EFFECTS

Period, or time, effects result from wholesale societal changes in circumstances or attitudes. For example, COVID-19 had an impact across society, including limitations on social engagement, curtailed education and loss of employment. Period effects can be difficult to differentiate from cohort effects. It is often hard to establish whether age, period or cohort differences or some combination of these is responsible for observed age differences. The simple observation of age differences, such as the reluctance of older people to engage digitally or learn to use computers, may reflect a real decrease in the ability of older people to learn new skills because of reductions in blood supply to the brain (age effect), the limited education received by older people (cohort effect) or the widespread availability and familiarity of computers within modern society, from which older people have been excluded (period effect).

Approaches to the Study of Ageing

What types of research design are used to determine and describe age differences? Irrespective of the research question (e.g., evaluating diet and health status, or describing attitudes toward retirement or grandparenting), two main types of study design are used in the study of ageing and the identification of age-based differences.

CROSS-SECTIONAL STUDIES

Cross-sectional studies involve comparing people of different ages at the same point in time on a variable of interest.

For example, you might investigate loneliness among different age groups. A cross-sectional study would survey people aged 45–54, 55–64, 65–74, and 75 years and over at a single point in time. This approach can demonstrate differences between age groups but not unambiguously determine whether they represent the result of ageing, as you would not be able to differentiate age, cohort or period differences. Numerous examples of cross-sectional studies have documented age differences within the population. An example from the United Kingdom is the Health Survey for England, which includes a wealth of health-related data about all age groups within the population.

LONGITUDINAL STUDIES

Longitudinal studies involve individuals who, after initial identification, are followed over time. Researchers take repeated measurements for the variables of interest. For example, you could first identify a group of 50-year-olds, then follow them every 5 years to collect further data. This very powerful research tool has been used to look at development, especially child development, over time (see NCDS website). It is the most scientifically rigorous way to study ageing but is expensive and difficult to administer. Loss to follow-up because of death, refusal or inability to trace subjects is a major methodological problem, as the sample may become less representative of the population or biased because of the systematic exclusion of particular groups, such as the very frail or very fit. Loss of follow-up limits the inferences that can be drawn from the study. There are more technical limitations to this approach, as study participants may become familiar with the testing regimen because of repeated exposure to the measurement techniques. Consequently, longitudinal studies can be compromised because of selection effects (i.e., loss of sample members), history effects (i.e., the events individuals experience between testing periods) and testing effects (i.e., the result of repeated exposure to the testing regimen). Further, it is not clear if longitudinal studies, which are usually based on a single cohort, are generalisable. To overcome selection effects, researchers can add refreshment samples. In the United Kingdom there are three longitudinal studies of ageing for England, Scotland and Northern Ireland. These are modelled on a health and retirement survey from the United States, thereby enabling comparison of ageing in different countries.

CONCLUSION AND LEARNING POINTS

The terms *OLD PEOPLE*, *OLDER* and *GERIATRICS* are widely used in popular and professional discourse. In this chapter we demonstrated the conceptual and methodological complexity that underpins these apparently simple, and highly pejorative, terms. There is no good, easily available definition of old age. Nurses and other health professionals need to recognise the highly arbitrary and socially constructed way such groups are defined and labelled. An influential view of older adults in the development of British gerontological research work is the concept of old age, and older people, as a social problem. At its most basic, this perspective has concentrated on identifying and enumerating the problems experienced in old age (a humanitarian approach) and on the burden this poses for society (an institutional perspective). Work in these areas has concentrated on looking at health and service issues, especially quality of life, health status and use of services, as well as retirement and employment. Viewing older people as a problem is concerned with determining the burden they pose for society as well as individuals. Numerous studies exist of who provides care and help to older people but comparatively few about how much help older people provide to other older people or younger family members (e.g., collecting children from school so their parents can work). The view of older people as a burden has influenced the types of questions posed and the knowledge base of British gerontology. For example, work on loneliness and old age has presumed loneliness is a problem unique to older people and has sought to establish the prevalence and risk factors for loneliness. It is only recently that researchers have sought to include the views of older people in investigating the factors that protect against loneliness. In fact, in cross-sectional analysis, older people are the least lonely group in the UK population (Hawkley et al., 2022).

KEY LEARNING POINTS

- The use of chronological age to identify the start of old age is highly arbitrary and often linked to pension policies rather than biological ageing.
- The meaning of chronological age varies over time and across populations and is culturally situated.
- Negative stereotyping of older people is linked with ageism—discrimination against people solely on the basis of age—and is one of the nine protected characteristics included in UK anti-discrimination laws.
- The observation of differences in, for example, health between people of different ages may be the result of ageing but could also reflect period and cohort differences.

REFERENCES

Abrams, D., Swift, H. J., Lamont, R. A., & Drury, L. (2015). *The barriers to and enablers of positive attitudes to ageing and older people, at the societal and individual level.* Government Office for Science Foresight Review.

Atchley, R. C. (1989). A continuity theory of normal aging. *The Gerontologist, 29*(2), 183–190.

Calment, J. https://en.wikipedia.org/wiki/Jeanne_Calment

Centre for Ageing Better. (2020). *Doddery but dear?* https://www.ageing-better.org.uk/sites/default/files/2020-03/Doddery-but-dear.pdf

Cumming, E., & Henry, W. (1961). *Growing old: The process of disengagement.* Basic Books.

Gilleard, C., & Higgs, P. (2020). *Social divisions and later life: Difference, diversity and inequality.* Bristol University Press.

Havighurst, R. J. (1961). Successful ageing. *The Gerontologist, 1,* 8–13.

Hawkley, L. D., Buecker, S., Kaiser, T., & Luhmann, M. (2022). Loneliness from young adulthood to old age: Explaining age differences in loneliness. *International Journal of Behavioral Development, 46*(1), 39–49.

Higgs, P., & Gilleard, C. (2015). *Rethinking old age.* Palgrave.

Kirkwood, T. B. (2005). Understanding the odd science of aging. *Cell, 120*(4), 437–447.

Laslett, P. (1991). *A fresh map of life: The emergence of the third age.* Weidenfeld and Nicolson.

Luszczyńska, M. (Ed.). (2020). *Researching ageing: Methodological challenges and their empirical background.* Routledge.

Marois, G., Muttarak, R., & Scherbov, S. (2020). Assessing the potential impact of COVID-19 on life expectancy. *PLoS ONE, 15.* https://doi.org/10.1371/journal.pone.0238678.

Nazroo, J. (2017). Class and health inequality in later life: Patterns, mechanisms and implications for policy. *International Journal of Environmental Research and Public Health, 14*(12), 1533. https://doi.org/10.3390/ijerph14121533.

NCDS website https://ncds.info/home/about/ accessed 20/10/22

Neugarten, B. L. (1974). Age groups in American society and the rise of the young-old. *The ANNALS of the American Academy of Political and Social Science, 415*(1), 187–198.

Phillipson, C. (1998). *Reconstructing old age.* Sage.

Peace, S. (2021). *Environments of ageing.* Policy Press.

Pickard, S. (2016). *Age studies: A sociological examination of how we age and are aged through the life course* (1st ed.). Sage.

Pickard, S., & Robinson, J. (2019). *Ageing, the body and the gender regime: Health, illness and disease across the life course* (1st ed.). Routledge.

Riley, M. W., Johnson, M., & Fones, A. (1972). *A sociology of age stratification.* Russell Sage.

Rowe, J. W., & Kahn, R. L. (1997). Successful ageing. *The Gerontologist, 33,* 433–440.

Sontag, S. (1978). The double standard of ageing. In V. Carver, & P. Liddiard (Eds.), *An ageing population* (pp. 72–80). Open University Press.

Strehler, B. L. (1982). Ageing: concepts and theories. In A. Viiditc (Ed.), *Lectures on gerontology* (pp. 1–57). Academic Press.

Torres, S. (2020). *Ethnicity and old age: Expanding our imagination.* Bristol Policy Press.

Townsend, P. (1981). The structured dependency of the older creation of social policy in the twentieth century. *Ageing and Society, 1,* 5–28.

Victor, C. R. (2005). *The social context of ageing.* Routledge.

Demographic and Epidemiological Trends in Ageing

Christina Victor

As noted in Chapter 2, the use of chronological age to determine the onset and definition of old age is highly arbitrary and subject to variation over time and across countries. In this chapter we consider individuals aged 65 and older be the older population, but the limitations of this approach are fully acknowledged. This chapter examines the size and composition of the older population, provides an overview of the key epidemiological data and provides a public health perspective on the health and social care needs of older adults.

POPULATION AGEING IN THE UNITED KINGDOM

Size of the Older Population

In examining demographic trends and population ageing, two separate dimensions are important: the absolute number of older people and the relative proportion of the total population represented by this group. The absolute number of people aged 65 and over in the current population reflects the interrelationship between births in 1955 or earlier and mortality rates, plus inward and outward migration. Fluctuations in the absolute number of older people in the population, or of other age groups, largely reflect variations in the original size of the birth cohort. For example, in the United Kingdom between 1900 and 1910, approximately 900,000 babies were born per year, compared with 600,000 in the 1930s (Grundy, 1995) and an estimated 680,000 in 2021. While we can estimate death rates with some accuracy, predicting the number of births is always more challenging.

The percentage of the population who are 65 and older—or any other age group—depends on both the absolute numbers of older people and the size of the other age groups. In 2019 the estimated population of the United Kingdom was 66,796,807, of whom 12.4 million were aged 65 or older (18.5%) (Office for National Statistics [ONS], 2020a). (See also the Government Office for Science's Foresight Future of an Ageing Population reports for 2016 and 2017.)

When we define the population aged 65 and above as older people, we identify a large subgroup of the population that encompasses a 40-year age span. Gerontologists are concerned not with treating this population as a single homogeneous group with an implied universal set of needs but with disaggregating this population into its relevant constituent parts. One important distinction is between the 'young old' (sometimes referred to as the third age; see Laslett, 1996) and the 'oldest old', paralleling the ideas of the third and fourth ages noted in Chapter 2. Put simply, the young old are under 75 years, while the oldest old are 85 and older. Nationally 2.5% of the population, or approximately 1.6 million people, are older than 85. When we identify the percentage of older people aged 85 and above as a factor likely to influence the demand for nursing care, we use age as a proxy measure for need. However, as we shall see in the sections on health, not all very old people are frail or in ill health. Therefore, in research, policy and practice, we must be careful not to treat all older people as a homogeneous group who present a common set of health problems to which we can respond with a common set of policy and practice responses (see Simmonds, 2021).

Population Ageing

The demographic structure of populations is not static but rather subject to constant change in terms of growth and age/gender composition. Demographers, using established trends, develop population projections based on assumptions about trends and the relationship between birth and death rates and inward and outward migration. This is not a precise science. One example of the influence of unanticipated events is that in 2021, births (683,000) outnumbered deaths (683,000) in the United Kingdom because of the impact of COVID-19 on mortality. This just cautions us to interpret statements about the certainty of specific population trends to take account of unpredictable events. Population projections suggest the UK population will increase to 69.6 million by 2029 and 72 million by 2041 (ONS, 2021), but these estimates are not revised for the impact of COVID-19 on mortality. Estimates for 2041 suggested there will be 19.8 million people aged 65 and older, accounting for 26% of the population. Compare this with 1901, when approximately 5% of the population were 65 and older. This large increase in the numbers of older people is often referred to as the demographic timebomb because of the presumed high levels of morbidity and disability among this population (discussed later in this chapter).

However, it is a matter of speculation as to whether future generations of older people will illustrate the same patterns of morbidity as today's cohorts of older adults, who have experienced considerable privation over their life course. Future generations of older adults may present a different set of needs because of the difference in experiences they will have had compared with older people we see today. One example is individuals ageing with lifelong physical or intellectual disability, a group that in previous times might not have lived long enough to enjoy old age (Leahy, 2021). See Chapter 33 for a discussion on older people with intellectual disabilities, new in this edition of *Nursing Older People*.

Key Demographic Characteristics of the Older Population

As well as variations in age, a number of key sociodemographic characteristics are relevant to the provision and need for health and social care.

Typically, these parameters are gender, civil status, socioeconomic status and household composition. However, as British society has become more diverse, we need to look at ethnicity; the next decades will see the ageing of post-1948 migrant communities.

A key feature of later life is that it is predominantly a female experience (see De Beauvoir, 1972; Sontag, 1978; Pickard & Robinson, 2019). Of individuals 65 and older, 55% are women. This increases with age, such that 70% of those aged 90 and above are female. In terms of civil marital status for individuals 65 and older, 72% of males and 50% of females are married, and 13% and 34%, respectively, are widowed. The majority of women aged 80 and older are widowed.

The increase in the proportion of older people who are divorced has approximately doubled since 2001 to 12%. For married couples, we cannot routinely differentiate between first or subsequent marriages. Changes in the civil status characteristics of older people serve to remind us these distributions are dynamic. In 2019 approximately 36% of individuals aged 65 and older lived alone (30% of males and 39% of females) (ONS, 2020b). This compares with 12% in 1945. Older people living alone are often characterised as an at-risk group. Again, we must cautious in the inferences we draw from these data. This statistic simply describes household composition; we cannot make inferences about social networks or other factors.

The British population aged 65 and older is predominantly White, with 3.5% identifying as belonging to minority communities. In 2011 it was estimated that 18% of individuals who described themselves as White were aged 65, compared with 6% Black/Black British and 5.7% Asian/Asian British (GOV.UK, 2020). However, the coming decades will see the ageing of minority communities, as the cohorts of individuals who came to this country for employment move into old age. This may result in the presentation of different types of health problems and require services to adapt to the cultural variety presented by an ageing ethnic-minority population (see Chapter 7).

EPIDEMIOLOGICAL ASPECTS OF AGEING

In this section we look at the major aspects of the epidemiology of health in later life (see Fried, 2000). Before we examine the empirical data concerning the health of older people, it is first necessary to provide a brief summary of the key concepts that underpin epidemiological analysis.

Incidence and Prevalence

In population-based, or epidemiological, health research, two key concepts are used to summarise the burden presented by different diseases: incidence and prevalence. Incidence describes the number of new cases of a specific disease, such as dementia, occurring within a defined population at risk of experiencing that disease, such as older adults during a given time period (e.g., a year). This statistic provides information about the rate of new cases being identified, from which we can determine if it is increasing or decreasing. Prevalence records the total number of cases of a specific disease (e.g., stroke or coronary heart disease) in a defined population at a specific time point. This gives us the total disease burden for specific diseases. For both concepts, a key issue is how cases are defined, which varies across studies and over time. For example, dementia could be defined by deaths, hospital admissions, diagnosis by a clinician, a score on a screening test or a performance on cognitive function tests. Consequently, when we look at trends in incidence and prevalence, we need to consider if any observed changes reflect changes in how cases are defined.

Measuring Health: Mortality

It remains a paradox of epidemiological research that our most comprehensive source of information about the health of the population relates to mortality data. Information about the numbers and causes of deaths is available for the United Kingdom, the four home nations, constituent regions and other local geographical areas.

Patterns of Mortality in Later Life: Death Rates and Life Expectancy

There were approximately 530,841 deaths in England and Wales in 2019, of which 85% were people aged 65 years and older. Life expectancy describes the average age an individual can expect to live. While it can be calculated from any age, typically life expectancy at birth is used as a summary index of the health of a population. Life expectancy at birth for women in England increased from 80.6 in 2000 to 83.6 in 2019 (and from 76 to 79.9 for males) (ONS 2020c; Welsh et al., 2021). As well as differences in gender, there are established life expectancy differences by socioeconomic status. Raleigh (2021) notes a 10-year difference in life expectancy at birth for males in the 10% least-deprived areas (84 years vs 74) and 8 years for women (86 vs 79 years) (see also Marmot, 2020; Gilleard & Higgs, 2021). Torres (2020) found approximate life expectancy differences at birth for individuals from Indian or Caribbean backgrounds as compared with the White British population of approximately 4 years. Wohland et al. (2015) also noted an 8-year difference in life expectancy for Pakistani individuals and a 10-year difference for Bangladeshi groups when compared with White British individuals.

What Are the Major Health Problems of Old Age?

As defined by mortality, the main health problems of later life are heart disease, which accounts for approximately 26% of deaths and dementia, and strokes, which account for 17% of deaths. However, these data expose the limitations of mortality data in identifying health priorities. Non-lethal but debilitating health problems such as osteoarthritis do not feature in the list despite their importance as a source of morbidity, disability and impact on the well-being of older adults.

Morbidity statistics focus on existing health problems rather than causes of death. Data about the national population are available from several sources. Since 1991 the decennial census has included a question about the number of individuals within households with 'long-term limiting illness'. This is a very broad indicator of the prevalence of chronic health problems within the population as it is concerned with measuring health problems of at least 12 months in duration that limit the ability of individuals to undertake normal activities. At both the local and national levels, it correlates very well with data about mortality.

There are a range of different sources of data about the health of older people. These include general surveys of the adult population that include health data (e.g., Understanding Society), general population surveys that focus on health (e.g., NHS, 2019a). However, these surveys limit their study population to adults who reside in the community. Excluded from the study are residents in institutions such as nursing and residential homes and prisons. This may limit the usefulness of data in determining the true health status of the total population. Examples of studies that focus on older people include the English Longitudinal Study of Ageing (ELSA, n.d.) and related studies in Northern Ireland and Scotland. These studies try to include participants who enter care homes, but it is challenging.

Prevalence of Chronic Illness and Disability

Mortality data show two distinct trends: (1) death rates increase with age; and (2) men illustrate higher mortality rates than women. Such analysis identifies older men as therefore having the poorest health in later life. Is this pattern replicated when we examine the distribution of chronic health problems in later life? If we look at long-standing limiting illness, a proxy measure for chronic long-term conditions, prevalence shows an age-related increase of 25% in individuals aged 16 to 24, and 74% for those 85 and older (63% for 65–74, 70% for 75–84) (NHS, 2019a). However, the gender difference observed for mortality is reversed. Thus, men are less likely than women to survive into old age. Those who do are generally in better health than their female contemporaries; females illustrate rates of chronic health problems approximately 20% higher than their male contemporaries. For older adults, musculoskeletal disorders and cardiovascular and circulatory diseases are the two biggest sources of chronic health problems. Hence a morbidity-based analysis reveals a different constellation of health problems from a mortality perspective.

Functional Ability: Activities of Daily Living

Another way of looking at the health of older people is to look at their ability to perform various activities of daily living that relate directly to their ability to live independently in the community. Such activities broadly cover two aspects of daily life: activities of daily living (feeding, washing, dressing, mobility) and instrumental activities (shopping, housework, managing bills and finances, getting out of the house). Overall, 74% of men and 63% of women aged 65 and older do not need help with activities, although this decreases with age (from 80% to 55% for men aged 65–74 to 85 and older, and 74% to 35% for women). The way these questions are asked enables us to determine unmet needs—in other words, where an individual needs help to undertake an activity, but it is not received. This increases with age, from around 10% for the 65–69 group to 40% for activities of daily living and 23% for instrumental activities of daily living for individuals 80 and older (NHS, 2019b).

Multimorbidity

Multimorbidity is recent development in research, policy and practice in terms of describing population health. Conceptually, multimorbidity is the presence of multiple diseases in a single individual. As such it is distinct from comorbidity, the presence of additional diseases in relation to an index disease in one individual (e.g., heart disease because of hypertension). The key approaches to the definition and measurement of multimorbidity are numerical indices, comparability of bodily systems involved and statistical clustering techniques (Johnson et al., 2019). Multimorbidity is frequently defined as the presence of two or more chronic conditions.

Another approach to multimorbidity is the generation of a weighted score based on mortality, quality of life and resource utilisation for specific disease combinations (e.g., Charlson Comorbidity Index). An alternative approach, based on the presumption of a common therapeutic management regimen, is to classify multimorbidity as either discordant—morbidities that span different bodily systems, such as arthritis and dementia, or concordant—morbidities that occur in the same bodily system, such as hypertension and heart failure. In practice and policy, a simple numerical count is the most commonly used measure, frequently with dichotomising scores of 0–1 and 2 or more conditions. This presupposes each condition is equally weighted in terms of the impact on the individual's health. Evidence to support that assumption is limited. As with chronic health, the prevalence of multimorbidity, defined as two or more conditions, is age-related and increases from approximately 45% in individuals aged 60–64 to 65% for those aged 85 and older (Age UK, 2019).

Frailty

Another perspective on the health of older adults is the concept of frailty (O'Caoimh et al., 2021). This is not disease-focused but is a clinical phenotype associated with increased vulnerability or risk of outcomes such as falls, disability, hospitalisation, admission to long-term care and death. (For more on frailty, see Chapter 6—another new addition in this edition). Numerous measures exist of frailty, but conceptually we can differentiate between those that focus on an accumulation of deficits and those defined by the presence or absence of specific characteristics (e.g., the Fried phenotype approach; see Dent et al., 2016). Studies differentiate between pre-frailty and frailty. Frailty is distinct from but related to disability and multimorbidity. Frailty, as measured by either approach, is age-related; the review by O'Caoimh et al. (2021) suggests 12% of individuals aged 50 and older are frail using the phenotype model, and 24% are frail using the deficit-accumulation model, with 46% and 49% estimated to be pre-frail using these two measures. O'Caoimh et al. suggest these differences reflect the different conceptualisation of frailty these measures represent. Hence although frail and frailty are terms in common clinical, policy and lay use, there are variations in how these concepts are defined and measured and in the design of interventions to address them (Travers et al., 2019; Liu et al., 2019)

Since 2017–2018, it has been mandatory in primary care to identify all individuals aged 65 and older who are moderately or severely frail. Frailty is assessed using a deficit-based approach, with the presence or absence of 36 components, with higher scores indicating increased frailty. Age UK (2019) reports that, as of autumn 2018, only a third of individuals aged 65 and older, or approximately 2.5 million people, had been assessed, with 34% classed as moderately or severely frail. It would be interesting to ask the older adults so defined how they evaluated their health status or whether they considered themselves frail.

Mental Health

Except for dementia, mental health problems are not a major source of mortality but are an important source of morbidity. Data about mental ill health are collected in a variety of different ways. The Health Survey for England uses an overall measure of psychological health—the General Health Questionnaire (GHQ-12)—on which a score of 4 and above is indicative of potential ill mental health. There is no clear age-related pattern. For women, there is a bell-shaped curve with the highest prevalence of ill health among individuals aged 45–54 (24%), but this decreases to 14% for those aged 85 and older. For men the prevalence is steady at about 14–16% up to age 65 and then increases to 19% for individuals 85 and above (National Health Service [NHS], 2017). This pattern may reflect sample size or representativeness issues, so we cautiously conclude there is little evidence of an age trend for men. The ONS well-being questions include one about anxiety. Before COVID-19, anxiety was highest in the 40–59 age group rather than the older and younger ends of the age distribution. Data from the 2016 adult psychiatric morbidity survey suggest around 11% of women and 6% of men aged 65 and older have symptoms of anxiety or depression and would benefit from treatment. The survey showed individuals aged 16–34 as having highest prevalence of anxiety, which declines with age (NHS, 2016).

Dementia is an important health problem that can result in a significant need for community care and other health care services. Enumerating the number of older people suffering from dementia is problematic, as it is particularly difficult to establish where along the continuum of cognitive functional changes dementia starts. The prevalence of clinically significant dementia (i.e., a degree of impairment of intellectual function that merits service interventions by health and social service agencies) approximately doubles every 5 years, from 0.5% of individuals aged 60–64 to 34% of those aged 90 and over. There is no consensus as to whether dementia is more common in men than women, and the pattern among minority communities remains to be established. Emerging evidence suggests incidence and prevalence of dementia is declining across Europe, Japan and North America (Wu et al., 2017). However, more evidence is required to confirm this finding.

Well-Being

One recent development in terms of measuring health status for a population is a new focus around well-being. We can identify two dimensions of well-being: eudemonic and hedonic. A eudemonic focus is on meaning and purpose in life; hedonic well-being emphasises happiness, pleasure and life satisfaction. There are several different measures and related concepts, such as life satisfaction and quality of life. Whichever measure is used, a broadly consistent pattern indicates older people report high levels of well-being. The 2017 Health Survey for England (NHS, 2018), using the Warwick-Edinburgh Mental Well-Being Scale, demonstrated that for men up to age 85, scores showed little variation by age. Women aged 65–84 reported the highest levels of well-being, and for both groups, individuals aged 85 and above had the lowest mean scores. The proportion of adults who reported being highly satisfied with their life was highest for those aged 70–74, at 38% (Centre for Ageing Better, 2020). Similarly, the ONS survey of national well-being shows that life satisfaction and happiness are generally highest in the 65–80 age group, with some decrease in late old age, although this is not substantial (ONS, 2018). There were some short-term reductions in well-being across the population during the COVID-19 pandemic, but this seems to have had a greater impact on younger adults (ONS, 2020d).

Healthy Life Expectancy

In this chapter we have looked at different measures of summarising the health status of the older population. Two broad approaches in terms of available data were identified: mortality and morbidity. The final measure we consider is healthy life expectancy, which combines the length of life with the proportion spent in good or bad health. The variation between these measures is in the definition and measurement of health as self-assessed health status or disability. However, the principle is the same, as we can estimate the duration and proportion of a life spent in good or bad health and draw comparisons across and within populations and over time. Welsh et al. (2021) report that for women in the United Kingdom, approximately 75% of life is spent as 'healthy'; 78% is healthy for men. Healthy life expectancy at birth in the United Kingdom decreased from 66 to 63 years between 2008 and 2016. There are differences in healthy life expectancy with socioeconomic status, area deprivation and ethnicity. In England and Wales, the disability-free life expectancy of approximately 62 years for key ethnic minority populations are as follows: Indian (–1 year), Caribbean (–2 years), Pakistani (–6 years) and Bangladeshi (–7 years) (Wohland et al., 2015).

CONCLUSION AND LEARNING POINTS

The UK population includes a substantial percentage of older people. Future decades will see a continuation of this trend of increasing numbers of older people, which is not unique to the United Kingdom but is a feature of most European countries. The nature of the older population is dynamic and reflects wider social trends. Old age is predominantly a female experience, and this seems unlikely to change in the near future. However, we expect to see an increase in the numbers of older people living alone and in the number of divorced and separated older people. It remains the subject of speculation as to how the changing pattern of family structure and relationships will influence the demands for care from older people and the role of the family in providing informal care. The ageing of minority communities remains another issue about which we can only speculate and draw attention to the need for further research. Older people are the main users of most of the elements of the health care system; however, there is little evaluative data about the most effective ways of providing for their care. It is vital such issues are addressed.

We have seen that, as measured by mortality and morbidity, health declines in later life. Men are less likely than women to achieve old age, but those who do are less likely to experience chronic illness and disability than their women contemporaries. It is unclear what the future patterns of health in old age will look like. Fries (1980) offers an optimistic view of the future health of older people. He argues, from the premise of a fixed biological limit to the human life span, that the onset of morbidity will be delayed, while age of death will remain fixed. People would die after a short period of ill health; morbidity and disability would be compressed into a short period at the end of life. While this view has been strongly challenged, it has served to draw attention to two important features of health in later life: (1) the length of time for which people experience disability before death; and (2) the relationship between healthy and unhealthy life expectancy.

The alternative view of the relationship between mortality and disability is more pessimistic. Greunberg (1977) has argued that reductions in late-age mortality have been achieved by medical interventions that result in the postponement of disability and disease and not their reduction or eradication. Following this line of argument would suggest that individuals who survive into old age are becoming frailer. A third, intermediate view is that older people are experiencing longer periods of disability than in the past, but the consequences of disability are less severe. Given

our current evidence, we cannot determine which of these suggestions about future patterns of late-age health status is correct. Discussions about the future health care needs are based on the projection of existing trends and evidence rather than being an exact science.

One issue of considerable policy relevance is the degree to which observed age-related variations in health status reflect the influence of ageing or are a reflection of cohort effects. Given the biography of the current generation of older adults (the experience of two wars and the privation of the interwar depression), we might speculate that much of the pattern of ill health seen in later life reflects these generational experiences. Future generations of older adults, because of their experiences, especially in early childhood, may show a pattern of better health in later life. There are insufficient available data to examine this hypothesis. We may therefore assume, for the present, that we are unlikely to see significant changes for the better in the immediate future in the health status of older people.

KEY LEARNING POINTS

- To measure health status, we require a suite of measures that include mortality, morbidity and physical, mental and social components.

- Socioeconomic and ethnic disparities in health status continue into later life.

REFERENCES

Age UK. (July 2019). *Briefing: Health and care of older people in England.* https://www.ageuk.org.uk/globalassets/age-uk/documents/reports-and-publications/reports-and-briefings/health–wellbeing/age_uk_briefing_state_of_health_and_care_of_older_people_july2019.pdf

Centre for Ageing Better. (2020). *State of ageing in 2020.* https://www.ageing-better.org.uk/summary-state-ageing-2020?gclid=CjwKCAiAhbeCBhBcEiwAkv2cY-ZrsP95GiLxOopBTGM7Xnxy11hejsOyTq9DrPoAXE6Sq3hYU2DwAhoCFaIQAvD_BwE

De Beauvoir, S. (1972). *Old age.* Penguin.

Dent, E., Kowal, E., & Hoogendijk, O. (2016). Frailty measurement in research and clinical practice: A review. *European Journal of Internal Medicine*, 31. doi: 10.1016/j.ejim.2016.03.007

English Longitudinal Study of Ageing (ELSA). (n.d.). https://www.elsa-project.ac.uk/

Fried, L. (2000). The epidemiology of aging. *Epidemiology Reviews*, 22(1), 95–106.

Fries, J. (1980). Ageing, natural death and the compression of morbidity. *New England Journal of Medicine*, 303, 130–135.

Gilleard, C., & Higgs, P. (2021). *Social divisions in later life.* Policy Press.

GOV.UK. (2020). *Focus on ethnicity.* https://www.ethnicity-facts-figures.service.gov.uk/uk-population-by-ethnicity/demographics/age-groups/latest#age-profile-by-ethnicity

Government Office for Science. (2016). *The future of an ageing population.* https://assets.publishing.service.gov.uk/government/uploads/system/uploads/attachment_data/file/816458/future-of-an-ageing-population.pdf

Government Office for Science. (2017). *Foresight project.* https://www.gov.uk/government/collections/future-of-ageing

Greunberg, E. (1977). The failures of success. *Millbank Memorial Quarterly*, 55, 3–24.

Grundy, E. (1995). Demographic influences on the future of family care. In I. Allen, & E. Perkins (Eds.), *The future of family care for older people* (pp. 1–17). HMSO.

Laslett, P. (1996). *A fresh map of life (2nd ed.).* Macmillan.

Leahy, A. (2021). *Ageing and disability.* Policy Press.

Liu, X., Ng, D. H.-M., Seah, J. W.-T., Munro, Y. L., & Wee, S.-L. (2019). Update on interventions to prevent or reduce frailty in community-dwelling older adults: A scoping review and community translation. *Current Geriatrics Reports*, 8, 72–86. https://doi.org/10.1007/s13670-019-0277-1.

Marmot, M. (2020). Health equity in England: The Marmot review 10 years on. https://www.health.org.uk/publications/reports/the-marmot-review-10-years-on

?gclid=Cj0KCQjwvaeJBhCvARIsABgTDM4TaNQ M4Lk9g0q0fUS_Y7Lxw6VWtnSVAQ9WiRwPeL_ VaJFP_3KYM2gaApRaEALw_wcB

National Health Service (NHS). (2016). Adult psychiatric morbidity survey 2014. https://digital.nhs.uk/ data-and-information/publications/statistical/adult-psychiatric-morbidity-survey/adult-psychiatric-morbidity-survey-survey-of-mental-health-and-wellbeing-england-2014#resources

NHS. (2018). Health Survey for England 2017. https://digital.nhs.uk/data-and-information/publications/statistical/health-survey-for-england/2017

NHS. (2017). Health Survey for England 2016: Well-being and mental health. http://healthsurvey.hscic.gov.uk/media/63763/HSE2016-Adult-wel-bei.pdf

NHS. (2019a). Health Survey for England 2018: Longstanding conditions. https://files.digital.nhs.uk/AA/E265E0/HSE18-Longstanding-Conditions-rep.pdf

NHS. (2019b). Health Survey for England 2018: Data tables. https://digital.nhs.uk/data-and-information/publications/statistical/health-survey-for-england/2018/health-survey-for-england-2018-data-tables

O'Caoimh, R., Sezgin, D., O'Donovan, M., Molloy, D. W., Clegg, A., Rockwood, K., & Liew, A. (2021). Prevalence of frailty in 62 countries across the world: A systematic review and meta-analysis of population-level studies. *Age and Ageing, 50*(1), 96–104. https://doi.org/10.1093/ageing/afaa219.

Office for National Statistics (ONS). (2018). Personal well-being estimates by age and sex. https://www.ons.gov.uk/people-population-and-community/wellbeing/datasets/personalwell-beingestimatesbyageandsex

ONS. (2020a). Population estimates for the UK, England and Wales, Scotland and Northern Ireland: Mid-2019. https://www.ons.gov.uk/peoplepopulationandcommunity/populationandmigration/populationestimates/bulletins/annualmidyearpopulationestimates/mid2019estimates#ageing

ONS. (2020b). People living alone aged 65 years old and over, by specific age group and sex, UK, 1996 to 2019. https://www.ons.gov.uk/peoplepopulationandcommunity/birthsdeathsandmarriages/families/adhocs/11446peoplelivingaloneaged65yearsoldandoverbyspecificagegroupandsexuk1996to2019

ONS. (2020c). Life expectancy at birth and selected older ages. https://www.ons.gov.uk/peoplepopulationandcommunity/birthsdeathsandmarriages/deaths/datasets/lifeexpectancyatbirthandselectedolderages

ONS. (2020d). Personal well-being in the UK: April 2019 to March 2020. https://www.ons.gov.uk/peoplepopulationandcommunity/wellbeing/bulletins/measuringnationalwellbeing/april2019tomarch2020

ONS. (2021). Overview of the UK population: January 2021. https://www.ons.gov.uk/peoplepopulationandcommunity/populationandmigration/populationestimates/articles/overviewoftheukpopulation/january2021#:~:text=The%20UK%20population%20is%20projected,%2C%20from%20mid%2D20191

Pickard, S., & Robinson, J. (2019). *Ageing, the body and the gender regime: Health, illness and disease across the life course* (1st ed.). Abingdon.

Raleigh, V. (2021). What is happening to life expectancy in England? *The King's Fund*. https://www.kingsfund.org.uk/publications/whats-happening-life-expectancy-england.

Simmonds, B. (2021). *Ageing and the crisis in health and social care*. Policy Press.

Sontag, S. (1978). The double standard of ageing. In V. Carver, & P. Liddiard (Eds.), *An ageing population* (pp. 72–80). Open University Press.

Torres, S. (2020). *Ethnicity and ageing*. Policy Press.

Travers, J., Romero-Ortuno, R., Bailey, J, & Cooney, M. T. (2019). Delaying and reversing frailty: A systematic review of primary care interventions. *British Journal of General Practice, 69*(678), e61–e69. doi:10.3399/bjgp18X700241.

Welsh, C. E., Matthews, F. E., & Jagger, C. (2021). Trends in life expectancy and healthy life years at birth and age 65 in the UK, 2008–2016, and other countries of the EU28: An observational cross-sectional study. *The Lancet Regional Health—Europe, 2*, Article 100023.

Wohland, P., Rees, P., Nazroo, J., & Jagger, C. (2015). Inequalities in healthy life expectancy between ethnic groups in England and Wales in 2001. *Ethnicity & Health, 20*(4), 341–353. https://doi.org/10.1080/13557858.2014.921892.

Wu, Y. T., Beiser, A. S., Breteler, M. M. B., Fratiglioni, L., Helmer, C., Hendrie, H. C., Honda, H., Ikram, M. A., Langa, K. M., Lobo, A., Matthews, F. E., Ohara, T., Pérès, K., Qiu, C., Seshadri, S., Sjölund, B. M., Skoog, I., & Brayne, C. (2017). The changing prevalence and incidence of dementia over time: Current evidence. *Nature Reviews Neurology, 13*(6), 327–339.

4

The Psychology of Human Ageing

Maria Teresa Ponto

CHAPTER OUTLINE

In order to understand the psychology of human ageing, it is necessary to consider the consequences of ageing on individuals. These are likely to be different for various people and depend on their state of health, both physical and mental, as well as on their individual, social, family and cultural circumstances. Psychological ageing is also likely to be influenced by individual life experiences and by societal expectations of age-graded behaviour. Because ageing is both an individual and a normative age-graded experience, it is a complex psychological phenomenon. Many developmental theories are concerned with the concept of age, but according to Kimmel (1980, p. 30), 'Age is merely a measure of a number of revolutions that the earth has made around the sun since a person's birth. Thus, chronological age by itself may not be a very meaningful indicator of development. At best, age provides a convenient index of the passage of *time*.'

This chapter examines psychological explanations of human ageing from many perspectives. Initially sociopsychological theories of ageing are explored, and thereafter ageing is considered from psychodynamic, humanistic, cognitive and behavioural perspectives. There is also a section

that evaluates the explanations and contributions made by these four psychological perspectives on the changes in mental health that occur in old age. The transitions and tasks of old age, life review and reminiscence among older people, and successful adaptation and adjustment to ageing are also debated. Finally, developmental approaches to ageing and satisfaction in later life are considered by examining work of several developmental theorists.

The complexity of ageing has been recognized by developmental theorists who consider getting old as part of human development. The notion of development implies growth, movement, progression and maturity, and human ageing can be considered from these perspectives. However, for the purpose of this chapter, ageing is considered in terms of sociopsychological theories and other major psychological perspectives.

PSYCHOSOCIAL THEORIES OF AGEING

There are two distinct and contrasting explanations of the processes involved in ageing: social disengagement theory (Cumming & Henry, 1961) and activity theory (Havighurst, 1963).

Social Disengagement Theory

Social disengagement theory proposes that, as individuals get older, they gradually withdraw or disengage from society. At the same time, there is a withdrawal of society from the individual. Social disengagement is influenced mainly by children leaving home, partners or friends dying and social circles decreasing. The theory is based on a longitudinal study of 279 individuals aged 50–90 and involved interviewing participants on issues related to health, general activities and interactions with others. Whether these findings were representative of the rest of the society in the 1960s is debatable. It is also difficult to speculate on whether the 50-year-old participants interviewed in 1961 continued to disengage 10 years later.

The theory of social disengagement was criticized severely almost from the moment it was introduced. It is true that, for most individuals, life revolves around work, and once an individual retires, it becomes difficult to maintain work relationships. However, it is not necessarily true that all individuals disengage from society once retired. Some continue to be active and remain involved with society. The theory tends to imply disengagement is desirable, thus almost condoning the separation of older people from mainstream society. Some people may choose to disengage in order to pursue a lifestyle that was not possible to adopt earlier because of family commitments. There is also a cultural dimension to disengagement. In Western society, retirement may impose disengagement for some people. This is not the case in China, where government ministers are often in their 80s. In some African tribes, elders become important members of the community who are valued for their life experience and wisdom.

The current views acknowledge that life-span development has an influence on how people adjust to old age and recognise that some older people may be more content with solitude after retirement than in earlier adulthood. This view is supported by a recent review of 31 longitudinal studies on social engagement in old age by Pinto and Neri (2017). They reported that results presented from 21 studies showed reduction of social-engagement levels in old age; only five studies found no change in levels of social involvement.

Activity Theory

Activity theory, proposed by Havighurst (1963), suggests for individuals to age successfully after retirement, they need to find substitutes for the activities and work of middle age. However, this theory is idealistic in nature, as the maintenance of activity is not possible for all older people and is influenced by personal, social, biological and economic circumstances. Furthermore, this theory is unidirectional. It implies people who are active are more likely to be happy, but there is evidence to the contrary that people who are happy are more likely to be active. A more modern approach to ageing considers developmental changes during the life span and also focuses on changes in social relationships and how people adjust to these changes as they age (Doyle et al., 2012). Other researchers (Kahlbaugh & Huffman, 2017) have examined human ageing from the perspective of personality. They state the style of ageing is influenced by an individual's personality, which is an important factor in successful ageing. This concept is examined in some detail below.

PSYCHODYNAMIC AND HUMANISTIC PERSPECTIVES

Psychodynamic Perspective

The psychodynamic perspective has its origins in the work of Sigmund Freud (1856–1939) and continues to be influential in psychology. It incorporates psychological systems and theories that emphasise the processes of change and development and considers motivation and drive theories as central to human development. The influence of unconscious forces on most aspects of human behaviour is also highlighted. The psychodynamic perspective offers a model of a person that is holistic, with behaviour and emotions resulting from the conflict of dynamic, unconscious forces. This model recognises human behaviour and experience may be driven by unconscious motives. The main concepts involve the development of personality and subsequent development of self. Freud considered development in late life to be similar to that of childhood. He believed the narcissistic tendencies of early childhood return to people in old age. Problems experienced by adults in later life may result in regression to the behaviour consistent with a stage of psychosexual development at which they fixated as children. Furthermore, adult neuroses could be the result of inadequate solutions to problems experienced during a particular stage of psychosexual development in childhood.

Although Freud's theory is difficult to confirm or refute, there has been some evidence to support it, as the types of personality described by Freud do appear to exist. There is evidence for the existence of oral personality; Perry et al. (2012) found characteristics associated with the oral personality tend to cluster in some individuals.

Freud offered interesting explanations for the structure of personality, in that it consists of three components: id (unconscious), ego (preconscious and conscious) and superego (conscious). Freud explained the ego constantly influences the id and its instinctual tendencies by bringing it back to reality (Gross, 2015).

The superego is influenced by the moral values of an individual's parents and is subdivided into conscience and ego-ideal. The development of the superego is shaped by the injunctions of significant others, parents, teachers and people in authority. If you behave badly, your conscience makes you feel guilty, but if you behave well, your ego ideal makes you feel good (Eysenck, 2018).

There is a continuous struggle to maintain a dynamic equilibrium between the id, ego and superego, and a degree of conflict is inevitable. Because it seems the id and super-ego constantly compete for dominance, the ego may use defence mechanisms for protection. According to Freud, the outcome of conflict can manifest in three ways: in dreams, in neurotic symptoms or in defence mechanisms.

A number of ego-defence mechanisms exist. Knowing about defence mechanisms may provide an insight into the behaviour of older people.

Denial occurs when the conscious mind refuses to accept the reality of a potential threat. For instance, a person may be diagnosed with cancer but refuse to accept it. *Repression* happens when a traumatic event is forced out of consciousness into the unconscious. *Regression* occurs when the individual is unable to deal with the current situation and reverts to an earlier stage of development—eating sweets when upset, for example, particularly if sweets were used to make things better in childhood. *Rationalisation* occurs when an individual finds an acceptable excuse for an unacceptable outcome in order to protect the self-image. For example, I forgot to take my pills, because the phone kept ringing. *Projection* is evident when people attribute their faults to others. *Displacement* occurs when an individual is not able to demonstrate real (often angry) feelings toward someone and uses another person, animal or object as a substitute. *Reaction-formation* happens when the repressed impulse is held in check by exaggerating the opposite tendency, and individuals display behaviour that contrasts with what they feel unconsciously—for example, being extra nice to someone they dislike. *Isolation* is evident when an individual dissociates thinking from emotion—for example, talking about an unpleasant personal experience without any evident emotion (Gross, 2015).

There are widely recognised methodological flaws in Freud's work. His sample—middle-class, middle-aged women in Vienna—was not representative of the rest of the population. Also, Freud's methods of collecting data would be considered unsound by today's standards. However, his ideas were original and have influenced not only developmental psychology but also Western culture (Gross, 2015).

Studies have been designed to investigate defence mechanisms in experimental settings, and weak empirical evidence was found in their support (Somerfield & McCrae, 2000). In spite of the weak evidence, clinical psychologists have developed methods for assessing defence mechanisms and continue to use the concept when introducing coping strategies (Cramer, 2000). To summarise, Freud's theories continue to be recognised as a major contribution to our understanding of ourselves and others, and his work has influenced other psychologists, particularly those working in the psychodynamic tradition—for example, Erikson, whose work is discussed later.

Humanistic Perspective

The humanistic perspective incorporates psychological theories that are concerned with higher human motives—self-development, self-awareness and understanding—with an emphasis on conscious experience. Humanistic theories utilise phenomenological and existentialist ideas, and are concerned with human experience, human needs, meaning and issues related to self-concept. Humanistic psychologists recognise all individuals have a potential for personal growth that can culminate in self-actualisation.

In order to evaluate the impact of humanistic perspective on old age, this section examines contributions made by Maslow and Rogers. Abraham Maslow (1908–1970) was a key proponent of humanistic psychology and is best remembered for his hierarchy of needs, introduced in 1954 (Box 4.1). According to Maslow (1954), all human beings are motivated by two forces, the survival force and the self-actualisation force, and have needs that reflect these forces. The survival force has a priority, and therefore the needs on the lower levels of the hierarchy must be met first. They include physiological needs, safety needs, love and belongingness, and esteem needs. Once the lower-level needs are satisfied, attention can be given to the self-actualisation force by striving for cognitive and aesthetic needs. These needs are much more difficult to achieve and are closely related to life experience.

BOX 4.1   Maslow's Hierarchy of Needs

- Self-actualisation
- Realising one's potential to find self-fulfilment
- *Aesthetic needs*
  - Beauty, order and symmetry
- *Cognitive needs*
  - To know, to explore and to search for meaning
- *Esteem needs*
  - To achieve respect from others, self-esteem, self-respect
- *Love and belongingness needs*
  - To be accepted, to be loved and to love
- *Safety needs*
  - To feel secure, safe and out of danger, physically and psychologically
- *Physiological needs*
  - Food, drink, rest, activity, survival needs

It is a fact that self-actualisation means different things to different people, and we all have needs that are individual and person-specific. Maslow accepts not everyone will self-actualise. However, the need for growth is widely recognised, and Maslow's hierarchy of needs model is suitable for nursing and can be successfully applied to nursing older people.

Carl Rogers (1902–1987), like Maslow, recognised the individuality of people and considered self-actualisation as an innate predisposition. According to Rogers (2002), people are predominantly good and have the potential to develop in every way. Rogers's main contribution to psychology was his theory on client-centred therapy and the concept of self. The concept of self can be explained in terms of self-image, or how you perceive yourself. When your self-image matches your ideal self, you have the potential to self-actualise. If, however, there is a mismatch between your self-image and the ideal self, the chances of anxiety and emotional dissatisfaction increase (Nolen-Hoeksema et al., 2014). Rogers's client-centred therapy has contributed considerably to counselling theory, and his ideas have also inspired groups in the personal-growth movement. Opportunities for personal growth in such groups can be achieved if participants interact freely and openly with each other (Gross, 2015).

COGNITIVE AND BEHAVIOURAL PERSPECTIVES

Cognitive Perspective

The cognitive perspective in psychology incorporates psychological theories that emphasise internal and mental processes. Mental processes or behaviours are often abstract in nature and may involve representation, belief, intention, expectancy, imagery and symbolising. The cognitive perspective in psychology is also concerned with cognitive abilities, which involve thinking, reasoning and problem-solving, among others. In essence, cognitive functioning depends on the ability to process information. The information-processing model involves several operational mental stages: input, coding, storing, retrieval, decoding and output of the information. To put it simply, information processing is about organising, interpreting and responding to incoming stimuli or information. To manipulate information successfully, you need to use language, memory, attention, perception and intelligence. The research into cognitive changes associated with ageing has found the speed with which people process information declines with age, thus leading to longer reaction times (Quigley & Müller, 2014).

Although an increase in reaction time in older people has been well documented, a number of explanations need considering. Often older people have difficulty maintaining readiness prior to reaction-testing tasks, particularly when distracting stimuli are present. Quigley and Müller (2014) propose that being exposed to competing information also interferes with reaction time, which demonstrates older people may find it difficult to divide their attention. However, focused testing used in studies quoted earlier assesses only one aspect of information processing. If participants are told where to focus their attention, differences are minimal. Providing the tasks are not complicated, older and younger people have a similar range of ability when attending to simultaneous activities—for example, having a conversation, watching TV and knitting.

Irrespective of the explanations offered on cognitive decline, it has to be remembered that inevitably there will be individual variations that result from differences in ability and motivation. These differences may also be influenced by biological and physiological changes—for example, by high blood pressure, cardiac or cerebrovascular disorders, and reduced activity in general. Apart from information processing, problem solving is another cognitive skill that has been reported to be affected by ageing (Hülür et al., 2016) . However, since problem-solving tasks are often confined to laboratory experiments, they may fail to demonstrate how individuals use a problem-solving approach in their everyday lives. Furthermore, most tests into problem solving rely on hypothetical, abstract-thinking activities, which may not be relevant to practical problem solving but are frequently assessed by intelligence tests.

The concept of intelligence has been debated by psychologists since intelligence testing began. The main arguments concern definitions of intelligence and the nature/nurture debate. The question is whether intelligence is innate—that is, genetically acquired—or dependent on environmental factors such as upbringing and education. In the early 1900s, when the first tests were being developed, research was concerned with improving and validating tests. Since then, intelligence testing has been used to predict educational performance and explain many different aspects of intelligence. The popularity of intelligence testing has not declined even though the predictive value of the intelligence quotient (IQ) score is highly debatable. In relation to older people, we have to consider whether ageing affects intelligence. This is a controversial issue that has attracted a considerable amount of research. Most intelligence tests rely on testing general knowledge, comprehension, arithmetic and vocabulary within a specific time. Therefore the speed of information processing is important for people to do well in such tests, but as previously stated, research evidence points to a slowing in the speed of information processing with age. This means older people are likely to be disadvantaged in standard intelligence testing, unless the tests are standardised for older age groups.

To explore this point further, the methods used for intelligence testing also need to be considered. Many studies use cross-sectional rather than longitudinal approaches to compare older and younger participants. The problem with the cross-sectional approach is it tests participants from different age groups on the same tests. Results from these groups are then compared, and generally the scores for older people compare unfavourably with those of younger people. To explain this, we need to consider differences in the educational opportunities that were available to a group of millennials as opposed to those available to the 70-year-old group. Without a doubt, research that uses longitudinal studies, where the same individuals are tested over a long period of time, is likely to offer more reliable information on changes in intelligence that occur with ageing. Hülür at el. (2016) reported on the Seattle Longitudinal Study, which tested the primary mental abilities of more than 582 adults aged 20–70 at 7 yearly intervals between 1956 and 2012. In the earlier data analysis, Schaie (1996) reported clear decreases in most primary abilities after the age of 60, although in relation to verbal intelligence, he found intellectual decline did not start until about 74 years of age. Schaie concluded the results were cohort specific, which could be explained in terms of differences in educational opportunities. The more recent data analysis (Hülür at el., 2016) of the Seattle Longitudinal Study focused on cognitive changes in primary mental abilities and processing speed in between-person and within-person associations. They found all primary mental abilities were linked to psychomotor speed and within-person associations, and took longer with age. However, within-person associations between primary mental abilities and cognitive flexibility were relatively stable with age.

Another way of looking at the concept of intelligence is to consider fluid and crystallised intelligence. Fluid intelligence is similar to abstract intelligence and characterised by the ability to solve unusual problems in a creative way. The speed of information processing as well as problem-solving abilities and mental agility all contribute to fluid intelligence. Crystallised intelligence is characterised by the ability to manipulate factual information, which is acquired through education and life experience. There is evidence fluid intelligence declines with age, whereas crystallised intelligence remains more static. A recent report (von Stumm & Deary, 2012) found differences in childhood and old-age IQ had a direct effect on differences in crystallised intelligence. These differences were particularly influenced by intellectual curiosity, defined as engaging in cognitive activities.

One of the factors that influence performance on intelligence tests is memory, and there has been considerable research on the ageing memory. Many older people notice some memory deterioration and complain about being forgetful. The majority of the research tends to make a distinction between short-term memory (primary memory), which involves holding information in consciousness, and working memory, which involves information processing while dealing with other information or cognitive tasks at a conscious level. Most tests on short-term memory require participants to hold information passively and recall it immediately—for example, recalling a name or a number of digits. Tests on working memory may involve tasks that require participants to process, transform, manipulate, reorganise and retain information.

Since the majority of short-term memory tests rely on laboratory experiments, this makes it difficult to apply findings to everyday life. However, if aspects of long-term memory are examined separately, more realistic findings result (Gross, 2015). It is now widely accepted that long-term memory could be divided into two long-term memory systems: declarative knowledge and procedural knowledge (Eysenck, 2018). Declarative knowledge is concerned with memory for personal experiences and memory about general knowledge; procedural memory involves memory for motor and cognitive skills such as playing the piano, driving or cycling (Fig. 4.1). The research into memory ageing has shown virtually no decline in semantic memory, although retrieval from semantic memory is slower. However, there are some exceptions to this, as reported by Zimprich (2020), who provided explanations on why popular songs from youth are remembered better than semantic knowledge tested in laboratory experiments. Well-learned motor skills such as typing (procedural memory) remain unaffected by ageing, although learning a new skill takes longer.

Findings from research into memory further elucidate cognitive functioning in late adulthood and enable us to understand the difficulties that can be experienced by older learners. Nowadays, access to education is possible for everyone, and some older people seek further education. Some people may want to learn about new technology, whereas others may wish to continue education as a means of self-actualisation. The evidence that older people can maintain their cognitive abilities into old age is demonstrated by the activities of members of the House of Lords, clergy and the judicial system. Imlach et al. (2017) found that older students who participated in cognitively stimulating activities during their lifetime were successful in academic pursuits. Furthermore, a recent study (Smith et al., 2020) showed that knowledge affects how well continuous information is chunked into multiple events. They found older adults, who previously demonstrated age-related declines in memory, may use their declarative knowledge acquired across the life span to enable more efficient encoding and memory of dynamic, everyday activities. The

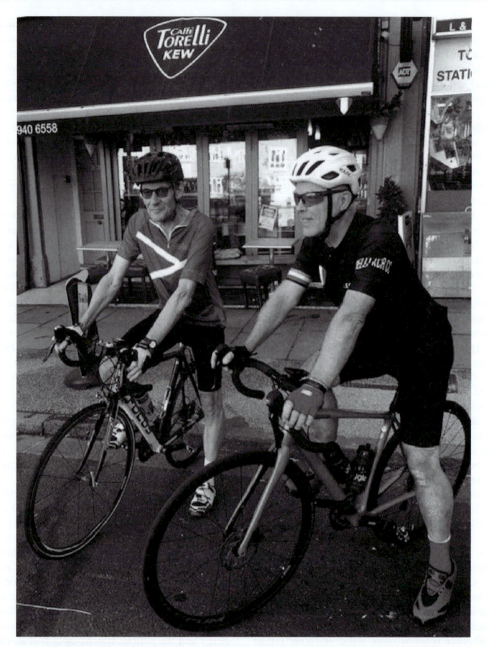

Fig. 4.1 Keeping fit into older age. (Copyright Fiona Ross, courtesy of John Tatam and Peter Kilby.)

results from both studies demonstrate the ability to learn and remember does not necessarily decline with age. It has to be recognised that both studies examined highly motivated older adults who were probably also very intelligent.

As we have seen, decline in cognitive competence affects older people, but this decline does not afflict everyone, may not be apparent until the mid-70s or 80s and may be reversible with training. When looking at the empirical evidence, it is important to acknowledge individual differences in education, occupation, lifestyle and nutrition as well as childhood influences on the individuals tested. Questions also need to be raised regarding the research tools used for testing cognitive abilities and, in particular, the suitability of general intelligence scales for older people. Finally, perhaps the research should focus on dimensions of practical intelligence, wisdom and creativity and on how age and experience interact to influence cognitive functioning rather than on laboratory intelligence testing.

Behavioural Perspective

The behavioural perspective in psychology incorporates psychological theories that are concerned with measurable and observable behaviour. The emphasis of the behavioural perspective is on explanations of learning and in particular on the conditions necessary for learning to take place. The main empirical concepts within the behavioural perspective centre on conditioning, which can be either classical or operant. Classical conditioning is considered a most basic form of learning that involves actions and reactions without conscious control. An example of this is when we salivate while going past a bakery or fish-and-chip shop. In relation to older people, we will consider another example. Mr Brown, who has meals on wheels, becomes very ill soon after eating his fish dinner. He may end up associating the meal with the illness, even if his illness was unrelated to the meal, and will consequently avoid such meals in the future. He has generalised the response from that particular situation to similar future situations. A slightly different example that still demonstrates conditioning is that of Mrs Smith, who is anxious about going upstairs at night and sleeps in the armchair downstairs. By sleeping downstairs, her fear is relieved, and that relief acts as a reinforcer, maintaining her response (sleeping downstairs). Another reinforcer using the same example could be illustrated differently. For instance, Mrs Smith may be anxious about going upstairs because her neighbour, who is the same age, fell down the stairs and broke her leg, ending up in hospital. These explanations demonstrate the concept of generalisation, which refers to the fact that once a response is learned, it may spread to similar situations.

Operant conditioning explains the second type of learning, in which the actions are voluntary and conscious. Here, the individual operates on the environment to cause an effect. For instance, Mrs Rogers, who has no relatives or friends living nearby, feels lonely and isolated as nobody visits her. One day she accidentally leaves her milk on the doorstep, and her neighbour calls to check on her that evening. She enjoys the chat as they have a cup of tea. In the weeks that follow, the neighbour notices the milk is not collected two or three times a week. For Mrs Rogers, the first visit was a reinforcer, and she is now reinforcing further visits from her neighbour by not collecting her milk. These examples illustrate the main claim made by behaviourist psychologists that any behaviour can be shaped by its consequences or that any behaviour that is rewarded is likely to be repeated.

This discussion highlights the point that our behaviour is very much influenced by other people—by their rewards or punishments. We learn if our behaviour is acceptable by observing how other people react to it, whether they approve or disapprove. The learning that takes place in this way is best explained by a theory that derives from the behavioural perspective—social learning theory, proposed by Bandura (1977). According to this theory, all behaviour is learned during interactions with others. While behaviourist psychologists consider both classical and operant conditioning as important to learning, social learning psychologists accept the importance of conditioning but do not believe conditioning can explain all aspects of learning. They stress the importance of observational learning, which occurs without any reinforcement.

Observational learning, or modelling, occurs spontaneously; the observer does not make any conscious effort to learn but is usually able to reproduce or imitate behaviour observed in others (Gross, 2015). Apart from explaining modelling behaviours in children, social learning theory can be used to explain differences between generations of people. The influence of parents, schools, peers and the media is powerful and has an impact on the behaviour of each generation. This also has an impact on the way various groups are seen by others in society. The image of old people presented on television may influence the way some viewers perceive them. This can be positive if older people are portrayed as active and helpful, but it can be negative if they are portrayed as difficult and rude. In terms of nursing, the modelling or observational aspect of social learning theory can be used to teach older clients particular aspects of care—for example, giving insulin injections.

MENTAL HEALTH AND AGEING

We now consider the contributions made by the main psychological perspectives toward our understanding of life-long human development and the changes in mental health that can result from ageing. The term *mental health* not only implies an absence of mental disorder but also refers to behavioural and emotional adjustment and adaptability in dealing with everyday life. Galderisi et al. (2015) offer a similar definition and state that mental health indicates the ability to deal with stress, grief, conflict and past failure as well as having good self-care and self-esteem. The ability to cope with stresses, the ability to introspect, being realistic about the world, and the ability to grow, develop and self-actualise are as fundamental to mental health as the absence of mental illness. Whether we can meet all these criteria all the time is highly debatable; for instance, it is widely accepted that not everyone will self-actualise (Gross, 2015).

Prevalent mental health changes in older people are depression and anxiety, delirium and dementia, but they are not universal and therefore not an inevitable consequence of ageing. All these changes can be detrimental to individual well-being, and they are addressed in greater detail in Chapters 28, 29 and 30. This chapter, however, considers anxiety from the psychological perspectives discussed earlier. Anxiety is a psychological disorder that produces an unpleasant emotional state, characterised by the inability to relax and (sometimes) trembling. Anxiety may also be characterised by hyperactivity, with symptoms of dizziness, a racing heart and perspiration as well as unreasonable apprehension, unexplained dread, distress and uneasiness (Gross, 2015). Anxiety is often seen as a symptom of depression, and consequently less attention is paid to it. However, according to Bryant et al. (2008), the incidence of anxiety in old age may be greater than previously thought and ranges from 12% to 15% in community samples. The prevalence of anxiety symptoms is much higher, ranging from 15% to 52.3% in community samples and 15% to 56% in clinical samples. Anxiety as a disorder may be underreported, as older people may misconstrue the symptoms they are experiencing by confusing them with ill physical health.

Older people may be anxious for a number of reasons. They may have a number of fears, such as a fear of falling in the house or in the street, fear of crime or fear of dying. The fear of falling is worrying to older people because of the consequences of a fall that could result in an individual being hospitalised and/or dependent on others. Hewston et al. (2018) found fear of falling to be the most common fear in the people they studied. The fear of crime is real for most people nowadays, with so much crime being reported on a daily basis. Older people see themselves as vulnerable because they perceive themselves as less fit physically than they once were. Fear of dying is another source of anxiety for some older people. Bowling et al. (2010) found older people may fear the pain and suffering related to dying. Older people are also likely to have suffered bereavement and loss as a result of spouses', friends' or neighbours' deaths, which could cause them anxiety. Anticipatory bereavement, when someone close is likely to die, can also contribute to generalised anxiety and grief. Loss, bereavement and grief can affect the mental health of the older people, leading to distress and depression. The ability to deal with loss and grief is individual; Spahni et al. (2015) found successful adaptation to spousal loss was associated with high scores in psychological resilience and extraversion and low scores in neuroticism. See Chapter 34 for more on bereavement and loss.

To appreciate the psychodynamic and humanistic explanations, we will use the contributions from both perspectives to explain anxiety. In terms of Freudian theory, anxiety in later life originates from earlier experiences, possibly from childhood. Anxiety arises from the conflict between demands made on the ego, which has to balance the instinctual needs of the id with the constraints of the superego (Gross, 2015). Humanistic theories, using existentialist ideas, see anxiety as characterised by notions of the meaninglessness and incompleteness of the world. Both psychodynamic and humanistic approaches suggest we should deal with anxiety by means of psychotherapy—psychoanalytic or client-centred.

In terms of mental health changes, both cognitive and behavioural perspectives can lead to successful psychotherapy. Behaviour therapy is generally sought when there is a need to change a maladaptive behaviour. Classical or operant conditioning can be utilised well in behaviour therapy, which focuses on treating the behaviour rather than causes of that behaviour. Behaviour therapy has been favourably used particularly with phobic anxiety. Gould et al. (2012) reported cognitive behaviour therapy can also be successful in treating anxiety disorders in older people.

DEVELOPMENTAL APPROACHES TO AGEING

Early developmental research in psychology centred mainly on childhood, but since the late 1960s and 1970s, the research has also addressed transitions and tasks in adulthood and old age. Although no distinct psychological theories concentrate solely on ageing, a number of human development theories consider the psychological changes during early and late adulthood and thus are relevant to old age (Erikson, 1973; Levinson et al., 1978; Gould, 1978).

Erikson's Theory of Development

Erik Erikson's work follows the psychoanalytic tradition but places greater emphasis on psychosocial development. Erikson proposed that human life follows a cycle of eight ages, from infancy to old age, as illustrated in Table 4.1. For each cycle there is an emphasis on ego development, which is underpinned by physical development and biological maturation. The stages are sequential, but no chronological age indicators are given for those in adulthood. Each cycle or stage is embedded in a social context, and the outcome for each stage results in personal growth. According to Erikson, ego development during each stage centres on a crisis that involves the struggle between two opposing polarities, culminating in a dynamic balance that is desirable for personal growth. Development during each stage also follows an epigenetic process, meaning the growth of the ego is gradual and progressive as well as unfolding.

To each stage, Erikson adds the lasting outcome, highlighting the basic advantages achieved: hope, will, purpose,

TABLE 4.1   A Cycle of Eight Ages

Stages of Development and Their Outcomes	Virtue	Age
8 Integrity vs despair, disgust	Wisdom	Old age
7 Generativity vs stagnation	Care	Maturity
6 Intimacy vs isolation	Love	Young adulthood
5 Identity vs role confusion	Fidelity	Adolescence
4 Industry vs inferiority	Competence	School age
3 Initiative vs guilt	Purpose	Play age
2 Autonomy vs shame, doubt	Willpower	Early childhood
1 Trust vs mistrust	Hope	Infancy

Based on Erikson (1973).

TABLE 4.2   Levinson's Stages of Development

Age (years)	Stage
17	Childhood and adolescence
22	Early adult transition
28	Entering the adult world
33	Age 30 transition
40	Settling down
45	Midlife transition
50	Entering middle adulthood
55	Age 50 transition
60	Culmination of middle adulthood

Based on Levinson et al (1978).

competence, fidelity, love, care, wisdom. Erikson views these advantages, which he terms *virtues*, as necessary and re-emerging from generation to generation. His last two stages extend over a long time. More recent views suggest Erikson's theory should be expanded, and his widow made an attempt to do that (Erikson & Erikson, 1997). Joan Erikson added a ninth stage, although not in the format of the eight stages. In essence Joan (Erikson & Erikson, 1997) proposed that in the ninth stage, individuals revisit all other stages and are challenged by negative outcomes such as mistrust and shame as well as doubt and guilt, mainly due to not being sure of their own capabilities. Although sensitively written, the chapter on the ninth stage lacks clarity when compared with the work on the eight stages of human. However, some recent evidence (Brown & Lewis, 2003) tentatively supports the existence of stage 9 in human psychosocial development.

Levinson's Transitions in Adult Life

Levinson et al. (1978), in the book *The Seasons of a Man's Life*, offer an explanation of transitions in adulthood. These stages offered are not separated by chronological age but concerned with transitions that occur as we move through the life-cycle. In pursuing their research, Levinson and his colleagues aimed to address the following questions: 'What does it mean to be an adult? What are the root issues of adult life—the essential problems and satisfactions, the sources of disappointment, grief and fulfilment?' (Levinson et al., 1978, p. ix). Levinson et al. interviewed 40 men aged 35–45 over a 2–3 month period and saw each subject for 10–20 hours. They also interviewed wives and, where appropriate, visited places

of work. On the basis of the data collected, they proposed nine stages of adult development (Table 4.2).

The main interest for Levinson's team was a focus on the changes in midlife, but they also described transitions in old age. Each period of adult development has developmental tasks that must be mastered during that stage.

Gould's Theory of the Evolution of Adult Consciousness

Gould (1978) took a different approach to adult development in his theory of the evolution of adult consciousness. Gould developed his theory while working as a psychiatrist and subsequently tested it on 524 people aged 16–50 (not his patients). He proposed growth and maturity involve a resolution of the separation anxiety that remains with us from childhood. This theory extends Freudian psychoanalytic theory, as it looks at adulthood but in terms of childhood influences. Gould's stages show approximate ages for each developmental stage, as is illustrated in Table 4.3.

Developmental Theories in Perspective

We now discuss the last two stages of Erikson's theory and the corresponding stages of Levinson's and Gould's theories, as they loosely reflect the mature time of life. Erikson did not use chronological age indicators against the eight stages, but many psychologists interpret stage 7 as corresponding with middle adulthood and stage 8 as late adulthood. The age span for stage 7 is interpreted as 40–65 years, and for many people, these are their most productive years (Nolen-Hoeksema et al., 2014). During this stage, which Erikson called maturity, people guide the next generation, either their own children or young people they work with. Through helping young people become responsible and knowledgeable adults, generativity—a valuable contribution to society—can be achieved. Some people who feel

TABLE 4.3 Gould's Stages of Adult Development	
Age (years)	Stage
16–18	Desire to escape parental control
18–22	Leaving the family; peer group orientation
22–28	Developing independence; commitment to a career and children
29–34	Questioning self; role confusion; marriage and career vulnerable to dissatisfaction
35–43	Period of urgency to attain life's goals; awareness of time limitation; realignment of life's goals
43–53	Settling down; acceptance of one's life
53–60	More tolerance; acceptance of past; less negativism; general mellowing

Based on Gould (1978).

they are stagnating in life may change the course of their life at this point.

Erikson's stage of 'generativity vs stagnation' is reflected in Levinson's 'middle adulthood' and Gould's stage of 'midlife decade'. Levinson's middle adulthood is a period of transition, when an individual is likely to review their life so far. This involves some disillusionment, which may provide an opportunity to modify life and its structure. Gould's stage of midlife decade also suggests the end of illusion as well as awareness of mortality and a sense of urgency in realigning life's goals.

Erikson refers to the eighth stage as old age, and this stage spans late adulthood, from 65 onward. The polarities for ego development at this stage are integrity vs despair. During this stage people can look back and reflect on what they have achieved during their lives. To experience ego-integrity, individuals must feel they have achieved their major life goals and have no regrets about the past. The resulting virtue is then wisdom. However, if on reaching this last stage of development, they find they lack a sense of fulfilment and regret many decisions they made in life, the outcome can be despair. Erikson's last two stages are reflected in Levinson's 'late adulthood transition' and 'late adulthood' stages. They concern transition to retirement and beyond. Levinson recognises this is a time for integrity vs despair but also asserts this could be a time for creative development.

In evaluating Erikson's, Levinson's and Gould's adult developmental theories, we are aware of the similarities between them and the ways they complement each other. Although these theories are old, they are seminal and have

generated research to test them. Some more recent studies will be briefly considered. For instance, Pittman et al. (2011) examined parallels between Bowlby's theory of attachment and Erikson's psychosocial stages of development with noteworthy suggestions. Erikson's stages of early adulthood—for example, identity vs role confusion and intimacy vs isolation—focus on psychosocial aspects of development, but lasting outcomes are similar to the outcomes proposed by Bowlby's attachment theory, as in order to achieve identity and intimacy, individuals need to have had secure attachments in their childhood.

An and Cooney (2006) examined the role of generativity across the life span and reported association with well-being. Interestingly, they found trusting relationships with parents influenced well-being in early and late adulthood.

Before concluding this section, it is useful to consider a more recent approach to explaining development proposed by Baltes (1987). According to Baltes, human development should be considered from the life-span perspective, and he suggests development is lifelong, multidimensional, multidirectional, plastic, embedded in history, multidisciplinary and contextual. Most of us will agree development follows a lifelong process, and we can develop in many dimensions and directions. By asserting development is plastic, Baltes (1987) implies flexibility and adaptation to different life conditions. It is a fact human development is embedded in history, as many world and societal events affect whole generations. The COVID-19 pandemic is a good example, as 6 months without formal schooling had an impact on the current generation of schoolchildren.

Human development during the life span is studied by many disciplines and thus is multidisciplinary. The final contention made by Baltes is development is contextual, meaning it is influenced by the contexts in which we grow and develop. These contexts are biological, psychosocial, environmental and cultural and are individually experienced as well as influenced by normative age-graded, history-graded and non-normative life events. Normative age-graded experiences are common to all, such as starting school, puberty and retirement. Normative history-graded experiences are associated with history, such as growing up during World War II. Non-normative life events provide individual experiences that influence development, such as the death of a parent, diagnosis with a terminal illness or moving to another country.

The Concept of Wisdom

Wisdom is an outcome and virtue of Erikson's last developmental stage. Wisdom is generally attributed to old age, and Erikson et al. (1986) suggest it is a desirable outcome of the tension between integrity and despair. The sense of integrity must prevail for wisdom to emerge. Erikson et al. define wisdom as a point in life when a person realises how little they know in spite of life experience and ability to resolve many life-related tasks. Baltes and Kunzmann (2003, p. 131) on the other hand, define wisdom as 'expert knowledge and judgement about important, difficult and uncertain questions associated with meaning and conduct of life. Wisdom related knowledge deals with matters of utmost personal and social significance'. Baltes and Kunzmann have designed a test for wisdom in which they present people with difficult hypothetical situations. Interestingly, they found wisdom-related knowledge emerges in late adolescence and early adulthood, and there is no further change in the level of wisdom during later adulthood beyond the level achieved in early adulthood. They also assert cognitive factors such as intelligence are not the most powerful predictors of knowledge-related wisdom, whereas personality factors are. These include having a sense of generativity, being creative and being open to new experience.

Baltes and Kunzmann (2003) also stated there is a link between wisdom-related knowledge and the emotional style of individuals. There is support for this assertion in a recent study (Thomas & Kunzmann, 2014) that examined age differences in wisdom-related knowledge across the adult life span. They found age differences in wisdom and reasoning on life issues are influenced by age-normative experiences such as marital discord, divorce or loss of job.

Perry et al. (2015) examined wisdom in relation to self-management of older adults. They reported on two qualitative studies that explored how older people manage major life transitions, chronic health conditions and disability. The findings from both studies showed older people used their previous life experience to adjust and adapt to new situations, using strategies that worked for them in earlier adulthood. They engaged in self-management activities that took longer to achieve than previously but were equally productive. They drew on their prior independence, autonomy and organisational skills to adapt to new situations.

Perry et al. (2015) stated their findings support assertions made by Erikson et al. (1986), who believed the possession of wisdom is about good judgement and ability to deal with difficult life problems, but also older adults develop a sense of wisdom by returning to earlier stages of development and adapting strategies that worked for them at that time.

Developmental Stages and the Adult Personality

Developmental stages provide a good framework for understanding development of the adult personality. However, we need to remember individual differences influence the meaning and timing of each developmental stage. When examining the concept of personality in relation to ageing, the main issue concerns the nature of stability and

change in personality. Approaches to the study of personality in ageing can be broadly divided into trait models, single-construct models and developmental models. Developmental models, discussed earlier, suggest development continues throughout adulthood, and changes that occur are reflected in the personality. On the other hand, single- and multitrait approaches show support for inter-individual stability (Eysenck, 2018), meaning some personality traits acquired early in life remain stable until old age. Single-construct models, instead of looking at traits, involve examining one construct of personality. An example of such a construct is locus of control (Rotter 1966), discussed in the next section, which has been used successfully to assess possible changes in the perception of control that may occur with ageing.

In the past most researchers were mainly concerned with testing stability of the personality using personality scales. More recent approaches focus on the individual variations that contribute to successful ageing and later-life resilience. Kahlbaugh and Huffman (2017) propose a better approach would be to explore how coping and self-evaluative processes within personality traits affect emotional well-being, satisfaction and adaptation in later life.

Locus of Control

The term *locus of control* is used to explain the perceived source of control over behaviour. An internal locus of control attributes outcomes in life to internal factors that are under a person's control. Conversely, if outcomes in life are attributed to external factors outside a person's control, the locus of control is external. Research shows stability in the locus of control construct, except for domain-specific scales of health and intelligence, where findings show a tendency to an increased external locus of control in older people (Helvik et al., 2016).

The external orientation in locus of control may affect coping processes in older people. A sense of control over our destiny is important and, if not perceived, may result in a passive rather than active way of coping with everyday problems. Depression in older people may influence coping further; Helvik et al. (2016) found negative correlation between external orientation on locus of control and coping in both depressed and non-depressed individuals. Acceptance of help from community services or admission to a nursing home may be perceived as admitting to incompetence, which can lead to loss of control. Passive acceptance of a situation can result in a state of 'learned helplessness' (Seligman, 1975) and lead to depression. Seligman argues depression can arise when individuals believe life events are beyond their control. By late adulthood many people have experienced illness, some role transitions, losses and changes. They may feel they are unable to influence events and therefore feel helpless. For example, people who move to a nursing home may judge their situation as unsatisfactory but as unavoidable and inescapable and may, therefore, act in a passive and helpless way. However, if they reappraise the situation, they may discover options do exist relating to how they cope.

Depending on the option chosen, outcomes may be negative or positive. This is particularly relevant to people with chronic illness; some individuals adapt and cope well, and others are more helpless, looking for constant support. A study by Bhat et al. (2010) examined the role of helplessness in older people with arthritis during an 8-week exercise-and-education randomised trial. They found helplessness was significantly related to disability, pain, fatigue and stiffness in both intervention and control groups. The authors concluded addressing helplessness in health promotion programmes and promoting positive outcomes would be desirable.

A positive outcome can be explained in terms of the concept of self-efficacy (Bandura, 1977). Self-efficacy requires a cognitive change toward positive beliefs regarding the outcomes of behaviour and involves efficacy expectations and outcome expectations. An example of this for a newly institutionalised person could be in contemplating the question: What are the chances I will be happy here? Believing social support resulting from participation in provided activities will lead to satisfaction and happiness can influence a reappraisal of the situation, which is then perceived as satisfying.

Interestingly, more recent research (Nafradi et al., 2017) has shown a link between empowerment and self-efficacy. In a comprehensive literature review, they also found most studies reported a link between internal locus of control and self-efficacy and better adherence to medication. The message here is that in order to improve patient compliance and sense of empowerment, nursing staff need to foster positive patient–nurse relationships that will improve not only compliance but also general well-being of patients and promote greater sense of control.

REMINISCENCE AND LIFE REVIEW AMONG OLDER PEOPLE

Recalling the past and reminiscing are popular mental activities among most groups of people, especially during family gatherings. We all have stories to tell about past experiences and reactions to various events. To engage in a life review is a normal activity and a psychological pursuit not exclusive to older people but open to all. Recalling stories can be a pleasurable experience for the person telling the story as well

as for the listener. Interestingly, according to Munawar et al. (2018), most autobiographical memories come from childhood and early adulthood, a period between 10–30 years old. Some recollections can be cathartic or therapeutic, and structured reminiscence has been reported to increase self-esteem and life satisfaction (Siverová & Bužgová, 2018). The term *reminiscence* is generally applied to a group activity that has a number of goals, including socialisation, communicating and entertainment. If sad memories emerge, the leader and group will act as a support. Reminiscence may be a starting point for contact and interest with older people in day centres or long-stay institutions and may contribute to life satisfaction. Reminiscence is often used in reality-orientation sessions and with depressed patients as well as with those who suffer from dementia.

Duru Asiret and Dutkun (2018) found reminiscence therapy had a positive impact on the quality of life of older adults and on their attitudes to old age and ageing. However, although reminiscence therapy reduced symptoms of depression, it had no effect on the cognitive function of participants in the study.

The term *life review* is used when a client is being offered assistance by a therapist to achieve a sense of integrity. This may involve recalling events and experiences in a one-to-one session that resembles counselling, with the therapist acting as therapeutic listener. This form of therapy sometimes involves working through painful memories and contains elements and principles of psychodynamic therapy. Lapsley et al. (2016) developed questionnaires to help structure a life review and found most participants in their study tended to view early life positively, and any challenges or adversities in early life were mitigated by support from the parents. The reliability of such data is questionable, but the richness of data from the study cohort, born in 1921, gives an interesting insight on life review and reminiscence of life in the early 1920s and how the impact of early childhood contributed to their well-being during their life.

SUCCESSFUL ADAPTATION, ADJUSTMENT AND SATISFACTION IN LATER LIFE

It was suggested earlier that an individual's personality is influential in determining adaptation and adjustment to ageing. There is also evidence some personality types may be better adapted to early adulthood than later adulthood and vice versa. For instance, individuals with Type A personalities who are very competitive, impatient and hard driving may find it difficult to adjust to a slower, more sedentary lifestyle with fewer responsibilities. Conversely, individuals with Type B personalities who are easygoing and carefree may find later adulthood much easier to adjust to than earlier adulthood (Stuart-Hamilton, 2012).

Some research evidence points to a possible link between cognitive and personality factors in later life (Kahlbaugh & Huffman, 2017). It seems older people who have intact cognitive abilities preserve their personality and consequently are more satisfied and able to adjust to old age. However, some older people have not adjusted well to old age and may therefore be cantankerous, withdrawn or hostile and shunned by their neighbours and families. Hostility is a personality trait characterised by having a negative orientation toward others. This attitude maybe less problematic in earlier adulthood, but in older age it may contribute to isolation. Hostility has been linked to increased coronary heart disease and other illnesses (Appleton et al., 2016).

Apart from the personality factors discussed above, the experience of negative life events and stresses also affects adjustment to ageing. The experience of life events and the ability to cope with stress may provide some answers as to why some people cope better than others. The first point to make is not all life events affect well-being in the same way. Normative life events, which affect most people during adult life, are often perceived as less stressful, whereas non-normative events tend to cause more stress. When life events defy the natural order of development, they may be perceived as more stressful. For instance, the death of a child may cause more psychological stress than the death of a spouse in old age. There is evidence older adults rate the death of a spouse as less stressful than do younger adults, particularly if the deceased suffered from a long term illness (Shah et al., 2013). The explanation for this may be linked to the social expectations for adult behaviour during each developmental stage in life, many of which involve some gains and some losses.

The concept of loss is often used to describe the experience of ageing. Older people experience many losses, such as loss of friends, neighbours, relationships, family, places, work and aspects of functioning, that may result in a loss of independence. Apart from the experience of loss and life events, there are other causes of stress. According to Graf et al. (2017), daily hassles may cause more psychological stress for people than major life events. Retirement may be stressful for some older people, especially through loss of income and meaningful activities. It could be argued that being involved in meaningful activities is desirable and satisfying at any time in life. However, this becomes more important in later life when work and family responsibilities no longer take up most of the time, and meaningful activities might help to structure time

and maintain particular identities and roles in life. Recent research shows workers in more physically demanding jobs retire earlier than those in less physically demanding jobs, whereas people employed in more cognitively demanding jobs are less likely to retire early (Collinson, 2019; Xue et al., 2018).

From this brief examination of literature, it becomes evident good adaptation and adjustment in late life may depend on a person's personality and ability to maintain a high level of self-esteem and self-acceptance. Self-esteem can be nurtured to become more resilient by maintaining interests not only in family members but also in other people. Having a perception of control over events boosts self-esteem and promotes better adjustment. However, the evidence from the motivational theory shows adults expect declines in control with advanced older age, and although control-striving remains active, individuals adjust their goals to changing opportunities (Heckhausen & Wrosch, 2016). Satisfaction in late life also seems to be correlated with personality. People who have a relaxed, emotionally stable personality have been found to be more satisfied in late life. Marital adjustment, involvement with social organisations and good health are also good predictors of later-life satisfaction. However, adjustment to ageing is a very individual experience, and therefore generalisations are inappropriate. This is evident in the individual variations and unpredictable emotional responses to the pandemic emergency.

In drawing this section to a conclusion, it is evident people do not age in the same way; nor do they necessarily have similar experiences of ageing. Some people enjoy the freedom of their years, as they have fewer responsibilities and more leisure time. Most advice for successful ageing suggests keeping active in body and mind (Fig. 4.2).

CONCLUSION AND LEARNING POINTS

This chapter examined human ageing from a number of psychological perspectives. The evidence suggests a developmental approach offers the best explanation for transitions that occur throughout the life span. This approach helps us understand adaptation and adjustment, which are part of normal and healthy ageing. The process of ageing should not be seen as a negative experience but as an opportunity to enjoy the freedom from constraints of work and family responsibilities. The psychological changes in ageing should not be considered in isolation but must be viewed from biological, social, environmental and historical contexts.

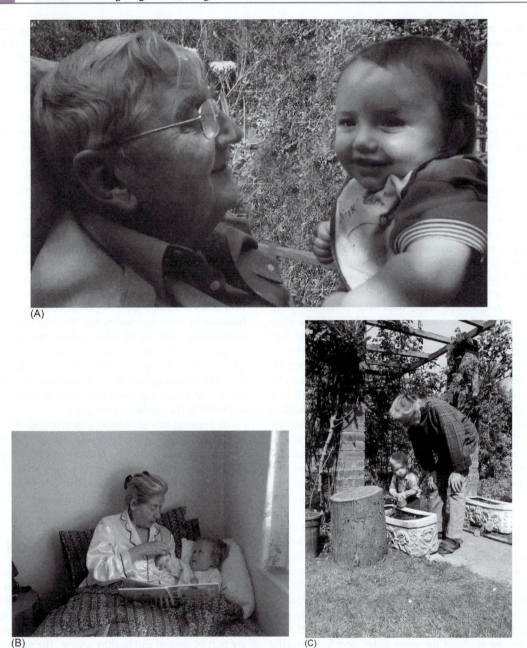

Fig. 4.2 Intergenerational relationships. (A: courtesy of Gian Brown and Fiona Ross; B: courtesy of Maria Ponto; C: courtesy of Fiona Ross.)

SUMMARY OF KEY POINTS

- Social disengagement theory proposes as individuals get older, they gradually withdraw or disengage from society, and there is a withdrawal of society from the individual. Activity theory, on the other hand, suggests for individuals to age successfully on retirement, they need to find substitutes for the activities and work of middle age. Both theories have been influential but have significant limitations.
- Freud believed the narcissistic tendencies of early childhood return to people in old age. Problems experienced by adults in later life may result in regression to the behaviour consistent with a stage of psychosexual development at which they fixated as children. According to Freud, knowing about ego-defence mechanisms may give us an insight into the behaviour of people.
- Maslow's hierarchy of needs is a suitable model for nursing and can be successfully applied when nursing older people. The need for growth is widely recognised and applies to people at every stage of development.
- Cognitive decline is inevitable in old age, but there are individual variations that result from differences in ability and motivation influenced by biological, physiological and environmental changes.
- Short-term memory declines in old age, but since testing relies on laboratory experiments, the application of such findings to everyday life is debatable. More realistic findings can be achieved by testing long-term memory systems such as declarative knowledge and procedural knowledge.
- Social learning and media may influence the way we perceive older people. This can be positive if older people are portrayed as active and helpful but negative if they are portrayed as difficult and rude.
- Anxiety and depression are underdiagnosed in old age. Anxiety is often seen as a symptom of depression, and consequently less attention is paid to it. However, according to recent research, anxiety is widespread in old people. Loss, bereavement and grief can affect the mental health of the older people, leading to distress and depression.
- To engage in a life review is a normal activity and a psychological pursuit not exclusive to older people. Some recollections can be cathartic or therapeutic, and structured reminiscence has been reported to increase self-esteem and life satisfaction.

REFERENCES

An, J. S., & Cooney, T. M. (2006). Psychological well-being in mid to late life: The role of generativity development and parent–child relationships across the lifespan. *International Journal of Behavioral Development, 30*(5), 410–421.

Appleton, K. M., Woodside, J. V., Arveiler, D., Haas, B., Amouyel, P., Montaye, M., Ferrieres, J., Ruidavets, J. B., Yarnell, J. W. G., Kee, F., Evans, A., Bingham, A., Ducimetiere, P., & Patterson, C. C. (2016). A role for behavior in the relationships between depression and hostility and cardiovascular disease incidence, mortality, and all-cause mortality: The prime study. *Annals of Behavioral Medicine, 50*(4), 582–591.

Baltes, P. B. (1987). Theoretical propositions of life-span developmental psychology: On dynamics of growth and decline. *Developmental Psychology, 23*, 611–626.

Baltes, P . B., & Kunzmann, U. (2003). Wisdom. *The Psychologist, 16*(3), 131–133.

Bandura, A. (1977). *Social learning theory*. Prentice-Hall.

Bhat, A. A., DeWalt, D. A., Zimmer, C. R., Fried, B. J., & Callahan, L. F. (2010). The role of helplessness, outcome expectation for exercise and literacy in predicting disability and symptoms in older adults with arthritis. *Patient Education and Counseling, 81*(1), 73–78.

Bowling, A., Iliffe, S., Kessel, A., & Higginson, I. J. (2010). Fear of dying in an ethnically diverse society: Cross-sectional studies of people aged 65 in britain. *Postgraduate Medical Journal, 86*(1014), 197–202.

Brown, C., & Lowis, M. J. (2003). An investigation into Erikson's ninth stage. *Journal of Ageing Studies, 17*, 415–426.

Bryant, C., Jackson, H., & Ames, D. (2008). The prevalence of anxiety in older adults: Methodological issues and a review of the literature. *Journal of Affective Disorders, 109*, 233–250.

Collinson, C. (2019). The unique retirement challenges of workers in physically demanding jobs. *Pension Benefits, 28*(5), 8–10.

Cramer, P. (2000). Defense mechanisms in psychology today: Further processes for adaptation. *American Psychologist, 55*, 637–646.

Cumming, E., & Henry, W. E. (1961). *Growing old: The process of disengagement*. Basic Books.

Doyle, Y. G., McKee, M., & Sherriff, M. (2012). A model of successful ageing in British populations. *European Journal of Public Health, 22*(1), 71–76.

Duru Asiret, G., & Dutkun, M. (2018). The effect of reminiscence therapy on the adaptation of elderly women to old age: A randomized clinical trial. *Complementary Therapies in Medicine, 41*, 124–129.

Erikson, E. H. (1973). *Childhood and society*. Penguin.

Erikson, E. H., & Erikson, J. M. (1997). *The life cycle completed*. Norton.

Erikson, E. H., Erikson, J. M., & Kivnick, H. Q. (1986). *Vital involvement in old age*. Norton.

Eysenck, M. W. (2018). *Simply Psychology* (4th ed.). Psychology Press.

Galderisi, S., Heinz, A., Kastrup, M., Beezhold, J., & Sartorius, N. (2015). Toward a new definition of mental health. *World Psychiatry, 14*(2), 231–233.

Gould, R. L. (1978). *Transformations: Growth and change in adult life.* Simon & Schuster.

Gould, R. L., Coulson, M. C., & Howard, R. J. (2012). Efficacy of cognitive behavioral therapy for anxiety disorders in older people: A meta-analysis and meta-regression of randomized controlled trials. *Journal of the American Geriatrics Society, 60*(2), 218–229.

Graf, A. S., Long, D. M., & Patrick, J. H. (2017). Successful aging across adulthood: Hassles, uplifts, and self-assessed health in daily context. *Journal of Adult Development, 24*(3), 216–225.

Gross, R. D. (2015). *Psychology: The science of mind and behaviour* (7th ed.). Hodder Education.

Havighurst, R. J. (1963). Successful ageing. In R. H Williams, C Tibbitts, & W Donahue (Eds.), *Process of ageing,* 1 (pp. 299–320). Atherton.

Heckhausen, J., & Wrosch, C. (2016). Challenges to developmental regulation across the life course. *International Journal of Behavioral Development, 40*(2), 145–150.

Helvik, A. S., Bjørkløfc, G. H., Corazzinid, K., Selbækc, G., Laksg, J., Østbyeh, T., & Engedalc, K. (2016). Are coping strategies and locus of control orientation associated with health-related quality of life in older adults with and without depression? *Archives of Gerontology and Geriatrics, 64,* 130–137.

Hewston, P., Garcia, A., Alvarado, B., & Deshpande, N. (2018). Fear of falling in older adults with diabetes mellitus: The IMIAS study. *Canadian Journal on Aging, 37*(3), 261–269.

Hülür, G., Ram, N., Willis, S. L., Schaie, K. W., & Gerstorf, D. (2016). Cognitive aging in the Seattle Longitudinal Study: Within-person associations of primary mental abilities with psychomotor speed and cognitive flexibility. *Journal of Intelligence, 4*(12), 1–17. doi:10.3390/jintelligence4030012.

Imlach, A. R., Ward, D. D., Stuart, K. E., Summers, M. J., Valenzuela, M. J., King, A. E., & Vickers, J. C. (2017). Age is no barrier: Predictors of academic success in older learners. *NPJ Science of Learning, 2,* 1–7.

Kimmel, D. C. (1980). *Adulthood and ageing: An interdisciplinary, developmental view.* Wiley.

Kahlbaugh, P., & Huffman, L. (2017). Personality, emotional qualities of leisure, and subjective well-being in the elderly. *The International Journal of Aging and Human Development, 85*(2), 164–184.

Lapsley, H., Pattie, A., Starr, J. M., & Deary, I. J. (2016). Life review in advanced age: Qualitative research on the "start in life" of 90-year-olds in the Lothian Birth Cohort 1921. *BMC Geriatrics, 16*(74). https://doi.org/10.1186/s12877-016-0246-x.

Levinson, D. J., Darrow, D. N., Klein, E. B., Levinson, M. H., & McKee, B. (1978). *The seasons of a man's life.* Knopf.

Maslow, A. (1954). *Motivation and personality.* Harper & Row.

Munawar, K., Kuhn, S. K., & Haque, S. (2018). Understanding the reminiscence bump: A systematic review. *PloS One, 13*(12). https://doi.org/10.1371/journal.pone.0208595.

Nolen-Hoeksema, S., Fredrickson, B., Loftus, G. R., & Lutz, C. (2014). *Atkinson & Hilgard's introduction to psychology.* Harcourt Brace Jovanovich.

Perry, T. E., Ruggiano, N., Shtompel, N., & Hassevoort, L. (2015). Applying Erikson's wisdom to self-management practices of older adults: Findings from two field studies. *Research on Aging, 37*(3), 253–274.

Pinto, J. M., & Neri, A. L. (2017). Trajectories of social participation in old age: A systematic literature review. *Revista Brasileira de Geriatria e Gerontologia, 20*(2), 259–272. https://doi.org/10.1590/1981-22562017020.160077.

Pittman, J. F., Keiley, M. K., Kerpelman, J. L., & Vaughn, B. E. (2011). Attachment, identity, and intimacy: Parallels between Bowlby's and Erikson's paradigms. *Journal of Family Theory & Review, 3,* 32–46.

Rogers, C. R. (2002). Client centred therapy. Constable.

Rotter, J. B. (1966). Generalized expectancies for internal versus external control of reinforcement. *Psychological Monographs, 30*(1), 1–26.

Quigley, C., & Müller, M. M. (2014). Feature-selective attention in healthy old age: A selective decline in selective attention? *Journal of Neuroscience, 34*(7), 2471–2476. https://doi.org/10.1523/JNEUROSCI.2718-13.2014.

Schaie, K. W. (1996). *Intellectual development in adulthood: The Seattle Longitudinal Study.* Cambridge University Press.

Seligman, M. E. P. (1975). *Helplessness. On depression, development and death.* WH Freeman.

Shah, S. M., Carey, I. M., Harris, T., Dewilde, S., Victor, C. R., & Cook, D. G. (2013). The effect of unexpected bereavement on mortality in older couples. *American Journal of Public Health, 103*(6), 1140–1145.

Siverová, J., & Bužgová, R. (2018). The effect of reminiscence therapy on quality of life, attitudes to ageing, and depressive symptoms in institutionalized elderly adults with cognitive impairment: A quasi-experimental study. *International Journal of Mental Health Nursing, 27*(5), 1430–1439.

Smith, M. E., Newberry, K. M., & Bailey, H. R. (2020). Differential effects of knowledge and aging on the encoding and retrieval of everyday activities. *Cognition, 196*(104159). https://psycnet.apa.org/doi/10.1016/j.cognition.2019.104159.

Somerfield, M. R., & McCrae, R. R. (2000). Stress and coping research: Methodological challenges, theoretical advances, and clinical applications. *American Psychologist, 55,* 620–625.

Spahni, S., Morselli, D., Perrig-Chiello, P., & Bennett, K. M. (2015). Patterns of psychological adaptation to spousal bereavement in old age. *Gerontology, 61*(5), 456–468.

Stuart-Hamilton, I. (2012). *The psychology of ageing: An introduction.* Jessica Kingsley Publishers.

Thomas, S., & Kunzmann, U. (2014). Age differences in wisdom-related knowledge: Does the age relevance of the task matter? *The Journals of Gerontology: Series B, 69*(6), 897–905.

von Stumm, S., & Deary, I. J. (2012). Typical intellectual engagement and cognition in the ninth decade of life: The Lothian Birth Cohort 1921. *Psychology and Aging, 27*(3), 761–767. https://doi.org/10.1037/a0026527.

Xue, B., Cadar, D., Fleischmann, M., Stansfeld, S., Carr, E., Kivimäki, M., McMunn, A., & Head, J. (2018). Effect of retirement on cognitive function: The Whitehall II cohort study. *European Journal of Epidemiology, 33*(10), 989–1001.

Zimprich, D. (2020). Individual difference in reminiscence bump of very long-term memory for popular songs in old age: A non-linear mixed model approach. *Psychology of Music, 48*(4), 547–563.

5

The Biology of Human Ageing

Brendan Garry, Laura Green, Jane Griffiths, Emma Stanmore

CHAPTER OUTLINE

Ageing is often considered to be synonymous with a reduction in biological, cognitive and social function. Further, ageing is associated with several diseases and disorders. However, it is important to distinguish between the process of 'normal' ageing and the development of pathology. Ageing itself is not a disease; it is a normal part of the life cycle (Kirkwood, 2003).

This chapter builds on the work of Rosamund A. Herbert in the 4th edition of *Nursing Older People*. Contemporary and seminal theories of ageing are addressed before we turn to the biological concept of homeostasis to demonstrate some of the ways an older person adapts over time. The focus then moves to specific systems to explore functional changes, with particular attention on aspects that have relevance for nursing practice.

STUDY OF HUMAN AGEING

The biology of ageing—biological gerontology—has been extensively researched over many decades. Much of the original work studied ageing cells in cultures: isolated groups of cells such as fibroblasts, artificially grown in vitro (literally, in glass). Increasingly, however, research is carried out on animals such as nematodes, fruit flies, rats/mice and sometimes primates. Data from these animal models are often extrapolated to humans. There are obvious inadequacies with cell cultures and animal studies in telling us about human ageing, but they are still invaluable in increasing general understanding of the ageing process.

In addition to animal studies, two main approaches have been used to study human ageing: cross-sectional and longitudinal studies. Both approaches have strengths and limitations, but combined data from these two methods have given us considerable knowledge about human ageing. Cross-sectional studies involve taking a sample of people in any one population at one time from a wide age range (e.g., 20-, 40-, 60-, 80-year-olds) and assessing their physiological function to look for changes that seem to occur with increasing age. Much of the early work on ageing in the 1950s and 1960s was done using this approach and produced findings that indicated a deterioration in function, such as hearing, sight, mobility, cognition and cardiovascular health. A limitation of looking at different age groups and directly comparing their responses is people from different age decades have lived through very different circumstances, including wars, economic depression, food shortages, changes in diet and access to health and medical care. If these factors affect the variable under consideration—called the cohort effect—differences may wrongly be attributed to ageing.

To avoid some of these pitfalls, longitudinal studies have followed the same individuals over a long time span. Several large-scale longitudinal studies have been underway for a long time in the United States (e.g., Baltimore Longitudinal Study of Aging), the United Kingdom and other parts of Europe. For example, the English Longitudinal Study of Ageing (2021) started in 2002. Interviews are conducted biannually with a cohort of 18,000 people over age 50. The Newcastle 85+ study (University of Newcastle, 2006) started in 2006 and follows a cohort of 1,000 people aged 85 from Newcastle and North Tyneside. An example from Europe are the Berlin Ageing Studies (BASE and BASE-II), multidisciplinary investigations that began in 1990 of older people aged 70 plus who lived in former Berlin (Steinhagen-Thiessen & Borcheltm, 1999).

The general conclusion from longitudinal studies is relatively few individuals follow predictable deterioration. Chronological age is a poor predictor of performance, and ageing is so highly individualised that averages give only an approximation of patterns of individual ageing. Gerontologists now appreciate the importance of lifestyle in the ageing process, but very little is understood about how critical events such as retirement, onset of pathology, loss of mobility and death of a spouse affect performance. The links between different psychological states and their effects on physiology—so-called mind–body links—are being increasingly recognised and acknowledged, especially their effects on the immune system, and may be very pertinent to studies of older people. The psychology of human ageing is discussed in Chapter 4.

In summary, different methods for studying ageing all contribute to our understanding but have their own advantages and disadvantages. By critically combining data from a variety of sources, a fuller picture of the biology of ageing can be gained. Research approaches to ageing are also discussed in Chapter 2.

THEORIES AND MECHANISMS OF AGEING

Why ageing occurs and what causes ageing are questions that have fascinated people for years. Much of the early interest in the ageing process was directed at finding the 'elixir' of life and ways of increasing longevity. Although progress has been made over the past 50 years in understanding the processes that underpin ageing, many competing theories and fundamental questions remain. We have to date been unable to extend the life of humans.

Many different theories have been proposed to explain ageing; some of these theories can be grouped together, as they incorporate similar approaches. For example, some theories have looked at the genetics of ageing and linked this with evolution. Some researchers have investigated changes in whole-body function or in one particular system, while others have concentrated on changes in cell structure and function. More recently, research has been directed at the molecular basis of ageing and changes in deoxyribonucleic acid (DNA), which may link to the genetics of ageing. It is not possible in a chapter of this nature to consider or do justice to all the theories of ageing; however, a few contemporary theories are considered briefly.

A dominant theory of ageing that held considerable sway for decades was that of wear and tear—in other words, as we age, we simply wear out through random molecular damage (Harman, 1981). The premise of this theory is we are complex organisms and, like complex machinery, have lots of moving parts that with overuse wear out or work less well. For instance, one small error in the long chain of reactions during protein synthesis would produce an imperfect structural protein or enzyme that in turn might interfere with cell function. There is evidence DNA, proteins and lipids accumulate damage during ageing. The theory was living in an oxidising environment, as we do, causes damage to DNA. An entire health industry selling antioxidants has thrived on this theory; you can still buy antioxidants in health-food shops. While attractive, the theory has been tested extensively over 20 years on animal models—specifically, the nematode worm *Caenorhabditis elegans*, the fruit fly drosophila and mice)—and been shown to be incorrect (Gems & Doonan, 2009). There is still interest in damage to DNA as a primary cause of ageing, but ideas have moved on.

Another recent theory of ageing that adds to the idea of damage processes is based on the work of George Williams, an evolutionary geneticist. The theory is called plieotropy (Williams, 1957). The premise is genes that are helpful when we are young can cause pathology as we age. Natural selection favours these genes, such as those that predispose fitness in a young person of reproductive age but cause damage as we get older. In other words, good genes create late-life pathology. This genetic explanation of the origins of disease has been researched extensively, again in animal models, and found to be robust and replicable.

Another compelling theory of ageing proposed by David Sinclair at Harvard University is we have built-in repair mechanisms that need to be activated to reverse damage to our cells (Sinclair & LaPlante, 2019). To use a car analogy, we are not just a vehicle that breaks down, but we have a repair shop that needs to be activated to repair the damage. It has been found through extensive laboratory research with *C. elegans* that a stress response leads to messages being sent to the repair shop, telling the mechanics to get to work (Gomes et al., 2013). In addition, researchers have found longevity genes that control the mechanics by tricking the body into thinking there's a stress response or damage (even though there isn't!). An example of a stressor is lack of food. It has been known for a long time that calorie restriction increases longevity in animal models, but the mechanism was unclear. It now appears perceived starvation triggers the cells to constantly repair themselves, reversing the effects of ageing. Application to humans is unclear, but in primate models, the effects have been far less dramatic than in less complex species such as nematodes (Harman, 1981).

A fascinating theory of ageing is a recent revision of the original mitochondrial theory (Jin, 2010). From age 50 and onward, there is known decline in our mitochondrial functioning. The mitochondria are the energy supply in our cells, producing chemical energy adenosine triphosphate (ATP). There are hundreds of them per cell. The amount of ATP produced declines dramatically with each decade but particularly in our 60s and 70s. Energy keeps the cells young. Fascinatingly, mitochondria have their own genome/DNA and are effectively a separate species in our cells. Their genome 'speaks' to the genome in the nucleus of the cell, and the messages are relayed through a protein messenger. In the early years of life, the conversation flows, and communication is excellent. Over time, however, the two genomes communicate less well, and messages become confused. In turn, less energy is produced. In mice models, communication has been restored using the protein nicotinamide adenine dinucleotide, and the reversal of biological ageing has been dramatic.

The final theory of ageing we consider here is the telomere theory (Kelly, 2011). Our strands of DNA (chromosomes) look like pieces of string. The ends of the strands can become damaged quite easily and frayed, and need to be protected, which is the role of the telomere. Telomeres, also made of DNA, sit at the ends of chromosomes and prevent them from becoming damaged. Each time the cell divides, the telomeres also divide, but in the process they become shorter. Longer telomeres mean less cell damage, and shorter ones more cell damage. Interestingly, telomeres in the skin cells of people with acne are longer, which delays the ageing process in later life! The shortening is a bit like a ticking clock that marks how many times the cell can divide before it dies. In contrast, the shortening mechanism is reversed in cancer cells, which have infinite capacity for cell division. Cancer cells maintain long telomeres, which silence the clock and allow the cells to continue dividing, even though they should be at the end of their life span.

HOMEOSTASIS IN OLDER PEOPLE

From a physiological perspective, the health of a person depends on the efficient functioning of individual cells and tissues in all systems of the body. Homeostasis is maintained through a complex series of physiological and biochemical changes and responses within those systems. The rate at which we age varies, and the physiological responses are heterogeneous; however, the hallmarks of ageing become progressively reliant on homeostatic reserves.

Homeostasis is maintained in older people. Older people can live a normal independent life, and most processes in the body appear to function adequately under basal or resting conditions. However, it is true to say most physiological processes in the body become less effective under certain circumstances with increasing age, and it is generally accepted that with ageing there is a decline in the functional competence of the individual. This decline in function may be due in part to the progressive loss of functioning body cells—in other words, there is a gradual loss of body tissue in many systems with age. The age-related deficits that exist are apparent only when the body or system is physiologically stressed, such as with illness, strenuous exercise or exposure to extreme environmental temperatures. For example, values for blood glucose do not change significantly under resting conditions, but if these values are increased for some reason, changes are often greater in older people, and more time is required to return the parameter to its original value (Lomeli et al., 2017).

Older people become more susceptible to disturbances of fluid and electrolyte balance. Reflexes that maintain blood pressure when going from lying to standing positions become less efficient, and some older people are prone to develop postural hypotension. Liver and renal function are less efficient, so metabolism and drug excretion are altered, and drugs can accumulate more easily, often reaching toxic levels in the body.

Ageing is also often associated with a decline in the physical function that affects habitual exercise, agility and mobility. These depend on coordination between many systems in the body; for example, muscles, joints, the cardiovascular and respiratory systems, balance, neural factors and skill all affect the ability to perform physical activity. The complexity of the interplay between this loss in function and ageing processes often complicates the actual aetiology of the decline. Often the maximum contraction many older people can generate in their quadriceps is just enough to get up from a chair without using their arms. If they use their arms to help push up, they need less strength in their quadriceps. The classic armless chair is the toilet; this is why handrails are so useful for some older people. Some of these changes are due to the ageing process itself, and some are due to the harmful or negative effects of inactivity. Changes in joints, cartilage and collagen, and an increase in osteoporosis and a decline in the number of muscle cells, could account for some of the observed changes. The cardiovascular system is not thought to be the limiting factor normally, and certainly, skill factors are retained and can often compensate for the decline in strength. However, structural and functional changes in the respiratory system are seen as important factors in restricting strenuous exercise (Roman et al., 2016). See Chapter 18 on mobility for a further discussion of these issues.

So often with the change in lifestyle that accompanies advancing age, physical activity in general declines, and cardiorespiratory and muscular systems in particular become deconditioned. Physical deconditioning accentuates age-related declines in performance, particularly in response to physiological stress (Smith et al., 2020). Appropriate activity and exercise—be it simply standing to do the washing up, walking upstairs to the toilet, attending appropriate keep-fit classes or hill-walking—should be encouraged for all older people. An overall decline in capacity is still likely, but it will be less if the individual is fitter. This is a message to all of us who tend to do things for older people, thinking we are helping them; we may not be helping at all.

Disorders of homeostasis with age are considered to arise not by virtue of changes in equilibrium levels but in the efficiency with which these steady states can be re-established once displacement has occurred. This is sometimes described as a decline in the adaptive ability of the body to cope with changes or stress. People who present with frailty who are compromised in several ways may be at greater risk. Thus, homeostasis is maintained but with increasing difficulty as the years pass.

It is characteristic of many biological systems that each has a certain amount of spare capacity, or functional reserve. An obvious example is we can manage perfectly well with one kidney, although we are born with two. This is an important concept because it relates to the decline in function shown by researchers to occur with ageing; because of this reserve, a decline in function may proceed for many years without lowering the functional capacity below what is required for homeostasis (Fig. 5.1).

Another example of reduction in functional capacity is coronary arteriosclerosis, or the thickening and loss of elasticity of the arterial walls. This steady loss of coronary vessel function usually goes unnoticed because there is still an adequate perfusion of the myocardium—in other words, because there is no effect on homeostatic function. System failure occurs only when the spare capacity or functional reserves are depleted below the levels required for homeostasis, and this may happen only after years of continual loss of function.

FUNCTIONAL CHANGES WITH AGEING

The previous section emphasised the importance of considering the interrelationships between ageing in the various systems of the body as a whole. It is still valuable to consider more discrete individual systems too. A decline in function may not mean impaired homeostasis. A detailed and comprehensive review of ageing changes is beyond the scope of this chapter; however, the discussion below selects some important aspects for further consideration.

NUTRITION AND GASTROINTESTINAL TRACT

The relationship between nutrition and the ageing process in humans is complex. Diet influences the maintenance of health and recovery of disease and plays an important role in brain function and mental health in older age

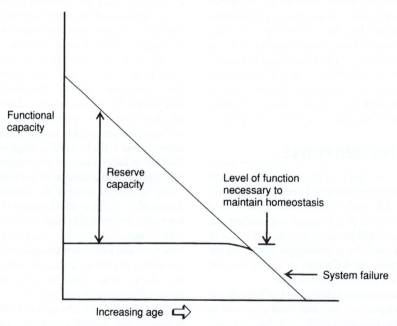

Fig. 5.1 System failure only occurs when functional reserve is depleted and homeostatic needs can no longer be met.

(Bourre, 2006; Jackson et al., 2016). Sense of taste and smell can also alter with age, which can affect appetite and enjoyment of food.

The physiological changes associated with advancing age may lead to older adults having difficulties in meeting their nutritional requirements, so nurses require specific knowledge and understanding to intervene as needed.

It is well established our body composition changes with ageing, and we tend to lose muscle and gain fat (Fig. 5.2). As fat requires less energy metabolism (needed for all cell functions), our energy requirements reduce. Studies indicate protein requirements may be higher in older adults in order to maintain muscle mass, with additional dietary protein, needed to build and repair tissues, particularly needed post-surgery and for those with fractures, frailty and gastrointestinal disease. The European Society for Clinical Nutrition recommends healthy older adults consume 1–1.2 grams of protein per kilogram of body weight daily, which is a 25% to 50% increase over the current recommended daily allowance (Deutz, 2014). Providing higher levels of protein in older individuals who have no pre-existing renal disease appears to be beneficial; however, a careful therapeutic regimen is needed for those with renal function problems.

Water intake is also important, as 70% of the body is made up of water. It is essential for older adults to drink adequately—approximately 2,000 ml for men and 1,600 ml for women per day—to keep the body functional (Association of UK Dieticians, 2021). This can be a challenge for older adults due to a reduction in thirst sensation (Kenny & Chiu, 2001) or concerns about nocturia. Inadequate fluid intake can lead to a multitude of problems such as dehydration, hypotension, confusion and constipation.

Dietary recommendations for fat, carbohydrate and dietary fibre are the same for older people as for the rest of the population, and similar healthy eating guidelines apply (Scientific Advisory Committee on Nutrition, 2021). However, a careful balance is needed to ensure the older person consumes essential fatty acids that are not made by the body (e.g., omega-3 found in oily fish) but also keep total fat and calorie intake within the recommended dietary range. The ability to absorb, metabolise and excrete vitamins and minerals changes with ageing, and this can be exacerbated by the use of medications (such as Metformin for type 2 diabetes mellitus) that reduce the ability of the small bowel to absorb micronutrients. For instance, vitamin B12 absorption is decreased when gastric acid production is reduced, which commonly occurs in older age. B12 absorption is necessary for the release of B12 from protein carriers. Older adults may also become deficient in fat-soluble vitamins (A, D, E, and K) due to reduced ability to store these vitamins in the liver.

Studies have also shown vitamin D, important for bone mineralisation and the immune system, is more likely to be deficient in older adults, particularly those who are homebound or living in care homes, as this vitamin is mainly synthesised in skin via exposure to sunlight (Royal Society of Osteoporosis, 2021). Calcium requirements have also generated much interest over recent years, with the National Health Service (2019) recommending a diet rich in calcium for older adults, resistance exercise and a vitamin D supplement to help prevent osteoporosis.

Malnutrition is common in older people and includes both under- and overnutrition. Reasons for older adults being at increased risk are multifactorial and include physiological, social and psychological factors that affect food intake and weight. This is further exacerbated by underlying medical illness. Assessment and recognition have improved with national guidance on screening (Wells et al., 2020). Excess weight, particularly around the waist, may increase the risk of developing cardiac disease, cancer and type 2 diabetes. Being underweight can predispose to frailty or developing pressure ulcers. In contrast, dietary restriction without malnutrition has been shown to increase life span, as discussed earlier in the chapter.

The nurse has an important role in supporting and educating older adults to eat a varied diet that contains plenty of fruit and vegetables to ensure an adequate supply of essential vitamins and minerals, including foods that contain vitamin D (e.g., oily fish, eggs and fortified cereals).

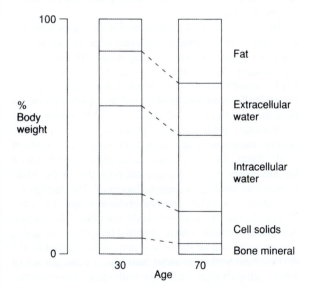

Fig. 5.2 Approximate changes in body composition with ageing. (Individual variations are large.)

For a fuller discussion of the nutritional requirements of older people and malnutrition, see the British Nutrition Foundation website (British Nutrition Foundation, n.d.).

The gastrointestinal tract is intricately involved in nutrition with its role in ingestion, digestion and absorption, so physiological changes due to ageing need to be considered. In the mouth, dental decay, bone loss and gum recession can lead to impaired chewing and digestion of food. Salivary flow decreases in individuals after the age of 50. In the small intestine, the villi shorten and become broader, which significantly reduces the surface area for absorption. Amino acid absorption does not appear to be impaired, although lipid absorption is reduced. The liver tends to reduce in mass and in the number of hepatocytes, which leads to some reduced storage capacity and function. The digestive functions of the pancreas are well conserved. In the colon there is atrophy of mucosa and muscle layers that leads to reduced and weaker peristaltic action. There is an increased incidence of diverticula and reduced elasticity of the rectal wall, which gives a reduced maximal tolerance to faeces.

Throughout the gut and associated organs (liver, pancreas, etc.), there is a reduction in perfusion and in the coordination of the enteric nerve reflexes, which synchronise events in the gut. Constipation is a common problem in older age and has a multifactorial aetiology: loss of muscle tone and motor activity in the colon, a low-fibre diet and inactivity may all contribute. Therefore, ensuring adequate hydration, dietary fibre and physical activity can reduce constipation in older adults.

IMMUNE SYSTEM

It is well established there is a general decline in immunocompetence with ageing, which could be an important contributor to senescence and to the development of chronic diseases and disorders. The decline in immunity in older people has largely been attributed to the impairment of T-cell mechanisms. The evidence of a role for the immune system in ageing is more convincing for the diseases of old age than it is for the normal processes of ageing. As immunological efficiency decreases, incidences of infections, autoimmune diseases and cancer increase. However, some theories suggest normal ageing is the consequence of a developing immunodeficiency; these are attractive theories, as they imply the process might then be potentially accessible to manipulation!

The immune system, which is distributed throughout the body and interacts with all other systems, provides a vital aspect of defence of the internal environment. The immune system recognises foreign molecules (antigens) and acts to immobilise, neutralise or destroy them. When it operates effectively, this system protects the body from a wide variety of infectious agents as well as from abnormal body cells. When it fails, malfunctions or is disabled, some of the most serious diseases, such as cancer, rheumatoid arthritis, acquired immune deficiency syndrome and COVID-19, may result.

Humoral and cell-mediated immunity are the two main components of a functioning immune system, and the responsiveness of both declines with increasing age. With ageing, lymphoid tissue is lost from the thymus, spleen, lymph nodes and bone marrow. One major change in the system is in the T cells or T lymphocytes that mature in the thymus gland. T cells are the non-antibody-producing lymphocytes that constitute the cell-mediated arm of immunity. These T cells directly attack and lyse body cells infected by viruses or other intracellular parasites, cancer cells and foreign grafts, and release chemical mediators that enhance the inflammatory response or help activate lymphocytes or macrophages. There is a blunted T-cell response with ageing and increased production of pro-inflammatory cytokines (Inoue et al., 2014). Changes in the B cells, which are responsible for the humoral response, are smaller and often secondary to changes in T-cell population.

The involution of the thymus gland during the first half of life may explain the altered formation and function of the immune system observed during the second half of life. The thymus gland is at its maximum size at sexual maturity, and after puberty its size decreases (Musi & Hornsby, 2021). The thymus is the site of differentiation of immature lymphocytes from the bone marrow; the lymphocytes then enter the cortex of the thymus gland and eventually become T lymphocytes.

The level of natural antibodies also decreases with age, and there is an increase in autoantibodies (i.e., antibodies that react against an antigenic component of the individual's own tissues). Autoantibodies to nucleic acids (e.g., DNA, RNA), smooth muscle, mitochondria, lymphocytes, gastric parietal cells, immunoglobulins and thyroglobulin have all been found with increased frequency in older people.

Abundant evidence exists to show how the immune system changes with age (Musi & Horsby, 2021; Weiskopf et al., 2009). To summarise, cell-mediated and humoral immune response to foreign antigens decreases, while response to autologous antigens increases. The changes are undoubtedly complex, and one problem is age-associated changes in the immune system do not always distinguish between an immune system impaired by age (i.e., an ageing change itself) and an immune system compromised by the environment within an older host (i.e., a consequence of other ageing changes within the individual). Environmental factors known to influence immune competence include disease, nutrition and exposure to ionising radiation.

An important consequence of the changes in the immune system is the dysregulation of the pro-inflammatory mediators such as cytokines and chemokines. These can induce a state of chronic inflammation, which plays an important role in a variety of diseases and conditions. The liver produces a protein known as C-reactive protein (CRP) in response to both acute and chronic inflammation, and blood levels of CRP can be used to indicate inflammatory processes in the body. CRP results are most useful as markers of chronic inflammation, for example in tracing the progression of a known disease such as chronic obstructive pulmonary disease or rheumatoid arthritis. In recent years it has become increasingly evident that chronic inflammation has a profound influence on health and well-being (Nowakowski, 2014). For example, it can affect adiposity and the development of insulin resistance, contributing to obesity, fatty liver and diabetes. It is also thought to contribute to the development of cardiovascular disease, particularly the process of atherosclerosis.

RESPIRATORY AND CARDIOVASCULAR SYSTEMS

The respiratory and cardiovascular systems work together to ensure an adequate supply of oxygen is delivered to the tissues and that carbon dioxide is removed from the body. The cardiovascular system also has a more general role in transporting heat and substances such as nutrients, hormones and waste products around the body.

A variety of structural changes occur in the thorax and lungs with ageing and have an adverse effect on function. For example, changes in lung volume and capacity result in a reduced surface area being available for gas exchange—for example, the fraction of lung volume occupied by the airways increases at the expense of alveolar space, and the alveoli become smaller. The lung tissue seems to lose its elasticity, primarily because of stiffening changes in collagen. Work that is more muscular is required to move air in and out of the lungs, because of the stiffening of ribs and other joints in the thorax and the structural changes in the lung tissue.

One of the main defence mechanisms in the lungs that protects against inhaled particulate matter is sometimes described as the mucociliary escalator. This depends on particles being trapped in the layer of mucus that lines the larger airways, after which the mucus is 'wafted' up to the larynx by beating movements of the cilia (hairlike projections) situated on the bronchial epithelium. With ageing, cilia are lost from the airways, and the vigour of the remaining cilia is reduced. Thus, the mucociliary escalator is less effective in removing debris. Macrophages that form the last line of defence farther down the airways, at the alveolar levels, also become less efficient.

The study of ageing changes in the cardiovascular system has been dogged by methodological problems. It is difficult to get a coronary artery disease–free population for study so ageing changes rather than disease-induced changes can be investigated. It is also particularly important when comparing the cardiovascular function of young and older subjects to ensure the level of physical conditioning or fitness is similar in subjects of all ages; heart rate, blood pressure and other cardiorespiratory parameters vary substantially according to the amount of physical activity normally undertaken.

Various components of the cardiovascular system change as part of the ageing process. The heart and blood vessels are highly dependent for their normal function on the physical properties of connective tissue and muscle, namely distensibility, contractility and elasticity, and these alter with ageing, leading to increased stiffness generally. Heart weight, as a fraction of body weight, tends to increase slightly. The blood vessels undergo changes with ageing, too. Major structural alterations in the arteries, due to an increase in collagen and smooth muscle, lead to increased arterial stiffness and reduced compliance with increasing age. As elsewhere in the body, collagen tends to become cross-linked, and calcium is deposited. Veins become increasingly tortuous, the walls become weaker due to loss of elastic tissue and varicosities occur in veins subjected to high pressure. The basement membrane of the capillary endothelium becomes thicker, and the fenestrations of the endothelium become fewer. These changes in the capillary structure, in association with the increased density of ground substance of connective tissues, impair the diffusion of gases and nutrients to and from the cells (Gude et al., 2018). Bruising is also more common due to the fragility and altered structure of the vessels and supporting tissues.

There is a tendency for perfusion of the organs in the body to be reduced with age, although the extent of this reduction varies considerably. Blood flow to the kidneys is reduced by up to 50%, and there are also large decreases in the splanchnic and cutaneous circulations. Cerebral blood flow is thought to reduce by 20%. Changes in resting blood flow to the myocardium and skeletal muscle are less marked; however, the ability to increase blood flow to these tissues when required, for example following tissue hypoxia, is reduced in older people.

Many of the factors mentioned above would be expected to increase arterial pressure. Both longitudinal and cross-sectional studies have shown an increase in systolic pressure with age (Wojciechowska, 2012). There is debate, however, as to whether this increase in blood pressure is an inevitable consequence of normal healthy ageing. It may be the age-related rise in pressure is a consequence of other factors such as diet and social stresses. Whatever the reasons behind its development, systolic hypertension is a known risk factor for developing coronary heart disease, and treatment now aims to ensure systolic pressures in middle-aged and older people are maintained at an optimal level.

THE ENDOCRINE SYSTEM

Both men's and women's endocrine systems show marked age-related changes. Some hormones remain unchanged or decrease only slightly, such as insulin and cortisol. However, this does not mean functions associated with them are unaffected, as sensitivity to hormones can decrease, which means circulating levels exert lower physiological effects (Fig. 5.3).

Although secretion of cortisol in response to stress is unchanged, the responsiveness of receptors within the negative feedback mechanism of the hypothalamus-pituitary-adrenal axis is altered. Usually, humans react to stress by producing corticoptrophic-releasing factor that leads to the release of glucocorticoids from the adrenal cortex. However, with advancing age, the negative feedback mechanism by which this process is halted can be disrupted. This leads to a prolonged stress response, which can result in changes in energy levels and mood, and alterations in the composition of body tissues. It can also lead to loss of tissue in the hippocampus, the part of the brain associated with declarative memory. This means recall of everyday facts and events can be impaired (Fig. 5.4).

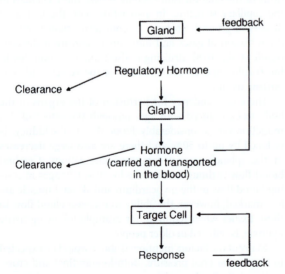

Fig. 5.3 The sequence of hormone action and regulation. Clearance refers to removal from the blood, and feedback is usually negative.

Some hormones actually increase in older people. Key examples are the catecholamines adrenaline and noradrenaline, which are associated with the stress response and can lead to reduced recovery from stressful stimuli (Yiallouris et al., 2019).

Altered cortisol metabolism raises the risk for problems in blood glucose homeostasis and may be associated with a rise in insulin resistance—often a precursor for the development of type 2 diabetes mellitus. Increased insulin resistance is thought to result primarily from increased adiposity rather than as a result of altered endocrine activity (Karakelides et al., 2010).

A range of changes take place in neuroendocrine function as a person ages, including reduced production of sex steroids and growth hormones.

THE REPRODUCTIVE SYSTEM

Women in particular experience adverse consequences of age-related changes in sex hormones. The early signs of reduced oestrogens include mood changes, increased body fat and reduced muscle mass. Later menopausal signs include greater propensity to cardiovascular disease, reduced bone density and cognitive impairment. For men, ageing leads to reduced serum levels of testosterone and oestrodiol, dehydroepiandrosterone, growth hormone and insulin-like growth factor (Chadwick & Goode, 2002). Testosterone exerts an anabolic effect, which means it plays an important role in muscle density and strength, sleep, energy and mood. Reduction in testosterone levels can therefore bring about global functional changes that in some ways mirror those experienced by women when oestrogen levels drop. This so-called andropause has received notably less attention than its equivalent in women, but there is ongoing debate as to the potential beneficial impact of androgen-replacement therapies as a means of preventing or mitigating osteoporosis and other negative sequelae such as sleep disturbance.

Women's ability to reproduce ceases with the menopause, defined as the absence of a menstrual period for 12 consecutive months along with a hypo-gonadotrophic state. The age at which this occurs depends on genetic, behavioural and environmental factors but globally takes place at a median age of 49–52 years. The aetiology of menopause is complex, but the most significant hormonal alteration appears to be a reduced sensitivity to oestrogen within the pituitary gland. Men exhibit a more gradual decline in fertility, with some retaining full reproductive capacity into extreme old age. The primary age-related change exhibited by men is the enlargement of the prostate gland with associated changes in micturition and altered levels of testosterone. For both men and women, these hormonal changes

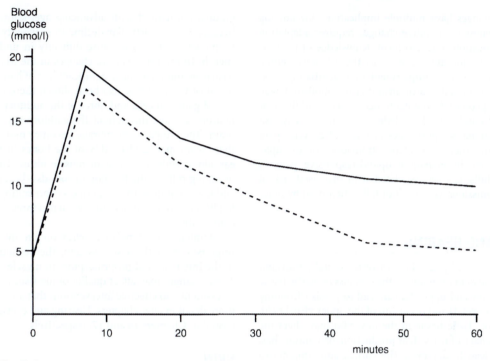

Fig. 5.4 Effect of glucose administration on young (———— age 20–30 years) and older (--- age 60–70 years) subjects.

may be accompanied by a variety of somatic and psychological symptoms such as sleep disturbance and cognitive changes, including depression, irritability and reduced muscle mass.

THE NERVOUS SYSTEM

Many people experience altered cognitive function as they age. Overall, the volume of the brain becomes smaller from mid to late life, but the impact on the individual is a complex interplay of these anatomical changes and environment. Patterns of cognitive decline, and its impact on individuals, show marked variability. Some aspects of cognitive function are maintained in the healthy older person, such as semantic memory (knowledge about the world) and emotional regulation. Other functions, such as processing speed, susceptibility to distracting stimuli and task-switching, show an age-related decline (Grady, 2012). Finally, there is an important distinction between healthy ageing and diseases of cognition that are common in old age, such as the dementias and neurological conditions like Parkinson's disease. As the blood vessels that supply the brain change, there may be increased risk of stroke or ischaemia.

The availability of neuroimaging technology, in particular functional magnetic resonance imaging (fMRI), has meant research into brain changes has developed apace in recent years. fMRIs offer a window into brain function, rather than solely its anatomy, by measuring activity that indicates use of a part of the brain. For example, fMRI experiments have demonstrated older adults appear to recruit more parts of the brain to complete the same tasks as a younger person. This is known as the compensation hypothesis (Reuter-Lorenz & Cappell, 2008). It is of interest to nurses because it suggests even though there is an overall depletion of brain tissue and volume with ageing, at the same time there is an adaptive process in which neural capacity is maintained by redistribution of resources within the brain. However, it is important to note some research has indicated this increased brain activity does not always lead to better task performance. The hippocampus is the part of the brain associated with declarative memory. It has been shown to reduce in size with age, with corresponding reduction in memory (Persson et al., 2006). Recent studies on the hippocampus have identified neurogenesis—the creation of new nerves and neural pathways—persists throughout ageing, which contradicts earlier assumptions the generation of new memories slows.

These changes have multiple implications for nursing care. Awareness of cognitive changes requires adaptation in communication style and form. Knowledge of medications and their side effects can reduce the risk of worsening any existing cognitive impairment or exacerbating existing effects of altered neurotransmitter metabolism. Given many older people take regular or occasional painkillers for a variety of conditions, knowledge of the nervous system can help rationalise approaches to safe and effective pain management. There is evidence tramadol, for example, while effective in managing opioid-responsive pain in younger adults, can be associated with increased risk of hospital admissions as a result of falls when used by older people.

VISION AND HEARING

Vision is affected by age. Loss of retro-orbital fat around the eye can lead to recession of the eye; loss of elastic tissue of the eyebrow and upper lid can lead to ptosis (drooping of the upper eyelid) and occlusion of the upper visual field, while loss of elastic tissue in the lower lid may affect the normal drainage of tears. Tear production also diminishes, which can lead to dry eyes. The cornea and conjunctiva become thinner. The diameter of the pupil gets smaller, to a minimum around the age of 60, and substantially impairs the amount of light admitted. This can significantly affect reading at night due to the resulting loss of light through the decreased pupil. An arcus senilis—a white ring encircling about 1 mm within the corneal margin—is a corneal degeneration that is often apparent but does not itself damage sight.

Presbyopia, the loss of ability to accommodate for near vision, is well known and is due to loss of flexibility of the lens, which becomes thicker with increasing age. The near point—the distance from the eye at which print can be read—begins to recede, which explains the common experience of having to hold books farther away in order to be able to read them. Cataracts, due to clouding of the lens, are also very common in older people, giving blurred vision.

Receptors are lost from the retina, and this reduces the size of the visual field, affecting peripheral vision. There are minor losses of receptors at the fovea or macula (the area of clearest vision), which lead to loss of visual acuity. Age-related macular degeneration is caused by deterioration to the macula in the retina. The chemical processes of vision that involve photochemical pigments become impaired, so that adaptation to dark/light conditions occurs more slowly and to a lesser extent.

Both auditory and vestibular structures within the inner ear can be adversely affected by ageing. Hearing becomes gradually impaired with advancing age, known as presbycusis, with a particular decline in sensitivity for higher frequencies, which can cause difficulty in understanding speech. In the inner ear are changes in the Reissner's and basilar membranes and a significant loss of hair cells in the organ of Corti. It has also been shown there is a gradual loss of ganglion cells and fibres of the auditory nerve, and neurons are lost throughout the auditory pathway in the brain. The tympanic membrane becomes more rigid, and there is an increased rigidity of the bones in the middle ear, along with some loss of muscle fibres. The auditory orienting reflex—the location of sounds—becomes slower and less accurate with age, perhaps contributing to the difficulty some older adults show when in a three- or four-way conversation.

Maintenance of balance relies on an integration of responses from the visual system, the vestibular system in the inner ear and proprioceptors in muscles and joints. These changes may affect quality of life issues and require assessment and effective interventions that are discussed in more detail in later chapters. Hearing and eyesight are discussed in Chapters 16 and 17, respectively.

SKIN

The skin is a complex organ that serves many functions in the body. It is vital as a defence against infection and in the process of thermoregulation and the regulation of fluids and electrolytes. It is also able to respond to the environment in order to protect itself—for example, through the production of melanin in response to exposure to ultra-violet radiation (Huang & Chien, 2020). Changes occur at both the molecular and cellular levels. An awareness of the anatomy and physiology of the skin is vital in nursing care of the older person. The topic of maintaining healthy skin is addressed fully in Chapter 24.

The process of intrinsic skin ageing resembles that seen in most internal organs and results from the reduced ability of cells to proliferate. This leads to skin becoming thinner, particularly in women, meaning it is more easily damaged. This fragility is thought to result from the loss of papillae responsible for the underlying contour of the layers of the skin in the dermo-epidermal junction (Farage et al., 2009). The characteristic wrinkling in older skin results from changes in collagen and elastin in the skin, the molecules responsible for structure and flexibility. This is the reason shearing forces—for example, during poor moving and handling techniques—can damage the epidermis. Advancing age is therefore an independent risk factor for the development of pressure damage and decubitus ulcers, although older people may also demonstrate other risk factors, such as reduced mobility, loss of sensation and cardiovascular impairment. Fig. 5.5A and B show the difference between young and old skin.

The reduced inflammatory response discussed earlier in the chapter impacts healing. Many older adults experience disorders associated with the skin. Older people have reduced lipid production and perspiration, which can lead to drier, coarse and itchy skin. Skin complaints such as eczema, contact and allergic dermatitis, and keratoses are common. Sweat glands become less effective, and blood flow through the skin diminishes, which reduces an individual's ability to lose heat. Sensitivity to the effects of the sun increases in older people; less melanin is produced, and the skin becomes paler. These natural patterns of ageing of skin can be accelerated through exposure to ultraviolet radiation, pollutants and microbes. Some of these environmental insults can cause molecular and subcellular alterations such as DNA mutation, leading to an increased risk of basal cell and squamous carcinomas and malignant melanomas.

MUSCULOSKELETAL SYSTEM AND CONNECTIVE TISSUES

The musculoskeletal system comprises bones, muscles, cartilage, ligaments, tendons, joints and other connective tissues that support and connect tissues and organs to provide form and stability and enable movement.

Connective tissue is the most common and widely distributed tissue in the human body and is made up of cells, fibres and ground substance. Ground substance is a clear, hydrated gel that fills the space between cells. Collagen, elastin and reticular fibres are the three types of protein fibres in connective tissues. Collagen fibres are the strongest and thickest fibres, found in cartilage, bones, tendons and ligaments. Elastin fibres are thinner fibres that can stretch and recoil and are found in skin and the ligaments of the spine. Reticular fibres are shorter, extensively branched fibres found in parts of the body such as the spleen and lymph nodes.

As connective tissue is so widespread, changes due to ageing can affect most parts of the body. As discussed earlier, skin loses its elasticity and becomes wrinkled, the lungs lose their elastic recoil and the costal cartilages become increasingly rigid, making breathing harder, and joints in the body become stiffened by the increase in fibrous tissue. The loss of hydration in the cartilage in the intervertebral discs leads to compaction of the vertebrae and shrinkage in stature. The cardiovascular system may also be adversely affected: the chambers of the heart become less distensible with reduced contractility, the valves of the heart become stiffer and the elastic arteries become more rigid.

In the ageing skeleton, bone volume and density declines, especially for women after menopause, which can lead to

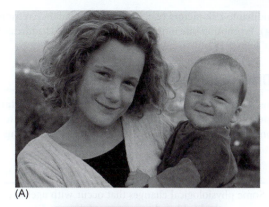
(A)

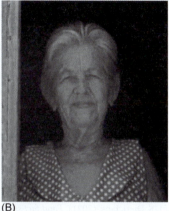
(B)

Fig. 5.5 (A) Young and (B) old skin.

an increased risk of osteoporosis and fracture. Peak bone mass is attained at around the age of 30, and a slow decline in bone mineral density, approximately 0.5% per year, begins from around the age of 40 (Clarke & Khosla, 2010). Many factors contribute to bone mineral loss, including hormonal changes (particularly reduced oestrogen levels), nutritional (calcium) and lifestyle factors (lack of weight-bearing physical activity and vitamin D deficiency due to low exposure to sunlight, smoking, excessive alcohol intake and certain medications such as corticosteroids).

Declining muscle mass, and therefore strength, also occurs with ageing and increases exponentially with age. Sarcopenia, a condition characterised by progressive loss of muscle mass and function, is an age-related process influenced by genetic and lifestyle risk factors (Cruz-Jentoft et al., 2019). Sarcopenia is associated with increased adverse outcomes, including falls, functional decline and frailty, but is potentially reversible. Greater understanding of the physiological processes and predictors for sarcopenia, falls and frailty have progressed over recent years, resulting in evidence-based interventions for the treatment of modifiable risk factors (e.g., strength and balance retraining). Promoting safe mobility for older people is addressed in Chapter 18.

CONCLUSION AND LEARNING POINTS

This chapter has considered some of the important aspects of the biology of human ageing and the implications of these physiological changes. Clearly, the changes observed in ageing are not all negative; quite the opposite—older people, in a biological sense, cope very adequately. What must be remembered is the enormous variability among older people; what is normal for one 80-year-old might be quite inappropriate for another, so we need to consider the individual. Similarly, there are ways of promoting or optimising the health and physical capacities of an older person, just as there are for a younger individual.

KEY LEARNING POINTS

- Some physiological changes that occur with ageing can increase the likelihood or severity of disease. For example, normal ageing is associated with a decline in pulmonary function, and this, together with reduced efficiency of the immune system, increases both the likelihood of a respiratory tract infection and the severity of subsequent loss of lung function. The same infection in a younger person may not have such a debilitating effect.
- It is sometimes difficult to differentiate the effects of physical deconditioning from those of ageing. Therefore, old age is often considered to be synonymous with disability, but there is much evidence to dispute this. A decline in levels of physical fitness is not inevitable.
- Although ageing results in physiological changes like declining muscle mass, good nutrition and sufficient exercise can be protective against a number of age-related conditions such as cardiovascular disease, frailty and cognitive decline.
- Ageing impacts all the body's organs and systems. Knowledge of the underlying pathophysiological processes can help direct evidence-informed nursing care of the older adult.

REFERENCES

Association of UK Dieticians. (2021). *Food fact sheet: Fluids (water and drinks)*. https://www.bda.uk.com/resourceDetail/printPdf/?resource=fluid-water-drinks

Bourre, J. (2006). Effects of nutrients (in food) on the structure and function of the nervous system: update on dietary requirements for brain. Part 1: Micronutrients. *Journal of Nutrition, Health, & Aging, 10*, 377–385.

British Nutrition Foundation. (n.d.). *Older adults*. https://archive.nutrition.org.uk/nutritionscience/life/older-adults

Deutz, N. E. P., Bauer, J. M., Barazzoni, R., Biolo, G., Boirie, Y., Bosy-Westphal, A., Cederholm, T., Cruz-Jentoft, A., Krznarič, Z., Nair, K. S., Singer, P., Teta, D., Tipton, K., & Calder, P. C. (2014). Protein intake and exercise for optimal muscle function with aging: recommendations from the ESPEN Expert Group. *Clinical Nutrition, 33*, 929–936. doi:10.1016/j.clnu.2014.04.007.

Chadwick, D., & Goode, J. A. (2002). *Endocrine facets of ageing*. Wiley.

English Longitudinal Study of Ageing (ELSA). (2021). *English longitudinal study of ageing*. https://www.elsa-project.ac.uk

Clarke, B. L., & Khosla, S. (2010). Physiology of bone loss. *Radiology Clinics of North America, 48*, 483–495. doi:10.1016/j.rcl.2010.02.014.

Cruz-Jentoft, A. J., & Sayer, A. A. (2019). Sarcopenia. *Lancet, 393*, 2636–2646. doi:10.1016/s0140-6736(19)31138-9.

Farage, M. A., Miller, K. W., Berardesca, E., & Maibach, H. I. (2009). Clinical implications of aging skin: Cutaneous disorders in the elderly. *American Journal of Clinical Dermatology, 10*, 73–86. doi:10.2165/00128071-200910020-00001.

Gems, D., & Doonan, R. (2009). Antioxidant defense and aging in *C. elegans*: Is the oxidative damage theory of aging wrong? *Cell Cycle, 8*, 1681–1687.

Gomes, A. P., Price, N. L., Ling, A. J. Y., Moslehi, J. J., Montgomery, M. K., Rajman, L., White, J. P., Teodoro, J. S., Wrann, C. D., Hubbard, B. P., Mercken, E. M., Palmeria, C. M., de Cabo, R., Rolo, A. P., Turner, N., Bell, E. L., & Sinclair, D. A. (2013). Declining NAD(+) induces a pseudohypoxic state disrupting nuclear-mitochondrial communication during aging. *Cell, 155*, 1624–1638. doi:10.1016/j.cell.2013.11.037.

Grady, C. (2012). The cognitive neuroscience of ageing. *Nature Reviews Neuroscience, 13*, 491–505. doi:10.1038/nrn3256.

Gude, N. A., Broughton, K. M., Firouzi, F., & Sussman, M. A. (2018). Cardiac ageing: Extrinsic and intrinsic factors in cellular renewal and senescence. *Nature Reviews Cardiology, 15*, 523–542. doi:10.1038/s41569-018-0061-5.

Harman, D. (1981). The aging process. *Proceedings of the National Academy of Science of the United States of America, 78*, 7124–7128. doi:10.1073/pnas.78.11.7124.

Huang, A. H., & Chien, A. L. (2020). Photoaging: A review of current literature. *Current Dermatology Reports, 9*, 22–29. doi:10.1007/s13671-020-00288-0.

Inoue, S., Suzuki, K., & Komori, Y. (2014). Persistent inflammation and T cell exhaustion in severe sepsis in the elderly. *Critical Care Journal, 18*, R130. doi:https://doi.org/10.1186/cc13941.

Jackson, P. A., Pialoux, V., Corbett, D., Drogos, L., Erickson, K. I., Eskes, G. A., & Poulin, M. J. (2016). Promoting brain health through exercise and diet in older adults: A physiological perspective. *Journal of Physiology, 15,* 4485–4498.

Jin, K. (2010). Modern biological theories of aging. *Aging and Disease, 1,* 72–74.

Karakelides, H., Irving, B. A., Short, K. R., O'Brien, P., & Nair, K. S. (2010). Age, obesity, and sex effects on insulin sensitivity and skeletal muscle mitochondrial function. *Diabetes, 59,* 89–97. doi:10.2337/db09-0591.

Kelly, D. (2011). Ageing theories unified. *Nature, 470,* 342–343.

Kenny, W., & Chiu, P. (2001). Influence of age on thirst and fluid intake. *Medicine & Science in Sports & Exercise, 33,* 1524–1532.

Kirkwood, T. (2003). The most pressing problem of our age. *BMJ, 326,* 1297–1299.

Lomeli, N., Bota, D. A., & Davies, K. J. A. (2017). Diminished stress resistance and defective adaptive homeostasis in age-related diseases. *Clinical Science (London), 131,* 2573–2599. doi:10.1042/cs20160982.

Musi, N., & Hornsby, P. (2021). *Handbook of the biology of aging* (9th ed.). Elsevier Academic Press.

National Health Service. (2019). *Osteoporosis—Prevention.* https://www.nhs.uk/conditions/osteoporosis/prevention

Nowakowski, A. C. (2014). Chronic inflammation and quality of life in older adults: A cross-sectional study using biomarkers to predict emotional and relational outcomes. *Health and Quality of Life Outcomes, 12,* 141. doi:10.1186/s12955-014-0141-0.

Persson, J., Nyberg, L., Lind, J., Larsson, A., Nilsson, L.-G., Ingvar, M., & Buckner, R. L. (2006). Structure-function correlates of cognitive decline in aging. *Cerebral Cortex, 16,* 907–915. doi:10.1093/cercor/bhj036.

Reuter-Lorenz, P. A., & Cappell, K. A. (2008). Neurocognitive aging and the compensation hypothesis. *Current Directions in Psychological Science, 17,* 177–182. doi:10.1111/j.1467-8721.2008.00570.x.

Roman, M. A., Rossiter, H. B., & Casaburi, R. (2016). Exercise, ageing and the lung. *European Respiratory Journal, 48,* 1471–1486. doi:10.1183/13993003.00347-2016.

Royal Society of Osteoporosis. (2021). *Vitamin D supplements and tests.* https://theros.org.uk/media/grija5r1/ros-vitamin-d-supplements-and-tests-fact-sheet-december-2018.pdf

Scientific Advisory Committee on Nutrition. (2021). *SACN statement on nutrition and older adults living in the community.* https://www.gov.uk/government/publications/sacn-statement-on-nutrition-and-older-adults

Sinclair, D. A., & LaPlante, M. (2019). *Why we age—and why we don't have to:* Atria.

Smith, T. O., Sreekanta, A., Walkeden, S., Penhale, B., & Hanson, S. (2020). Interventions for reducing hospital-associated deconditioning: A systematic review and meta-analysis. *Archives of Gerontology and Geriatriatrics, 90,* Article 104176. doi:10.1016/j.archger.2020.104176.

Steinhagen-Thiessen, E., & Borcheltm, M. (1999). *Morbidity, medication and functional limitations in very old age.* Cambridge University Press.

University of Newcastle. (2006). *The Newcastle 85+ study.* https://research.ncl.ac.uk/85plus

Wells, J. C., Sawaya, A. L., Wibaek, R., Mwangome, M., Poullas, M. S., Yajnik, C. S., & Demaoi, A. (2020). The double burden of malnutrition: Aetiological pathways and consequences for health. *The Lancet Global Health, 395,* 75–88.

Weiskopf, D., Weinberger, B., & Grubeck-Loebenstein, B. (2009). The aging of the immune system. *Transplant International, 22,* 1041–1050. doi:10.1111/j.1432-2277.2009.00927.x.

Williams, G. (1957). Pleiotropy, natural selection, and the evolution of senescence. *Evolution, 11,* 398–411.

Yiallouris, A., Tsioutis, C., Agapidaki, E., Zafeiri, M., Agouridis, A. P., Ntourakis, D., & Johnson, E. O. (2019). Adrenal aging and its implications on stress responsiveness in humans. *Frontiers in Endocrinology (Lausanne), 10,* 54. doi:10.3389/fendo.2019.00054.

Wojciechowska, W., Stolarz-Skrzypek, K., Tikhonoff, V., Richart, T., Seidlerová, J., Cwynar, M., Thijs, L., Li, Y., Kuznetsova, T., Filipovský, J., Casiglia, E., Grodzicki, T., Kawecka-Jaszcz, K., O'Rourke, M., & Staessen, J. European Project on Genes in Hypertension. (2012). Age dependency of central and peripheral systolic blood pressures: Cross-sectional and longitudinal observations in European populations. *Blood Pressure, 21,* 58–68. doi:10.3109/08037051.2011.593332.

6

Nursing the Older Person Living With Frailty

Caroline Nicholson, Abigail Barkham

CHAPTER OUTLINE

FRAILTY: A WORLDWIDE NURSING CHALLENGE

Frailty is a complex medical syndrome, combining the effects of natural aging with the outcomes of multiple long-term conditions and loss of fitness and reserve. Evidence is conclusive that frailty is independently predicative of many adverse events, including disability, falls, delirium, hospitalisation and mortality. Frailty has been termed "the most problematic expression of population ageing" (Clegg et al., 2013, p. 752) and as such is an increasingly important consideration for nurses in any area of practice worldwide.

Globally, the number of people living into old age is growing; by 2050 22% of the world's population—approximately 2 billion people—will be over 60. Population ageing is happening most quickly in low- and middle-income countries, and the effects of long-term illness, coupled with socioeconomic disadvantage, present challenges and opportunities for nurses to lead and shape the care of older people with frailty. While biological frailty is not directly correlated with chronological ageing, the older you are, the more likely you are to be frail (Turner & Gregg, 2014). It is estimated a quarter to half of older people over 85 are living with frailty, and these people have significantly increased risk of falls, disability, long-term care need and death (Fried et al., 2001). People living into late old age are the fastest growing sector of the population, particularly in more economically developed regions, where the number of people aged 80 and older is growing at twice the rate of people over 60 years (World Health Organization, 2022).

Perhaps one to the greatest opportunities nurses need to realise in care for older people with frailty is that frailty is not a single disease. Therefore the identification, assessment and care of older people with frailty needs to move beyond disease as the focus of care (Tinetti & Fried, 2004) along a spectrum of capability and capacity. Frailty has biological, psychological and social dimensions. Crucially enabling people to live well with frailty requires an understanding of the individual and their social strengths and networks to optimise quantity and quality of life. Frailty is not a predictable process of decline; instead a person's level of frailty fluctuates with potentially reversible elements, that if managed well can delay adverse frailty responses.

This chapter looks at the implications and interventions for nurses caring for people with frailty across the three frailty stages: pre- to mildly frail, moderately frail and severely frail. Although these stages are not linear, they offer the nurse, in the context of a multidisciplinary team, a focus for assessment and intervention. The reversibility of frailty presents important opportunities for nurses.

Gill et al. (2006), in their prospective cohort study, noted transitions occurred between frailty states, and these transitions were in both directions—in other words, there was reversibility particularly in the milder levels of frailty. Thus the dynamic nature of frailty provides nurses many opportunities to facilitate frailty prevention and rehabilitation where possible. What is of central importance at all times, however, is for nurses to see the person behind the patient (Goodrich & Cornwell, 2008) and in so doing support optimal quality of life for an individual living with frailty.

FRAILTY: MORE THAN VULNERABILITY

Frailty is often described clinically as a state of vulnerability where a person is at increased risk of adverse outcomes, including recurring falls, injuries, frequent hospitalisation or progressive disability and morbidity (Vermeiren et al., 2016). However, for older people, *frailty* is often a pejorative term (Nicholson et al., 2016); older people often do not describe themselves as frail. Although they recognise their physical decline, they often focus on capability and striving to maintain connections (Nicholson et al., 2012). It is rare that people see themselves as frail but may describe slowing down or modifying their activities to maintain their capacity to carry on. Health-care professionals, including nurses, need to recognise these subtleties and sensitivities and avoid reinforcing negative stereotypes of frailty and dependency (Richardson et al., 2011). Care for people with frailty needs to be situated within a picture of what older people can do and what support structures, including their own individual and community assets, can support living well. The Frailty Fulcrum model of frailty by Moody (see 'Resources' at the end of the chapter) articulates the multidimensional nature of frailty and the need in care to understand the interactions between vulnerability and resilience in frailty and how these domains balance and interact to influence a person's quality of life. Shibley Rahman's book *Living with Frailty* (2018) argues for a move by health professionals and policy makers to more positive approaches to frailty that develop an individual's self-activation and strengths in relation to living with frailty. While such an approach is multidisciplinary and crosses sectors, nurses are uniquely placed to establish and maintain a therapeutic relationship underpinned by values of respect, understanding and self-determination.

FRAILTY: A PUBLIC HEALTH ISSUE

Although genetics play a part in the ageing process, it is estimated less than 25% of the variability in population longevity is attributed solely to genetic factors. There is increasing evidence that frailty in older age is directly associated with socioeconomic factors during the life course, including low birth weight (Haapanen et al., 2018), lower educational opportunities and insecure housing and job opportunities (Garrett et al., 2020). Frailty is associated with multimorbidity, certain long-term conditions, socioeconomic deprivation, smoking and obesity (Hanlon et al., 2018). Frailty is a public health issue and one nurses need to be aware of in any encounter with people of any age with socioeconomic and multiple physical vulnerabilities. Readdressing the lack of understanding of the term *frailty* is key in the public health and social care domains. There is a need to maximise the public health agenda regarding early opportunities to identify frailty and to signpost for interventions. The publication *Frailty: A Framework of Core Capabilities* (see 'Resources') includes knowledge and interventions specifically written for the person with frailty, their family and the public as well as capabilities more tailored to care providers across social and health settings.

All health professionals need to identify and understand frailty as a concept and a long-term condition for which to provide the best care and advice to individuals and families. The fundamentals of making every contact count (MECC; see 'Resources') is simple. It recognises care providers across health, local authorities and voluntary sectors have thousands of contacts every day with individuals and are ideally placed to promote health and healthy lifestyles. MECC relies on the opportunistic delivery of consistent and concise healthy lifestyle information and enables individuals to engage in conversations about their health at scale across organisations and populations. Public-health interventions include discussions on exercise, diet and remaining socially engaged and can be individual and system wide. The World Health Organization and United Nations are proactively working to support older people to live well at all levels of the system, including promoting age-friendly cities. The UN Decade of Healthy Ageing (see 'Resources') has a strong emphasis on fostering agency and enablement. Part of nurses' role is to look beyond the care context—hospital, community or outpatients—to the world of the people they care for. Many countries have national bodies and charities dedicated to supporting ageing well with useful advice on incorporating health-promoting activities into daily life, such gardening, walking and other social activities.

FRAILTY: A CLINICAL MEDICAL SYNDROME

It is important to distinguish between the word *frailty* in everyday language—which is often used to describe a quality of weakness, or fragility, or a physical or moral failing—and *frailty* as discussed in this chapter as a complex medical syndrome. This is an essential distinction, because the complex medical syndrome of frailty can never be identified by looking at or describing an individual without a clear understanding of the syndrome of frailty, how frailty can be diagnosed and crucially what interventions will be offered to support an older person with frailty. The medical syndrome of frailty is now recognised in some countries as a long-term condition among older people.

There is no overarching single clinical definition of frailty. Morley et al. (2013, p. 2) report on an international consensus definition of physical frailty and conclude it "is a medical syndrome with multiple causes and contributors that is characterized by diminished strength, endurance, and reduced physiologic function that increases an individual's vulnerability for developing increased dependency and/or death." Clegg and colleagues' (Clegg et al., 2013, p. 752) definition is widely used. "Frailty is a state of vulnerability to poor resolution of homoeostasis after a stressor event and is a consequence of cumulative decline in many physiological systems during a lifetime." This cumulative decline depletes homoeostatic reserves until minor stressor events trigger disproportionate changes in health status. This increased vulnerability contributes to increased risk for multiple adverse outcomes, including procedural complications, falls, institutionalisation, disability and death. Although different emphases are noted, there is consensus that frailty puts individuals who have it at higher risk of an adverse reaction or change in health status following a relatively minor stressor, such as constipation. It is recognised older people living with frailty have a reduced reserve in their ability to manage an acute change in condition with resilience. There is a rapidly expanding evidence base related to the pathophysiology of frailty.

How does this translate to nursing care of the older person living with frailty? In this chapter we discuss the importance of frailty identification, assessment and planning, and the nurse's role in supporting older people with frailty to live well across a variety of care settings and at different stages of frailty. The settings in which nurses may come across frailty are varied and not always obvious. When you apply a frailty lens to nursing care, it allows you to freely address frailty in your service users' care outcomes across all settings. The nurse who works in primary care may link with areas of mild frailty through routine care check-ups, with the opportunity to address preventative measures in frailty, for example, at 50-plus reviews and long-term condition reviews. The hospital and community nurse may have the opportunity to work with older people with moderate to severe frailty toward restorative and reactive care and advance planning. The nurse working in a care-home setting may have the opportunity to care for older people living with severe frailty and lead with aspects of advance care planning. See Chapter 34 for a larger discussion of end-of-life care.

With more people living with mild, moderate and severe frailty attending emergency departments and over 4,000 admissions a day for people living with frailty, it has never been more important to understand the care needs of individuals living with frailty. By gaining a wider knowledge and understanding of frailty in nursing care, there is the potential to improve patient-care outcomes. Nurses working toward preventative and restorative care can potentially reverse early signs of frailty and work toward avoiding unnecessary hospital admissions.

Strong evidence suggests older people living with frailty are more likely to experience delays in care outcomes. The concept of frailty decompensation is highlighted through the international End PJ Paralysis campaign (see 'Resources'). Its aim is to reduce immobility and muscle deconditioning. Nurses have a key role as the patient's advocate to avoid lost days or delays in care outcomes. For the individual in hospital, immobility leads to deconditioning, loss of functional ability and cognitive impairment, all of which have the potential to increase a patient's length of stay. The complications this can cause for the individual are more obvious in, but not exclusive to, the hospital setting. The way nurses care for service users living with frailty who are experiencing a hospital admission can affect their length of stay. The story of Mrs June Andrews presented in an educational film (see 'Resources') shows how long periods of physical inactivity can lead to physical decompensation and how multiple bed moves and changes of environment can impact cognition, ultimately delaying social-care planning and discharge.

In community, primary care and nursing home settings, nurses can work in various ways to improve the outcomes of older people living with frailty. Working proactively to avoid unscheduled admission could involve identifying early warning signs through fall identification, polypharmacy, medication reviews, encouraging engagement in exercise groups and ensuring shared care-planning across the health care system. Home-first options that encourage early discharge schemes from hospitals and continued nursing care at home can avoid lengthy hospital stays. Early discharge schemes or admission avoidance provide a multidisciplinary approach to rehabilitation at home rather than in hospital. Schemes such as virtual ward at home can exist. A Virtual Ward is a time-limited service enabling people who have an acute condition or exacerbation of a chronic condition requiring hospital-level care to receive this care in the place they call home, either as an alternative to hospital admission or by facilitating an earlier discharge from hospital (BGS, 2022).

It is important to understand the individual's journey when they come into a care setting. The key aspect is to ensure all assessment and planning is completed with the older person and with individuals who know them the best. It is important to understand and consider what happened prior to admission or referral to an acute service for the older person. Gaining collateral information is important because it helps you gain a richer assessment of what was normal for the older person prior to the acute episode and current level of frailty. Prioritise this aspect of assessment by involving the older person and the individuals who know them the best.

Frailty can be made better or worse. It's important to understand if this is the first frailty presentation for the individual or they have a history of repeated problems such as falls, acute admissions, delirium, etc. The importance of looking back helps you understand how frailty impacts the individual and therefore what plans can be put in place to reverse the frailty trajectory and support the person to achieve their goals.

For the older person living with severe frailty, an acute deterioration in frailty or a slow decline will have life changing impact. At this point it becomes essential for the nurse to work with the individual and those who know them the best to discuss and plan future medical interventions. This is referred to as the patient's ceilings of treatment. Encourage the individual or their friends and family to ascertain the maximum level of care they would like to see provided. An example is an older person with severe frailty who opts to be treated conservatively at home with oral medication, avoiding inpatient treatment. This is often a complex and sensitive decision reached between the patient, their family and their health care team.

WHY DOES FRAILTY OCCUR?

The pathology of frailty is one of cumulative molecular and cellular damage that leads to reduced physiological reserve across multiple body systems (see Fig. 6.1). While no single process can be identified as the cause of frailty, the most significant changes seen at cellular and organ levels are related to muscle mass and strength and a reduction in type II muscle fibres—which generate more power and force of contraction than type I. Replacement with connective and adipose tissues contributes to sarcopenia, or muscle weakness. A reduction in bone mass and density leads to altered mobility and osteoporosis. Frailty is associated with a decline in efficiency in major organs such as the heart and lungs. It is also linked with reductions in hormones such as the gonadal (sex) hormones and insulin-like growth hormones and an increase in inflammatory cytokines, reducing capacity for cell repair as well as suppressing the body's immune and stress responses. Frailty is also associated with an increased incidence of dementia (Petermann-Rocha et al., 2020). Currently the association between the two is not clearly understood but may be related to confounding factors such as pre-existing health conditions. Thus frailty can exist independent of long-term conditions like diabetics, cardiovascular disease and dementia, but the presence of these conditions increases the likelihood and severity of frailty (Turner & Clegg, 2014).

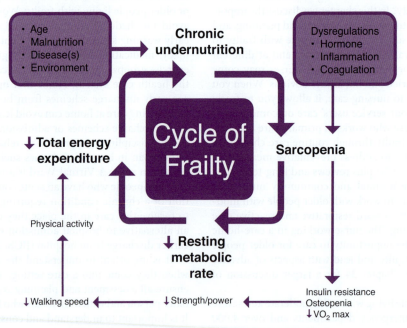

Fig. 6.1 The cycle of frailty. (British Geriatrics Society.)

Frailty Prevalence

The prevalence of frailty in the worldwide population is currently unclear. O'Caoimh et al.'s (2018) systematic view of physical frailty prevalence in 62 countries notes variation related to the classification of frailty and calls for a standardised method of frailty classification. Frailty increases with age independent of the assessment instrument used. Its prevalence is between 4% and 59% in community-dwelling older people and higher in women than in men. Long-term diseases, depression, socioeconomic status and education are also important predicators of frailty. There is increasing evidence of an association between frailty and dementia, such that individuals who are pre-frail or living with frailty are more at risk of dementia (Petermann-Rocha et al., 2020). However, not all people with frailty will have dementia. The multifactorial nature of frailty underlines the importance of robust clinical assessment.

Frailty Models

There are two principle models of frailty (Fig. 6.2): the phenotype model (Fried et al., 2001) and the cumulative deficit model (Rockwood et al., 2005). These models are used to identify frailty and are distinct and complementary. The phenotype model describes a group of patient characteristics comprising unintentional weight loss, reduced muscle strength, reduced gait speed, self-reported exhaustion and low energy expenditure that are indicative of frailty. The presence of these characteristics in an individual can predict poorer outcomes. Generally, individuals with three or more of these characteristics are said to have frailty. Examples are an individual who has gradually withdrawn from activities they used to enjoy such as clubs or going out with friends and family, or a person who reports falls, unsteadiness and loss of confidence in functional ability.

The cumulative deficit model assumes an accumulation of deficits that can occur with ageing. This has been identified as a decline in specific biological, psychosocial and social domains. The domains are medical conditions, functional decline, depression, cognition, nutrition and social vulnerability and express the concept of the graduation of frailty. An accumulation of deficits in all identified domains can indicate levels of frailty, and when combined, these deficits increase the frailty index. This introduces the idea that a greater number of deficits increases the severity of the frailty experienced, in turn increasing the risk of an adverse outcome.

Assessment is important to identify and understand how frailty affects an individual. Interventions can then be discussed with the person to optimise outcomes.

Identifying Frailty

A variety of tools exist to identify frailty at population and individual levels. International guidelines recommend routine identification of frailty. At a population or caseload level, the electronic frailty index (eFI; Clegg et al., 2016) uses routinely collected data from electronic primary-care record systems. The index applies a cumulative deficit approach by

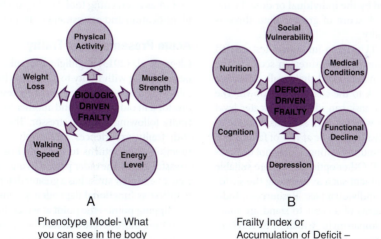

A

Phenotype Model- What you can see in the body
Freid et all 2001

B

Frailty Index or Accumulation of Deficit – across Biological, Psychological and Social Domains
Rockwood et al 2005

Fig. 6.2 Identification and assessment of frailty—Phenotype and accumulation of deficit. (Based on Fried, L. P., Tangen, C. M., Walston, J., Newman, A., B., Hirsch, C., Gottdiener, J., Seeman, T., Tracy, R., Kop, W. J., Burke, G., & McBurnie, M. A. (2001). & Cardiovascular Health Study Collaborative Research Group. Frailty in older adults: evidence for a phenotype. *The Journals of Gerontology Series A: Biological Sciences and Medical Sciences, 56*(3), M146–M157. Rockwood, K., Song, X., MacKnight, C., Bergman, H., Hogan, D. B., McDowell, I., & Mitnitski, A. (2005). A global clinical measure of fitness and frailty in elderly people. *Canadian Medical Association Journal, 173*(5), 489–495.)

identifying 36 biological, psychosocial and social deficits. The more deficits are identified, the higher the frailty index, indicating worsening frailty. The eFI enables understanding of frailty prevalence in a population, which is vital for future health and social care planning. The eFI also has robust predictive validity for the outcomes of nursing home admission, hospitalisation and mortality.

At an individual level, frailty needs to be clinically validated, and early identification is imperative. Levels of frailty can increase or decrease. Through active identification, steps can be taken to reverse frailty and improve individual outcomes. Increasing levels of frailty result in worsening health outcomes, such as falls, acute admissions to hospital and potentially death. Equally, reversing frailty results in maintenance of meaningful function across activities of daily living and healthy ageing.

The British Geriatric Society (Turner & Clegg, 2014) provides guidance on the identification of frailty (Fit for Frailty; see 'Resources") and a range of tests that can be applied to the patient should frailty be suspected: the Edmonton Frail Scale, PRISMA and Timed Up and Go Test (TUGT; Turner & Clegg, 2014).

Edmonton frail scale. The Edmonton Frail Scale is a multidimensional frailty measure that can be used for case-finding, to estimate severity, and to enhance care planning. It includes a set of nine domains. The clinician can score the individual at presentation and determine the level of frailty.

PRISMA. PRISMA is a simple validated tool to identify frailty in older adults that consists of seven questions that can be self-completed by the individual or done by the health-care professional. A score of greater than three is considered to identify frailty.

Timed up and go test. TUGT is a functional test carried out by the health professional. It measures, in seconds, the time taken to stand up from a standard chair, walk a distance of 3 metres, turn, walk back to the chair and sit down. The time taken to perform the task can identify a greater level of fall risk. An older adult who takes 12 seconds or more to complete the TUCT is considered to be at risk of falling. For nurses working in the community setting, it may not be practical to implement a TUGT. Other options are more suitable to the community environment such as assessing the sit-to-stand functionality of the individual (see 'Resources'). Individuals who require the arms of a chair to stand are more likely to have lower-limb impairment, which in turn relates to poorer balance and an associated risk of falls.

Clinical frailty scale. The clinical frailty scale (CFS) is an inclusive nine-point scale developed to summarise the overall level of fitness or frailty of an older person. A higher score equates to greater risk (Rockwood et al., 1999, A copy of the CFS can be accessed at the following link: https://www.england.nhs.uk/south/wp-content/uploads/sites/6/2022/02/rockwood-frailty-scale_.pdf). The CFS is a judgement-based tool completed by professionals. It is suggested in the guidance the scale should not be applied when the individual is acutely unwell. In practice, it's important for the clinician to adhere to this. An acute presentation of frailty comes with a decline in function and is not a true representation of the baseline health state. Scoring in the acute phase may result in an overinflated and inaccurate score. The baseline health state is what the person was like before they were unwell (e.g., 2 weeks ago). Understanding their baseline is essential in planning their care. If the person cannot tell you about their health over the past two weeks, you should speak with someone who can. The more information you have about someone, the better you can score them on the scale.

The CFS is not a standalone tool. If frailty is suspected through the presentation of a frailty syndrome or identification using one of the suggested tools, the clinician needs to complete a comprehensive geriatric assessment (CGA). Following the CGA, the CFS should be applied, followed by a plan of care for the individual. It is essential frailty is not diagnosed in isolation. The four key elements are to identify frailty, assess the individual using a CGA approach, apply a CFS, then implement a collaborative plan with the individual and their carers. It is recognised that in clinical practice health professionals apply the CFS as a screening tool prior to a CGA, often in acute settings. The CFS is validated for application in the non-acute phase of frailty; however, it is recognised that more recently it is applied before a CGA as a screening tool. See Fig. 6.3 for a flow diagram of identification and assessment of frailty.

Acute Presentation of Frailty

Clegg et al. (2013) highlight the vulnerability of an older person living with frailty to a sudden change in health status following a minor illness. Fig. 6.4 represents two trajectories, one for a fit older person and another for a person living with frailty following a minor stressor. The individual not living with frailty experiences a relatively small deterioration in function, then returns to their level of activity prior to the stressful event. The older person living with frailty who experiences a similar stress has a greater deterioration, which may manifest as functional dependency. This could be described as a tipping point—the point at which frailty is advancing, is becoming more severe and may be irreversible.

It is important for the clinician not to see these events in isolation. Frailty can be made better and made worse. The older adult who presents with an acute frailty syndrome may present with their first acute episode, or they may continually present in an acute state and not have time to recover from the previous event. Often, repeated acute frailty presentations indicate the individual is moving from moderate to severe frailty and has inadequate reserves to recover fully.

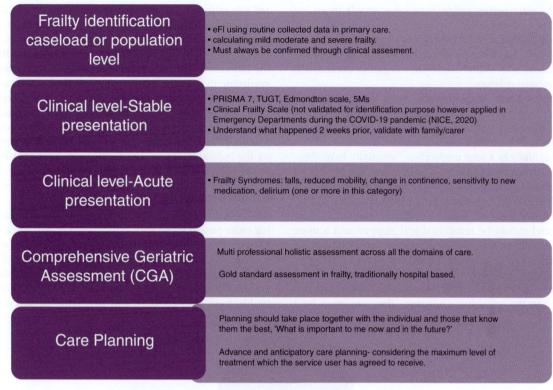

Frailty identification caseload or population level	• eFI using routine collected data in primary care. • calculating mild moderate and severe frailty. • Must always be confirmed through clinical assesment.
Clinical level-Stable presentation	• PRISMA 7, TUGT, Edmondton scale, 5Ms • Clinical Frailty Scale (not validated for identification purpose however applied in Emergency Departments during the COVID-19 pandemic (NICE, 2020) • Understand what happened 2 weeks prior, validate with family/carer
Clinical level-Acute presentation	• Frailty Syndromes: falls, reduced mobility, change in continence, sensitivity to new medication, delirium (one or more in this category)
Comprehensive Geriatric Assessment (CGA)	Multi professional holistic assessment across all the domains of care. Gold standard assessment in frailty, traditionally hospital based.
Care Planning	Planning should take place together with the individual and those that know them the best, 'What is important to me now and in the future?' Advance and anticipatory care planning- considering the maximum level of treatment which the service user has agreed to receive.

Fig. 6.3 Flow diagram of identification and assessment of frailty.

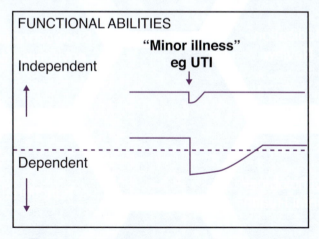

Fig. 6.4 Tipping point of frailty. (From Clegg et al., 2013.)

Frailty syndromes. Five frailty syndromes are recognised and frequently referred to as acute presentations. They should be regarded as red flags for frailty. It is important to recognise these are acute presentations and often mean a sudden change in an individual's physical health function and mental capacity.

Falls. A fall can be clinically demonstrated as a new fall but does not have to be the first fall. It indicates some new acute presentation may have caused functional decline.

Reduced mobility. Reduced mobility can present as a sudden change in an individual's usual functional ability, e.g., the older person suddenly becomes unable to get out of bed or mobilise safely.

New confusion. New confusion can present as either a new state of confusion or an accelerated state of confusion in someone with underlying organic cognitive decline. It is often termed *delirium*.

Acute change in continence. Acute change in continence can present as a new episode of incontinence that previously didn't exist and can be in bowel or bladder function, including constipation.

Sensitivity to a new medication. Sensitivity to medication can present with an acute change in function that can be isolated and identified through a change in medication. It is usually due to the introduction of a new medication. Opiate-based medications can induce a sudden reaction in an older adult and should be recognised and stopped and a more suitable alternative agreed on. Comprehensive guidance on this aspect can be found in STOPP and START (Gallagher et al., 2008). See Chapter 31 for additional information.

These syndromes represent a sudden and significant change in the individual's function. They can often be a red flag in frailty; the clinician should be vigilant to these presentations. It is important to understand an older person could present with one or more frailty syndromes, and that is enough to highlight questions regarding frailty in the individual. The individual who presents with a frailty syndrome may be the first person with frailty, that health professional has come into contact with. It is therefore important to have an understanding of frailty syndromes, their impact and how they can be avoided through care planning. Each syndrome can have an immediate impact on the individual living with frailty, with a tangible effect on the person's function in a short period.

Comprehensive Geriatric Assessment

The CGA is widely accepted as the gold standard for assessing older people living with frailty (see Fig. 6.5). (See also Chapter 10 for more information.)

The CGA is a multidimensional and usually interdisciplinary diagnostic process designed to determine an older person living with frailty's medical conditions, mental health, functional capacity, and psychological and social

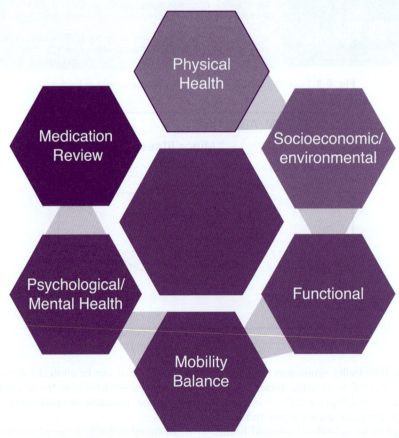

Fig. 6.5 Domains of the Comprehensive Geriatric Assessment.

circumstances. The purpose is to develop a holistic plan for treatment, rehabilitation, support and long-term follow-up.

The CGA should be a combined assessment with input from all professionals involved in the care of the individual working in partnership with the older person and their family and carers. The British Geriatrics Society provides resources to enable use of the CGA across all care settings. The CGA is not the sum of its parts or a checklist; it is about being holistic while focusing on the parts that matter and will affect change for the patient. The CGA should always link to a plan of care or intervention but balance the need for onward over referral and also the individual's wishes with regard to their ceilings of care. A diagnostic component must exist where the diagnosis is unclear.

The benefits of the CGA approach and associated care planning in the hospital setting are compelling. Ellis et al. (2017) showed that by taking a CGA, there was a greater likelihood of the individual being alive and living in their own home at 6 and 12 months post-assessment. There was also a lower likelihood of institutionalisation, death and functional decline and a greater likelihood of improved cognition.

The importance of comprehensive assessment is captured in Molnar et al.'s (2017) 5 Ms of geriatric medicine—mind, mobility, medications, multicomplexity, matters most (see Table 6.1). This helpful framework can be adapted for use in difference clinical settings and is useful where staff are not familiar with the CGA.

Post CGA planning

As with the CGA, the plan of care post CGA should be achieved collaboratively and meaningfully for the individual. The individual's goals and aspirations should be included as part of the overall plan.

Applying an assets vs deficits approach at this point is essential. Rahman (2018) highlights that often frailty assessment focuses on the individual's deficits and can be overmedicalised. The opposite of this is an assets approach, which requires the nurse to understand the life lived by the older person with frailty, taking time to understand the person, how they live, who they live with, what they still enjoy doing and what they can still achieve. It is the nurse's role to elicit this information without making assumptions based on the presenting picture or current care setting. Recognition of what can still be achieved forms a positive base for planning and developing lifestyle changes that are meaningful for the individual.

Assessment and Management of Different Frailty States

The condition of frailty can be made better or worse by the care given. In this chapter a case study is used to demonstrate the different stages of frailty—mild, moderate and severe—and the appropriate nursing care across the frailty continuum. See Case Studies 6.1, 6.2 and 6.3 respectively.

Nursing care of an older person living with mild frailty: Commentary on case study. Nurses might meet Edith in a variety of settings and need to be aware of the preventative measures they can signpost Edith to and instigate as part of nursing care. Older people living with mild frailty have a good chance of reversibility. The underlying principle in managing frailty is early recognition in combination with population-based preventive measures (see "Frailty: A public health issue"). Key areas of change in Edith move beyond the physical—reduced function and

TABLE 6.1   Geriatric 5 Ms

MIND	Mentation, dementia, delirium, depression
MOBILITY	Impaired gait and balance, fall injury prevention
MEDICATIONS	Polypharmacy, deprescribing, optimal prescribing, adverse medication effects and medication burden
MULTICOMPLEXITY	Multimorbidity, complex bio-psychosocial situations
MATTER MOST	Each individual's own meaningful health outcome goals and care preferences

CASE STUDY 6.1   Edith, Living with Mild Frailty

Edith is an 80-year-old lady who lives with her husband in an urban area in a two-storey home. They have been married for 58 years and have three children who live locally. Edith spent her married life bringing up her children and later enjoyed working in the local supermarket. Edith has been managing all her activities of daily living and enjoying social contact with her friends and groups. Since her husband's recent illness, her focus has been on him, leading her to withdraw from groups she previously attended and limiting the possibilities of her and her husband going out. Although she still manages her daily activities in the home, she reports feeling weaker and slower and is also noticing fatigue. She has been putting this down to the worry over her husband. Edith feels disconnected from her previous social contacts. While her mobility is safe in the home, she feels less stable than she did 12 months ago. She feels as if her 'world has shrunk' in the past 6 to 12 months and that she is less connected to her once-established life.

feeling less stable on her feet—to a wider assessment of her social and emotional needs. She is experiencing increased anxiety due to her husband's diagnosis, reduced social contact and reduced confidence. Therefore, along with giving tailored advice on nutrition, hydration and exercise that takes account of Edith's wishes and quality of life goals, it is vital to think about interventions to support Edith's social and psychological health. There is a virtuous cycle between increased social interaction (including keeping connections with meaningful places and people) and mental health, and between increased fitness and decreased depression. The use of volunteers from charities and voluntary and community groups, to support home-based exercise training and provide nutrition and social support is increasingly crucial in meeting health needs in the community. In the United Kingdom, social prescribing is an initiative based in community health care to support these linkages. Early evidence suggests benefits in clinical outcomes and social participation, but more work is needed to understand the effectiveness of social prescribing. Wider models of connecting with communities are emerging in concert with a call to be more flexible and creative with partnerships across sectors in the local community.

The focus for Edith at this point is on enabling her to stay well. Part of this intervention is for nurses to connect beyond their immediate work colleagues to a wider understanding with range of local resources and connections: social workers, age-related charities and health connectors. All can support nurses to give Edith the best care at this point in her life.

Nursing care of an older person living with moderate frailty: Commentary on case study. Edith has always expressed a preference to remain at home; this is important to her. A person living with moderate frailty may present with an acute need that may or may not require hospitalisation. It is important for Edith to remain as independent as possible wherever she receives acute care.

If Edith were to remain at home with a 'keeping well' focus, the nurse assessing Edith can take a CGA approach to her assessment, looking at each of the six domains. It is important for the nurse to work collaboratively with health and social care professionals, taking an integrated approach to the interventions required. We previously discussed the asset-based approach, so questions about what Edith can do at home, what is important to her and what can be done to help her achieve this are important. Following a CGA, coproduced plans can be implemented. Immediate needs regarding function can be addressed in collaboration with multidisciplinary colleagues. It is important to ensure care planning with Edith includes the proactive aspects of care that could help prevent acute admission in the future by applying the domains discussed below. The British Geriatric Society has a suite of resources for assessing a patient with frailty in primary care (See 'Resources': Fit for Frailty).

Some key physical, mental and environmental changes were identified through the nurse's assessment:

- Constipation: Edith has not had a bowel movement for 7 days
- Frequency of micturition and pain on micturition
- Poor hydration
- Poor nutrition
- Confusion/delirium
- Low mood
- Reduced mobility and poor balance
- High risk of falling again in the next 24 to 48 hours
- Evidence of environmental neglect.

Edith needs immediate nurse intervention. In the United Kingdom, crisis and rapid response services have been introduced to enable home management of crisis care. Such services often take a multiprofessional approach to care in

---

CASE STUDY 6.2   Edith, Living with Moderate Frailty—Keeping Well and Crisis Intervention

Edith is now 82 years old and living alone, having lost her husband 14 months ago. It has been a very difficult two years for Edith; alongside her family, she cared for her husband at home until the end of his life. Edith misses her husband and since his death has become low in mood and often finds herself forgetting things or not finding the right word. Her world has continued to shrink, and she is more withdrawn from social activity and no longer has the enthusiasm for it. In the past 6 months she suffered two falls at home. Edith put the falls down to 'slipping' and 'not looking where I was going,' but her unsteadiness has increased, and she is holding on to the furniture when she walks around the home. More recently Edith has been falling asleep in the chair downstairs and not going to bed; she finds it hard to sleep without her husband. Her nutritional intake is poor as she has lost her appetite and has little motivation to cook.

In the past week Edith has become more confused and fatigued and has not been eating or drinking. Her neighbour found her on the floor; her fall-sensing device had detected a change and alerted her contact. The ambulance was called, and Edith was assessed as having a National Early Warning Score (NEWS) of 6 as urinary sepsis was suspected. The few days before the fall, Edith reported not eating or drinking. She also reported no bowel movements for 7 days.

the home, responding within a specified time, such as 0 to 2 hours. Advanced clinical practitioners, including nurses working at this level, often lead care in an acute phase at home. Appropriate management in the first 24 hours at home or in hospital is crucial for people living with frailty. Optimal care should be established that includes considering whether community or primary care options are more appropriate than hospital care. The following are required: a full physical assessment; history taking; immediate review of care needs; assessment of function; treatment for constipation; review of medications, including whether to prescribe antibiotics for a urinary tract infection without relying on urine dipping (Public Health England, 2018); and assessment for delirium. A psychological and spiritual assessment should include consideration of Edith's husband's death and the ongoing effects of bereavement—emotional, social and physical. Loneliness after bereavement is associated with an increased risk of depression; a cycle of fatigue, loss of activity, appetite and increased depression can ensue.

It is imperative out-of-hospital care is developed for older people living with frailty. If Edith is cared for at home, the nursing care maybe at an advanced level of practice. Advanced clinical practice is a defined level of practice within clinical professions such as nursing, pharmacy, paramedics and occupational therapy. It is designed to transform and modernise pathways of care, enabling the safe and effective sharing of skills across traditional professional boundaries.

Whether care is provided in an acute setting or at home, it is essential to commence effective rehabilitation at the earliest opportunity to decrease the impact of deconditioning. Using the skills of the multidisciplinary team, especially allied health professionals, is key.

How care is transferred from a hospital to other settings after the acute phase is important. Optimising this key interface within the system provides integrated support for patients while supporting efficiency in health and care services. It is vital the nurse understands the patient's immediate future and long-term care requirements. Aspects of environment and function are to be considered. The nurse is key to ensuring timely transfer back to the agreed-on care setting and that the wishes of the individual are listened to when planning transfer.

It was agreed Edith needed to be reviewed at home by the community team. Edith's wish was to remain at home and enjoy some time in her garden. She also wanted to be able to get out of the house and needed support to do so. Edith thought she might like to try another club or meeting where she could once again begin to engage with others and liked the look of a local lunch club. Using the goals Edith set, a plan was implemented to help her to stay well at home and prevent further unscheduled hospital admissions. Through the planning process for Edith's care, the community nursing team was able to broach early discussion of advance planning and ceilings of treatment for the future, as determined by Edith.

For the older person living with frailty, advance planning and ceilings of treatment are important considerations. Nurses need to develop skills so they can discuss these issues with patients. Advance planning is discussed later in this chapter. Ceilings of treatment refer to patient choices about future wishes with regard to medical intervention at times of acute health crises. Ultimately, all ceilings of treatment decisions result in one of three patient pathways: full escalation, limited escalation or maintenance of current care with the option of palliative care initiation.

Regardless of their place of work or speciality, nurses have a hugely important role to play in supporting older people like Edith to live and die well. Coordinating care and supporting other care providers is part of this, as is supporting family and friends who often provide most of the day-to-day end-of-life care (see Chapter 34).

Nursing care of an older person living with severe frailty: commentary on case study. This section looks at Edith' and her family's specific needs related to advancing frailty. It assumes the shared goal is to maximise comfort and provide support and treatment founded on what matters most to the person and their family. Nurses are often in the privileged position of being with the person for longer and are uniquely placed to connect with them and the individuals who matter to them most.

CASE STUDY 6.3   Edith, Living with Severe Frailty

Edith now lives in residential care accommodation. For the past 3 years she managed with assistance from carers twice a day. However, following a series of falls at home, a CT brain scan was performed that showed significant cerebral atrophy. This along with the presentation of further-reduced cognition led to Edith being diagnosed with dementia. Edith's family had to stay with her at night. Her confusion was worsening, and being cared for at home was becoming impossible. She now requires 24-hour care. Her mobility has significantly declined; she can slowly complete an independent sit-to-stand function and walk 5 metres with the use of her wheeled walking frame. As the day goes on, her functional ability worsens. With the decline in Edith's cognitive and functional state and the impact of advancing frailty, Edith is in the last phase of her life.

LIVING AND DYING WELL WITH FRAILTY

In people with frailty, a palliative care approach is often started in a crisis or when dying is imminent, but this needs to be integrated earlier into routine practice. Knowing when end of life is near is often limited to the last days of life. It is important to understand an individual's increased risk of end of life and likely benefit from palliative person-centred care focused on improving quality of life. Dolan and Holt suggest a person with advancing frailty is likely to be in their last 1,000 days of life; this should guide intervention decisions to enable people to live well until they die (see "Resources).

Life expectancy for residents in long-term care facilities is on average 2 years in the United Kingdom and shorter for nursing-home residents. People with advancing frailty are five times more likely to die in a year than those without frailty. In recognition of this, the British Geriatrics Society commissioned a multidisciplinary team to explore aspects of end-of-life care with tips for clinicians (see "Resources").

Achieving a balance between loss and continuity is crucial for older people's well-being and is supported—or undermined—by the quality of their interactions with health and social care and the assumptions that are made about their preferences and capabilities: what they can and cannot do (Nicholson et al., 2013). Goals of care need to be both future-looking and situated in the immediate, and nurses are key to supporting this endeavour, thinking with a person about what and who matters most to them. The question 'What makes today a good day?' can help people focus on living well now. Evidence suggests immediate goals of care for many older people in the last years of life often centre round remaining mobile and as independent as possible (Nicholson et al., 2018). Although Edith's mobility is declining, a rehabilitative potential and assessment must link to goals of care that optimise her physical function and emotional well-being to the highest extent possible.

Clinical Uncertainty Is Common

Identifying someone is moving toward the end of life is necessarily based on individual need rather than a clear prognosis. This is particularly the case for older people with frailty. The functional trajectory of frailty describes a progressive decline or prolonged dwindling over several months or years, punctuated by episodes of acute illness. This unpredictable trajectory makes it difficult to know for certain when people are nearing the end of life (see Fig. 6.6). Health-care professionals may be reluctant to identify a person with frailty as approaching end of life when there is no clear underlying pathology (Elliott et al., 2017). This means using time until death as the sole indicator of end of life. The identification and communication of entering the end of life for older people with frailty requires attention to the realities of living and dying over time. Identification of end of life is important; it allows for an optimal clinical response and gives the older person and their family a sense of security and control despite a changing condition. It enables older people with frailty to both live and conclude their lives well.

Revisiting Advance Care Planning

Advance care planning is a helpful way to discuss an older person's wishes and desires at the end of life and guide care. Combes et al.'s (2019) work on older people with frailty notes such conversations need to start early, focus on living well now and in the future, and seek to involve people who matter to the person while ensuring the older person with frailty and their choices are centre stage. Edith's worsening condition means it is imperative to revisit previous support and enable her to continue to express her choices and work with her family to ensure everyone agrees about what is going to happen as Edith enters the last months of life. Of equal importance is that future care wishes are known,

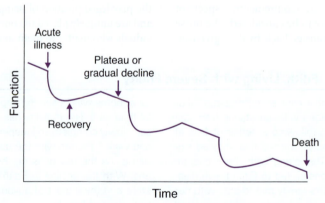

Fig. 6.6 Expected trajectory of decline in older people with frailty at the end of life. (British Geriatrics Society.)

documented and communicated widely across the whole care team, including Edith's family. Electronic palliative care coordination systems have been shown to be helpful in ensuring care coordination, reducing unplanned hospital admissions and ensuring patient's wishes are met, although rigorous evaluation is limited (Leniz et al., 2020).

Symptoms and Concerns Are Common

The last months of life are often associated with increasing physical symptoms and psychological, spiritual and practical concerns. Key symptoms and concerns related to people with frailty include pain, breathlessness, psychological distress (e.g., anxiety and depression), spiritual distress, incontinence and fatigue (Stow et al., 2019). Delirium has a poor prognosis; patients who develop delirium while on older people's medicine wards have an increased risk of death within 6 months (Kiely et al., 2009). (See also Chapter 28.)

It may be harder to communicate and assess Edith's symptoms due to cognitive decline. It it is important to work with residential care staff and family to understand how Edith can be the best she can be. Specific assessment tools that use observation of changes in behaviour rather than self-report are useful. Carers concerns often relate to the ability for their loved one to eat or drink toward the end of life. Edith's family are also important to assess for needs and support and to inform and support them to give best care.

Support for Carers

Supporting carers is critical to sustain this resource and reduce the potentially negative impact of caring on their health. Assessment of carer support needs is an important part of end-of-life care. In some counties, including England, all carers have the right to a carers' needs assessment. One tool that might help nurses identify the needs of Edith's family is the Carer Support Needs Assessment Tool, which was developed from evidence and carers and evaluated for community palliative care (Ewing et al., 2013). Part of the nurse's role within the wider multidisciplinary team includes knowing what local and national resources might be available to signpost people to.

Bereavement

Loss and grief: A normal part of dying

Living bereavement is a term that highlights the numerous losses older people with frailty experience before they physically die. Supporting older people with frailty to talk about their life and legacy and stay connected to people and places that give meaning and comfort is a vital role for the nurse. (See Chapter 34.)

Loss after death

Most bereavement reactions are not complicated, and the necessary support is provided by family, friends and various societal resources. It is important not to medicalise normal grief. However, the impact of bereavement on older people is often minimised as a universal experience that is expected in old age. It affects all older people differently and can leave the bereaved feeling alone and isolated. Not everyone needs or wants connection with a formal bereavement service, but for many there is a need for their grief to be recognised. Bereaved spouses are particularly at risk of a significant rise in mortality and morbidity in the year following death. This risk is greater if the spouse died in a sudden or unpredictable manner (Morin et al., 2017).

SUMMARY OF KEY NURSING CONCEPTS ACROSS FRAILTY

- Person driven
- Goals of care
- Quality of life for the older adult
- Nurse as advocate
- Multidisciplinary team
- Bringing in family's/friends' wider community perspectives, with the nurse as a bridging person
- Competence
- All patients consistently offered the opportunity to make the choice for or against independence and participation

DEVELOPING FRAILTY CAPABILITY: EVERYBODY'S ROLE

A framework of core frailty capabilities was launched in 2019 (Skills for Health, 2018). The aim of the core capabilities is to provide three tiers of frailty skills and knowledge, setting out the guidance to improve and standardise the understanding and educational requirements at three tiers of intervention. This framework aims to identify and describe the skills, knowledge and behaviours required to deliver high-quality, holistic, compassionate care and support. It provides a single, consistent, comprehensive framework on which to base review and development of staff.

We would like this chapter to inspire nurses to see frailty as core business and one where nursing has a central leadership role. The future of nursing in the field of frailty holds some exciting opportunities. The development of the advanced clinical practice role and the future accreditation of this role in practice is an example. Consultant nursing practice has developed, with new roles such as the consultant practitioner in frailty. These roles serve as examples in the way nurses are working to encompass advanced practice, research, education and system leadership. An application of these roles in the out-of-hospital setting can result in individuals like Edith remaining at home through acute phases of care.

The combined focus on senior clinical nursing roles and the acknowledgement of nurses' vital roles in research provides the perfect platform for the continued development of the clinical academic in practice. Clinical academics are clinical professionals who work across health-care providers and academic institutions. They have a dual role that combines their clinical career with a research career. They work in health and social care while researching ways to improve patient outcomes.

As well as advanced and consultant practice opportunities, the nurse has a crucial role in education across multidisciplinary forums in health and social care as well as for service users/carers and families. Although this is an opportunity, it can also be faced as a challenge for the nurse striving to work and navigate across different and non-traditional boundaries. However, in practice, this serves only to strengthen nurses' level of frailty understanding and improves their levels of integrated working.

Nurses need to ensure integrated approaches are normalised in health and social care settings and recognise the roles all professionals can bring to the care of the older person living with frailty. As with the CGA, an approach whereby all professionals work to provide the best outcome through assessment must be applied when caring for individuals living with frailty. Other professionals bring a different but complementary 'lens' through which to provide frailty care.

CONCLUSION AND KEY LEARNING POINTS

This chapter invites nurses to see the opportunities for nursing in supporting older people with frailty and the individuals who matter to them—at whatever stage of their illness. Clinical nurses can both lead and be an integral part of a multidisciplinary and multisector response. The complex care needs of older people with frailty require truly holistic care. The educational role of the nurse is vital in enabling older people, their families and communities to enhance quality and quantity of life.

Frailty has ramifications across all care settings. The nurse has a leading role in evidence generation and ensuring practice is guided by best available evidence. As we continue to research frailty, we understand the strong socioeconomic determinants and the importance of frailty in younger age groups. The importance of strong social networks, strength-based exercise, good nutrition and patient activation are policy and nursing considerations. Nursing must always centre on the person. Our care can positively impact the quality and experience of older people with frailty.

Frailty is a long-term condition, and as Edith's case study illustrates, older people's circumstances and needs change. Core at every stage is to identify what matters most to the person and to recognise and support their personal and social strengths in achieving as good a quality of life as possible at every stage of frailty.

KEY LEARNING POINTS

- Frailty is a complex medical syndrome with physical, psychological and social determinants that requires a holistic multidisciplinary approach where the nurse's role is central.
- Early identification and assessment increases reversibility of frailty.
- Frailty is on a continuum and can be made better or worse by the interventions given.
- Care must be tailored to the individual to enable maximum quality of life for as long as possible.

- Focusing on exercise, nutrition, ensuring a strong support network and education all empower older people and prevent adverse outcomes associated with frailty.
- The role of the nurse is key in giving safe and compassionate care and in supporting the delivery of specific treatments.
- The role of the nurse is important in identifying and addressing needs across the stages of frailty.

RESOURCES

- Frailty Fulcrum: https://www.england.nhs.uk/blog/dawn-moody
- Frailty Framework of Core Capabilities: https://skillsforhealth.org.uk/info-hub/frailty-2018
- MECC: http://makingeverycontactcount.co.uk
- Decade of Healthy Ageing: https://www.who.int/initiatives/decade-of-healthy-ageing

- End PJ Paralysis: https://endpjparalysis.org
- Story of Mrs. Andrews https://www.bing.com/videos/search?q=June+Andrews+story+delayed+transfers+of+care&ru=%2fvideos%2fsearch%3fq%3dJune%2bAndrews%2bstory%2bdelayed%2btransfers%2bof%2bcare%26FORM%3dVDVVXX&view=detail&mid=969474E9469F014E4769969474E9469F014E4769&rvsmid=BF4F054199A659F8139CBF4F054199A659F8139C&FORM=VDRVRV

- Fit for Frailty: https://www.bgs.org.uk/sites/default/files/content/resources/files/2018-05-14/fff2_short.pdf
- Last 1,000 days: https://www.last1000days.com/
- British Geriatrics Society "End of Life Care in Frailty" series: https://www.bgs.org.uk/resources/resource-series/end-of-life-care-in-frailty

REFERENCES

British Geriatrics Society (2022). Bringing hospital care home: Virtual Wards and Hospital at Home for older people | British Geriatrics Society. Available at: www.bgs.org.uk/virtualwards (accessed 17 August 2022)

Clegg, A., Bates, C., Young, J., Ryan, R., Nichols, L., Teale, E. Z., Mohammed, M. A., Parry, J., & Marshall, T. (2016). Development and validation of an electronic frailty index using routine primary care electronic health record data. *Age and Ageing, 45*(3), 353–360.

Clegg, A., Young, J., Iliffe, S., Rikkert, M. O., & Rockwood, K. (2013). Frailty in elderly people. *The Lancet, 381*(9868), 752–762.

Combes, S., Nicholson, C. J., Gillett, K., & Norton, C. (2019). Implementing advance care planning with community-dwelling frail elders requires a system-wide approach: An integrative review applying a behaviour change model. *Palliative Medicine, 33*(7), 743–756.

Elliott, M., & Nicholson, C. (2017). A qualitative study exploring use of the surprise question in the care of older people: perceptions of general practitioners and challenges for practice. *BMJ Supportive & Palliative Care, 7*(1), 32–38.

Ellis, G., Gardner, M., Tsiachristas, A., Langhorne, P., Burke, O., Harwood, R. H., Conroy, S. P., Kircher, T., Somme, D., Saltvedt, I., Wald, H., O'Neill, D., Robinson, D., & Shepperd, S. (2017). Comprehensive geriatric assessment for older adults admitted to hospital. *Cochrane Database of Systematic Reviews, 9*(9), Article CD006211.

Ewing, G., Brundle, C., Payne, S., & Grande, G. (2013). The Carer Support Needs Assessment Tool (CSNAT) for use in palliative and end-of-life care at home: A validation study. *Journal of Pain and Symptom Management, 46*(3), 395–405.

Fried, L. P., Tangen, C. M., Walston, J., Newman, A., B., Hirsch, C., Gottdiener, J., Seeman, T., Tracy, R., Kop, W. J., Burke, G., & McBurnie, M. A. (2001). & Cardiovascular Health Study Collaborative Research Group. Frailty in older adults: evidence for a phenotype. *The Journals of Gerontology Series A: Biological Sciences and Medical Sciences, 56*(3), M146–M157.

Gallagher, P., Ryan, C., Byrne, S., Kennedy, J., & O'Mahony, D (2008). STOPP (Screening Tool of Older Person's Prescriptions) and START (Screening Tool to Alert Doctors to Right Treatment): Consensus validation. *Internationl Journal of Clinical Pharmacology and Therapeutics, 46*(2), 72–83.

Garrett, J., Worrall, S., & Sweeney, S. (2020). *Reducing health inequalities for people living with frailty.*

Gill, T. M., Gahbauer, E. A., Allore, H. G., & Han, L. (2006). Transitions between frailty states among community-living older persons. *Archives of Internal Medicine, 166*(4), 418–423.

Goodrich, J., & Cornwell, J. (2008). *Seeing the person in the patient.* The Point of Care Review Paper.

Haapanen, M. J., Perälä, M. M., Salonen, M. K., Kajantie, E., Simonen, M., Pohjolainen, P., Eriksson, J. G., & von Bonsdorff, M. B. (2018). Early life determinants of frailty in old age: the Helsinki Birth Cohort Study. *Age and Ageing, 47*(4), 569–575.

Hanlon, P., Nicholl, B. I., Jani, B. D., Lee, D., McQueenie, R., & Mair, F. S. (2018). Frailty and pre-frailty in middle-aged and older adults and its association with multimorbidity and mortality: A prospective analysis of 493 737 UK Biobank participants. *Lancet Public Health, 3*(7), e323–e332.

Kiely, D. K., Marcantonio, E. R., Inouye, S. K., Shaffer, M. L., Bergmann, M. A., Yang, F., M., Fearing, M., A., & Jones, R. N (2009). Persistent delirium predicts greater mortality. *Journal of the American Geriatrics Society, 57*(1), 55–61.

Leniz, J., Weil, A., Higginson, I. J., & Sleeman, K. E. (2020). Electronic palliative care coordination systems (EPaCCS): A systematic review. *BMJ Supportive & Palliative Care, 10*(1), 68–78.

Morin, L., Aubry, R., Frova, L., MacLeod, R., Wilson, D. M., Loucka, M., Csikos, A., Ruiz-Ramos, M., Cardenas-Turanzas, M., Rhee, Y., Teno, J., Öhlen, J., Deliens, L., Houttekier, D., & Cohen, J. (2017). Estimating the need for palliative care at the population level: A cross-national study in 12 countries. *Palliative Medicine, 31*(6), 526–536.

Morley, J. E., Vellas, B., van Kan, G. A., Anker, S. D., Bauer, J. M., Bernabei, R., Cesari, M., Chumlean, W. C., Doehner, W., Evans, J., Fried, L. P., Guralnik, J. M., Katz, P. R., Malmstrom, T. K., McCarter, R. J., Gutierrez Robledo, L. M., Rockwood, K., von Haehling, S., Vandewoude, M. F., & Walston, J. (2013). Frailty consensus: A call to action. *Journal of the American Medical Directors Association, 14*(6), 392–397.

Nicholson, C., Davies, J. M., George, R., Smith, B., Pace, V., Harris, H., Ross, J., Noble, J., Hansford, P., & Murtagh, F. E. M. (2018). What are the main palliative care symptoms and concerns of older people with multimorbidity?—A comparative cross-sectional study using routinely collected Phase of Illness, Australia-modified Karnofsky Performance Status and Integrated Palliative Care Outcome Scale data. *Annals of Palliative Medicine, 7*, S164–S175.

Nicholson, C., Gordon, A. L., & Tinker, A. (2016). Changing the way "we" view and talk about frailty…. *Age and Ageing, 46*(3), 349–351.

Nicholson, C., Meyer, J., Flatley, M., & Holman, C. (2013). The experience of living at home with frailty in old age: A psychosocial qualitative study. *International Journal of Nursing Studies, 50*(9), 1172–1179.

Nicholson, C., Meyer, J., Flatley, M., Holman, C., & Lowton, K. (2012). Living on the margin: Understanding the experience of living and dying with frailty in old age. *Social Science & Medicine, 75*(8), 1426–1432.

O'Caoimh, R., Galluzzo, L., Rodríguez-Laso, Á., Van der Heyden, J., Hylen Ranhoff, A., Lamprini-Koula, M., Ciutan, M., López-Samaniego, L., Carcaillon-Bentata, L., Kennelly, S., Liew, A., & Work Package 5 of the Joint Action ADVANTAGE. (2018). Prevalence of frailty at population level in European ADVANTAGE Joint Action Member States: A systematic review and meta-analysis. *Annali dell'Istituto superiore di sanita, 54*(3), 226–238.

Molnar, F., Huang, A., & Tinetti, M. (2017). *Update: The public launch of the geriatric 5Ms.* http://canadiangeriatrics.ca/wp-content/uploads/2017/04/UPDATE-THE-PUBLIC-LAUNCH-OF-THE-GERIATRIC-5MS.pdf

Petermann-Rocha, F., Lyall, D. M., Gray, S. R., Esteban-Cornejo, I., Quinn, T. J., Ho, F. K., Pell, J. P., & Celis-Morales, C. (2020). Associations between physical frailty and dementia incidence: prospective study from UK Biobank. *The Lancet Healthy Longevity, 1*(2), e58–e68.

Public Health England. (2018). *Diagnosis of urinary tract infections.* PHE Publications.

Rahman, S. (2018). *Living with frailty: from assets and deficits to resilience.* Routledge.

Richardson, S., Karunananthan, S., & Bergman, H. (2011). I may be frail but I ain't no failure. *Canadian Geriatrics Journal, 14*(1), 24–28.

Rockwood, K., Stadnyk, K., MacKnight, C., McDowell, I., Hèbert, R., & Hogan, D. B. (1999). A brief clinical instrument to classify frailty in elderly people. *Lancet, 353*(9148), 205.

Rockwood, K., Song, X., MacKnight, C., Bergman, H., Hogan, D. B., McDowell, I., & Mitnitski, A. (2005). A global clinical measure of fitness and frailty in elderly people. *Canadian Medical Association Journal, 173*(5), 489–495.

Skills for Health. (2018). Frailty: The frailty framework for core capabilities. https://www.skillsforhealth.org.uk/info-hub/frailty-2018

Stow, D., Spiers, G., Matthews, F. E., & Hanratty, B. (2019). What is the evidence that people with frailty have needs for palliative care at the end of life? A systematic review and narrative synthesis. *Palliative Medicine, 33*(4), 399–414.

Tinetti, M. E., & Fried, T. (2004). The end of the disease era. *The American Journal of Medicine, 116*(3), 179–185.

Turner G., & Clegg A. British Geriatrics Society; Age UK; Royal College of General Practitioners (2014). Best practice guidelines for the management of frailty: a British Geriatrics Society, Age UK and Royal College of General Practitioners report. *Age Ageing, 43*(6):744–747.

Vermeiren, S., Vella-Azzopardi, R., Beckwee, D., Habbig, A.-K., Scafoglieri, A., Jansen, B., & Bautmans, I. (2016). Frailty and the prediction of negative health outcomes: a meta-analysis. *Journal of the American Medical Directors Association, 17*(12), 1163. e1–1163.e17.

World Health Organization. (2022). Ageing and health. https://www.who.int/news-room/fact-sheets/detail/ageing-and-health

People, Policy and the Place of Care

7

Policy Context of Nursing in Health and Social Care

Fiona M. Ross

CHAPTER OUTLINE

INTRODUCTION

As governments come and go, the top lines of policy change, but the big questions endure, often largely unsolved. Over 40 years there have been energetic policy debates about the best way to fund and support an ageing population. What is affordable? What is the optimum balance of responsibility between individuals and the government? In what ways can people be given choice of where and how they best age? This chapter centres on policy for older people, focusing on the organisation of care and financial support for older people in health and social care with a brief outline of the differences in England, Wales, Scotland and Northern Ireland. It is particularly geared toward what nurses need to know for their work with older people in a variety of health and social care settings. The coronavirus pandemic exposed weaknesses in the health and social care system but also demonstrated the compassion, resilience and courage of front-line staff dealing with an onslaught of critically ill patients suffering from a disease we had to learn about as we went along.

The chapter also considers nursing workforce policy and discusses some of the reasons why care of older people is still seen as a Cinderella service. It addresses other key themes in government responses to an ageing population and policy hot spots, notably around difference and diversity. The chapter ends with an analysis of the potential power and influence of older people in the policy-making process, since it is often forgotten that many older people are highly active in social and political debates and have much to say about what they think is wrong and what should be done. New policy debates will have to acknowledge older people's human rights and their expression of them.

A BRIEF HISTORY

The building blocks of today's system of health and social care in the United Kingdom, and some parts of pension provision and housing, owe much to the legislation laid down in the 1940s and the compromises made to implement the welfare state. Older people's needs and circumstances became starkly visible in the aftermath of the Second World War, which influenced the design of the welfare state. Many current services have their origins in the thinking of that time and in ideas developed as wartime stopgaps. These include the development of meal services, home help and local organisations and charitable initiatives to meet needs and promote independence at home—for example, age concern groups. A familiar issue of post-war policy was the pressure to remove older people from occupying hospital beds, now often discussed in pejorative terms of 'bed blocking'. Community care policies over the past 30 years have similar roots in government concern that older people were posing a social problem in their excessive consumption of the welfare budget, particularly residential care. The charging, or fining, of local authorities for failing to arrange hospital discharge for patients reflects similar concerns.

Government policy—both Labour and Conservative administrations—over the past 30 years has argued for the extension of patient choice, establishing better quality standards for older people and partnership work, including with the private sector. While the internal market has been criticised and officially discontinued in health care, there is still an emphasis on contracting with private agencies, now called commissioning. Reorganisation of the National Health Service (NHS) is beloved of governments both left and right. Current policy suggests the state-run health system is bureaucratic, bloated, slow and overregulated (Kwartang et al., 2012). By contrast the private sector is cast as innovative and efficient. Assumptions drawn from political ideology have often led to questioning, challenging and radical change of structures, rationalised using a narrative of choice, quality and efficient use of a resource-strapped system.

PLACE-BASED CARE

A consensus over the years is the structural divide between health and social care needs fixing, particularly in England. The King's Fund (2021) has been influential in shaping solutions and offering practical ideas for place-based systems, which are about bringing organisations together around the population they serve. The King's Fund identified 10 principles to inform the design of place-based care:

- Define the population group and the system's boundaries.
- Identify the right partners and services.
- Develop a shared vision and objectives.
- Develop an appropriate governance structure.
- Identify the right leaders and develop a new form of leadership.
- Agree how conflicts will be resolved.
- Develop a sustainable financial model.
- Create a dedicated team.
- Develop systems within systems.
- Develop a single set of measures.

The current changes in health and social care are being shaped by the *Five Year Forward View* (NHS, 2014), the NHS's long-term plan and the idea of integrated care (NHS, 2020) draw on the King's Fund principles of place-based care to develop integrated care systems (Department of Health and Social Care [DOH], 2021). The direction is toward exploiting the existing relationships and partnerships between NHS trusts, general practice, local authorities and independent and charitable sectors to create new entities that work together for the benefit of the local population. Themes of this structural change are to extend patient choice, provide value for money and encourage care being provided in the right place and at the right time and out of hospital. These changes are driven by the view the internal market has had unintended consequences of waste and inefficiencies—for example, the complexity of contracting across multiple partners with sometimes conflicting values, such as private-sector contracts for social care with local authorities. Outcomes too often have been poor quality care, poor performance, failures of communication and inefficiencies. The new Integrated Care Boards (ICBs) were established as statutory bodies in July 2022.

But what do we mean by integration? The Canterbury initiative in New Zealand has been influential in current policy thinking and was designed around the core principles of 'one system and one budget', service delivery focused on 'right care, right place, right time by the right person', and responsibility of the system to achieve the best outcomes rather than these being attributed to a person or organisation (Timmins & Ham, 2013). It is emphasised that successful integration takes time, which is true in the Torbay and South Devon model, seen as an early adopter of integration. It built on the success of the Torbay Care Trust, which in 2005 incorporated adult and social care into the NHS. The project has pooled a budget of £400 million, bring together 6,000 members of staff from acute and community social care to develop a unique risk-sharing agreement that satisfies governance and regulation. Another example of integration is the Greater Manchester model, which set out a collaborative vision for the region that emphasises well-being and alternative approaches to service delivery. In practice this means the local councils work together with the health-care providers in a neighbourhood model that brings services to a local level and co-locates professionals, thus improving communication and care planning across health and social care services.

Arguably England is late to the integration game and has a lot to learn from similar partnership arrangements reaching maturity in Scotland, Wales and Northern Ireland. The Scottish and Welsh commitment to integration is embedded in political devolution of health care. They are on different journeys to reform but share a rejection of competition in health care in favour of collaboration, merging commissioning with provision, pooling budgets and having clear governance and regulatory frameworks. In Scotland health and social care integration was launched in 2016 with the purpose to improve support and care for patients, carers and families by joining up services and focusing on anticipatory and preventive care. Northern Ireland has had a structurally integrated system of health and social care since 1973, which developed against the backdrop of political uncertainty, instability and at times bitter sectarian violence. The integration authorities are required to work with their local communities and providers of care to ensure care is responsive to need. In practice and on the ground, programme managers or team leaders are open to a range of professions. For example, a social worker may lead a team that includes nurses in mental health, or a nurse may lead a team that includes social workers in the care of older people. As Chris Ham (2013) notes, this management structure enables teams to make the most of all the talents and opens up management opportunities more broadly.

Integration across systems with long histories of rivalry, competition and in some cases mistrust is a huge challenge. Creating a government department of health and social care with a matching ministerial title in England may provide a cosmetic appearance of unity and direction, but the proof of the pudding will be in whether the experiences and outcomes of care for patients and their families are different and better. There are some early positive signs in England, as lessons from an evidence review suggests integrated care leads to improved quality and patient satisfaction with access, but the impact on costs are not clear (Baxter et al., 2018). The experience in Scotland and Wales shows it takes time and patience to enthuse partners to work differently and develop the shared understanding and language necessary for cultural change.

Leadership is critical to success. A new realist review of the evidence of leadership in integrated health and social care systems exposes the mismatch between the rhetoric with the lack of practical guidance about how to lead. The review found leaders have a tendency to fall back on familiar networks rather than brokering new ones, evidence of a preoccupation with the notion of hero leadership and who the person is rather than what they do and how they do it, and finally that there is little evidence of leaders making the most of the patient and carer perspectives (Sims et al., 2021).

SOCIAL CARE

This section offers an overview of social care and support available for older people in care homes and their own homes. More detail is covered in Chapters 9 and 11.

Here the focus is on the policy that underpins social care provision and its possible future as a result of the lessons learned during the global coronavirus pandemic that shook the world in 2020. Under section 2 of the Care Act 2014 (DOH, 2014), councils must provide or arrange to provide services, facilities or resources, or take other steps, that contribute to preventing, delaying or reducing need or the development of need for care. Anyone can request an assessment for care from the local council. The reality of provision is inevitably stretched by the resources available, as since 2010 local councils have experienced serious budget cuts, and choices have to be made between schools, libraries, parks, waste disposal and other essential services. While assessment is a requirement of local authorities and councils, the delivery of care is assessed against eligible needs. Social care, unlike health, is not free in England; local authorities have always been able to charge for services. A recent proposal caps care costs at £86,000 (at the time of writing) as the maximum contribution anyone may need to make toward their care costs over their lifetime. When that cap is reached, the state pays. For individuals unable to pay, a means test ensures the state helps with fees.

Assessment of Need and Priority

Some have argued assessment and case management is part of the solution to make sure older people with high health needs receive a proactive service that can prevent continual readmission to hospitals, crises in care and support, and optimise rehabilitation and quality of life. The Wanless (2002) report, for example, considered 'properly targeted assessment and active care management' would promote independence, prevent deterioration of long-term conditions, manage risk and even potentially reduce service demand.

Much has been written about assessment and care planning—for example using the National Institute for Clinical Excellence (NICE, 2015) as a mechanism to overcome reports of fragmentation, difficulties in access and the unfortunate consequences of an individual being treated as a collection of conditions or systems rather than as a whole person. A list of principles often cited as underpinning health and social care is set out below.

Eligibility and priority setting through professional assessment of need is fundamental to being allocated to a service in social care, in contrast to health care, which enshrines the principle of universal, equitable, comprehensive high-quality care that is free at the point of delivery. In social care, eligibility criteria define who gets care, advice and information. The Care Act of 2014 introduced six principles to guide social care providers. These aim to put the individual at the centre and provide services that are empowering, protective, preventive, proportional, partnership-based and accountable. New eligibility criteria for adults with care and support needs replaced the former risk-based system. Now social care seeks to help people meet their needs to achieve the outcomes that matter to them in their lives and in turn promote their well-being. Prioritisation of high needs often includes the 'housebound' criteria, which is critical to being offered support, although in practice there are ambiguities around it. Questions are asked by assessors—for example, is someone considered housebound if they can go out in a wheelchair but only with help?

Assessment is vital to making the system of social care fair. But the pinch point is inevitably the demand for assessment is greater than the resources available to support services. Assessments are typically carried out by social care practitioners, such as occupational therapists employed by social services. They aim to assess needs, target resources and coordinate care by setting up and reviewing individual care packages. Such packages include input from family members and services such as home care, day care and care homes. Service provision varies from one area to another, with local authorities having contracts with a range of care providers from independent to charitable.

Social Care Providers

Social care in England is mostly run by private providers, from small employers that run one or two care homes to agencies that provide social care in a person's home through contracts, for example for home care. In the public imagination care homes are sometimes seen as a place for older relatives to move to when home is no longer managable or sustainable. Standards are variable, but in many cases have improved despite workforce shortages. Many care homes provide outstanding care overseen by regulators that publish inspection outcomes for public view, attitudes remain that are hard to break. Ninety per cent of all care homes are in the independent sector—private or voluntary organisations providing care for 85% of people. Levels of disability in most care homes are high, with many residents having multiple morbidities, increasing frailty and often mental health problems such as dementia and depression. The pandemic was a wakeup call to policy makers that although it may be possible to separate social from health care on paper and in the minds of policy makers, in practice it is all one system as older people and caregivers move between them. Two service user stories of living in a care home follow, and more discussion of nursing care in care homes is provided in Chapter 8.

CASE STUDY 7.1

Mrs Dunne lives in a care home that was previously owned and run by a local authority in England. It is now under the ownership and management of an independent not-for-profit trust. The local authority has a contract with this trust for 25 places and pays a set fee for each place. Mrs Dunne pays part of the cost, her Attendance Allowance pays for some and the local authority makes up the remainder. If she were in Scotland, she would receive further financial assistance to pay for the personal care provided by the home but would have to contribute to her food and living costs. The home is part of a group of homes, and considerable sums have been borrowed to modernise the building. Now most residents do not have to share a bedroom. Staff receive training, and over half have a basic qualification. Since 2009 the care home has been inspected by the Care Quality Commission (CQC). Prior to that it was regulated by the Commission for Social Care Inspection.

CASE STUDY 7.2

Mrs Eden lives in a nearby residential care home that is owned and run by a former nurse. It is a small home with only seven residents, and the owner wonders how long she will keep the business, as staff have left since the pandemic, and she has the financial challenges of rising costs to the minimum wage and national insurance, which are increasing prices of energy and food bills. She has had to make extensive changes to comply with new standards, and it is hard in a small business to release staff for training. All the residents have their fees paid by the local authority, which has assessed everyone financially and calculated the amounts they must pay, but there is little contact between their care managers and the homeowner. Local community nurses are regular visitors to the home to help the staff with end-of-life care, treatment of leg ulcers and other conditions.

During the pandemic we bore witness to the pain that care homes experienced in terms of a torrent of infection and exponential increase in end-of-life care through COVID-19 deaths that were not only difficult to manage but were also exacerbated by the pain of separation as the outside world was kept away. Families were separated from loved ones by personal protective equipment, having to say last goodbyes through a window, deprived of human touch. Figure 7.1 shows an independently minded care home

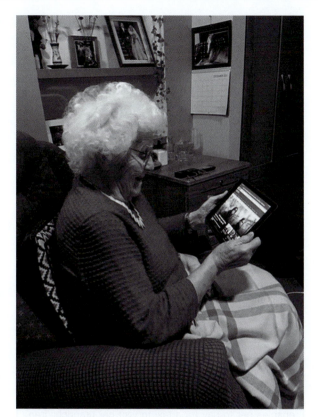

Fig. 7.1 Care home resident using her iPad.

resident in her nineties missing the physical visits of her supportive family but using technology to communicate during the pandemic.

The challenges facing social care are commonly raised in the media and policy papers such as the British Geriatrics Society (2021). Some of the common issues raised are as follows:

- Complicated mixture of agencies (commercial, some voluntary-sector and some social services provision)
- Lack of continuity of care-home workers (high turnover and problems with quality)
- Continued restrictions of availability over the time of day and days of the week for home visits
- Lack of access to experienced or specialist workers
- Continued problems with coordination of people and services
- Limited short-break care services at home (e.g., sitting services)
- Lack of useful information about service users to inform care staff

In England the CQC and in Scotland the Care Inspectorate register and inspect care providers, including NHS Trusts, care homes, general practices and home-care agencies. In England the CQC inspection framework sets out five domains to assess providers on whether they are safe, effective, caring, responsive to people's needs and well led.

Despite efforts to promote community care policies, the attempts to shift funding from the acute to community sectors has proved formidable. Integrated care systems might offer a new opportunity with strategic commissioning and pooled budgets that focus on individuals and communities rather than providers. This might enable individually designed support that could 'wrap around' people wherever they are.

Admission and Transfer From Hospital

In England in 2017 there were 16.6 million hospital admissions, and of these 3.5 million (22%) were people 75 years and older, despite being only 8.2% of the population (Public Health England [PHE], 2020). We know under a quarter of all admissions are people in the last year of their life, and a staggering 81% of people aged 75 years and older have at least one hospital admission in the last year of life (PHE, 2020). This matters, as the disruption and disorientation experienced by frail older people in a strange and unfamiliar environment can exacerbate confusion and other problems such as incontinence, which add to distress and might be avoided with proper investment in community services that support families to provide care without becoming exhausted and stressed.

For decades problems have been identified in discharge or transfer from hospital. For example problems may arise when older people are discharged from hospital at night or over the weekend and have no one to support them. Delays in leaving hospital have resulted in the development of services such as intermediate care. Leaving hospital without sufficient or appropriate support may result in a person's rapid return to hospital, with needless distress or disability, or precipitate a move to a care home as a community care 'failure'. Naturally, not all hospital discharges result in problems. However, both admissions and discharges have been put under the spotlight in attempts to respond to the problems that may arise if they are inappropriate and the suffering felt by older people who need treatment in hospital and whose health is deteriorating while they wait. Chapter 9 discusses care in the community and initiatives such as intermediate care that attempt to reduce the need for hospital admission; rehabilitate older people on their return home; implement hospital-at-home schemes where care, treatment or observation can be provided in place; and continue care funding that enables people to receive free nursing care outside hospital settings.

Levers and Penalties

In England the Community Care (Delayed Discharges etc.) Act of 2003 established a system of cross-charging or reimbursement for cases where a local authority is judged to have delayed a person's transfer by not setting up social care to enable a safe discharge home or to another setting when the patient has been as assessed as fit and ready to go by the multidisciplinary team. This last point is important as readiness to go home means assessing the patient and their home environment and the capacity to function safely. The effects of this system have been looked at by the King's Fund (2018), which highlighted delays may be caused by multiple factors and not just local authorities or councils, despite the tendency of the media to shift blame in that direction. Delays may be due to families and the patient being unable to agree about the best solution and where to go.

Although this chapter concentrates on England, it is important to note older people's experiences are affected by political devolution. Private or commercial care, for example, is far more common in England than in Scotland and Wales. Scotland has prioritised 'free' personal care, at considerable government cost, following the recommendations of the Royal Commission on the Funding of Long-Term Care (Scottish Executive, 2002). Scotland has also reformed its law in respect of mental capacity with the Adults with Incapacity Act in 2000, which has particular importance for people with dementia, well in advance of England's Mental Capacity Act of 2005. The Adults with Incapacity Act requires anything done on behalf of adults with incapacity must benefit them. For example, spending their money must take account of the person's wishes, current or past, and those of family or appointed guardian, and must be as minimally restrictive as possible. For full details, see the legal statute and regulations.

Benefits and Personalisation

The principle behind the benefits system is older people should not live in poverty; therefore, universal entitlements are allocated on the basis of age. Examples are the state pension and the £100 winter fuel allowance, which are essential for individuals without an occupational pension and for many older women who were never employed. There is also a complicated system of discretionary benefits that are intended to provide supplementary support for individuals who can demonstrate need—for example, the Attendance Allowance. The Attendance Allowance and other benefits

such as the winter fuel payment have been devolved to the Scottish Parliament. This chapter offers a brief overview. Readers are directed to additional resources available from the relevant local authority. It is never possible to be up to date in a book of this kind, because the time lag between writing and publication inevitably means some things like benefits quickly become of date.

Attendance Allowance provides a flexible, highly valued national entitlement that helps with the costs of living for individuals with a disability and promotes independence for people above pension age. It is not means tested, so it does not matter how much you have in savings or other income. There are two levels; the higher level is provided for dependent older people with significant caring needs, for example who need help to get out of bed, get dressed and manage incontinence. If the person is in receipt of a Personal Independent Payment, Attendance Allowance is not payable. The application form is long and daunting, and often people need help to complete it. A local citizens advice office can help.

CASE STUDY 7.3

Muriel has mild dementia. She is 85 and lives in her own home in a small town. She has help from social services. Her standard-rate Attendance Allowance allows her to pay her bills and keep the heating on. It enables her to pay for a taxi to visit her grandchildren. When the taxi arrives, she likes the driver to ring on the door and helps her on with her coat. As she gets very anxious and confused on public transport, the money for occasional taxis makes her feel independent, and she loves the social contact with family.

Carers allowance varies across the four countries, with Scotland having a more generous system. This is intended to recognise the cost of caring and the loss of earnings.

NHS continuing care payments are available for people with a serious physical or mental health condition who need ongoing care in the community. Funding is provided by the NHS for those who are eligible and is normally accessed through a general practitioner or social worker and in practice may be nurse-led. The assessment process can be daunting and time consuming. The criteria are strict and defined by the primary health need. Put simply, eligibility rests on whether an individual's need is primarily a health one and specifically the nature of the need, its intensity or seriousness, the complexity of care support required and the unpredictability—in other words, how the needs fluctuate and the difficulty of managing them.

CASE STUDY 7.4

Richard is 75 and has end-stage fibrosis of the lungs. He is rapidly becoming more dependent on his daughter as he struggles to deal with breathlessness and fatigue, for which he receives continuous oxygen at home. His GP has had a conversation about planning for the future and put him in contact with the local hospice, which has a team of specialist nurses and medical practitioners who support people at home. On the first visit, the team leader asked about benefits and organised the completion of the application form for NHS continuing health care. This was based on her expert assessment of his needs and his preference, supported by his daughter, to die at home. The extra money was helpful to pay a sitter to stay with Richard while his daughter went to the shops or visited her grandchildren.

NHS continuing health care is similar in Northern Ireland and Wales but different in Scotland, which has its own scheme called hospital-based complex clinical care. Under this scheme, NHS funding is limited to patients who need to be in hospital to have their care needs properly met. Scotland enjoys an integrated system of health and social care, which supports people to live independently as far as possible in their own homes. This includes intermediate care services, hospital at home and intensive home-care services.

Direct Payments

The introduction of direct payments was part of a general move toward personalisation in adult social care policy. Direct payments offer older people the option of receiving a cash payment in lieu of receiving community-based social services. The cash enables them to choose, manage and pay for their own social care in a way that is appropriate and targeted (see Case Study 7.5). Originally, older people were not eligible for direct payments, which were designed to empower people with disabilities using services to support them at home. There was initially a good deal of policy nervousness that direct payments would be expensive to the public purse, but contrary to expectations this has not happened, as savings are accrued elsewhere and waste avoided. Crucially these are benefits that are popular and well regarded as they enable people to live independently and have a better quality of life. Most commonly, people with disabilities employ someone to act as a personal assistant, providing help with activities of daily living and a range of other activities the person sees as important, such as going on visits or participating in leisure activities. A recent evaluation of direct payments for older people shows that

uptake of personal care and household support has been slow and the interpretation by local authorities has lacked consistency (Davey, 2021).

CASE STUDY 7.5

Ann is 82 and lives alone with chronic musculoskeletal problems that limit mobility and moderate cardiac failure. She is housebound, her husband died five years ago and she lives in the family home surrounded by memorabilia and memories of her large family, who live overseas. Supported by her social worker, she has received direct payments for 4 years. She is very positive about their value as they have allowed her to employ a personal assistant to manage the post, pay bills, write emails and oversee deliveries. She prefers to use the payments in this way rather than having support for personal care, which she just about manages. Her main worry is leaving a jumble of family papers and photos in boxes for her children to sort out after she dies. Having someone to help with sorting is hugely important and has done away with some of her anxiety and improved her self-image as someone who is independently making her own decisions about the kind of care she receives and when.

CASE STUDY 7.6

Mrs Fox just celebrated her 100th birthday. Her family are looking after her at home with the help of a live-in carer, who goes home on the weekends. They have had support from social services with adaptations to the house such as rails and equipment, a hospital bed, a wheelchair and other aids such as a commode. Mrs Fox goes to a care home occasionally for respite care to give the family a break. Mrs Fox has savings and pays for her private carer.

THE IMPORTANCE OF HOME

We often forget in the health policy narrative that other things contribute to well-being, such as housing, heating and outside space like parks and gardens. The home is important as a place where individuality, choice and relationships can be nurtured, but not everyone has the privilege of their own home, and some live in crowded environments among strangers (see Chapter 12). Since the Second World War major changes in housing have occurred. The current cohort of older people have witnessed immense growth and then decline in local-authority, or council, housing, and they have been beneficiaries of home ownership and the sale of council houses. The most common type of housing in the United Kingdom is owner occupancy. Older people have seen policy attention oscillate from residential care to sheltered housing to very sheltered housing, or 'extra care housing', which has augmented care services to support individuals who may experience sudden or gradual health and/or mental health problems. Some older people may have been excluded from housing improvements and remain in poor facilities in the private sector or face homelessness. As nurses recognise, the home of an older person is inextricably linked to personal dignity, the memories that matter and independence. For these reasons it is an important factor to consider in assessment and delivery of treatment, care and support.

Many older people live in housing that is unsuitable for a variety of reasons, and this has an impact on their quality of life and their ability to cope with disability. Equality and safeguarding policies place responsibility on local authorities to accommodate older homeless people over 55 years as well as those with young families, pregnant women and disabilities. Generally local-level housing advice agencies, often in the voluntary sector, are helpful for advice. In practice social workers tend to liaise with housing departments, which are often part of the local authority, to resolve housing issues or concerns. For more information, visit https://www.gov.uk and search for guidance on housing for older people and individuals with disabilities.

Three new developments that illustrate the importance of linking housing and health care are briefly described below to indicate the potential for thinking about accommodation and its links to health.

The Smart Home

A smart home provides individuals, carers and professionals with technology to assist people with disabilities. In the situation of a person with dementia, for example, technology can switch off gas cookers, monitor the level of bath water to avoid flooding and provide prompts to check door chains are on or medication is due. Even simple technologies such as large clocks and calendars can be very beneficial. Such adaptations can be expensive, but funding may be available through the use of direct payments, carers' support monies or sums for aids to independent living that are joint-funded between health and social services partnerships. See Chapter 35 for more discussion on technology that supports independence for older people.

The Safe Home

Many older people report feeling crime and disorder in their communities make their lives difficult and sometimes miserable. Community safety initiatives, often linked to regeneration programmes, are locally led partnerships that aim to provide visible demonstrations it is safe to go outside the house, and harassment of older people, or anyone else, is not tolerated. Research has found that particularly in inner-city areas, many older people do not feel safe and think the community is dangerous and out of control. Evidence of environmental neglect, such as rubbish and graffiti, is being targeted by joint initiatives that sometimes include seeking the views of older people.

The Home With Care

The view there is nothing between living independently and life in residential care has been challenged by the development of 'extra care' or 'very sheltered' housing. Although this has been promulgated for some time, new developments have only recently occurred that make use of complex funding systems that involve grant aid to housing associations in the voluntary sector, funds from individuals' benefits and rents, and assistance from local authorities. In such accommodation, tenants may have the ability to draw on support as their needs change, for example, receiving extra hours of home care on returning from hospital or taking their meals in a restaurant if they are no longer able to cook or eat without support. Other possible changes may emerge with greater development of different types of housing with care, such as very sheltered housing as alternatives to care homes. Here, older people have the status of tenants, not residents, and although many are likely to have disabilities, they continue to have control over important aspects of their daily life, such as having the key to their door. In addition they potentially have greater involvement in determining who works in their homes rather than whether they are considered suitable for entry into a care home.

Staying Put' at Home

Older people mostly live in their own homes; as mentioned, in many areas of the United Kingdom, owner occupancy is the majority form of housing tenure. This has advantages; older people often wish to grow older at home, in familiar neighbourhoods, in familiar surroundings. Figures 7.2 and 7.3 show older people successfully living independently in their own homes and enjoying meaningful and quality existence. For many the advantage of owner occupancy is it provides capital that can be passed to younger generations. The disadvantages are also evident, especially if disability occurs. Homes may be difficult or expensive to adapt, and maintenance and repairs may be hard to afford when income is low and capital diminishes. In response, private-sector schemes offer people the ability to raise money on the basis of the capital of their home, while other agencies at the local level can assist older people to take advantage

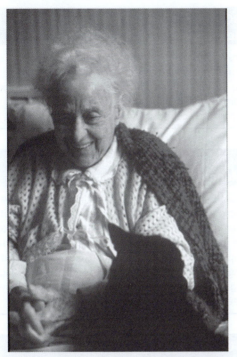

Fig. 7.2 Living at home. (Courtesy Fiona Ross.)

of loans and grants to repair their homes or make adaptations—for example, housing improvement agencies or staying-put schemes. While in the past such schemes concentrated on alterations and facilities to help people with physical disabilities, some schemes now consider ways they can provide support to people with long-term conditions such as dementia. As with most voluntary-sector activity, there is much local variation, and nurses may find information on specific local resources is best obtained from groups such as the local branch of Age UK. The principles of health and social care are summarised in Boxes 7.1, 7.2 and 7.3 identify common issues encountered and debated in social care.

Self-Management

Self-management is defined as the systematic process of learning and practising skills that enable individuals to manage their health condition on a day-to-day basis and make informed decisions. This is important, as research shows older people welcome help to manage their conditions. For example, Abdi et al. (2019) undertook a scoping review to understand the care and support needs of older people with long-term conditions living at home in the United Kingdom. The evidence shows older adults require first care and support in social activities and relationships, second support for

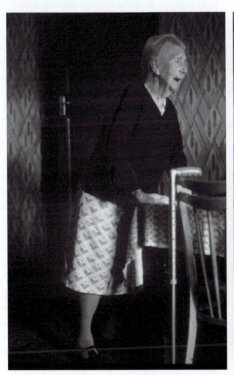
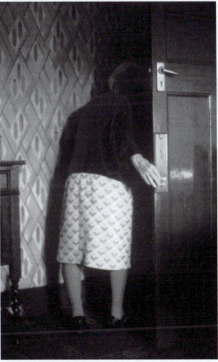

Fig. 7.3 Living at home. (Courtesy Fiona Ross.)

BOX 7.1   Principles of Health and Social Care

- Continuity of care: Valued highly by patients and service users and normally describes an ongoing relationship with a clinician or the smooth transition between different parts of the health and social care system.
- Integrated care: Health and social care inputs are organised and delivered in the same care package consistently over time and working toward jointly agreed objectives and outcomes.
- Coordinated care: Services are linked together to ensure continuity within a pathway of care with jointly agreed objectives and outcomes and a single, named care coordinator.
- Parallel care: Where two or more services provide care to the same users or client groups but pursue their own objectives and outcomes. It can be assumed the user does not require integrated or coordinated care and not that there has been a failure to set up integrated or coordinated care so that parallel care is the accidental and inappropriate result.
- Service user involvement: Taking patients' strengths, needs and preferences into account in planning, decision making and evaluating the outcomes of care.
- Digital solutions to support self-management: Becoming more common and discussed later in this chapter.

BOX 7.2   Summary of Issues Often Encountered in Social Care

- Help is prioritised for those in most need.
- Intention is to enable people to stay at home.
- Support needs of carers are integral to assessment.
- Resources are limited and hard decisions have to be made.
- Many people manage well without high levels of services.

However, other views suggest targeting leads to the following:

- A focus on crisis help
- Limited ability to prevent problems getting worse
- Pressure on families
- Too great an emphasis on assessment and the threshold for services rather than delivery
- The removal of professional discretion
- A focus on risk that is perceived as negative and controlling

BOX 7.3   Further Information on Benefits and Resources

Care Information Scotland: https://www.careinfoscotland.scot
Age UK information and advice: https://www.ageuk.org.uk/information-advice
Citizens Advice: https://www.citizensadvice.org.uk

BOX 7.4   Good Practice in Self-Management of Chronic Arthritis Pain

ESCAPE-pain is a group rehabilitation programme for people with chronic joint pain that integrates educational self-management and coping strategies with an exercise regimen individualised for each participant. It helps people understand their condition, teaches them simple things to help themselves and takes them through a progressive exercise programme so they learn how to better cope with pain (Hurley et al., 2021).

BOX 7.5   Good Practice in Self Management of People With a Stroke

Bridges is a social enterprise that exists to make a difference to the lives of people with acute and long-term conditions by working with teams from health, social care and the third sector to define and deliver best practices in self-management support. The Bridges model has its origins in stroke recovery, is evidence-based and tailors self-management and working alongside patients using co-production methods (Jones et al., 2016).

psychological health, and third activities related to mobility, self-care and domestic life. The review also highlighted many old people demonstrate a desire to manage themselves and maintain independence but are hampered by the lack of infrastructure, including professional advice on self-care, information on services, and communication and coordination. The concept of self-management is familiar to nurses as they are trained to explore with patients how they can best help themselves through education and health promotion. This is now supported in government policy in the NHS's *Long Term Plan* (2019), which is committed to the idea of personalisation and sees supported self-management as the way health and care services encourage, support and empower people to manage their ongoing physical and mental health conditions themselves, for example through health coaches. Examples of good practice in self-management are described in Boxes 7.4 and 7.5.

Social prescribing is a key component of personalisation. It was introduced in 2019 in the NHS's (2019) *Long Term Plan*. It is targeted at people with one or more long-term conditions who may be lonely and isolated or have complex social and mental health conditions. The ideas were influenced by a progressive primary care model and general practice in Bromley by Bow that believed in holistic care and that often problems presented in the GP surgery may be ameliorated by non-pharmacological activities such as gardening, befriending and physical activity. It works by general practitioner or practice nurse referral to a link worker, typically based in general practice or the primary care network, who prescribes a social intervention—for example, connection to a community group, respite care, neighbourhood support or bereavement help.

DIFFERENCE AND DIVERSITY

Policies for an ageing population need to reflect the increasing diversity of older people, including race, religion and gender identity. This section outlines some of the emergent issues related to divergence of identity, experiences, preferences, values, beliefs and ethnicity, which are important for nurses to understand. Diversity exists between older people of different gender identities, age cohorts, socioeconomic classes and places or geographies. These different identities are not mutually exclusive and often intersect and connect in many complex ways. Identity politics refers to the thinking and political activities that focus on the experiences of injustice shared by different and often excluded social groups. It is dangerous to generalise, but for some people ageing means horizons shrink as opportunities and physical fitness diminish. Some individuals may have a sense of alienation from contemporary and youth culture, resulting in deepening of conservative views and perceptions of widening of the generation gap.

Race, ethnicity and culture became centre stage in the United Kingdom following Black Lives Matter and the George Floyd murder in 2019. Terminology in this space is evolving and somewhat confusing as terms used are often emotionally loaded and may be contested. Aspinall (2002) suggests certain descriptors are so imprecise as to lose meaning or utility, such as pan-ethnic terms like 'Asian' or 'mixed-race', and that binary terms such as Black or White make White minorities, such as older people from Irish or Polish backgrounds, invisible.

Ethnic minority populations do not form a homogenous group, and their experience of ageing may differ in several ways. However, in the past the narrative in health and social care services has rested on assumptions of sameness that arguably lead to disadvantage and often racism. First, the assumption is often made practitioners lack confidence and experience working with people from minority ethnic groups, because only small numbers of older people from minority ethnic groups are represented in some communities. The second assumption, which is now questioned, is minority groups 'look after their own'. Although this may be true for some individuals who live with extended families, it cannot be taken for granted. The 2011 Census showed ethnic minority communities are concentrated in London and other large metropolitan areas, where Black Caribbean elders, for example the Windrush generation who arrived in the 1950s and 1960s, are becoming old. It is right their voices should be more prominent.

There is a belated acceptance that large health inequalities are experienced in Black, Asian and minority ethnic communities. In the largest ever study of health inequalities of Black, Asian and minority ethnic people in England, it was shown the health impact of belonging to some ethnic minority groups is the equivalent of being 20 years older than your actual age (Watkinson et al., 2021). The shocking outcomes from COVID-19 amplify this racial disadvantage; you are four times more likely to die of COVID-19 if you are from an ethnic minority group, exposing a bigger crisis of inequality that as a society and as health professionals we have not been paying attention to.

Strategic or policy responses to older people's experiences of racism are limited, resources are scarce and targets are unclear. Local initiatives often focus on a narrow range of activities, such as advocacy, translation and interpreting services. It is the duty of public bodies to promote equality and eliminate racial discrimination. Strategies for older people need to reflect this legal imperative but also need to be aware of local contexts and overall global influences. This can extend to the support given to relatives abroad and the wishes of many older people to spend time overseas with families as well as in their homes in the United Kingdom.

Cultural competence may be a way for nurses to acquire skills and confidence in working with older people and to fully understand that older people from ethnic minority groups are not homogenous, and difference should be accepted and respected. As a nurse, reflection on your own attitudes to ageing, difference and inequalities is important in shaping relationships and positive communication with older people. The policy response to older people from Black and minority ethnic groups must increasingly tackle disadvantage and recognise there are more differences within ethnic groups (intra) than between them (inter). The poverty of older people from Bangladeshi backgrounds, for example, may be far greater than that of other migrant groups even in similar areas, and specific public health measures may be needed to assist this group along with greater attention by nurses to ensure welfare benefits are maximised in such communities.

WORK IN LATER LIFE

Much emphasis in health and social care is on the minority of older people who are major users of services, so it is sometimes easy to forget many older people make significant contributions to society and the economy through running charities, volunteering, caring, grandparenting, continuing paid roles and contributing in local or national politics as elected members of local councils. There are some magnificent role models worldwide of older people doing extraordinary things, carrying massive roles and responsibilities, such as President Joe Biden of the United States, age 79 at the time of writing; Nancy Pelosi, a formidable figure in United States politics as the speaker of the House of Representatives, age 81; David Attenborough, an internationally renowned campaigner for the natural world who is vigorous and influential in his mid-90s; and Queen Elizabeth the Second who recently died aged 96, but was active and fulfilling her duties until the end.

There is no longer a retirement age in the United Kingdom, and age is a protected characteristic in equality legislation, so employers are not able to discriminate on account of a person's age, as age plays no part in influencing capability to do a job. However, as Age UK (2019) notes, older people face barriers that include ageism, poor transport links and digital exclusion, which can contribute to feelings of social isolation.

Some interesting facts from Age UK (2019) about the older workforce are as follows:

- The United Kingdom has an ageing workforce. Over a million people are working past the age of 64 and contributing to the economy.
- It needs to be recognised older people are not just engaged in formal paid work; over 3 million people over 50 care for a spouse, parent or other, and 3 million combine caring with paid work.
- A quarter of families rely on grandparents for child care; in this way older people make significant contributions to the economy.

Barriers do not just exist in getting work but are experienced by older people who access training and are considered 'past it' when other opportunities arise. Research into the experiences of nurses over 50 (Watson et al., 2003) found, even in a profession where it is widely acknowledged there are significant shortages of staff, ageist attitudes exist, and more attention is given to recruiting younger people than to retaining older nurses or providing ways for older nurses to return to their profession.

Phased or flexible retirement is being slowly introduced, along with changes in employment practices to allow older people with health or disability-related needs to stay in work or retrain. However, Age UK (2020) recommends more should be done and flexible working promoted, which would be good for the wider workforce and not just for older people. Nurses who work in health promotion and who work with people with long-term conditions may play a greater part in supporting older people to maintain their roles in employment; such roles may require close collaboration with professionals allied to medicine who have experience in occupational settings.

However, work in later life is unlikely to resolve the growing divides between older people who have adequate or substantial resources and those who are poor, have worked in low-paid jobs or have been unemployed or made redundant. People with long-term health problems or who have provided care for family members are more likely to enter retirement on low incomes and often experience old age as a time of poverty, disadvantage and exclusion from social activities and community life.

OLDER PEOPLE IN THE POLICY-MAKING PROCESS

Recent British elections have seen increasing polarisation along age lines, with older voters more likely to vote for political parties on the right (British Election Study, 2019) and more likely to vote to leave the European Union. Thus the 'grey vote' is significant. Older people are not only involved as voters but also often play an important part in local democracy (Fig. 7.4). In the health service, where democratic structures are not developed, older people may be appointed to membership of trust boards, and some have used their own and their family's experiences as ways of thinking about and influencing older people's provision.

The voices of older people are also important in the policy-making process. Over the past 20 years there has been considerable progress toward greater engagement and involvement of older people in health services research and related activities such as co-production and participating as equal partners in the redesign of health services with a view to improving care (Morrow et al., 2012; Ross et al., 2014).

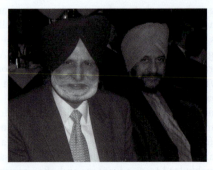

Fig. 7.4 Local democracy and participation of Sikh elders as council members. (Courtesy Fiona Ross.)

The notion of increasing citizen participation is a challenge to health and social care services, but there are examples of good practice. Participation may encompass first consultation with older people and senior citizens' or older people's community groups; second the experiences of patients and former patients, for example through annual national surveys of patient experiences; and finally concerns raised with patient advice and liaison services and independent complaints advocacy services. Some older people have taken on roles as advisors or as critical friends in research and development to bring their perspectives and ideas to the area of health care in co-creation or co-production initiatives. The Expert Patient Programme was constructed to encourage people to help themselves by breaking the cycle of symptoms, trying pain management techniques and improving their health generally—this too may have potential for people to tell service commissioners and providers how they can provide better support.

As part of the inspection process of health and social care services, the CQC has made some moves to include older people as lay observers. Other means of having influence and control include membership in governing bodies of NHS Trusts in England and innovative ways of seeking the views of individual older people. For example, a recent evidence review showed true involvement of people with multiple long-term conditions requires person-centred approaches with face-to-face interactions that offer authentic opportunities and space to discuss care options and make shared decisions (Bunn et al., 2018). This work suggests there is more room for older people, even with significant disabilities, to set out their feelings and for them to be considered and reflected on. There is, however, a notable gap in how services can better engage with Black and minority ethnic communities. A recent systematic review of available evidence suggests people from Black, Asian and minority ethnic groups are underrepresented in public engagement initiatives and health services research (Dawson et al., 2018). This came to the fore during the pandemic, when people from Black, Asian and ethnic minority communities experienced a disproportionately higher risk for COVID-19 and were slow to come forward for vaccination.

It is unusual to end a chapter on older people and policy with observations that older people are major contributors to society rather than problems, and their citizenship should be a key theme in policy debates rather than their status as patients or service users. In exercising more control over their own health and social care, quality of life and participation, older people need to challenge practitioners, managers and politicians with their views, perspectives and demands.

NURSING WORKFORCE

As noted, the nursing workforce is ageing. It is estimated one in six (17%) nurses around the world are 55 or older and expected to retire within the next 10 years, as set out in the World Health Organization's *State of the World's Nursing* report (World Health Organisation, 2020). The replacement of retiring nurses with newly qualified ones is not expected to keep up or match those leaving. Therefore, workforce shortages are made worse by nurses leaving with fatigue and the hopelessness reported anecdotally by some nurses on the frontline of the COVID-19 pandemic. Buchan et al. (2020) argue for a 10-point plan to support the retention of older nurses, which includes among other things flexible job planning, a pay-and-benefits system that rewards experience and advanced skills and succession planning. However, some earlier work that explored the views of older nurses suggested achieving flexibility in a rigid system is not easy and recommended pivots on the willingness and readiness of nurse managers to be creative with bespoke part-time roles and rotas that support improved work–life balance (Harris et al., 2010).

These macro challenges in the nursing workforce are amplified when you consider the field of care for older people. Historically, care of older people—or geriatrics, as it used to be called—was regarded a Cinderella service and not an area for the ambitious doctor or nurse. High-status areas are traditionally acute specialities and intensive care, while the community and care of older people are seen as low-status areas. Over the past 30 years in particular, there have been vigorous attempts to change attitudes, led by academic departments of nursing and expansion of nurse-led research on practice improvements and person-centred care in the United States, Europe and United Kingdom. The expansion of specialist and advanced leadership roles, such as nurse consultants, also increases the standing and authority of nursing and contributes to better patient outcomes in hospital and community settings—for example, for patients with frailty (see Chapter 6). There is encouraging growth in post-graduate and applied programmes that focus on innovations and improving care for older people.

CONCLUSION AND LEARNING POINTS

Writing about policy in nursing and health care is challenging, as the macro landscape moves rapidly. This chapter retains its currency and relevance by focusing on principles and explaining trends that will inform the future. It is important for nurses to understand the policy context of their work so they can better influence decisions and be future leaders of change to improve the culture and practice of nursing older people.

KEY LEARNING POINTS

- Health and social care is organised differently across the four countries of the United Kingdom.
- Northern Ireland, Wales and Scotland have adopted integrated health and social care, and England is moving in the same direction from 2021.
- In England social care is the responsibility of local government and is means tested, while health care is free at the point of use. There is political debate about the balance of responsibility between the state and the individual, including what is affordable and to whom.
- Care in the community and at home form a long-standing policy goal and the place most people want to die, given the choice. However, the funding of community care in England is contested, and there has been a lack of investment in community nursing and social care services.
- Social care assessment targets individuals with the highest needs and tends to give lower priority to those with fewer assessed needs, thus compromising prevention.
- Self-management and personalisation are central strategies in current health policy, encouraging greater involvement and empowerment.
- The health needs of older people from Black and minority ethnic groups have been overlooked, and big inequalities exist. Services are designed for the White majority, so it is not surprising that people from Black, Asian and minority ethnic communities feel invisible and not a priority.
- Many older people contribute to society and the economy after formal retirement. Nurses must avoid making generalisations about the needs of older people or seeing them as a homogenous group.
- Respecting and valuing difference and individual needs must be central to the nursing care of older people.

REFERENCES

Abdi, S., Spann, A., Borilovic, J., de Witte, L., & Hawley, M. (2019). Understanding the care and support needs of older people: a scoping review and categorisation using the WHO international classification of functioning, disability and health framework (ICF). *BMC Geriatrics, 19*, 195.

Age UK. (2019). *Employment: Policy position paper*. https://www.ageuk.org.uk/our-impact/policy-research/policy-positions

Age UK. (2020). *A means to many ends: Older workers' experiences of flexible working*. https://www.ageuk.org.uk/our-impact/policy-research/policy-positions

Aspinall, P. J. (2002). Collective terminology to describe the minority ethnic population. *Sociology, 36*, 803–816.

Baxter, S., Johnson, M., Chambers, D., Sutton, A., Goyder, E., & Booth, A. (2018). The effects of integrated care: A systematic review of UK and international evidence. *BMC Health Services Research, 18*, 350.

British Election Study. (2019). *Age and voting behaviour at the 2019 General Election*. https://www.britishelectionstudy.com/bes-findings/age-and-voting-behaviour-at-the-2019-general-election/#.YtXVvcHMLrA

British Geriatrics Society. (2021). *Ambitions for change: Improving healthcare in care homes*. https://www.bgs.org.uk/resources/ambitions-for-change-improving-healthcare-in-care-homes

Buchan, J., Catton, H., & Shaffer, F. A. (2020). *Ageing well? Policies to support older nurses at work*: International Council of Nurses. https://www.icn.ch/sites/default/files/inline-files/Ageing%20ICNM%20Report%20December%209%202020.pdf.

Bunn, F., Goodman, C., Russell, B., Wilson, P., Manthorpe, J., Rait, G., Hodkinson, I., & Durand, M. (2018). Supporting shared decision making for older people with multiple health and social care needs: a realist synthesis. *BMC Geriatrics*(165), 18. https://doi.org/10.1186/s12877-018-0853-9.

Davey, V. (2021). Influences of service characteristics and older people's attributes and outcomes from direct payments. *BMC Geriatrics, 21*, 1.

Dawson, S., Campbell, S., & Cheraghi-Sohi, S. (2018). Black and minority group involvement in health and social care research: a systematic review. *Health Expectations, 21*(1), 3–22.

Department of Health. (2014). *The Care Act and whole family approaches*. https://www.local.gov.uk/sites/default/files/documents/care-act-and-whole-family-6e1.pdf

Department of Health. (2020) The NHS Choice Framework: what choices are available to me in the NHS?

Department of Health and Social Care. (2021). *Integration and innovation: Working together to improve health and social care for all*. https://www.gov.uk/government/publications/working-together-to-improve-health-and-social-care-for-all/integration-and-innovation-working-together-to-improve-health-and-social-care-for-all-html-version

Ham, C. (2013). Successful integrated care. A Canterbury tale: An invaluable education. *Health Service Journal, 123*(6367), 18–19.

Harris, R., Bennett, J., Davey, B., & Ross, F. (2010). Flexible working and the contribution of nurses in mid-life to the workforce: a qualitative study. *International Journal of Nursing Studies, 47*(4), 418–426.

Hurley, M., Sheldon, H., Connolly, M., Carter, A., & Hallett, R. (2021). Providing easier access to community-based healthcare for people with joint pain: Experiences of delivering ESCAPE-pain in community venues by exercise professionals. *Musculoskeletal Care, 20*(2), 408–415.

Jones, F., Gage, H., Drummond, A., Bhalla, A., Grant, R., Lennon, S., McKevitt, C., Riazi, A., & Liston, M. (2016). Feasibility study of an integrated stroke self-management programme: A cluster randomised controlled trial. *BMJ Open, 6*(1), Article e:008900.

King's Fund. (2018). Delayed transfers of care: A quick guide. https://www.kingsfund.org.uk/publications/delayed-transfers-care-quick-guide

King's Fund. (2021). Developing place-based partnerships: The foundation of effective integrated care systems. https://www.kingsfund.org.uk/publications/place-based-partnerships-integrated-care-systems

Kwartang, K., Patel, P., Raab, D., Skidmore, C., & Truss, E. (2012). *Britannia unchained: Global lessons for growth and prosperity.* Palgrave Macmillan.

Morrow, E., Boaz, A., Brearley, S., & Ross, F. (2012). *Handbook of service user involvement in nursing and healthcare research.* Wiley Blackwell.

National Health Service (NHS). (2014). *The five year forward view.* https://www.england.nhs.uk/wp-content/uploads/2014/10/5yfv-web.pdf

NHS. (2019). *The NHS long term plan.* https://www.longtermplan.nhs.uk

NHS. (2020). *Integrating care: Next steps to building strong and effective integrated care systems across England.* https://www.england.nhs.uk/publication/integrating-care-next-steps-to-building-strong-and-effective-integrated-care-systems-across-england/

National Institute of Clinical Effectiveness. (2015). *Older people with social care needs and multiple long term conditions.* https://www.nice.org.uk/guidance/ng22.

Public Health England (PHE). (2020). *Older people's hospital admissions in the last year of life.* https://www.gov.uk/government/publications/older-peoples-hospital-admissions-in-the-last-year-of-life/older-peoples-hospital-admissions-in-the-last-year-of-life

Ross, F., Smith, P., Byng, R., Christian, S., Allan, H., Price, L., & Brearley, S. (2014). Learning from people with long term conditions: New insights for governance in primary healthcare. *Health and Social Care in the Community, 22*(4), 405–416.

Scottish Executive. (2002). *Adding life to years: Report of the expert group on healthcare of older people.* Edinburgh.

Sims, S., Fletcher, S., Brearley, S., Ross, F., Manthorpe, J., & Harris, R. (2021). What does success look like for leaders of Integrated Health and Social Care Systems? A Realist Review. *International Journal of Integrated Care, 21*(4), 26.

Timmins, N., & Ham, C. (2013). *The quest for integrated health and social care: A case study in Canterbury: New Zealand.* Kings Fund.

Wanless, D. (2002). *Securing our future health: Taking a long-term view.* HM Treasury.

Watkinson, R., Sutton, M., & Turner, A. J. (2021). Ethnic inequalities in health-related quality of life among older adults in England: Secondary analysis of a national cross-sectional survey. *Lancet Public Health, 6*(3), e145–e154.

Watson, R., Manthorpe, J., & Andrews, J. (2003). *Nurses over 50: Options, decisions and outcomes.* Policy Press.

World Health Organization. (2020). *State of the world's nursing 2020.* https://www.who.int/publications/i/item/9789240003279

8

Public Health: Healthy Ageing and Well-Being

Sarah Ann Cowley, Vasiliki Tzouvara, Tiago Manuel Horta Reis da Silva

CHAPTER OUTLINE

INTRODUCTION

In developed countries, the majority of infants are born healthy and well, with the prospect of reaching a ripe old age. Those prospects are not equally divided, however. There are wide inequalities in both how long people can be expected to live—called life expectancy—and how healthy and well they might expect to be as they age. These inequalities are not inevitable, but they follow what (Marmot et al., 2010) call a 'social gradient'. They explain that inequalities are not about poor health for poor people and good health for everyone else. Instead, everyone below the wealthiest group has worse health than those above them. When mortality rates and most indicators of ill health are plotted on a graph according to socioeconomic group or the extent of deprivation in an area, there is a stepwise difference between each centile, showing a clear gradient on a range of social factors. These also tend to accumulate over the life course, for better or worse, so many of the acts or omissions that contribute to a healthy old age begin much earlier (Kuruvilla et al., 2018). While this has implications for the promotion of healthy ageing, there is never a time when it is too late to start health promoting preventive actions, explained later in this chapter.

This chapter is divided into three broad sections. We begin by explaining the nature of public health, which provides a context for preventive and promoting activities, and some of the wider determinants that contribute to health and well-being. This first section also explains how *social*

determinants can lead to healthy or unhealthy ageing and also to health inequalities across the life course. There is a vast literature about a multitude of significant factors that contribute to inequalities in the older population, but this chapter aims only to raise awareness of how they may connect to the concepts of healthy ageing. The middle section of the chapter links the idea of healthy ageing across the life course to different views of health and well-being. The many definitions and concepts embedded within these different views are explored, with specific reference to the older population. In the final section, two overarching models are provided that show how the many different and interconnected concepts come together. They combine to offer a unified approach to healthy ageing and well-being or, using the example of COVID-19, to illustrate how health challenges reinforce inequalities established over a lifetime. The models each provide nurses with some practical ideas for working with older people to improve their health and well-being.

PUBLIC HEALTH

Public health can be defined as the 'science and art of promoting health, preventing disease and prolonging life through the organised efforts of society' (Acheson, 1998). Public health is a social and political concept aimed at improving health, prolonging life and improving the quality of life among whole populations through health promotion, disease prevention and other forms of health intervention. The World Health Organization (WHO, 1998) pointed to the distinction between public health and a new public health to emphasise significantly different approaches to the description. As with the old and new divisions in many other aspects described in this chapter, there is an expanded understanding in the more modern approach, with an analysis of the determinants of health in the methods of solving public health problems.

Ashton and Seymour (1998) described four phases of public health, starting with a focus on environmental change early in the 19th century, then moving to personal preventive measures by the end of that century. As the 20th century progressed, therapeutic interventions seemed to hold much promise, before their limitations were realised and the new public health emerged with a focus on more holistic, humanistic philosophy and a broad, socially based belief in the value of health. Eventually, the need for all four approaches became clear, as knowledge about the relevance of social factors and health inequalities increased. In the current century, the importance of health inequalities and implications of disadvantage were highlighted in a review by Marmot et al. (2010). That review, and the authors' more recent update (Marmot et al., 2020a), showed the whole life course has a cumulative effect on health in old age, much of which is mediated by social conditions and living experiences, including lifestyle.

A great deal of public health effort is expended in seeking a comprehensive understanding of these impacts, including the ways in which lifestyles and living conditions determine health status. Public health is concerned with the development of plans, policies, programmes, services and actions for every sector in order to advocate health equity in all stages of life (Marks et al., 2020). Strategic global action plans prioritise interventions that promote healthy ageing and create age-friendly environments, which demonstrate a shift toward public health interventions in relation to older people, due to the increased life span throughout the 20th century (WHO, 2018). At the start of this century, the WHO warned that, while population ageing is one of humanity's greatest triumphs, it is also one of our greatest challenges. As we entered the 21st century, WHO said, 'Global ageing will put increased economic and social demands on all countries' (2002, p. 6). New concerns have been expressed, because former gradual, but persistent, improvements have not been maintained in the past decade. Increases in life expectancy have begun to falter in the United Kingdom, and there are now widening health inequalities in the anticipated life span of different socioeconomic groups (Marmot et al., 2020a).

HEALTHY AGEING

The WHO designated 2021–2030 the Decade of Healthy Ageing—explained further below—largely to focus attention on the growing older population across the world (WHO, 2020a). In 2020 there were more than 1 billion people over 60 years old, mainly living in low- and middle-income countries where there may be limited access to organised or freely available health care. This lends some urgency to the need for prevention, especially as the number is expected to rise to 2 billion worldwide by 2050. In the United Kingdom and much of the developed world, the same preventive priorities arise for different reasons. Increased life expectancy is a huge achievement and human benefit, but the costs of health care for an ageing population are vast and increasing, with a relatively smaller number of working-age people to pay for it.

Health in older age, as throughout life, is affected by a wide range of factors known as the determinants of health. Health services are one aspect of this, but the way society is organised has a greater impact, with social and economic factors being particularly influential. The range of factors were visualised by Dahlgren and Whitehead (1991) in their classic rainbow diagram, designed to encapsulate the multiple interconnected factors in a single picture (see Fig. 8.1). It illustrates the way individual lifestyle is influenced strongly by immediate social and community networks, but these in turn are influenced by wider issues that stem from general, cultural and environmental conditions.

Conditions, choices and chances occur, recur and recede throughout life and have a cumulative effect on health throughout the life course. Ideally, the life course is one that enables healthy ageing and an active older age, but this is far from the case for everyone. It has been estimated around 70% of preventable deaths from noncommunicable diseases in adults have been linked to risks encountered, and behaviours that started, during adolescence (Kuruvilla et al., 2018).

Healthy ageing is defined as the process of developing and maintaining functional ability that enables well-being in older age. Functional ability is about having the capabilities that enable all people to be and do what they have reason to value (WHO, 2020a). In an earlier policy framework, the WHO (2002) identified the positive determinants of active ageing (see Box 8.1).

The WHO (2002) framework identifies culture and gender as cross-cutting determinants, as they surround all individuals and populations, shaping the way we age. Because of this, it is said they influence all the other factors that influence active ageing. In reality, all the determinants apply at all ages and interact to such an extent that it

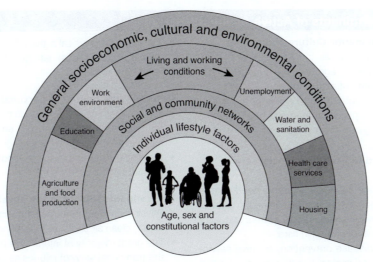

Fig. 8.1 Determinants of health (Dahlgren & Whitehead, 1991).

is seldom possible to identify any particular factor which predicts how well an individual or population will age. The idea that any one factor can determine an outcome is a little misleading, as they all intertwine and interconnect at different points across the life course. There is rarely a single harmful issue or event that cannot be improved by making a different life choice, seizing an opportunity or receiving appropriate health care. Likewise, positive health can be readily undermined by taking unwise risks or experiencing an adverse life-changing event from external forces. Having said that, it is clear life chances are unequally distributed throughout society, and individual choices are highly influenced and constrained by a range of factors that lie beyond individual control (see Thinking Point 1).

Someone who was born in the Depression of the prewar years, known as the Hungry Thirties, and grew up in a society where formal schooling ended at the age of 14 (which was raised to 15 years old in 1947) would have had far less opportunity to further their education than today's young people. This was particularly true for girls, who were not expected to have careers, with gender affecting future plans and choices. Career choices were more limited across the board, with young men often expected to follow in their father's footsteps, whether to be a miner or a physician. In turn, choice of occupation dictates income and the potential to save for a pension in later years. Family culture, faith and community networks all affect such decisions, sometimes encouraging and sometimes limiting the choices people make. Some choices may seem like small, immediate decisions—perhaps what to eat for tea, whether to go

to a particular social event—but taken over the life course, they accumulate to affect health and ageing. Think about diet, smoking, friendships, marriage and civil status, for example.

All these are affected by what Worthman (1999) identified as wider determinants, sometimes called 'root causes' or even 'causes of the causes' (Sadana et al., 2016). These are social conditions such as economic inequality, urbanisation, mobility, cultural values, attitudes and policies related to discrimination and intolerance on the basis of race, gender and other differences. Social conditions have an impact on the choices made by individuals but are outside their control. Major sociopolitical shifts, such as recession, war and governmental collapse, have been experienced by older adults in the population and had an impact on the extent to which they were able to control decisions that affected their life course. Other significant factors identified by Worthman (1999) include access to transportation, water and sanitation, housing and other dimensions of urban planning and the built environment. Chapter 7 explores benefits.

Wider environmental issues and links between so-called behavioural determinants, physical environments and personal factors (see Box 8.1) are also heavily influenced by culture, income and opportunities, so they cannot be regarded as truly driven by individual choice alone. Instead, choices are heavily mediated by the extent to which society offers opportunities; in turn, these are affected by policies that might enable life chances that can be seized by individuals—or not. Health inequalities

---

BOX 8.1   Determinants of Active Ageing (WHO, 2002)

Cross-cutting determinants: Culture and gender

- Culture, which surrounds all individuals and populations, shapes the way we age because it influences all the other determinants of active ageing.
- Gender is a lens through which to consider the appropriateness of various policy options and how they will affect the well-being of men and women.

Determinants related to health and social service systems

- To promote active ageing, health systems need to take a life-course perspective that focuses on health promotion, disease prevention and equitable access to quality primary health care and long-term care.
- Health promotion, disease prevention, curative services, long-term care and mental health services all need considering.

Behavioural determinants

- The adoption of healthy lifestyles and actively participating in your own care are important at all stages of the life course. One of the myths of ageing is that it is too late to adopt a healthy lifestyle in the later years.

- Tobacco use, physical activity, healthy eating, oral health, alcohol, medications, iatrogenesis and adherence all need considering.

Determinants related to personal factors

- While genes may be involved in the causation of disease, for many diseases the cause is environmental and external to a greater degree than it is genetic and internal.
- Biological, genetic and psychological factors need considering.

Determinants related to the physical environment

- Physical environments, safe housing, avoiding falls, clean water, clean air and safe food all need considering.
- The great majority of injuries are preventable; however, the traditional view of injuries as accidents has resulted in historical neglect of this area of public health.

Determinants related to the social and economic environment

- Social support, violence and abuse, education and literacy are all relevant.
- Income and social protection are significant economic determinants of active ageing.

Thinking Point 1: Life Stories

Bob and Joe were born in 1940, the year after the Second World War started. Both had fathers who were in the armed forces and away from the family home for most of their preschool years. Their mothers had to contend with strict rationing, which affected Bob's and Joe's early diet and food experience. Both remember it, as it went on well into the 1950s. Both boys began their formal education at their local infants' school just as the war ended and both their fathers came home from the war. That is where their similarities ended.

Bob's mum lived in a small tenement with her parents in Glasgow while her husband was conscripted and sent off to fight on the front line. He was injured and 'suffered from his nerves' for the rest of his life, so his work was intermittent and poorly paid. The family had moved into a new council home by the time Bob started at the local secondary modern school, which he left when he was 15 years old.

Joe's mum moved to a small house in the Mendips just before Joe was born, to be 'safe' away from the big cities, although she didn't know anyone there. Joe's dad had been an engineer until he joined the RAF at the start of the war. He

spent the war on secret aircraft design and was rarely able to get home or say where he had been. The family moved to a larger home in Bristol, where Joe went to the grammar school before going to university when he was 18 years old.

- What sort of work do you think Bob and Joe did after leaving education? And later in their lives?
- What if the stories had been about Mary and Jean—girls instead of boys? How would they differ?
- Think about the different chances each might have had and the choices they might have made.
- What risks, behaviours and habits might the boys have formed during adolescence—for example, smoking, illicit drug use, drinking alcohol and sensation-seeking activities like extreme sports, fast cars or motorbikes and fairgrounds?
- What kind of food might they each have eaten as they grew up, and how that might have affected their weight and health in the long term?
- Which choices and pressures to take one option or another might have been the same for both boys as they reached adulthood, and which different?

Make a few notes to use with the next Thinking Point.

are mainly driven by variation in the wider social determinants, with measurable disparities between and within nations and socioeconomic and ethnic groups. The extent to which individual nurses are able to influence these wider determinants of health is limited as well, although they are a legitimate and important focus for public health. Many nurses choose to work in public health, sometimes because they are driven by the sense of injustice occasioned by health inequities. *Inequity* describes avoidable—and therefore unfair or unjust—inequalities that can be remedied, although it often requires political will and community action. Health and care services are a significant mechanism for reducing health inequalities and enabling healthy ageing. The way this provision is organised and delivered is explored in more detail in Chapters 7 and 9.

To mitigate some of the health inequalities in older age, the WHO (2002; 2020a) promotes the idea of a *life course perspective* that focuses on health promotion, disease prevention and equitable access to quality health care, including primary care and long-term care. Life course approaches are examined in greater depth later in this chapter. First, we present some examples about key concepts encompassed within a framework set out by Kuruvilla et al. (2018) (see Fig. 8.2). This conceptual framework for a life course approach to health depicts functional ability and intrinsic capacity as idealised arcs across the life course. Intrinsic capacity, they say, follows a biologically determined trajectory of physical and mental capacities. In contrast, functional ability can be optimised throughout life by an environment that is supportive of good health.

This way of describing a life course approach to health includes ideas that are also incorporated in the Meikirch model (Bircher & Hahn, 2016; Bircher & Hahn, 2017; Bircher, 2020), which is explained in later sections.

PHYSIOLOGICAL AND ENVIRONMENTAL FACTORS

Determinants of active ageing related to personal factors include genetic and environmental issues (WHO, 2002); the biology of ageing is explored in Chapter 5. The three major types of requirements of life include physiological, environmental and psychosocial demands (Bircher & Kuruvilla, 2014; Bircher & Hahn 2017). In order to fulfil physiological demands that change over time and situations, people cope with various conditions. For example, most food eaten in the United Kingdom comes from industrialised agriculture and manufacturing with food supplies that require external networks, such as small stores or supermarkets, for packaging

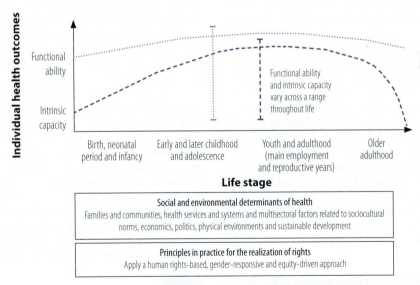

Fig. 8.2 Life course approach to health (Kuruvilla et al., 2018).

and delivery. Older people have had to contend with major changes in the way food is produced, packaged and sold since they were children, which affects their dietary choices.

Environmental factors encountered across the life course may also accumulate to affect an older person's health as they age. Some of them are readily evident, while others may have been dormant for several years—for example, exposure to carcinogens from tobacco smoke or pollutants or the impact of poor air quality. Concerns about preservation of the environment are also about establishing circumstances conducive to the promotion of both health and sustainable growth (Bircher & Kuruvilla, 2014).

Psychosocial Determinants: Cross-Cutting Factors

Psychosocial requirements contribute to personal growth and societal inclusion of people, including involvement in social, economic and political bodies. The impact of neighbourhoods on social capital and social inclusion for older people is explored in more detail in the second part of this chapter, but personal health is influenced greatly by the cross-cutting issues identified above. We highlight the examples of racial and ethnic disparities in health (also covered in Chapter 3), spirituality and marital status ageism, loneliness and social networks. These all affect individuals throughout their life course, with a cumulative impact on ageing and health in later life.

Racial and Ethnic Disparities in Health

Black and minority ethnic elders are more likely than White British elders to claim restricted well-being and low self-rated health. Evandrou et al. (2016) explain the 'health downside' tends to be most pronounced among elders of South Asian descent, with Pakistani elders showing the worst health outcomes. In terms of the life course, older people from minority groups are more likely than the younger population to have migrated to the United Kingdom than to have been born here, so their formative experiences may have been significantly different to the British-born population. Older people from ethnic minority groups show worse health effects even after data are adjusted for social and economic disadvantages. This finding illustrates the difficulty of measuring health inequality between various ethnic groups in the United Kingdom and the need to implement health strategies that take account of gaps in social and economic opportunities between different ethnic groups (Evandrou et al., 2016).

Spirituality

Spirituality is a known component of wellness in the area of health education and public health (Scriven, 2010). Interestingly, while spirituality and spiritual health are widely regarded as essential to health and well-being, they do not appear in main models of health determinants, such as the classic rainbow diagram of Dahlgren and Whitehead (1991) (Fig. 8.1) or even in Kuruvilla et al's (2018) more recent conceptual framework (Fig. 8.2). Nor is spirituality used in prominent discourses about health determinants and improvement of health, which appears to be a significant omission (Talley, 2016). Notions of meaning that may come from faith are included in some theories of well-being (e.g., Seligman, 2011) and health (e.g., Antonovsky, 1979) that are explored in the second part of this chapter. Faith groups are often a significant source of support for older people and need to be taken into account in planning either long-term care or health promotion.

Marital Status

Living conditions and marital status have been found to have a substantial impact on individual well-being and mortality. Research has reliably established an adverse mortality risk for men who remain unmarried or have undergone marital dissolution (Robards et al., 2012). Shifts in marital status and living arrangements that take place at middle and older age may have a significant impact across the life course and on long-term health and mortality. Murphy et al. (2007) established the growing number of cohabiting partners at older ages would entail wider recognition of informal, rather than legal, declarations of marital status in the future.

Even so, marriage, rather than cohabitation or civil partnership, remains far more common among the over-70-year-old population of England and Wales (Office for National Statistics, 2020a). Longitudinal living arrangements and partnership status of older people need to be considered within the context of their life course to fully account for the health and mortality outcomes of different living arrangements (Robards et al., 2012). Zueras et al. (2020) explored the growing diversity in family constellations, marital status and living arrangements in mid- and later life in two regions of Europe—the northwest and the southeast, which represented different levels of welfare state. While they confirmed being partnered is associated with lower mortality, especially for middle-aged men, their analysis also showed marital status and family living arrangements are complementary variables in what they called the 'complex associations between family and mortality' (Zueras et al., 2020, p. 635). These relationships have a particularly important bearing on health and mortality in countries where state welfare provision is limited.

Ageism

Ageism refers to the stereotypes (how we think), prejudice (how we feel) and discrimination (how we act) directed toward people on the basis of their age. It affects all aspects of older people's health and has been called 'a social determinant of health that has come of age' (Mikton et al., 2021). Ageism is implicated in shortening people's life span, potentially worsening physical and mental health, hindering recovery from disability and accelerating cognitive decline (WHO, 2021). It also exacerbates social isolation and loneliness, which are keys concern for the health and well-being of older people.

Loneliness and Social Networks

Increased life expectancy, improved life conditions and higher longevity have resulted in a growth in the older population. There is a misconception that old age equals isolation, lack of social networks and loneliness. Unquestionably, a large proportion of older adults are able to live fulfilled lives and continue to be integrated members of our communities, despite their old age. However, older adults are at high risk of experiencing emotional and health challenges that can lead to estrangement of social networks that, in turn, triggers the occurrence of isolation and loneliness. Loneliness and social isolation are two concepts close to each other yet unique and equally important. Although the concepts have largely been used interchangeably, the focus of this section is on loneliness and social networks as key determinants for healthy ageing and public health in old age (also discussed in Chapter 2).

Loneliness is a subjectively unpleasant experience that results when desired relationships do not meet, both quantitatively and qualitatively, an individual's actual relationships (Perlman & Peplau, 1982; De Jong Gierveld et al., 2015; Chana et al., 2016; Tabue Teguo et al., 2016; Bandari et al., 2019). Loneliness is different from living alone or being alone. In fact, you may feel lonely even when surrounded by others. In contrast, you may live alone but not experience feelings of loneliness (Holwerda et al., 2014; Wilson et al. 2015; Tzouvara et al., 2015). Prevalence of loneliness in old age among various European countries ranges between 3% and 34%, with studies reporting lower levels of loneliness in North European countries such as Denmark, Germany, Sweden and Britain compared to other countries in Eastern and Southern Europe (Stickley et al., 2013). Yet estimates of levels of loneliness reveal one-third of the older population experiences it to some degree toward the end of their life (Hauge & Kirkevold, 2010; Ayalon & Shiovitz-Ezra, 2011; Yan et al., 2014).

Loneliness is higher among the older old population (Dykstra, 2009), with studies revealing 50% of individuals age 80 and over are frequently lonely (Pinquart & Sörensen, 2003). Studies have also revealed the adverse effects of loneliness on the mental and physical health of older adults. For example, psychiatric conditions such as depressive and anxiety disorders can lead to social withdrawal and loneliness, and reciprocally, loneliness can also lead to clinically significant depression and anxiety (Donavan & Blazer, 2020). Loneliness relates to poor physical health in old age, such as impaired daytime functioning, reduced physical activity, lower subjective well-being, increased rates of mortality, impaired cognitive performance, dementia progression, significant likelihood of nursing home admission and multiple disease outcomes such as hypertension, heart disease and stroke (Ong et al., 2016). There is increased use of primary care and emergency departments, particularly for older women who feel lonely (Burns et al., 2020). Estimates and effects of loneliness on older people's heath highlight the significance of the condition and demonstrate it must be taken seriously.

Several factors have been found to contribute to loneliness in older age. A review of the literature revealed loss of a spouse, declining health, reduced social networks and hospitalisation are some of the factors that contribute to loneliness in older adults (Valtorta & Hanratty, 2012; Squires, 2015). In addition, studies showed loneliness in older adults results from increasing functional disabilities such as loss of mobility and reducing social contacts such as a minimised social network (Rico-Uribe et al., 2016; Niedzwiedz et al., 2016). Finally, a meta-analysis by Pinquart and Sörensen (2001) found loneliness is correlated with age and gender, with older women tending to feel lonelier. Also, older people with lower socioeconomic status tend to feel lonelier, as do older people who live in care homes.

Research revealed the composition of social networks is also a key indicator for loneliness, with the more restricted types of network indicating a greater risk of feeling lonely. Where people depend mainly on close family ties for support, with few neighbourhood and friend links, or conversely, where they have a more private support network with no relatives and few nearby friends, along with low levels of community involvement, then loneliness is far more common (Wenger, 1997; Wenger & Tucker, 2002).

Studies in old age showed older adults have reduced social networks and fewer social interactions compared to their younger counterparts (Tang & Lee, 2011; Weijs-Perrée et al., 2015). This reduction in the size of social networks is mainly due to life events, including retirement and loss of family members, friends and neighbours (Wrzus et al., 2013; Kemperman et al., 2019). It is worth highlighting here a reduced number of social interactions does not necessarily mean an individual feels lonelier or less satisfied with their social network (Bonsang & Soest, 2010; Delmelle et al., 2013). Nevertheless, older people seem to value the quality in their relationships and social interactions more than the quantity.

Loneliness and reduced social networks are aspects of the life of older people, which are key social determinants for their health. Yet older adults—particularly post-war baby boomers, who grew up with welfare provision and educational opportunities denied to earlier generations—are generally more active, healthy, wealthy and highly educated compared to previous generations (Patterson, 2002). However, today's older adults are increasingly likely to be single and childless (Office for National Statistics, 2020b). In addition to the major life cycle changes mentioned above (retirement, bereavement and so on), a higher proportion of older adults experience health declines and mobility limitations along with loneliness. Therefore, it is important to consider how to improve these social aspects of health in order to increase the quality of life in this population. Social participation and integration are important determinants of healthy ageing. Activities that increase social opportunities are likely to reduce feelings of loneliness and improve a sense of well-being and satisfaction.

Thinking Point 2: Wider Determinants and the Life Course

Think about Bob and Joe again.
- Now they've reached pension age, are either—or both—likely to have a secure, private pension or to depend solely on a state pension?
- What about housing? What might their living conditions be like? Who might they live with?
- Think about neighbourhoods and their chances of having friends and family nearby.
- Are there any choices during their lives that might have led them to be lonely in older age? To what extent were those choices really free or part of the culture in which they lived?
- Which opportunities, or unplanned stresses, in life might have affected their current situations?
- How might these issues differ for women?
- What if Bob had been born in Jamaica instead of Glasgow and travelled to Britain on HMS *Windrush* in 1948 with his parents? What difference would his ethnicity have made to his life experiences and his sense of security in old age?

Add to your earlier notes to use with the next Thinking Point.

HEALTH AND WELL-BEING

Health is a complex concept. At one level, everyone understands and uses the word quite readily without causing confusion or needing recourse to a dictionary. On closer inspection, it becomes apparent *health* is a word that rarely stands alone. It is much easier to explain what is meant by health care or a health club, or to use the adjective to describe things such as a healthy diet or healthy living, than it is to consider what is meant by *health* in an abstract sense. Even attaching descriptors, as in phrases like good health or poor health, seems to make the term easier to grasp. However, each addition alters the meaning of the word, demonstrating the huge diversity of understanding and the multitude of very different connotations and underlying assumptions associated with the term.

The idea of well-being is equally complex. In the past it seemed synonymous with health, according to the changing definitions listed in Box 8.2. In practice a focus on

---

BOX 8.2   Defining Health and Well-Being

- Health is a state of complete physical, mental and social well-being and not merely the absence of disease or infirmity (WHO, 1946).
- Health is a resource for everyday life, not the object of living. Health is a positive concept that emphasises social and personal resources as well as physical capabilities (WHO, 1986).
- A person's health is equivalent to the state of the set of conditions that fulfil or enable them to fulfil their realistic and chosen biological potentials (Seedhouse, 1986).
- Health is the ability to adapt and self-manage. It consists of three domains of physical, mental and social health and, for purposes of research and practice, a set of dynamic features and dimensions that can be measured (Huber et al., 2011).
- Health is a state of well-being emergent from conducive interactions between individuals' potentials, life's demands, and social and environmental determinants (Bircher & Hahn 2017).
- Well-being is a subjective state that can be evaluated across three domains: perceived life satisfaction, emotions experienced, and self-realisation and a sense of purpose or meaning (Kuruvilla et al., 2018).
- Healthy ageing is the process of developing and maintaining the functional ability that enables well-being in older age (WHO, 2020b).

physical health and health care has long overshadowed the broader understandings of health as a form of well-being. Many descriptions of health subsume well-being without focusing on it in any shape or form.

Partly as a counterpoint to what has been termed the 'deficit-centred, repair-shop' conception of health, Jayawickreme et al., described an 'engine of well-being' (2012, p. 328). In this model health is not seen as synonymous to well-being, although it is encompassed within it. Instead, notions of happiness and well-being are seen as similar, with a great deal of theorising and research that focuses on which elements of either are the most important. The engine of well-being is presented as a way of clarifying concepts to enable better research about subjective well-being, which is implicated in a range of positive outcomes, including better health (Jayawickreme et al., 2012).

The engine of well-being explains the inputs (i.e., the resources needed to enable well-being) and processes (i.e., the internal states or mechanisms that influence well-being) needed to produce desirable outcomes, which are behaviours characteristic of well-being. Input variables, according to Jayawickreme et al. (2012), are either external, such as environment, education, income, political freedom and adequate nutrition, or internal, such as a particular personality type or abiding values, talents and capabilities. The processes required to turn inputs into outcomes are described as internal states that influence the choices people make, including their specific beliefs or the way they understand those choices. Outcomes include intrinsically valuable behaviours such as good social relationships and highly engaged work, which reflect the attainment of well-being. The authors draw on Seligman (2011) and Sen (1999) to define well-being outcomes in terms of what people, when free from coercion, would choose to do for their own sake—that is, the described behaviours are motivating in their own right.

Subjective well-being has been linked to a wide range of positive outcomes, including better physical and mental health and possibly even longer life (Danner et al., 2001; Diener & Tov, 2007; Diener & Chan, 2011), so it deserves a clear place in any concept or definition of health. Some of the different understandings are explored below, followed by how they inform the various approaches—such as health education, health promotion and health literacy—to enabling better health and well-being through the life course and into older age.

Concepts of Health and Well-Being

An international review of health promotion practices and concepts (Anderson, 1984) was commissioned to inform the Ottawa Charter, a major review into how health promotion was understood and practiced, which was published

---

BOX 8.3 Different Views of Health (Anderson, 1984)

- As an outcome or product—a state or end point: The archetypal or traditional medical formulation, in which health is viewed as a product, bound up with notions of disease and measurable deviations from a biological norm.
- As a potential or capacity—a starting point: Links health with an ability to cope with, or adapt to, environmental challenges as well as an ability to realise personal goals and aspirations.
- As a process—an ongoing, continuous part of life: Relating to optimum physical growth and body development, it may be cumulative in relation to learning and development or cyclical in phases of creation and destruction.

---

two years later (WHO, 1986). Since that review, the spiritual, social and mental dimensions of health have been more widely recognised (WHO, 1998). The concepts Anderson identified are summarised in Box 8.3, and their relevance to older people's health and well-being are expanded on below.

Health as a Product

In the traditional medical formulation, health tends to be viewed as a product, bound up with notions of disease and measurable deviations from a biological norm. Such biomedical measurements give rise to the widely accepted idea of health as a state, as suggested in the WHO's original (1946) definition (see Box 8.2). That definition has been criticised for seeming static and fixed as well as being far too idealistic and unattainable for most people. Also, despite the specific mention of mental and social well-being in the definition, the standalone term *health* is routinely assumed to mean physical health. In particular, the idea of mental illness was even more widely stigmatised in years past than it is now, so older people may be simply unaware questions about health could encompass wider concerns.

However, the WHO definition remains useful in drawing attention to the fact health is not the same as an absence of disease, an idea that still has wide currency. Often, this is presented by describing a continuum, with absolute health placed at the positive end and total disease, or even death, at the negative extreme. It is easy to see how readily such a linear view could portray health as associated with youth and fitness, with any deterioration toward the disease end of the continuum being almost inevitably linked in people's minds with ageing and a pessimistic outlook.

Such an all-or-nothing view of health would be quite detrimental to older people who may be healthy in some respects but not others. People living at home with a well-managed long-term condition like diabetes or arthritis, for example, may not wish to characterise themselves as ill. It is entirely possible for a person of any age to be healthy in one aspect of their lives and unhealthy in another. This suggests health is a characteristic of the whole person, which may be affected in part without being radically changed by a single unhealthy element.

Concentrating on health as an end-state, or product, is closely aligned to the emphasis on the outcomes stressed in much health policy. Equating health with a series of clearly definable and measurable qualities, even if they are health measures, like blood pressure or cholesterol levels, can imply the elements of health, if not health itself, can be obtained from others by being bought, sold or somehow acquired. This is a particular risk in countries where health care is a lucrative business. Restoring health might be viewed as little more than a technical matter, with control for it being removed from the person (Aggleton, 1990). Perhaps the most negative point about viewing health as a product is its association with the idea health is best owned and controlled by health care professionals or organisations rather than the people whose health is under discussion. This is a particular problem for older people or those with disabilities, as their views may be disregarded in favour of views expressed by doctors, nurses or other professionals. In turn, this is linked with a tendency to underplay the importance of the practical, social and cultural contexts for health.

Having said that, the view of health as an end-state underpins a great deal of valuable medical research and most of the surveys that illustrate the extent of ability and disability within the older age group. These continue to provide very helpful information to discredit stereotyping perceptions of older people. Moreover, the traditional view of health that underpins the biomedical approach remains significantly useful when illness occurs. The clarity that can be lent to a confusing or frightening situation by identifying a specific diagnosis or measurable basis for reassurance should not be underestimated. Alternatively, such data can be used to demonstrate clear risks and enable safety measures to be put in place. This happened when epidemiological data demonstrated a clearly greater risk to the older population from COVID-19, leading to a nationwide plan to protect them, first by isolation, then by prioritising them for vaccines.

Health as Potential

Anderson (1984) linked the idea of health as a potential with an ability to cope with, or adapt to, environmental challenges as well as an ability to realise personal goals and aspirations. Seedhouse's (1986) ideas popularised this view a few decades ago; he described health as the 'foundation for achievement'. He explained how regarding health as a potential could integrate a number of different ways of looking at health, including the ideas described above—that it can be regarded as an ideal state or as a commodity that can be bought or given. He incorporated two other groups of theories: those that hold health is a personal strength or ability, whether physical, metaphysical or intellectual, and those that see health as the physical and mental fitness to do socialised daily tasks.

Seedhouse (1986) described a vision of health as the potential to grow, develop and experience different things, which fits with an emphasis on personal control, understanding and autonomy. He suggested people may continue to develop new potentials throughout life, even in the face of quite serious disabilities or illnesses. He explained it in terms of maintaining a positive balance between liabilities and obstacles that threaten health—particularly adverse living conditions and diseases—and central conditions for maintaining health.

These ideas were expanded more recently by Bircher and Hahn (2017), who described the 'demands of life' and two forms of potential: one that is biologically given and one that is personally acquired. These potentials have opposite trajectories, but they continuously interact with each other. *Biologically given potential* (BGP) has a finite value at the time of birth and decreases continuously throughout life, reaching zero when the person dies. Conversely, *personally acquired potential* (PAP) is small at the time of birth, increasing most rapidly at the start of life, then more slowly as the person grows older. Survival depends on fulfilling the demands of life, which may be physiological, psychological or environmental, using either BGP or PAP, which can compensate for each other, according to Bircher and Hahn (2017). If demands outweigh the person's overall capacity, then disease, or ultimately death, results (see Fig. 8.3).

Kuruvilla et al. (2018) (see Fig. 8.2) developed these ideas to refer to intrinsic capacity and functional ability, terms that were also used in the WHO's (2020b) baseline report for its Decade of Healthy Ageing. Functional ability, which is central to the WHO's description of healthy ageing (see Box 8.2), 'combines the intrinsic capacity of the individual, the environment a person lives in and how people interact with their environment' (WHO, 2020b, p. 12). The report explained that functional ability enables people to be and do whatever they have reason to value, which is key to overall health and well-being.

Health as a Process

The continuing interactions between life's demands and the potential to cope or thrive with them is a process, which is

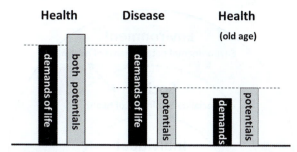

Fig. 8.3 Distinction between heath and disease (Bircher & Hahn, 2016).

a third way of looking at health. Process theories emphasise health as an ever-changing, dynamic phenomenon. In this view, health is a continuing pattern of change that occurs over the lifetime in all dimensions of the individual (Anderson, 1984). Choices are greatly influenced by self-concept, environment and culture and likewise the ability (or not) to cope with stress or flow with experience. Regarding health as a process emphasises seeing it as a means rather than an end in itself. Although this has become integral to descriptions of health as potential, a key difference lies in the fact that processes require context and meaning to make sense of them, so linkages, patterns, interconnections and actions are emphasised more than separate factors or events.

One of the most significant process theories stresses the importance of starting from a positive consideration of how health is created and maintained rather than focusing on the negative aspects of illness and disorder (Antonovsky, 1979; 1987). This health-creating, salutogenic theory—which is the opposite of pathogenic theories that focus on causes of disease—can be particularly useful for promoting older people's health (Koelen et al., 2017). All human beings face pathogens, psychosocial stresses and risks from disease, but by virtue of having survived the challenges for a greater number of years than their young relatives, older people have demonstrated their salutogenic ability. Antonovsky (1993) considered ageing to be a process of human development rather than one of biological and mental degradation

of the body. His theory proposed life experiences produce *'generalised resistance resources'* (explained further in Idan et al., 2017), which are positive methods of responding and adapting to situations. These may be complemented by *'specific resistance resources'* developed for particular situations (Mittelmark et al., 2017).

The various resistance resources promote the development and maintenance of a strong sense of coherence, which is described as the extent to which an individual has a pervasive, enduring and dynamic feeling of confidence that things will work out as well as can reasonably be expected. This explanation locates the theory very closely in the person's own context, expectations and culture, but it incorporates practical and physiological aspects as well. The sense of coherence, which is closely linked with health and well-being, can continue to develop well into old age, according to Koelen et al. (2017), and is explained through three central components: manageability, meaningfulness and comprehensibility.

Manageability refers to the extent to which people feel they have the resources to meet demands that arise in their daily lives. This includes resources under direct individual control and those accessible from family, friends or the community. For older people, this may involve having the confidence they can obtain suitable treatment or learn coping strategies for dealing with a chronic disorder or distressing symptoms, for example. Health care professionals may serve as resources if they are able to help in practical ways or teach ways of coping. The idea of manageability depends quite closely on people experiencing a practical and physical sense of self-empowerment in coping with their own biology and threats to health.

Comprehensibility refers to the extent to which sense and order can be drawn from the situation, and the world seems understandable, ordered, consistent and clear. In translating an exceptional experience such as illness, disability or unpleasant symptoms into the normal context of their everyday lives, people make sense of what is happening to them and can gain strength to deal with the situation. Helping an older person understand their illness can enhance comprehensibility of the situation they are in.

Thinking Point 3: Life Course and Its Impact

Revisit the notes you made for the earlier Thinking Points.
- Can you identify the factors related to social, cultural and environmental determinants that might have influenced Bob's and Joe's life courses? And the other imagined men and women?
- What about personal/individual capacity, or PAP?
- Are health and well-being two sides of the same coin, or do you think they are different?

- How might understanding these interconnected aspects affect the approaches you use when nursing older people in hospital? At home?
- Can you think of approaches nurses might use to help an older person develop their functional ability, PAP, or some salutogenic resistance resources?

The sense of *meaningfulness* individuals can gain from a situation refers to their ability to participate fully in the processes shaping their future. To be fully engaged in the health-creating processes of their own lives, people need to make sense of events in an emotional as well as a cognitive sense, possibly drawing on faith and cultural beliefs. This means setting symptoms, experiences, treatments and coping mechanisms in the context of their own family, friends, personal contacts and reasons for living. Social relationships are significantly implicated in enhancing health, as explained in the earlier section about loneliness and social networks. Loneliness may affect the extent to which life continues to hold a positive meaning for older adults.

BRINGING TOGETHER THE DIFFERENT CONCEPTS OF HEALTH

Two significant publications summarise and combine the many different elements that contribute to health and well-being or to disease and less positive outcomes.

The Meikirch model, named after the Swiss village in which it was conceptualised, was devised by doctors who described it as 'not only a unifying theoretical framework for health and disease but also a scaffold for the practice of medicine and public health' (Bircher & Hahn, 2017, p. 1). They described a complex adaptive system that consists of five component—BGP and PAP, social and environmental determinants and demands of life—and ten complex interactions, shown as arrows in Figure 8.4. Health is viewed as a lifelong process, defined as a 'dynamic state of well-being emergent from conducive interactions between an individual's potentials, life's demands, and social and environmental determinants' (p. 3). The demands of life may be physiological, psychological or environmental, varying between individuals and contexts.

The constant interactions between life's demands and a person's potentials, along with their individual social and environmental determinants, said Bircher and Hahn (2017), lead to either health or disease, depending on how the interaction is balanced (see Fig. 8.3). Health requires that individual resources—including their potentials and those available from their environment, such as health care, support, advice and so on—match the demands of life. The BGP represents the whole basis of human existence; it is at its highest at birth and decreases throughout life, until it reaches zero at the time of death. PAP represents all the physical, mental, social and spiritual abilities a person can acquire; it can develop throughout life and is also the site of an individual's responsibility for their own health.

In the Meikirch model, the social and environmental setting, including government policies, is regarded as responsible

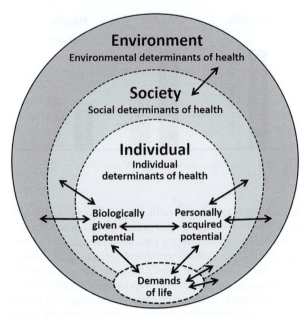

Fig. 8.4 Meikirch model (Bircher & Hahn, 2017).

for ensuring individuals can access the resources they need to develop and reach their full potential and therefore good health. This includes the wider determinants outlined earlier in the chapter, like education, accessible health care, clean air and safe food, for example. Some of these determinants may be cultural or based in faith and family traditions, which are often the site of inspiration or confidence. And, as explained earlier, they may also act as barriers or stressors, which create demands on an individual's personal capacity.

The WHO's (2020b) baseline report describes environments as simply where people live their lives, noting they shape what older people, with a given intrinsic capacity, can be and do, including how they can develop and maintain their functional ability. Environments include the home, community and broader society and all the factors within them. They note five key domains for each of the three elements—intrinsic capacity, functional ability, environments—that contribute to healthy ageing, summarised in Box 8.4.

Together, these two publications help to make sense of the multitude of different factors and issues outlined in this chapter. The Meikirch model (Bircher & Hahn 2016; 2017) incorporates a wide range of theoretical and research perspectives on health and well-being. The baseline report prepared for the WHO's Decade of Healthy Ageing (WHO, 2020b) clarifies key domains and concepts, concentrating on identifying key measures and practical suggestions for governments about how to develop their public health policies to achieve improvements in the health of their older populations. Taken together, they demonstrate how

---

BOX 8.4 Three Components of Healthy Ageing (WHO 2020b, pp. 12–13)

Functional ability combines the intrinsic capacity of the individual, the environment a person lives in, and how people interact with their environment. To optimise functional ability, input is required from multiple sectors and a whole-of-government response to population ageing in order to:

- Meet their basic needs to ensure an adequate standard of living, such as being able to afford an adequate diet, clothing, suitable housing, health care and long-term-care services, including medication.
- Learn, grow and make decisions to strengthen a person's autonomy, dignity, integrity, freedom and independence.
- Be mobile for completing daily tasks and participating in activities.
- Build and maintain relationships with children and family, intimate partners, neighbours and others.
- Contribute to society, such as by assisting friends, mentoring younger people, caring for family members, volunteering, pursuing cultural activities and working.

Intrinsic capacity comprises all the physical and mental capacities a person can draw on. Important domains include the following:

- Locomotor capacity (physical movement)
- Sensory capacity (such as vision and hearing)
- Vitality (energy and balance)
- Cognition
- Psychological capacity

Environments include the home, community and broader society and all the factors within them. Key domains include the following:

- Products, equipment and technology that facilitate movement, sight, memory and daily functioning
- The natural or built environment
- Emotional support, assistance and relationships provided by other people and animals
- Attitudes, which can influence behaviour both negatively and positively
- Services, systems and policies that may or may not contribute to enhanced functioning at older ages

---

the multiple, separate aspects encountered across the life course—and described in this chapter—can combine to support and encourage healthy ageing. Conversely, they help explain how adverse environments and wider social and economic determinants can create stress, demands and challenges, which ultimately undermine the potentials and capacity of individuals, thwarting the possibility of a healthy old age and creating health inequalities. The two models also offer a basis from which to develop policies or interventions to help improve the health of people who are already in the older age range. Person-centred care is a key area for action invoked by the WHO's (2020b) baseline report as a means of overcoming unhelpful attitudes and approaches in health care and nursing.

Person-Centred Care

Person-centredness has roots in psychotherapy and the work of psychologist Carl Rogers, who, in the 1950s, wrote about how a therapist might engage with a client in a non-directive, client-focused (as opposed to therapist-focused) way that acknowledges the potential of the person to self-direct and reach their own sense of fulfilment. Rogers (1980) later explained this approach is based on the assumption people have within themselves resources for self-understanding, for shifting their self-concept and for self-directing their behaviour. This is very strongly in

tune with the WHO's (2020b) Decade of Healthy Ageing baseline report, which repeatedly emphasised the need to release and strengthen the older person's intrinsic capacity and resources. Rogers described unconditional positive regard as the foundation of person-centredness, which also depends on empathy, willingness to suspend judgement and an appreciation of the service user's perspective.

Four key elements of person-centred care highlighted by the Health Foundation (2016) are as follows:

- Affording people dignity, compassion and respect.
- Offering coordinated care, support or treatment.
- Offering personalised care, support or treatment.
- Supporting people to recognise and develop their own strengths and abilities to enable them to live an independent and fulfilling life.

The Health Foundation maintains when people are better informed, they may choose different and potentially less costly or invasive treatments. Also, people who are supported to manage their own care more effectively are less likely to use emergency hospital services, and those who take part in shared decision making are more likely to stick to their treatment plan and take their medicines correctly (Health Foundation, 2016). Person-centred care is, therefore, a health-promoting approach. It is well established in nursing and discussed further in Chapter 10. An example is given in Case Study 8.1.

CASE STUDY 8.1   Person-Centred Care

Mr Brown had been attending outpatient services on and off for more than 20 years, so he had seen some changes, especially when his old specialist left and the new one came. His rheumatism started before he retired, but now it was getting to be more of a problem; he supposed it was what you had to expect when you were nearly 80.

It was different at the hospital now, though; instead of always seeing the doctor, he sometimes saw a nurse specialist. He was a bit uncertain about that at first, but now he had got to know her, he was very happy about it. She really seemed to understand what he needed. She always put him through his paces, checking his tablets and how well he could walk, and got him moving joints he didn't know moved anymore! It wasn't just that, though; he could talk to her. He didn't know how she knew which questions to ask, but she did. Like this morning, he wasn't going to mention getting to the toilet—it was too embarrassing, like a child always with a dribble on his trousers. Perhaps that was why she asked him about how he was managing but in such a matter-of-fact way it just seemed natural to answer and not difficult at all. It might be easier to use a urinal, as she said; at least then he wouldn't be worn out with pain by the time he got to the toilet. He could give it a try, as she had arranged for him to borrow one from the hospital store. He wasn't too sure about having a home assessment; he would think about it and let her know next time, like she suggested. Perhaps it would be a good idea, but he would take his time to decide.

PROMOTING HEALTH AND WELL-BEING IN OLDER PEOPLE

Health promotion is the process of enabling people to increase control over the determinants of health and thereby improve their health (WHO, 1998). Modern approaches to health promotion place a high value on citizen participation and collectivism, rejecting professional dominance in favour of common understanding between lay and professional spheres of knowledge (WHO, 1986). Health promotion includes attention to *health literacy*, which is the combination of personal competencies and situational resources needed for people to access, understand, appraise and use information and services to make decisions about health. Health literacy includes the capacity to communicate, assert and act on these decisions (International Union for Health Promotion and Education, 2018).

The ideals embedded in the term health promotion were developed in part to challenge the supremacy of the rather didactic approach to health education that was prevalent in the middle years of the last century. Health education had developed before and after the Second World War; during this period people were expected to respect authority and obey orders without question. It was a great age of discovery, as countless new so-called wonder drugs such as antibiotics, steroids and effective immunizations were developed. This led to a growing belief in the almost magical power of medicine to prevent, treat and cure an ever-increasing range of illnesses.

In keeping with this period of history, the traditional approach to health education assumed people should obey a doctor's orders to become healthy. In the context of this chapter, it is worth bearing in mind that many of the present older population grew up in the time when this kind of directive approach was expected. That is not to say they either approved of it or felt it to be a benefit, although some might have done. However, they may not voice objections to being told what to do by professionals as much as younger people who have grown up in a consumerist society, expecting to be consulted and have their views taken into account. Didactic attitudes and approaches are far less prevalent now and would usually be considered rather arrogant and judgemental, possibly based in ignorance of the challenges older people might face now or overcame in the past.

However, recent calls to respect older people and ensure their dignity is maintained (Bircher & Hahn, 2017; WHO, 2020b) demonstrate there is still room for improvement. Consider the way COVID-19 vaccinations were rolled out during 2021. It was an emergency situation, (detailed further below), with wonderful examples of good, supportive practice, such as vaccine buses delivering an accessible local service or nurses delivering injections at home. All too often, though, there were distressing tales of older people queuing outside in the wind and rain, perhaps with inadequate support or even seating for those who were too frail to stand.

Health education is now defined as comprising 'consciously constructed opportunities for learning, involving some form of communication designed to improve health literacy, including improving knowledge, and developing life skills which are conducive to individual and community health' (WHO, 1998, p. 14). Approaches may aim to help people by enabling them to develop the resistance resources (Antonovksy, 1987) detailed earlier in the chapter, for example by increasing understanding (comprehensibility), developing skills or focused support (manageability) and enabling people to make sense of challenging diagnoses and situations (meaningfulness). Such activities may focus on individuals or whole groups and communities (see Case Study 8.2).

CASE STUDY 8.2   **Different Styles of Health Education in Practice**

When the district nurse visited 82-year-old Mrs Mary Davies to follow up her visit to the accident and emergency department, she found her upset, miserable and in pain. She had been walking back home from the paper shop when her bad knee gave way. She fell and could not get up; someone called an ambulance. At first Mrs Davies felt silly, then relieved, because they were kind and checked her over, which made her feel safe. But then the nurse told her she was far too heavy and must lose weight or she might not be so lucky next time; she should do more exercise, the nurse said. She didn't know how she was supposed to exercise when she could hardly move. Her bad knee was swollen and bruised, and the bandages they had put on felt too tight.

At times like this she missed her first husband, who had always been very practical and would have known what to do. Not that he liked skinny women; he used to say he liked a bit of meat to get hold of! Bert, her second husband, was kind in his way as well and had made some sausages and bacon for her dinner before he went out. Fried food gave her indigestion, but she had always done all the cooking, so he didn't know how to make stews and pies like she did. She had always been on the large side and never had time for exercise, what with having to walk all the way to shops and carry the things back two or three times a week. It used to be better when there was a greengrocer at the end of the road. You couldn't get fresh vegetables now like you used to, and she missed having a natter to her neighbours while she waited to be served. Her old friends had nearly all moved away or were in homes now. She didn't like to think about when that would happen to her. The paper shop sold most of what you needed, but they cost a fortune, and it was a struggle to walk to the shops at the other end of the estate.

Mary felt much better by the time this nurse left and Bert came home. She couldn't really recall the nurse had said much, but she had stayed some time and put the bandage on Mary's leg right, which eased the pain. Mary wasn't sure why she had told the nurse so much about herself—just nattering, she supposed. She had never thought of walking to the shops as exercise before; it was just what you had to do. Of course, she had always known about good home cooking, and she was sure she could find some of her old mother's recipes that used less fat from when she was a child after the war, when you couldn't get it anyway. She said she would look up some of them for the nurse, who was too young to remember rationing but was interested in it. It'd be good to be able to get some fresh vegetables again if that new greengrocer the nurse told her about would deliver this far away. She could get a bus to choose what she wanted, then the nurse said they'd deliver what you ordered. Although she said there's always a queue! That'd be like the old days, chatting to folks while you waited, and if you could get a whole batch of vegetables in one go, you would save money there. It did make sense to think her bad knee might not hurt so much if she was less heavy, and she wouldn't mind talking to that nurse about her weight when she came again.

COVID-19

The coronavirus pandemic provides a contemporary case study of the global and British state of public health. A warning to the world came in 2003, when sudden acute respiratory syndrome (SARS) made international headlines. SARS was a newly identified human infection caused by a coronavirus, SARS-CoV-1, and transmitted during face-to-face exposure through infected droplets expelled during coughing or sneezing. The disease spread rapidly, with the international outbreak eventually causing more than 8,000 cases and 900 deaths in 30 countries before largely burning itself out. Overall, around 11% of individuals infected died, with mortality much higher in the older population (WHO, 2003).

The novel coronavirus that emerged in China late in 2019, called SARS-CoV-2, is responsible for the new disease known as COVID-19. Highly infectious, the disease swept across the world in 2020, causing almost 200 million cases, with over 6.7 million deaths in 192 countries at the time of writing (January 2023) (Johns Hopkins University, 2022). The pandemic shows little sign of abating worldwide, despite the existence of a raft of effective vaccinations. The disease reached Britain in January 2020; by early March, 100 people had tested positive, and the country went into its first lockdown later that month. Given the severity of the disease, both existing public health legislation and new health protection laws were used to enforce social distancing, quarantine and financial recompense for individuals affected by business closures.

From the start it was clear the mortality rate from COVID-19 was much higher for older groups. It is particularly serious for people over 80 years old and affects men more than women. Individuals with long-standing health conditions are the most vulnerable (Marmot et al., 2020b). There is also a clear socioeconomic gradient, the more deprived the area, the higher the mortality rate (see Fig. 8.5).

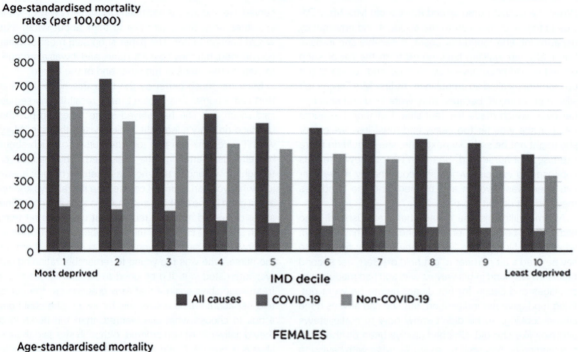

MALES

Age-standardised mortality
rates (per 100,000)

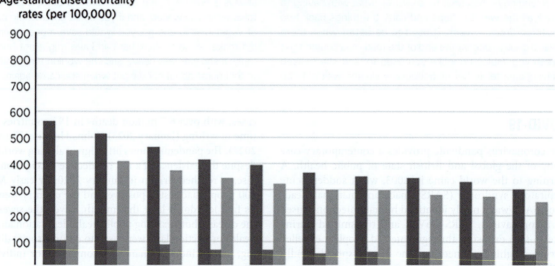

FEMALES

Age-standardised mortality
rates (per 100,000)

Note: Deaths involving COVID-19 include those with an underlying cause, or any mention, of (COVID-19) virus.

Source: ONS. Deaths involving COVID-19 by local area and socioeconomic deprivation, 2020 (30).

Fig. 8.5 Age-standardised mortality rates from all causes, COVID-19 and other causes, by sex and deprivation deciles in England and Wales between March and July 2020 (Marmot et al., 2020b); (Office for National Statistics, 2020c).

The high mortality and morbidity of the disease makes it a serious 'demand of life', to use a term employed by Bircher and Hahn (2017). It affects individuals differently depending on where they live, their intrinsic capacity and the resources they have to draw on within their immediate environment, including from family, friends, neighbours and local services.

Compared to the least-deprived communities, people in the most-deprived areas experience more than twice the number of hospital admissions for intensive care and almost double the risk of dying (Pagel, 2021). Among the 20% of poorest UK households, 7% live in overcrowded housing, which is a risk factor for respiratory infections. Living in a household with more than six occupants doubles the risk of catching the virus (Patel et al., 2020). Furthermore, the mental stress of poverty and uncertain employment reduces the effectiveness of the immune system, which also increases the risk of succumbing to serious disease (Patel et al., 2020).

People from Black and minority ethnic groups also face a greater risk of severe disease and death from COVID-19. These groups are more likely to be living in overcrowded conditions, possibly in multigenerational households, with family members working in high-risk occupations, including health and care staff, transport and other public-facing work, and with pre-existing conditions. An older person living in a deprived area and from a minority group faces a cumulative risk of mortality. According to Marmot et al. (2020b), this reflects a lifetime of often adverse experiences, including long-standing inequalities and structural racism.

Early in the pandemic, older people were classed as vulnerable by virtue of their age and any pre-existing conditions, with those considered most at risk being advised to shield by staying at home. This was the source of further self-reinforcing inequalities. People who already lived in already overcrowded conditions were at greater risk of catching the virus, and those in low-wage employment were at greater risk of losing their work, further reducing household income and adding to the stressful nature of living through a pandemic.

Although loneliness was on the rise prior to the pandemic, confinement to home reduced opportunities to have meaningful conversations with neighbours and friends, increasing feelings of loneliness for almost 30% of individuals 70 years and older (Marmot et al., 2020b). People who lived alone faced an increased risk of loneliness and isolation, with poorer people generally having less opportunity than their wealthier neighbours to mitigate this through online access to remote social activities or services.

Overall, as Pagel (2021) suggested, there is a very real danger that COVID-19 will become entrenched as a disease of poverty, with social and health inequalities set to increase as a result of the pandemic.

Thinking Point 4: COVID-19 and the Impact of a Public Health Emergency

The WHO's (2020b) Decade of Health Ageing baseline report points to the importance of where people live, noting it shapes what older people, with a given intrinsic capacity, can be and do.

- Which environmental factors can you identify that contributed to the social gradient in deaths from COVID-19?
- How could society have helped reduce the risk for older people from the direct effects of COVID-19 or the impact of isolation caused by shielding or lockdown?
- What activities could help strengthen individuals' intrinsic capacity or their PAP in the face of this public health emergency?
- Do you agree with Bircher and Hahn (2017) that responsibility for health is shared between individuals, who need to develop their PAP, and wider society, which is responsible for providing the resources, including education, health care, safe food and clean air, and opportunities for development?
- How far did society meet its responsibility to the health of older people during the COVID-19 pandemic?

CONCLUSION AND LEARNING POINTS

An understanding of public health provides a fundamental basis for the Decade of Healthy Ageing (2021–2030) being sponsored by the WHO (2020b). Its baseline report offers a series of starting points for action, drawing on the key concepts of intrinsic capacity and functional ability and set within the environments in which older people live. This chapter explained how those environments contribute to health and well-being across the life course, as embedded social determinants can lead to either healthy ageing or greater difficulties in older age. Social and cultural environments contribute hugely to health inequalities, but adverse outcomes are not inevitable.

A great deal of health service attention is focused on acute and severe episodic care, but more low-key promotive and preventive actions can have a long-lasting impact. As indicated in this chapter, it is never too early to begin the process of developing personal capacities for health, whether viewed as resistance resources (Antonovsky, 1987) or PAP (Bircher & Hahn, 2017). Equally, it is never too late, or more important, than in the later years of life. Nurses have a large role in helping individuals to develop these capabilities during their everyday practice and, through their work in public health departments, contributing to health-enhancing policies for the life course.

KEY LEARNING POINTS

- Understand the relevance of public health, including the wider determinants that contribute to health and well-being.
- Be able to explain how social determinants affect health across the life course, leading to health inequalities and a social gradient in outcomes in older age.
- Be able to identify significant factors that contribute to healthy ageing.
- Explain how nurses can support functional ability, intrinsic capacity and the environments in which older people live.

- Explain how nurses can help with the key challenges, or demands of life, that might undermine active lifestyles and healthy ageing in the longer term.
- Explore any differences between health and well-being, including whether it is useful to distinguish between the concepts in practice.
- Be able to give examples to show how public health thinking, including social determinants, life course events and healthy ageing, can explain why different people experience similar diagnoses and disorders in very different ways.

REFERENCES

Acheson, D. (1998). *Public health in England*. HMSO.

Aggleton, P. (1990). *Health*. Routledge.

Anderson, R. (1984). Health promotion: An overview. *European Monographs in Health Education Research, 6*, 4–119.

Antonovsky, A. (1979). *Health, stress and coping*. Jossey-Bass.

Antonovsky, A. (1987). *Unraveling the mystery of health*. Jossey-Bass.

Antonovsky, A. (1993). The structure and properties of the sense of coherence scale. *Social Science and Medicine, 36*(6), 725–733.

Ashton, J., & Seymour, H. (1998). *The new public health*. Open University Press.

Ayalon, L., & Shiovitz-Ezra, S. (2011). The relationship between loneliness and passive death wishes in the second half of life. *International Psychogeriatrics, 23*(10), 1677–1685.

Bandari, R., Khankeh, H. R., Shahboulaghi, F. M., Ebadi, A., Keshtkar, A. A., & Montazeri, A. (2019). Defining loneliness in older adults: Protocol for a systematic review. *Systematic Reviews, 8*(1), 26.

Bonsang, E., & Soest, A. (2010). Satisfaction with job and income among older individuals across European countries. *SSRN Electronic Journal, 105*, 227–254.

Bircher, J. (2020). Meikirch model: New definition of health as hypothesis to fundamentally improve healthcare delivery. *Integrated Healthcare Journal, 2*(1), Article e000046.

Bircher, J., & Hahn, E. G. (2016). Understanding the nature of health: New perspectives for medicine and public health. *Improved wellbeing at lower costs F1000Research, 5*, 167.

Bircher, J, & Hahn, E. G. (2017). Will the Meikirch model, a new framework for health, induce a paradigm shift in healthcare? *Cureus, 9*(3), e1081.

Bircher, J., & Kuruvilla, S. (2014). Defining health by addressing individual, social, and environmental determinants: new opportunities for health care and public health. *Journal of Public Health Policy, 35*(3), 363–386.

Burns, A., Leavey, G., Ward, M., & O'Sullivan, R (2020). The impact of loneliness on healthcare use in older people: Evidence from a nationally representative cohort. *Journal of Public Health, 30*, 675–684.

Chana, R., Marshall, P., & Harley, C. (2016). The role of the intermediate care team in detecting and responding to loneliness in older clients. *British Journal of Community Nursing, 21*(6), 292–298.

Dahlgren, G., & Whitehead, M. (1991). *Policies and strategies to promote social equity in health*. Institute for Futures Studies.

Danner, D. D., Snowden, D. A., & Friesen, W. V. (2001). Positive emotions in early life and longevity: Findings from the Nun Study. *Journal of Personality and Social Psychology, 80*, 804–813.

De Jong Gierveld, J., Van der Pas, S., & Keating, N. (2015). Loneliness of older immigrant groups in Canada: Effects of ethnic-cultural background. *Journal of Cross-Cultural Gerontology, 30*(3), 251–268.

Delmelle, E. C., Haslauer, E., & Prinz, T. (2013). Social satisfaction, commuting and neighborhoods. *Journal of Transport Geography, 30*, 110–116.

Diener, E., & Chan, M. Y. (2011). Happy people live longer: Subjective well-being contributes to health and longevity. *Applied Psychology: Health and Well-Being, 3*, 1–43.

Diener, E., & Tov, W. (2007). Subjective well-being and peace. *Journal of Social Issues, 63*, 421–440.

Donovan, N. J., & Blazer, D. (2020). Social isolation and loneliness in older adults: Review and commentary of a national academies report. *The American Journal of Geriatric Psychiatry: Official Journal of the American Association for Geriatric Psychiatry, 28*(12), 1233–1244.

Dykstra, P. A. (2009). Older adult loneliness: Myths and realities. *European Journal of Ageing, 6*(2), 91–100.

Evandrou, M., Falkingham, J., Feng Z., & Vlachantoni, A. (2016). Ethnic inequalities in limiting health and self-reported health in later life revisited. *Journal of Epidemiology and Community Health, 70*, 653–662.

Hauge, S., & Kirkevold, M. (2010). Older Norwegians' understanding of loneliness. *International Journal of Qualitative Studies on Health and Well-being, 5*(1), 10.3402/qhw.v5i1.465410.3402/qhw.v5i1.4654.

Health Foundation. (2016). Person-centred care made simple. https://www.health.org.uk/publications/person-centred-care-made-simple

Holwerda, T. J., Deeg, D. J. H., Beekman, A. T. F., van Tilburg, T. G., Stek, M. L., Jonker, C., & Schoevers, R. A. (2014). Feelings of loneliness, but not social isolation, predict dementia onset: results from the Amsterdam study of the elderly (AMSTEL). *Journal of Neurology, Neurosurgery, and Psychiatry, 85*(2), 135–142.

Huber, M., Knottnerus, J. A., Green, L., von der Horst, H., Jadad, A. R., Kromhout, D., Leonard, B, Lorig, K, Loureiro, M. I., van der Meer, J. W. M., Schnabel, P., Smith, R., van Weel, C., & Smid, H. (2011). How should we define health? *British medical journal, 343*, d4163. doi:10.1136/bmj.d4163.

Idan, O., Eriksson, M., & Al-Yagon, M (2017). The Salutogenic model: The role of generalized resistance resources. In M. B. Mittelmark, S. Sagy, M. Eriksson, G. F. Bauer, J. M. Pelikan, B. Lindström, & G. A. Espnes (Eds.), *The Handbook of Salutogenesis* (pp. 57–69). Springer Nature.

International Union for Health Promotion and Education. (2018). https://www.iuhpe.org/index.php/en

Jayawickreme, E., Forgearde, M., & Seligman, M. (2012). The engine of well-being. *Review of General Psychology, 16*(4), 327–342.

Johns Hopkins University. (2022). COVID-19 dashboard by the Centre for Systems Science and Engineering at Johns Hopkins University. https://coronavirus.jhu.edu/map.html

Kemperman, A., van den Berg, P., Weijs-Perrée, M., & Uijtdewillegen, K. (2019). Loneliness of older adults: Social network and the living environment. *International Journal of Environmental Research and Public Health, 16*(3), 406.

Koelen, M., Eriksson, M., & Cattan, M (2017). In. In M. B. Mittelmark, S. Sagy, M. Eriksson, G. F. Bauer, J. M. Pelikan, B. Lindström, & G. A. Espnes (Eds.), *The Handbook of Salutogenesis* (pp. 138–147). Springer Nature.

Kuruvilla, S., Sadana, R., Montesinos, E. V., Beard, J., Vasdeki, J. F., de Carvalho, I. A., Thomas, R. B., Drisse, M.-N. B., Daelmans, B., Goodman, T., Koller, T., Officer, A., Vogel, J., Valentine, N., Wootton, E., Banderjee, A., Magar, V., Neira, M., Bele, J. M. O., & Bustreo, F. (2018). A life-course approach to health: Synergy with sustainable development goals. *Bulletin of World Health Organization, 96*, 42–50.

Marks, L., Hunter, D. J., & Alderslade, R. (2020). *Strengthening public health capacity and services in Europe*. World Health Organization and Durham University. https://www.euro.who.int/__data/assets/pdf_file/0007/152683/e95877.pdf.

Marmot, M., Allen, J., Goldblatt, P., Boyce, T., McNeish, D., Grady, M., & Geddes, I. (2010). *Fair society, healthy lives: The Marmot review. Strategic review of health inequalities in England post-2010*. Institute of Health Equity.

Marmot, M., Allen, J., Boyce, T., Goldblatt, P., & Morrison, J. (2020a). *Health equity in England: The Marmot review 10 years on*. Institute of Health Equity.

Marmot, M., Allen, J., Goldblatt, P., Herd, J. E., & Morrison, J. (2020b). *Build back fairer: The COVID-19 Marmot review. The pandemic, socioeconomic and health inequalities in England*. Institute of Health Equity.

Mikton, C., de la Fuente-Núñez, V., Officer, A., & Krug, E. (2021). Ageism: A social determinant of health that has come of age. *Lancet, 397*, 1334.

Mittelmark, M. B., Bull, T., Daniel, M., & Urke, H (2017). Specific resistance resources in the salutogenic model of health. In M. B. Mittelmark, S. Sagy, M. Eriksson, G. F. Bauer, J. M. Pelikan, B. Lindström, & G. A. Espnes (Eds.), *The handbook of salutogenesis* (pp. 71–76). Springer Nature.

Murphy, M., Grundy, E., & Kalogirou, S. (2007). The increase in marital status differences in mortality up to the oldest age in seven European countries, 1990–99. *Population Studies, 61*(3), 287–298.

Niedzwiedz, C. L., Richardson, E. A., Tunstall, H., Shortt, N. K., Mitchell, R. J., & Pearce, J. R. (2016). The relationship between wealth and loneliness among older people across Europe: Is social participation protective? *Preventative Medicine, 91*, 24–31.

Office for National Statistics. (2020a). Population estimates by marital status and living arrangements, England and Wales: 2019. Office for National Statistics. https://www.ons.gov.uk/peoplepopulationandcommunity/populationandmigration/populationestimates/bulletins/populationestimatesbymaritalstatusandlivingarrangements/2019

Office for National Statistics. (2020b). Living longer: Implications of childlessness among tomorrow's older population. https://www.ons.gov.uk/peoplepopulationandcommunity/birthsdeathsandmarriages/ageing/articles/livinglonger/implicationsofchildlessnessamongtomorrowsolderpopulation

Office for National Statistics. (2020c). Tables that accompany the article 'Deaths involving COVID-19 by local area and socioeconomic deprivation: deaths occurring between 1 March 2020 and 31 July 2020.

Ong, A., Uchino, N. B., & Wethington, E. (2016). Loneliness and health in older adults: A mini-review and synthesis. *Gerontology, 62*, 443–449.

Pagel, C. (2021). A very real danger that COVID-19 will become entrenched as a disease of poverty. *BMJ Opinion*. https://blogs.bmj.com/bmj/2021/04/09/christina-pagel-a-very-real-danger-that-covid-19-will-become-entrenched-as-a-disease-of-poverty.

Patel, J. A., Neilson, F. B. H., Badiani, A. A. S., Assi, S., Unadkat, V. A., Patel, B., Ravindrane, R., & Wardle, H. (2020). Poverty, inequality and COVID-19: The forgotten vulnerable. *Public Health, 183*, 110–111.

Patterson, I. (2002). Baby boomers and adventure tourism: The importance of marketing the leisure experience. *World Leisure Journal, 44*, 4–10.

Perlman, D., & Peplau, L. A. (1982). *Theoretical approaches to loneliness*. John Wiley & Sons.

Pinquart, M., & Sörensen, S. (2001). Influences on loneliness in older adults: A meta-analysis. Influences on loneliness. *Basic and Applied Psychology, 23*(4), 245–266.

Pinquart, M., & Sörensen, S. (2003). *Risk factors for loneliness in adulthood and old age: A meta-analysis*: Nova Science Publishers.

Rico-Uribe, L. A., Caballero, F. F., Olaya, B., Tobiasz-Adamczyk, B., Koskinen, S., Leonardi, M., Haro, J. M., Chatterji, S., & Ayuso-Mateos, J. L. (2016). Loneliness, social networks, and health: A cross-sectional study in three countries. *PLoS One, 11*(1), Article e0145264.

Robards, J., Evandrou, M., Falkingham, J., & Vlachantoni, A. (2012). Marital status, health and mortality. *Maturitas, 73*(4), 295–299.

Rogers, C. (1980). *A way of being*: Houghton Mifflin Company.

Sadana, R., Blas, E., Budhwani, S., Koller, T., & Paraje, G. (2016). Healthy ageing: Raising awareness of inequalities, determinants, and what could be done to improve health equity. *Gerontologist, 56*(S2), S178–S193.

Seedhouse, D. (1986). *Health. The foundations for achievement*: John Wiley & sons.

Seligman, M. (2011). *Flourish*: Free Press.

Sen, A. K. (1999). *Development as freedom*: Oxford University Press.

Squires, S. E. (2015). To a deeper understanding of loneliness amongst older Irish adults. *Collegium Antropologicum, 39*(2), 289–295.

Stickley, A., Koyanagi, A., Roberts, B., Richardson, E., Abbott, P., Tumanov, S., & McKee, M. (2013). Loneliness: Its correlates and association with health behaviours and outcomes in nine countries of the former Soviet Union. *PLoS One, 8*(7), e67978.

Tabue Teguo, M., Simo-Tabue, N., Stoykova, R., Meillon, C., Cogne, M., Amiéva, H., & Dartigues, J.-F (2016). Feelings of loneliness and living alone as predictors of mortality in the elderly: The PAQUID study. *Psychosomatic Medicine, 78*(8), 904–909.

Talley, J. (2016). Spirituality as a determinant of health—a health promotion perspective. In *2nd International Sprituality in Healthcare Conference: Nurturing the Spirit*, 22 Jun 2016, Dublin, Ireland. http://oro.open.ac.uk/47736/

Tang, F., & Lee, Y. (2011). Social support networks and expectations for aging in place and moving. *Research on Aging, 33*, 444–464.

Tzouvara, V., Papadopoulos, C., & Radhawa, G. (2015). A narrative review of the theoretical foundations of loneliness. *The British Journal of Community Nursing, 20*(7), 329–334.

Valtorta, N., & Hanratty, B. (2012). Loneliness, isolation and the health of older adults: Do we need a new research agenda? *Journal of the Royal Society of Medicine, 105*(12), 518–522.

Weijs-Perrée, M., Van den Berg, P., Arentze, T., & Kemperman, A. (2015). Factors influencing social satisfaction and loneliness: A path analysis. *Journal of Transport Geography, 45*, 24–31.

Wenger, G. C. (1997). Social networks and the prediction of elderly people at risk. *Aging and Mental Health, 1*, 311–320.

Wenger, G. C., & Tucker, I. (2002). Using network variation in practice: Identification of support network type. *Health & Social Care in the Community, 10*, 28–35.

Wilson, R. S., Boyle, P. A., James, B. D., Leurgans, S. E., Buchman, A. S., & Bennett, D. A. (2015). Negative social interactions and risk of mild cognitive impairment in old age. *Neuropsychology, 29*(4), 561–570.

World Health Organization (WHO). (1946). *Constitution*. Geneva.

WHO. (1986). *Ottawa charter for health promotion*. Ontario, Canada.

WHO. (1998). *Health promotion glossary*. Geneva.

WHO. (2002). *Active ageing: a policy framework*. Geneva.

WHO. (2003). *World health report*. Geneva.

WHO. (2018). Ageing & health. https://www.who.int/newsroom/fact-sheets/detail/ageing-and-health WHO. (2018). Ageing & health. https://www.who.int/news-room/fact-sheets/detail/ageing-and-health

WHO. (2020a). Decade of Healthy Ageing 2021–2030. https://www.who.int/westernpacific/news/q-a-detail/ageing-healthy-ageing-and-functional-ability#:~:text=Healthy%20ageing%20replaces%20the%20World,their%20families%2C%20communities%20and%20economies

WHO. (2020b). Decade of healthy ageing: Baseline report. Geneva. https://www.who.int/publications/i/item/9789240017900

Worthman, C. M. (1999). Epidemiology of human development. In C. Panter-Brick, C. M. Worthman (Eds.), *Hormones, Health, and Behavior: A Socio-Ecological and Lifespan Perspective* (pp. 47–104). Cambridge University Press.

Wrzus, C., Hänel, M., Wagner, J., & Neyer, F. J. (2013). Social network changes and life events across the life span: A meta-analysis. *Psychological Bulletin, 139*, 53–80.

Yan, Z., Yang, X., Wang, L., Zhao, Y., & Yu, L. (2014). Social change and birth cohort increase in loneliness among Chinese older adults: A cross-temporal meta-analysis. *International Psychogeriatrics, 26*(11), 1773–1781.

Zueras, P., Rutigliano, R., & Trias-Llimo, S. (2020). Marital status, living arrangements, and mortality in middle and older age in Europe. *International Journal of Public Health, 65*, 627–636.

9

Health and Social Care for Older People in the Community

Caroline McGraw

CHAPTER OUTLINE

To secure the best outcomes for older people and reduce the financial costs associated with old age, the United Kingdom pursues an ageing in place agenda. This is where people live in their own homes and communities safely, independently and comfortably, regardless of age, income or disability (Centers for Disease Control and Prevention, 2009). Today, most older people live at home, with support from family, friends and community networks. Yet as people grow old, especially as they grow very old, they experience increasing frailty and susceptibility to illness and disability, which, combined with high levels of carer burden, create demand for high-quality health and social care services in community settings.

According to the Kings Fund (2014), the key functions of health and social care provision for older people include the following:

- Promoting healthy active ageing and supporting independence
- Helping people live well with stable long-term conditions as well as complex co-morbidities, dementia and frailty
- Providing rapid support close to home in times of crisis
- Facilitating good discharge planning and post-discharge support

- Providing rehabilitation and re-ablement after acute illness or injury
- Ensuring choice, control and support toward the end of life.

However, despite their contribution to successful ageing in place, community care services are poorly understood, partly because they are delivered out of sight and partly because of the complexity of different models of provision and commissioning.

This chapter explores the organisation of health and social care services and the use of these services by older people and their carers. It also examines the experiences of service users and evaluates strategies to engage older people and carers in the planning, design and evaluation of community services. Additionally, the chapter raises questions about how changes in service delivery during the COVID-19 pandemic impacted service users. But first it defines health and social care needs and explores the distinction between health and social care systems in the United Kingdom from a historical perspective. The chapter primarily focuses on service provision in England; it should be noted the devolved nations of Scotland, Wales and Northern Ireland have their own health and social care systems that work independently and differently to England and to one another.

SEPARATE HEALTH AND SOCIAL CARE SYSTEMS

The 1946 National Health Service (NHS) Act and the 1948 National Assistance Act distinguished between older people who were sick and in need of constant nursing and medical attention and those who were infirm and in need of care and attention (NHS Act, 1946; National Assistance Act 1948). Older people who were sick were the responsibility of the hospital sector, where they would be either treated in geriatric departments or classified as chronically sick and nursed in long-stay annexes. In contrast, older people who were infirm were the responsibility of local government. The 1948 National Assistance Act recognised the principle that while hospital and nursing services should be delivered free, charges for residential care and welfare services in the home were acceptable as long as they were reasonable.

There was little explicit provision for older people, and community services received little attention. It is conceivable this was due to concerns such services might erode the responsibilities of families and neighbours. The focus was instead on hospital and specialist services. Long-stay hospital beds and residential care homes were the main forms of provision for older people who could not be cared for by families and neighbours. The subordination of community services to hospital and specialist services meant welfare services in the home were developed in a piecemeal fashion, and they and community nursing services were subject to strong regional variations.

By the 1960s there was growing disillusionment with long-stay hospital and residential care homes as the main forms of provision for chronically sick and frail older people, due to the escalating cost of residential and nursing home provision and people increasingly believing the well-being of older people was better served by supporting them at home. The 1990 NHS and Community Care Act saw the focus shift from hospital provision to care in the community (NHS and Community Care Act, 1990). It radically altered the organisation and delivery of community services to enable people to live as normal a life as possible in their own homes. Local government became the lead agency for assessing individual need for personal social services, designing care arrangements and securing their delivery within available resources.

Today health care in both hospital and community settings is the responsibility of the NHS and remains publicly funded by central government. Access to NHS services is now based on health need rather than ideas about sickness vs infirmity. While there is no legal definition of a health need, contemporary government guidance contends it is one 'related to the treatment, control or management of a disease, illness, injury or disability, and the care or after-care of a person with these needs (whether or not the tasks involved have to be carried out by a health professional)' (Department of Health and Social Care, 2018, p. 17).

Since the implementation of the 2012 Health and Social Care Act, funding for health care has moved from the Department of Health and Social Care to the NHS Commissioning Board to local clinical commissioning groups (CCGs) (Health and Social Care Act, 2012). In April 2020 there were 135 CCGs in England (NHS Clinical Commissioners, 2020). These organisations are responsible for buying services to meet the needs of their local community, including hospital services and targeted community health services such as palliative care, physiotherapy, podiatry, speech and language therapy, district nursing and wheelchair services. In addition, some CCGs have responsibility for the commissioning and contract management of primary care services, including community pharmacy, community dentistry and general practice. To give patients more choice over their care and make greater use of competition to improve outcomes, services can be purchased from any provider who meets NHS standards and costs.

CCGs are also responsible for funding social care services to individuals with significant health-related care needs and who are eligible for NHS continuing health care. However, most state-funded social care is commissioned and paid for by local governments, who have a duty to ensure people in their areas are able to access and afford the care services they need. Like health needs, there is no legal definition of social care needs. However, the 2014 Care Act set out national eligibility criteria for care and support to judge when someone has eligible needs the local authority must address, subject to means where applicable (Care Act, 2014). These criteria propose an individual has eligible needs where their needs arise from or relate to a physical or mental impairment or illness that results in them being unable to achieve two or more of the following outcomes that have or are likely to have a significant impact on their well-being:

- Managing and maintaining nutrition
- Maintaining personal hygiene
- Managing toilet needs
- Being appropriately clothed
- Being able to make use of the home safely
- Maintaining a habitable home environment
- Developing and maintaining family or other personal relationships
- Accessing and engaging in work, training, education or volunteering
- Making use of necessary facilities or services in the local community
- Carrying out any caring responsibilities the adult has for a child

To fund means-tested support, local governments rely on a combination of grant funding from central government, council tax, business rate revenues and funding streams such as parking charges. This means some councils have more money to dedicate to social care than others. Prior to the COVID-19 pandemic, a number of local councils were reportedly close to financial collapse and feared social care provision for older adults was no longer sustainable (National Audit Office, 2018).

Social care services are commissioned from the independent sector. Local governments are also responsible for contracting public health services, including most sexual health services, services aimed at reducing drug and alcohol use and services allied to health such as sports and recreation.

While CCGs and local authorities are the two main commissioners of health and social care services, there are also opportunities for some service users to commission their own care using personal health budgets and direct payments. Personal health budgets are relatively new in the NHS, but direct payments in social care have a longer history. In social care, a personal budget is the overall cost of the care and support the local authority provides or arranges for a service user. Direct payments are a funding choice and allow service users to purchase their own care and support services. Initially, people aged 18–65 years who were assessed as needing community services were eligible. Services were then extended to older people and carers in 2001. Personal health budgets operate in much the same way and allow patients to manage their own health care and to purchase treatments, equipment and nursing care. Eligible individuals include adults who receive NHS continuing health care.

The distinction between health and social care systems and the concomitant need to define areas of responsibility has led to both inefficiencies and a fragmented system of care. Timely and safe transitions are imperative to ensure older people receive the support they require in the right place and at the right time, moving quickly and seamlessly across services and settings as their needs change. This includes changeovers between hospital and community settings and changeovers between health and social care providers. In relation to the former, research has consistently demonstrated the transfer of older patients from hospital to the community can be problematic, with older people sent home without adequate arrangements for their continuing medical, nursing and personal care (Age UK, 2019). Similarly, evidence suggests older people often find the experience of moving between health and social care providers confusing, with duplicated assessments and visits from multiple different providers (Ellins et al., 2012).

Successive governments have introduced initiatives to break down the boundary that exists between hospital and community providers and the health and social care systems. For example, to facilitate transition across the hospital

and community interface, attempts have been made to strengthen out-of-hospital provision and develop services to reduce hospital admission and facilitate timely discharge. These services include walk-in centres, minor injuries units and urgent care centres. They also include intermediate care services, which were developed as part of the 2000 NHS Plan (Department of Health, 2000) and were one of the national standards in the 2001 National Service Framework for Older People (Department of Health, 2001). Meanwhile, in 2015, NHS England invited individual organisations and partnerships to apply to become 'vanguards' for a new models of care programmes as a step toward delivering improvement and integration of services (NHS, 2016a).

Despite these efforts, many commentators argue boundary issues will be resolved only by wholesale change involving parity of funding and the merger of the two systems. At the time of writing, the 2020 Coronavirus Act remained in effect (Coronavirus Act, 2020). This temporary emergency legislation was enacted to enable public bodies to respond to the pandemic in the context of reduced capacity due to staff sickness and a surge in social care demand. It suspended and modified some of the duties of local governments under the 2014 Care Act and allowed them to prioritise care and support packages for people with the most urgent and serious social care needs (Care Act, 2014). The pandemic worsened the financial situation of many local councils, leading to concerns there will be limited reintroduction of duties suspended or modified by the Coronavirus Act and an attendant risk older people will not get the care they need to live safely, independently or comfortably at home or that family and friends will be called on to shoulder more of the burden as eligibility shifts to older people assessed as having the most severe needs. At the time of writing, the consequences of the pandemic on the funding and organisation of health and social care services are not known. However, government plans for improved integration and increased political control were announced in early 2021.

THE HEALTH AND SOCIAL CARE NEEDS OF OLDER PEOPLE LIVING AT HOME

In 1948, 48% of the United Kingdom population died before the age of 65 (Kings Fund, 2014), and life expectancy at birth was 66 years for men and 70 years for women (Office of Health Economics, 2008). In contrast, in 2017, 14% of the population died before the age of 65 (Office for National Statistics, 2018a), and life expectancy at birth reached 79.6 years for men and 83.2 years for women (Public Health England, 2018).

Increasing longevity is undoubtedly a public health success story; however, not everyone experiences a healthy and independent old age. Improvements in healthy life expectancy and disability-free life expectancy have failed to keep pace with increases in life expectancy. For example, in the period 2015–2017, across the United Kingdom, men could expect to live only 63.1 years in good health and women to 63.6 years; similarly, disability-free life expectancy for men was 62.7 years and women 61.9 years (Office for National Statistics, 2018b). Furthermore, healthy life expectancy across local authority areas varied by 21.5 years for women and 15.8 years for men (Office for National Statistics, 2018b).

There is a strong link between years not in good health and/or years with a disability and social inequalities. The life course approach suggests an individual's health as they grow older is largely dependent on their health throughout their lives. This is influenced by the cumulative effect of social, economic and environmental conditions in which people are born, grow, live, work and age (Marmot, 2010). Individuals who experience the worst health are often those living in marginalised communities, such as Black, Asian and minority ethnic older people, people with cognitive impairment, and people living in areas where there are high levels of socioeconomic deprivation.

Nurses who work in community settings need to be able to provide care and support to older people with diverse health care needs and differing personal and social circumstances. This section examines the nursing needs of older people with multimorbidity and/or frailty. The rationale for selecting these conditions for special consideration was twofold; first because they are associated with high levels of morbidity and mortality, and second because they are affected by socioeconomic status. The section also explores loneliness among older people. While research has shown loneliness is prevalent throughout society, its health impacts on older people are widely acknowledged.

Multimorbidity and Frailty: Implications for Community Nursing Practice

Multimorbidity refers when two or more conditions exist in the same person at the same time (British Geriatric Society, 2012). It is estimated 50% of older people have at least two chronic conditions (Salive, 2013); however, prevalence rates are disputed due to the cut-off point taken for the number of diagnoses and the range of health conditions considered. Some comorbidities happen entirely by chance; at other times one condition directly effects the onset of the other. For example, the stresses associated with a diagnosis of diabetes can predispose a person to anxiety or depression. Multimorbidity is associated with increased risk of hospital admission, reduced quality of life, decline in the ability to perform activities of daily living, polypharmacy and increased mortality (National Institute for Health and Care Excellence [NICE], 2017). An association has also

been found between multimorbidity and frailty and high levels of social isolation and loneliness.

Attempts to improve the care of patients with long-term conditions have centred on developing guidelines to implement standardised care for each disease. While people with single conditions benefit from a highly specialised but isolated approach, strengthening person-centred care, multidisciplinary teamwork and care coordination have been identified as the preferred approaches to managing multimorbidity. Researchers, practitioners and policy makers agree care for people with multimorbidity should be overseen by a single individual case manager to ensure it is integrated and activity managed. This person can be a nurse, social worker or allied healthcare professional. The Case Management Society of America (2017) described case management as a collaborative process of assessment, planning, facilitation, care coordination, evaluation and advocacy for options and services to meet a patient's and family's comprehensive health needs through communication and available resources. Key domains within the case management competencies framework include leading complex care coordination; proactively managing complex long-term conditions; managing cognitive impairment and mental well-being; supporting self-care and self-management and enabling independence; professional practice and leadership; identifying high-risk patients, promoting health and preventing ill health; managing care at the end of life; and interagency and partnership work (NHS Modernisation Agency and Skills for Health, 2005).

Frailty is defined as a distinctive health state or syndrome related to the ageing process in which multiple body systems gradually lose their in-built reserves (British Geriatric Society, 2014). Around 10% of people over 65 years old have frailty, rising to between 25% and 50% of those aged over 85 (British Geriatric Society, 2014). Older people living with frailty report fatigue, unintended weight loss, diminished strength, reduced ability to recover from illness and adverse reactions to new medication. Like multimorbidity, it is associated with disability, hospitalisation and death. New perspectives on frailty are discussed in more detail in Chapter 6.

Identifying older people living with frailty is key to ensuring those at risk are supported on the basis of their needs. Contact between a health-care practitioner and an older person should include a frailty assessment. Various frailty assessment tools are available, such as PRISMA, the Edmonton Frail Scale and the clinical frailty scale. The latter defines someone who is moderately frail as someone who experiences difficulty with stairs, bathing and housekeeping and who needs help with all outside activities (Rockwood et al., 2005). Such patients would have once been identified as being infirm and in need of the care and attention of local government. Today frailty is recognised as a health need and one that benefits from an integrated response that involves general practice, community nursing services, allied health care professionals and social care providers. Interventions to reduce the impact of frailty include strength and balance training to increase muscle strength and functional abilities, nutritional interventions to address impaired nutrition and weight loss, strengthening community networks and identifying patients at the end of life.

Loneliness: Implications for Community Nursing Practice

Loneliness has been identified as a significant risk to the quality of life of older people and an important field for public health intervention. Loneliness is defined as a subjective negative feeling that can encompass emotional loneliness (e.g., the absence of a significant other such as a partner or close friend) and social loneliness (e.g., the absence of a social network such as a wider group of friends and neighbours). Between 2016 and 2017, the Community Life Survey found one in nine people aged 55 years and over reported feeling lonely always or often, and an additional four in nine reported feeling lonely some of the time (Office for National Statistics, 2018c). Risk factors include limited opportunities for meaningful work post retirement, income poverty, fear of crime in local neighbourhoods, difficulty accessing public transport, impaired mobility, sensory difficulties such as hearing loss, cognitive impairment, reduced access to information technology and old age discrimination/stigma.

Loneliness is associated with premature mortality and excessive morbidity (Neigh-Hunt et al., 2017). (See Chapter 2 for an in-depth discussion of loneliness and older people.) The reasons are multifactorial and include poor treatment adherence, depression, smoking, excessive alcohol consumption, obesity, high cholesterol, high blood pressure, raised stress hormones and poor immune function. Loneliness is also associated with increased visits to general practitioners. Given these adverse outcomes, nurses have a role to play in the identification of loneliness and in connecting older people to community groups and services. In some areas, CCGs commission social prescribing schemes, which employ link workers to introduce patients to non-clinical support services. These might include group interventions such as day centres, luncheon clubs and groups that focus on shared interests; individual interventions such as befriending programmes or animal companion schemes; or computer-based interventions such as computer training or the provision of tablets to provide older people with virtual contact with family and friends.

Evaluations of interventions to address loneliness show there is no one-size-fits-all approach, and interventions need to be tailored to suit the needs of individuals, specific groups or the degree of loneliness experienced.

An alternative to individual or group interventions is the population health or social-ecological approach, where emphasis is placed on improving the health outcomes of an entire population (i.e., local, regional or national) and the idea behaviours both shape and are shaped by the environment. One such approach is the Age Friendly Cities initiative (World Health Organization, 2007), where people of all ages are able to actively participate in all aspects of community life and can stay connected to people who are important to them. The creation of such an environment requires action on the part of individuals, organisations and local and national governments. It also requires a commitment to listening to and engaging with older people to understand their needs and preferences. Such preferences might be for more green spaces, toilets and seating in public spaces; affordable and accessible housing and transport; and flexible paid job opportunities.

THE HEALTH AND SOCIAL CARE NEEDS OF CARERS FOR OLDER PEOPLE LIVING AT HOME

As the situation of older people changed over the past 70 years, so too did the situation of their carers. Despite concerns the rise of the welfare state would result in the decline of care by families and neighbours, both still play a major role in meeting the needs of older people. However, the circumstances under which many carers meet these needs have changed. These include declining family size, rising mobility and the increased participation of women in the labour market. While women remain more likely than men to be carers, older people themselves often provide care as spouse/partner carers. Other groups with increased propensity to care include Bangladeshi, Pakistani and Indian people, due to socioeconomic factors such as differing levels of employment, cultural factors such as three-generation households and higher levels of ill health and disability among older dependents. This section explores the effect of caring on the health and well-being of carers and considers the implications of increasing levels of carer burden for community nursing practice. For further discussion of family carers, see Chapter 13.

Carer Burden: Implications for Nursing Community Practice

The care provided by family and friends for older people ranges from keeping an eye on and keeping company to assistance with housekeeping, laundry, shopping and paperwork. It can also involve the provision of personal care, such as assistance with washing and dressing. Family and friends often provide a substantial number of hours of care per week. According to data from the Family Resources Survey 2013–2014 (New Policy Institute, 2016), 26% of carers provided less than 5 hours a week care, and a further 19% provided fewer than 10 hours a week. At the opposite end of the scale, 38% provided at least 20 hours per week of support. However, the COVID-19 pandemic had a significant impact on carers and the care they provide. For example, many carers increased the level of care and support they provide to protect the older person from being exposed to service providers who might carry the virus. In other cases, they increased the level of care and support they provide due to workforce shortages. For instance, there is anecdotal evidence of carers who would not otherwise have wished to administer subcutaneous injections for symptom management at the end of life feeling obligated, as nurses could not attend due to sickness.

For many, caring can be a positive experience; however, the role can be challenging and can negatively impact on many aspects of the carer's life. First, it can have financial consequences. Combining work and caring responsibilities is often difficult due to problems with the coordination of care and inflexibility in employment. Second, caring can have health and well-being consequences. In terms of health, carers report problems such as tiredness due to interrupted sleep, physical injury from patient moving and handling, anxiety and depression, increased susceptibility to illness and deterioration in existing health conditions. In terms of well-being, caring can lead to social isolation as it can be difficult to leave the house, sustain friendships and maintain activities previously enjoyed. Feelings of loneliness were likely to have been intensified by the COVID-19 pandemic.

Carers are not a homogenous group. Different backgrounds, personal situations and relationships with the person being cared for result in different needs and priorities. However, research suggests carers value support to keep a normal home routine; being spoken to about their needs; help with their mental health; information about carer breaks and respite; help identifying, anticipating, and preventing crises; and help accessing support to manage care alongside paid employment and child care responsibilities (Department of Health, 2014a).

Self-identification as a carer can be difficult, as many see their relationship with the person they care for as being that of a child, sibling, neighbour or spouse/partner. Therefore, identification by community nurses is especially important. Once someone is identified and recorded as a carer, their expert knowledge about the person they care for is more likely to be acknowledged, and they can begin to access different forms of support. For example, their GP practice should register them as a carer to ensure they get appointments at convenient times and are offered annual health checks and free influenza vaccinations. Carers may also be eligible for a range of benefits, including Carer's Allowance, Carer's Credit, Carer's Premium and Pension Credit.

The 2014 Care Act strengthened the rights and recognition of adult carers in England, giving them specific rights to personal budgets, direct payments, information and advice, assessment and support to maintain their health and well-being (Care Act, 2014). Dame Philippa Russell, chair of the Standing Commission on Carers, said of the legislation, 'At last, carers will be given the same recognition, respect and parity of esteem with those they support. Historically, many carers have felt that their roles and their own wellbeing have been undervalued and under-supported. Now we have a once in a lifetime opportunity to be truly acknowledged and valued as expert partners in care' (Department of Health, 2014b, p. 1).

Anyone can request a statutory carer's assessment. The local authority area where the person who receives care lives is responsible for assessing the needs of the carer and providing support to them. After the assessment, the local authority confirms whether they have eligible care and support needs. If eligible, help might include the following:

- Money to pay for things that make caring easier
- Respite care and short breaks
- Referral to local support groups
- Support to attend medical appointments
- Support if the carer needs to go into hospital
- Training (e.g., moving and handling)
- Help with housework or gardening
- Buying a laptop so they can keep in touch with family
- Membership at a gym so they can look after their own health

However, there are a number of reasons why carers may decline an assessment: they may not see the point; they might think their fitness to be a carer is being tested; they may not understand what is on offer to them as carers; and they may feel uncomfortable talking about themselves rather than the care recipient. These barriers have important implications for nurses, who have a role to play in explaining why a formal conversation about their need for support is a valuable exercise. Prior to the assessment, nurses can also encourage carers to think about various aspects of their caring role: whether they have enough information about being a carer, if they feel physically capable of caring, whether caring causes them sleepless nights or feelings of loneliness or being overwhelmed, and what types of support might make things a little easier.

HEALTH AND SOCIAL CARE SERVICES

Older adults access health and social care services more frequently than younger individuals. This section provides an overview of some of these services and describes how they are organised, funded, accessed and resourced. Like younger people, most older people do not want to simply sit back and let others do what they think is best. They have their own views and priorities. We explore the experiences and preferences of service users and examine the extent to which services respond to and focus on the needs of older people and their carers.

General Practice

In England the vast majority of the population are registered with a general practice. Roles performed by general practitioners (GPs) include consultations, prescriptions, treatments, referrals, screening and immunisations, management of long-term conditions and health promotion. To become a GP, doctors need to complete a 3-year specialist training course in general practice in addition to their 5-year degree in medicine and 2-year foundation course of general training.

The 1948 NHS Act divided the medical profession into salaried employees (i.e., hospital specialists and consultants) and independent contractors (i.e., GPs). As independent contractors, the NHS or CCGs specify what work GPs are required to undertake and fund this work through arrangements known as the general medical services (GMS) contract, which is negotiated nationally, or a personal medical service contract, which is negotiated locally. Independent contractors can be single-handed, partnerships or other types of limited companies. GP partnerships comprising four to six GPs, each with a practice list of approximately 1,800 patients, are the most common configuration. After qualification, GPs apply to become a GP partner, meaning they are self-employed and receive a share of the partnership, or a salaried GP, meaning they are employed by GP partners.

In England general practice provides over 300 million consultations every year compared with 23 million emergency visits (NHS, 2017a). However, it is a service under growing pressure from increasing demand and funding shortages. While data from the National Centre for Social Research's British Social Attitudes survey suggests general practice is consistently the most popular part of the NHS, satisfaction with GP services fell to 65% in 2017, the lowest level since the survey began in 1983 (Robertson et al., 2018). Important drivers of satisfaction among older people include doctor communication and the helpfulness of reception staff (Paddison et al., 2015).

The General Practice Forward View (NHS, 2016b) set out a road map for reinvention, including an expanded and upskilled workforce, greater investment in technology and extended access to out-of-hours and urgent care services. In terms of an expanded and upskilled workforce, general practice is increasingly introducing non-medical roles. These include physicians' associates, practice nurses and advanced nurse practitioners.

The physicians associate is a relatively new role. They are health care practitioners who have undergone education and training to diagnose, treat and refer patients with a range of acute and long-term conditions. In contrast, the practice nurse is the longest standing non-medical member of the general practice team. Their main areas of responsibility include long-term conditions management, cervical cytology, screening for disease risk factors, travel health, immunisation, smoking cessation, wound care, ear care and contraceptive care. In addition to practice nurses, some general practices also employ advanced nurse practitioners. Advanced nurse practitioners are educated at master's level in generalist clinical practice and have been assessed as competent in practice using their clinical knowledge and skills. They have freedom and authority to act, making autonomous decisions in the assessment, diagnosis and treatment of patients. Key competencies for the general practice workforce include business acumen and a clear understanding of the practice's commitments under the Quality and Outcomes Framework (QOF). The QOF is a fundamental part of the GMS contract and is designed to financially reward practices for providing good quality patient care. Non-medical practitioners have a vital role in meeting QOF targets that pertain to diabetes and other long-term conditions.

In terms of technology, the use of phone triage has been commonplace in general practice for many years. However, in order to meet the demand for faster access to healthcare, NHS (2016b) encouraged the use of remote systems to conduct full consultations. Online video use grew exponentially in general practice during the COVID-19 pandemic. However, a formal physical examination cannot be performed during a video consultation, which poses a potential threat to patient safety. Risks need to be identified and managed. Furthermore, there is a paucity of research exploring the acceptability of video consultations among older people.

To extend access to out-of-hours and urgent care services, the General Practice Forward View proposed the creation of local clinical hubs, but it did not address the controversial issue of GP home visits. The GP-led home visit is well established in current practice and highly valued by older people and their carers. However, research into the effects of GP-led home visits on physical functioning, hospital avoidance and mortality among older people has shown inconsistent results (Mitchell et al., 2019). GPs also often argue they are too busy to conduct them. To that end, at the Local Medical Committee Conference in November 2019, a motion was passed to instruct the General Practitioners Committee to remove home visits from core contract work. Currently, it seems unlikely they will disappear, but they might be increasingly delegated to another health care professional such as an advanced nurse practitioner or community paramedic or in some instances substituted with video consultations.

District Nursing Services

Approximately 20% of NHS spending on community health services is on district nursing services, which equates to about 2% of the total NHS budget (Department of Health and Social Care, 2015). These services are commissioned by CCGs to deliver a wide range of nursing interventions to people living in their own homes: bowel care and continence management, end-of-life care, intravenous therapy, enteral feeding, wound care, urinary catheterisation and ongoing catheter management, and support for self-management. Some district nursing services are provided by standalone community NHS trusts, some are provided by combined community and acute or mental health trusts, and others are provided by charities, social enterprises or private sector providers. District nurses work in skill-mixed teams, which comprise district nurses (i.e., nurses with an adult nursing qualification and an additional specialist practitioner qualification in district nursing recordable with the Nursing and Midwifery Council), community staff nurses and health care support workers. Teams work geographically and/or by GP attachment. As well as a core daytime offer, many provide evening and overnight nursing care, for example for the very old.

Patients are usually eligible for district nursing care only if they are housebound due to a physical or psychological illness. Referrals are received from hospitals, health and social care professionals and patients and carers. Their caseloads are mostly made up of patients over 65. As generalists, district nurses are competent in several different fields and activities and are well placed to undertake the case management and care coordination of older people with multimorbidity and frailty. This includes interacting with clinical specialist nurses, including palliative care nurses, tissue viability nurses, admiral nurses, diabetes nurses and respiratory nurses. They also have an important role to play supporting carers.

At their best, district nurses are experts in delivering person-centred care in the home, adapting care according to the patient's condition and preferences, the home environment and the equipment available. For example, circumstances may be such that during the period of active dying, while pressure ulcer prevention is important,

comfort and the patient's and carer's preferences may override implementation of active prevention strategies. Suggesting or making too many changes at once, particularly in a new, complex and personal situation, may be stressful for the patient. It may also be interpreted as interference of a painful reminder of the loss of independence and deterioration in health, or it may threaten the balance of a relationship where the carer's role is sustained by looking after a dependent member of the family. Improvisation and the imaginative use of available equipment and resources are also important—for example, using a wire coat hanger to make a catheter stand—and a willingness to go the extra mile for patients, such as going to the local shop to buy bread and milk for individuals whose cupboards are unexpectedly empty or charging electricity metre keys when accommodation is found to be dangerously cold and damp.

In 2016 the Kings Fund published the findings from an investigation into district nursing care from the perspectives of patients, carers and staff. On the one hand, it painted a picture of services that delivered an ideal model of person-centred, preventative and coordinated care that reduced hospital admissions and helped people to stay at home. On the other, it highlighted concerns about increased activity levels and decreased staff numbers and evoked an image of a task-focused and solely reactive service where there was a lack of continuity of care and where staff were rushed and brusque with patients. The authors recommended greater recognition of the vital strategic importance of community health services in transforming the health and social care system, the creation of a sustainable district nursing workforce and the development of strategies for monitoring resources, activity and workforce (Kings Fund, 2016).

One promising approach to improving the delivery of community nursing is the Buurtzorg model, an approach founded in the Netherlands in 2006 in response to increasing levels of disillusionment among the nursing workforce, declining patient experiences and concerns about fragmentation of care. The Buurtzorg model has four key missions: to take a holistic approach, to bring a neighbourhood approach, to maximise patient independence and to rely on the professionalism of nurses. The first mission is pursued by nurses taking a person-centred approach to assessing patients' nursing and personal/social care needs and providing a full range of services from meal preparation to intravenous therapy. The second mission is pursued through the establishment of small caseloads and a focus on building community capacity. In terms of the latter, the microscale of the teams allows members to know and use local resources and to build and support informal networks such as voluntary services and/or good neighbouring schemes. The third mission is achieved through front loading care—intensively teaching and supporting patients from the first visit. The final mission is achieved through the avoidance of all forms of central management and the creation of self-governing teams where individuals work on the basis of consent.

In the Netherlands, evaluations of the Buurtzorg model found patient satisfaction scores were 30% above the industry average, episodes of care were 2 months shorter than the industry average and staff turnover was 5% less than the industry average (Centre for Public Impact, 2020). These achievements provoked interest among policy makers in other countries, including in the United Kingdom. Findings from an evaluation of an early pilot project in an NHS trust in South London indicated an improved patient experience when comparing a variant of the Buurtzorg model to routine community nursing services. However, while staff reportedly enjoyed the autonomy afforded in clinical decision making, they highlighted challenges pertaining to the extent to which the wider organisation recognised the concept of the self-governing team (Drennan et al., 2017). Similarly, an evaluation of the implementation of a community nursing approach based on the Buurtzorg model in East London found patient experience of the service was largely positive; however, nurses felt their ability to exercise professional autonomy was constrained by the wider organisation's reluctance to delegate responsibility for aspects of the service management (Lalani et al., 2019). Despite these limitations, application of the Buurtzorg model in East London serves as an example of integrated commissioning in a vanguard site.

Allied Health Care Professionals

Allied health care professionals in community settings include speech and language therapists, occupational therapists and physiotherapists. Speech and language therapists work with people to help them communicate effectively. They also work with people who have eating and swallowing problems. Occupational therapists help people overcome the effects of disability caused by physical or psychological illness; for an older person, this may include working together to find ways of having more social contact or recommending changes to the home environment to promote independence. Physiotherapists use skills such as manual therapy and therapeutic exercise. Together with occupational therapists, physiotherapists have an important role to play in fall prevention for older people who live at home. Speech and language therapists and physiotherapists are employed by health care organisations. In contrast, occupational therapists are employed by health care organisations and by local governments; depending on a patient's situation and needs, they receive a health occupational therapist or a local government occupational therapist.

Community Pharmacy

The NHS Community Pharmacy Contractual Framework consists of three levels of services: essential services, advanced services and enhanced and locally commissioned services. Essential services include the dispensing of medication, advanced services include medicine-use reviews, and enhanced and locally commissioned services include NHS Health Checks for people aged 40–74 years and seasonal influenza vaccination services. In addition, many pharmacies provide repeat prescription delivery services, whereby they contact the prescriber and obtain the repeat prescription and then send them to the patient when they need them. Others supply medicines in blister packs or monitored dosage systems to promote medication adherence and concordance. There are also examples of clinical pharmacists working in GP practices to resolve issues with medicines, including liaising with hospitals to ensure correct medicine follow-up on discharge and leading on high-risk prescribing (e.g., methotrexate and warfarin) to ensure patient safety.

Community Care Assessors

Community care assessors are responsible for assessing whether someone has eligible care and support needs the local authority must address, subject to means where appropriate. These roles are usually undertaken by either a social worker or occupational therapist. Where possible, the assessor diverts people to existing community resources; however, when eligible needs are identified, the assessor devises a personalised care and support plan with the individual that describes how these needs may be met—for example, through the provision of traditional services such as care homes, day centres, equipment and adaptations, community meals and home care or more novel approaches such as gym membership, art therapy, personal assistants and classes or courses. The assessor also calculates the sum of money to be allocated by the local authority for services to meet their care needs. This is referred to as a personal budget. The individual can choose to have their personal budget managed by the local authority, who will arrange all the care and support based on the agreed care plan. Alternatively, the individual can ask that the money be paid to another organisation, such as a care provider, or be paid directly to them or to someone they choose to purchase their own care and support services.

Home Care Services

Home care services were introduced as part of the 1990 NHS and Community Care Act (NHS and Community Care Act 1990). They replaced home help services, whose role had been to provide domestic assistance such as cleaning, making beds, lighting fires and washing laundry. Home carers perform the types of personal care activities that would previously have been provided in care homes or long-stay hospitals; for example, assistance with personal toilet (i.e., washing, bathing, skin care and grooming), eating and drinking (i.e., preparing and serving meals), maintaining continence and managing incontinence, managing problems associated with immobility, managing prescribed treatment (e.g., prompting medication) and ensuring personal safety. To access publically funded home care services, the individual must have a community needs assessment and the need for home care added to the care and support plan. For those who choose to have their personal budget managed by the local authority, the local authority commissions independent sector home care providers on a rate per hour or time-and-task approach. In 2015 it was estimated 350,000 older people were in receipt of home care services in England, of whom 257,000 had their care paid for by the local government (Kings Fund, 2018).

Home care quality is far from uniform. According to a literature review conducted by the National Institute for Health and Care Excellence (NICE, 2015), service users valued home carers who demonstrated kindness, friendliness and gentleness and who were competent and professional. However, service users also raised concerns about 15-minute appointments, which meant home carers were rushed and had little time to meet their needs. In response to concerns about attitudes, some providers introduced values-based recruitment strategies. However, given many home carers are employed on zero hours contracts and paid only the minimum wage, the impact of such strategies is potentially limited. In relation to flying visits, the NICE (2016) recommended visits should be at least 30 minutes in duration to ensure outcomes can be achieved in a way that does not compromise the dignity of the service user. However, in 2017, a survey suggested up to 20% of local authorities were still commissioning 15-minute visits (Leonard Cheshire, 2018).

Some alternatives to home care have been identified. For example, telecare has a potential role to play in minimising risk and providing urgent notifications of adverse events. Telecare technologies include personal alarms, bed and chair occupancy sensors, bogus caller buttons, carbon monoxide monitors, fall detectors, fire and smoke alarms, flood detectors, gas shut-off valves, incontinence sensors, medication prompt devices and property exit sensors. Shared lives and home share models have also been identified as alternatives to home care. The former matches an older person with an approved carer, who then shares their home, family and community network and gives care and support to the older person in return for a weekly fee. The latter is when an older person with a spare room is matched with someone who is in need of low-cost accommodation in return for help with household tasks.

Intermediate Care Services

Intermediate care is an intensive form of non-means-tested, short-term support. It is offered when an older person is assessed as having potential to improve and live more independently—for example, someone who has been in hospital and needs help to recover their independence or someone who is experiencing increasing difficulty with activities of daily living through illness or disability. Intermediate care services can be commissioned by either health or social care or jointly as part of an integrated approach.

There are four types of intermediate care. The first is reablement, which provides support in the home to improve the person's self-confidence and ability to live independently. Service user goals are usually related to personal care activities or engagement in social activities. Specially trained support staff, akin to advanced home carers, focus on observing, guiding, and encouraging the service user rather than on delivering hands-on care. The second is home-based intermediate care, which includes the provision of multidisciplinary health and social care team interventions—for example, a physiotherapist to deliver tailored strength-based exercises, an occupational therapist to recommend home adaptations and a nurse to administer a short course of intravenous antibiotics. The third is bed-based intermediate care, which involves a temporary stay in a care home or community hospital and interventions much like those offered in home-based intermediate care. For patients who receive reablement, home-based intermediate care and bed-based intermediate care, interventions are provided for up to 6 weeks. Finally, crisis response offers prompt assessment of people who experience an urgent increase in their health and social care needs, and the cause of the deterioration has been identified. Crisis response teams are usually comprised of health care professionals who may provide short-term interventions up to 48 hours.

During the COVID-19 pandemic, as hospital wards were turned into intensive care units, intermediate care services came under intense pressure. For example, HM Government (2020) published guidance requiring hospitals to discharge all patients as soon as it was clinically safe to do so in order to free up at least 15,000 beds by March 27, 2020. The guidance also asked health and social care providers to free up community hospital and intermediate care beds that could be used flexibly for non-invasive respiratory support during the height of the pandemic. At the time of writing, intermediate care services have not returned to a normal way of working.

To work effectively in intermediate care, nurses need to possess the right attributes and skills. According to NICE (2018), the key principles that underpin the delivery of an effective intermediate care service include building an equal partnership with patients (i.e., discovering what motivates them and what goals they want to achieve), concentrating on patient strengths (i.e., what the person is able to do and optimising these abilities), building resilience and confidence (i.e., identifying interventions that will help the person feel more able to complete activities of daily living), observing and encouraging even when the person finds an activity difficult and wants the practitioner to take over, and supporting positive risk-taking (i.e., recognising the benefits of taking risks and the harm associated with their avoidance). In terms of skills, nurses who work in intermediate care need to be able to perform a holistic and patient-centred assessment, considering areas that might previously have been the preserve of one professional group: physical and mental health and emotional well-being; protection from abuse and neglect; education, training and recreation; domestic, family and personal relationships; contribution made to society; securing rights and entitlements; and social and economic well-being.

INVOLVEMENT OF OLDER PEOPLE IN PLANNING AND DESIGNING SERVICES

Patients, carers, parents and advocates of the sick and vulnerable should have input into the kind of health services we have. They should be involved in the design of those services. They should help to set the standards by which services are judged, and help to assess whether a particular aspect of the service meets those standards. At every stage, the users of the health service should be offered the opportunity to play an active part in developing, delivering and evaluating their service. After all, it is their (i.e., our) taxes which pay for it and their (our) lives which are at stake if things go wrong. (Greenhalgh et al., 2011, p 1).

Patient-centred care is where nurses consciously adopt the patient's perspective and mainstream them through all aspects of the health care system and its processes. To help navigate the system through the patient's eyes, nurses need to involve older people and carers in planning and designing community services. The preceding section highlighted how service users should be involved at an individual level in planning and designing their own care. In this section we explore the ways in which older people and carers can have a direct voice in decisions about service provision at strategic and community levels.

It has long been held that citizen participation is a key component of democracy. Given approaches led by professionals are often limited by a lack of understanding of the lived experiences of service users and carers, the primary benefit of service user engagement is the development of more appropriate services. Service user involvement also offers health and well-being benefits by increasing social capital and developing new skills and confidence among those involved.

Under the Health and Social Care Act of 2012, CCGs and the NHS have duties to involve the public in commissioning decision making (Health and Social Care Act, 2012). Service user engagement can be used to

- Identify and assess what people want and need from health and social care.
- Decide priorities and develop strategies and plans (e.g., through feedback on joint strategic needs assessments).
- Design pathways and services (e.g., service specifications).
- In tendering and contracting processes, provide feedback on existing services (e.g., through surveys and inspections). (NHS, 2017b)

It can also include lay involvement in governance, including formal assurance processes and performance management (e.g., through sitting as lay members of CCG governing boards).

Effective engagement requires high levels of commitment from organisations, older people and carers. Statutory requirements have driven the establishment of independent forums, older citizens' panels and supported groups to capture the views of older people. However, older people who are housebound, whose first language is not English and who experience sensory impairments, together with carers juggling employment and caring responsibilities, remain seldom-heard voices. At the same time, a recurrent theme in the service user involvement literature is a sense of tokenism (Ocloo & Matthews, 2016). This is where there is an appearance of engagement and involvement in decision making, but service users do not actually have much influence or feel patronised by health and social care professionals. Furthermore, there is a paucity of research exploring what impact service user involvement has on health and well-being outcomes for communities, particularly for older members of a community. To that end, some authors suggest older people's groups might better dedicate their time and resources to scrutiny and campaigning, independent of service providers, rather than to participating in formal activities that pertain to commissioning (Wistow et al., 2011).

CONCLUSION

Responding to the needs of older people and carers remains one of the biggest challenges faced by health and social care systems in the community. During the pandemic in 2020, the NHS was mobilised to respond to the acute needs of people infected with the virus at the same time as delivering scaled-down non–COVID-19 health care. At the time of writing, government attention is focused on minimising the risk of a second coronavirus wave and on restarting hospital health care, particularly surgical and cancer services. In general practice, digital technologies have already become part of the new normal. However, there remains no coherent plan for the social care sector, which is now reeling from the impact of the virus, with paid carers experiencing difficulties obtaining personal protective equipment, older people dying prematurely, family caregivers grieving in isolation and others unable to access community-based services. For years, social care has been positioned as the underdog in policy decisions about health and well-being. An important legacy of the pandemic must be to secure the status of social care as one equal to the NHS.

KEY LEARNING POINTS

- Health and social care for older people living at home is delivered by a wide range of organisations and professionals. To manage changeovers between hospital and community, and health and social care, nurses must span the boundaries that exist between these organisations and professionals.
- More older people are living at home with multimorbidity and frailty than ever before. Both conditions require nurses to adopt a person-centred, multidisciplinary teamwork and coordinated approach to care.
- Loneliness is a substantial threat to the health and well-being of older people living at home. Nurses play a significant role in the identification of loneliness and in connecting older people to community groups and services.
- Family caregivers play a major role in meeting the needs of older people living at home. Nurses must recognise family caregivers and engage them in discussions about the types of support that might enable them to provide optimal care.

- Historically, social care has been positioned as the underdog in policy and funding decisions about health and well-being. At an individual level, social care practitioners have not always been treated with respect for the work they do. Nurses must maintain a positive vision of social care, valuing and celebrating the contribution their social care colleagues make to successful ageing in place.
- Clinical Commissioning Groups, and their successor bodies Integrated Care Boards, are required to involve members of the public in developing, delivering and evaluating healthcare services. Nurses should contribute to developing strategies to engage older people in planning and designing services, including those who are housebound, whose first language is not English, and who experience sensory impairment, as well as carers juggling employment and caring responsibilities.

REFERENCES

Age UK. (2019). Briefing: Health and care of older people in England 2019. https://www.ageuk.org.uk/globalassets/age-uk/documents/reports-and-publications/reports-and-briefings/health--wellbeing/age_uk_briefing_state_of_health_and_care_of_older_people_july2019.pdf

British Geriatric Society. (2012). Morbidity—Comorbidity and multimorbidity. What do they mean? https://www.bgs.org.uk/resources/morbidity-comorbidity-and-multimorbidity-what-do-they-mean

British Geriatric Society. (2014). Introduction to frailty, fit for frailty (Part 1). https://www.bgs.org.uk/resources/introduction-to-frailty

Case Management Society of America. (2017). What is a case manager? https://www.cmsa.org/who-we-are/what-is-a-case-manager

Centers for Disease Control and Prevention. (2009). Healthy aging and the built environment. https://www.cdc.gov/healthyplaces/healthtopics/healthyaging.htm

Centre for Public Impact. (2020). Buurtzorg: Revolutionising home care in the Netherlands. https://www.centreforpublicimpact.org/case-study/buurtzorg-revolutionising-home-care-netherlands

Department of Health. (2000). The NHS plan: A plan for investment. A plan for reform. https://webarchive.nationalarchives.gov.uk/20130123203940/http://www.dh.gov.uk/en/Publicationsandstatistics/Publications/PublicationsPolicyAndGuidance/DH_4010198

Department of Health. (2001). National service framework for older people. https://assets.publishing.service.gov.uk/government/uploads/system/uploads/attachment_data/file/198033/National_Service_Framework_for_Older_People.pdf

Department of Health. (2014a). Carers strategy: Second national action plan 2014–2016. https://assets.publishing.service.gov.uk/government/uploads/system/uploads/attachment_data/file/368478/Carers_Strategy_-_Second_National_Action_Plan_2014_-_2016.pdf

Department of Health. (2014b). Factsheet 8: The care act—The law for carers. https://assets.publishing.service.gov.uk/government/uploads/system/uploads/attachment_data/file/268684/Factsheet_8_update__tweak_.pdf

Department of Health and Social Care. (2015). NHS reference costs 2014 to 2015. https://www.gov.uk/government/publications/nhs-reference-costs-2014-to-2015

Department of Health and Social Care. (2018). *National framework for NHS continuing healthcare and NHS-funded nursing care.* https://assets.publishing.service.gov.uk/government/uploads/system/uploads/attachment_data/file/746063/20181001_National_Framework_for_CHC_and_FNC_-_October_2018_Revised.pdf

Drennan, V., Ross, F., Saunders, M., & West, P. (2017). The Guy's and St Thomas' NHS Foundation Trust neighbourhood nursing team test and learn project of an adapted Buurtzorg model: An early view (project report). https://eprints.kingston.ac.uk/40416

Ellins, J., Glasby, J., Tanner, D., McIver, S., Davidson, D., Littlechild, R., Snelling, I., Miller, R., Hall, K., Spence, K., & the Care Transitions Project co-researchers. (2012). Understanding and improving transitions of older people: A user and carer centred approach. Final report. NIHR Service Delivery and Organisation programme.

Greenhalgh, T., Humphrey, C., & Woodward, F. (2011). *User involvement in health care*: John Wiley and Sons, Incorporated.

HM Government. (2020). *COVID-19 hospital discharge service requirements.* https://assets.publishing.service.gov.uk/government/uploads/system/uploads/attachment_data/file/880288/COVID-19_hospital_discharge_service_requirements.pdf

Kings Fund. (2014). *Making our health and care systems fit for an ageing population.* https://www.kingsfund.org.uk/sites/default/files/field/field_publication_file/making-health-care-systems-fit-ageing-population-oliver-foot-humphries-mar14.pdf

Kings Fund. (2016). *Understanding quality in district nursing services: Learning from patients, carers and staff.* https://www.kingsfund.org.uk/sites/default/files/field/field_publication_file/quality_district_nursing_aug_2016.pdf

Kings Fund. (2018). *Home care in England: Views from commissioners and providers.* https://www.kingsfund.org.uk/sites/default/files/2018-12/Home-care-in-England-report.pdf

Lalani, M., Fernandes, J., Fradgley, R., Ogunsola, C., & Marshall, M. (2019). Transforming community nursing services in the UK: Lessons from a participatory evaluation of the implementation of a new community nursing model in East London based on the principles of the Dutch Buurtzorg model. *BMC Health Services Research*(945), 19. doi.org/10.1186/s12913-019-4804-8.

Leonard Cheshire. (2018). 15-minute personal care is destroying lives. https://socialcare.leonardcheshire.org

Marmot, M. (2010). *Fair society, healthy lives: The Marmot review.* http://www.instituteofhealthequity.org/resources-reports/fair-society-healthy-lives-the-marmot-review/fair-society-healthy-lives-full-report-pdf.pdf

Mitchell, S., Hillman, S., Rapley, D., & Dale, J. (2019). GP home visits: More evidence is urgently needed to inform debate. *BJGP Life.* https://bjgplife.com/2019/12/03/gp-home-visits-more-evidence-is-urgently-needed-to-inform-debate.

National Audit Office. (2018). *Financial sustainability of local authorities 2018: Report by the comptroller and auditor general.* https://www.nao.org.uk/wp-content/uploads/2018/03/Financial-sustainabilty-of-local-authorites-2018.pdf

National Institute for Health and Care Excellence (NICE). (2015). *Home care: Delivering personal care and practical support to older people living in their own homes.* https://www.nice.org.uk/guidance/ng21/evidence/full-guideline-pdf-489149252

NICE. (2016). *Home care for older people: Quality standard [QS123].* https://www.nice.org.uk/guidance/qs123/chapter/Quality-statement-4-Length-of-home-care-visits

NICE. (2017). *Multimorbidity and polypharmacy: Key therapeutic topic (KTT18).* https://www.nice.org.uk/advice/ktt18/chapter/evidence-context

NICE. (2018). *Promoting independence through intermediate care: A quick guide for staff delivering intermediate care services.* https://www.nice.org.uk/Media/Default/About/NICE-Communities/Social-care/quick-guides/promoting-independence-through-intermediate-care.pdf

Neigh-Hunt, N., Bagguley, D., Bash, K., Turner, V., Turnbull, S., Valtorta, N., & Caan, W. (2017). An overview of systematic reviews on the public health consequences of social isolation and loneliness. *Public Health, 1152,* 157–171. doi.org/10.1016/j.puhe.2017.07.035.

New Policy Institute. (2016). *Informal carers and poverty in the UK: An analysis of the Family Resources Survey.* https://www.npi.org.uk/files/2114/6411/1359/Carers_and_poverty_in_the_UK_-_full_report.pdf

NHS Clinical Commissioners. (2020). About CCGs. https://www.nhscc.org/ccgs

NHS. (2016a). *New care models: Vanguards—developing a blueprint for the future of NHS and care services.* https://www.england.nhs.uk/wp-content/uploads/2015/11/new_care_models.pdf

NHS. (2016b). *General practice forward view.* https://www.england.nhs.uk/wp-content/uploads/2016/04/gpfv.pdf

NHS. (2017a). *Next steps on the NHS five year forward view.* https://www.england.nhs.uk/wp-content/uploads/2017/03/NEXT-STEPS-ON-THE-NHS-FIVE-YEAR-FORWARD-VIEW.pdf

NHS. (2017b). *Patient and public participation in commissioning health and care: Statutory guidance for clinical commissioning groups* and NHS England. https://www.england.nhs.uk/wp-content/uploads/2017/05/patient-and-public-participation-guidance.pdf

NHS Modernisation Agency and Skills for Health. (2005). *Case management competencies framework for the care of people with long term conditions.* Skills for Health.

Office of Health Economics. (2008). *Sixty years of the NHS: Changes in demographics, expenditure, workforce and family services.* https://www.ohe.org/system/files/private/publications/312%20-%20Sixty_Years_NHS_9-2008.pdf

Office for National Statistics. (2018a). Deaths registered in England and Wales: 2017. https://www.ons.gov.uk/peoplepopulationandcommunity/birthsdeathsandmarriages/deaths/bulletins/deathsregistrationsummarytables/2017#age-standardised-mortality-rates-continued-to-decrease-in-2017

Office for National Statistics. (2018b). Health state life expectancies, UK: 2015 to 2017. https://www.ons.gov.uk/peoplepopulationandcommunity/healthandsocialcare/healthandlifeexpectancies/bulletins/healthstatelifeexpectanciesuk/2015to2017

Office for National Statistics. (2018c). Loneliness—What characteristics and circumstances are associated with feeling lonely? https://www.ons.gov.uk/peoplepopulationandcommunity/wellbeing/articles/lonelinesswhatcharacteristicsandcircumstancesareassociatedwithfeelinglonely/2018-04-10

Ocloo, J. & Matthews, R. (2016). From tokenism to empowerment: progressing patient and public involvement in healthcare improvement. BMJ Quality and Safety, 1–7. https://doi.org/10.1136/bmjqs-2015-004839

Paddison, C., Abel, G., Roland, M., Elliott, M., Lyratzopoulous, G., & Campbell, J. (2015). Drivers of overall satisfaction with primary care: evidence from the English General Practice Patient Survey. *Health Expectations, 18*(5), 1081–1092.

Public Health England. (2018). *A review of recent trends in mortality in England.* https://assets.publishing.service.gov.uk/government/uploads/system/uploads/attachment_data/file/827518/Recent_trends_in_mortality_in_England.pdf

Robertson, R., Appleby, J., & Evans, H. (2018) *Public satisfaction with the NHS and social care in 2017: Results and trends from the British Social Attitudes survey.* https://www.nuffieldtrust.org.uk/files/2018-02/nut-kf-bsa-2018-web.pdf

Rockwood, K., Song, X., MacKnight, C., Bergman, H., Hogan, D., McDowell, I., & Mitnitski, A. (2005). A global clinical measure of fitness and frailty in elderly people. *Canadian Medical Association Journal, 173*(5), 489–495. doi.org.1503/10.1503/cmaj.050051.

Salive, M. (2013). Multimorbidity in older adults. *Epidemiologic Reviews, 35,* 75–83.

Wistow, G., Waddington, E., & Davey, V. (2011). *Involving older people in commissioning: More power to their elbow?* https://www.jrf.org.uk/sites/default/files/jrf/migrated/files/older-people-service-commissioning-full.pdf

World Health Organization. (2007). Global age-friendly cities: A guide. https://apps.who.int/iris/handle/10665/43755

ACTS OF PARLIAMENT

Care Act (2014): https://www.legislation.gov.uk/ukpga/2014/23/contents/enacted

Coronavirus Act (2020): https://www.legislation.gov.uk/ukpga/2020/7/contents

Health and Social Care Act (2012): https://www.legislation.gov.uk/ukpga/2012/7/contents/enacted

National Assistance Act (1948): https://www.legislation.gov.uk/ukpga/Geo6/11-12/29

NHS Act (1946): https://www.legislation.gov.uk/ukpga/1946/81/pdfs/ukpga_19460081_en.pdf

NHS and Community Care Act (1990): https://www.legislation.gov.uk/ukpga/1990/19/contents

10

Nursing Older People in Hospital

Antony Arthur

With the obvious exceptions such as children's wards and maternity units, older people increasingly account for a significant proportion of inpatients cared for by nurses who work in hospital wards. Reflecting wider demographic changes, in England the rate of hospital admission is growing, with disproportionately higher increases among older people, particularly those aged 85 years and over (Wittenberg et al., 2014). Simultaneously, the number of hospital beds has halved in the past 30 years (King's Fund, 2019).

These seemingly paradoxical shifts in demand and supply of hospital beds are partly explained by a long-standing policy to provide more treatment outside hospitals and dramatic declines in the average length of hospital stays. The time spent in hospital is longer for older people, which means older people account for a large proportion of hospital bed days. Individuals aged 65 and older occupied nearly two-thirds of all non-elective hospital bed days in England in 2013 (Wittenberg et al., 2014). Nonetheless, the increasing demand for hospital care outweighs the capacity of both hospital beds and the staff to care for them. This is felt acutely by patients, their families and carers, and the nursing teams and other health professionals responsible for their care.

Nursing older people in hospital is both highly challenging and intensely rewarding. It requires a high level of skill to care for people who are acutely unwell with pre-existing comorbidities likely to be chronic and complex. With more older patients being admitted with a greater number of comorbid conditions, frailty is likely to be highly prevalent among older people in hospital (Steventon et al., 2018). It requires empathy, resourcefulness and creativity to overcome the barriers of communication difficulties that are highly prevalent in a population at increased risk of hearing, visual and cognitive impairment. There are few areas of hospital care where effective liaison with colleagues both within and beyond the hospital is so critical in supporting patients through a complex system of interrelated acute, community and social care services.

This chapter examines the care of older people in hospital and the role of nurses in managing and delivering that care. It describes the context of acute hospital services for older people within the broader provision of health and social care services. I also explore alternatives to hospital care and describe interventions for minimising the risk of adverse outcomes of hospital admission for older people. In addition, the chapter covers good practice in assessment and discharge processes as well as the importance of, and challenges to, providing nursing care that respects the individual older person at a time when they are most vulnerable.

ADMISSION AVOIDANCE

Older people are particularly vulnerable to hospital-associated complications (Mudge et al., 2019). These include delirium from hospital-acquired infections, inpatient falls, hospital-acquired pressure ulcers and functional impairment from deconditioning. These are serious adverse events. While it is vital to avoid unnecessary hospital admissions, it is important to remember the vast majority of hospital admissions are necessary, and acute-care hospital is often the right place to treat certain conditions regardless of age. Using chronological age as a basis for rationing hospital care means making ageist assumptions about the rights and expectations of older people with health care needs.

It has been estimated from an observational study conducted in the Netherlands that around one in six admissions are preventable (van den Broek et al., 2020). The alternatives to hospital can be broadly considered under the umbrella term of 'hospital at home', whereby coordinated multidisciplinary care is provided at home with the twin goals of reducing demand on acute-care beds and reducing the risk of functional decline through the maintenance of home-based activities of daily living that cannot be undertaken in a hospital. In a systematic review of 16 randomised controlled trials, there was some evidence to suggest hospital at home, with the option to transfer to a hospital if needed, is a safe and effective alternative to acute hospital admission (Shepherd et al., 2016).

While hospital at home may be a viable alternative, other interventions may reduce the risk of hospital admission. However, the evidence for these interventions is weaker and often from studies undertaken in younger age groups. In primary care, patients who receive continuity of care by their GP may be less likely to be admitted to hospital (Tammes et al., 2017). The case-management model on which the introduction of community matrons was based in 2004 does not appear to reduce hospital admissions (Oeseburg et al., 2009), although it is valued by patients and their families and perceived as fulfilling needs that are unmet by other care services (Sandberg et al., 2014). Self-management interventions for conditions such as asthma (Hodkinson et al., 2020) and heart failure (Toukhsati et al., 2019) may also reduce admissions to hospital.

OLDER PEOPLE'S EXPERIENCES OF HOSPITAL CARE

The Challenge of Providing Compassionate Care

The long-held perception that nurses and nursing are the very embodiment of compassionate caring was rocked by the scandal at Mid-Staffordshire Hospital in England that came to light in 2008. The subsequent inquiry (Francis, 2013) found that patients, vulnerable and mostly older, had been neglected and left for long periods without being given hydration, kept clean or provided with the most basic dignity and exposed to a culture lacking in compassion. This was not a failing of nurses alone; it was a failure of leadership and systems, but it asked important and difficult questions of all levels within the profession of nursing.

What happened at Mid-Staffordshire Hospital was an extreme case of care failure, but it drew attention more broadly to the issue of older people receiving suboptimal care in hospitals. Although 81% of surveyed NHS inpatients report being always treated with dignity and respect, this still means one in five patients experience a lack of respect or a feeling of having their dignity compromised at some point during their hospital stay (Care Quality Commission, 2020). Dignity and respect are arguably more important for older patients than those in younger age groups as they are likely to be more reliant on care staff for help in maintaining their dignity.

Nursing Interventions to Improve the Care of Older People in Hospitals

A number of interventions are designed to improve the way nurses and other care staff relate to the older patients in their care and, by extension, enhance the care experience of patients themselves. A systematic review of such interventions suggests their use is often underpinned by evidence from weak study designs, and a lack of specific detail makes them difficult to deliver consistently (Blomberg et al., 2016). Nonetheless, initiatives to improve the experiences of older people inevitably require nurses and other groups to look critically at the way they communicate and care for older patients and ways in which this might be improved. Some examples of hospital-based interventions are described here.

Creating Learning Environments for Compassionate Care

Creating Learning Environments for Compassionate Care (CLECC) is a workplace learning intervention whereby the ward, as a learning environment, provides the context for building the capacity of nursing teams to deliver compassionate care (Bridges & Fuller, 2015). It draws on evidence that staff well-being is critical to the delivery of high-quality nursing care. CLECC is implemented over 4 months but designed to lead to long-term improvement. The intervention is targeted at both the team itself and the team leader and includes practice development facilitation of action learning sets, team learning, cluster discussions and peer observations of practice. An evaluation of CLECC found staff felt it improved their capacity to be compassionate, but embedding it in practice required resources and commitment from senior nurse managers (Bridges et al., 2018).

Intentional Rounding

Intentional rounding is a timed, planned intervention that sets out to address fundamental elements of nursing care by means of a regular bedside ward round by nursing staff (Harris et al., 2019). Originating in the United States, intentional rounding is a proactive form of care that aims to anticipate needs of patients rather than react to them. The content of the round may vary both within and between hospitals, but they typically include ensuring comfort through physical positioning, assessing personal needs such as toileting, checking whether the patient is in pain and making sure drinks and other items are in easy reach.

Since the publication of the Francis report, there has been widespread uptake of intentional rounding. A large evaluation study suggested intentional rounding has been inconsistently implemented (Harris et al., 2019). It may meet the need for organisations, and individuals working within them, to protect themselves against charges of insufficient staff/patient contact through systematic documentation of patient contact time, but there is little evidence it improves relationships between care staff and patients.

Older People's Shoes

Older People's Shoes is a two-day training programme for health-care assistants who work in hospitals, designed to improve the relational care they provide to older people (Wharrad et al., 2020). This two-day programme includes three elements: experiencing what it is like for older people in hospital, ways of getting to know older people better and learning from customer care practices in other sectors. It is led by in-house clinical trainers or practice development nurses using a 'train the trainer' model. The programme is based on the assumptions that care staff bring a breadth of experience, skills and knowledge about individuals they care for (i.e., asset-based) and that good relational care should be threaded through both physical and non-physical care interactions.

While the training programme has relevance beyond this particular section of the workforce, it recognises the crucial contribution health-care assistants make to the nursing teams who care for older people, and they may have specific learning needs. It uses elements of experiential learning to enable the learner to 'get into older people's shoes' and biographical approaches for staff to learn more about the lives of the individuals they care for. The programme is well received by care staff, but as with other interventions designed to facilitate compassionate care, it requires commitment by senior hospital staff to ensure staff are enabled to attend training (Arthur et al., 2017).

SAGE and THYME

The SAGE and THYME model (Connolly et al., 2010) is a mnemonic for use by health professionals to structure conversations and communication to provide emotional support for patients when they are distressed. The structured conversation is broken down into a series of components: setting, ask, gather, empathy (SAGE); and talk, help, you, me, end (THYME). The model is implemented through facilitated workshops. Although it is predominantly used in palliative care settings, it is also used more broadly to assist any care worker to listen and respond in a way that is patient or client-centred rather than staff-centred. This makes it a potentially useful communication model with older people in hospitals, although the authors of the model do not recommend it for use with people with cognitive impairment. It appears staff members' knowledge and confidence improve from the facilitated SAGE and THYME workshop, but similar to other interventions designed to improve the relational care of people in hospitals or the way staff communicate, there is little evidence as to whether it achieves improvements over the longer term.

Compassionate Care: A Critique

It is important to note the drive for more compassionate care, particularly by nurses looking after older people in hospitals, is neither new nor without its critics. Tierney et al. (2019) argue it has been wrongly assumed compassionate care comes without cost in terms of time and to the individual nurse, and historically it has been seen solely as the responsibility of the individual rather than the organisation or wider care system. Notwithstanding these points older people are at risk of being treated generically rather than as individuals, which in turn makes it easier to lose a sense of identity. Hospital nurses can and do make a huge difference to the experience of an older person during a hospital stay, both directly and by example (Bridges et al., 2020, Nicholson et al., 2017). In examining hospital ward culture older people are cared for within the NHS, Patterson et al. (2010) highlighted the pervading culture of pace and a focus on quick-fix solutions. They argued interventions targeted at ward leadership are likely to have the greatest benefit for patients, their relatives and staff.

ASSESSING NURSING NEEDS

Comprehensive Geriatric Assessment

The National Institute for Health and Care Excellence (NICE) recommends older people with complex needs have a comprehensive geriatric assessment on admission to hospital (NICE, 2016). The term *comprehensive geriatric assessment* (CGA) emerged in the 1990s when concerns were first expressed that for older people admitted to hospital, assessment tended to narrowly focus on the immediate health problem that prompted the admission rather than the person's broader health and social needs. A CGA is a multidimensional process to determine an older person's medical, functional, mental and social problems and resources. NICE recommends CGAs for individuals with one or more specified need or problem (e.g., falls, immobility, delirium and dementia, polypharmacy, incontinence and end-of-life care). The evidence to support the use of CGAs is strong (Ellis et al., 2017). They can increase the likelihood of an older person living independently in their own home up to a year later and reduce the probability of care home admission.

Nursing Assessment

While the concept of the CGA is multidisciplinary, and nurses play an essential part, there are certain assessment areas where nurses are likely to take the lead. Three of these—pressure ulcers, malnutrition and falls—are described in more detail below and also in Chapters 18, 21 and 24, on promoting safe mobility, eating and drinking, and maintaining healthy skin, respectively. Importantly, any assessment is essentially an assessment of need, and it therefore follows a plan should be put in place for those needs to be met. If not, the assessment becomes simply a tick-box exercise that, perhaps unethically, raises an expectation problems identified will be addressed. There are other benefits to careful nursing assessment. Assessments require close contact between the nurse and patient, which allows both parties to get to know each other better. Good assessment should be carefully documented in order to monitor progress and can indicate whether interventions put in place are having the hoped-for effect. Below are some examples of assessment domains and commonly used tools nurses caring for older people in hospitals are likely to come into contact with.

Assessment of Malnutrition Risk

Although there is wide variation in estimates of the prevalence of undernutrition in hospitals, ranging from 11% to 45% (Ray et al., 2014), it is a particular challenge for older people who may be malnourished on admission or at risk of malnourishment during their hospital stay. For older people, malnutrition is associated with frailty and poor health outcomes. It is perhaps unsurprising an older person's nutritional status often worsens while in hospital, where their appetite is likely to be low. They are, by definition, acutely unwell and are often prescribed a number of medications. Prevalence of cognitive impairment, whether due to delirium or dementia, is high. Nurses have a responsibility to identify individuals at risk of malnutrition and put in place the appropriate care interventions to ameliorate that risk.

The Malnutrition Universal Screening Tool (MUST) is the most frequently used tool for identifying individuals at risk of malnutrition in hospital settings (Stratton et al., 2004). It is relatively quick to use and consists of five steps. Step one is assessing height and weight to calculate body mass index. Step two determines whether and what percentage weight loss has occurred. Step three notes whether the patient is acutely ill. Step four brings each of the previous steps together to determine a risk score that places the individual at a low, medium or high risk of malnutrition. Step five presents guidelines for an appropriate care plan based on risk category. Importantly, the MUST contains alternatives to body mass index due to the challenges of measuring weight, particularly in patients who are bed bound.

Assessment of Pressure Ulcer Risk

In 2018 NHS Improvement recommended a standardisation to the definition and measurement of pressure ulcers (NHS Improvement, 2018). It noted each year around 25,000 patients develop a pressure ulcer during their stay in hospital with a cost to the NHS of around £4 million. Older patients are far more susceptible to developing pressure ulcers. Pressure ulcers are defined as 'localised damage to the skin and/or underlying tissue, usually over a bony prominence (or related to a medical or other device), resulting from sustained pressure (including pressure associated with shear). The damage can be present as intact skin or an open ulcer and may be painful' (NHS Improvement, 2018, p. 7). Hospital-acquired pressure ulcers should no longer be categorised as avoidable or unavoidable to ensure they are all investigated fully.

While NICE suggests considering use of an assessment scale, the evidence for their use in prevention is weak, and there exists some debate as to whether they are more effective than a nurse's clinical judgement (NICE, 2014). Nonetheless a tool allows a structured process to be undertaken and provides documentary evidence a risk assessment has taken place. The widely used Waterlow pressure ulcer risk assessment tool (Waterlow, 2005) consists of a series of items that are predictive of developing pressure ulcers—age, sex, body mass index, continence, mobility, nutrition, tissue malnutrition risk factors, neurological deficit and major surgery or trauma. A score is then constructed and categorised according to level of pressure ulcer risk.

Assessing Risk of Falls

In older people, falls are one of the most common reasons for non-elective hospital admission, with around 150,000 of people aged 80 years and over admitted to English hospitals each year as a result of a fall (Public Health England, 2020b). Causes of falls are multifactorial and include muscle weakness, poor balance, visual impairment, cognitive impairment, the number and type of medications, certain health conditions and environmental hazards (Public Health England, 2020a). Clearly many of these factors are present for older people in hospital and compounded by being in an unfamiliar environment. Hence falls are highly common occurrences in hospital for older people. In NHS hospitals, falls are the most frequently reported safety incident, with over 200,000 inpatient falls reported each year. Falls in acute settings that involve older people and are likely to cause the most serious harm incur an estimated annual cost to the NHS of £630 million (NHS Improvement, 2017). Nurses who care for older people in hospitals have a key role to play in assessing the risk of falls, putting interventions in place to prevent falls and responding quickly and appropriately when a fall occurs.

In contrast to pressure ulcers and malnutrition, NICE guidelines recommend not using a fall-risk assessment tool due to a lack of evidence they are sensitive or specific enough to effectively identify individuals at risk (NICE, 2013a). In the absence of a formal tool, any assessment of risk calls on nurses' clinical judgement and takes account of known risk factors, input from other professions such as physiotherapy, individual patient history and discussions with a patient's family and friends. Nurses are also responsible for reviewing risk assessments regularly as a patient's condition changes during their hospital stay and should always be reviewed when an inpatient fall has taken place.

THE TEAM-BASED NATURE OF HOSPITAL CARE FOR OLDER PEOPLE

The Multidisciplinary Team

In caring for older people in hospital, nurses work as part of a multidisciplinary team. The nature of frailty and new health problems faced by older people already affected by other chronic conditions means a range and depth of skills and expertise are required to address the physical, emotional and social needs of older patients. Nurses have both a unique and generic role to play within this team. Their unique contribution stems from their close and firsthand knowledge of patients in their care. Having responsibility for skin care, assisting with washing and elimination, and often being the first to respond to patients in need means there is often a closeness and immediacy in the way nurses provide care that gives insights other professionals are unlikely to have. Their generic contribution lies in the fact they are the only professional group who are present on the ward throughout a 24-hour period. They observe patients around the clock when, for example, diurnal variability of behaviour is a known issue for older people (Johnson, 2001). Nurses therefore play a central role in coordination, assessment, communication and implementation of decisions agreed on by the multidisciplinary team.

The multidisciplinary team has been described as the 'engine room' of the provision of acute care for older people (Ellis & Sevdalis, 2019). Central to the work of this team is the multidisciplinary meeting, which takes many forms. Its functions include establishing goals of care within specific time frames, allocating responsibility for agreed actions, reviewing patient progress and communicating decisions to patients and carers. Successful working requires leadership, clear processes and shared values across the team. Such is the importance of a high-functioning multidisciplinary team, Ellis and Sevdalis question why there is a lack of multidisciplinary training. In a narrative review of seven trials of multidisciplinary team working, high levels of specialist expertise in the team reduced the risk of readmission, and a strong focus on transitional care arrangements was key for successful discharge planning (Hickman et al., 2015).

With an increasing pace of turnover in hospital care for older people, the multidisciplinary team is likely to meet at least once daily during the week and at other ad hoc times. The composition of the team likely varies but typically includes a number of core members. The ward manager or nurse on duty with oversight of the ward has the most up-to-date information on each patient, including changes in condition, how they are responding to care decisions, communication with relatives and responsibility for acting in the patient's best interests if the patient is unable to express them. A consultant in older people's medicine has overall responsibility for the medical management of the patient, including the goals of treatment, deciding on and responding to diagnostic investigations and other tests, and the need for input from other medical specialties. Physiotherapy input includes the provision of suitable walking aids, tailored rehabilitation plans that focus on strength and balance, and education on reducing the risk of falls. Contributions from ward occupational therapists are based around a patient's ability to conduct daily tasks and include functional assessment and the provision of equipment and education to help compensate against physical and/or cognitive impairments. A discharge coordinator is also key, liaising with outside services to facilitate safe discharge at home or placement in another care setting. Depending on the way the local multidisciplinary team is organised, other essential professions such as speech and language therapy, pharmacy, social work and dietetics have core or as-required input. Furthermore, nurse specialists in areas such as tissue viability, palliative care, diabetes and mental health, who operate at an organisational rather than ward level, are needed to provide expertise for the particular needs of particular patients. One study found the breadth of the multidisciplinary team was associated with better functioning, and nurses score more highly than their medical colleagues in their ability to facilitate relational co-ordination—that is, communication and relationships to achieve shared tasks (Hartgerink et al., 2014). Below are two case studies of new hospital initiatives for older people where the nursing contribution is pivotal to the multidisciplinary effort required to make these innovations work.

CASE STUDY 10.1 Older People's Emergency Department

What Is It?
The Older People's Emergency Department (OPED) at the Norfolk and Norwich Hospital was set up in 2017 in response to rising emergency admissions, a local ageing population and recognition of the particular challenges in providing optimal emergency care for older people (Arie, 2020). The unit takes patients aged 80 years and over, directly on arrival by ambulance. A CGA is initiated that includes advance care planning, medication review and social care needs.

What Are the Underlying Principles?
The aim of the unit is to provide a service that can fully assess and treat multiple needs in an environment that caters to people who may have decreased mobility, problems with continence and sensory or cognitive impairment. The area is much quieter than the main emergency department. It has wide corridors, more space to assist patients getting to the toilet, a meal service and large clocks in prominent places.

By being directly transferred from ambulance to the OPED decreases the number of unnecessary moves an older person may experience in hospital. Rather than a generic emergency assessment undertaken in a large department, there is rapid access to assessment from specialists in older people's medicine with a multidisciplinary team on hand to coordinate care. The aim is to avoid hospital admission wherever possible due to the risks inherent for older people who are frail.

What Is the Nursing Contribution?
Key to the success of the OPED is the close working of nurses with expertise in older people's medicine and those with experience in emergency care. This provides learning opportunities for both groups and an ideal environment to share skills and knowledge. Patients are seen by advanced clinical practitioners of varied professional backgrounds. This includes not just nurses but also physiotherapists, pharmacists and paramedics, reflecting the need for providing a highly specialised service rooted in holistic care.

CASE STUDY 10.2 Medical and Mental Health Unit What Is It?

What is it?
The Medical and Mental Health Unit (MMHU) at Nottingham University Hospitals NHS Trust is designed to provide the best hospital care for people with delirium and dementia. The MMHU was created to meet the needs of older people with confusion admitted to the acute hospital by offering acute medical care alongside mental health expertise.

What Are the Underlying Principles?
People with delirium and dementia constitute a large patient group with complex needs in general hospitals. The challenges associated with their care may result in unnecessary time spent in hospital, and they are at risk of worse outcomes and poor care experiences. Multidisciplinary in approach, the MMHU aims to assess and treat specific syndromes associated with older adulthood, both physical and mental. The unit is characterised by staffing of both medical and mental health professionals; enhanced training for staff in delirium, dementia and person-centred care; organised purposeful activities; environmental modification that reflects the needs of individuals with cognitive impairment; and an inclusive approach to family carers.

What Is the Nursing Contribution?
The key element of the MMHU is the close working of general nurses and mental health nurses. This occurs at all levels, including ward managers and clinical nurse specialists. Mental health nurses are seconded from the specialist mental health trust, creating a positive environment for liaison across organisational boundaries. Mental health assessment and care planning becomes routine rather than a response to a crisis because of the nursing expertise available, and interventions for defusing severe distress behaviours can be implemented promptly, drawing on experience learned in other settings. In an evaluation of the MMHU, the benefits were shown to be inpatient experience and carer satisfaction (Goldberg et al., 2013). These are the outcomes where the nursing contribution is likely to be felt the most.

The Role of Health-Care Assistants

Nearly all health systems employ a large health-care support workforce that works closely with nurses. In the United Kingdom, health-care assistants (HCAs) are the bedrock of the provision of care for older people in hospitals. Their role is to undertake direct and essential patient care and free registered nurses to focus on clinical activities. HCAs spend approximately 60% of their time in direct contact with patients, around twice the proportion of that spent by nurses (Kessler & Heron, 2010). In most hospital wards where older people are being cared for, a registered nurse is likely to have responsibility for a set number of patients and work with one or more HCAs to deliver that care. While the nurse remains responsible for the care provided, much of that care, including personal care and recording of observations, is delivered directly by HCAs. It is therefore vital nurses work closely with HCAs, are confident in their competence and can delegate tasks as and when appropriate. This requires leadership skills and good working relationships and often gives rise to particular learning needs for newly qualified and experienced nurses (Dahlke & Baumbusch, 2015).

IMPROVING OUTCOMES

While older people are vulnerable to adverse outcomes associated with hospital admission, there remains much nursing teams can do to limit this risk. Examples of this are given below in three areas: deconditioning, falls and delirium.

Deconditioning

For most older patients, the overwhelming majority of their time spent in hospital is spent in bed. Even for those able to walk prior to admission, it is estimated less than 45 minutes per day in hospital is spent standing or walking (Brown et al., 2009). This is a problem with very real consequences because after only a few days of immobilisation, muscular atrophy occurs with weakness in the legs, arms and back that slow an individual's recovery or create avoidable problems not directly related to the original admission (Knight et al., 2018).

It is unclear why nurses are sometimes reluctant to encourage mobility for older patients. Suboptimal staffing levels may be one factor. The immediate risks of collapse due to postural hypotension or the risk of falling may discourage nurses and their teams from helping older people get out of bed early on in their hospital stay. There may also be a reluctance to help patients out of bed until after a review by a physiotherapist. However, this may not happen until a few days after admission. There is good evidence active mobilisation that occurs early in an older person's hospital stay can increase physical functioning, reduce hospital stay and prevent pulmonary embolus (Cortes et al., 2019). Increased awareness of the problem of deconditioning underpins the End PJ Paralysis campaign, which highlights the benefits of helping patients get out of bed, get dressed and mobilise (Dolan, 2021). The other clear advantage to helping older people wear their own clothes in the hospital is they are afforded greater individuality and, by extension, dignity.

Prevention of Falls

Falls are a frequent occurrence in hospital, with potentially highly significant consequences, including hip and other fractures, delayed discharge and an increased risk of mortality. Other indirect harms may include loss of confidence and social isolation after discharge (NHS Improvement, 2017). Although falls are unlikely to ever be 'engineered out of the hospital system' and are not necessarily an indication of poor care (Oliver, 2018), reducing the risk of falls can have important positive effects for both individual older patients and the organisation itself.

If falls among older people are multifactorial, it is perhaps unsurprising that single-component interventions delivered generically, such as low-rise beds, chair/bed alarms or specific medicines, have not been found to be effective (Centre for Reviews and Dissemination, 2014). While multifactorial interventions are likely to be far more effective, the optimal combination of components and how these are targeted are yet to be determined (Morris & O'Riordan, 2017). However, nurses can and should ensure simple checks are in place so older patients have easy and unobstructed access to their call bells and appropriate walking aids, hearing and visual aids are in place and toileting needs are anticipated. One group of researchers put together a package of six components—'fall alert' sign, supervision of patients in the bathroom, ensuring patients' walking aids are within reach, a toileting regimen, use of a low-low bed and use of a bed/chair alarm—but although this combination appeared to improve practice, they did not find any evidence it reduced inpatient falls (Barker et al., 2016). As with other nursing interventions, commitment from ward managers through to the hospital board is likely to be essential in the priority placed on addressing the issue of hospital falls and ensures accurate and meaningful fall data are collected (Centre for Reviews and Dissemination, 2014).

Identification and Prevention of Delirium

Although delirium, or acute confusional state, in older people is covered in depth elsewhere (see Chapter 28), it is particularly pertinent for older hospitalised patients who are not only at far greater risk of delirium but also of the poor outcomes associated with delirium. Nurses who care for older people in hospitals need to be vigilant in the prevention, detection and treatment of delirium, as it is preventable and, if dealt with promptly, treatable. Hyperactive delirium is characterised by confusion, restlessness, agitation and sometimes aggression. Patients with hypoactive delirium tend to be withdrawn and sleepy.

Prevalence of delirium in hospitals is estimated to be around 28% (Schubert et al., 2018), with around a quarter each having hypoactive and hyperactive delirium, with the remainder having a mixed form of the two (Sandberg et al., 1999). Although nurses are well placed to recognise delirium in a patient whose condition is deteriorating, it can often be missed. This is a particular problem for hypoactive delirium and among patients who are older or have dementia (Rice et al., 2011).

The causes of delirium include infection, dehydration, poor nutrition and medications. Individuals with dementia, or who are particularly frail, or who have undergone surgery are at particular risk (Collier, 2012). Prevention strategies are therefore based on addressing these risk factors with good infection control, adequate nutrition and hydration, and close monitoring of patients. Where doubt exists as to whether the cause of behavioural symptoms is dementia or delirium, the serious immediate consequences of the latter means delirium should be treated in the first instance (NICE, 2013b).

EFFECTIVE DISCHARGE FROM THE HOSPITAL

Worsening delays in discharge from the hospital are of concern to politicians and policy makers. It is predominantly an issue for older rather than younger patients, and delays tend to occur at the transition point between hospital care and social care. This is the point whereby a domiciliary package of care or residential care placement, typically provided by the social care sector, may not be available in a timely manner, thereby delaying discharge from the hospital. Delays in discharge cost the NHS an estimated £820 million pounds each year, with over a million bed days occupied by somebody at the point of their hospital stay where care is likely to be more suitable outside of hospital (National Audit Office, 2016). Beyond the financial cost of older patients being delayed in hospitals when home or another care setting is likely to be more appropriate, the physical and emotional cost is felt by patients and their families. Although funding constraints are clearly an issue, particularly for social care, some delays may be due to poor communication between professionals within and between organisations and hospital discharge mechanisms not fit for purpose (Oliver, 2016). With older people in hospital facing complex health problems, the discharge of an older patient is likely to be multidisciplinary and based on reliable and up-to-date information about care needs, with nurses deeply involved throughout.

Hospital stays should be no longer than necessary, and successful discharge from a hospital should be patient-centred. It requires early planning in the patient's hospital stay, which can potentially reduce the risk of readmission (Zhu et al., 2015). Broadly speaking, older patients fall into one of four categories for discharge purposes: those who require minimal or no support, those who require short-term support for recovery at home or in a residential setting where a clearer idea of long-term needs can be assessed, those who are unlikely to benefit from short-term support and require care in a nursing or residential home, and those with rapidly deteriorating health who are nearing the end of life. When working within a busy ward environment, where a shortage of beds brings with it pressure to discharge patients quickly, it is perhaps easy to forget decisions around discharge destination have a dramatic effect on an older person's life. Although many patients return to the home or care home they were living in prior to their admission, many whose support needs have changed temporarily or permanently leave the hospital for a new living arrangement. Options are finite and constrained, but nurses are in a position to gain insights into patients' and carers' preferences and an understanding of their social circumstances. A patient needs the discharge process explained in a format they can engage with (Age UK, 2020).

While it is helpful for patients, their families and staff to be clear about what criteria need to be met to determine when a patient is ready for discharge, there is evidence that only half of NHS hospitals do this consistently (National Audit Office, 2016). Such criteria provide transparency around care decisions, ensure everybody has a sense of a shared and defined goals and allow discharge planning to take place in anticipation of, rather than at the point of, the patient becoming medically fit for discharge. Preparing older people for discharge reduces the risk of readmission, with evidence that patients who feel unready for discharge, particularly those being discharged with greater support needs than on admission, are more likely to be readmitted (Coffey & McCarthy, 2013). Across all age groups, readmission to hospital within 30 days of discharge is around 14% (Nuffield Trust, 2020). Risk factors for readmission among older people include greater frailty, being on a high number of medications, longer hospital stays and being discharged on a Friday (Glans et al., 2020).

Coordination with services is essential, and a ward discharge coordinator leads on this, but the passing on of clinical information requires direct communication between a ward nurse and, for example, a care home manager or district nursing team. Here good quality documentation is essential to ensure information flows easily and safely to individuals with a legitimate need for the information within and outside the hospital. It is the nurse's responsibility to ensure medications, of which there may be many and a regime that may be unfamiliar to the patient, are checked, and the patient or carer is aware of what the medications are for and how and when they should be administered.

If ongoing blood tests are needed for monitoring medications or any other reason, these should be booked prior to discharge and explained to the patient or carer.

NHS services for older patients are provided free of charge, but services outside the NHS that are required to assist with independent living may not be. Most of these services are based on eligibility criteria and/or are means-tested. These costs may be significant and require careful explanation to patients and relatives. The discharge coordinator or hospital social worker is able to assist here to highlight what financial support may be available. At the time of writing, patients who would benefit from time-limited support in the form of intermediate care for reablement to gain confidence and maximise the ability to live independently were entitled to funding of this service for up to 6 weeks.

An overview of the evidence of discharge interventions suggest what works best are integrated systems between the hospital and community that are multidisciplinary and highly tailored to individual patient need (Coffey et al., 2019). Box 10.1 outlines the principles of good practice for effective hospital discharge for older people.

BOX 10.1	Principles Of Good Practice for Effective Hospital Discharge for Older People
Planning	Early discharge planning helps prepare older patients and may avoid unnecessary delays.
Timeliness	Explicit criteria for discharge make it easier to determine when a patient is medically fit for discharge.
Collaboration	Collaboration between members of the multidisciplinary team, patients, carers and community services is vital for smooth transition on leaving the hospital.
Coordination	Any home-based care services need to come into effect at agreed-on time points following discharge. This may require coordination across multiple service providers.
Safety	Medications need to be checked and explained to patients/carers, and referrals for drug monitoring and dressings need to be made, prior to discharge.

NURSING ROLES

It is only relatively recently that nursing older people has been considered a specialist skill. Nursing older people in hospitals and elsewhere has often been considered a Cinderella service, characterised by a lack of status, being physically rather than intellectually demanding and an area of nursing without any obvious clear career pathway. One study of nurses who cared for older people in hospitals between 1955 and 1980 concluded that, historically, the structure and regimentation of care dehumanised staff and by extension the people they cared for (Brooks, 2009). Although there has been progress in the United Kingdom with new nursing roles developed for the care of older people (Fitzpatrick et al., 2021), it has lagged behind that of other clinical specialties and behind established pathways in North America (Mezey & Fulmer, 2002).

Attitudes remain difficult to shift and are not restricted to the United Kingdom. In a survey of Israeli nursing students, most said they had no intention of working within the specialty of nursing older people until there was a more recognisable career structure for it (Haron et al., 2013). One longitudinal study of health-care staff found the recognition of the care of older people as a specialism had not altered between 1999 and 2009 in spite of policy changes in pre- and post-registration nurse education (Kydd et al., 2013). Survey respondents identified the working conditions and working environment, and the perceived lack of value placed on the care of older people by staff in other areas, as the main barriers to recruitment.

Nurse consultant roles were introduced in the NHS in 1999 (Department of Health, 1999). These new clinical leaders were expected to be experts in their field of practice, professional leaders and consultants, educators and trainers, and actively developing practice and research. Their role was anticipated to be more strategic in focus than that of clinical nurse specialists with a greater focus on leadership and the development of others. Since then evaluation of the nurse consultant post has been patchy, generating little robust evidence (Kennedy et al., 2012), although one large survey of nurse consultants found high levels of reported impact were associated with engagement in a broad range of activities, perceived competence in the role and strong medical support (Coster et al., 2006).

For nurse consultants who work predominantly within the acute care of older people, there remains a lack of clarity as to what defines a specialist and a lack of agreement about clinical expertise (Reed et al., 2007). In recent years frailty has become the focus for some consultant nurse posts. In Norway, advanced geriatric nurses felt their skills were not always utilised and their colleagues were sometimes unclear about the scope of their role, suggesting a need for greater work around adaptive organisational work (Henni et al., 2019). The need to prepare the work environment for changes in the structure of a workforce is true irrespective of the level the change occurs. In 2017 the nursing associate role was created to bridge the perceived gap between registered nurse and the support workforce and ease the pressure from significant nursing post vacancies. It is too early to tell how successful this workforce innovation will be, but it requires a clear understanding by the team and wider organisation of the scope of the role and how it can be supported and utilised most effectively.

CONCLUSION AND LEARNING POINTS

This chapter described some of the problems faced by older people in hospitals and the challenges of providing the highest level of nursing care. Many of these challenges were made much more acute after the COVID-19 pandemic dramatically shifted the way hospital care was organised and delivered. COVID-19 disproportionately affected older people. At the time of writing, the legacy of this remains to be seen, although lasting changes are anticipated. Changes to family and friend visiting policies and the barriers of personal protective equipment increase the risk of isolation for older hospital patients. Strong nurse leadership and creativity at all levels of the hospital organisation are needed to ensure the experience of hospital admission for older people is positive, care is optimised and adverse events are avoided.

KEY LEARNING POINTS

- Two-thirds of non-elective hospital inpatient days are occupied by those aged 65 years and older.
- Avoidable delays in discharge from hospital put older patients at greater exposure to adverse events including falls, hospital acquired infections, and deconditioning.
- Meaningful comprehensive assessment on admission and updated throughout a hospital stay forms the basis of hospital nurses' care of their older patients.

- Higher prevalence of sensory, cognitive and functional impairment among older hospital patients mean that older people are particularly vulnerable to the effects of poor communication in busy hospital settings.
- Nurses are key members of multi-disciplinary and multi-sector teams required to meet the complex needs of older patients.

REFERENCES

Age UK. (2020). *Factsheet 37: Hospital discharge.* https://www.ageuk.org.uk/globalassets/age-uk/documents/factsheets/fs37_hospital_discharge_fcs.pdf

Arie, S. (2020). Welcome to the emergency department exclusively for the over 80s. *BMJ, 368,* m931.

Arthur, A., Aldus, C., Sarre, S., Maben, J., Wharrad, H., Schneider, J., Barton, G., Argyle, E., Clark, A., Nouri, F., & Nicholson, C. (2017). *Can Health-care Assistant Training improve the relational care of older people? (CHAT) A development and feasibility study of a complex intervention. Health Services Delivery Research, 5.*

Barker, A. L., Morello, R. T., Wolfe, R., Brand, C. A., Haines, T. P., Hill, K. D., Brauer, S. G., Botti, M., Cumming, R. G., Livingston, P. M., Sherrington, C., Zavarsek, S., Lindley, R. I., & Kamar, J. (2016). 6-PACK programme to decrease fall injuries in acute hospitals: cluster randomised controlled trial. *BMJ, 352,* h6781.

Blomberg, K., Griffiths, P., Wengstrom, Y., May, C., & Bridges, J. (2016). Interventions for compassionate nursing care: A systematic review. *International Journal of Nursing Studies, 62,* 137–155.

Bridges, J., Collins, P., Flatley, M., Hope, J., & Young, A. (2020). Older people's experiences in acute care settings: Systematic review and synthesis of qualitative studies. *International Journal of Nursing Studies, 102,* Article 103469.

Bridges, J., & Fuller, A. (2015). Creating learning environments for compassionate care: a programme to promote compassionate care by health and social care teams. *International Journal of Older People Nursing, 10,* 48–58.

Bridges, J., Pickering, R. M., Barker, H., Chable, R., Fuller, A., Gould, L., Libberton, P., Mesa-Eguiagaray, I., Raftery, J., Sayer, A. A., Westwood, G., Wigley, W., Yao, G., Zhu, S., & Griffiths, P. (2018). *Implementing the Creating Learning Environments for Compassionate Care (CLECC) programme in acute hospital settings: A pilot RCT and feasibility study. Health Services Delivery Research, 6.*

Brooks, J. (2009). 'The geriatric hospital felt like a backwater': Aspects of older people's nursing in Britain, 1955–1980. *Journal of Clinical Nursing, 18,* 2764–2772.

Brown, C. J., Redden, D. T., Flood, K. L., & Allman, R. M. (2009). The underrecognized epidemic of low mobility during hospitalization of older adults. *Journal of the American Geriatrics Society, 57,* 1660–1665.

Center for Reviews and Dissemination. (2014). Effectiveness matters: Preventing falls in hospitals. University of York.

Coffey, A., Leahy-Warren, P., Savage, E., Hegarty, J., Cornally, N., Day, M. R., Sahm, L., O'Connor, K., O'Doherty, J., Liew, A.,

Sezgin, D., & O'Caoimh, R (2019). Interventions to promote early discharge and avoid inappropriate hospital (re)admission: A systematic review. *International Journal of Environmental Research and Public Health*, 16.

Coffey, A., & McCarthy, G. M. (2013). Older people's perception of their readiness for discharge and postdischarge use of community support and services. *International Journal of Older People Nursing*, 8, 104–115.

Collier, R. (2012). Hospital-induced delirium hits hard. *Canadian Medical Association Journal*, 184, 23–24.

Care Quality Commission. (2020). 2019 Adult inpatient survey. https://www.cqc.org.uk/publications/surveys/adult-inpatient-survey-2019

Connolly, M., Perryman, J., McKenna, Y., Orford, J., Thomson, L., Shuttleworth, J., & Cocksedge, S. (2010). SAGE & THYME: A model for training health and social care professionals in patient-focussed support. *Patient Education and Counseling*, 79, 87–93.

Cortes, O. L., Delgado, S., & Esparza, M. (2019). Systematic review and meta-analysis of experimental studies: In-hospital mobilization for patients admitted for medical treatment. *Journal of Advanced Nursing*, 75, 1823–1837.

Coster, S., Redfern, S., Wilson-Barnett, J., Evans, A., Peccei, R., & Guest, D. (2006). Impact of the role of nurse, midwife and health visitor consultant. *Journal of Advanced Nursing*, 55, 352–363.

Dahlke, S., & Baumbusch, J. (2015). Nursing teams caring for hospitalised older adults. *Journal of Clinical Nursing*, 24, 3177–3185.

Department of Health. (1999). *Making a difference: Strengthening the nursing, midwifery and health visiting contribution to health and healthcare*. Department of Health.

Dolan, B. (2021). End PJ paralysis. https://endpjparalysis.org

Ellis, G., Gardner, M., Tsiachristas, A., Langhorne, P., Burke, O., Harwood, R., Conroy, S., Kircher, T., Somme, D., Saltvedt, I., Wald, H., O'Neill, D., Robinson, D., & Shepperd, S. (2017). Comprehensive geriatric assessment for older adults admitted to hospital. *Cochrane Database of Systematic Reviews*. doi:10.1002/14651858.CD006211.pub3.

Ellis, G., & Sevdalis, N. (2019). Understanding and improving multidisciplinary team working in geriatric medicine. *Age and Ageing*, 48, 498–505.

Fitzpatrick, J. M., Hayes, N., Naughton, C., & Ezhova, I. (2021). Evaluating a specialist education programme for nurses and allied health professionals working in older people care: A qualitative analysis of motivations and impact. *Nurse Education Today*, 97, Article 104708.

Francis, R. (2013). Report of the Mid Staffordshire NHS foundation trust public enquiry. The Stationery Office.

Glans, M., Kragh Ekstam, A., Jakobsson, U., Bondesson, A., & Midlov, P. (2020). Risk factors for hospital readmission in older adults within 30 days of discharge: A comparative retrospective study. *BMC Geriatrics*, 20, 467.

Goldberg, S. E., Bradshaw, L. E., Kearney, F. C., Russell, C., Whittamore, K. H., Foster, P. E., Mamza, J., Gladman, J. R., Jones, R. G., Lewis, S. A., Porock, D., & Harwood, R. H. Medical Crises in Older People Study. (2013). Care in specialist

medical and mental health unit compared with standard care for older people with cognitive impairment admitted to general hospital: randomised controlled trial (NIHR TEAM trial). *BMJ*, 347, f4132.

Haron, Y., Levy, S., Albagli, M., Rotstein, R., & Riba, S. (2013). Why do nursing students not want to work in geriatric care? A national questionnaire survey. *International Journal of Nursing Studies*, 50, 1558–1565.

Harris, R., Sims, S., Leamy, M., Levenson, R., Davies, N., Brearley, S., Grant, R., Gourlay, S., Favato, G., & Ross, F. (2019). *Intentional rounding in hospital wards to improve regular interaction and engagement between nurses and patients: A realist evaluation*. University of Southampton Science Park.

Hartgerink, J. M., Cramm, J. M., Bakker, T. J., van Eijsden, A. M., Mackenbach, J. P., & Nieboer, A. P. (2014). The importance of multidisciplinary teamwork and team climate for relational coordination among teams delivering care to older patients. *Journal of Advanced Nursing*, 70, 791–799.

Henni, S. H., Kirkevold, M., Antypas, K., & Foss, C. (2019). The integration of new nurse practitioners into care of older adults: A survey study. *Journal of Clinical Nursing*, 28, 2911–2923.

Hickman, L. D., Phillips, J. L., Newton, P. J., Halcomb, E. J., Al Abed, N., & Davidson, P. M. (2015). Multidisciplinary team interventions to optimise health outcomes for older people in acute care settings: A systematic review. *Archives of Gerontology and Geriatrics*, 61, 322–329.

Hodkinson, A., Bower, P., Grigoroglou, C., Zghebi, S. S., Pinnock, H., Kontopantelis, E., & Panagioti, M. (2020). Self-management interventions to reduce healthcare use and improve quality of life among patients with asthma: Systematic review and network meta-analysis. *BMJ*, 370, m2521.

Johnson, M. H. (2001). Assessing confused patients. *Journal of Neurology, Neurosurgery, and Psychiatry*, 71(1), i7–i12.

Kennedy, F., McDonnell, A., Gerrish, K., Howarth, A., Pollard, C., & Redman, J. (2012). Evaluation of the impact of nurse consultant roles in the United Kingdom: A mixed method systematic literature review. *Journal of Advanced Nursing*, 68, 721–742.

Kessler, I., & Heron, P. (2010). NHS modernisation and the role of HCAs. *British Journal of Healthcare Assistants*, 4, 318–320.

King's Fund. (2019). *The number of hospital beds*. https://www.kingsfund.org.uk/projects/nhs-in-a-nutshell/hospital-beds

Knight, J., Nigam, Y., & Jones, A. (2018). Effects of bedrest 1: Introduction and the cardiovascular system. *Nursing Times*, 114, 54–57.

Kydd, A., Wild, D., & Nelson, S. (2013). Attitudes towards caring for older people: Findings and recommendations for practice. *Nursing Older People*, 25, 21–28.

Mezey, M., & Fulmer, T. (2002). The future history of gerontological nursing. *The Journals of Gerontology: Series A, Biological Sciences and Medical Sciences*, 57, M438–M441.

Morris, R., & O'Riordan, S (2017). Prevention of falls in hospital. *Clinical Medicine (London)*, 17, 360–362.

Mudge, A. M., Mcrae, P., Hubbard, R. E., Peel, N. M., Lim, W. K., Barnett, A. G., & Inouye, S. K. (2019). Hospital-associated complications of older people: A proposed multicomponent outcome for acute care. *Journal of the American Geriatrics Society*, 67, 352–356.

National Audit Office. (2016). *Discharging older patients from hospital*. Department of Health.

National Institute for Health and Clinical Excellence (NICE). (2013a). Falls in older people: Assessing risk and prevention. https://www.nice.org.uk/guidance/cg161

NICE. (2013b). *Quality standards and indicators briefing paper: Delirium*. https://www.nice.org.uk/guidance/qs63/resources/delirium-briefing-paper

NICE. (2014). *Pressure ulcers: prevention and management*. https://www.nice.org.uk/guidance/cg179

NICE. (2016). *Transition between inpatient hospital settings and community or care home settings for adults with social care needs*. https://www.nice.org.uk/guidance/qs136/resources/transition-between-inpatient-hospital-settings-and-community-or-care-home-settings-for-adults-with-social-care-needs-pdf-75545422401733

NHS Improvement. (2017). *The incidence and costs of inpatient falls in hospitals*. https://improvement.nhs.uk/uploads/documents/Falls_report_July2017.v2.pdf

NHS Improvement. (2018). *Pressure ulcers: revised definition and measurement*. https://www.england.nhs.uk/wp-content/uploads/2021/09/NSTPP-summary-recommendations.pdf

Nicholson, C., Morrow, E. M., Hicks, A., & Fitzpatrick, J. (2017). Supportive care for older people with frailty in hospital: An integrative review. *International Journal of Nursing Studies, 66*, 60–71.

Nuffield Trust. (2020). *Emergency readmissions*. https://www.nuffieldtrust.org.uk/resource/emergency-readmissions

Oeseburg, B., Wynia, K., Middel, B., & Reijneveld, S. A. (2009). Effects of case management for frail older people or those with chronic illness: A systematic review. *Nursing Research, 58*, 201–210.

Oliver, D. (2016). *Why is it more difficult than ever for older people to leave hospital?*https://www.kingsfund.org.uk/blog/2016/05/older-people-leave-hospital

Oliver, D. (2018). David Oliver: Do bed and chair sensors really stop falls in hospital? *BMJ, 360*, k433. https://www.bmj.com/content/360/bmj.k433

Patterson, M., Nolan, M., Rick, J., Brown, J., & Adams, R. (2010). *From metrics to meaning: Culture change and quality of acute hospital care for older people*: University of Sheffield.

Public Health England. (2020a). *Falls: Applying all our health*. https://www.gov.uk/government/publications/falls-applying-all-our-health/falls-applying-all-our-health

Public Health England. (2020b). *Falls: Applying all our health*. https://www.gov.uk/government/publications/falls-applying-all-our-health/falls-applying-all-our-health

Ray, S., Laur, C., & Golubic, R. (2014). Malnutrition in healthcare institutions: A review of the prevalence of under-nutrition in hospitals and care homes since 1994 in England. *Clinical Nutrition, 33*, 829–835.

Reed, J., Inglis, P., Cook, G., Clarke, C., & Cook, M. (2007). Specialist nurses for older people: Implications from UK development sites. *Journal of Advanced Nursing, 58*, 368–376.

Rice, K. L., Bennett, M., Gomez, M., Theall, K. P., Knight, M., & Foreman, M. D. (2011). Nurses' recognition of delirium in the hospitalized older adult. *Clinical Nurse Specialist, 25*, 299–311.

Sandberg, O., Gustafson, Y., Brannstrom, B., & Bucht, G. (1999). Clinical profile of delirium in older patients. *Journal of the American Geriatrics Society, 47*, 1300–1306.

Sandberg, M., Jakobsson, U., Midlov, P., & Kristensson, J. (2014). Case management for frail older people: A qualitative study of receivers' and providers' experiences of a complex intervention. *BMC Health Services Research, 14*, 14.

Schubert, M., Schurch, R., Boettger, S., Garcia Nunez, D., Schwarz, U., Bettex, D., Jenewein, J., Bogdanovic, J., Staehli, M. L., Spririg, R., & Rudiger, A. (2018). A hospital-wide evaluation of delirium prevalence and outcomes in acute care patients: A cohort study. *BMC Health Services Research, 18*, 550.

Shepherd, S., Iliffe, S., Doll, H., Clarke, M., Kalra, L., Wilson, A., & Gonçalves-Bradley, D. (2016). Admission avoidance hospital at home. *Cochrane Database of Systematic Reviews*. doi:10.1002/14651858.CD007491.pub2.

Steventon, A., Deeny, S., Friebel, R., Gardner, T., & Thorlby, R. (2018). *Emergency hospital admissions in England: Which may be avoidable and how?* The Health Foundation.

Stratton, R. J., Hackston, A., Longmore, D., Dixon, R., Price, S., Stroud, M., King, C., & Elia, M. (2004). Malnutrition in hospital outpatients and inpatients: Prevalence, concurrent validity and ease of use of the 'malnutrition universal screening tool' ('MUST') for adults. *British Journal of Nutrition, 92*, 799–808.

Tammes, P., Purdy, S., Salisbury, C., Mackichan, F., Lasserson, D., & Morris, R. W. (2017). Continuity of primary care and emergency hospital admissions among older patients in England. *Annals of Family Medicine, 15*, 515–522.

Tierney, S., Bivins, R., & Seers, K. (2019). Compassion in nursing: Solution or stereotype? *Nursing Inquiry, 26*, e12271.

Toukhsati, S. R., Jaarsma, T., Babu, A. S., Driscoll, A., & Hare, D. L. (2019). Self-care interventions that reduce hospital readmissions in patients with heart failure: Towards the identification of change agents. *Clinical Medicine Insights Cardiology, 13*, Article 1179546819856855.

van den Broek, S., Heiwegen, N., Verhofstad, M., Akkermans, R., van Westerop, L., Schoon, Y., & Hesselink, G. (2020). Preventable emergency admissions of older adults: An observational mixed-method study of rates, associative factors and underlying causes in two Dutch hospitals. *BMJ Open, 10*, Article e040431.

Waterlow, J. (2005). *The Waterlow pressure ulcer risk assessment*. http://www.judy-waterlow.co.uk/index.htm

Wharrad, H., Sarre, S., Schneider, J., Maben, J., Aldus, C., Argyle, E., & Arthur, A. (2020). In-PREP: A new learning design framework and methodology applied to a relational care training intervention for healthcare assistants. *BMC Health Services Research, 20*, 1010.

Wittenberg, R., Sharpin, L., McCormick, B., & Hurst, J. (2014). *Understanding emergency hospital admissions of older people*.

Zhu, Q. M., Liu, J., Hu, H. Y., & Wang, S. (2015). Effectiveness of nurse-led early discharge planning programmes for hospital inpatients with chronic disease or rehabilitation needs: A systematic review and meta-analysis. *Journal of Clinical Nursing, 24*, 2993–3005.

11

Care Home Nursing Is 'Maxi-Nursing': The Value and Contribution of Nursing Older People in Long-Term Care Settings

Richard Adams, Karen Spilsbury

CHAPTER OUTLINE

As the life expectancy of older people worldwide continues to rise, especially in high-income countries, 'deep and fundamental reforms of health and social care systems will be required' (Beard, 2014) to meet the increasing demands of an ageing population living with multiple complex health conditions and care needs. Living a longer life does not necessarily equate to living a healthier life. Although various public health policy initiatives, such as the reduction in tobacco use and subsequent reduction in cardiovascular disease, have resulted in a decline in deaths, the incidence of long-term chronic conditions in people over 60 years old, such as chronic respiratory conditions, diabetes and musculoskeletal diseases, pose a significant challenge to health and social care systems and to promoting healthy ageing. In many countries this requires a structural change to health and social systems. Not least, there is a requirement for a shift from the dominant and traditional condition-focused model of cure and hospital-based medicine to one of person-centredness and care provided in the most appropriate setting for the individual and to best meet their needs.

Many countries are being forced to look for more efficient and scalable primary care service models, where people with long-term conditions receive effective and comprehensive care in a community setting. For many older people, this is in their own home. However, for a proportion of older people, their physical, psychological and/or cognitive care needs are significant and better met in a long-term social care environment or care home (Kingston et al., 2018). However, if these structural changes are to be effective and acceptable for society, there needs to be greater parity of esteem between the models of cure and care as well as greater understanding and value accorded to the important contribution of care homes and individuals who work in these environments to meet the complex health and care needs of the population.

Historically, work in long-term social care settings, and the art and science of nursing older people, was not perceived as skilled or high value. It has lacked the kudos accorded areas of nursing associated with a high level of technical skill or popularised on national television, such as emergency and trauma nursing. As a result of this lack of appeal, older people's services have struggled to attract and retain staff, especially newly registered or early career nurses (Devi et al. 2021; Thompson et al., 2016). The image of nurses working in older people's services, and nursing homes in particular, is that of a nurse at the end of their career playing out their time until they reach retirement or a nurse who has no career ambition or can't get a 'proper' nursing position. The reality could not be further from the truth. More recently there has been greater recognition of the value and contribution of social care nursing (Cornes & Manthorpe, 2022). In the United Kingdom, for example, a number of statements have been made by statutory and representative bodies about the important contribution of adult social care nurses. This coincides with an emerging narrative that cites nursing homes, in particular, as nurse-led units, where nurses are able to practice with greater autonomy and as advocates for the people in their care. Very recent changes in practice related to the COVID-19 pandemic have meant increasing recognition of both the clinical and leadership skills of nurses who work in care homes.

Despite these endorsements, the art and science of older people's nursing, especially in long-term care settings, needs to overcome a number of obstacles to become the career of choice for newly registered and experienced nurses. Although some of these obstacles are political or require significant system change, many lie within the fabric of the profession perpetuated by rumour and myth. It is our view two main myths loom large in the discourse of care-home nursing. The first is care-home nursing is not regarded as proper nursing. Often characterised as the last resort for nurses who couldn't get a job anywhere else, it is regarded as having less value than other nursing specialisms and lacking in any readily identified clinical or technical expertise. This belief leads directly to the second myth: there is no possibility for a career of any description, or worth, for individuals who find themselves working in the sector. Our aim in this chapter is to explore, discuss and dispel these myths through demonstrating the value, contribution, potential and expertise associated with the art and science of nursing older people in long-term care settings. It is our view care-home nurses are 'maxi-nurses' who use the breadth and depth of nursing skills, knowledge and expertise to promote high-quality care for care-home residents.

At this juncture we would like to clarify terms we use in this chapter. We refer to people using long-term care as *residents*. This is deliberate on our part for a number of reasons. First, the long-term nature of people's admission means they reside at the home. Also, care homes tend to have a philosophy of care that means they strive to provide a home to the people they look after. Third, by using *resident*, we can neatly differentiate from the curative model's use of the term *patient*. We also wish to clarify use of *care home*, a generic term that refers to long-term care facilities where a number of older people live together and staff are available 24 hours a day to provide personal care (e.g., residential care or assisted living/supportive housing facilities) and facilities where a registered nurse is required on duty 24 hours a day to provide additional nursing care for more dependent residents (e.g., nursing homes or skilled nursing facilities).

A LITTLE SOCIAL HISTORY

To understand the origins of these myths, and the reasons health and social care systems are not geared toward meeting the present and future demands of an ageing population, it is important to have an appreciation of the history of geriatrics and the pervasive belief only a curative model of health care constitutes successful treatment. Nolan et al. (2006) discussed the factors that led to a prevalent view of the hospital as the bedrock of modern health care. Historically, the voluntary hospitals of the 1800s became the centres of medicine founded on science and as a result the place of training for the medical and later other clinical professions and the treatment of acutely ill patients. At the same time these hospitals and the culture of modern medicine was developed, the old and chronically ill were termed *incurables*, destined for workhouses and their infirmaries. The workhouse infirmaries had to accept the patients refused by voluntary hospitals, becoming long-stay institutions for individuals marginalised by society.

The success of the hospital model in the treatment and cure of conditions, and the subsequent esteem awarded the senior doctors, later consultants, saw the establishment of a medical elite and reinforced the supremacy of a health care system focused on cure and the superiority of medical practitioners and the hospital. Even within medicine there was resistance, and often antagonism, to the recognition of geriatric medicine as a specialism by acute physicians and surgeons who could see 'no value in spending time, money, energy and bed space on redundant senior members of society' (Felstein, 1969, p. 15). Even at the inception of the much-vaunted National Health Service (NHS) in the United Kingdom, which inherited all these infirmaries, warnings were issued about the implication of being 'lavish to old age' (Beveridge, 1942). From the outset, health care systems were inherently ageist.

There is an argument to suggest geriatric medicine, when it was eventually recognised, came about only as it provided a mechanism by which the acute specialisms could move chronically sick patients through the hospital system. The cruel and pejorative term *incurable* had by now been replaced with the equally inhuman but all too familiar *bed blocker*. Rather than being seen as individuals with complex health and social care needs in a system that wraps around and supports them, older people were instead seen as a blockage in the hospital system and impeding its ability to function well. The hospital system was neither designed nor equipped to meet the social care needs of older people, and therefore these individuals were stripped of their identities as individuals—their personhood—and seen simply as taking up beds that could be better used by someone else.

Increasing life expectancy and morbidity levied an ever-increasing pressure on health care systems. In the 1980s in the United Kingdom, the NHS began a process of withdrawal from long-term care and invited the private and charitable sectors to own, manage and deliver care in these settings. The pressures of patient turnover and rapid discharge meant consultant geriatricians became more involved in acute medicine and withdrew from continuing care and rehabilitation. This had significant implications for nursing. As far back as the 1960s, nurse academics argued the care of the *irredeemable patient* (note again the hopelessness associated with such a term) was true nursing (Norton et al., 1962) and highlighted the need for a new approach to nursing older people that would help nursing realise its potential. Sadly, successive studies over the past six decades have demonstrated nursing's approach to development remains 'uncritically rooted in a curative model' (Kelly et al., 2005, p. 17).

Further studies in the 1980s and 1990s explored the role of the nurse in the long-term care system and characterised nurses as being left with the work no one else wanted to do, lacking the authority to change things and defining good care by the process of getting things done (Kitson, 1991). This led to care that was often depersonalised, task orientated and needing direction (Kitson 1991). These studies highlighted nursing older people as a field of nursing perceived negatively by the majority of nurses not just with regard to choosing to work in this field of practice but also negatively reporting on colleagues who worked in such settings. This view persists today, despite significant changes over the past two decades in the practice of the art and science of nursing older people.

THE SOCIOPOLITICAL CONTEXT

Since the start of the 21st century, the delivery of health and social care has changed in fundamental ways. Most notably this was the result of greater availability of and access to information and the subsequent desire and power of people to have a greater say in their care and to make decisions based on shared knowledge and experience rather than a blind trust in medical expertise. A significant number of health and social care policies have focused on creating partnerships between service providers, older people and their families and the rights of the latter two groups to have a say in treatment plans and decisions. More recently this focus has moved to one of co-design, not just in respect of individual options but in the structural and systemic changes in health and social care as they adapt to the health challenges and personal expectations of an ageing population.

Globally, health and social care policy has taken as its central tenant the right for individuals to live and die in their chosen environment. Such a policy approach is underpinned by an increasing argument that prolonging life at any cost, a legacy of the curative approach to care, is less important than quality of life lived (Clark, 1995). For many older people, their chosen environment is their own home, and help and support to enjoy a good quality of life are accommodated. However, a significant number of older people require a level of care and support that needs to be provided in other settings and ensures the level of input and expertise required to safely meet an individual's needs. For many older people this involves a move to a residential long-term care facility or a new and more supportive home environment.

As a result of changes in policy, and to meet the higher expectations of the newly informed and empowered older generation, a significant shift in thinking about care provision and care environments has been demanded of long-term care providers. Material changes are evident in the proliferation of newly built care homes opened over the past 20 years. The emphasis on the quality and design of these environments, and the impact they have on the health of the people living and working in them, has led to a whole field of expertise and industry being established.

CARE HOMES: ONE SIZE DOES NOT FIT ALL

Sociopolitical and demographic changes over the past 50 years led to development of the care-home sector; care homes come in all shapes and sizes. At one end of the scale are small converted houses with 15 to 20 residents and at the other are large multisite developments with 100 or more bedrooms. As the need for long-term care increased, particularly during the past decade, a significant amount of capital was invested in the care-home sector. Many new, purpose-built care homes have come into use that focus on the design to provide high-quality environments for care and support, particularly for people with dementia. A number of institutions consider the whole home environment, such as the Dementia Services Development Centre at the University of Stirling (https://dementia.stir.ac.uk). These institutions have strong design principles specifically developed to help people live successfully in the care-home environment. Through a better understanding of the lived experiences of ageing and dementia, and impact on the senses (e.g., hearing and taste), environments are now designed to take these issues into account. Some elements are relatively simple, such as ensuring carpets continue in the same pattern through doorways so there is no border that may be seen by someone with visual disturbances as a boundary to jump over or simply painting handrails a colour that makes them stand out from the wall so they can be easily seen. Other schemes are hugely ambitious, with the construction of cinemas, spas and in some cases a street of shops and the feeling of living in a village setting (see Case Study 11.1).

As environments have developed to allow for greater mixing and socialising, there has been an increasing focus on health and well-being. Traditionally care homes have been located on the outside of communities; in the 1990s it was not unusual to find care homes on the edges of industrial and commercial estates where land was cheap, somewhat underlining the value placed on older people by society. Many of the large providers were accused of warehousing older people, and care of older people was something that happened and was not seen. More recently there has been a significant shift in thinking. Society is beginning to recognise the value older people bring to their communities through their life experiences. Care homes have become more open to the outside world, inviting people in and sharing more information than ever before. As care services have become more community focused, many care homes are positioning themselves to become community hubs, running services like a dementia café and day care alongside their residential operation. Now there is a much greater focus on care homes becoming part of the community. Recent TV programmes in the United Kingdom, such as Channel 4's *Old People's Home for 4-Year Olds*, have focused on connecting care homes to communities and

the oldest generation to the youngest. Many care providers have now started similar programmes of work with local schools, and some have a nursery adjacent to the care home to promote intergenerational care and activities.

The thought and investment that goes into turning these design ideas into reality leads in turn to the creation of buildings built for people to thrive in. This has advantages for the people who work in them. There are many more newly built care homes than there are hospitals, all designed around the practicalities of caring for the people living in them. As a result of such great design features, making care delivery easier and being better able to work in a high-quality environment potentially make care homes more attractive places to work.

As well as structural and design changes, care homes have witnessed significant service-level changes, with greater acuity and complexity of need for people using these services. Although initially this change posed a challenge to the social care workforce, the innovation, creation of new roles and new levels of knowledge, skill and nursing expertise required have transformed the provision of care in the sector. These changes have been documented and celebrated within social care itself, but the historical perception of the work in these environments as low skilled and low value persists and perpetuates the myth we are about to tackle: that care-home nursing is not proper nursing.

WHAT DO CARE HOMES DO?

First, people need to understand what care homes do—or more specifically what services and care they provide and for whom. Care homes provide a range of services,

---

CASE STUDY 11.1   The Chocolate Works

The Chocolate Works Care Village, which opened in 2017 in York (UK), provides a very good example of a contemporary and well designed, if somewhat unique, care village. Housed in a former chocolate factory, the design makes the best use of the original art-deco features and the size of the space afforded by the former factory floor. The Chocolate Works has won multiple awards, not just for the sensitive restoration of a treasured and highly valued building, but also for the way in which design maximises the health and well-being of the residents.

Located in a prominent position in the city, next to the racecourse, the Chocolate Works is very much in heart of the local community. This means that residents are able to maintain community links and a real sense of connection to the area in which they live.

The centrepiece of the village is a large central atrium that houses a café, sweet shop, gym, spa, hairdressers and pub – everything that you would expect to find in a village centre. There are comfortable seating areas and park benches where people can relax or meet up with others. This creates a sense of community that residents can be part of and belong to, enabling them to continue to be socially active, meet people and make new friends.

The Chocolate Works provides residential, nursing and dementia care services, located in different parts of the village, but all with access to this amazing space. Nursing people in such an environment requires a special set of skills and knowledge. This is very much caring for people in their own home, in an environment that is designed around them. Nurses need to know the residents well in order to maximise their abilities to live and thrive in this environment.

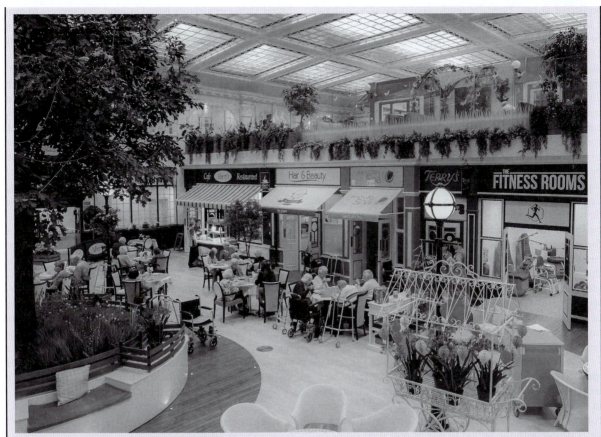

Permission to use image granted by Steph Simmons Photography (www.stephsimmonsphotography.co.uk) and Springfield Healthcare (https://www.springfieldcarevillages.com/).

including care for older people, people with learning disabilities, poor mental health and other long-term conditions such as acquired brain injury. The range of services and people are represented in many of the services that make up the care-home sector today. It is important to highlight people often connect care homes with care for older people and largely ignore other populations, such as care for people with learning disabilities or mental health needs. However, as seen in all parts of the population, better health care and improvements in medicine mean people with learning disabilities are living longer into old age. It is important to reflect this population when talking about long-term care for older people in a way that has not been the case before. For more on nursing approaches to care for people with intellectual disabilities, see Chapter 33.

Broadly speaking, the different types of services care homes provide can be categorised to reflect residents' needs, levels of dependency and complexity caused by multiple morbidities, some of which require nursing input. Often, a care home provides care in a number of these categories and usually, but not always, in different parts of the care home. By doing this, care homes are able to provide care to a resident for a longer period of time, providing continuity for them and for their families as their care needs change. Other care homes exercise much stricter criteria when looking at care need and provide care for only a narrow segment of care need. As a result, if a resident's needs change, and they fall outside the criteria set by the care home, they need to move to another care home that can meet their needs. We expand on these care needs below and reflect on the range of care-home environments.

Residential care homes generally do not employ registered nurses, so where a health care need emerges that requires care by a nurse, it is provided by local primary and community care nursing teams. Nursing homes provide both social and health care to people who need it and employ registered nurses. Typically, residents of these services have a health care or nursing need that goes beyond what could be reasonably met by primary or community nursing teams. Often these individuals don't have a single health care need but multiple morbidities that require consistent nursing input and oversight due to their complexity (Gordon et al., 2014). Dementia care is an expanding area of care that has perhaps developed the most in the past few decades. Many care homes provide specialist dementia care and have environments and training programmes specifically designed to support people living with dementia. Dementia care can be both residential and nursing in nature. Dementia nursing may be due to either a physical or mental health need, depending on the presentation and progression of the dementia. Often physical needs become more pressing as the person reaches the end of life. End-of-life care has become the mainstream work of care homes. Historically, the average length of stay for residents in nursing homes was 3 years, but this is now closer to 12–14 months, and length of stay for residents in residential care homes has reduced from 5 years to around 2.5 to 3 years (LangBuisson, 2020). Across the range of settings and populations they serve, care homes have an important and significant role in providing end-of-life care (see Chapter 34).

Recent years have seen significant growth in the retirement-living sector. Retirement living was historically seen more in North America but has become more common in recent years in the United Kingdom. Often retirement communities offer a village-style environment that provides people with the option to buy or rent their home or apartment and buy in care as required, which might include help around the home, personal care or emotional support. Larger villages often have a residential and/or nursing home on-site and are able to provide nursing care to people in their own homes, or residents are able to move into the care home in the village for respite or long-term care.

In recent years models of service provision have also changed, with many care homes now fulfilling specific contracts with primary and secondary care organisations. Numerous models are in practice. For example, one care home might have a contract with a local hospital to provide beds for older people as a step down from the hospital before going to another destination, whether a return to their home or another care environment. In this type of model, the care home provides the nurses, carers and hotel services, and the hospital provides the therapists and medical staff to cover the home. With better information technology infrastructures and locations close to hospitals, this has become a tried-and-tested model and one that can better meet individual care needs (NHS England and NHS Improvement, 2020) while creating capacity for acute-care focus in the hospital and providing income for the care home. Other models are based around step-up care to provide care for people with increased need but who may not need acute-care services. Usually these services are wholly staffed by the care home, and people are referred by primary care services. Referred individuals often require support or help for a short period of time or for treatment, such as administration of antibiotics before being discharged home. In the future there will be more demand for delivery of complex care that has traditionally occurred in hospital. The NHS Long Term Plan (NHS, 2019) sets out a vision for health care in England that puts greater emphasis on health care being delivered in the community. This will require significant uplift in the provision of the number of nursing beds and the skill set of the workforce. There is also the potential for areas of care delivery to become more specialist as population health needs change, with greater need for specialist care, such as bariatric care, as well as greater provision of end-of-life care supported, for example, by charities such as local hospices with reach into the community.

Care homes provide a range of complex and diverse services to health and social care communities. This includes fundamental care for older people through to complex interventions such as managing people on long-term ventilation or with complex mental health needs. It requires a knowledgeable and competent workforce and dispels the myth that care-home nursing is not skilled and demands a rethink of the value of nurses who work in the sector.

A DIFFERENT WAY OF NURSING

Nursing in a care-home setting (i.e., in a person's home) requires an approach that focuses on how to support the individual to live well and provide care to help manage their condition so it has minimal impact on their day-to-day life. The focus is not the individual's condition—the basis of the cure model. Nurses in care homes focus on the person, not the disease.

In the late 1980s, Tom Kitwood (1997), a pioneer in the field of dementia care, used the term *person-centred care* as a description of bringing together ideas about care that focused on communication and relationships. Fundamental to the model of person-centred care as defined by Kitwood was the rejection of the standard approach to managing dementia as defined by the medical model and its associated negative implications. Kitwood (1998) further developed this model, asking nurses and caregivers to think about what they did according to principles that reinforce or support personhood and well-being rather than simply providing care in accordance with tasks organised around staff routines. Does person-centred care provide nurses with a model that articulates long-term care? Person-centred care became a popular discourse in the gerontological nursing

---

CASE STUDY 11.2   An Example of Person-Centred Care

Let us consider this example of a resident's care plan around a bathing routine: Ron had dementia and had been living in the care home for a number of weeks since his wife, who was his main carer, had died. Although he was sad, Ron was very settled and had built good relationships with the staff and other residents. However, every time the care staff tried to help Ron with a bath, he became very distressed and his behaviour changed from his usual congenial manner to a state of high anxiety and distress. The more care staff tried to encourage and support Ron with the bath, the more distressed he became. The nurses had spoken to his (adult) children about this, but they could not explain the behaviours, and said that their father had never shown any distress about bathing in the past.

One day Ron was visited by a long-time friend who the family wanted to be involved in Ron's care. The nurses took the opportunity to discuss with his friend Ron's anxiety about bathing. Ron's friend explained that Ron had been in the navy during World War 2. This the staff knew. Ron's friend then went on to explain that one of the ships Ron had served on had been hit by a torpedo and that Ron had been trapped for a period of time under the deck of the ship before he was able to get out and swim to the boats. This had affected Ron deeply at the time and for a long time afterwards Ron would only wash at a sink or have the occasional shower. As Ron got older, he did bathe but always during the day when the bathroom was well lit by daylight.

The bathroom near Ron's bedroom was on the inside of the home, and so had no natural light, and could be quite dark. Armed with this new knowledge about Ron, the staff took him to a bathroom on a different floor that had a window to the outside. In this room, Ron's anxiety considerably reduced, and the carers were able to help Ron bath without the distress he had experienced previously.

This case study demonstrates the power and importance of understanding the person, and of getting to know them through those who know them best—in this case a long-time friend. The person-centred approach meant that Ron's distress was treated, not as a problem to overcome or cure, but as something to understand so that Ron could be cared for in a way that worked for him.

---

literature, and there was an increase in descriptive accounts of attempts to develop and deliver person-centred practice by the profession. However, McCormack (2004) argued nurses were uncritically adopting this model of care, and systematic research into the practice of person-centred care was not sufficiently developed. Further work by McCormack and McCance (2007) developed the concept of person-centred care as a model of nursing care, and later multidisciplinary care, and is now a well-established concept in nursing and health care (McCormack et al., 2021). There is still a limited evidence that explores the outcomes of implementing person-centred care, but it provides a useful alternative to the curative model.

Putting person-centred care into practice means each resident is seen as a unique individual who is a valued member of the community in which they live. Person-centred care planning places the resident at the centre of the assessment and planning process. Such a care plan is different from the predetermined treatment and care pathways often seen in the acute and short-term care environment and requires a different approach to solving care issues (Corazzini & Anderson, 2014) (see Case Study 11.2). Care planning in long-term care is a detailed and informed process through which residents, their relatives and friends and nurses must work together and form strong, trusting relationships. This is achieved by nurses working with the resident, their relatives and friends using a biographical approach to gather information about the resident that informs nurses how to support the resident in maintaining a high quality of life. A person-centred care plan underpins this approach, providing a format through which the information gathered can be shared among all who care for the resident. For many nurses, person-centred planning is more about adopting a different way of thinking about how care is planned rather than learning an entirely new technique. Although there are many ways of developing a person-centred care plan, there are key features at the core of the planning process (see Fig. 11.1).

Person-centred care has been embraced by long-term care settings as a model of care. As such, nurses working in care homes can articulate the value of care and the role of nursing within long-term care settings. Surely this is proper or maxi-nursing.

TECHNOLOGY AND INNOVATION FOR CARE

For many reasons the care-home sector has often been perceived as lagging behind in terms of technology and the infrastructure to support innovation. There is some truth in this for a number of reasons, such as challenges of securing good network coverage in older buildings or

1. The resident is at the centre and the nurse engages with the resident, and their family and friends where appropriate and as chosen by the resident. A good person-centred plan will balance what is important to the resident, their aspirations and the support that they require. to ensure a sound understanding of the resident and their situation. Nurses need to consider how to support the resident to participate proactively in planning their own care and also how to include relatives, friends and other people that the resident would like to involve in planning their care.

2. The focus is on the capacities and capabilities of the resident to promote community participation and meaningful engagement. Person-centred care planning focuses on what a resident can do – their capacities and capabilities, and not on their deficits, or what they can no longer do. This shift in focus is key to person-centred care and to ensure inclusion in the community in which they live, and to participate as fully as possible in community life and in a meaningful way.

3. The resident has authority and control and nurses recognise this when ensuring person-centred care. Residents and the people who care about them (family and friends) decide what is important, which opportunities should be taken and what the future will hold. Nurses are therefore 'problem solvers' rather than 'decision-makers'. They continue to give professional advice and care but support the resident by providing the care the resident feels they need, rather than dictating what care the resident can have.

4. The care plan results in actions that are about life, not just services, and reflects what is possible, not just what is available. This requires commitment shared by the residents and all people involved in their care. It identifies what is important to the resident now, i.e. the small things every day that will make a difference for the person, but also prompts people to consider what they can do to help the resident have a better quality of life.

Relationships form the basis of everyday lives: we want to belong and be a part of other people's lives and vice versa. Older people, and particularly those living with dementia, often only spend time with people who are paid to be with them. This segregates them from the 'real' world and deprives them of the chance to meet new people and develop new relationships. Person-centred planning aims to help people create and maintain meaningful relationships with people who are not paid to be with them and beyond the care home doors.

5. People change, and person-centred care recognises this through listening, observing and learning from the resident and their family and friends. Person-centred planning should not be a one-off event: a care plan written today will not be fit for purpose in the future. People change, as will their aspirations and goals. A person-centred plan will evolve and change with that resident, and continue to reflect their changing capacity, capability and aspirations.

Fig. 11.1 Key features of person-centred care planning.

staff reluctance to engage with technology. Traditionally, technology in care homes focused on the nurse call system and little else! However, as technology has become more widely adopted by the population, there is a greater expectation it will be used in the workplace. Digital technology has multiple potential applications in care homes (Hanratty et al., 2019). As in many care settings, there has been a major shift in care homes to use electronic platforms for record-keeping, time management and quality improvement. There is also increased demand from people who use these services too, with a proliferation of tablets, smartphones and smart devices becoming part of everyday activities. Digital communication was a lifeline for many during the successive lockdowns of the COVID-19 pandemic, when visiting was restricted and socially distanced.

One of the most significant technological innovations is electronic care plans. Increasing numbers of electronic care platforms are being developed. Although there are some clear market leaders, this is an area that continues to grow as the capability of the technology and confidence and competence of the workforce increases. Such developments have been able to support changes in how services are delivered, especially where there is capability to link the home with the general practitioner (GP) or other nursing and support services. Electronic medication records have been in existence for a number of years and have evolved from being self-contained record-keeping systems to multifunctional platforms that connect the home, GP and pharmacy. This means medication reviews, medication ordering and good stock control have become much more effective, saving time and improving medicine management. Some homes have been reluctant to take up such systems, and there are challenges with regard to ensuring the information technology systems used by the home, GP and pharmacy have the ability to communicate with one another. However, where these systems are implemented well, the ability to improve care and the experience of the people involved is significant (Digital Social Care, 2020).

This capability through technology to connect people in different parts of the health and social care system led to a number of changes in how these systems work together and promotion of cross-sector and interdisciplinary working for the benefit of resident care. More effective use of video technology means care homes can have much more direct contact with hospital and community services. As the technology to support telecare develops, nurses in care homes are able to send health data direct to health care professionals and get advice and treatment plans without the need to wait for an appointment, minimising travel for residents. When assessed at the start of the decade, telecare to improve social and health care was not considered cost effective (Henderson et al., 2014). Commissioning of technology was therefore limited to pilot sites. However,

the wider use of wearable technology in everyday life and the impact of COVID-19 means telehealth technologies are more readily adopted and put into practice at a pace previously unseen across a wide range of care homes.

Real-time data collection driven by developments in wearables and other forms of telemonitoring such as movement sensors will enable health-care professionals to provide timely and appropriate treatment and support for patients and carers while generating large data sets that, with appropriate permissions, could drive forward research in many areas such as prevention and early detection. A growing body of evidence indicates off-the-shelf smart technologies are already being used effectively, helping people maintain a degree of independence where previously they needed assistance (Hanratty et al., 2019; Digital Social Care, 2020). For example, smart technology can be used to turn lights on and off, open and close blinds and change the television or radio station. The next generation of care-home residents will be more familiar with technology and with using it in everyday life, so there is an expectation this will continue when they move into a care home. Widespread adoption of digital technologies has lead to the building of smart homes with technology infrastructures built into the fabric of the building. The use of technology to support care delivery and connect health-care professionals more closely has the potential to transform care. Although the technology used may be different to the technology more closely associated with acute and critical care, this does not mean it is absent. It is simply different. Rather than saving lives at a point in time, it enables people to live their lives. As with so much of what we discuss in this chapter, it is about viewing the technology through a different lens—the lens of care rather than the lens of cure. For more on technology and digital tools, see Chapter 35.

Technology and innovation for care relies on a workforce with the skills, knowledge and competence to promote person-centred care and embrace and lead innovation.

WHO CARES? UNDERSTANDING THE CARE-HOME WORKFORCE

The quality of care and life experienced by care-home residents is influenced by the staff who lead, manage and deliver care. Accepting that staff influence quality necessitates consideration of what is known about the care-home workforce and how they influence quality. Scrutiny of quality in care-home contexts is often associated with scrutiny of staffing levels, recruitment and retention and whether the right kind of staff with the right skills are employed. There are important differences in the makeup of the workforces that provide care in different types of long-term residential-care settings in the United Kingdom and global variations in long-term residential care provision and workforces. Capturing this international diversity is beyond the scope of this chapter but important to acknowledge.

In recent years the status of the workforce in care homes has emerged as a matter of public and policy concern. We wrote this chapter during the COVID-19 pandemic, which threw into sharp focus the important role of care homes and the workforce they employ to care for the most vulnerable members of our society. Care for older people in care homes requires staff who can build and maintain relationships with the people they support, including their families and friends, and who can coordinate and build connections with wider teams of health and social care professionals involved with a resident's care. As the most important asset, care homes need to employ staff with the right knowledge, attitudes and approach to ensure staff are competent, appreciate the challenges of working in the sector and understand how to promote quality of care and quality of life for residents.

In this section we focus on factors that influence the supply of the care-home workforce and its makeup, then examine the critical role of nurses within care homes, the importance of nursing leadership and promoting evidence-based practices and cultures of learning and teaching. By challenging the misconceptions associated with the role of care-home nurses and considering the career opportunities and role fulfilment offered by care homes, we amply demonstrate care-home nursing can be a rewarding and fruitful career. We tackle the myth nurses cannot have a successful career working in a care home.

THE CHALLENGE OF NURSING SUPPLY FOR THE SECTOR

There are about three times as many care-home beds for older people as there are NHS hospital beds in England. This proportion of residential long-term care to acute-care beds is replicated globally (Organisation for Economic Cooperation and Development, 2015), although some countries, such as Sweden and the Netherlands, have gradually reduced numbers of residential long-term care beds and focused on community care provision. In England care homes employ about 465,000 direct care staff, and care homes with nursing employ approximately 33,000 registered nurses (Organisation for Economic Cooperation and Development, 2015). An additional 42,000 staff are employed in managerial roles in the sector; some of these staff are also registered nurses (Skills for Care, 2020). This makes care homes a significant employer of staff who meet the health and care needs of residents. However, the sector

faces challenges in recruiting and retaining its workforce and, in particular, attracting registered nurses. The vacancy rates for registered nurses and care staff in care homes in England during 2019–2020 were high, at 12.3% and 8.2%, respectively (Skills for Care, 2020). This is a cause for concern: any mismatch between demand and supply impacts quality of care. A global shortage of registered nurses impacts the sector, a situation that will be exacerbated in the United Kingdom by Brexit. Another significant challenge for the sector relates to attracting nurses and other care staff to work in care homes. United Kingdom campaigns like Every Day Is Different (https://www.adultsocialcare.co.uk/getinvolved.aspx) and Care for Others: Make a Difference (https://www.adultsocialcare.co.uk/resources/Care-for-others-Make-a-difference.aspx) were launched to attract people with values suited to the sector and generate interest in roles and a career in the sector.

Nurse education may not always focus on care for older people or care homes. Repeated analyses of nursing curricula highlighted limited gerontological content needed to prepare nurses to meet the complex needs of older people (Garbrah et al., 2017). These curricula echo the early foundations of medical training and focus predominantly on nursing models enthralled by cure, with insufficient focus on care for older people, frailty, co-morbidities, complex long-term conditions, dementia, end-of-life care, health and social care partnerships and the political landscape of care homes (Spilsbury et al., 2015). However, some notable improvements in recent years tried to address these deficiencies (Berman et al., 2005). Ensuring older people can access good nursing care in care homes is crucial. There is considerable overlap in dependency levels and care needs among residents in care homes with and without nursing but important differences in the ways care is provided.

NURSING ROLES WITHIN CARE HOMES AND MEETING THE NEEDS OF OLDER PEOPLE

When considering workforce, it is important to acknowledge the makeup of the care-home workforce and how it differs across different types of care homes. In the United Kingdom in homes with nursing care, or nursing homes, registered nurses are employed around the clock to supervise care delivery, which is mainly provided by a large workforce of non-registered care staff. In care homes without nursing, or residential homes, the workforce is comprised solely of social care staff, and the NHS provides nursing input on an as-required basis. Registered nurses who work for the NHS may also be involved in supporting specialist care for residents in both types of care homes, for example palliative care or dementia care. Care staff in both of these settings are employed at different levels and have different levels of preparation for their roles. We recognise international differences in the organisation and structure of long-term care provision and the roles employed in these settings. Regardless, the role of the care-home nurse is broad and multifaceted.

Care-home nurses require particular skills, knowledge, competencies and experience to provide high-quality care and meet the complex and wide-ranging needs of residents while working in a highly regulated environment. Describing the care-home nurse role in this way may not be recognised in society or by nurses who work in other settings for reasons we have already discussed. Yet caring for these populations is both challenging and rewarding. The care-home nurse has overall responsibility for the care of residents, often working as the only registered nurse on duty, supervising care delivery by a range of care staff and without on-site medical cover. Perhaps we need different language to describe this role if it is to be more widely recognised. If nurses in the sector were described as working in nurse-led units or were called advanced practitioners in complex care, would this change perceptions? Let's consider the role in more detail and why it should not be dismissed as the role nurses have when they can't get a job elsewhere or where they work prior to retirement.

The main roles and responsibilities of care-home nurses include providing day-to-day fundamental care for residents; promoting person-centred care, including personal choice and meaningful, purposeful activities; engaging with family members and providing appropriate support; clinical care treatments and interventions; preventing adverse events and ensuring resident safety; assessing and monitoring residents' physical, mental, emotional and social well-being; making appropriate and timely referrals to other professionals; managing long-term conditions and acute episodes of illness; providing specialist care such as end-of-life or dementia care; counselling; managing; acting as a role model for other staff; leading; coordinating; educating; advocating; maintaining accurate and complete records of care; keeping up to date and ensuring services comply with relevant sector regulation and legislation (Skills for Care, 2019; Spilsbury et al., 2015). This list is not exhaustive and not presented in any order of priority but highlights the diversity of nurses' roles in this setting and the high level of skills and knowledge required. Importantly, care-home nurses must be able to make decisions, know the boundaries of their knowledge and skills and know when to seek help to ensure the needs of residents are met. They are truly autonomous practitioners. The role is far from boring or repetitive, and it is much more than administering medicines.

Nurses in this setting might also be described as the conductors of care. It is important they promote partnership working with other health and social care professionals to ensure the best quality care for care-home residents (Goodman et al., 2017). Examples of opportunities to promote partnership working include in-reach link specialist nursing roles (e.g., in pressure ulcer care or palliative care) or joint reviews of resident care by care-home nurses, GPs or other community or hospital health-care professionals. A whole-systems approach to care for the older person is required. The care-home nurse is pivotal for this ambition to be realised. During the COVID-19 pandemic, the critical role of care-home nurses was thrown into the spotlight as they responded to the crisis, demonstrating resourcefulness and innovation to ensure the physical, cognitive and emotional needs of residents were met (Spilsbury et al., 2020). The need for recognition and reward of these critical staff was also highlighted by this international crisis in addition to ensuring they have the necessary support for their own, resilience, well-being and physical, psychological and mental health.

Our earlier description of the care-home sector described the breadth and diversity of services care homes provide not only focused on care of older people but also in specialised care, such as support of people with dementia or learning disabilities. There are a range of opportunities for nurses in the sector to progress and tailor their career ambitions. Studies revealed existing undergraduate pre-registration nursing-degree programmes do not adequately prepare the future nursing workforce with the skills, knowledge, competencies and experience to deliver high-quality care to older care-home residents or profile care-home nursing as a fulfilling career option (Cooper et al., 2017). This is a significant omission and one that needs to be addressed. One solution often offered is to deliver a specialist gerontological qualification for care-home nurses (Adams, 2019). This may also be helpful in highlighting a career pathway and ensuring staff are adequately trained post-registration for this area of practice. Training courses are available for nurses in the sector, although there is scope to increase and expand these opportunities.

Nurses can progress their careers working in care-home nursing with roles such as senior care home nurse, specialist nurse, clinical lead, clinical development manager or practice development facilitator. Some nurses pursue a management career, moving into the care-home manager role, and depending on the size of the care organisation, there may be opportunities at a regional level, such as operations manager or divisional nurse. The largest organisations have quite large central quality-assurance teams led by a director of nursing or director of quality. While this list is not exhaustive, it challenges commonly held assumptions no career framework exists for care home nurses (see Case Study 11.3). By example, one of the authors of this chapter, Richard Adams,

CASE STUDY 11.3   Erskine: Caring for Veterans

Erskine is a charity providing support for nearly a thousand veterans in Scotland every year. Erskine's model of care provides an excellent example of a modern care provider, operating multiple services, including 4 care homes and a Veterans Village comprising cottages, an activity centre assisted living apartments and single living apartments.

The scale and size of the organisation requires the many different knowledge and skills that we have discussed in this section. Erskine have been using a nursing career ladder to demonstrate to staff the value and importance of each of these roles in the organisation.

Each rung of the career ladder provides a stepping stone to the next level, and encourages staff to build career within Erskine. The ladder image helps staff visualise the other roles that they might aspire to and the different routes available to them from registered nursing roles into practice development, advanced practice or management roles.

The ladder has proved to be of great benefit to the organisation, both as a recruitment tool and a means of improving staff retention, demonstrating to prospective staff the dynamic and progressive nature of the organisation. Numerous staff have progressed from carer roles to preparation for nursing, and nurse training programmes. The ladder also plays a role in showcasing careers in care to those outside of the sector, clearly illustrating the complex and multiskilled nature of care home nursing.

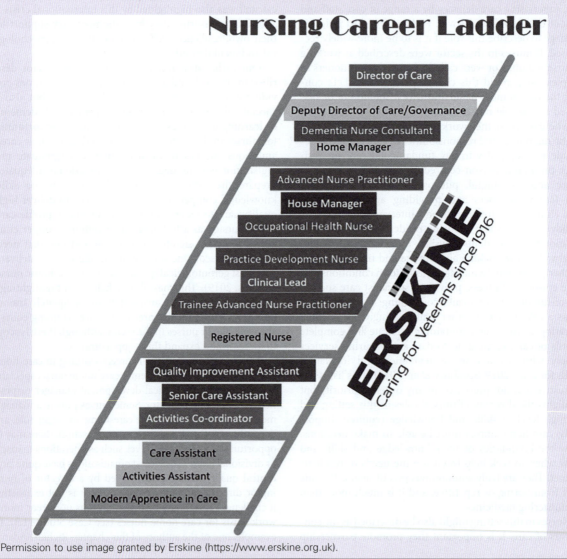

Nursing Career Ladder

- Director of Care
- Deputy Director of Care/Governance
- Dementia Nurse Consultant
- Home Manager
- Advanced Nurse Practitioner
- House Manager
- Occupational Health Nurse
- Practice Development Nurse
- Clinical Lead
- Trainee Advanced Nurse Practitioner
- Registered Nurse
- Quality Improvement Assistant
- Senior Care Assistant
- Activities Co-ordinator
- Care Assistant
- Activities Assistant
- Modern Apprentice in Care

ERSKINE Caring for Veterans since 1916

Permission to use image granted by Erskine (https://www.erskine.org.uk).

started his career as a care-home carer and is now chief executive officer for a care organisation. Opportunities and rewards exist in the sector, and as the population ages, care-home nurses will become increasingly important to manage the needs of some of the most vulnerable members of society and provide strong leadership for care staff at different levels. Roles for all staff in care homes are not static but evolve in response to resident demands for care, skills shortages, quality improvement, technological innovation and cost containment. Within the care-home sector, this has led to the expansion of roles for registered nurses through role diversification and specialisation and new roles for non-registered care staff who come under the direction and supervision of the nurse. There has been particular growth in the number and range of roles to take on work previously within the domain of registered nurses. In care homes, the senior carer, nursing associate and associate practitioner are members of the care team who provide valuable support and care for residents alongside care staff. As the workforce diversifies, nursing leadership has an increasingly important role.

THE IMPORTANCE OF NURSING LEADERSHIP

Nursing leaders have a key role in promoting quality of care for care-home residents and creating positive work environments for staff (Haunch et al., 2021). Evidence reveals the relationship between good leadership and its positive impact on resident experience and outcomes, staff satisfaction and retention, and there is a suggestion that positive staff experiences at work influence resident care and outcomes (Anderson et al., 2003; Havig et al., 2011). Leading is different to managing and can occur at different levels in a care team. Leadership may be provided by the care-home manager, who may or may not be a registered nurse. Clinical or frontline registered nurses may also provide active leadership and influence the care team. Care-home leaders facilitate cultures, relationships and the context in which groups of people work and approach care delivery, including working across care systems and influencing policy and practice at local and national levels. This is especially important where care homes are not integrated into local primary and secondary care systems.

Importantly, leaders in care homes enable person-centred care and cultures to thrive by encouraging and supporting staff to place residents' values and preferences first, considering the resident as a whole person rather focusing on their functional limitations and promoting core values of dignity, choice, privacy and independence. Eliciting resident preferences and values and incorporating them into the provision of care is a dynamic process that demands adaptive leadership at all levels to encourage and support the work of care staff for residents (Corazzini & Anderson,

2014). Strong active nursing leadership in this environment is essential and an important area for investment and development to ensure the coordination and delivery of care, clarification of roles and responsibilities of the care team, and monitoring and evaluation of the impact on care for resident experiences and outcomes.

Nurse leaders in care homes require skills and competence in clinical excellence and critical thinking. Evidence-based practice is important in this context. Poor staff knowledge and competence lead to suboptimal outcomes for residents and increased referrals to other primary and community care services—for example, community nurses or general practitioners—or unscheduled acute-hospital attendance (Cooper et al., 2017; British Geriatrics Society, 2011). It is essential for nurses in care homes to ensure they keep up to date to meet the complex health and care demands of residents. Care-home organisations provide an important environment for learning, teaching and research.

PROMOTING EVIDENCE-BASED PRACTICES AND CULTURES OF LEARNING AND TEACHING

Enhancing and promoting quality in long-term care through clinical innovation, new technologies and new ways of delivering services and deploying the caring workforce are imperatives. Any innovation, independent of care setting, should be evidence based. There are examples of models for promoting evidence-based practice and creating cultures of learning and teaching that involve structural collaborations between care homes and academia.

In the 1980s teaching nursing homes were promoted internationally to better prepare the workforce, foster research cultures and improve resident outcomes. The principles of these models have been described as follows:

- Quality of care and quality of life for residents
- An ethical learning collaborative/partnership
- Mutual accountability
- Shared resources
- Valuing, supporting, and disseminating of best practices
- Reciprocity
- Research
- Commitment to transparency and quality improvement. (Mezey et al., 2008)

In recent years teaching care homes have been implemented in England (see the Foundation of Nursing Studies website at https://www.fons.org) alongside other approaches for supporting care homes to promote quality and evidence-based solutions for their context.

NICHE-Leeds, or **N**urturing **I**nnovation in **C**are **H**ome **E**xcellence in Leeds (https://niche.leeds.ac.uk), builds on the successful Academic Collaborative Centre on Care for Older People (ACC-COP) in the Netherlands (Verbeek et al., 2013). ACC-COP has proven its feasibility, acceptability and sustainability to care-home residents, workers and policy makers over 20 years (Verbeek et al., 2020). At the core of these models is generating and undertaking relevant research and effective implementation of findings and evidence-based innovation alongside promoting cultures of learning and teaching in care homes (Fig. 11.2). There are two key principles:

- A resident-centred focus that ensures research and development concentrates on clinical and/or organisational areas that promote quality of life, quality of care, choice and autonomy, and/or meaningful activities for residents or focus on quality of work for staff, which has a direct influence on residents' care
- Interdisciplinary collaboration between care, policy, education and research

NICHE-Leeds is the first team in the United Kingdom to replicate and develop the ACC-COP model. Both teams are focused on mobilising and translating established research evidence for care-home practice and policy and, where research evidence is lacking, generating new evidence through competitively funded research studies where both universities and care homes agree these are important (Griffiths et al., 2021). In addition, they aim to improve the quality of education by incorporating scientific knowledge in educational programs, offering opportunities for students to work on innovative projects and encouraging enthusiasm for work in this important field of practice.

CONCLUSION

This chapter addressed two significant myths about care-home nursing: that care-home nursing is not proper nursing and that nurses cannot have a career in care-home nursing.

We started by considering the evolution of social care from the workhouse through long-stay wards and hospitals to the current provision in the private and charitable sectors. In doing so we highlighted the dominance and prestige of the cure model and the corresponding perceived lack of value of a model of practice based on care.

We challenged commonly held perceptions about the range of services care homes provide in terms of types of service provision and the level of acuity and complexity of people who use these services. Care homes are now a place where care and the emerging discipline of care-home design combine to create environments in which people, supported by technology, can thrive rather than simply survive.

Our exploration of the different roles and skills required to meet and represent the wide-ranging and complex needs of the care-home population at local and national levels put to bed (we hope!) the myth nurses cannot have a career in care-home nursing.

We concluded by reiterating the care home is a nurse-led unit and the home of the person first that seeks to support people to live a full, meaningful, engaging life while managing a range of physical, psychological, cognitive or mental health needs. We described care-home nurses as critical thinkers, autonomous practitioners and dynamic leaders. Care-home nurses are without doubt proper nurses and are in fact maxi-nurses.

PURPOSE
To facilitate:
- Collaboration across care homes, university, local and national authorities
- Development of initiatives for improving quality of care, life and work
- Cultures of learning and development
- Stimulation of knowledge exchange across the sector

MAIN GOAL
NICHE-Leeds is a driving force for enhancing knowledge and quality in care homes in Leeds
To promote:
- Quality of care and services in local and national prioritised areas
- Continued development of clinical practice for staff and students
- Confidence and development among care home staff
- Research and development in care and services

Fig. 11.2 NICHE-Leeds purpose and goals.

KEY LEARNING POINTS

- The emergence of care-home nursing provides opportunities for nursing, and an initial reluctance to move away from models based on cure faded as the person-centred care framework was widely adopted by the sector. This framework required a shift in thinking from cure to one of helping individuals continue to achieve their ambitions and live well within their capabilities and their own home.
- Care-home nurses are autonomous practitioners who function as conductors of care, with many options for progression not just into management but also advanced practice and practice development roles—all of which require strong, adaptive leadership and a commitment to clinical excellence in highly regulated environments.
- The ongoing challenge for the sector is to promote understanding about the rewarding and challenging careers available for nurses in care homes at any stage of their careers and ensure undergraduate nursing curricula include the appropriate gerontological content needed to prepare nurses to meet the complex needs of older people, particularly in long-term care environments.
- Care-home nursing requires representation at local and national levels to ensure the needs of care-home residents are represented and reflected in local care systems and national health and social care policy.

REFERENCES

Adams, R. (2019). Opinion: A specialist qualification in older people's nursing is needed. *Nursing Times*. https://www.nursingtimes.net/opinion/a-specialist-qualification-in-older-peoples-nursing-is-needed-12-04-2019.

Anderson, R. A., Issel, L. M., & McDaniel, R. R. (2003). Nursing homes as complex adaptive systems: Relationship between management practice and resident outcomes. *Nursing Research, 52*(1), 12–21. doi:10.1097/00006199-200301000-00003.

Beard, J. (2014). 'Ageing well' must be a global priority. *World Health Organization*. https://www.who.int/mediacentre/news/releases/2014/lancet-ageing-series/en.

Berman, A., Mezey, M., Kobayashi, M., & Fulmer, T. (2005). Gerontological nursing content in baccalaureate nursing programs: Comparison of findings from 1997 and 2003. *Journal of Professional Nursing, 21*(5), 268–275. doi.org/10.1016/j.profnurs.2005.07.005.

Beveridge, W. (1942). *Social insurance and allied services*: His Majesty's Stationery Office.

British Geriatrics Society. (2011). *British Geriatrics Society joint working party inquiry into the quality of healthcare support for older people in care homes—Quest for quality: A call for leadership, partnership and quality improvement*. https://www.bgs.org.uk/sites/default/files/content/attachment/2019-08-27/quest_quality_care_homes.pdf

Clark, P. G. (1995). Quality of life, values and teamwork in geriatric care: Do we communicate what we mean? *Gerontologist, 35*(3), 402–411.

Cooper, E. C., Spilsbury, K., McCaughan, D. M., Butterworth, T., Thompson, C. A., & Hanratty, B. (2017). Priorities for the care home nursing workforce: A Delphi study. *Age and Ageing. 46*(1), 39–45.

Corazzini, K., & Anderson, R. (2014). Adaptive leadership and person-centered care: A new approach to solving problems. *North Carolina Medical Journal, 75*(5), 352–354. https://doi.org/10.18043/ncm.75.5.352.

Cornes, M., & Manthorpe, J. (2022). *The role and contribution of registered nurses in social care: A rapid evidence review*. NIHR Policy Research Unit in Health and Social Care Workforce, The Policy Institute, King's College London. https://doi.org/10.18742/pub01-071.

Devi, R., Goodman, C., Dalkin, S., Bate, A., Wright, J., Jones, L., & Spilsbury, K. (2021). Attracting, recruiting and retaining nurses and care workers working in care homes: The need for a nuanced understanding informed by evidence and theory. *Age and Ageing, 50*(1), 65–67. doi:10.1093/ageing/afaa109.

Digital Social Care. (2020). *The Hubble project: Technology-enabled care*. https://www.digitalsocialcare.co.uk/social-care-technology/the-hubble-project

Felstein, I. (1969). *Later life: Geriatrics today and tomorrow*: Routledge and Kegan Paul.

Garbrah, W., Välimäki, T., Palovaara, M., & Kankkunen, P. (2017). Nursing curriculums may hinder a career in gerontological nursing: An integrative review. *International Journal of Older People Nursing, 12*(3). doi:10.1111/opn.12152.

Goodman, C., Davies, S. L., Gordon, A. L., Dening, T., Gage, H., Meyer, J., Schneider, J., Bell, B., Jordan, J., Martin, F., Iliffe, S., Bowman, C., Gladman, J. R. F., Victor, C., Mayrhofer, A., Handley, M., & Zubair, M. (2017). Optimal NHS service delivery to care homes: A realist evaluation of the features and mechanisms that support effective working for the continuing care of older people in residential settings. *Health Services and Delivery Research, 5*(29). https://www.journalslibrary.nihr.ac.uk/programmes/hsdr/11102102/#/.

Gordon, A. L., Franklin, M., Bradshaw, L., Logan, P., Elliot, R., & Gladman, J. R. F. (2014). Health status of UK care home residents: A cohort study. *Age and Ageing, 43*, 97–103. doi:10.1093/ageing/aft077.

Griffiths, A., Devi, R., Cheetham, B., Heaton, L., Randle, A., Ellwood, A., Douglas, D. V. A., Csikar, J., Vinall-Collier, K., Wright, J., & Spilsbury, K. (2021). Maintaining and improving mouth care for care home residents: A participatory research project. *International Journal of Older People's Nursing, 16*(5), e12394. doi:10.1111/opn.12394.

Hanratty, B., Craig, D., Brittain, K., Spilsbury, K., Vines, J., & Wilson, P. (2019). Innovation to enhance health in care homes and evaluation of tools for measuring outcomes of care: Rapid evidence synthesis. *Health Services and Delivery Research, 7*(27). https://www.journalslibrary.nihr.ac.uk/programmes/hsdr/157705/#/.

Haunch, K., Thompson, C., Arthur, A., Edwards, P., Goodman, C., Hanratty, B., Meyer, J., Charlwood., A., Valizade, D., Backhaus, R., Verbeek, H., Hamers, J. P. H., & Spilsbury, K (2021). Understanding the staff behaviours that promote quality for older people living in long term care facilities: A realist review. *International Journal of Nursing Studies*. May, 117. https://doi.org/10.1016/j.ijnurstu.2021.103905.

Havig, A. K., Skogstad, A., Kjekshus, L. E., & Romøren, T. I. (2011). Leadership, staffing and quality of care in nursing homes. *BMC Health Services Research*(327), 11. http://www.biomedcentral.com/1472-6963/11/327.

Henderson, C., Knapp, M., Fernandez, J. L., Beecham, J., Hirani, S. P., Beynon, M., Cartwright, M., Rixon, L., Doll, H., Bower, P., Steventon, A., Rogers, A., Fitzpatrick, R., Barlow, J., Bardsley, M., & Newman, S. P. (2014). Cost-effectiveness of telecare for people with social care needs: The Whole Systems Demonstrator cluster randomised trial. *Age and Ageing, 43*, 794–800.

Kelly, T. B., Tolson, D., Schofield, I., & Booth, J. (2005). Describing gerontological nursing: An academic exercise of prerequisite for progress. *International Journal of Older People Nursing in association with Journal of Clinical Nursing, 14*(3A), 13–23.

Kingston, A., Robinson, L., Booth, H., Knapp, M., & Jagger, C. (2018). Projections of multi-morbidity in the older population in England to 2035: Estimates from the Population Ageing and Care Simulation (PACSim) model. *Age and Ageing, 47*(3), 374–380. doi:10.1093/ageing/afx201.

Kitson, A. (1991). *Therapeutic nursing in the hospitalized elderly*. Scutari Press.

Kitwood, T. (1997). *Dementia reconsidered: The person comes first*. Open University Press.

Kitwood, T. (1998). Toward a theory of dementia care: Ethics and interaction. *Journal of Clinical Ethics, 9*, 23–34.

LaingBuisson. (2020). *Care homes for older people UK market report*. LaingBuisson.

McCormack, B. (2004). Person-centredness in gerontological nursing: An overview of the literature. *Journal of Clinical Nursing, 13*(3a), 31–38. doi:10.1111/j.1365-2702.2004.00924.x. PMID: 15028037.

McCormack, B., & McCance, T. (2007). Development of the person-centred nursing framework. *Journal of Advanced Nursing, 56*(5), 472–479. doi:10.1111/j.1365-2648.2006.04042.x.

McCormack, B., McCance, T., Bulley, C., Brown, D., McMillan, A., & Martin, S. (2021). *Fundamentals of person-centred healthcare practice*. Wiley Blackwell.

Mezey, M. D., Mitty, E. L., & Burger, S. G. (2008). Rethinking teaching nursing homes: Potential for improving long-term care. *Gerontologist, 48*(1), 8–15. doi:10.1093/geront/48.1.8.

NHS. (2019). *The NHS long term plan*. https://www.longterm-plan.nhs.uk

NHS England and NHS Improvement. (2020). *The framework for enhanced health in care homes 2020/2021, Version 2*. https://www.england.nhs.uk/wp-content/uploads/2020/03/the-framework-for-enhanced-health-in-care-homes-v2-0.pdf

Nolan, M., Brown, J., Davies, S., Nolan, J., & Keady, J. (2006). The Senses Framework: Improving care for older people through a relationship centred approach. Getting Research into Practice: University of Sheffield. http://shura.shu.ac.uk/280.

Norton, D., McClaren, R., & Eyton-South, A. N. (1962). *An investigation of geriatric nursing problems in hospital Research Report NCCOP*. Churchill Livingstone.

Organisation for Economic Cooperation and Development. (2015). *Health at a glance 2015: Long-term care beds in institutions and hospitals*. https://www.oecd-ilibrary.org/social-issues-migration-health/health-at-a-glance-2015/long-term-care-beds-in-institutions-and-hospitals_health_glance-2015-78-en

Skills for Care. (2019). *Registered nurses recognising the responsibilities and contribution of registered nurses within social care*. Skills for Care. https://www.skillsforcare.org.uk/Documents/Learning-and-development/Regulated-professionals/Registered-nurses-recognising-the-responsibilities-and-contribution-of-registered-nurses-within-social-care.pdf

Skills for Care. (2020). *The state of the adult social care sector and workforce in England. Skills for Care*. https://www.skillsforcare.org.uk/adult-social-care-workforce-data/Workforce-intelligence/documents/State-of-the-adult-social-care-sector/The-state-of-the-adult-social-care-sector-and-workforce-2020.pdf

Spilsbury, K., Devi, R., Daffu-O'Reilly, A., Griffiths, A., Haunch, K., Jones, L., & Meyer, J (2020). *Less COVID-19: Lessons from the frontline*. University of Leeds. https://niche.leeds.ac.uk/news/niche-leeds-and-national-care-forum-publish-less-covid-19-report.

Spilsbury, K., Hanratty, B., & McCaughan, D. (2015). *Supporting nursing in care homes*: University of York. https://rcnfoundation.rcn.org.uk/funded-projects/improving-patient-care/supporting-nursing-in-care-homes.

Thompson, J., Cook, G., & Duschinsky, R. (2016). Experiences and views of nursing home nurses in England regarding occupational role and status. *Social Theory & Health, 14*(3), 372–392.

Verbeek, H., Zwakhalen, S. M. G., Schols, J. M. G. A., & Hamers, J. P. H. (2013). Keys to successfully embedding scientific research in nursing homes: A win-win perspective. *Journal of the American Medical Directors Association, 14*, 855–857.

Verbeek, H., Zwakhalen, S. M. G., Schols, J. M. G. A., Kempen, G. I. J. M., & Hamers, J. P. H. (2020). The living lab in ageing and long-term care: A sustainable model for translational research improving quality of life, quality of care and quality of work. *Journal of Nutrition, Health & Aging, 24*(1), 43–47. https://europepmc.org/backend/ptpmcrender.fcgi?accid=PMC6934630&blobtype=pdf.

12

Meeting the Health Needs of Older People Experiencing Homelessness and Other Inclusion Health Groups

Samantha Dorney-Smith, Caroline Shulman, Briony F. Hudson, Fenella Jolly, Elizabeth Keat, Raphael Rogans-Watson, Krishna Misra

CHAPTER OUTLINE

INTRODUCTION

What Is Inclusion Health?

Inclusion health is a research, service and policy agenda that aims to prevent and redress the health inequalities experienced by the most vulnerable and marginalised people in our society (Aldridge et al., 2018). This includes a variety of people living on the margins, for example people experiencing homelessness; Gypsy, Roma, Traveller and Boater communities; asylum seekers; refugees and vulnerable migrants; people living within the prison system; and sex workers. Much of what follows is relevant for all these vulnerable or marginalised groups, but in view of the specific cultural considerations, we have included a section on Gypsy, Roma, Traveller and Boater communities and vulnerable migrants. It is important to note the challenges experienced by individuals in inclusion health groups can worsen as they get older.

Morbidity and Mortality in Inclusion Health Groups

It is well known people living in the most deprived areas in the United Kingdom suffer poor health outcomes, and health inequity has worsened over the past 10 years (Marmot, 2020; Marmot et al., 2020). All-cause standardised mortality rates are approximately twice as high for people who live in deprived areas compared with the least deprived. The social determinants of health, such as income, education, employment, food security, housing and social inclusion, have very important roles to play.

Inclusion health groups specifically are known to suffer the very worst health outcomes. For example, Aldridge et al. (2018) showed all-cause standardised mortality ratios in people experiencing homelessness, people in prison, sex workers and individuals with addictions were 11.86 times higher in women and 7.88 times higher in men than in the general population (see Fig. 12.1). This was mirrored by a recent Office for National Statistics study that showed the average age of death of people identified as homeless in 2019 was 45.9 for men and 43.4 for women (Office for

National Statistics, 2020). Similarly, life expectancy across the Gypsy and Traveller population is estimated to be 10 to 12 years less than that of the non-Traveller population (Traveller Movement, 2012).

In addition, inclusion health groups are known to suffer worse physical health morbidity during their lifetimes. For example, people experiencing homelessness are 2.5 times more likely to have asthma, five times more likely to have a stroke, six times more likely to have heart disease and 12 times more likely to have epilepsy than the general population (Story, 2013). Similarly, 42% of English Gypsies and Travellers are affected by a long-term condition, as opposed to 18% of the general population (Royal College of General Practitioners, 2013). Rogans-Watson et al. (2020) identified 33 people living in a homeless hostel with a mean age of 55.7 years had an average level of frailty comparable to 89-year-olds in the general population, and the average number of long-term conditions per person was 7.2. Frailty among inclusion health groups is discussed further in this chapter.

Lack of Access to Care Experienced by Inclusion Health Groups

Barriers to accessing primary and secondary health care for inclusion health groups are considerable (Gunner et al., 2019; Elwell-Sutton et al., 2017), and this is one reason for such poor outcomes. Individual barriers can include lack of an address, language, literacy, mental health, addictions, cognitive issues, poverty (e.g., no money to get to appointments or pay for phone service), digital exclusion and practical issues, such as who will look after pets.

Systemic issues include the fact patients are often stigmatised (Rae & Rees, 2015), and health care issues are often addressed in silos using a medical reductionist model, particularly in hospitals (McCartney, 2016). National Health Service (NHS) charging regulations also put many non–United Kingdom nationals off accessing secondary health care (British Medical Association [BMA], 2019a), and patients without identification are frequently wrongly turned away from GP registration (Doctors of the World, 2017, 2018). Many GP practices do not allow patients without proof of address to register, despite the fact it is clearly indicated in NHS guidance there is no requirement to provide a personal address or immigration ID to access GP registration (NHS, 2019). GP registration issues have in some cases recently been exacerbated by the move of general practice during COVID-19 to a model of 'total triage' and 'remote by default'. The resultant demise of drop-in services and reception meant many patients found it harder to access GP registration and GP appointments (Groundswell, 2020).

Palliative and end-of-life care is also an area inclusion health groups may miss out on due to health conditions not

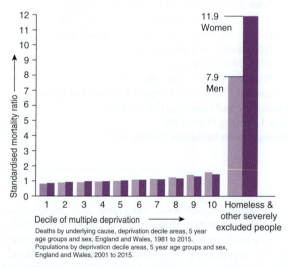

Fig. 12.1 Mortality in people experiencing homelessness and other inclusion health groups (Aldridge et al., 2018).

fitting the mainstream criterion for palliative care (e.g., end-stage liver disease rather than cancer) or to deterioration being quick and unexpected although arguably still predictable. Later in the chapter we discuss ways to promote better access to palliative and end-of-life care for inclusion health groups. See also Chapter 34 for end-of-life care.

Cultural Competence

When health care practitioners meet people from inclusion health populations, they may lack understanding of the way these populations normally live. For example, Gypsies, Roma, Traveller and Boater communities; asylum seekers; undocumented migrants; and vulnerable migrants often have specific cultural norms related to their backgrounds practitioners may be unaware of. Even people experiencing homelessness, prisoners and sex workers are likely to have their own social norms, for example, related to language or expectation of services, that are unlikely to be fully understood by someone living outside these communities.

Cultural competence is the ability to understand, communicate with and effectively interact with people from a wide variety of backgrounds. It encompasses being aware of your own worldview, then developing a positive attitude toward cultural differences and gaining knowledge of different cultural practices and worldviews. Cultural competence in health care refers to the ability for health care professionals to communicate and interact effectively, demonstrating integrity, compassion and professionalism when working with patients with different values, beliefs and feelings.

This chapter includes content from practitioners who work with Gypsy, Roma, Traveller and Boater communities, asylum seekers and vulnerable migrants to help you build cultural competence in these areas. However, this is just an introduction; further cultural competence training can be accessed free via the NHS's elearning for healthcare resource (https://www.e-lfh.org.uk/programmes/cultural-competence). Friends, Families and Travellers also provides specific cultural training online (https://www.gypsy-traveller.org/training-packages).

What Makes Up Person-Centred Care?

Person-centred care is about focusing care on the needs of the individual by ensuring people's preferences, needs and values guide clinical decisions and providing care that is respectful of and responsive to them (https://www.hee.nhs.uk/our-work/person-centred-care). This kind of approach is vital to engaging with inclusion health groups.

Principles of person-centred care include the following:
- Care and support are personalised, coordinated and empowering.

- Services are created in partnership with patients and their communities.
- There is a focus on equality and narrowing inequalities.
- Relevant carers and/or support workers are identified, supported and involved.
- Voluntary and housing sector services are involved as key partners.
- Volunteering and social action are considered as part of the solution.

Starting Where the Person Is

A key concept in inclusion health is starting with the patient's own priorities. Patients from inclusion health groups often present with a multitude of social issues as well as health issues and come with a history of mistrust in services due to having faced poor attitudes or poor care in the past. Sometimes they have years of personal traumatic experiences to combat. As health care professionals it is important to invest time to build relationships with individuals who find it difficult to engage in order to bring them into services, particularly if there are risks associated with non-engagement.

In a recent systematic review that identified good practices in inclusion health, Luchenski et al. (2018) underlined the importance of initial engagement work and meeting people where they are both psychologically and geographically. This chapter outlines how the need to engage with individuals from inclusion health populations may necessitate service providers going beyond what might usually be expected from their role, such as actively reaching out to individuals from these communities.

Luchenski et al. (2018) outlined the following key principles for services:
- Provide ample time and patience to really listen.
- Strive to develop trust and acceptance.
- Provide supportive, unbiased, open, honest and transparent services in inclusive spaces and places.
- Encourage clients to accept personal responsibility for health.
- Allow clients to take ownership, have choices and participate in decisions.
- Promote accessibility, fairness and equality.

Case studies in this chapter draw out many of these principles.

Service Acceptability

As well as initial engagement, it is important to work with patients in a collaborative way to understand what is acceptable to them in terms of service provision. For example, some people who have been sleeping rough find the concept of being inside challenging, and others may reject certain types of accommodation due to bad past experiences. Good practice ideally encompasses open-ended, persistent, flexible and coordinated support (Cornes et al., 2011) and moves away from institutionalisation wherever possible such that people have the option of staying in ordinary housing with support rather than being offered only a hostel or refuge. Whole-person (Terry & Cardwell, 2015), strengths-based approaches, in which individuals' strengths and abilities are emphasised, are also appropriate.

Managing Complexity

The Challenge of Tri-Morbidity

People experiencing homelessness, prisoners and sex workers are commonly described as suffering from tri-morbidity (Himsworth et al., 2020; Player et al., 2020). Tri-morbidity is the intersection of physical health, mental health and addiction conditions. This intersection of conditions can make the treatment of each element more challenging (Hewett et al., 2012), particularly in a siloed health care system. The role of nurses is to advocate to ensure all health needs are met.

Complex Psychological Trauma and the Intersectionality of Mental Health, Addictions, Brain Injury and Neurodiversity

Tri-morbidity can be further exacerbated by complexity in mental health. A high incidence of adverse childhood experiences (Grey & Woodfine, 2019) and traumatic events means levels of personality disorder (Maguire et al., 2009) and post-traumatic stress disorder (Yeonwoo et al, 2017) are high in inclusion health communities. Associated issues with anxiety, hypervigilance, trust, impulse control and emotional regulation can make it hard for some individuals to communicate effectively, prioritise well and be calm in the face of adversity. It can also lead to some people coming across as obstructive or aggressive when what they actually feel is threatened or unsafe. Trauma-informed services and communication skills can help reduce conflict and increase trust and engagement. For useful training and tips, see the online training video provided by Fulfilling Lives South East (2020).

Psychological trauma can be combined with a high prevalence of other mental illnesses (Homeless Link, 2014), brain injury (Topolovec-Vranic et al., 2014) and neurodiversity (McCarthy et al., 2016). Research into this area is still developing, but a recent academic paper found 12% of a group of people experiencing homelessness showed strong signs of autism (Churchard et al., 2019) as opposed to the prevalence of autism in the general population, which is estimated to be 1.1%. This combination of factors

that affect cognition can ultimately mean people's ability to take in and process health information may be limited and decision making potentially impaired. However, mental capacity assessments can be difficult to undertake because patients are suspicious about their necessity.

Ensuring a Safe Approach

It is vital that even if it is difficult to assess mental capacity, if a patient is making decisions that are likely to put them at risk, every effort should be made to ensure a mental capacity assessment is undertaken. Clinicians with senior expertise in work with inclusion health groups may be needed.

Self-discharge from hospital, care refusal and self-neglect are common issues that need close attention. In some cases concerns may lead to requests for inherent jurisdiction even if someone has mental capacity.

CULTURAL CONSIDERATIONS

Cultural competence in health care refers to the ability for health care professionals to demonstrate awareness, understanding and respect of the cultural contexts of patients' lives. In particular it is important for health care professionals to demonstrate cultural competence toward patients with a different background to their own and to embrace it. Cultural competence leads to a better understanding of the screening and specific health care needs of certain populations.

Gypsy, Roma and Traveller Communities

Gypsy, Roma and Traveller communities are not a single homogenous group but a number of distinct ethnic groups. This includes a range of people with different backgrounds, beliefs, cultures and languages that often stretch back over hundreds of years. Such groups may share things in common, but other cultural norms and beliefs may be very different. Gypsy, Roma, and Traveller groups include Irish Travellers, Scottish Gypsy Travellers, Welsh Gypsies and Romany Gypsies. These groups are all recognised as distinct ethnic minority groups and are protected under the Equality Act of 2010. Other Traveller groups that may be considered cultural minority groups include New Age Travellers, Barge Travellers and Showmen, who may share cultural traits with Gypsies and Travellers.

Of all ethnic minorities, Gypsies and Travellers are reported to have the worst health outcomes. The average life expectancy of Gypsies and Travellers is 10–20 years less than the general population, but there is a wide range; a study in Leeds in 2005 found it to be as much 28 years less (Baker, 2005). The health outcomes of Gypsies and Travellers are known to be adversely affected and determined by socioeconomic position over the life course (Nazroo, 2003).

Romany Gypsies have been in Britain since around 1515. The name *Gypsy* comes from Egyptian, as settled people believed this was where they originated due to their darker skin. In fact, the Romani language demonstrates their origins are northern India. Other groups of Travellers in Britain, such as Scottish, Welsh and English Travellers, trace their groups' nomadism for many generations. Nomadic people were already in Britain when Romany Gypsies arrived, and in some ways the different ethnicities and cultures may have merged. Irish Travellers originate from Ireland and trace their heritage back hundreds of years. They may be known as Parvee or Minceirs. For more information on Gypsy, Roma and Traveller culture and history, visit the Traveller Movement website at https://travellermovement.org.uk.

Gypsies and Travellers historically honed traditional skills they could take on the road, often related to seasonal agricultural industry, smithing or scrap metal collection. Some Gypsies and Travellers still work in these trades today. Some Gypsies and Travellers live in caravans, travel for work and live nomadically. Others now live in brick-and-mortar structures and travel for only part of the year, and some do not travel at all. People of Gypsy and Traveller heritage are seen in our communities and workplaces and are often fully integrated into non-travelling society. The ethnic identity of Gypsies and Travellers is not affected by whether they are travelling or currently in settled accommodation.

Family networks are very important to the Gypsy and Traveller way of life. Family anniversaries, births, weddings and deaths are often marked by extended family or community gatherings. Gypsies and Travellers generally marry young and respect their older generation. Contrary to frequent media depictions, Traveller communities value cleanliness and tidiness. Many Gypsies and Travellers have a strong focus on their religion, which is often Catholic or other Christian denominations.

People from Gypsy, Roma or Traveller backgrounds may have experienced poorer access to education, leading to lower literacy and lower health literacy. Community members report experiencing bullying and racism in school, and their culture is not recognised within the education system (Friends, Families and Travellers). Gypsy, Roma and Traveller community members have the lowest educational attainment of all ethnic groups in childhood (Equality and Human Rights Commission, 2019).

Older People in Gypsy, Roma and Traveller Communities

Although Gypsies and Travellers can have poorer health and lower life expectancy than the general population, there are many assets to being an older person in Gypsy and Traveller communities. The Leeds Gypsy and Traveller Exchange is a grassroots, community-led organisation that tries to build on community assets (LeedsGate, 2000). This organisation identified that older or frail community members or those with disabilities are often treasured in families and are usually cared for in the family home by extended family members as unpaid family carers. They are less likely to be socially isolated, and they remain important and loved elders in their community.

The specific needs of older Gypsies and Travellers is often not considered by statutory services, particularly if they do not live in permanent accommodation or are travelling and living in roadside camps. Additionally, health and social care services can have barriers that restrict access, particularly if someone does not have a permanent address or local GP. Gypsies and Travellers who are no longer be able to travel due to old age, poor health or disability are generally not considered in local authority accommodation provision planning. As a result, when they need to be placed in culturally appropriate accommodation with their extended family, there may be no provision for this, leading to inappropriate accommodation and causing isolation and loneliness (Equality and Human Rights Commission, 2019). In general, some services lack awareness of the importance of family and community considerations in care delivery to Gypsy, Roma and Traveller communities.

Case Study: Key Points

Case Study 12.1 underlines the importance of starting where the patient is and working with specific access barriers (in this case, literacy) and cultural issues (involving the family) when working with Gypsy, Roma and Traveller populations. These principles can be applied to other inclusion health populations.

Key points to draw from Case Study 12.1 include the following:

- Start with yourself. People connect with a person, not a job.
- Consider any pre-existing biases you may have, think how they will affect your care and actively mitigate against them.
- Ensure you ask about literacy and that services record any literacy challenges and use accessible standards. Lack of literacy is a particularly common challenge in Gypsy, Roma and Traveller communities and other inclusion health groups.
- Challenge access decisions that may be made due to underlying stigma. Advocate for your patient while exploring and considering what barriers need to be broken down. Do rules make sense and meet the needs of all patients? Which groups in the community are missing from your team?

CASE STUDY 12.1   Case Management of Mary by Liz Keat, Gypsy, Roma and Traveller Nurse

Mary is a 78-year-old woman of Irish Traveller heritage. She lives on a local authority site but in an adapted chalet-style property rather than caravan. She has eight children, four of whom live on-site nearby. She has rheumatoid arthritis, chronic obstructive airway disease (COPD), previous bowel cancer, type 2 diabetes and depression. Mary has no literacy and was not taught to read as a child.

Liz says, 'I met Mary on outreach, not through any formal referral process. She invited me in after hearing through family members there was a nurse doing outreach to the site where she lived.

'Our first meeting was not really about health at all. It was the start of a relationship. She told me about her family and asked about mine. She told me a lot about the history of the site, her family and what it was like travelling with her eight children, and how poor health had eventually led to needing to live on a site. She told me about past difficulties of her children receiving an education while travelling and the racism they had all experienced.

'She also told me about how she used to love listening to the rain on the roof of the trailer and of always having the caravan gleaming and the children around her. Mary also told me she used to enjoy sewing but was now unable to do so. Before any discussion about health, I learned what mattered to her.

'Over a period of time, I developed warm and trusting relationship with Mary. It was clear there were many assets to build on; she was actively cared for and surrounded by her extended family in the community, she was important to them and they consulted her on decisions.

'Eventually she revealed her health was a concern to her, and it became clear her health conditions were not being well managed. Over a period of time, she had some significant falls and recent hospital admissions due to exacerbations of her COPD. Mary frequently borrowed other people's inhalers if she ran out. She was given inhaler information in leaflet form and wasn't able to read the information, which had led to poor compliance overall.

'It also transpired that Mary had missed six invitations for diabetic eye screening and multiple follow-ups by primary care for COPD and diabetes reviews because she wasn't able to respond to text invites or letters. This happened despite the fact her lack of literacy was documented as an accessibility issue on her records, and there had been no investigation as to why she wasn't responding to invitations. She was also struggling with broader medication compliance.

'Mary had significant debt from electricity bills, causing anxiety and reluctance to heat her property. There was also an observed carer strain on Mary's sons.'

What Was Achieved—and Some Challenges

In Leeds there is an established outreach model for visiting Gypsy and Traveller communities that has been well evaluated (Warwick-Booth et al, 2018). Its aims include building relationships with Gypsy and Traveller communities and looking at health systems to address barriers.

Mary was referred to the community respiratory team, and information was given to her in a way she understood, with appropriate support. This included the use of YouTube videos and videos from Asthma UK to demonstrate correct inhaler technique.

Mary was referred to the local neighbourhood rehabilitation team due to frequent falls. There was a delay in her being seen as her GP was out of area, and initially they refused the referral. They needed to be encouraged to come to a local arrangement for access. Mary was then seen for her initial assessment but discharged following a reported no-access visit (i.e., they reported her as not being there) despite Mary being housebound. This was then successfully challenged.

The neighbourhood team also documented that Mary should be visited only in twos, because she lived on a Gypsy and Traveller site. There was no rationale given for this discriminatory decision, and it was also challenged. System-level work was then done with the neighbourhood team to increase their awareness of the community and to look at how Gypsy and Travellers could be responded to in an equitable way.

A dosette box was trialled for Mary, which she didn't like, but a solution was found that she preferred—essentially her recognising the tablets better. A nurse now regularly reviews her medication to check her ongoing understanding and concordance.

Finally, an electronic device was applied for with a screen reader, so Mary will be able to have digital health appointments if needed, and the local Gypsy and Traveller third-sector organisation supported her with the debt. They arranged for her bills to be reviewed and applied for a grant to dissolve it.

Throughout this time, her family, and in particular her elder sons, were involved.

As a result of all these interventions, Mary reduced her hospital admissions and has felt less anxious and more in control at home, and her sons feel better able to support her.

- Patients are part of a family, community and culture. Look at their assets first. How can your care complement what is already being provided?
- Consider carer roles and what carers need in terms of support. Look to local carers' charities and organisations.

Vulnerable Migrant Groups

Vulnerable migrants (see Table 12.1 for definition) are another inclusion health group who are highly stigmatised and affected by lack of access to care. They are not a homogenous group, but the population is often linked by a shared experience of emotional and psychological trauma.

Globally in 2019, the population of individuals forcibly displaced due to persecution, conflict or violence stood at 79.5 million, with more than 3 million over the age of 60 (United Nations High Commission for Refugees [UNHCR], 2019). In the United Kingdom in 2019, it was estimated there were approximately 200,000 refugees, asylum seekers and displaced persons, and 4% were over 60 years of age (UNHCR, 2019). Although this

figure means the number of older migrants is relatively low, at around 8,000 in the United Kingdom, it may be an underestimation due the dynamic nature of migration (Bolzman, 2014).

Forced migration as a result of fleeing from war, torture, violence or trafficking is likely to result in physical injury, trauma, psychological distress and loss of family members. The subsequent journey of migration continues to pose significant challenges to physical and psychological well-being as people travel across regions and spend prolonged periods in temporary settings awaiting immigration processes. The toll of these experiences combined with poor nutrition and exposure to disease can cause forced migrants to age more quickly than settled populations and present with chronic diseases of ageing earlier (UNHCR, 2021).

Assessment of the challenges faced by these groups to accessing health care and understanding their specific health needs allows for greater engagement with this vulnerable group and better health outcomes.

TABLE 12.1 Terminology: Vulnerable Migrants

Refugee: A person who has fled their country and is unable to return due to well-founded fear of being persecuted due to race, religion, nationality, political opinion or membership of a particular social group as defined by the 1951 United National Refugee Convention (United Nations General Assembly, 1950).

Asylum seeker: A person who has fled their country and made an application to be recognised as a refugee under the 1951 UN convention but has not yet been granted this status. While awaiting the outcome, they may be housed in temporary accommodation with access to minimal-subsistence financial support.

Refused asylum seeker: A refused or failed asylum seeker has been refused asylum under Article 3 of the European Convention on Human Rights, and any subsequent appeals have been unsuccessful. Unsuccessful asylum seekers are often referred to as appeals rights exhausted. Some refused asylum seekers voluntarily return home; others are forcibly returned. Others remain in the country. For some it is not safe or practical to return until conditions in their country change.

Undocumented migrant: A person who may be in a country without required documentation to enter, live and work within that country. This can result in long-term temporary accommodation or homelessness.

Trafficked person: Human trafficking is generally understood to refer to the process through which individuals are placed or maintained in an exploitative situation for economic gain. Trafficking can occur within a country or involve movement across borders. Women, men and children are trafficked for a range of purposes, including forced and exploitative labour in factories, farms and private households; sexual exploitation; and forced marriage. Trafficked people are recognised as such through the national referral mechanism. Some go on to seek asylum.

Forced migrant: A person subject to migratory movement in which an element of coercion exists, including threats to life and livelihood, whether arising from natural or humanmade causes (European Commission, n.d.).

European Economic Area (EEA) nationals: Some EEA nationals who have never worked formally in the United Kingdom (i.e., paid tax and national insurance) may have no rights to welfare or benefits and may thus be vulnerable through destitution.

No recourse to public funds: A person has no recourse to public finds when they are subject to immigration control as defined at Section 115 of the Immigration and Asylum Act of 1999. This includes groups who have been granted leave to remain with certain conditions. As a result they may have no access to financial or housing assistance. In these circumstances access to support can be available through local authority and third-sector support.

Barriers to Health Care Access

It well recognised vulnerable migrant groups have significant unmet health needs that are compounded by barriers to health care access (Burnett & Peel, 2001). These barriers are often significant and are summarised in Table 12.2.

It is important to note confusion exists about who is eligible for NHS treatments free of charge, which causes significant barriers to accessing health for this group. Primary care, emergency care and certain conditions of public health concern such as tuberculosis can be accessed by everyone free of charge, regardless of immigration status. Secondary care services deemed urgent and necessary should also be accessible to all; this important decision is made by the clinical team. The legal responsibility of deciding who is eligible for NHS care falls to the NHS trust, not the clinical team. All asylum seekers with an active asylum claim or appeal in place are eligible for free NHS secondary care services.

Health Needs

The experience of forced migration can result in specific physical and mental health risks that and need to be considered in a specific comprehensive health needs assessment (Pavli & Maltezou, 2017). These health risks are outlined below. Some considerations are also relevant to other inclusion health groups.

Physical Health

Communicable Diseases

Infectious diseases, including bloodborne viruses, sexually transmitted infections, parasitic infections and tuberculosis, are more prevalent in newly arrived migrant groups (Pavli & Maltezou, 2017; Lebano et al., 2020). Screening is recommended during initial health assessment. Vaccination against infectious diseases such as measles and tetanus may also have been missed due to lack of access or disruption of schedules in the country of origin; ascertaining immunisation status and offering immunisation needs to be prioritised (European Centre for Disease Prevention and Control, 2018).

Non-Communicable Diseases

Older forced migrants have higher levels of non-communicable diseases than the same-aged host population (Hynie, 2018). For example, a review of older Syrian refugees in 2018 reported 60% with hypertension, 47% with diabetes and 30% with some type of cardiovascular disease (Strong et al., 2015). Continued displacement, financial difficulties and lack of knowledge of health services resulted in delayed diagnosis, interrupted monitoring and poor management of chronic conditions (Hynie, 2018). Supporting the management of chronic conditions requires accessibility to medication, transport to appointments and culturally appropriate and accessible health information to reduce the associated health burden (BMA, 2019b; Frost et al., 2019).

Soft tissue and bone injuries caused by experiences of violence or conflict can result in long-term disabilities and symptoms of chronic pain, especially in older populations (Strong et al., 2015). These require significant social, practical and medical support (Burnett & Ndovi, 2018), which may be lacking for older vulnerable migrants who lack a voice to advocate for themselves. Skin conditions

TABLE 12.2 Main Barriers to Accessing Health Care for Vulnerable Migrant Groups (British Medical Association, 2019b; Doctors of the World, 2018)	
Communication	- Limited access to interpreters and translated information sources - Untreated visual and auditory hearing impairments - Lack of access to mobile phones, data, video technology
Information and knowledge	- Misunderstanding around eligibility to access health services by health professionals and fear of being charged for care* - Lack of information on how to access services - Incorrect requests for information and documentation to register with health services
Trust	- Mistrust in government organisations due to previous experiences - Reticence to share personal information due to fear of being exposed
Sociocultural differences	- Differences in organization of health service delivery - Different expectations of patient journey - Acceptability of clinician gender, assessment settings, cultural norms of the host setting

*Eligibility to health services for vulnerable migrant groups is clear in the United Kingdom: universal entitlement to emergency, immediately necessary and primary care for all, including refugees, asylum seekers and undocumented migrants.

and nutritional deficiencies may also be common due to the ongoing social deprivation (Burnett & Peel, 2001), and visual and hearing impairments may go untreated, further limiting engagement in health and social support services (Burnett & Ndovi, 2018).

Mental Health

Refugees and victims of forced migration have higher rates of mood disorders, psychotic illness and post-traumatic stress disorder relative to non-migrant host populations (Hynie, 2018), and it is now recognised that as well as the trauma experienced in the country of origin, experiences during the migration journey and subsequent ongoing immigration processes significantly increase mental health vulnerabilities (Porter & Haslam, 2005).

The impact on mental health of forced migration in the older age group is reflected in higher rates of depression and anxiety (Hynie, 2018). Older men were found to have a higher prevalence of experiences of torture and a related prominence of medically unexplained symptoms such as headaches, chronic pain and gastric symptoms (Burnett & Ndovi, 2018).

Presentation of mental distress can be variable and includes extreme sadness, insomnia, anxiety and nightmares. These symptoms in migrants should trigger further screening for mental health diagnosis. Consideration should also be given to the additional impacts of social isolation, racial discrimination, homelessness and destitution on mental health and social function migrants often face when considering support services (Burnett & Ndovi, 2018).

Social Factors

The social determinants of health, such as income, nutrition, housing and access to health care, have a particular cumulative impact for older forced migrants that results in increased and unmet health needs that need to be carefully considered (Lebano et al., 2020). Forced migration and the subsequent sudden removal from an individual's country of origin result in significant social, emotional and financial disruption. Older adults may feel these changes acutely, having lived for longer in a particular area and being less flexible to adaptation (Bolzman, 2014).

Loss of status and disruption of family and community networks result in marked social isolation and loneliness (Bolzman, 2014). This not only increases mental health needs but also impacts care needs. Resistance to accepting carers can occur due to cultural differences and can increase the potential for neglect in the older adult.

Assessing and Managing the Health Needs of Older Vulnerable Migrants

Table 12.3 outlines a framework for assessing and managing the health needs of older vulnerable migrant adults. Although the considerations in Table 12.3 apply to all ages, some are particular concerns for the older population of vulnerable migrants. Any robust health needs assessment must consider engagement of the patient in management

---

TABLE 12.3   Migrant Health Assessment Framework

	Assessment of Needs	Support Strategies
Migration history	- Country of origin - Reason for leaving - Journey to current location - Victim of previous violence, torture, trafficking	- Referral to non-governmental support agencies, charities
Physical health	- Screen for communicable and non-communicable diseases - Assess physical effects of previous injuries - Determine immunisation status	- Infectious diseases follow-up - Immunisation catch-ups - Patient education about access to health services and interpreters - Chronic disease follow-up
Mental health	- Screen for depression and anxiety, post-traumatic stress disorder - Determine functional impacts of mental health symptoms and somatisation	- Patient education around impacts of trauma on mental health. - Referral for psychotherapy
Social history	- Establish previous social identity - Identify current social networks - Family support - Access to culturally appropriate support - Consider loneliness	- Signpost to local ethnic minority support groups - Enable family contact - Collaborate to ensure patient-centred approach

of their condition with access to culturally appropriate and translated information (BMA, 2019b).

In summary, vulnerable migrant groups, including refugees, asylum seekers and undocumented migrants, are at increased risk of chronic diseases, mental health conditions and some infectious diseases. Taking time to understand previous experiences and journeys builds trust and rapport and informs the health needs assessment. Consideration of the social determinants of health in this group is particularly relevant to mitigate inequalities in access to health services and to improve outcomes.

FRAILTY IN INCLUSION HEALTH GROUPS

The importance of understanding frailty in older people is discussed in Chapter 6. However, in this section we discuss the example of frailty in people experiencing homelessness. Frailty is defined as a state of health that results from cumulative decline across multiple physiological systems over a person's lifetime. Looking at people through a lens of frailty presents a 'practical, unifying notion in the care of elderly patients that directs attention away from organ-specific diagnoses towards a more holistic viewpoint of the patient' (Clegg et al., 2013, p. 759).

Frailty in People Experiencing Homelessness

Mainstream secondary health services are primarily organised according to single-organ diseases such as respiratory and cardiology, which poses a challenge for the care of many older people with multi-organ problems. This can be even worse for inclusion health groups, who more frequently experience comorbidities as well as the previously described barriers to accessing health care.

Frailty has traditionally been identified only in older people; the prevalence increases with age, affecting 4% of the United Kingdom population between 65 and 69 years of age and 26% of those aged 85 and over (Clegg et al., 2013). However, the wider determinants of health accelerate the development of frailty in the same way they have a cumulative effect on older forced migrants. Thus, there are associations between lower financial income, fewer years of education, neighbourhood deprivation and frailty in later life (Hale et al., 2019). The impact of social and economic factors on people experiencing homelessness and multiple social exclusion is crucial, and there is growing recognition these experiences put people at much higher risk of developing frailty and of developing it earlier in life (Garrett et al., 2020).

Two studies in the United States assessed frailty using different definitions in people experiencing homelessness with average ages in the 50s and found more than half of participants were frail (Hadenfeldt et al., 2017; Salem et al.,

2013). In the United Kingdom, a study of people in a homeless hostel with an average age of 56 found 55% were frail, and average frailty scores were comparable to 89-year-olds in the general population (Rogans-Watson et al., 2020). This suggests efforts to identify frailty from a younger age than in the general population are needed to avoid missed opportunities to intervene early.

Frailty is characterised by low energy and low strength, slow walking speed and low levels of physical activity (British Geriatrics Society, 2015). People with frailty are less able to recover from physical illnesses and accidents, which are more likely to result in falls, delirium, disability and deterioration in health status, including even death (Clegg et al., 2013; Fried et al., 2001). However, there is good evidence frailty has greater reversibility than disability and that important outcomes may be improved through holistic interventions targeted across the frailty spectrum (Beswick et al., 2008; British Geriatrics Society, 2015; Ellis et al., 2017). As such, it is vital to identify frailty in inclusion health groups, even in younger adults. A needs-based rather than an age-based approach is essential to ensure at-risk groups are reached by efforts to manage frailty.

Tools for identifying frailty have not been validated in younger people, but existing screening tools can be used or adapted for clinical practice (Rogans-Watson et al., 2020). The appropriate frailty scale depends on the setting and purpose. The Fried frailty phenotype is useful in research and to compare to population data but impractical for routine clinical use since it requires time-consuming physical assessments. This approach to assessing frailty involves the observation of five elements of health and performance (Fried et al., 2001). The Rockwood scale relies heavily on appraisal of physical functional abilities sometimes preserved in younger people with frailty and accounts less for other aspects of frailty, potentially resulting in lower sensitivity for frailty identification (Rockwood et al., 2005). However, the Edmonton Frail Scale can be administered by non-clinical staff and has the advantage of highlighting specific areas for intervention in subsequent care plans (Rolfson et al., 2006). Some of the questions may have to be adapted to be more relevant for younger people or those experiencing homelessness.

Frailty identification in people who have experienced homelessness should direct you to look for conditions more commonly associated with older age, such as cognitive impairment, falls, mobility problems, sensory impairment (e.g., hearing and vision), continence problems (e.g., bladder and bowels), malnutrition and social isolation. These conditions are often known as geriatric syndromes and are surprisingly common even in younger people with frailty, but they are often underrecognised and undiagnosed (Brown et al., 2017; Depaul Health Initiative, 2018; Rogans-Watson et al., 2020). Screening for and managing these conditions when they arise can in turn contribute to reversing the extent of frailty and improving quality of life (British Geriatrics Society 2015).

Identification of frailty should act as a trigger to adapt care and provide enhanced support. Guidance for managing older people with frailty indicates they should be prioritised for comprehensive holistic assessment and person-centred care, management of long-term conditions and opportunities to consider advance care planning (British Geriatrics Society, 2015; Turner & Clegg, 2014).

It is important to acknowledge the multiple barriers to accessing primary care services many disadvantaged groups have faced and that the previous negative experiences resulted in many losing trust and disengaging from health and social care systems (Bradley 2018; Eavis, 2018). Consequently, a proactive patient-centred approach, particularly suitable for individuals with frailty or multiple comorbidities, is lacking in many encounters homeless patients have with mainstream services, which frequently take the form of crisis-driven hospital attendances. To ensure these underserved groups are reached, health care providers must move beyond an open-door approach to offer services tailored to the needs and priorities of individuals (Garrett et al., 2020). Health care providers can offer extended appointments that enable holistic reviews for long-term conditions (Turner & Clegg, 2014).

Reducing the complexity of care schedules and number of appointments for people with frailty can improve the quality and continuity of care (British Geriatrics Society, 2015). Co-location of services in the community and information sharing across organisations also improves engagement. Social prescribing can connect people to community groups and statutory services in order to access the practical and emotional support needed to help them manage their health care conditions. It is important to note a one-size-fits-all approach is unlikely to address the needs of the most disadvantaged. The key principles listed in the section titled 'Starting where the person is,' from the review by Luchenski et al. (2018), are of particular importance. This requires flexibility in the way services are delivered both in time and space, with a great emphasis on rebuilding trust and confidence with patients and enabling them to play a key role in shaping services to be inclusive and welcoming (Garrett et al., 2020).

THE ROLE OF SPECIALIST INCLUSION HEALTH SERVICES

Although the principles described apply to all services for people from marginalised backgrounds, specialist services can help meet the health needs of inclusion health groups. In many areas around the country, community specialist inclusion health services have developed to help meet the unmet health needs of some inclusion health groups. The overall aim of a health inclusion team is to provide a wide range of targeted clinical and support services to vulnerable adults from marginalised groups (Schiffer & Schatz, 2008). The following section outlines an example of a specialist inclusion health service and a case study of how the service works with older adults.

Guy's and St Thomas' NHS Foundation Trust Health Inclusion Team

The Guy's and St Thomas' NHS Foundation Trust Health Inclusion Team (HIT) works across the three South London boroughs of Lambeth, Southwark and Lewisham. The service has evolved over the past three decades from smaller multidisciplinary teams that targeted specific groups—refugees, asylum seekers, people experiencing homelessness and addictions clients—to become the much larger, multiskilled HIT. The team is nurse-led by a team of 18 clinical nurse specialist nurses, including a paediatric nurse and a health visitor. The team also hosts specialist GPs, an occupational therapist, a well-being support worker, high-intensity user leads and case workers.

The key aims of the HIT are to:
- Reduce inequalities by enabling access to all necessary primary and secondary care health services.
- Offer specialist advanced holistic health assessments and interventions on outreach (e.g., screening, vaccination, treatment for minor ailments, chronic disease management, dressings, etc.).
- Case manage clients to achieve maximised physical and mental health, taking into account social circumstances.
- Avoid unnecessary use of emergency secondary care wherever possible.
- Promote the wider well-being, health and safety of vulnerable groups.
- Empower individuals to take responsibility for their own health and self-care.

The HIT strives to find innovative ways to provide health care that is safe, accessible and tailored to meet clients' needs. Nurse-led clinics are held in a wide variety of settings in the community, including homeless and migrant day centres, hostels, temporary accommodations (e.g., bed-and-breakfasts and hotels), home office accommodations and addiction centres, and outreach is provided on the street to rough sleepers. For street homeless clients, the HIT developed a model called HITPlus, which works in collaboration with street outreach teams in each borough. Anyone who sleeps rough is engaged with on the street and their health needs identified, and a nurse plans how their needs can be met.

Inclusion health groups can be transient and stigmatised and have complex and multiple morbidities. This impacts how they receive health care and respond to professionals who offer help. Therefore, the team believes it is important to have an opportunistic and adaptive approach, offering a comprehensive range of health care interventions, treatments, screening tests and vaccinations at the point of access and aiming to make every contact count. The team also works to ensure clients feel empowered and listened to as part of every interaction.

The HIT works in many non-NHS sites in partnership and collaboration with third-sector services and other statutory/government organisations, including:

- Homelessness and migrant support charities, church groups, specialist interest groups and advocacy groups
- Hostel providers, local authority housing officers and private accommodation providers
- Social services, home offices, specialist health and safeguarding teams

These partnerships are vital to providing effective outreach.

Permanent clinic rooms are often set up on-site at hostels, day centres and hotels where health needs are ongoing. Where these outreach clinics are provided, NHS clinical standards of infection control and safety are maintained, and the rooms are equipped with basic equipment and hand-washing facilities. Clinic rooms are used as safe clinical spaces if clients need to have clinical interventions such as wound assessments, dressings, blood tests, vaccines or further investigations. If a client on outreach needs these services, the outreach team can transport them to the nearest hub, where a nurse can safely administer the required care.

HIT clinics have an open-door walk-in policy, and staff assertively reach out to residents of concern, knocking on doors with the support of the staff who run the different projects. This accessibility facilitates engagement and acceptability and builds trust with clients.

Health Inclusion Team Management Approach for Older Homeless Adults

Only a small percentage of HIT clients fall into the older person age group (i.e., older than 65). However, as per the earlier frailty discussion, many homeless clients present as *young olds*—younger people who experience health problems more associated with older people. Such health problems include poor tissue viability, vascular impairment (i.e., leg ulcers), incontinence, COPD, cardiac damage, renal damage and brain damage/dementia, including head injuries and alcohol dementia. Pressure ulcers are a common problem for both older and young homeless clients.

Relevant factors include being underweight or malnourished, being a wheelchair user, alcohol/drug dependence, incontinence and poor hygiene.

It is necessary for all the nurses on the HIT to have a variety of skills and knowledge to be able to offer competent, comprehensive care. All HIT nurses have advanced assessment and chronic disease assessment skills and a skill set that is both generic and specialist. For example, the team offers specialist care for the management of leg ulcers in people who use drugs, including completing ankle-brachial pressure index assessments and establishing a layer bandaging regime and care plan.

There are many challenges to nursing the young old and older person homeless cohort. Most clients are housed in non-clinical settings such as hostels or temporary accommodations where on-site staff, if they exist, do not provide direct care or health support. Inclusion health services may visit, but this might be only once a week. Although continuing care needs may be applied for and awarded, there are often few residential and nursing home places for people who are younger and/or have challenging behaviour and drug/alcohol dependence. In some cases, clients decline both care and care assessments, which keeps them in less suitable accommodation. Working with individuals who decline interventions and care is difficult. In these situations it is important to assess the individual's capacity (Mental Capacity Act, 2005) to make the decision to decline care. It is important it is clearly recorded in the client's nursing notes, and their capacity is assessed for each decision that may impact their health and social care outcomes.

Case Study 12.2 is an example of the complex challenges inclusion health teams meet every day and how suboptimal choices on accommodation are sometimes the only ones available. However, such challenges do not mean many or most health care and support needs cannot be met.

It is important to note inclusion health services are not provided everywhere, and there can be a postal code lottery of provision around the country. In addition, even if an inclusion health service exists, not all day centres or hostels in a local area may receive support. It is vital to find out what provisions exist locally and to never make assumptions about the level of health support that exists before discharging a client to a hostel or hotel. In addition, if an inclusion health service doesn't exist, it may be worth considering what your service can do differently to plug this gap. Case Study 12.2 provides an excellent example of specialist care provided in the community, but all mainstream services can and should consider whether they can provide outreach to vulnerable communities to support them to access care.

CASE STUDY 12.2   Case Management of 'Peter' by a Health Inclusion Team Nurse

Peter was an 82-year-old male with a history of living in Cardiff, but he became homeless when his partner died due to destitution. He travelled to Bristol and Oxford before coming to London. When he was identified by the street outreach service, he had already slept on the street for 6 months.

He was immediately placed in a hotel as an emergency measure in order for housing workers to establish his eligibility for housing (i.e., whether he was entitled to welfare support in the United Kingdom) and if so where he had a local connection. A local authority may not have a duty to house someone who does not have a local connection to their area, which means a proven history of living in an area for 6 of the past 12 months or 3 of the past 5 years). Peter was found to have no recourse to public funds, being from Africa, with no history of work in the United Kingdom.

A full health assessment was undertaken as soon as he was in the emergency accommodation. It was found Peter had type 2 diabetes that required insulin, but he had not been able to register with a GP to get a prescription for the insulin and had not had insulin for a year as he said he had to pay for prescriptions. Peter also reported blurred vision and that he should wear glasses, but he did not have them. He reported some generalised weakness, although he had no obvious mobility issues, and due to his destitution and not being familiar with the area he had been placed in, he was struggling to provide food for himself. He also had dental issues.

Interventions

- Peter was given a full health assessment, including screening for bloodborne viruses, liver and kidney function, cholesterol, hemoglobin A1C, thyroid function and infection markers. A urine dipstick revealed high levels of glucose and ketones, and MSU samples were sent.
- He was given both seasonal influenza and pneumococcal vaccinations.
- He was registered with a local GP.
- His blood results the next day showed his diabetes was out of control. He was advised of the findings and the need to attend Accident and Emergency (A&E) for treatment. He was accompanied to A&E by the outreach team manager.
- He spent 5 days in hospital having his insulin titrated and his diabetes stabilised. Nurses and outreach workers advocated for Peter not to be discharged back to the street and, although medically fit, to be kept in the ward until more suitable emergency accommodation was found (the previous bed had been closed). On discharge he was provided with other emergency accommodation for a limited period. During his stay he was found to be not eligible for welfare support or local authority housing and was assessed not to have any care needs, so this period of accommodation was required to work on his existing health and support needs to attempt to find a resolution.
- After discharge he was provided with food-bank vouchers for ongoing support.
- Peter was referred to an immigration lawyer for ongoing support.
- The team supported him to apply for an receive an HC2 certificate to receive free prescriptions.
- He was referred to a dentist for treatment.
- Appointments were made with a GP for immediate follow-up, diabetic eye screening and the practice nurse for ongoing diabetic care and foot checks.
- He was referred for bereavement support.
- He was referred to ophthalmology, then later for cataract surgery.
- He was referred to the winter night shelter scheme to ensure no further nights of sleeping rough.

Other professionals involved: Street population outreach team, local GP service, ROBES winter night shelter, and Guy's and St Thomas' NHS Foundation Trust's homeless team, ophthalmology and endocrinology departments.

Feedback from client: 'I'm very grateful', Peter said. 'Without them, access to the right treatment, medication and monitoring would have been impossible for me'.

SAFER HOSPITAL DISCHARGE

High levels of morbidity mean many inclusion health groups use secondary care more than the general population. For example, one study showed people experiencing homelessness are admitted to hospital three times as often and stay three times as long as do the general population, with annual costs of unscheduled care for homeless patients estimated to be eight times as much (Department of Health and Social Care, 2010).

However, hospitalisation presents an opportunity to support or help someone to turn their life around and get on the road to recovery. This section of the chapter discusses how you can contribute to making a difference in hospital and ensuring individuals are discharged safely.

The Statutory Duty to Refer

Since April 2018 the Homelessness Reduction Act has conveyed a duty to refer on various statutory bodies, including health care (Ministry of Housing, Communities and Local Government, 2018). This duty requires people experiencing homelessness are referred to the local authority for assistance with their consent. In health this duty explicitly applies to A&Es and inpatient services and includes the responsibility to refer people at risk of homelessness within the next 56 days, for example those likely to be evicted. The duty provides a reason to proactively ask patients about their housing status to identify those at risk of eviction.

Most local authorities have an dutytorefer@xcouncil.gov.uk email for referrals, and some have signed up to the Jigsaw system, which enables rapid referral. The National Homelessness Advisory Service has guidance on the duty to refer and may be able to provide in-house training to health organisations. Hospitals should consider including the duty to refer in their mandatory training.

Discharge Checklists

In rare cases you may be asked to discharge someone who is currently homeless, even if they are older. This might be because they have no welfare eligibility—in other words, they are not entitled to benefits or housing support in the United Kingdom.

If this happens, think carefully about the reasons it is being considered, and ask yourself the following questions:
- Is the background situation of this patient fully understood?
- Does this person have any care and support needs, and have they been assessed? Even if someone has no eligibility for benefits or housing support, if they have care and support needs, social services have a duty to undertake a Care Act assessment and possibly a duty to provide them with support, including accommodation.
- Are there any safeguarding concerns, including self-neglect?
- Does the person have the mental capacity to understand any risks their homelessness situation will present to them in their current health status?
- Does this person have outstanding medical needs on discharge? If so, can they be met while the person is homeless? Have all relevant referrals been made to enable this?
- Is this person going to be able to manage safely in their current homelessness situation, be it the streets, a hotel, a car or a caravan?

- Does this person have underlying frailties? Would you be surprised if this person died in the next 6 months?
- Are there any specialist health services or voluntary-sector organisations that might know the patient that can help you make the discharge safer?
- Does this person have any existing health support, voluntary-sector support, family and/or connections outside the hospital? If so, have people been informed of the impending discharge?
- Is this person able to independently get where they want to be?
- Has everything possible been done to attempt to resolve this person's situation?

These questions should be explored fully on *every* occasion a patient attends hospital. An example of a safe discharge tool—Safe and Effective Discharge of Homeless Hospital Patients—is available on the Healthy London Partnership website (Healthy London Partnership, 2019).

Hospital-Based Interventions That Can Improve Care

It is important to note some inclusion health patients who might benefit from additional support to achieve a safe discharge may not naturally reveal their inclusion health status when they come into hospital. This particularly applies to older people, who may feel embarrassed about their circumstances.

Better identification of inclusion health groups within hospital systems and by hospital clinicians is needed. Clinical nurse histories should always include an open assessment of home circumstances and discharge destination. Routine questions like 'Do you have any concerns about where you will go on discharge?' or 'Where do you live at the moment? Are you okay to go there on discharge?' are hopefully open enough to illicit honest responses. Often patients with initial embarrassment about their homelessness status do not immediately see the relevance of their homelessness to their recovery. Asking questions in an open way helps. Picking up homelessness early allows for the consideration of homelessness as a context for the initial assessment and any health care plan prepared.

The creation of specialist inclusion health nurse roles on wards, and linking these nurses together to form collaborative networks, can improve care across acute trusts for all inclusion health groups. Such champions can take responsibility for making links with relevant statutory and voluntary-sector organisations, including local authority housing and social care, mental health and addiction services, day centres, peer support and befriending organisations, food banks and advice agencies, then teaching and advising other staff. They can also improve intranet information available to staff and leaflets for patients in various languages and easy-to-read formats. These nurses can work to set up local GP registration processes that enable people to be registered from inside the hospital.

Medical Respite and Step-Down Care

There is a huge need for medical respite care on discharge, with the purpose of an immediate solution to housing problems and the continuation necessary for medical treatment and recovery work. Inclusion health patients may be excluded from step-down care if they don't have an onward address. This is a serious inequity issue that needs local discussion, but it may be appropriate to have local specialist provision. An example of specialist provision is provided in Box 12.1.

BOX 12.1   Bradford Respite and Intermediate Care Support Services

Bevan Healthcare provides a range of fully integrated services to support people in inclusion health groups in Bradford. This includes a Pathway homeless hospital discharge team, a street medicine team and a 14-bed medical respite project for discharged patients called Bradford Respite and Intermediate Care Support Services (BRICCS). The Pathway charity sets up and supports specialist teams in many hospitals around the country that aim to maximise the benefit of hospital stays and provide safe, appropriate and sustainable discharges for people experiencing homelessness.

BRICCS is delivered in partnership with Horton Housing and local social care services and is managed via a weekly multidisciplinary team meeting. The health support element of the project is nurse-led and funded jointly by the clinical commissioning group and public health. Beds are paid for by housing benefits. Clients have to be eligible although not actually in receipt of housing benefits when they are admitted. Social services also have funded beds for no recourse to public funds clients with care needs.

The service provides comprehensive intermediate care and end-of-life care and ensures patients access a wide range of other services, including screening, vaccination, dental, optician services, mental health support, English as a second language classes if needed and a variety of recovery courses. Patients can stay up to 6 months. An independent analysis from the BRICCS identified annual secondary care cost savings of £280,000 and high levels of client satisfaction with services (Lowson & Hex, 2014). The project won both a housing and a community impact award and is an example of a highly successful, truly integrated service.

GAINING INPUT FROM SOCIAL SERVICES, CARE REFUSAL AND CONCERNS OVER SELF-NEGLECT

Accessing Care Act assessments

Since 2014 the Care Act has mandated local authorities must carry out an assessment of anyone who appears to require care and support, regardless of their likely eligibility for state-funded care. However, there are occasions when it is difficult to access Care Act assessments for inclusion health groups. This may be related to concerns over ordinary residence, broader eligibility, a lack of understanding regarding the potential care and support needs (e.g., dementia concerns in younger-age clients), active addictions and generally high thresholds for care. Ordinary residence is a complex concept. A person is ordinarily resident in an area if they normally reside in the United Kingdom, apart from temporary or occasional absences, and their residence in that area has been adopted voluntarily and for settled purposes as part of the regular order of their life, whether for short or long duration.

Voices of Stoke produced a toolkit to support referrers to clearly specify how the presenting needs of inclusion health patients can be mapped onto the requirements of the Care Act 2014. These requirements are important to know, because they trigger the legal duty for the local authority to meet a person's needs. The Voices of Stoke team recognised many referrals to adult social care provided a narrative account but did not hit some of the key triggers. Care needs were then not immediately identified by adult social care. The tool helps a referrer negotiate the initial customer screening process and to secure an assessment for their customers. Hostel staff and other frontline homelessness staff often struggle to get support from social services for people who are self-neglecting or have high care and support needs, particularly if they have an active addiction. Using the Voices of Stoke toolkit can help secure much-needed support.

Why People Might Refuse Various Interventions

Many people, including in the general population, refuse various types of health and social care, but it is felt this happens more in inclusion health groups. Anecdotally, people experiencing homelessness, for example, self-discharge from A&E at considerably higher rates than the general population. Immediate reasons include a lack of feeling welcomed into services, competing priorities that make waiting difficult, uncontrolled anxiety, poor impulse control, addictions, other mental health difficulties, neurodiversity and wanting to remain independent. This may be complicated by cultural issues; cultural competence is definitely needed.

It is always important to explore care refusal and understand why it is happening and whether the person has the mental capacity to make the decision, and if they do, does it constitute self-neglect? Spending time talking with someone, building trust and exploring their insights in a person-centred way can enable a deeper understanding about what is important to them and the motivation for their decisions.

Mental Capacity Assessment Refusal or Lack of Engagement

A person lacks mental capacity if they are unable to make or communicate a decision because of an 'impairment of, or a disturbance in the functioning of mind or brain'. The impairment or disturbance may be caused by a variety of factors, including mental illness, learning disability, dementia, brain damage or intoxication (Mental Capacity Act, 2005, p. 2).

However, a variety of factors impact their willingness or ability to engage with a mental capacity assessment:
- Language and literacy
- Cultural norms
- Level of relationship and trust
- Beliefs about the purpose of the assessment
- Mental health conditions
- Addictions
- Brain injury or dementia processes
- Neurodiversity
- Behavioural issues

At the most basic level, excellent communication in a person's first language is essential to ascertain capacity. A full assessment of mental capacity may require a considerable amount of time spent with a patient to build a relationship that enables you to explore an issue. A number of visits may be required, and even then it may not be possible. It is important that inability to undertake a mental capacity assessment because a patient refuses is not inappropriately recorded as a patient either having or lacking mental capacity.

If it is not possible to undertake a capacity assessment, a multidisciplinary discussion should take place, and a plan should be put in place to gain the trust of the patient to be able to proceed and to gain external evidence about them. Although anyone can undertake a mental capacity assessment, it may be appropriate to involve a clinician with clear expertise in this area and people who know the person best, such as frontline workers.

Mental capacity decisions are situation- and time-specific and in homelessness often relate to a person's decision to not seek treatment or leave a health care environment before completing treatment. They may relate to whether a person is genuinely able to care for themselves while homeless (e.g., to take medication effectively), particularly if they are unwell. Fluctuating capacity can be

particularly important in the presence of an addiction, so the time of day an assessment is undertaken is an important consideration.

Safeguarding and Self-Neglect

Self-neglect is a safeguarding issue under the Care Act of 2014 if the person also has care and support needs alongside or as a result of self-neglect. Self-neglect is an extreme lack of self-care that may be a result of many issues, including worsening physical health, psychological trauma, brain injury, mental health, addictions, neurodiversity and cultural norms. Self-neglecting behaviour is common in homelessness populations and may be associated with hoarding behaviour.

It is important to offer all the support available and to understand the possible limitations to interventions if the person does not wish to engage. However, if a person is believed to be unable to protect themselves because of their care and support needs, regardless of whether a person has capacity, it may be necessary to seek permission to act through a court. If the person does not have mental capacity, this is through the Court of Protection. If the person does have capacity, this is through inherent jurisdiction.

Inherent Jurisdiction

The High Court has an inherent jurisdiction to protect adults at risk whether or not they lack capacity. The court can exercise this jurisdiction where it is lawful, necessary and proportionate to do so. Intervention seeks to minimise risk while respecting an individual's choices.

It is important to note the operation and implications of any hoped-for remedy may amount to a deprivation of the person's liberty and infringement of their human rights, and it is unlikely to be a quick fix. Applying for an inherent jurisdiction order is likely to a time-consuming and costly process and needs to be the result of in-depth multidisciplinary discussion.

END-OF-LIFE CARE

Most people, when asked about where they want to be cared for when they are unwell or nearing the end of their lives, say they would like to be cared for at home. This is challenging for inclusion health groups and in particular individuals who do not have a home.

Palliative and End-of-Life Care for People Experiencing Homelessness

If someone has been living in a homeless hostel or another form of temporary accommodation for a number of years, they may consider that place to be their home. However, even when people have accommodation, it is known the majority of people with palliative care needs who are experiencing homelessness end their lives without adequate support, with very little in the way of choices or access to palliative care services (Hudson et al., 2016; Shulman et al., 2018). In addition, people experiencing homelessness may like support to be reunited with family or friends or to find an alternative place of care; in many cases they do not get this chance.

Why Are People Who Are Homeless Rarely Referred to Palliative Care Services?

Uncertainty about when someone needs palliative care due to their illness trajectory, young age, substance use or barriers to accessing health care are key reasons why people experiencing homelessness do not get referred to palliative care services in a timely manner (Shulman et al., 2018). Often, people who have been homeless for many years present with a combination of substance use disorder, mental health difficulties and profound physical health difficulties. They are at higher risk of sudden death, for example from overdose, accidents and suicide. For any given age, they are also at higher risk than the rest of the population of dying from many long-term conditions, including COPD, strokes and heart disease, with a particularly high risk of dying from liver disease (Aldridge et al., 2019). Death from conditions such as advanced liver disease and severe COPD have uncertain trajectories (see Fig. 12.2).

It is notoriously difficult to predict from these conditions when someone is nearing the end of their life. Someone's last years or months are often punctuated by severe deterioration and hospital admissions, each one of which could be the episode of illness that leads to their death. This uncertainty in prognosis results in often very late referral to palliative care (Low et al., 2018).

When this unpredictable illness trajectory is coupled with barriers to accessing services and continuing substance use, predicting when someone is in the last months of life is very difficult. These reasons contribute to people experiencing homelessness not being considered for referral to palliative care services. In addition, people experiencing homelessness

are often quite young, making it hard for everyone to consider they may be dying (Hudson et al., 2016; Klop et al., 2018; Shulman et al., 2018).

Where Are People Currently Cared for?

Currently, there is often a lack of options around place of care. People who have complex needs often remain in homeless hostels they were placed in when they left the streets. These environments have key workers or support workers but not health or care workers. Key and support workers are not trained in health and social care, yet are often left to support people who are dying, including with their personal care. They often struggle to get adequate social services or health professionals to provide care. Other people may be in temporary accommodation with access to even less support (Cornes et al., 2020). As discussed, the Voices of Stoke toolkit may be useful in advocating for people to get appropriate care.

Advanced Care Planning

People experiencing homelessness often do not have the opportunity to consider their advanced care plans for the reasons considered above. If no one considers someone may be dying, their wishes around care and support for their last months are unlikely to be explored. In addition, the lack of options for place of care can make it difficult to discuss someone's wishes if there is little to offer in the way of choice. There is a real and appropriate concern about how to discuss death and dying with someone who may be in denial about their situation or who may be using substances to blank out previous trauma (Hudson et al., 2017). It's important to consider how discussions about current and future care preferences and wishes could be framed in such a way as to not remove hope or make someone feel they have been given up on.

What Needs to Change?

More support needs to be provided to people with advanced ill health who have complex needs and who are experiencing homelessness. This support needs to be delivered wherever the person who needs it is, be it a hostel or temporary accommodation.

No one professional group can necessarily deal with the range of complexity that surrounds palliative care for people experiencing homelessness. It needs a multidisciplinary, multiagency approach that includes people from addiction services, social services and health and palliative care services working together. Different models work extremely well, such as where nurses provide in-reach care to homeless hostels and then connect other agencies to share information and provide person-centred support to people with complex needs.

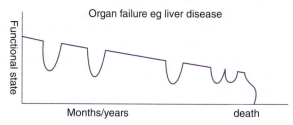

Fig. 12.2 Unpredictable illness trajectory of long-term conditions. (Adapted from Lunney et al., 2002.)

Working With Uncertainty

Rather than using the traditional routes into palliative care, such as considering if a person may die from their illness in the next 6 to 12 months, when supporting someone experiencing homelessness, consideration of a notable deterioration in health may be a more appropriate trigger for a referral to palliative care services. Parallel planning in a person-centred way—hoping for the best but planning for the worst—can be an extremely helpful lens through which to consider palliative care needs for this group (Hudson et al., 2017).

Parallel Planning and Person-Centred Care

Fundamental to all this is developing a trusting relationship and putting the person at the centre of decisions. Conversations should be led by the person supporting an individual experiencing homelessness to explore their insights into their illness and identify their priorities and what living well means to them. This includes exploring what is important in different scenarios.

People who have experienced significant trauma during their lives often use substances to blank out past experiences or as a way of self-soothing. They may not want to have discussions related to their death, and they may not be able to face life without substances. It is important to enable them to be in control of conversations with the focus being about what is important to them and what living well means to them. Conversations should be flexible and repeated. It is important, particularly where there are reversible causes to someone's illness, they do not lose hope and recognise the health care system is always there to support them if they want help with changing direction

(Hudson et al., 2017). For many people it is important to reflect on whether they would like to reconnect with family and what they would like to happen should their health continue to deteriorate.

The homeless palliative care toolkit can help with person-centred care planning and conversation openers (http://www.homelesspalliativecare.com/wp-content/uploads/2018/09/Questions-to-consider-tool.pdf).

SUMMARY AND LEARNING POINTS

Proportionate universalism is the resourcing and delivering of universal services at a scale and intensity proportionate to the degree of need. Services should therefore be universally available, including for the most disadvantaged, and able to respond to the level of presenting need.

Supporting an older person from an inclusion health group with deteriorating health and/or complex health needs requires a multiagency, multiprofessional and sometimes expert specialist response. At the core is the need for a person-centred approach to care and support planning. Conversations need to be led by the patient to explore their insights into their health and illness.

Health care practitioners also need to support people to explore what living well means to them. Nurses need to be able to accept what they may consider as unwise choices, such as supporting someone to continue drinking alcohol or using substances, but also recognise when they have a responsibility to intervene due to self-neglect. Only through these approaches are people be enabled to live and die with respect and dignity.

KEY LEARNING POINTS

- People experiencing homelessness; Gypsy, Roma, Traveller and Boater individuals; asylum seekers; refugees and vulnerable migrants; and individuals from other inclusion health groups suffer poorer health and worse health outcomes than the general population.
- Inclusion health groups often have difficulty accessing health care. They may also present with clinical complexity, early onset frailty, complex safeguarding concerns and difficulty communicating their needs.
- It may take time to build a relationship with a patient from one of these groups due to cultural and other

barriers, and effort needs to be put in to understand the person's health and social care needs.
- Referring someone to specialist inclusion health, social care and voluntary-sector services or connecting with pre-existing specialist support the person has been accessing is beneficial in designing a package of care.
- People from inclusion health groups should have equal access to palliative and end-of-life care services. Usual approaches to referral may need to be considered, particularly where the likely end point of someone's life may be hard to predict due to chaos and a related uncertain disease course.

RESOURCES ON INCLUSION HEALTH

- Public Health England—Inclusion health: Applying all our health: https://www.gov.uk/government/publications/inclusion-health-applying-all-our-health/inclusion-health-applying-all-our-health
- The Queen's Nursing Institute Homeless and Inclusion Health Programme: https://www.qni.org.uk/nursing-in-the-community/homeless-health-programme

- Pathway Healthcare for Homeless People Faculty of Homeless and Inclusion Health: https://www.pathway.org.uk/faculty

RERERENCES

Aldridge, R. W., Menezes, D., Lewer, D., Cornes, M., Evans, H., Blackburn, R. M., Byng, R., Clark, M., Denaxas, S., Fuller, J., Hewett, N., Kilmister, A., Luchensk, S., Manthorpe, J., McKee, M., Neale, M., Story, A., Tinelli, M., Whiteford, M., Wurie, F., & Hayward, A. C. (2019). Causes of death among homeless people: A population-based cross-sectional study of linked hospitalisation and mortality data in England. [version 1; peer review: 2 approved]. *Wellcome Open Res, 4*, 49. https://doi.org/10.12688/wellcomeopenres.15151.1

Aldridge, R. W., Story, A., Hwang, S. W., Nordentoft, M., Lucheski, S. A., Hartwell, G., Tweed, E. J., Lewer, D., Katikireddi, S. V., & Hayward, A. C. (2018). Morbidity and mortality in homeless individuals, prisoners, sex workers, and individuals with substance misuse disorders in high-income countries: A systematic review and meta-analysis. *Lancet, 391*(10117), 241–250.

Baker, M. (2005). *Leeds Racial Equality c. Gypsies and Travellers: Leeds Baseline Census 2004–2005* (pp. RP78524). Leeds Racial Equality Council.

Beswick, A. D., Rees, K, Dieppe, P., Ayis, S., Gooberman-Hill, R., Horwood, J., & Ebrahim, S. (2008). Complex interventions to improve physical function and maintain independent living in elderly people: A systematic review and meta-analysis. *Lancet, 371*(9614), 725–735.

Bolzman, C. (2014). Older Refugees. In E. Fiddian-Qasmiyeh, G. Loescher, K. Long, & N. Sigona (Eds.), *The Oxford handbook of refugee and forced migration studies* (pp. 409–417). Oxford University Press.

Bradley, J. (2018). Health of homelessness. Rapid response to V. Adebowale (2018), There is no excuse for homelessness in Britain in 2018. *BMJ, 360*, k902.

British Geriatrics Society. (2015). *Fit for Frailty—Part 2: Developing, commissioning and managing services for people living with frailty in community settings.* https://www.bgs.org.uk/sites/default/files/content/resources/files/2018-05-23/fff2_full.pdf

British Medical Association. (2019a). BMA says charging regulations for overseas patients are threatening the quality of NHS care. https://www.bma.org.uk/news/media-centre/press-releases/2019/april/bma-says-charging-regulations-for-overseas-patients-are-threatening-the-quality-of-nhs-care

British Medical Association. (2019b). *Refugee and asylum seeker health resource.* https://www.bma.org.uk/media/1838/bma-refugee-and-asylum-seeker-health-resource-june-19.pdf

Brown, R. T., Hemati, K., Riley, E. D., Lee, C. T., Ponath, C., Tieu, L., Guzman, D., & Kushel, M. B. (2017). Geriatric conditions in a population-based sample of older homeless adults. *Gerontologist, 57*(4), 757–766.

Burnett, A., & Peel, M. (2001). Asylum seekers and refugees in Britain: Health needs of asylum seekers and refugees. *BMJ, 322*(7285), 544–547.

Burnett, A., & Ndovi, T. (2018). The health of forced migrants. *BMJ, 363*, k4200.

Churchard, A., Ryder, M., Greenhill, A., & Mandy, W. (2019). The prevalence of autistic traits in a homeless population. *Autism, 23*(3), 665–676. https://doi.org/10.1177/1362361318768484

Clegg, A., Young, J., Iliffe, S., Rikkert, M. O., & Rockwood, K. (2013). Frailty in elderly people. *Lancet, 381*(9868), 752–762.

Cornes, M., Joly, L., Manthorpe, J., O'Halloran, S., & Smyth, R. (2011). Working together to address multiple exclusion homelessness. *Social Policy and Society, 10*(04), 513–522.

Cornes, M., Rice, B., Shulman, C., & Hudson, B. (2020). *Tenancy sustainment team health research: Morbidity and mortality amongst people with experience of rough sleeping.* Thames-Reach and St Mungos. https://thamesreach.org.uk/wp-content/uploads/2020/01/TST-Executive-Summary.pdf

Department of Health and Social Care. (2010). Healthcare for single homeless people. https://www.dh.gov.uk/en/Publicationsandstatistics/Publications/PublicationsPolicyAndGuidance/DH_114250

Depaul Health Initiative. (2018). *Premature ageing in the homeless population.*https://ie.depaulcharity.org/sites/default/files/Depaul%2C%20Premature%20Ageing%20Report%20Feb%202018_0.pdf

Doctors of the World. (2017). Registration refused: A study on access to GP registration in England, an update. https://www.doctorsoftheworld.org.uk/wp-content/uploads/import-from-old-site/files/Reg_Refused_2017_final.pdf

Doctors of the World. (2018). Registration refused: A study on access to GP registration in England, update 2018. https://www.doctorsoftheworld.org.uk/wp-content/uploads/2019/08/Registration-Refused-final.pdf

Eavis, C. (2018). The barriers to healthcare encountered by single homeless people. *Primary Health Care, 28*(1), 26.

Ellis, G., Gardner, M., Tsiachristas, A., Langhorne, P., Burke, O., Harwood, R. H., Conroy, S. P., Kircher, T., Somme, D., Saltvedt, I., Wald, H., O'Neill, D., Robinson, D., & Shepperd, S. (2017). Comprehensive geriatric assessment for older adults admitted to hospital. *Cochrane Database of Systematic Reviews, 19*(9), Article CD006211.

Elwell-Sutton, T., Fok, J., Albanese, F., Mathie, H., & Holland, R. (2017). Factors associated with access to care and healthcare utilization in the homeless population of England. *Journal of Public Health, 39*(1), 26–33. https:doi:10.1093/pubmed/fdw008.

Equality and Human Rights Commission. (2019). Disabled, elderly and ill gypsies and travellers forgotten in site provision. https://www.equalityhumanrights.com/en/our-work/news/disabled-elderly-and-ill-gypsies-and-travellers-forgotten-site-provision

European Centre for Disease Prevention and Control. (2018). *Public health guidance on screening and vaccination for infectious diseases in newly arrived migrants within the EU/EEA.* https://www.ecdc.europa.eu/sites/default/files/documents/Public%20health%20guidance%20on%20screening%20and%20vaccination%20of%20migrants%20in%20the%20EU%20EEA.pdf

European Commission. (n.d.). Migration and home affairs glossary: Forced migrant. https://ec.europa.eu/home-affairs/what-we-do/networks/european_migration_network/glossary_search/forced-migrant_en

Fried, L. P., Tangen, C. M., Walston, J., Newman, A. B., Hirsch, C., Gottdiener, J., Seeman, T., Tracy, R., Kop, W. J., Burke, G., & McBurnie, M. A. Cardiovascular Health Study Collaborative Research Group. (2001). Frailty in older adults: evidence for a phenotype. *Journals of Gerontology Series A: Biological Sciences and Medical Sciences, 56*(3), M146–M157.

Frost, C. J., Morgan, N. J., Allkhenfr, H., Dearden, S., Ess, R., Albalawi, W. F., Berri, A., Benson, L. S., & Gren, L. H. (2019). Determining physical and mental health conditions present in older adult refugees: A mini-review. *Gerontology, 65*(3), 209–215.

Friends, Families and Travellers. Getting a fair deal for Gypsies, Roma and Travellers. https://www.gypsy-traveller.org/our-vision-for-change/education/

Fulfilling Lives South East. (2020). https://www.youtube.com/watch?v=UR66jiGVjcg

Garrett, J., Worrall, S., & Sweeney, S. (2020). *Reducing health inequalities for people living with frailty: A resource for commissioners, service providers and health, care and support staff.* https://www.gypsy-traveller.org/wp-content/uploads/2020/10/health_ineq_final.pdf

Grey, C., & Woodfine, L. (2019). Homelessness and childhood adversity, Public Health Wales. *Feantsa.* https://www.feantsa.org/public/user/Resources/magazine/2019/Winter/Homeless_in_Europe_Winter_2019_-_Article_8_-_Homelessness_and_childhood_adversity_-_Charlotte_Grey_and_Louise_Woodfine.pdf

Groundswell. (2020). *Monitoring the impact of COVID-19 on people experiencing homelessness.* https://groundswell.org.uk/wp-content/uploads/2020/12/Monitoring_Impact_COVID_Groundswell-FINAL-REPORT.pdf

Gunner, E., Chandan, S. K., Marwick, S., Saunders, K., Burwood, S., Yahyouche, A., & Paudyal, V. (2019). Provision and accessibility of primary healthcare services for people who are homeless: A qualitative study of patient perspectives in the UK. *British Journal of General Practice, 69*(685), e526–e536. https://doi.org/10.3399/bjgp19x704633

Hadenfeldt, C. J., Darabaris, M., & Aufdenkamp, M. (2017). Frailty assessment in patients utilizing a free clinic. *Journal of Health Care for the Poor and Underserved, 28*(4), 1423–1435.

Hale, M., Shah, S., & Clegg, A. (2019). Frailty, inequality and resilience. *Clinical Medicine, 19*(3), 219–223.

Healthy London Partnership. (2019). *Safe and effective discharge of homeless hospital patients.* https://www.healthylondon.org/wp-content/uploads/2019/01/190124-GUIDANCE-Safe-and-effective-discharge-of-homeless-hospital-patients.pdf

Hewett, N., Halligan, A., & Boyce, T. (2012). A general practitioner and nurse led approach to improving hospital care for homeless people. *BMJ, 345,* e5999.

Himsworth, C., Paudyal, P., & Sargeant, C. (2020). Risk factors for unplanned hospital admission in a specialist homeless general practice population: Case–control study to investigate the relationship with tri-morbidity. *British Journal of General Practice, 70*(695), e406–e411. https://doi.org/10.3399/bjgp20x710141

Homeless Link. (2014). *The unhealthy state of homelessness.* https://www.homeless.org.uk/sites/default/files/site-attachments/The%20unhealthy%20state%20of%20homelessness%20FINAL.pdf

Hudson, B.F., Flemming, K., Shulman, C., & Candy, B. (2016). Challenges to access and provision of palliative care for people who are homeless: a systematic review of qualitative research. *BMC Palliat Care, 15,* 96. https://doi.org/10.1186/s12904-016-0168-6

Hudson, B. F., Shulman, C., Low J, Hewett, N., Daley, J., Davis, S., Brophy, N., Howard, D., Vivat, B., Kennedy, P., & Stone, P. (2017). Challenges to discussing palliative care with people experiencing homelessness: A qualitative study. *BMJ Open, 7*(11):e017502.

Hynie, M. (2018). The social determinants of refugee mental health in the post-migration context: A critical review. *Canadian Journal of Psychiatry, 63*(5), 297–303.

Klop HT, de Veer AJE, van Dongen SI, Francke AL, Rietjens JAC, Onwuteaka-Philipsen BD. Palliative care for homeless people: a systematic review of the concerns, care needs and preferences, and the barriers and facilitators for providing palliative care. *BMC Palliat Care.* 2018 Apr 24;17(1):67. doi:10.1186/s12904-018-0320-6. PMID: 29690870; PMCID: PMC5914070.

Lebano, A., Hamed, S., Bradby, H., Gil-Salmerón, A., Durá-Francis, E., Garcés-Ferrer, J., Azzedine, F., Riza, E., Karnaki, P., Zota, D., & Linos, A. (2020). Migrants' and refugees' health status and healthcare in Europe: a scoping literature review. *BMC Public Health, 20*(1039).

LeedsGate. (2000). Roads bridges, and tunnels. https://www.leedsgate.co.uk/roads-bridges-and-tunnel

Low, J., Marshall, A., Craig, R., Davis, S., Gola, A., Greenslade, L., Henawi, N., Stone, P., Vickerstaff, V., Wilson, J., & Thorburn, D. (2018). Why do we offer palliative care so late to patients with liver disease? *Lancet Gastroenterol Hepatol, 3*(4), 225–226.

Lowson, K., & Hex, N. (2014). *Evaluation of Bradford homeless health Interventions*: York Health Economic Consortium.

Luchenski, S., Maguire, N., Aldridge, R. W., Hayward, A., Story, A., Perri, P., Withers, J., Clint, S., Fitzpatrick, S., & Hewett, N. (2018). What works in inclusion health: Overview of effective interventions for marginalised and excluded populations. *Lancet, 391*(10117), 266–280.

Lunney, J. R., Lynn J., Hogan C. (2002). Profiles of older medicare decedents. *Journal of the American Geriatric Society. 50*, 1108–1112.

Maguire, N. J., Johnson, R., Vostanis, P., Keats, H., & Remington, R. E. (2009). *Homelessness and complex trauma: A review of the literature*. University of Southampton.

Marmot, M. (2020). *Health equity in England: The Marmot review 10 years on*. Institute of Health Equity.

Marmot, M., Allen, A., Goldblatt, P., Herd, E., & Morrison, J. (2020). *Build back fairer: The COVID-19 Marmot review*: The Health Foundation.

McCarthy, J, Chaplin, E., Underwood, L., Forrester, A., Hayward, H., Sabet, J., Young, S., Asherson, P., Mills, R., & Murphy, D. (2016). Characteristics of prisoners with neurodevelopmental disorders and difficulties. *Journal of Intellectual Disability Research, 60*(3), 201–206.

McCartney, M. (2016). Breaking down the silo walls. *British Medical Journal, 354*, i5199.

Mental Capacity Act. (2005). Chapter 9. London, HMSO. https://www.legislation.gov.uk/ukpga/2005/9/pdfs/ukpga_20050009_en.pdf

Ministry of Housing, Communities and Local Government. (2018). A guide to the duty to refer. https://www.gov.uk/government/publications/homelessness-duty-to-refer/a-guide-to-the-duty-to-refer

National Health Service. (2019). How to register with a GP surgery. https://www.nhs.uk/nhs-services/gps/how-to-register-with-a-gp-surgery/

Nazroo, J. Y. (2003). The structuring of ethnic inequalities in health: Economic position, racial discrimination and racism. *Public Health Matters, 93*(2), 277–284.

Office of National Statistics. (2020). Deaths of homeless people in England and Wales: 2019 registrations. https://www.ons.gov.uk/peoplepopulationandcommunity/birthsdeathsandmarriages/deaths/bulletins/deathsofhomelesspeopleinenglandandwales/2019registrations

Pavli, A., & Maltezou, H. (2017). Health problems of newly arrived migrants and refugees in Europe. *Journal of Travel Medicine, 24*(4), 1–8.

Player, E., Clark, E., Gure-Klinke, H., Walker, J., & Steel, N. (2020). A case study of tri-morbidity. *Journal of Public Mental Health*. https://www.emerald.com/insight/content/doi/10.1108/JPMH-05-2020-0047/full/html

Porter, M., & Haslam, N. (2005). Predisplacement and postdisplacement factors associated with mental health of refugees and internally displaced persons: A meta-analysis. *JAMA, 294*(5), 602–612.

Rae, B., & Rees, S. (2015). The perceptions of homeless people regarding their healthcare needs and experiences of receiving health care. *Journal of Advanced Nursing, 71*(9), 2096–2107.

Rockwood, K., Song, X., MacKnight, C., Bergman, H., Hogan, D. B., McDowell, I., & Mitnitski, A. (2005). A global clinical measure of fitness and frailty in elderly people. *CMAJ, 173*(5), 489–495.

Rogans-Watson, R., Shulman, C., Lewer, D., Armstrong, M., & Hudson, B. (2020). Premature frailty, geriatric conditions and multimorbidity among people experiencing homelessness: A cross-sectional observational study in a London hostel. Housing, Care and Support. https://www.emerald.com/insight/content/doi/10.1108/HCS-05-2020-0007/full/html

Rolfson, D. B., Majumdar, S. R., Tsuyuki, R. T., Tahir, A., & Rockwood, K. (2006). Validity and reliability of the Edmonton Frail Scale. *Age and Ageing, 35*(5), 526–529.

Royal College of General Practitioners. (2013). Improving access to health care for gypsies and travellers, homeless people and sex workers. https://www.basw.co.uk/system/files/resources/basw_110405-3_0.pdf

Salem, B. E., Nyamathi, A. M., Brecht, M.-L., Phillips, L. R., Mentes, J. C., Sarkisian, C., & Leake, B. (2013). Correlates of frailty among homeless adults. *Western Journal of Nursing Research, 35*(9), 1128–1152.

Schiffer, K., & Schatz, E. (2008). Marginalisation, social inclusion and health. Colophon. https://www.drugsandalcohol.ie/11927/1/Correlation_marginalisation_web.pdf

Shulman, C., Hudson, B. F., Low, J., Hewett, N., Daley, J., Kennedy, P., Davis, S., Brophy, N., Howard, D., Vivat, B., & Stonel, P. (2018). End-of-life care for homeless people: A qualitative analysis exploring the challenges to access and provision of palliative care. *Palliative Medicine, 32*(1), 36–45. doi:10.1177/0269216317717101.

Story, A. (2013). Slopes and cliffs: Comparative morbidity of housed and homeless people. *Lancet, 382*, S1–S105.

Strong, J., Varady, C., Chahda, N., Doocy, S., & Burnham, G. (2015). Health status and health needs of older refugees from Syria in Lebanon. *Conflict and Health, 9*(12).

Terry, L., & Cardwell, V. (2015). Understanding the whole person: What are the common concepts for recovery and desistance across the fields of mental health, substance misuse and criminology? http://www.revolving-doors.org.uk/file/1845/download?token=3jprn2sc

Topolovec-Vranic, J., Ennis, N., Howatt, M., Ouchterlony, D., Michalak, A., Masanic, C., Colantonio, A., Hwang, S. W., Kontos, P., Stergiopoulos, V., & Cusimano, M. D. (2014). Traumatic brain injury among men in an urban homeless shelter: observational study of rates and mechanisms of injury. *CMAJ Open, 2*(2), E69–E76.

Traveller Movement. (2012). Gypsy and traveller health briefing, March 2012.

Turner, G., & Clegg, A. (2014). Best practice guidelines for the management of frailty: A British Geriatrics Society, Age UK and Royal College of General Practitioners report. *Age and Ageing, 43*(6), 744–747.

United Nations General Assembly. (1950). Resolution 429(V). https://www.unhcr.org/en-lk/3b66c2aa10

United Nations High Commissioner for Refugees (UNHCR). (2019). Global trends: Forced displacement in 2019. https://www.unhcr.org/globaltrends2019

UNHCR. (2021). UNHCR Emergency handbook: Older persons. https://emergency.unhcr.org/entry/113765/older-persons

Warwick-Booth, L., Woodward, J., O'Dwyer, L., & Di Martino, S. (2018). *An evaluation of Leeds CCG gypsy and traveller health improvement project report*: Leeds Beckett Univerisity. http://eprints.leedsbeckett.ac.uk/id/eprint/5410/1/AnEvaluationofLeedsCCGGypsyandTravellerHealthImprovementProject-WARWICK-BOOTH.pdf.

Yeonwoo, K., Bender, K., Ferguson, K., Begun, S., & DiNitto, D. M. (2017). Trauma and posttraumatic stress disorder among homeless young adults: The importance of victimization experiences in childhood and once homeless. *Journal of Emotional and Behavioural Disorders*. https://doi:10.1177/1063426617710239

13

Informal, Unpaid Carers

Nan Greenwood

CHAPTER OUTLINE

INTRODUCTION

The roles undertaken by unpaid informal adult—often family—carers or caregivers continue to grow and change as worldwide populations age and people live longer, often with several long-term complex conditions. This chapter focuses on unpaid caring provided by families and friends to people living at home, not the care provided by statutory and voluntary services or institutions. It draws on international evidence, often using findings from systematic reviews, and describes adult carers, their enormous diversity and their challenging but also satisfying multidimensional roles. We discuss carers' experiences and support needs and the interventions for supporting carers. Throughout, the chapter highlights the limitations and gaps in the research and possibilities for future studies. Although an important, growing group, young carers aged 18 or younger are not in the focus of this chapter, as their experiences and support needs are recognised as different from those of adult carers.

BACKGROUND

Ageing Populations and an Ever-Changing Picture

Caring and supporting ageing, elderly or unwell partners, family members or friends is common across all cultures throughout the world. Although research on informal carers began only toward the end of the 20th century, this form of support has been undertaken for centuries.

Many people are informal carers at some time, but their individual experiences as carers are influenced by multiple factors, including where they are in their lives when they take on the role and the course and nature of the illness or condition of the person being cared for. Taking the United Kingdom as an example, three in five people will be carers at some point, and it is estimated every year approximately 2.1 million people become carers, and a similar number relinquish the role. Estimates of numbers of carers vary, but in the United Kingdom it is clear the numbers have been growing steadily. A commonly cited report suggests there were nearly 9 million carers in 2019 (Carers UK, 2019a), but by 2037 this figure is expected to grow to 9.9 million (Carers UK, 2014). However, a study undertaken in May 2020 during the COVID-19 pandemic for Carers Week put the numbers of carers across all age groups much higher, at over 13 million (Carers UK, 2020a). The report did not explain why numbers rose so quickly or whether they will remain high after the pandemic, but such findings highlight the ever-changing, fluid nature of caring.

There are several reasons why carer numbers are growing worldwide. Increasing longevity and improved health care adds significantly to growing carer numbers, as more people need support to continue living at home. Ageing often brings increased opportunities for leisure activities and, for example, volunteering, but despite improved health care, it also frequently brings greater disability and dependency. Data show problems increase with age; about one-third (32%) of people aged 60–64 years describe themselves as having disabilities, compared with, for example, nearly two-thirds (60%) of people over 80 (Department of Work and Pensions, 2020). Added to this, the increased emphasis on care in the community in the latter half of the twentieth century means the carer role has expanded in terms of both the tasks performed and the time spent caring. In contrast, the part played by statutory services has reduced.

In many parts of the world, understanding the caring role and carers' experiences is complicated by altering population structures. Such changes are important for a variety of reasons. Especially in the West, women, who traditionally undertook much of this caring, are now in paid work, and although some balance both roles, this can be very challenging. Another change is the increasing tendency for extended families to no longer cohabit or live in close proximity. Living farther apart alters who is close at hand to provide care regularly, with an associated impact on who else in the family might have to take on the role, whether other family members, voluntary or statutory services, or a mixture. This too has an impact on caring experiences. Evidence suggests cohabiting carers often have different caring experiences from those not living in the same households. For example, carers of people with dementia who live with them report poorer quality of life than those who live apart (Farina et al., 2017).

The Extent of the Caring Role

The length and trajectory of caring varies enormously. It can be short-term and very intense or longer term and less intense. It can also be episodic—for example, when caring for someone with heart failure, or longer-term and continuous—for example, when caring for someone with post-stroke disabilities or dementia. Generally, the role comes to an end only when the person being cared for recovers, moves into an institution or dies.

Some carers support their loved ones for only a few hours per week, but others have little time for anything other than caring. Reports show almost 15% of carers care for between 50 and 100 hours a week, and over one-third (36%) care for more than 100 hours a week. By taking on the caring role, carers save economies vast amounts of money. In the United Kingdom this is estimated at £132 billion annually (Carers UK, 2019b), but it is important to remember most people prefer to remain at home, living in the community and maintaining their independence and autonomy but supported by those who know them best—families and friends—rather than living in an institution. Most carers take on their role willingly, but many require support to do so.

Carers' experiences are influenced by the support and interactions they have with health and social care providers. A recent review of the literature (Ris et al., 2019) identified 26 relevant studies that looked at how families saw their caring role and revealed carers usually want to be involved in decision making and care planning of their loved ones, but they need to be supported. Often many services are involved, with the carer acting as a central role coordinating services, organising transport to and from services and medication provision. As a result, many carers are experts in the care of their loved ones and remain a key point of contact and information for service providers. Ris et al. (2019) identified several themes that highlight the importance of relationships and working with and interacting with professionals, including relationship building, negotiating professional care, being professionally supported, managing role expectations, knowledge sharing and working together. The authors concluded carers regard collaboration and being part of the health care team as very important, but in order for services and carers to work together successfully, nurses and other professionals need an understanding of individual caring contexts. For example, it cannot be assumed a carer's only responsibility is caring. Many are also parents, grandparents and perhaps in paid employment, meaning they constantly juggle various obligations with an impact on their ability and capacity to care.

The Term *Informal Carer*

The term *informal carer*, or *caregiver* as carers are often referred to in international literature, is not without critics from both the public and research communities. Among the public, adopting the term *carer* is not always automatic and is sometimes contested by individuals who provide and receive informal care. Often, especially among older people, the caring role develops gradually and increases with age-related disability, making it difficult to identify when caring begins. Furthermore, particularly among older people, informal care is frequently mutual, with couples supporting each other and their roles being determined by each partner's strengths. Many in this situation regard caring as part of their expected and natural marital or family roles. They often do not see themselves as carers but simply as wives, husbands, partners or other family members. Added to this, the term *informal carer* can be regarded as devaluing the role because of the implicit comparison with formal or statutory services provided by paid 'experts' (Nolan et al., 1996).

In some cultures the term *carer* is not recognised. Some Asian languages such as Bengali, Gujarati, Urdu and Punjabi do not have an equivalent word. Here caring is not seen as distinct from other family relationships, which may influence whether carers ask for support for their role. It is therefore important that any considerations of carers' experiences and support needs are situated within the cultural context they occur.

However, the term *carer* is adopted here as it is frequently used in policy and research and helps distinguish unpaid carers from paid care workers.

CARERS, THEIR DEMOGRAPHIC CHARACTERISTICS AND WHAT THEY DO

Gender, Age, Ethnicity and Health

The estimated 8.8 million adult carers in the United Kingdom (Carers UK, 2019a) are more likely to be women (58%) than men (42%). Similar proportions are reported worldwide, with the same gender split in Hong Kong and very similar proportions (61% women and 39% men) in the United States (AARP and National Alliance for Caregiving, 2020).

Carers are not equally distributed across all age groups, with a peak age for caring between 50 and 64 years, but notably numbers of carers in older age groups are growing most rapidly. Not only do many older carers have

disabilities or health conditions themselves, but also they are more likely to be caring for someone with dementia, which is generally regarded as one of the most challenging caring roles. For example, over half of carers over 85 care for someone with dementia, who may also have multiple physical disabilities. Given their age, the carers' own health cannot be ignored (Carers UK, 2019a).

Worldwide, older people from Black, Asian and minority ethnic communities are among the most disadvantaged groups, with higher rates of physical and mental illness compared with majority populations (Bécares et al., 2020). Even after controlling for economic and social disadvantage, evidence from the United Kingdom and internationally shows disparities in health related to ethnicity. For example, in the United Kingdom, Black, Asian and minority ethnic carers often live with greater ill health and also provide disproportionately more care than their White British counterparts. The COVID-19 pandemic highlighted the inequalities, where several demographic groups, including older people and people from Black, Asian and minority ethnic groups, experienced worse outcomes compared to younger people and those from majority White ethnic groups. Thus, older people from minority groups were doubly disadvantaged. Although slightly dated, findings from the Health Survey for England (2004) are revealing (Bécares et al., 2020). Close to one-third (34%) of individuals aged 61–70 years who described themselves as White English people rated their health as 'bad' or 'fair', but for the same age group of Bangladeshi respondents, this figure was 86%, and for Pakistani respondents, it was 69%. Similar comparatively high percentages with 'bad' or 'poor' health were reported by Indian and Black Caribbean communities. Put another way, the self-rated health of White English respondents aged 61–70 was similar to Pakistani people in their late 30s and Bangladeshi respondents in their late 20s or early 30s (Bécares et al., 2020). In Britain, people from Black, Asian and minority ethnic populations are younger than the White majority population, and the next generations will see a significant increase in the numbers of older people who need support from informal carers.

Caring Tasks and Time Taken

The amount of time taken up by caring is variable, ranging from a few hours a week—perhaps including tasks such as collecting prescriptions or food shopping—to continuous 24-hour care. Differences in time spent caring and whether carers live nearby or at a distance are reflected in the tasks undertaken and the hours spent with the individuals they care for.

Overall, as a group, carers most frequently provide practical, day-to-day support, with four in five (82%) providing help with shopping, preparing food and laundry.

Three-quarters of carers say they keep an eye on their loved one (75%), and similar numbers keep them company (68%). Around half support someone with finances (49%) or dealing with statutory services (47%). Caring activities vary in relation to the total time spent caring. For example, if individuals who care for more than 20 hours a week are compared with those who care for fewer hours, they are more likely to provide help with personal care (57% vs 21%), physical care (54% vs 23%) and support taking medicines (54% vs 17%). Similar differences are found with cohabiting carers. Carers who live with the person they support are more likely to provide personal care, physical help and support with taking medication (Carers UK, 2019a).

CARER HETEROGENEITY AND CARING EXPERIENCES

Carer Heterogeneity

One concern about the term *carer* is it could imply carers are a homogenous group who undertake similar caring activities and therefore benefit from the same types of support. However, the caring role covers an enormous range of situations and tasks and often depends on the needs of the person being supported. For example, if the focus is on only the potential differences for carers of people with different health conditions or symptoms, it is immediately apparent that caring for someone with only physical disabilities post-stroke is different from caring for someone post-stroke with no physical disabilities but with cognitive or communication difficulties. Similarly, caring for someone at the end of their life is different from caring for someone with a long-term condition such as heart disease or diabetes. In addition, there are cultural differences in what constitutes caring. This relates not only to the expectations that surround the tasks to be undertaken but also who should take responsibility for the caring role in terms of gender and relationship with the person being cared for. In many cultures it is expected that female relatives—frequently wives, daughters and daughters-in-law—will automatically take on the role. This in turn is associated with different motivations for being a carer and potentially very different experiences in the role. For some people, caring is primarily regarded as a duty, especially for female relatives, while others regard it as a voluntary role rooted in love and respect for family members. It is important to stress there are usually multiple motivations for caring, and individuals who take on the role out of duty may simultaneously care out of love and respect for the person being cared for. There appear to be more similarities than differences between cultures in motivations for caring (Greenwood & Smith, 2019).

One of the main criticisms of research about carers is the failure to adequately recognise variations in carer demographics and the implications differences might have on carers' experiences and support needs. For example, even if this information is recorded by researchers, the impact of differences in carer gender, age and relationships with the cared for are seldom investigated or reported. Failure to recognise and respond to differences with a one-size-fits-all approach hampers research and may also account for the frequently reported low success rate of carer interventions. This is discussed in greater detail below.

The following is a brief description of the impact of demographic differences on the caring experience by the broad demographic groups frequently recorded in the literature. It is worth bearing in mind demographic characteristics do not exist in isolation; people have multiple interacting characteristics. Carers are not just from a particular age or ethnic group or gender; rather, demographic characteristics combine and interact. The combination of characteristics is sometimes referred to as *intersectionality*, a term used to emphasise that characteristics such as ethnicity, sexuality and gender are not isolated but combine to give multiple social identities. These in turn produce unique experiences and sometimes social injustice and discrimination.

Gender

In most age groups female carers outnumber male carers, and it might therefore be expected female carers outnumber male carers in research. In fact, female carer participants are considerably overrepresented in research samples, but this limitation is seldom highlighted, despite the fact it may bias understanding of male carers' experiences and has led to the concern much of what we know about caring is largely from a female perspective.

Nevertheless, there is a small but growing body of research into the relationship between gender and carers' experiences. Overall, it appears that although there are many similarities in male and female carers' experiences, there are some important differences. For example, evidence suggests male carers' approach to caring is more task-orientated than female carers, who tend to adopt emotion-orientated coping. Some authors have reported male carers struggle more to adapt to their role because of its 'feminine' nature (Greenwood & Smith, 2015). Generally, female are more likely to report higher carer burden and greater psychological distress and depression than male, and male carers are less likely to ask for help or access services than their female counterparts. However, it is also possible male carers are more reluctant to admit feelings of distress and burden because of traditional perceptions of masculinity (Greenwood & Smith, 2015).

Sexuality

Although there is growing recognition of care undertaken by members of lesbian, gay, bisexual and transgender (LGBTQ+) communities, caring among these groups has often been described as 'invisible' (Shiu et al., 2016). Older LGBTQ+ carers especially may fear discrimination when interacting with services, particularly if they care for a same-sex partner. Some research suggests they may be excluded from decision making if they are not married (Alba et al., 2020).

Across all types of caring for older people, caring undertaken by a partner is the most common, but older LGBTQ+ carers generally have fewer informal support systems, such as adult children and wider family members. As a result they usually rely more heavily on their friends and peers for support. There is also some evidence that carers are less likely to use formal services and may report poorer mental and physical health than heterosexual carers. The difficulties of using health and social care services can be compounded for carers without formalised relationships, as they do not have the rights of next-of-kin carers and may not feel they fit in with services designed primarily for heterosexual partners or biological family members (Shiu et al., 2016).

Age

Although carer age is frequently recorded in the research literature, it is often reported only as an average, which fails to show the diversity of carer participant ages and neglects to acknowledge the potential impact of age differences. This hampers understanding of the relationship between age and caring experiences, but evidence is growing there are differences linked to age. Research suggests carer age is related to carers' assessment of the impact of caring on their lives and on feelings such as guilt; younger adult carers describe both greater impact and more guilt. However, studies also demonstrate the challenges of understanding these relationships (Springate & Tremont, 2014). Many of the older carers in Springate and Tremont's (2014) study were spouses, and the younger carers tended to be adult children. Therefore, the differences may not be due to age alone but may reflect different life situations, with younger carers more often trying to balance the demands of child care and paid employment with their caring role (Springate & Tremont, 2014).

Despite their growing importance and the fact older carers frequently have their own health concerns and are often in difficult caring roles, researchers have only recently begun to look at the experiences of older carers specifically. de Oliveira et al. (2015) reviewed the available quantitative literature investigating older carers' quality of life and concluded increasingly older people care for others with dementia, and as they age, carers have poorer perceived quality of life. Another systematic review that included both quantitative and qualitative literature related to carers

aged 75 and older (Greenwood & Smith, 2016) found that overall, quantitative studies generally identified the challenges of caring for older people, while qualitative studies were more likely to emphasise caring satisfaction and carers' active responses to their situations. Other work by the same authors (Greenwood et al., 2019) highlighted that although carers over 75 have many similar experiences and challenges to younger adult carers, their own often declining health makes it especially hard to maintain social contacts and access support. Loneliness among older carers was very common, especially if they were housebound or caring for someone with conditions such as dementia that make leaving the house difficult. A huge source of concern for older carers concerned the future: What would happen to their loved ones if they became unable to maintain their caring role or if they died before their loved ones? This anxiety applied to individuals who cared for others of similar ages but was particularly striking for individuals who cared for adult children with disabilities. The findings suggested any support for older carers needs to be tailored for their often isolated situations, with specific support for the emotive issues around their own mortality.

Although not the focus of this chapter, young carers, under 18 years old, are an important group who often require different types of support to adult carers. Estimates vary hugely, but according to a Department for Education (2016) report, using statistics from 2011, there were approximately 166,000 young carers aged 5–17 in the England alone, and there was good evidence of the negative effects of caring on their health, social activity, education and later employment. Like adult carers, young carers are also entitled to an assessment. Many organisations that focus on supporting carers in general, such as Carers Trust network partners, have specialised support for young carers. Nurses who work with families need to ensure they look out for and are aware of young carers and can signpost them to assessment and appropriate support.

Ethnicity

Earlier we saw evidence for the potentially greater role played by carers from Black, Asian and minority ethnic communities. Evidence also shows numbers of carers from minority ethnic groups are increasing, especially in developed countries, as these populations age and their demographic profiles change.

There is growing evidence that Black, Asian and minority ethnic carers' experiences are different and may be more challenging than for White carers. In the United Kingdom, for example, carers from Black, Asian and minority ethnic groups provide proportionally more care than the White British majority, are more likely to struggle financially and are more likely to care for 20 hours or more per week (56%

vs 47%) (Carers UK, 2011). Understanding Black, Asian and minority ethnic carers' experiences and support needs is therefore essential.

Spending longer hours caring may increase Black, Asian and minority ethnic carers' risks of poor health, making it harder to remain in paid employment and increasing the chances of social exclusion and emotional health problems. Furthermore, some research suggests higher levels of isolation among Pakistani and Bangladeshi carers (Carers UK, 2011). Greater anxiety and depression have also been identified for British Indian carers (Manning et al., 2014). These facts demonstrate the importance of recognising carer cultural diversity and potentially tailoring support services for their specific needs. Historically, service providers assumed strong kinship networks meant Black, Asian and minority ethnic families would look after their own, and professionals did not always offer much-needed support (Katbamna et al., 2004). This perception may be changing, but it still remains in some areas.

Caring Towards the End of Life

An important group of carers support someone toward the end of their life. This is a particularly challenging time for many, but research that focuses on this period is surprisingly limited. Most people say they would prefer to spend the end of their life at home, and families usually want this as well. Where possible these wishes should be respected, but the emotional and physical costs to families should always be acknowledged and support provided. Equally, it should not be assumed all carers and their loved ones want to remain at home until the very end of life; some may prefer to move to a hospice, for example. In all situations, families should be supported in their decision making. The available studies suggest caring at this time is very stressful, with greater anxiety, depression and physical burden, but supportive interventions can have positive outcomes for carers (Chi et al., 2015). However, more longitudinal research is needed to improve our understanding of how caring changes over this important time. Caring toward the end of life was even more challenging during the COVID-19 pandemic (Aker et al., 2021).

Evidence for the impact of COVID-19 on carers is gradually accumulating. According to Carers UK, (2020b), the majority of carers had to provide more care than previously, and millions more people took on the caring role. Many carers were unable to access respite and their usual forms of support with a resultant negative impact on their mental health. Some carers also reported reduced access to health care (Carers UK, 2020b). It also seems likely that because of fear of the virus, many carers were less willing to have paid carers visit for domiciliary support. Further work is needed to understand the impact of the pandemic on unpaid carers, but this work is essential if we are to support carers in any future pandemics.

IMPACT OF CARING–NEGATIVES AND POSITIVES

Research, both quantitative and qualitative, into informal caring has proliferated over the past three decades. A considerable amount is now known about carers' experiences and support needs, and there is a much better understanding of the challenges and satisfactions of their role. However, it is important to highlight common limitations of the studies in this area, which need careful consideration when looking at research that investigates the impact of caring and research that focuses on interventions to support carers.

First, these studies often have small samples, are not representative of carers as a whole, are often not theoretically grounded, are cross-sectional and do not always employ suitable outcome measures. Considering who takes part in the research, generally participating carers are not representative of carers; female carers and those from White or majority ethnic backgrounds are often overrepresented (Greenwood et al., 2018). Concerns are being raised that the carers who are willing to take part in research may not be typical of carers as a whole, and individuals who spend the most time and greatest involvement in caring may be more likely to participate. Furthermore, the context of caring is often not considered—for example, in terms of wider family support and availability of statutory or voluntary services. Strikingly, the research tends to treat carers as an homogenous group and fails to consider carer diversity in terms of age, gender or ethnicity, despite the growing evidence of differences in the experiences among these groups. Even if carer demographics are recorded and described, these characteristics are often not included in the analysis. In addition, research generally fails to recognise and explore intersectionality and its potential impact on findings by treating carer demographics in isolation. A further issue is although it is generally claimed carers often experience emotional distress such as anxiety and depression, researchers seldom include matched comparison groups of participants not in caring roles. They often conclude carers' mental health is worse than that of non-carers, but without a direct comparison as part of the research design, it is clearly unwise to assume this.

The dominance of cross-sectional studies does not capture the dynamic nature of caring or show how much it can change from day to day and week to week. This fluidity is frequently associated with changing carer well-being and support needs. Even so, longitudinal studies are rare, and as a result the varying nature of caring is seldom depicted.

Finally, some authors (for example Greenwood et al., 2018) argue the outcomes selected in quantitative research fail to represent the entirety of caring experiences, and the negative focus of some studies may lead to misrepresentation of the caring experience as a whole. It is worth considering in some depth one of the most frequently applied concepts in carers research—carer burden. Measurement of carer burden is common in research and is used to describe a range of negative experiences, including aspects of emotional health such as anxiety and depression. It is also often incorporated as an outcome measure when trying to understand the impact of supportive interventions for carers. Nonetheless, the concept is increasingly criticised as ill-defined, vague and too inclusive to be of real value either to our understanding of carers' lives or in clinical practice and policy making (Mosquera et al., 2016). It is important for nurses to be able to question and think about the impact of caring in relation to their patients. In addition, carer burden's negative connotations mean it fails to recognise the complexity of caring, the balance of which is influenced by relationships prior to caring and the nature of the caring role. Furthermore, it may offer a harmful depiction of the person being cared for with potentially an adverse impact on them, as the term *burden* can make caring sound one-sided without giving recognition to its often mutual nature. However, it seems interventions intended to ameliorate the negative impact of caring increasingly include more specific outcomes such as reductions in anxiety and depression or increases in caring confidence, resilience and self-efficacy.

Despite these criticisms of carer research, it is now recognised caring can be both rewarding and challenging, and at times carers need support from services such as district nurses. The overlapping and interrelated nature, complexity, fluidity and variety of these experiences must be recognised, but for simplicity here, the impact of caring and its associated needs are classified into positive and negative. The negative impact is further subdivided into emotional, social, physical and financial areas. To help bring carers' experiences to life, anonymous quotes from older carers over 70 collected in the course of earlier research are included in the following sections (Greenwood et al., 2019).

Negative Impacts

Emotional Impact

It is generally acknowledged caring can result in adverse changes in emotional health with consequences for the carer. This in turn may have a detrimental effect on the carer's ability to care and therefore on the individual they care for. These negative impacts are the most commonly investigated effects of caring. Researchers frequently identify and measure depression, anxiety, stress and carer burden. Improvements in carer emotional health and well-being are therefore often the intended outcomes of interventions for supporting carers.

A plethora of studies report high levels of anxiety and depression in carers. A recent systematic review that looked at the causal impact of caring rather than only identifying correlations concluded there was evidence of a negative effect of caregiving on the mental and physical health of carers. The presence and strength of this impact varied with different carer groups, with married female carers and those who provided more intensive care more likely to experience negative effects (Bom et al., 2019).

Highlighting the relationship between mental and physical health, one carer described the relationship between her emotional well-being and her physical health: 'I had a fall just before Christmas, I fell down the stairs…and it's a lack of sleep in that situation, that's what I really noticed, because I had in pain with my legs, I was full of tension and anxiety for my daughter… You don't have that same energy level'.

A less frequently reported but very important aspect of caring is guilt. Some carers feel guilty whatever they do, because despite their best efforts, they believe they are not doing enough: 'You're doing your best, but you're guilty all the time'.

An individual with neurological conditions such as dementia may have changed significantly and can be challenging to look after. Carers describe losing their patience and, as a consequence, often feel guilty. They may constantly have to remind themselves of the person before their illness. This carer had been married for over six decades: 'He'll do something stupid, and I'll shout at him and then I feel terrible, because he tries all the time, and every night he tells me how he loves me and how pleased he is he married me'.

Physical Impact

Caring can have both short- and long-term impact on carers' physical health. A survey in the United Kingdom reported more than four in five (83%) carers said caring had an adverse effect on their physical health (Carers UK, 2012). Caring can lead to tiredness from providing around-the-clock care and the day-to-day demands of dealing with statutory services. Typical comments from older carers include: 'I get very tired, very, very tired, and I don't sleep a lot in the night, worried about him, and I have a lot to do'.

Feeling constantly in demand from many directions and a sense of hypervigilance can lead to exhaustion: 'You feel totally responsible for everything all the time. You have to do everything. There are so many hats to wear'.

To support their loved ones, carers frequently have to work with statutory services. Although the support is generally valued, engaging with these services can be very time consuming and frustrating, adding to carers' overwhelming tiredness. One carer was unsure whether employing paid carer workers was worth the effort she put into it because of the tension it created between her and her husband: 'As good as some of them [care workers] were, we still had all the problems of me on the phone, constantly... "Have we got a carer today?" Because nobody came, and then my husband would shout (that's the only thing he could do), so then I'd get called up... Part of me said, "Is it, is it worth having carers?" Because to me it was more stressful'.

Furthermore, carers often neglect their own health and do not have sufficient time to look after themselves, for example, by getting enough exercise or eating healthily. Reports of back strain and injuries from lifting are also common. Two out of five carers say they have delayed medical treatment for themselves because of their caring role (Carers UK, 2012).

Social Impact—Isolation and Loneliness

Carers frequently refer to their loneliness and social isolation, which increases as their caring role continues. There are many possible reasons for the loss of social contact, including physical restrictions. For example, if the cared for is confined to a wheelchair, it creates challenges when using public transport or gaining access to buildings. Embarrassment over the cared-for person's condition can lead to isolation. Challenging behaviour and incontinence can mean carers are unwilling to venture out into public. Many carers are afraid to leave their loved one alone and do not want to entrust their care to others. As a result their own friendships and social activities dwindle. Added to this, the carers' physical health may restrict where they can take the person they care for. The following quotes from older carers illustrate these difficulties and their shrinking social contacts.

'Your so-called friends disappear, because they don't want to have to be involved. They perceive they could be called on, and so you're left with perhaps two or three people who've got problems of their own'.

'You are very isolated as an older person. I have lost most of my friends that I used to meet up with and go out with... I can't do anything like that because I can't leave him'.

One carer worried about what other people would think of her husband's behaviour: 'I used to do lots of things before, but you do withdraw a little... I don't invite people to the house that much, especially if I think my husband is not very well'.

Financial Impact

Evidence of the huge financial impact of caring on families has been growing steadily and is largely the result of loss or reduced employment but also due to the costs of care, including equipment, extra heating, laundry and paying for support such as respite care. Financial concerns add to carers'

stress and anxiety. Importantly, financial impact does not affect all groups equally; evidence shows Black, Asian and minority ethnic carers are more often financially disadvantaged (Carers UK, 2011). Giving up paid work or reducing hours worked may have longer-term consequences for carers with poorer career opportunities and reduced pensions and retirement security. Over one-third (37%) of working-age carers say they had to give up paid work entirely (Carers UK, 2012). The tension between paid employment and unpaid caring is growing, as more women in Europe and other high-income countries enter the labour market and as retirement ages increase. Leaving employment has an impact not only on carers and their families but also on employers and society more widely. The effect on government income is striking; it is estimated carers leaving paid employment in England costs the government £2.9 billion annually. This includes £1.7 billion in social security benefits paid to people who have left their jobs and another £1.2 billion in taxes forgone on carers' lost earnings. Supporting people to be able to combine caring and paid work is therefore important for both carers and economies (Pickard et al., 2017).

Positives, Satisfactions and Rewards of Caring

One major criticism of caring research is the general focus on the negative and challenging aspects of caring, which potentially provides an unbalanced picture of caring and carers' lives and does not acknowledge how many carers, at least some of the time, enjoy the reciprocal benefits from caring and can identify rewards from their role. Satisfaction from caring is reported in a variety of cultures and countries, and it is increasingly recognised that caring is a mixture of challenging and rewarding experiences.

Investigations into the satisfaction derived from caring have grown significantly since the 1990s. With early work by authors such as Nolan et al. (1996) and Kramer (1997), we now have a fairly comprehensive picture of the positives of caring. Rewards include feelings of pride in reducing deterioration of loved ones, improved self-worth, personal growth, closer relationships, an improved sense of meaning, warmth and pleasure (Kramer, 1997).

Echoing earlier studies, Yu et al. (2018) reviewed 41 studies on the satisfaction of caring for someone with dementia. The authors concluded the positive aspects of caring are multidimensional and cover four main themes: a sense of personal accomplishment and gratification, feelings of mutuality in dyadic relationships, an increase in family cohesion and functionality, and a sense of personal growth and purpose in life.

Carers' sense of purpose—the feeling life has meaning and direction—seems to be an important aspect of the rewards of caring. Many carers eloquently describe their sense of purpose and pride:

'I think of a tree, my branches that I support, and that gives me a purpose in life, and that's the main thing I get from caring is a purpose'.

'You feel a sense that you've achieved a sense of vocation as well, dedication, pride in what you're doing'.

Another typical comment from an older carer reflects rewards and satisfactions: 'They say you grow from the difficult experiences of life and not from the good things that happen to you, and I, yeah, I've grown, and I've learnt coping strategies'.

Carers talk about how caring has opened doors or is a journey of discovery. Some would not have chosen different lives. One 80-year-old carer described how she was grateful for her decades of caring responsibilities. Her quote demonstrates how caring is neither always stressful nor always rewarding: 'My daughter has brought me a lot of worry and a lot of joy. You're never free, but I'm happy with life, and I've got a happy family life. So I just think she is a blessing because she's made me a nicer person'.

Quinn and Toms (2019), in a systematic narrative review of the relationship between the positive aspects of caregiving and the well-being of carers of people with dementia, identified 53 relevant studies. They reported positive aspects of caring were associated with better mental health, quality of life and self-efficacy but were not related to perceived health or strain and stress. The authors concluded identifying positive aspects of caring is associated with carer well-being, and interventions that help carers gain and identify more positive experiences from caring could help promote them.

SUPPORTING CARERS

Importantly for nurses, the vital role played by carers was clearly recognised in recent English legislation: 'Carers need to be recognised and valued. Carers need access to information and support to provide the best care they can. Carers need to be helped to balance their caring responsibilities with their own employment and to preserve their personal health and wellbeing' (Department of Health and Social Care, 2018, p. 5). Part of this action plan is intended to support health and social care professionals to be better at identifying, valuing and working with carers and to help employers recognise carers' roles. This directive has led to the development of a wide range of support for carers, and nurses need to play their part in supporting carers to enable older people to live independently.

However, it has been repeatedly shown carers in general frequently do not engage with support services, despite the fact many report unmet needs, and using services can delay the transfer of individuals being supported to long-term care. Many researchers have attempted to understand carers' failure to access and engage with services. Findings

suggest carers' reasons are varied and individual but include, for example, not seeing the need for support, poor previous experiences with services, lack of time, lack of information about available support and concerns about its suitability for them and the person they care for (Greenwood et al., 2015). Carers' own personal characteristics such as their coping style and sense of personal duty have also been demonstrated to have an impact. Other research has highlighted unwillingness on the part of the person being cared for to have strangers involved in their care or to have them in their homes. Perceived stigma associated with the health condition of the person being cared for, such as dementia, addictions or mental illness, may also deter carers from coming forward for help (Janevic & Connell, 2001).

Looking closely at service uptake by diverse groups can help explain this low engagement more generally. For example, evidence shows service usage is related to carer demographic characteristics such as ethnicity and gender. Despite the important role played by Black, Asian and minority ethnic carers, evidence repeatedly shows they are even less likely than White majority carers to use statutory services . A review of relevant studies (Greenwood & Smith 2015) found most of the issues described by Black, Asian and minority ethnic carers were applicable to carers of all ethnic groups and tended to be a mixture of attitudinal and structural barriers. These included carers not seeing the need for support, not wanting to involve people outside the family, and low awareness and poor availability of services. Some challenges were more specific to Black, Asian and minority ethnic groups and included language barriers and carers' concerns about cultural sensitivity or religious appropriateness (Greenwood et al., 2015).

In relation to gender, it is often reported male carers are less likely than female carers to use services. A review of reasons highlighted that many barriers such as poor awareness of services and insufficient information apply across carers of all genders. However, male carers were more likely to emphasise their reluctance to use services because of their sense of responsibility, duty and unwillingness to pass on the responsibility of caring to services or other family members. Poor previous experiences with services were also highlighted (Greenwood & Smith, 2015).

Support Needs

It is clear many carers find their role challenging, and many say they would like more support. Similar themes have emerged in inquiries into what carers want from services going back over three decades. Nolan and Grant (1989) argued what carers feel is missing can be divided into insufficient information, skills training, emotional support and respite. More recent evidence shows in addition to wanting acknowledgment of their expertise and respect for their role, carers say they want timely information and signposting to support services, flexible care to suit themselves and their loved ones, and recognition they need support with maintaining their own health and well-being (Carers UK, 2012). Interventions to support carers generally reflect these needs and primarily focus on information, education and training, and interventions to support their emotional and physical well-being (Brimblecombe et al., 2018). Unsurprisingly, given the diversity of needs, interventions are hugely variable in length, scale, scope and content. Some are multicomponent interventions with many different strands; others have only one element. Many are offered in the voluntary sector, but others are offered by health care providers.

To gain a more detailed sense of the assistance available for carers, the following are some examples of specific types of support for carers. Much of the evidence provided comes from systematic reviews. Increasingly, researchers and service providers rely on such reviews to understand what interventions have a demonstrable impact on carers. Systematic reviews identify studies, undertake quality assessments, synthesise relevant research and summarise the findings. Very recently researchers have explored this further, undertaking meta-reviews, or reviews of reviews. Some relate to carers in general; others focus on carers of people with particular health conditions, on specific types of support or on certain demographic groups of carers, such as those from Black, Asian and minority ethnic groups.

Information

Carers say they need information on a wide range of areas and topics. They would like to know about the health condition of the person they care for and more about treatments and support services. In terms of information about available support, carers want advice and to know about financial and legal support and information about the physical aspects of caring. It is essential any information offered is given at an appropriate time, and carers are not overwhelmed because of the nature of the timing—for example, given too early or too late in their caring role. It must be provided in a suitable format, for example in a language carers are familiar with, in hard copy, online or both. Often information needs to be offered on several occasions until the carer is ready to receive it.

In a typical review of interventions aimed at providing information for carers of people with stroke, Forster et al. (2012) identified 21 studies and concluded although it was unclear how best to deliver information, possibly actively involving patients and carers was most effective. Overall, there was evidence that providing information increased both groups' knowledge of stroke, patient satisfaction and reduced patient depression.

Respite or Carer Breaks

Many carers say they need a break from their caring role, but the evidence for the benefits of respite are mixed. This may in part be because of the variety of types of breaks available; they can be a few hours or several days and can take place at home or in residential care. Vandepitte et al. (2016), in a review of respite for carers of people living with dementia, concluded day services could decrease both carer burden and challenging behaviour in a person with dementia, but perhaps surprisingly, individuals who received day care often moved earlier to nursing homes. The evidence for the impact of respite in residential care is more mixed and shows negative effects on both carers and the individuals they care for. There is less evidence for community-based respite, but qualitative studies suggest benefits (Vandepitte et al., 2016).

Training for the Caring Role

Many carers feel inadequately prepared for their role and want to learn how better to support the people they care for. One of the most well-known attempts at providing carers with training focused on carers of people with stroke in the United Kingdom (Kalra et al., 2004). In this study with 300 patients and their carers during rehabilitation, investigators evaluated the effectiveness of carer training in reducing stroke costs and improving patient and caregiver outcomes. Using a single blind randomised controlled trial, the investigators looked at the impact of a programme that provided information about, for example, statutory benefits, community and voluntary-sector services, and encouragement to learn about basic nursing and personal care techniques, including facilitating transfers and mobility, with encouragement to attend nursing and therapy activities. At 1 year, the training programme resulted in reduced costs and carer burden and improved psychosocial outcomes for carers and patients but had no impact on stroke survivors' rates of institutionalisation or levels of disability or mortality (Kalra et al., 2004).

Problem-Solving Training

There is growing evidence training carers in problem-solving can be beneficial. Overall research suggests such interventions are a promising means of reducing carer depression, anxiety and burden (Garand et al., 2019). However, there is considerable diversity in the intended recipients of the intervention—for example, carers of people with stroke or carers of people living with dementia, the content of the interventions, session numbers and in administration—for example, whether face-to-face, on the telephone, online or a mixture. It appeared problem-solving interventions for carers, whether face-to-face, via video conferencing, over the telephone or in combinations of these methods improve caregiving skills, reduce stress and give carers a sense of increased mastery or control, which in turn helps their mental health (Nezu et al., 2004). Problem-solving training can be particularly helpful for carers who live a long way from services or have limited time and resources. However, problem-solving is often provided as part of a multicomponent intervention, making it impossible to detect effects specific to this approach.

Peer Support

Many carers say they want peer support from current or former carers. Research shows they benefit from talking to others in similar situations or those who with previous similar experiences (Greenwood et al., 2017). Some receive peer support without engaging in statutory or voluntary services. Family members and friends with caring experience may provide support, and other carers become involved more formally in group or one-to-one peer support, often provided by the voluntary sector. Support groups of carers may meet regularly with or without any particular structure. Some organisations provide information sessions, but there is usually a social element with the provision of light refreshments and opportunities to interact informally (for example dementia cafes). The quantitative evidence for the benefits of these groups is mixed, but qualitatively many carers report enjoying attending and say these meetings provide valuable peer support and much needed social contact (Dickinson et al., 2017; Greenwood et al., 2017).

A good example of a growing type of support that offers a range of benefits for people living with dementia and their carers are Alzheimer's, dementia and memory cafés. They originated in the Netherlands in the 1970s but are now offered globally. They have been available in the United Kingdom for over 2 decades and provide a place where people living with dementia and their carers can meet others in similar situations. The intention is to have social, café-style atmospheres where carers and people with dementia can come and go as they please and talk to others but also have refreshments and maybe take part in activities or listen to talks. Venues vary. Some are held in local cafés, but more often they are hosted by the voluntary sector in community halls and libraries with a mixture of paid and volunteer staff. There are usually some organised activities, refreshments and support from staff. Activities vary but include music, singing, quizzes, gardening and information provision. Evidence suggests these events are well received by carers; many feel the cafés not only provide peer support but also somewhere carers and their loved ones can be themselves, normalise their experiences and meet others familiar with the symptoms of dementia and the challenges of the caring role (Greenwood et al., 2017).

Technology-Based Interventions

There is some growing evidence of the value of technology in helping, for example, reduce social isolation. However, the age of many carers means some are unable or unwilling to engage with it. Added to this, the cost of technology makes it unavailable to many demographic groups.

Interventions based around technology were already a growing area of interest, but the COVID-19 pandemic highlighted the importance of support that does not require face-to-face contact between carers and service providers. Many organisations that support carers moved activities online, including support groups, coffee mornings and exercise and yoga classes. They were generally well received, and providers reported housebound carers who had previously been unable to physically attend classes often joined the activities (Lorenz-Dant & Comas-Herrera, 2021).

Sin et al. (2018) reviewed the evidence for technology-based interventions and identified 78 studies that fit their inclusion criteria. Many interventions were aimed at carers of people living with dementia, and most were intended to increase self-efficacy and knowledge and reduce physical illness. Psychoeducation delivered online that included network support with peers and professionals was most common. Carers valued the flexibility and the fact they could control the pace of the intervention and were generally very satisfied with this support.

Another review of the impact of internet-based interventions on carer mental health (Sherifali et al., 2018) concluded they can be helpful in improving depression, anxiety and stress. The most effective interventions included education and information with or without psychological support. The study also noted more research is needed in this relatively new field. Further discussion of the role of technology in care of older people is found in Chapter 35.

OVERVIEW OF THE EVIDENCE FOR THE EFFECTIVENESS OF SUPPORT FOR CARERS

Overall Evidence

A selection of systematic reviews and meta-reviews of carer interventions is provided below. Despite often having slightly different foci, these reviews demonstrate although there are some similarities in their findings and conclusions, there are also considerable divergences and discrepancies.

Brimblecombe et al.'s (2018) review of the international evidence for carer interventions concluded evidence was mixed, but it was strongest for psychological therapy, training or education interventions, support groups, and replacement or substitution care that allows flexible working. They also argued often the greatest impact comes with a combination of or multicomponent interventions.

In a large, comprehensive meta-review of supportive interventions for carers, Dalton et al. (2018) identified 61 relevant reviews. The authors found study quality was variable, and most focused on carers of people with specific health conditions such as dementia or stroke. Many included multicomponent interventions with psychosocial or psychoeducational content. A range of carer outcomes were investigated—primarily carer mental health, burden, stress, quality of life and well-being. The authors concluded there is no one-size-fits-all approach to interventions for carers, but contact with people outside carers' usual social networks can be helpful. They also reported specific types of intervention are more beneficial for certain carer groups. For example, carers of people living with dementia are more likely to benefit from shared learning, cognitive reframing, meditation and computer-delivered psychosocial interventions. Carers of people with stroke may be helped by counselling, as can carers of people with cancer, who may also benefit from art therapy and psychosocial interventions. Despite the fact respite, whether at home or in an institution, is frequently offered as a supportive intervention and carers tend to be very positive about it, evidence for its effectiveness was mixed. Quantitative, empirical evidence generally showed limited benefits.

Carers of people living with dementia have received particular attention. To synthesise and evaluate studies that looked at interventions to help this group, Dickinson et al. (2017) undertook a meta-review. They identified 31 reviews fitting inclusion criteria, but only 13 rated as high or moderate quality were included in the analysis. The authors concluded well-designed, structured multicomponent interventions can not only help maintain the psychological well-being of carers but also delay institutionalisation of the person with dementia. It was suggested interventions need therapeutic and educational components, and delivery in groups can increase their effectiveness.

Cheng and Zhang (2020) reported on a meta-review of non-pharmacological support for carers of people with dementia that focused on outcomes rather than types of interventions. They identified 60 reviews, and although the quality of the reviews was variable, the conclusions reached by the authors appeared unrelated to study quality. Carer depression seemed most readily changed using a range of interventions—for example, psychoeducation, counselling or psychotherapy, mindfulness-based interventions or multicomponent interventions. Quality of life, mastery and communication skills training were also modifiable, but weak or no impact was reported for changing anxiety, social

support and carer burden. Respite and support groups were mostly ineffective. The researchers also found no evidence delivering support to carer-cared for dyads or groups was any more effective than interventions provided for carers alone. In agreement with some other reviews, they concluded multicomponent interventions are generally more effective than single component interventions.

Evidence Specifically for Black, Asian and Minority Ethnic Carers

Ethnicity may be regarded as creating a context for carers' caring experiences, which leads to differences in coping. Some ethnic groups provide less social support, and differences in familism—defined as the subordination of the personal interests and prerogatives of an individual to the values and demands of the family—may influence how carers appraise and approach their role and their overall well-being. In turn, this influences perceptions of interventions and outcomes such as depression or stress. Differences in carers' health status also contribute to differences in well-being in these groups.

In recognition of their sometimes more challenging situations, for Black, Asian and minority ethnic carers, some recent attempts have been made to explore the impact of supportive interventions. However, finding evidence is very difficult in part because of poor reporting of participant demographics in carer research. Many do not report carer ethnicity, and cultural tailoring is unusual (Gilmour-Bykovskyi et al., 2018).

A few studies have investigated culturally tailored support. In a rare United Kingdom study of South Asian families who support someone living with dementia, Parveen et al. (2018) investigated the impact of a culturally adapted carers' information programme about dementia for South Asian families. Several benefits were identified that went beyond the study participants to the wider family and the person with dementia. Knowledge of dementia increased, and it also helped carers recognise the need to look after themselves and accept that peer support could be beneficial.

End-of-Life Caring

It is important to consider nursing interventions for carers who look after someone at home at the end of their life. A recent systematic review (Becqué et al., 2019) identified nine studies. The four main components of interventions were psychoeducation, needs assessment, practical support and peer support, which had a beneficial effect on carers' sense of competence, preparedness, rewards and burden. Again, multicomponent interventions were found to be most effective. More on end-of-life care is found in Chapter 34.

The Role of General Practice in Supporting Carers

General practice teams are frequently one of the earliest points of contact for services for carers. Visits to GPs are common, making them well placed to recognise and support carers. Evidence suggests carers and the individuals they care for want regular contact with their GPs, and GPs and others in their teams believe they have an important role to play, although their support is limited by time and resources. Despite their clear potential role, little research has investigated carer support provided in general practice. Findings from a survey published in 2015 that included 195,364 informal carers, reported that compared to non-carers, carers experienced a double disadvantage of worse health-related quality of life and poorer patient experience in primary care (Thomas et al., 2015). The authors recommended GPs should identify and treat carer-related health problems such as pain, anxiety and depression, particularly in carers from deprived areas and those who spending longer hours caring (Thomas et al., 2015). A recent interview study with health and social care providers, commissioners and policy makers in the United Kingdom (Peters et al. 2020) described their perceptions of support provision to carers in primary care. Three main themes emerged: identifying carers, carer support, and assessing and responding to carer needs. It was recognised neither primary care nor other services were doing enough for carers, but they could play an important part in identifying and supporting them. Although these groups recognised service providers were often not sufficiently proactive in identifying carers, they also highlighted many carers do not self-identify as such. Supporting carers was seen as requiring collaboration between health, social care and voluntary sectors, which has important implications for nursing services, especially in the community.

The Role of the Voluntary Sector

In the United Kingdom a range of organisations in the voluntary or third sector support informal carers. Some are specifically for informal carers, such as the Carers Trust, an umbrella organisation with over 100 network partners, while others include carers but have a wider brief, such Age UK, which supports older people, or the Stroke Association, which supports people with stroke and their carers. The help offered varies and includes one-to-one counselling and peer support; form filling; respite; group education, including healthy eating, exercise and coping strategies; mindfulness training; and group support. Many organisations emphasise enjoyable activities such as day trips, exercise or arts and crafts. The specific help can be tailored to the needs of the local community. For example, in areas with large numbers of Black, Asian and minority ethnic carers, there may be support with language, form filling and for certain groups only, such as Asian Muslim women.

Often the support offered is time and fund-limited, meaning there is little capacity for evaluation of services. However, internal audits and satisfaction surveys among carers suggests they are highly valued; some carers regard them as life changing.

CHAPTER CONCLUSIONS

Informal carers play a vital role in looking after older people, including those living with frailty and other conditions. Health professionals who work with older carers and the individuals they support need to be aware of the satisfying yet often difficult nature of their role. Nurses need to bear in mind many carers may prefer to refer to themselves as partners or family members, and they may be unwilling to accept support. Furthermore, health practitioners need to consider the diversity of carers and the individuals they care for, their caring situations and their challenges but also the fluid nature of caring, which means support needs constantly change. In addition, nurses should recognise carers' expertise and the fact carers often wish to be involved in decision making and care planning. Equally, individuals who work with carers should not assume all carers have the capacity or desire to take up or continue in their caring role.

Meeting the needs of older people and their carers has to be a balance between available statutory and voluntary-sector support and recognising the unique part played by families and friends. This increasingly requires blurring of boundaries between formal and informal care and ever more knowledgeable carers. Furthermore, not all partners wish to be carers; some prefer to remain in a spousal rather than care or nursing role. Nurses who work with such families should not make assumptions about who wants to be or is equipped for caring. In addition, early on, families may be both happy and able to take on this role, but as the person they care for deteriorates and their care needs increase, they may no longer be able to undertake the care without increasing support. Countries vary hugely in the amounts and types of support available to carers and in the affordability and availability of institutional care. Importantly, any conversations about whether the carer can no longer cope and whether the needs of the cared for may be best met in institutional care clearly require skill and sensitivity on the part of nurses and other health and social care professionals. While professionals have a difficult path to tread, they can learn and benefit hugely from working with and listening to this important group: the carers themselves.

KEY LEARNING POINTS

- As our populations age, the role played by unpaid carers is increasing.
- Nurses who work with older people and their families and others who support them need to recognise the vital role played by these carers.
- Carers generally know more about the individuals they support than anyone else. Nurses and social care professionals need to acknowledge this and work in partnership with them to provide optimal care.
- Carers are diverse, and their individual characteristics and circumstances need to be recognised. Supportive interventions should be tailored to meet their requirements.
- Carers can be supported in a variety of ways, but the diversity of carers, situations and experiences means not all support works for all carers.
- The caring role can be both challenging and rewarding and is constantly changing. Nurses and allied health professionals who work with carers need to be sensitive to this and able to signpost carers to support from statutory and voluntary services.

BACKGROUND READING ON CARERS

General background reading about carers:

Twigg, J., & Atkin, K. (1994). *Carers perceived: Policy and practice in informal care.* Open University Press.

Background reading about Black, Asian and minority ethnic carers:

Greenwood, N. (2018). *Better health briefing 48: Supporting Black and minority ethnic carers.* Briefing paper for the Race Equality Foundation. https://raceequalityfoundation.org.uk/wp-content/uploads/2018/10/REF-Better-Health-484.pdf

Parveen, S., & Oyebode, J. R. (2018). *Better health briefing 46: Dementia and minority ethnic carers.* Briefing paper for the Race Equality Foundation. http://raceequalityfoundation.org.uk/wp-content/uploads/2018/07/REF-Better-Health-463.pdf

Background reading about caring during a pandemic:

International Long-Term Care Policy Network. (2021). The impact of the COVID-19 pandemic on informal carers across Europe (Eurocarers). https://ltccovid.org/2021/06/09/the-impact-of-the-covid-19-pandemic-on-informal-carers-across-europe-eurocarers

REFERENCES

AARP and National Alliance for Caregiving. (2020). Caregiving in the United States 2020. https://www.aarp.org/ppi/info-2020/caregiving-in-the-united-states.html

Aker, N., West, E., Davies, N., Moore, K. J., Sampson, E. L., Nair, P., & Kupeli, N. (2021). Challenges faced during the COVID-19 pandemic by family carers of people living with dementia towards the end of life. *BMC Health Services Research, 21,* 996. doi:10.1186/s12913-021-07019-6.

Alba, B., Lyons, A., Waling, A., Minichiello, V., Hughes, M., Barrett, C., Fredriksen-Goldsen, K., & Edmonds, S. (2020). Health, well-being, and social support in older Australian lesbian and gay caregivers. *Health and Social Care in the Community, 28,* 204–215.

Bécares, L., Kapadia, D., & Nazroo, J. (2020). Neglect of older ethnic minority people in UK research and policy. *BMJ, 368.* doi:10.1136/bmj.m212 https://doi.org/.

Becqué, Y. N., Rietjens, J. A., van Driel, A. G., van der Heide, A., & Witkamp, E. (2019). Nursing interventions to support family caregivers in end-of-life care at home: A systematic narrative review. *International Journal of Nursing Studies, 97,* 28–39.

Bom, J., Bakx, P., Schut, F., & Van Doorslaer, E. (2019). The impact of informal caregiving for older adults on the health of various types of caregivers: A systematic review. *Gerontologist, 59*(5), e629–e642. doi:10.1093/geront/gny137.

Brimblecombe, N., Ferandez, J.-L., Knapp, M., Redhill, A., & Whittenberg, R. (2018). Review of the international evidence on support for unpaid carers. *Journal of Long-Term Care, 1,* 25–40.

Carers UK. (2011). Half a million voices: Improving support for BAME carers. http://www.carersuk.org/forprofessionals/policy/policy-library/half-a-million-voicesimprovingsupport-for-bame-carers

Carers UK. (2012). In sickness and in health. https://www.carersuk.org/for-professionals/policy/policy-library/in-sickness-and-in-health#:~:text=Based%20on%20a%20survey%20of,the%20causes%20of%20deteriorating%20health

Carers UK. (2014). Facts about carers. https://www.carersuk.org/for-professionals/policy/policy-library/facts-about-carers-2014

Carers UK. (2019a). Facts about carers. https://www.carersuk.org/for-professionals/policy/policy-library/facts-about-carers-2019

Carers UK. (2019b). *State of caring. A snapshot of unpaid care in the UK.* http://www.carersuk.org/images/News__campaigns/CUK_State_of_Caring_2019_Report.pdf

Carers UK. (2020a) *Carers week (2020) research report: The rise in the number of unpaid carers during the coronavirus (COVID-19) outbreak.* https://www.carersuk.org/images/CarersWeek2020/CW_2020_Research_Report_WEB.pdf

Carers UK. (2020b). *Caring behind closed doors: Forgotten families in the coronavirus outbreak.* https://www.carersuk.org/images/News_and_campaigns/Behind_Closed_Doors_2020/Caring_behind_closed_doors_April20_pages_web_final.pdf

Cheng, S. T., & Zhang, F. (2020). A comprehensive meta-review of systematic reviews and meta-analyses on nonpharmacological interventions for informal dementia caregivers. *BMC Geriatrics, 20,* 137. doi:10.1186/s12877-020-01547-2.

Chi, N. C., Demiris, G., Lewis, F. M., Walker, A. J., & Langer, S. L. (2015). Behavioral and educational interventions to support family caregivers in end-of-life care: A systematic review. *American Journal of Hospice and Palliative Medicine, 33*(9), 894–908.

Dalton, J., Thomas, S., Harden, M., Eastwood, A., & Parker, G. (2018). Updated meta-review of evidence on support for carers. *Health Services and Delivery Research, 5*(12), 1–12.

de Oliveira, D. C., Nurse, C. V., & Aubeeluck, A. (2015). Ageing and quality of life in family carers of people with dementia being cared for at home: A literature review. *Quality in Primary Care, 23*(1), 18–30.

Department for Education. (2016). *The lives of young carers in England.* https://assets.publishing.service.gov.uk/government/uploads/system/uploads/attachment_data/file/498116/DFE-RB499_The_lives_of_young_carers_in_England_brief.pdf

Department of Health and Social Care. (2018). *Carers action plan 2018–2020: Supporting carers today.* https://assets.publishing.service.gov.uk/government/uploads/system/uploads/attachment_data/file/713781/carers-action-plan-2018-2020.pdf.

Department of Work and Pensions. (2020). Family resources survey: Financial year 2018/19. https://www.gov.uk/government/statistics/family-resources-survey-financial-year-201819

Dickinson, C., Dow, J., Gibson, G., Hayes, L., Robalino, S., & Robinson, L. (2017). Psychosocial interventions for carers of people with dementia: What components are most effective and when? A systematic review of systematic reviews. *International Psychogeriatrics, 29*(1), 31–43.

Farina, N., Page, T. E., Daley, S., Brown, A., Bowling, A., Basset, T., Livingston, G., Knapp, M., Murray, J., & Banerjee, S. (2017). Factors associated with the quality of life of family carers of people with dementia: A systematic review. *Alzheimer's and Dementia, 10.* doi:10.1016/j.jalz.2016.12.010.

Forster, A., Brown, L., Smith, J., House, A., Knapp, P., Wright, J. J., & Young, J. (2012). Information provision for stroke patients and their caregivers. *Cochrane Database Systematic Reviews, 11,* Article CD001919. doi:10.1002/14651858.CD001919.pub3.

Garand, L., Morse, J. Q., Chia, L., Barnes, J., Dadebo, V., Lopez, O. L., & Dew, M. A. (2019). Problem solving therapy reduces subjective burden levels in caregivers of family members with mild cognitive impairment or early-stage dementia: Secondary analysis of a randomized clinical trial. *International Journal of Geriatric Psychiatry, 34*(7), 957–965. doi:10.1002/gps.5095.

Gilmore-Bykovskyi, A., Johnson, R., Walljasper, L., Block, L., & Werner, N., (2018). Underreporting of gender and race/ethnicity differences in NIH-funded dementia caregiver support interventions. *American Journal of Alzheimer's Disease and Other Dementias, 33*(3), 145–152. doi: 10.1177/1533317517749465.

Greenwood, N., Habibi, R., Smith, R., & Manthorpe, J. (2015). Barriers to access and minority ethnic carers' satisfaction with social care services in the community: A systematic review of qualitative and quantitative literature. *Health and Social Care in the Community, 23*(11), 64–78. doi:10.1111/hsc.12116.

Greenwood, N., & Smith, R. (2015). Barriers and facilitators for male carers in accessing formal and informal support: A systematic review. *Maturitas, 82*(2), 162–169. doi:10.1016/j.maturitas.2015.07.013. https://www.maturitas.org/article/S0378-5122(15)30020-7/pdf.

Greenwood, N., & Smith, R. (2016). The oldest carers: A narrative review and synthesis of the experiences of carers aged over 75 years. Invited publication for *Maturitas.* 94, 161–172. doi.org/10.1016/j.maturitas.2016.10.001

Greenwood, N., Smith, R., Akhtar, F., & Richardson, A. (2017). A qualitative study of carers' experiences of dementia cafés: A place to feel supported and be yourself. *BMC Geriatrics, 17*(1), 164.

Greenwood, N., McKevitt, C., & Milne, A. (2018). Time to rebalance and reconsider: Are we pathologising informal, family carers? *Journal of the Royal Society of Medicine, 111,* 253–254.

Greenwood, N., Pound, C., Brearley, S., & Smith, R. (2019). A qualitative study of older informal carers' experiences and perceptions of their caring role. *Maturitas, 124,* 1–7. https://www.maturitas.org/article/S0378-5122(19)30087-8/pdf.

Greenwood, N., & Smith, R. (2019). Motivations for being informal carers of people living with dementia: A systematic review of qualitative literature. *BMC Geriatrics, 19,* 169. https://doi.org/10.1186/s12877-019-1185-0

Janevic, M. R., & Connell, C. M. (2001). Racial, ethnic, and cultural differences in the dementia caregiving experience: Recent findings. *The Gerontologist, 41*(3), 334–347.

Kalra, L., Evans, A., Perez, I., Melbourn, A., Patel, A., Knapp, M., & Donaldson, N. (2004). Training carers of stroke patients: randomised controlled trial. *BMJ, 328,* 1099–1101.

Katbamna, S., Ahmad, W.I.U., Bhakta, P., Baker, R. & Parker, G. (2004). Do they look after their own? Informal support for South Asian carers. *Health and Social Care in the Community, 12*(5), 398–406.

Kramer, B. J. (1997). Gain in the caregiving experience: Where are we? What next? *Gerontologist, 37,* 218–232.

Lorenz-Dant, K., & Comas-Herrera, A. (2021). The impacts of COVID-19 on unpaid carers of adults with long-term care needs and measures to address these impacts: A rapid review of evidence up to November 2020. *Journal of Long-Term Care.* http://doi.org/10.31389/jltc.76.

Manning, L., Katbamna, S., Johnson, M., Mistri, A., & Robinson, T. G. (2014). British Indian carers of stroke survivors experience higher levels of anxiety and depression than white British carers: Findings of a prospective observational study. *Diversity and Equality in Health and Care, 11*(3–4), 187–200.

Mosquera, I., Vergara, I., Larrañaga, I., Machón, M., del Rio, M., & Calderón, C. (2016). Measuring the impact of informal elderly caregiving: A systematic review of tools. *Quality of Life Research, 25,* 1059–1092.

Nezu, C. M., Palmatier, A. D., & Nezu, A. M. (2004). Problem-solving therapy for caregivers. In E. Chang, T. J. D'Zurilla,

& L. J. Sanna (Eds.), *Social problem solving: Theory, research and training* (pp. 223–238). American Psychological Association. doi:10.1037/10805-013.

Nolan, M. R., & Grant, G. (1989). Addressing the needs of informal carers: A neglected area of nursing practice. *Journal of Advanced Nursing, 14,* 950–961.

Nolan, M., Grant, G., & Keady, K. (1996). *Understanding family care: A multidimensional model of caring and coping.* Open University Press.

Parveen, S., Blakey, H., & Oyebode, J. R. (2018). Evaluation of a carers' information programme culturally adapted for South Asian families. *International Journal of Geriatric Psychiatry, 33,* e199–e204.

Peters, M., Rand, S., & Fitzpatrick, R. (2020). Enhancing primary care support for informal carers: A scoping study with professional stakeholders. *Health and Social Care in the Community, 28,* 642–650. doi:10.1111/hsc.12898.

Pickard, L., King, D., Brimblecombe, N., & Knapp, M. (2017). Public expenditure costs of carers leaving employment in England, 2015/2016. *Health and Social Care in the Community, 26*(1), e132–e142. doi:10.1111/hsc.12486.

Quinn, C., & Toms, G. (2019). Influence of positive aspects of dementia caregiving on caregivers' well-being: a systematic review. *Gerontologist, 59*(5), e584–e596.

Ris, I., Schnepp, W., & Imhof, R. M. (2019). An integrative review on family caregivers' involvement in care of home-dwelling elderly. *Health and Social Care in the Community, 27*(3), e95–e111.

Sherifali, D., Ali, M. U., Ploeg, J., Markle-Reid, M., Valaitis, R., Bartholomew, A., & McAiney, C. (2018). Impact of internet-based interventions on caregiver mental health: System-

atic review and meta-analysis. *Journal of Medical Internet Research, 20*(7), e10668. doi:10.2196/10668.

Shiu, C., Muraco, A., & Fredriksen-Goldsen, K. (2016). Invisible care: Friend and partner care among older lesbian, gay, bisexual, and transgender (LGBT) adults. *Journal of the Society for Social Work and Research, 7*(3), 527–546. doi:10.1086/687325.

Sin, J., Henderson, C., Spain, D., Cornelius, V., Chen, T., & Gillard, S. (2018). eHealth interventions for family carers of people with long term illness: A promising approach? *Clinical Psychology Review, 60,* 109–125.

Springate, B. A., & Tremont, G. (2014). Dimensions of caregiver burden in dementia: Impact of demographic, mood, and care recipient variables. *American Journal of Geriatric Psychiatry, 22*(3), 294–300.

Thomas, G., Saunders, C., Roland, M., & Paddison, C. (2015). Informal carer' health-related quality of life and patient experience in primary care: Evidence from 195,364 carers in England responding to a national survey. *BMC Family Practice, 16,* 62.

Vandepitte, S., Van Den Noortgate, N., Putman, K., Verhaeghe, S., Verdonck, C., & Annemans, L. (2016). Effectiveness of respite care in supporting informal caregivers of persons with dementia: A systematic review. *International Journal of Geriatric Psychiatry, 31,* 1277–1288. doi:10.1002/gps.4504.

Yu, D. S. F., Cheng, S.-T., & Wang, J. (2018). Unravelling positive aspects of caregiving in dementia: An integrative review of research literature. *International Journal of Nursing Studies, 79,* 1–26.

14

Abuse and Safeguarding

Bridget Penhale

CHAPTER OUTLINE

In November 1965 three members of the House of Lords and several other concerned people sent the following letter, which appeared in the correspondence column of *The Times*:

> *Sir, We, the undersigned, have been shocked by the treatment of geriatric patients in certain mental hospitals, one of the evils being the practice of stripping them of their personal possessions. We have now sufficient evidence to suggest that this is widespread.*
>
> *The attitude of the Ministry of Health to complaints has merely reinforced our anxieties. In consequence, we have decided to collect evidence of ill-treatment of geriatric patients throughout the country, to demonstrate the need for a national investigation. We hope this will lead to the securing of effective and humane control over these hospitals by the Ministry which seems at present to be lacking.*
>
> *We shall be grateful if those who have encountered malpractices in this sphere will supply us with detailed information which would of course be treated as confidential.*
>
> *(Martin, 1984)*

This was one of the earliest mentions in the United Kingdom of what is now known as elder abuse. Much has changed since then, and the detection and prevention of abuse in the care of older people has become a central concern for dignified and safe ageing. This chapter offers an overview of the key issues, debates and potential solutions.

The Nursing and Midwifery Council (NMC) professional code of conduct provides nurses with unambiguous guidance about professional standards, although there have been variations over the years.

The current version of the code, from 2018, introduces the core standards all nurses and midwives must adhere to under the following broad headings:

- Prioritise people
- Practise effectively
- Preserve safety
- Promote professionalism and trust

Each standard contains a series of statements and requirements, between five and seven each, for registrants (Nursing and Midwifery Council, 2018). The third standard, which relates to safety, has the most focus on protecting individuals who are at risk of or have experienced harm from violence, abuse and/or neglect. This version builds on the code published in 2004, which emphasised the need to protect and support the health of individual patients and clients as well as wider public health and promoted both the duty of care and the need to provide safe and competent care (Nursing and Midwifery Council, 2004).

The NMC code sets the framework for the profession's response to abuse, as it does to any other condition professionals face in the course of work. It is therefore essential nurses recognise the code's relevance to knowing, understanding and contributing to the management of abuse in an older person as well as efforts to prevent it. However, it is clear any abuse of an older person contradicts the standards contained in the code.

The hospital setting provides opportunities for the identification and prevention of abuse. Nurses who work in Accident and Emergency departments may be among the first to encounter cases of physical abuse and neglect and to distinguish non-accidental from accidental injury (Kingston & Penhale, 1995). Nurses who contribute to decisions about discharge of patients may understand, and are well placed to explore, the nature of the home circumstances to which an older person is returning—circumstances that may be critical concerning possible abuse and the potential need to intervene.

In the community nurses are also on the front line of identifying abuse (Kitchen et al., 2002; Richardson et al., 2002). It is important, therefore, that in whatever position they hold, nurses are aware of the existence of abuse and its possible effects and consequences. Community nurses may visit older peoples' homes on a regular basis. Their knowledge of the older person, their social network, the relationships in the family, the way people come and go, and the older person's state of mind, including some amount of their history, makes them among the foremost experts on their family circumstances. As a regular visitor, the observant and listening nurse may come to know things other professionals involved on a less regular basis never get to know (Phair & Goodman, 2003).

Nurses are often managers or even owners of residential or nursing homes as well as members of staff in such locations. Community nurses may visit nursing and care homes on a regular basis to attend to treatment needs of some residents. Nurses may thus be expert on the communal household and what is happening within it. They may know where quality of care is doubtful, about staff's difficulties and stresses, the personalities and disabilities of residents and the demands that can be made, and the way that staff respond to these demands. In the context of communal settings, nurses are often instrumental in promoting good practice and high standards of care. Historically, care homes have found it difficult to get adequate input and support from primary care such as GPs, other community health professionals and pharmacists (Goodman et al., 2017). Finally, nurses are active in the registration and inspection of communal settings, are involved in the training and supervision of students and junior nurses, and undertake key management tasks such as appointments and the letting of contracts for nursing-home placements.

In all these contexts, knowledge and awareness of issues related to abuse and neglect are important.

This chapter begins by examining definitions of abuse, then looks at prevalence and research in different settings where older people live. Wherever possible, we draw on research that specifically involves nurses. The chapter discusses issues around intervention largely in the context of the community, reflecting the lack of research into abuse in communal settings. However, for nurses who work in acute wards, the reality is their patients are discharged to community settings, and they can potentially play a crucial role in being alert to the safety of those settings. We explore intervention with particular reference to assessment of older people, legal and professional issues, and multidisciplinary working. The chapter also covers financial abuse, confidentiality, and education and training. The issues that arise in communal settings are considered in the sections that voice concerns about abuse and the regulation of residential and nursing homes. The chapter concludes with a brief consideration of policy development. Although written from the perspective of developments in the United Kingdom, these developments have been substantially influenced by research from abroad, notably the United States but including interesting literature from Canada, Australia and continental Europe. Much can be learnt, along with proper recognition of differences in service provision, culture and legal systems between countries.

Although there have been several overview articles about elder abuse in the nursing literature (e.g., Baker & Heitkemper, 2005; Phelan, 2018), relatively little research on elder abuse with nurses has been undertaken. However, several small studies (e.g., Kitchen et al., 2002) and some helpful research has been done in Sweden. The latter examined how district nurses defined abuse (Saveman et al., 1993a; 1995), the nature of the cases they encountered (Saveman et al., 1993b; 1996) and the problems they faced in addressing abusive situations (Saveman et al., 1992). Although these studies were undertaken several decades ago, they are still of interest and we can learn from them.

DEFINITIONS

The word *abuse* has no legal meaning, and older people may not naturally use it. Some kinds of behaviour defined as abuse are criminal acts, such as assault and theft; others, such as verbal abuse or the restraint of someone who is aggressive or displays behaviour challenging to manage, may seem much more contingent on particular circumstances. The tensions that arise from workload pressures in institutional settings may include a conflict between the need to get a care task done and respect for the autonomy of the patient, who may not, for example, wish to have a bath. What is abuse in these circumstances?

Psychological abuse, in the form of infantilisation, demeaning and humiliating attitudes, and ignoring patient/resident requests, especially if they are seen as troublesome, is often found in care settings (e.g., Francis, 2013). Further, when is restraint abuse, given the patient or resident may be violent, the patient or someone else may need protection and the reality of care in communal settings may be a shortage of staff? If someone is oversedated or given inappropriate medication, is this abuse? See Case Study 14.1.

Under the general umbrella of elder abuse, therefore, a great many different situations may be subsumed. There is some room for debate about where to draw the line in distinguishing abuse from poor-quality care, unkindness, mistaken strategies for coping, poor relationships or even keeping the change from an older person's shopping.

In the *No Secrets* guidance document (Department of Health, 2000), abuse is defined as 'the violation of an individual's

CASE STUDY 14.1

Ethel was widowed 10 years earlier, lived alone and was regularly visited by her three children. She managed to get out and do some shopping every day but was increasingly feeling tired and weak and sometimes complained of tightness in the chest. The GP was asked to visit, found some evidence of early heart failure and prescribed digitalis and a diuretic. Relatives who visited a few months later thought her condition had deteriorated, and the GP was asked to visit again. She was somewhat tremulous, and he prescribed medication for early parkinsonism. Soon after Ethel became rather more agitated, had a few falls in the house and was put on a daytime tranquilliser. Her children were still concerned, and she went to stay with her oldest daughter in a small house with much loved but boisterous grandchildren. The move unsettled her, and she became depressed. The local GP was asked to call. He prescribed antidepressants as well as her other medication, and when she did not improve, the dose was increased. She then developed some nocturnal restlessness, which was very hard for the daughter, who was finding it hard to cope with her mother's care needs as well as the children and her own work. Ethel was given sedatives at night. A visit from the district nurse revealed a fraught and anxious daughter at the end of her tether who admitted to outbursts of frustration and occasional roughness when she tried to urge Ethel to eat and drink and dealt with occasional falls and incontinence. The daughter felt enormous guilt when she lost her temper but said it was becoming more difficult to control her reactions at such times.

How should the district nurse respond?

human or civil rights by any other person or persons' (p. 9). This is a broad definition not now in general use. The Care Act of 2014, referred to later, does not contain a definition of abuse in either the legal statute or the guidance that accompanied the law. The definition used by the World Health Organization (WHO) is probably the closest to a standard definition, although it is not universally or consistently used: 'Elder abuse is a single, or repeated act, or lack of appropriate action, occurring within any relationship where there is an expectation of trust, which causes harm or distress to an older person' (World Health Organisation, 2022).

Despite the lack of universal or standard definitions, it is easier to be clear about the meaning of abuse if the different types are spelt out. There is now widespread agreement about five types of abuse (Bonnie & Wallace, 2003):

- Physical abuse
- Psychological abuse
- Financial abuse
- Sexual abuse
- Neglect

Sometimes sexual abuse is subsumed under physical abuse, although it is increasingly recognised as a form of abuse in its own right and usually appears thus in discussion and documentation about abuse. The Care Act of 2014, which provides the legal position in England pertaining to adult safeguarding, added several other types, including domestic violence, organisational or institutional abuse, modern slavery, discriminatory abuse and self-neglect.

Abuse involves both behaviour by someone and the effect it has on another person. That is, it generally occurs in the context of a relationship. Self-neglect was previously regarded as a distinct phenomenon in the United Kingdom; in the United States it is included in consideration of elder abuse and adult protective services. However, with the introduction of the Care Act of 2014 in England, implemented in 2015, self-neglect is included within the remit of adult safeguarding. This is the generic term now used to cover the field of what was previously known as adult protection, or protection of vulnerable adults. It covers adults who might be known to health and care organisations due to their care and support needs who are considered to be at risk of harm from abuse.

It is helpful to consider some dimensions of abuse, particularly the impact and severity on individuals and the extent of their distress and harm. It may also be useful to consider how frequently abuse occurs and for how long. Some answers to these questions may provide clues to the nature of the abusive situation and the appropriateness of any intervention. For the practitioner, however, definitions provided for the purposes of academic research have limited value. Real life is far more complicated, and the practitioner faces complex situations, particularly when they suspect abuse. As seen elsewhere, the search for standard definitions applicable to all settings and situations is unlikely to be easily achieved. It is probably better to recognise a number of different definitions exist and acknowledge the differences that exist between them in an open manner that means appropriate actions can be taken (Penhale, 1993). It is also important to recall the requirements and standards of the NMC code.

Further, what this means in practice is practitioners must know about safeguarding policy, local practice guidelines that relate to abuse, and to whom and at what point they should report concerns or suspicions. Health and social care providers are accountable to the Care Quality Commission (CQC) for complying with safeguarding responsibilities and providing mandatory training for staff.

NURSES' EXPERIENCES OF WORKING WITH ABUSE

Abuse can be one of the most difficult problems encountered by nurses, including the fact labels such as abuse or mistreatment that may be applied to observed interactions or communications between individuals can be inexact and unreliable. It may also lead to misunderstandings, as they can be open to different interpretations.

In the Swedish research referred to earlier, 21 district nurses, all with experience of a case of abuse, were asked in interviews to describe one from their own experience. They were asked about how they defined abuse and how they recognised it when it was occurring (Saveman et al., 1993a). The authors suggested the four salient factors in defining abuse were as follows:

- The actual act of abuse (i.e., the behaviour)
- The relationship between the two parties
- The impact of the abuse on the abused person
- The intention of the abuser

Acts of abuse appeared to range on a continuum in terms of behaviours. In terms of relevant relationships, abusers were not just carers but could be relatives living together without family responsibilities or professional caregivers, or the abuse could result from the way in which services were run. This is an important point, as it is quite common in the literature to see the word *carer* used as though only carers can be abusers. In this study the nurses were asked to think themselves into the situation of the abused person so they could consider the likely impact of abuse and provide examples of the effects of lack of respect and humiliation as forms of psychological abuse.

Finally, the nurses referred to the intentions or motivations of the abuser. This was sometimes seen as a deliberate act to inflict harm, but sometimes it consisted of actions the abuser knew harmed the older person but did not want to believe was the case. Although intention is clearly relevant to understanding the abusive situation and the nature of any intervention, generally it is not considered part of a definition of abuse, as essentially the effect and impact on the person who is abused is what is considered important.

The authors of the Swedish report noted, 'The district nurses had no distinct, easily formulated definition of abuse…instead they reasoned around it using intuition, concrete descriptions, sometimes with examples and abstract terms to explain the abuse' (Saveman et al., 1993a, p. 1397).

The nurses' replies reflect the rather blurred nature of the boundaries of abuse. This is where the existence of a definition helps in delineating the scope of the field. The Swedish authors suggested, however, the common theme through all the examples cited was of 'overriding the boundaries of a person's integrity/autonomy' (Saveman et al., 1993a, p. 1397). This chimes with findings from research by the WHO and the International Network for Prevention of Elder Abuse (INPEA) across eight countries, not including the United Kingdom, in which older people indicated lack of respect and dignity and having decisions taken from them were very much seen as elements of elder abuse (WHO & INPEA, 2002). See Case Study 14.1, where medical decisions and interventions made in best interests of the patient over time can contribute to creating difficult situations for families to manage and result in challenging consequences.

PREVALENCE

In view of the increasing amount of research from around the world on the prevalence of abuse in the past two decades, the WHO undertook a systematic review and meta-analysis to determine a global prevalence rate (Yon et al., 2017). The pooled prevalence rate from the 52 studies included in the review was 15.7%. This included all types of abuse, therefore establishing overall prevalence. When translated to the global population, the WHO estimated one in six older people across the world is affected by elder abuse in community settings.

There has been limited research on the prevalence of abuse in institutions and scarcely any in hospital settings. This may seem surprising and reflect some element of denial or underreporting, despite a greater focus on safeguarding and external scrutiny. There have been, however, a few studies of restraint use in care and nursing home settings and professional perceptions as well as reports about abuse and neglect. Recent research in care homes has been undertaken in Norway (Harris & Benson, 2008; Malmedal et al., 2009a; 2009b; 2020).

As a follow-up to the review of prevalence studies in community settings, the WHO undertook another systematic review and meta-analysis of relevant prevalence studies of abuse in communal settings to determine a global prevalence rate (Yon et al., 2019). Only nine studies met the inclusion criteria. From these studies, based on reports by staff members, overall abuse estimates indicated almost two-thirds of staff (64.2%) admitted abuse of an older resident in the past year. However, there were insufficient studies to determine a pooled prevalence rate based on self-reports by residents due to the lack of robust studies in this area. From the limited rigorous research, individual rates for abuse subtypes were high: over one-third (33.4%) of self-reports indicated psychological abuse, followed by physical abuse (14.1%), financial abuse (13.8%) and neglect (11.6%). Self-reports of sexual abuse were much lower at 1.9%. The WHO's conclusion was the prevalence rate of abuse in institutional settings was high, and much more needs to be done in monitoring and surveillance of abuse to improve prevention and intervention in institutional forms of elder abuse (Yon et al., 2019).

Understanding Abuse in the Community

An early prevalence study undertaken in Boston (Pillemer & Finkelhor, 1988) produced some interesting findings. Abuse was not related to age or to ethnic, religious, educational or economic background. Risk of physical and verbal abuse was higher for coresident older people, an obvious but important point when it comes to awareness of risk of abuse by others. Rates of physical and verbal abuse toward men were higher than toward women. This partly reflected the fact there are fewer older men overall in populations; in absolute terms, the numbers of abused were similar at 52% men and 48% women. However, the difference in relative risk appeared to result from the fact older men are more likely to live with someone than are older women. In this study, the difference was 83% men vs 58% women. This was qualified by a further finding from follow-up data that women appeared to be more seriously abused. Another striking finding was related to health. There were no statistically significant associations between health status and physical and verbal abuse, although highly significant ones ($P = 0.0001$) for neglect. Clearly this is just as likely to be an effect of the neglect as it is to be its cause. Finally, contrary to the stereotype of elder abuse that prevailed during the 1980s—as behaviour perpetrated by an adult child who was the main carer of the older person—the research showed a somewhat higher prevalence of marital abuse in old age, thereby reflecting the fact older people, if they are living with anyone, are more likely to live with their spouse. A similar finding about abuse by a spouse or partner was found in a United Kingdom prevalence study in 2005 (O'Keeffe et al., 2007).

Several studies included some suggestion abuse is gendered but not always in the direction you might expect; for example Podnieks's (1990) data showed abuse was gendered but again in an unexpected way. In the Podnieks study, more men were found to be victims of physical violence, although not of other forms of abuse, while substantially more women were victims of neglect. Considerable differences occurred between the different types of abuse; the risk of financial abuse increased markedly for individuals living on their own, just as the risk of physical and verbal abuse declined. In terms of health, it is notable the health of non-victims was in general better than that of victims, but, as found in the Boston study, there were differences between the types of abuse. More than half of victims of verbal aggression, and just under half those who reported physical violence, reported their health was good to excellent. In contrast to non-victims, victims also reported greater unhappiness and a greater sense of hopelessness, and nearly one-third of victims of all types of abuse had wished their life might end (Podnieks, 1990).

However, these large prevalence studies mainly report about one side in the abusive relationship —the victim's. It is necessary to turn to the smaller and more intensive pieces of research to learn about the wider household and the factors that seem to discriminate abusive from non-abusive situations. They display considerable consistency in relation to physical and verbal abuse, the types of abuse that have been the subject of most research (McCreadie, 1996). Apart from the importance of coresidence, abusive situations appear, on accumulated knowledge, to be discriminated from non-abusive situations in two ways: first, the characteristics of the abuser and most notably any problems they have in their own right, and second, the quality of the long-term relationship between the two parties. Abuse is therefore not a product of the illnesses and disabilities that occur in later life as much as a manifestation of longer-term problems in personalities and relationships that may be exacerbated by behaviour that arises from illness or disability. The picture that prevailed for some time of the implicitly well-meaning and younger carer who is stressed by the demands of caring and hits out at the dependent and implicitly demanding older person is a drastically simplified and to a large extent inaccurate picture of the complexities of abusive situations. See Case Study 14.2.

An early study by Homer and Gilleard (1990) illustrates this, as does the Swedish research (Saveman et al., 1996). Homer and Gilleard examined the factors that distinguished carers who admitted abuse (i.e., physical or verbal abuse or neglect) from those who did not. They found all carers who admitted abuse were coresident with their relative. The factors most significantly associated with abuse were alcohol consumption by the carer and abuse by the patient toward the caregiver. The circumstances that triggered physical violence in the seven carers who admitted to

CASE STUDY 14.2

William was in his 90s, living at home and supported by a live-in carer. He had four adult children, who were very caring but lived some way away. They took turns looking after William at the weekends when the carer went away for a break. William was frail and had some mental confusion. One of the daughters had a very close relationship with her father and loved him dearly but also was conflicted at seeing her 'best friend' become increasingly dependent and no longer there to support her. She struggled with the role reversal of being the one he looked after to having to look after him. She was a 'high flyer' in the city and at the weekend was exhausted from work and the demands of her own family. Sometimes if William was incontinent or refused to get up or take his medication, she got angry. After her weekends caring for him, the other siblings noticed their father often had bruises and abrasions on his legs, which they were told came about from being knocked when he was lifted off the commode.

What should the carer and the family do?

it were physical abuse or threats of violence by the patient in four cases, incontinence in one, and both in one. One carer 'could not identify the trigger' (Homer & Gilleard, 1990, p. 1361). In this study it appeared disruptive behaviour by the patient was a key factor rather than presence or absence of cognitive impairment, although cognitive impairment, particularly dementia, remains an important recognised risk factor.

Several studies looked specifically at the relationship between dementia and abuse. What emerged strongly from this research was the carer, who may also be older and in poor health, in some circumstances is most at risk. An example is seen in an early study by Compton and his fellow psychiatrists in Northern Ireland (Compton et al., 1997), in which 38 carers were asked about abuse toward a patient with dementia. One-third admitted to verbal abuse, and 10% to physical abuse. Significant factors that predicted the abuse were coresidence, poor carer health status, poor premorbid relations, abuse or problem behaviour by the patient, and carer dissatisfaction with the help received.

Understanding Abuse in Communal Settings

Communal settings comprise care homes, including homes that provide nursing and are registered to provide such care, hospitals and day cares. In these settings, there is an organisational context to the delivery of care, so in relation to mistreatment, something more may be at issue than the behaviour or lack of care of a particular individual toward

a resident or patient (Ash, 2014). There have been many reviews and inquiries into major deficiencies in institutional care over decades; one common feature is abuse can flourish within a culture that allows it to be acceptable (e.g., Clough, 1999; Flynn, 2015; Francis, 2013). Regrettably, the situation appears to have changed little in recent years. The abuse and neglect that occurs in health and care settings may be referred to as institutional abuse or as mistreatment to denote abuse and/or neglect. Institutional abuse can refer to policies and practices that happen at the organisational/institutional level. In addition, it may occur due to the actions, or lack of actions, of staff and volunteers in the setting but may also be perpetrated toward individual residents/patients by relatives, friends or other visitors (Sethi et al., 2011). However, even in institutional settings. much of the abuse or neglect that happens occurs behind closed doors so is not either visible or necessarily open to external scrutiny.

In the absence of research in institutional settings of prevalence, a great deal of the information about aspects such as risk factors has been developed from analysis of policy and practice documents that relate to incidents. Thus, relevant factors at the institutional level seem to be related to the broader level of the institution, such as poor management and lack of staff supervision as well as the care or lack of care provided to residents or the existence of a regime or inflexible routines designed for organisational purposes rather than care. There also seems to be a tolerance of aggression in the environment.

Characteristics concerned with staff involved in mistreatment in institutional settings include a lack of knowledge, training and qualifications in health or care; negative attitudes toward older people and ageing; stress in personal circumstances; and staff burnout. Some of these factors might be resolved by provision of staff training and targeted resources designed to reduce staff burnout. For example, environments with high levels of stress, including due to poor design features, are likely to increase risk of staff burnout; tackling and resolving these aspects is likely to be beneficial to staff and resident well-being.

Intervention in the Community

Elder abuse undoubtedly presents nurses with some of their most difficult professional dilemmas (Miller, 2005). Yet, as suggested earlier, due to their position in the community and their role within it, community nurses are in an ideal position to detect abuse. Nurses are generally very well placed to observe and be aware of the potential for abuse to occur in the community setting. With major growth in independently supplied home care since the implementation of community care policies, nurses are in a position of visiting older people in situations where there

BOX 14.1 Key Issues for Nurses to Consider When Assessing Risk of Abuse:

- Demands from one party, which the other is unwilling or unable to meet, that may lead to abuse of one person, the other, or both.
- Demands and perceived burden often implicit in a caring situation that could lead to abuse of the patient, carer, or both.
- When a filial, parental or other personal relationship is distorted by unhealthy use of power exercised over the older person, which results in abusive behaviour.
- A previous history of violence in the relationship, graphically described by Homer and Gilleard (1990, p. 1361) as the 'elderly graduates of domestic violence'.

is no involvement from other statutory agencies. They are in an ideal position to monitor situations carefully and to report abusive situations to adult social care services as the lead agency in coordinating local responses to abuse (Department of Health, 2014).

The over-75 health assessment is a component of the GP contract and an annual assessment of the factors that affect health in older people (see also Box 14.1). It offers an important opportunity to members of the primary care team to assess possible risks of abuse (Amiel & Heath, 2003; Phair & Goodman, 2003). In the United States, Shugarman and colleagues (2003) evaluated the incorporation of routine screening for potential abuse within more standardised health assessments of older people and found it to be successful. A helpful and practical guide to the United Kingdom health assessment process recognised the assessment serves as an opportunity for more than a health check and should be used to prevent difficulties and examine carer needs. This includes asking who the older person sees in the course of a week and whether the person can do what they wish socially and recreationally. If they are not able to, what are the difficulties? It is also helpful to know if the person can manage their own affairs at home, including finances and bill payments. Family relationships are a central aspect of social functioning, and it is important to be sensitive to varying family structures and the roles assumed within them. The needs of carers may be different from those of the older person. Carers should ideally be seen alone so they can raise any problematic issues. It is also important to recognise family dysfunction, which may precede inadequate care or abuse.

Under the terms of the Carers (Recognition and Services) Act of 1995, if an individual is in receipt of community care services or having an assessment or reassessment of need, the carer is eligible in their own right to an assessment of needs for assistance. This right was reaffirmed in the Care Act of 2014 but with an adjustment, so where a carer appears to have their own care and support needs irrespective of the person they care for, they have a right to an assessment and should be entitled to support if relevant eligibility criteria are met.

A policy briefing by Carers UK that included analysis and comparison of national census data from 2001 and 2011 showed although in overall terms by the 2011 census more women than men were carers (58% vs 42%) and more women provided 50 or more hours of care each week (60%), more men over 85 provided care (59% vs 41%), the majority of whom were caring for their spouses/partners (Carers UK, 2019). This trend is expected to continue for the foreseeable future. Further information on carers is discussed in Chapter 13.

It should be added here that, as part of good practice, it is important to see the older person alone. In any situation that may involve abuse, separate interviews for the older person and others involved in the situation are not just good practice but likely to be essential. If there is any reluctance on the part of carers, it should be noted and, if possible, further explored. Bennett (2000) maintained if this situation arose in practice, it was always likely to provide helpful clues that would be useful in the assessment. Nurses need to be open and alert to body language or a dropped comment in a conversation. As community nurses know, it is often the last-minute exchange with a carer on the doorstep that can be a signal all is not well.

PROFESSIONAL AND LEGAL ISSUES

A difficult issue for nurses and other health professionals is the professional and legal framework that exists to protect individuals who may be at risk or who have experienced abuse. In the majority of cases narrated by the district nurses in Sweden, the abused party did not want to change the situation. This could be attributed to a variety of reasons, including the powerful one of protection for the perpetrator or not wishing them to be punished. There are several reasons why an older person might not wish to report or acknowledge an abusive situation (e.g., Penhale, 1993).

One of the most obvious and important factors about abuse of an older person is it occurs in the context of a person's history. The follow-up study to the Canadian prevalence research considered how older people coped with their situation and established the individual's whole life experience was relevant to their ability to cope (Podnieks, 1992).

The legal issues around abuse are considerable. Although in most of the United Kingdom, there is no standalone law that relates to abuse and protection of older people or vulnerable adults, particularly in England, sections from a large number of laws in different fields, including domestic violence, community care and mental health legislation, might apply to situations of elder abuse. A number of specialised books offer guidance concerning this aspect. The Mental Capacity Act 2005 revised the law in relation to people who are not competent to make their own decisions in England and Wales. However, apart from one section (44) that concerns 'mistreatment or wilful neglect of the person who lacks capacity' (Mental Capacity Act, 2005), this law does not cover issues of abuse and protection further.

In Scotland the Adults with Incapacity Act was passed in 2000, which contains helpful material related to older people as well as clear guidance to be followed concerning incapacity. It was followed by the Adult Support and Protection (Scotland) Act 2007, implemented in 2008, which provides a framework for responding to allegations of abuse and neglect of adults at risk of harm and their protection, but it applies only to Scotland.

In Wales, the Social Services and Well-being Act of 2014 is similar to the Care Act in England in that it consolidates legislation in relation to social care and includes specific sections that relate to adult safeguarding. Northern Ireland is the only jurisdiction in the United Kingdom that does not have legislation that includes adult safeguarding as an area of concern. Codes of practice related to both capacity legislation and the Adult Support and Protection (Scotland) Act were produced to support professional staff in Scotland. In addition, the Care Act of 2014 contains several sections related to adult safeguarding. The sections on safeguarding provide what is known as framework legislation, which details the structure and processes of safeguarding but does not include a provision for enforced entry to a premises to ascertain if someone is at risk or removal of a person from their home who is experiencing harm from mistreatment and/or neglect. The Scottish legislation includes this provision. In Wales a comparable code of practice to help professional staff relates to the sections of the 2014 act about safeguarding (Welsh Government, 2019).

In practice, nurses should always ensure they are up to date on the latest safeguarding policy and practice and consult with their manager about the best course of action in a situation. They also need to consider what the local procedures and guidance for their agency require them to do. It is likely adult social care services mandated locally to be the lead agency for coordinating responses to abuse (Department of Health, 2000; 2014) need to be involved. Involvement may be needed from the police and other agencies such as housing or the registration and inspection units of the CQC if the situation concerns a residential or nursing home. Therefore, nurses should be aware of and prepared for the possibility of involvement and liaison with different organisations when dealing with abusive situations and actively seek out opportunities for multi-agency working.

Importantly, the conclusions drawn from the Swedish research (Saveman et al., 1996) indicate district nurses need support to deal with situations where they think or know abuse is happening. In general, respondents were prone to side with the weaker party in the relationship rather than being able to assess with some objectivity the moral and ethical issues they needed to address. The result was their intervention risked making the situation worse. Saveman et al. (1996) argued it is a strength to view the abusive family system from a wider perspective and to analyse the situation to understand its complexity and find suitable interventions. Nurses must be able to step outside the system and reflect on it as a whole to find the most appropriate solutions. Good supervision and management support help with this.

The conflict between respecting the expressed wishes of patients and protecting them from harm is one of the most difficult issues encountered. Health-care practitioners need to remember older people have the right to reject offers of help and can say no to interventions. This right may be ignored only in certain circumstances, for example if the person is mentally incapable of making a decision, within the remit of the Mental Capacity Act and where the situation is assessed as very serious.

However, it is necessary to recognise at times an older person may be intimidated or coerced into a position of rejecting help. Although it can be difficult to assess this type of situation, the involvement of other professionals in the assessment can be helpful. Even in these situations, it is not likely the individual can be forced to accept help, but a system of ongoing monitoring or even periodic review can be agreed on with the person or possible avenues can be established for them to make contact if they decide they want assistance or action.

Even in the most intractable circumstances, when parties state they do not want help, nurses should play their part to ensure trust, openness and transparency in communication. In sensitive situations there may be feelings of guilt and inadequacy mixed up with wanting to do the best thing. It is important to remember situations can and do change over time. A person who is reluctant to accept help at one point in time may accept it later. Older people therefore need to know it is possible to change their mind, and if they initially refuse, the possibility of help remains open to them should they need it in future. They need information about how to access help in future and who to contact. This information should be provided in a sensitive way; a leaflet that announces services for abused people may not be appropriate for a vulnerable person who lives in a difficult and unsafe situation.

Interprofessional and Inter-Agency Approaches to Managing Abuse

No single professional is likely to have a complete or comprehensive picture of an older person's household. Moreover, a wide range of resources and expertise is available, and services for support and assistance are found in a variety of agencies. The number and types of agencies and services vary from area to area. Nurses need to work closely with colleagues in other services in both the statutory and the voluntary sectors. The point of discharge from hospital of older people offers a clear, if demanding, opportunity to collaborate and develop open communication with other professionals. The appropriateness of providing a particular service depends on the type of abuse, the reasons for the abuse, and the views and decision-making capacity of the parties involved. There is a danger victims of abuse may be provided with the same services as other frail older people without proper regard for the wider household perspective, which the research suggests is so important. In many cases it is necessary to think in terms of services to both abuser and abused.

There is comparatively little robust evidence for successful interventions in elder abuse (Sethi et al., 2011). The Violence Prevention Unit of the WHO developed gold standards for evaluating evidence from intervention studies on violence. At the time of the *Global Status Report on Violence Prevention* (Mikton et al., 2014), none of the interventions that had been developed for elder abuse met the criteria for these standards; unfortunately, this is still the case. Some of the promising interventions in terms of evidence concern intergenerational programmes to improve attitudes toward and perceptions of older people and ageing, and provision of support to carers (Mikton et al., 2014; Sethi et al., 2011), but they are somewhat tangential to direct programmes of intervention with older people with regards to elder abuse.

Examples of the types of interventions developed range from victim support services to mediation (McCann-Beranger, 2014) and volunteer support via telephone helplines run by charities (e.g., Hourglass, Age UK, Independent Age). However, not all initiatives have been subject to robust evaluation. Where physical or psychological abuse occurs in a relationship that involves the care of a dependent person, education or anger management may be an appropriate form of intervention (Reay & Browne, 2002). Research indicates psychological stress in carers of people with dementia can be reduced by an intensive training programme (Brodaty & Gresham, 1989; Mental Health Foundation, 1995). Although short stay or respite care can be beneficial for carers, its impact on the individual who has the respite stay may be noteworthy (Homer & Gilleard, 1994), and the overall effect in reducing physical and psychological abuse is not fully known.

For nurses to respond appropriately to abuse, they need three kinds of support: from education and training, from the setting where they work and from their professional body.

Financial Abuse

Lasting powers of attorney are available in relation to both property and financial affairs (also known as financial decisions) and health and welfare (also known as health and care decisions); however, these are legal instruments that must be registered with the Office of the Public Guardian prior to use by designated and approved attorneys.

In communal care settings there is an important range of issues around the handling of older people's finances, particularly for residents who have cognitive impairment or dementia. They include the extent to which proprietors of homes take responsibility for the older person's financial affairs and financial abuse of some older people by their relatives, which may be a continuation of abuse while the person was living at home or occurring for the first time in the care setting. See Case Study 14.3.

Confidentiality

A major issue to be addressed in any guidance for nurses is confidentiality. It is a basic precept of the professional code of conduct for nurses they respect any information given to them in confidence by a patient. Dimond (1995) listed the exceptions to the code as consent of the patient, interests of the patient, court orders, statutory duty to disclose, the public interest and where the police can require information. Abuse perpetrated by family members can at first sight present the nurse and other professionals with difficult

---

CASE STUDY 14.3

Mary was in hospital following a stroke that had left her with limited mobility and unable to return home. While she waited for a suitable care placement, she was visited regularly by her daughter Jean. Each week the ward sister noticed Jean brought the pension book in for her mother to sign. However, Mary never seemed to have any money for purchases from the ward trolley, and if the ward had not supplied her with fruit squash, tissues and soaps, she would not have access to any of those items. Janice, the ward sister, mentioned it to Jean, who flushed a little and said she did not really have anything to do with her mother's money, and by the time she had paid for the bus fare to the hospital, she did not have any funds for such purchases. Jean said in any case, the hospital provided such items, did it not?

What should the ward sister do?

issues of confidentiality. Since it is invariably bound up with relationships and dispositions in a whole household, often vital information may be held by another professional, or the nurse may hold a piece of this essential information that is lacking elsewhere, the possession of which would make it easier to assess the best course of action in the interests of the patient and the wider household. However, the data protection act (Data Protection Act, 2018) does not prevent or limit the sharing of information for the purposes of safeguarding and protecting vulnerable adults. Thus, sharing information with individuals who may need to know about it can be an important consideration, and discussion with managers and/or supervisors can help to determine whether and when this should happen.

The duty to share information can be as important as the duty to confidentiality. In 2013 the Health and Social Care Information Centre, now NHS Digital, issued guidance for staff on confidentiality (Health and Social Care Information Centre, 2013). The guide established for health and care staff what they should do and why in order to safely share information while maintaining confidentiality. The guide covers the five rules of confidentiality, including point two in the guide: that members of a care team should share confidential information when it is needed for care of a person to be safe and effective. This is the so-called need-to-know basis.

Additionally, guidance developed alongside the Care Act of 2014 provides useful direction on information sharing between agencies, which can be of particular importance and use in situations of mistreatment. Moreover, at local area level there are likely information-sharing protocols in existence between different agencies and organisations, including the health care sector, that provide detail about when information should be shared and with whom.

Education and Training

It is now recognised it is essential for nurses, whether in communal or community settings, to have some training around issues of elder abuse. Basic awareness training about the different forms of abuse and neglect is fundamental for all health and social care practitioners, together with more advanced courses for those who specialise in work with older people who may be vulnerable to abuse. An introductory level of knowledge and awareness for all practitioners increases the likelihood abuse, when and wherever it occurs, is detected and reported within local guidelines and procedures so appropriate action can be taken. Nurses are central within this and a key professional group to include in such training. Educational curricula at pre- and post-registration levels also need to include relevant modules that concern abuse and neglect. NHS trusts and other health care providers provide mandatory introductory-level training as part of induction and refresher programmes for staff.

However, it is important nurses should join other professionals in training initiatives as part of a holistic interprofessional approach for health and social care provision. The Department of Health has consistently advocated for education and training about abuse to be provided on a multi-agency, multidisciplinary basis (Department of Health, 2014).

Research on the effect of education on knowledge and management of elder abuse suggests although educational courses for professionals assist in improving the identification and reporting of abusive situations, courses need to be planned and targeted to take into account baseline knowledge about abuse, which appears to affect receptiveness to training courses and the amount of learning that takes place (Pike et al., 2011; Richardson et al., 2002).

Voicing Concerns About Abuse

Legislation exists about whistle-blowing and the duty of candour. The Employment Rights Act of 1996, as amended by the Public Interest Disclosure Act of 1998, provides the right for an employee to take a case to an employment tribunal if they are victimised at work or lose their job due to whistle-blowing. So some protection is provided for individuals who whistle-blow about practices in their workplace or organisation, which include abusive or unsafe practices. The legislation covers employees, including of the NHS, and trainees such as student nurses. Concerns can be raised about an incident that happened in the past, one that is happening now or one that is believed will happen in future. In 2015, following a review undertaken by Sir Robert Francis, the *Freedom to Speak Up* report was published, enabling staff to speak out about concerns within the NHS (Francis, 2015). As a result of the review, a confidential telephone line was established for NHS staff to use to report concerns, including whistle-blowing; it was extended to cover social care staff as well.

Support for individuals in raising concerns and using the law is also available from the legal charity Protect, which provides assistance to individuals who wish to raise concerns but do not know how best to do so and require some support. The organisation also provides information about the act and other form of assistance via its website. For details, see the useful resources listed at the end of this chapter.

The duty of candour was introduced as a regulation (Regulation 20) of the Health and Social Care Act (Regulated Activities) Regulations of 2008. It relates to a situation when a 'notifiable safety incident', as defined in the act, has occurred (Health and Social Care Act, 2008). The duty concerns promoting cultures of openness and transparency in relation to safe care and treatment of individuals who are subject to regulated activity, as is the case within communal settings. The registered person must notify relevant individuals an incident has happened and provide support to the person in relation to the incident. The account must be truthful and include all facts about the incident known at that point. It should include information about whether further enquiries will be undertaken and an apology, and the information should be recorded in a written form and kept securely by the registered person. Situations of abuse and neglect in communal settings often fall within the remit of the duty of candour, so it is important that nursing and other staff know about the provisions of the regulations and how and when they are applied.

Placing concern about the well-being of patients first can be extremely difficult for nurses as for other staff. Voluntary-sector organisations issued early advice to people concerned about the possible abuse of an older person and who wanted to do something about it (Action on Elder Abuse, 1994[1]; Counsel and Care, 1994[2]). These may be members of the public or professionals in contact with older people in their own homes, or a member of staff in a hospital, nursing home or other communal setting who might be worried about a fellow staff member's or relative's behaviour toward a resident. The dedicated telephone line and the fact most professionals now have training on abuse and safeguarding held on a regular basis, much of which is mandatory, may mean staff use of helplines run by charities has diminished, but contact with independent helpline might be useful on occasion and is clearly of use to relatives and the general public.

Regulation

The wider context in which care is provided is also of crucial importance to the prevention of abuse. As far as nursing homes are concerned, authorities involved in registration and inspection are at the forefront of this wider context. In England this is the CQC; there are comparable bodies in other nations of the United Kingdom. It is their responsibility to make sure homes reach certain standards before they are opened, and they are maintained. This includes checks to establish owners and managers of homes are fit to run care establishments. Some nurses work for the CQC (formerly the Commission for Social Care Inspection and prior to that the National Commission for Care Standards). The role of nurses as registration and inspection officers therefore provides the opportunity to make sure care settings provide the safest possible environment for residents.

---

[1]The charity Action on Elder Abuse is now called Hourglass.
[2]The charity Counsel and Care is now called Independent Age.

> **BOX 14.2** **Commentary on the Relationship Between Regulation, Organisational Culture and Quality:**
>
> 'The relationship of regulation to the quality of care is unclear. At the least it establishes a minimum standard—a safety net below which care standards should not be able to fall...but in the end some of the most important factors are outside the direct scope of regulation—the motivation of providers, the attitudes of care staff, the supportive involvement of friends and relatives. Regulation can never substitute for these but at its best it can serve to encourage and reinforce them' (Burgner 1996, p. 117).

Care homes are now expected to have policies and procedures on safeguarding and abuse that comply with the policies and procedures on safeguarding that exist at local level developed by the Safeguarding Adults Board.

Regulation of standards is recognised as central to good-quality services in health and social care. However, an interesting report on the regulation and inspection of social services concluded with the commentary in Box 14.2. Although the comments were made 25 years ago, they are relevant in the current context.

The CQC is a non-departmental public body, independent of government, that regulates and inspects health and care provision in England. The regulatory bodies for health care, hospitals and primary care/GP services, mental health services and social care services were amalgamated when CQC was formed. The standards services must adhere to in order to maintain registration are stipulated by CQC and equivalent organisations elsewhere in the United Kingdom, and several of them relate to safeguarding and abuse. Core standards are that services should be safe, effective, caring, responsive and well led; the main standard relevant to abuse is the one that pertains to safety. A new strategy developed and issued in 2021 contains four themes, of which one, safety through learning, is concerned with developing stronger cultures of safety within services.

Legislation in the form of the Registered Homes Act of 1984 and the Care Standards Act stipulates the requirements for registration (i.e., effectively licensing) of care homes. The grounds on which homes may be de-registered are also included. Registration includes provision for emergency action to be taken, if necessary, to provide protective measures for residents. Clearly abusive situations are likely to be covered. Generally, however, actions such as home closures are not undertaken lightly, due in part to the distress they almost inevitably cause for residents who are already frail and vulnerable. At times, via CQC actions, experienced health and care staff are seconded to support and work with care homes to improve the quality of care provision and avoid the need for closure of the home.

It is still the case some care homes are closed either due to regulatory or inspection failures or to the private care home provider or company going out of business. When this happens, careful and sensitive planning and coordination between a number of agencies are necessary to try and ensure, if residents have to be moved, the transition period runs as smoothly as possible and traumatic effects are minimised.

POLICY DEVELOPMENT

The development of appropriate policies related to abuse and protection is a difficult and problematic area. Certainly, from 1990 onward, there was considerable development, particularly by social services departments, and to a lesser extent by health purchasers and providers, of policies to address the abuse of older people. These were increasingly framed in terms of adult protection, initially by the publication of the government guidance document *No Secrets* (Department of Health, 2000). This clearly stated abuse in communal settings was to be included and addressed within local policies related to abuse and protection. Within the community, a policy that is framed only in terms of protection may not adequately recognise older people may be at risk of harm, although not necessarily frail and vulnerable, and they may need the help of services because the person they live with has the capacity to inflict harm on them. This needs to be clearly reflected in local policies.

A review of the *No Secrets* guidance was undertaken by the Department of Health between 2008 and 2012. Issues related to what was by then termed *adult safeguarding* were included in the consolidating legislation, the Care Act of 2014. Since then adult safeguarding has more legal standing, as it is part of the law that governs adult social care, and the sections related to safeguarding detail the structure, processes and statutory requirements that now exist in this area. The legislation includes, for example, the establishment of safeguarding boards in local areas, with high-level/senior representatives from health, social care services, the police and other agencies attending the regular meetings; statutory agencies such as health, police and social care are mandated to attend. The guidance is regularly updated and available from the website for the Department of Health and Social Care. The CQC (2019) and the equivalent organisation in Scotland (Care Inspectorate, 2020) have also developed and issued policies; in Northern Ireland, the Health and Social Care Board (2016) Adult Safeguarding Partnership produced operational guidance for staff.

The Royal College of Nursing (RCN) guidelines for nurses made valuable points, including suggestions for nurses to keep accurate written records and record telephone conversations with other professionals (RCN, 1996). The RCN also contributed to guidelines on the abuse of older people in the community with several other concerned organisations, including the Royal College of General Practitioners. They provided guidance on what to do if a nurse is concerned about a possible case of abuse (Action on Elder Abuse, 1996). Following further updates, the RCN developed additional guidance on adult safeguarding in 2018 (RCN, 2018a), together with resources for health care assistants (RCN, 2018b). Additional separate guidance is also available in relation to children, domestic abuse and specific areas such as modern slavery and trafficking, which can affect adults at risk of harm (RCN, 2020).

It is essential nurses who work with older people, from the range of possible settings, are aware of and familiar with the national framework provided in the Care Act and, perhaps more crucially, with the local policies and procedures in their areas. Familiarity means not just awareness but also knowledge and understanding of the guidance and relevant roles and responsibilities within the processes established at the local level to deal with abuse and neglect. This includes knowing when and how to take appropriate action—for example, how and who to make a report to, if necessary.

CONCLUSION AND LEARNING POINTS

'The challenge is to make sure efforts on behalf of mistreated older persons do more good than harm and do not lead to the neglect of other societal needs' (Wolf, 1992, p. 429). Rosalie Wolf was a leading campaigner against elder abuse in the United States in the 1980s and 1990s. Her words here are profoundly important. The unease of many nurses and other professionals in intervening in abusive situations is generally connected to the fear of making things worse. It is probably the first rule of professional practice that older people must be listened to, whether they are the carer or the cared-for, the abuser or the abused, in hospital or in community settings, including communal settings such as care homes and those that provide nursing care. Second, awareness that abuse and neglect can and does exist is essential to dealing with these harms, although it is always important to raise concerns with the safeguarding lead, who will undertake an independent assessment. Finally, the current legitimate and necessary interest in the mistreatment of older people should have the effect of making us all think about the general way society treats elders and how discrimination against older people might exacerbate situations of abuse and neglect, as was regrettably seen during the COVID-19 pandemic. Prevention of abuse should be nurses' main priority, although we need well-developed interventions to assist when prevention does not work or is not possible. Abuse, whether by paid staff or by family members, is the extreme end of a continuum that covers the care of older people. It is most likely to be prevented by strengthening a whole range of other services that bear on household and family relationships and the provision of communal health and social care.

KEY LEARNING POINTS

- The term *abuse* has a professional construction. It may mean different things to different people and to professionals from different disciplines. It is always important to clarify meaning so understanding about abuse is clear.
- Understanding the context and circumstances of abuse is vital, as is acknowledging ambiguity and confusion in personal and family relationships around alleged abuse.
- Real life is complicated, and the standard definitions of abuse do not necessarily fit. Individuals may experience several types of mistreatment, at the same time or

separately, so awareness is needed, and monitoring of situations can be helpful.
- Nurses need to make sure they know the boundaries of their accountability, understand confidentiality, know when they should communicate with other professionals or agencies and ensure they are up to date on safeguarding regulations and their responsibilities in relation to providing safe, quality care.
- Cultures of trust and openness in organisations are vital for prevention and for raising concerns in the spirit of making a difference to the well-being and care of older people.

RECOMMENDED FURTHER READING

A general text on family violence, including five chapters specifically about older people. Although written for general practitioners, nurses might find it useful:

Amiel, S., & Heath, I. (2003). *Family violence in primary care.* Oxford University Press.

Guidance documents produced on aspects of safeguarding for nursing and related health care professionals:

Royal College of Nursing (RCN). (2018a). *Adult safeguarding: Roles and competencies for nursing staff.* Royal College of Nursing.

RCN. (2018b). *First steps for healthcare assistants: Key principles of safeguarding.* Royal College of Nursing.

RCN. (2020). *Modern slavery and trafficking: Guidance for nurses and midwives.* Royal College of Nursing.

A useful text on adult safeguarding with some helpful chapters and useful case studies on such aspects as the Mental Capacity Act and how it relates to safeguarding, assessment and management of risk, self-neglect and hoarding:

Cooper, A., & White, E. (Eds). (2017). *Safeguarding adults under the Care Act 2014: Understanding good practice.* Jessica Kingsley Publishers.

This edited volume predates the changes introduced by the Care Act but includes some helpful chapters on elder abuse in minority ethnic communities and institutional abuse:

Pritchard, J. (Ed.). (2008). *Good practice in safeguarding adults: Working effectively in adult protection.* Jessica Kingsley Publishers.

USEFUL RESOURCES

Hourglass England (previously Action on Elder Abuse): https://www.wearehourglass.org

Independent Age (previously Counsel and Care): https://www.independentage.org

International Network for the Prevention of Elder Abuse: https://www.inpea.net

Protect (previously Public Concern at Work): https://www.protect-advice.org.uk

REFERENCES

Action on Elder Abuse. (1994). *Elder abuse in care homes: Who to contact and what to do*. Action on Elder Abuse.

Action on Elder Abuse. (1996). *The abuse of older people at home: Information for workers*. Action on Elder Abuse.

Amiel, S., & Heath, I. (2003). *Family violence in primary care*: Oxford University Press.

Ash, A. (2014). *Safeguarding older people from abuse*: Policy Press.

Baker, M., & Heitkemper, M. (2005). The roles of nurses on interprofessional teams to combat elder mistreatment. *Nursing Outlook, 53*, 253–259.

Bennett, G. (2000). Personal communication to B. Penhale.

Bonnie, R., & Wallace, R. (2003). *Elder mistreatment*. National Academies Press.

Brodaty, H., & Gresham, M. (1989). Effect of a training programme to reduce stress in patients with dementia. *British Medical Journal, 299*, 1375–1379.

Burgner, T. (1996). *The regulation and inspection of social services*. Department of Health/Welsh Office.

Care Inspectorate. (2020). *Adult support and protection*. Care Inspectorate.

Care Quality Commission (CQC). (2019). *Safeguarding people*. CQC.

Carers UK. (2019). *Policy briefing 2019: Facts about carers*. https://www.carersuk.org/for-professionals/policy/policy-library

Clough, R. (1999). Scandalous care: Interpreting public enquiry reports of scandals in residential care. *Journal of Elder Abuse and Neglect, 10*, 13–28.

Compton, S. A., Flanagan, P., & Gregg, W. (1997). Elder abuse in people with dementia in Northern Ireland: Prevalence and predictors in cases referred to a psychiatry of old age service. *International Journal of Psychiatry, 12*, 632–635.

Counsel and Care. (1994). *Older people at risk of abuse in a residential setting: Fact sheet 2*. Counsel and Care.

Data Protection Act. (2018). https://www.legislation.gov.uk/ukpga/2018/12/contents

Department of Health. (2000). *No secrets: Guidance on developing and implementing multi-agency policies and procedures to protect vulnerable adults from abuse*. Department of Health.

Department of Health. (2014). *Care Act guidance*. TSO.

Dimond, B. (1995). *Legal aspects of nursing* (2nd ed.). Prentice-Hall.

Flynn, M. (2015). *In search of accountability: A review of the neglect of older people living in care homes investigated as Operation Jasmine*. TSO.

Francis, R. (2013). *Report of the Mid-Staffordshire NHS Foundation Trust public inquiry*. https://assets.publishing.service.gov.uk/government/uploads/system/uploads/attachment_data/file/279124/0947.pdf

Francis, R. (2015). *Freedom to speak up: An independent review into creating an open and honest reporting culture in the NHS*. TSO.

Goodman, C., Davies, S. L., Gordon, A. L., Dening, T., Gage, H., Meyer, J., Schneider, J., Bell, B., Jordan, J., Martin, F., Iliffe, S., Bowman, C., Gladman, J. R. F., Victor, C., Mayrhofer, A., Handley, M., & Zubair, M. (2017). Optimal NHS service delivery to care homes: A realist evaluation of the features and mechanisms that support effective working for the continuing care of older people in residential settings. *Health Services and Delivery Research, 5*(29).

Harris, D., & Benson, M. (2008). *Maltreatment of patients in nursing homes*. Haworth Press.

Health and Social Care Act. (2008). Health and Social Care Act 2008 (Regulated Activities) Regulations 2014—Part 3 Section 2 Regulation 20. https://www.legislation.gov.uk/ukdsi/2014/9780111117613/regulation/20

Health and Social Care Board. (2016). *Northern Ireland adult safeguarding partnership: Adult safeguarding operational procedures*. RQIA.

Health and Social Care Information Centre. (2013). *A guide to confidentiality in health and social care*. https://digital.nhs.uk/data-and-information/looking-after-information/data-security-and-information-governance/codes-of-practice-for-handling-information-in-health-and-care/a-guide-to-confidentiality-in-health-and-social-care/a-guide-to-confidentiality

Homer, A., & Gilleard, C. J. (1990). Abuse of elderly people by their carers. *British Medical Journal, 301*, 1359–1362.

Homer, A., & Gilleard, C. J. (1994). The effect of inpatient respite care on elderly patients and their carers. *Age and Ageing, 23*, 274–276.

Kingston, P., & Penhale, B. (1995). Elder abuse and neglect: Issues in the accident and emergency department. *Accident and Emergency Nursing, 3*, 122–128.

Kitchen, G., Richardson, B., & Livingston, G. (2002). Are nurses equipped to manage actual or suspected elder abuse? *Professional Nurse, 17*, 647–650.

Martin, J. P. (1984). *Hospitals in trouble*. Blackwell.

Malmedal, W., Hammervold, R., & Saveman, B.-I. (2009a). To report or not to report: Attitudes held by Norwegian nursing home staff on reporting inadequate care carried out by colleagues. *Scandinavian Journal of Public Health, 37*(7), 744–750.

Malmedal, W., Ingebrigtsen, O., & Saveman, B.-I. (2009b). Inadequate care in Norwegian nursing homes—as reported by nursing staff. *Scandinavian Journal of Caring Sciences, 23*(2), 231–242.

Malmedal, W., Kilvik, A., Steinsheim, G., & Botngad, A. (2020). A literature review of survey instruments used to measure staff to resident elder abuse in residential care settings. *Nursing Open, 7*(6), 1650–1660.

McCann-Beranger, J. (2014). *Exploring the role of elder mediation in the prevention of elder abuse*. http://www.justice.gc.ca

McCreadie, C. (1996). *Elder abuse: An update on research*. Age Concern Institute of Gerontology.

Mental Capacity Act. (2005). *Section 44 Ill-treatment or neglect*. https://www.legislation.gov.uk/ukpga/2005/9/section/44

Mental Health Foundation. (1995). *Making life better: Mental health for older people*. Mental Health Foundation.

Mikton, C., Butchart, A., Dahlberg, L., & Krug, E. (2014). *Global status report on violence prevention*. WHO.

Miller, C. (2005). Elder abuse: The nurse's perspective. In G. Anetzberger (Ed.), *The clinical management of elder abuse*. Haworth Press.

Nursing and Midwifery Council. (2004). *The NMC code of professional conduct: Standards for conduct, performance and ethics*. London.

Nursing and Midwifery Council. (2018). *The NMC code of professional conduct: Standards for conduct, performance and ethics*. London.

O'Keeffe, M., Hills, A., Doyle, M., McCreadie, C., Scholes, S., Constantine, R., Tinker, A., Manthorpe, J., Biggs, S., & Erens, B. (2007). *UK study of abuse and neglect of older people: Prevalence survey report*. King's College London and National Centre for Social Research.

Penhale, B. (1993). Abuse of elderly people: Considerations for practice. *British Journal of Social Work, 23*, 95–112.

Phair, L., & Goodman, W. (2003). The role of the community nurse. In S. Amiel & I. Heath (Eds.), *Family violence in primary care* (pp. 391–395). Oxford University Press.

Phelan, A. (2018). *The role of the nurse in detecting elder abuse and neglect: Current perspectives*: Dove Press.

Pike, L., Gilbert, T., Leverton, C., & Indge, R. (2011). Training, knowledge and confidence in safeguarding adults: Results from a postal survey of the health and social care sector in a single county. *Journal of Adult Protection, 13*(5), 259–274.

Pillemer, K. A., & Finkelhor, D. (1988). The prevalence of elder abuse: A random sample survey. *Gerontologist, 28*, 51–57.

Podnieks, E. (1990). *National survey on abuse of the elderly in Canada: The Ryerson study*. Ryerson Polytechnic Institute.

Podnieks, E. (1992). Emerging themes from a follow-up study of Canadian victims of elder abuse. *Journal of Elder Abuse and Neglect, 4*, 59–111.

Reay, A., & Browne, K. (2002). The effectiveness of psychological interventions with individuals who physically abuse or neglect their elderly dependents. *Journal of Interpersonal Violence, 17*, 416–431.

Richardson, B., Kitchen, G., & Livingston, G. (2002). The effect of education on knowledge and management of elder abuse: a randomized controlled trial. *Age and Ageing, 31*, 335–341.

Royal College of Nursing (RCN). (1996). *Combating abuse and neglect of older people: Royal College of Nursing guidelines for nurses*. Royal College of Nursing.

RCN. (2018a). *Adult safeguarding: Roles and competencies for nursing staff*. Royal College of Nursing.

RCN. (2018b). *First steps for healthcare assistants: Key principles of safeguarding*. Royal College of Nursing.

RCN. (2020). *Modern slavery and trafficking: Guidance for nurses and midwives*. Royal College of Nursing.

Saveman, B.-I., Norberg, A., & Hallberg, I. R. (1992). The problems of dealing with abuse and neglect of the elderly: Interviews with district nurses. *Qualitative Health Research, 2*, 302–317.

Saveman, B.-I., Hallberg, I. R., & Norberg, A. (1993a). Identifying and defining abuse of elderly people, as seen by witnesses. *Journal of Advanced Nursing, 18*, 1393–1400.

Saveman, B.-I., Hallberg, I. R., & Norberg, A. (1993b). Patterns of abuse of the elderly in their own homes as reported by district nurses. *Scandinavian Journal of Primary Health Care, 11*, 111–116.

Saveman, B.-I., Norberg, A., Anders, G., & Oden, B. (1995). The trustworthiness of the stories of elder abuse narrated by district nurses. *Scandinavian Journal of Caring Sciences, 9*, 29–34.

Saveman, B.-I., Hallberg, I. R., & Norberg, A. (1996). Narratives by district nurses about elder abuse within families. *Clinical Nursing Research, 5*, 220–236.

Sethi, D., Wood, S., Mitis, F., Bellis, M., Penhale, B., Marmalejo, I., Lowenstein, A., Manthorpe, J., & Karki, F. (2011). *European report on preventing elder maltreatment*. WHO.

Shugarman, L. R., Fries, B. E., Wolf, R. S., & Morris, J. N. (2003). Identifying older people at risk of abuse during routine screening practices. *Journal of the American Geriatrics Society, 51*, 24–31.

Welsh Government. (2019). *Social Services and Well-being (Wales) Act 2014: Working together to safeguard people. Volume 6: Handling individual cases to protect adults at risk*. Cardiff.

Wolf, R. S. (1992). Making an issue of elder abuse. *Gerontologist, 32*, 427–429.

World Health Organization (WHO), & International Network for the Prevention of Elder Abuse (NPEA). (2002). *Missing voices: Views of older persons on elder abuse*. https://apps.who.int/iris/handle/10665/67371HO

World Health Organisation (WHO). (2022). *Abuse of older people—Factsheet*. https://www.who.int/news-room/fact-sheets/detail/abuse-of-older-people

Yon, Y., Mikton, C., Gassoumis, Z., & Wilber, K. (2017). Elder abuse prevalence in community settings: A systematic review and meta-analysis. *Lancet Global Health, 5*(2), E147–E156.

Yon, Y., Ramiro-Gonzalez, M., Mikton, C., Huber, M., & Sethi, D. (2019). The prevalence of elder abuse in institutional settings: A systematic review and meta-analysis. *European Journal of Public Health, 29*(1), 58–67.

SECTION 3

Independence and Maintaining Function

15

Communication Challenges and Skills

Andrée C. le May, Heather M. Fillmore Elbourne

CHAPTER OUTLINE

This chapter starts by defining communication and discussing its continuing importance in older age. We also highlight reasons for communicating and discuss some of the factors that shape and influence communication between older people and the nurses and others who care for them in acute, community and long-term care facilities. The central part of the chapter focuses on some of the most commonly occurring communication challenges older people face, including challenges associated with the natural course of ageing, such as altered hearing and seeing; illnesses such as stroke or dementia; sensory deprivation such as the communication challenges posed by the COVID-19 pandemic; and challenging behaviours. Communication strategies and pointers for good communication are detailed for each of these challenges, usually targeted toward the nurse. In many instances they are also useful for informal carers, volunteers, relatives and friends. The chapter concludes by reminding readers of the therapeutic value of communication with older people. Throughout the chapter we use a blend of original seminal works and contemporary references to support our propositions and show that some of the challenges and their associated solutions have a long and relevant history.

Communication is often described as a two-way process, involving the transmission and comprehension of a message. This complex interaction is so well integrated into our daily lives most of us take it for granted, and it is only when the effectiveness of the process is challenged

its importance becomes clear. Growth in the field of electronic devices such as tablets and smartphones and technologies such as videoconferencing and speech-to-text may provide greater opportunities for people to communicate either directly through these devices or through helping one another use them.

WHAT IS COMMUNICATION?

Communication is a complex process that involves passing a message intentionally or unintentionally between two or more people. This process is often explained using a simple model that suggests four essential features required for communication:

1. A source from which the message is communicated
2. A message to be sent
3. A channel for communicating the message
4. A receiver of the message

Once the message is received, another message—feedback or a response—is usually sent to the source, creating a dynamic and ongoing process between the interactors (Monaghan, 1995). Although this seems to be a relatively old definition, it still works today in the virtual *and* face-to-face worlds we work and live in.

In order to convey a message, the source, or sender, needs to determine the content and purpose of the message as well as target a recipient for the message. The message usually arises from stimulation of a sensory or cognitive nature. Therefore an interruption in the usual functioning of these processes, for instance a cognitive impairment, leads to the disruption of communication at an early stage. Any alteration in the ability to recognise the transmission or content of messages also has an impact on the effectiveness of the communication, as does the receptiveness of the receiver of the message.

Although this model forms a useful basis for understanding the theory that underlies communication, it does not acknowledge the complexity of the process or show how impairment of communication channels has an impact on the effective transmission and interpretation of messages. To understand how growing older challenges communication, it is necessary to consider the mechanisms for conveying and recognising messages more closely.

Each message is transmitted in a unique way through a series of sensory, motor and cognitive channels. The meaning of a message is shaped by each interactor's perception, which is unique to that interactor and formed by their indivudual psychological and social status and experiences (Fig. 15.1). In unimpaired communication the complexity of this process may make messages hard to decipher and lead to misinterpretation, which may be compounded when ageing or illness compromises sensory, motor or cognitive functioning or a person's psychological or social condition. Alteration in any of these five key areas impinges on communication, with the neurological site of damage or the underlying illness or deficit determining the effects on communication.

Message transmission, recognition, comprehension and interpretation are primarily learnt behaviours that incorporate a variety of coordinated activities in relation to achieving a goal. Any alteration to these activities results in a challenge to communication. Message transmission occurs through the use of verbal, graphic and non-verbal cues. Their use is situation-specific, individually determined, socially constructed and a basis for judging the interpersonal effectiveness of the communicator (Hargie, 2018). Verbal and non-verbal cues are complementary, often working together to augment messages. However, where communication is undertaken in writing or electronically through emails and text messages, it is difficult to pick up the more subtle cues passed on non-verbally; a text message or email lacks the emotional context present when face-to-face communication occurs. Recognition, comprehension and interpretation of messages are primarily associated with the sensory and cognitive processes of sight, hearing, touch, smell, taste and cognition. Any impairment may result in ineffective communication through misunderstanding the message and/or giving inappropriate feedback to the sender. Sensory and cognitive processes are closely linked to the use of verbal and non-verbal cues. Increasingly, graphic forms of communication, such as drawings, photographs and sketches, are used in healthcare situations to enhance or replace traditional verbal and non-verbal cues.

REASONS FOR COMMUNICATING

We spend most of our time communicating with people we live, work or socialise with (Argyle, 1994). We communicate to 'be approved of and to make friends, to dominate or to depend on others, to be admired, to be helped or given social support, [and] to provide help to others' (p. 1).

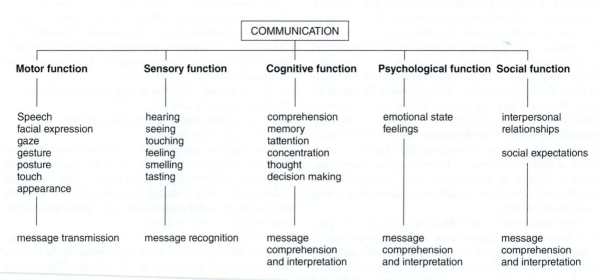

Fig. 15.1 Conveying and receiving messages.

Communicating is one of our principal pastimes, so to be deprived of it or have it inhibited in any way has a major impact on quality of life, regardless of age. Recently we saw and experienced the impact unpredicted disturbances such as social distancing and the prolonged use of personal protective equipment had on people's usual communication patterns. For example, for nurses, the use of touch and facial expresions to convey compassion and reassurance were mimised. We had to find alternative ways to build relationships and communicate with people.

Worrall and Hickson (2003) emphasised the 'everydayness' and pervasiveness of communication for older people, asserting communication, in some form, occurs in almost everything from taking money out of the bank to playing bingo. Worrall and Hickson (p. 12) also highlighted several reasons why effective communication is important for older people, who use it as a means of:

- Exerting influence and power
- Relieving loneliness, depression and anxiety
- Receiving high-quality care
- Establishing and maintaining friendships
- Participating in activities of living
- Facilitating adaptation to change
- Involvement in decision-making
- Stimulating thinking
- Maintaining social networks
- Enhancing well-being

It's hard to find research that focuses on who older people communicate with. However, we get an idea from Worrall and Hickson (2003), who quoted an unpublished study of older people's communication partners; the study reported the most frequently occurring communications were between older peers (50%), and the next most common were with family members (25%). Increasingly, anecdotal evidence suggests formal carers form the only avenues for face-to-face communication for some older people. Typical topics of communication include discussions of past life experiences, family matters, health, politics and financial and other practical daily-living concerns. More recently Yuan et al. (2016) explored the mechanisms through which older people communicate, noting face-to-face communication was still the most commonly used and preferred medium, but phone and internet communications were also popular. During the COVID-19 pandemic, we noted a change to our communication strategies, with the internet becoming increasingly popular and accessible. Many nursing consultations moved into the virtual world.

Communicating becomes increasingly important for older people if they are dependent on others for care. Isolation may make older people feel vulnerable and increase their need to maintain social interaction and gain support through various communication networks. Communication

possibilities may be actively sought and maximised through, for example, interacting with friends and family, seeking advice from health-care professionals or attending day centres or clubs, either face-to-face or virtually, that are run within formal care services or informally in the community (e.g., Age Exchange). Conversely, with the increased likelihood of very old people communally living in nursing or residential homes, opportunities that minimise communication with others may be welcomed in order to promote privacy and solitude. In these situations nurses are in a key position to facilitate a more equal balance of social interaction with opportunities for privacy and solitude that meet each resident's needs.

In the nursing context, communication is of vital importance, helping nurses establish, define and maintain relationships between themselves, members of their multidisiplinary team and older people. Through the use of skilled communication, nurses can do the following:

- Obtain information about the older person's physical, social, emotional and psychological well-being and understand better their usual communication environments
- Assess any deficits in communication skills
- Assess any opportunities for communication that may increase feelings of support and the development of rapport
- Assess an older person's requirements for increased privacy and solitude or increased involvement
- Determine how communication deficits may be overcome (e.g., by using glasses, hearing aids, specialised communication aids, interactive technologies or interpreters)
- Monitor and explain change in relation to altered communication skills or general health status
- Provide appropriate information through the most effective communication channels
- Evaluate progress and the impact of care on the person's general condition and ability to communicate
- Make referrals to other relevant health-care professionals (e.g., speech and language therapists, audiologists, opticians)

It is also essential—particularly when older people experience long hospital stays, need continuing care or are socially distanced from their friends or family, such as during the recent pandemic or as a result of moving into a long-term care facility—that nurses consider ways in which they might facilitate communication between older patients or residents in order to ensure social distancing does not result in social isolation and the negative outcomes that may accompany it (van der Roest et al., 2020). They may consider, for instance, encouraging story-telling between individuals (e.g., Andrews et al., 2020) or more formally in designated groups or instigating a peer-mentoring system among older patients or residents (e.g.,

Dorgo et al., 2013). Singing and arts-based actitivites are also increasingly popular and have been shown to have positive effects on well-being while encouraging communication and skills development about and around the activity (e.g., Batt-Rawden & Stedje, 2020; Vogelpoel & Jarrold, 2014).

SHAPING THE MEANING OF COMMUNICATION

Several mediating factors are associated with message interpretation and feedback. Hargie and Marshall (1993, p. 31) defined these mediating factors as 'internal states, activities or processes within [each] individual which mediate between the feedback which is perceived, the goal which is being pursued and the responses that are made'. These variables affect the ways in which all messages are interpreted and include age, gender, sociocultural background, the context of the communication, the way we think and feel, and the roles we play. They are all important in the context of nursing older people, as communicators bring with them to every interaction a unique set of variables that influence the transmission and interpretation of each message. Older people are not a homogeneous group, and while it is acknowledged age-related changes are variable and cannot be generalised, the following summary of the likely impact of ageing and its effects on communication may help readers identify some of their actual or potential communication challenges.

Dowd (1986, p. 183) reminded us older people had 'been socialized at a different time and to a different set of cultural imperatives' compared with those in younger age groups, and this influences their communication abilities and strategies. This holds true today and resonates with discussion in Christina Victor's earlier chapter in this book where she talks about understanding cohort differences in old age (Chapter 3). Since then many others have suggested people of different ages have different hopes, fears and activities to perform, leading to intergenerational differences that may affect communication.

These differences raise several issues nurses, as naturally of a different generation to older patients, should be aware of:

- The undertakings of the young and the old may be different and have differing associated societal values.
- The organisation of people into age-specific groups may reduce opportunities for intergenerational communication. Generally people prefer interacting with others they see as equals in some way, which may result in, as Dowd (1986, p. 152) put it, 'an eventual outcome [of] disinclination toward cross-age social interaction'.
- The need for care may throw people together who would not usually interact.
- Younger people may find it hard to concur with older people's views and feelings because they have not had the same experience of ageing. Conversely, older people have had the experience of being younger but in a different culture and time, thereby minimising the potential for shared experiences. The mismatch of experiences may make the establishment of an empathetic rapport difficult or result in misinterpretation of messages between people.
- Generations may not share the same 'language'; athough the same words are used, they may hold different meanings, and conversations may take on different structures and functions between generations.

Biggs (1993) and Armstrong and McKechnie (2003) maintain all these factors influence the quality of interaction and development of a relationship between a younger and an older person. Biggs also suggests, owing to age-related changes, communication becomes increasingly reliant on the sensitivity and goodwill of others who need to adjust their communication styles and channels to meet the needs of older people who have deficits in communication.

The idea of intergenerational communication differences became prominent in the 1980s. Nussbaum et al. (1989), though acknowledging people of all ages generally communicate in the same way, proposed some characteristics unique to older people. They suggested older people might be more cautious in their willingness to communicate with younger people, be more reluctant to suggest specific courses of action or ask for information, and take longer to react during interactions. For some people these differences are manifest today and have important repercussions for nurses and other health-care professionals when skilled communication is a contributor to high-quality care.

Older people may place more value on talk, particularly small talk and banter, seeing it as a more vital component of relationship-building than younger people, who may be sceptical about the value of this type of verbal interchange (Andrews et al., 2015; Giles & Coupland, 1991). Dissimilar values may limit social interactions between people of different generations. Nurses need to consider these factors so they are able to distinguish between normal age-related changes, societal distancing between generations and changes associated with illness, such as the early stages of dementia. The impact of societal distancing may be exaccerbated further in health-related situations where social distancing is enforced, such as during infectious-disease outbreaks, resulting in greater isolation, which may contribute to the onset of depression, feelings of despair and, in people with dementia, further cognitive decline.

There are, however, many examples in the literature of positive intergenerational communication. For example, Armstrong and McKechnie (2003) studied intergenerational communication by interviewing schoolchildren, care home staff and older women about what it meant to grow old and the value of communication with older people. They concluded all three groups held generally positive views about old age and older people, although some gender stereotyping was evident in the children's views; older men were perceived as being grumpy, whereas older women spoilt children. More recently, the Intergenerational Foundation succssfully spearheaded campaigns to bring younger people and children together with older people living in care homes (e.g., the Apples and Honey nursery in the Nightingale House care home in south London). Ford and Sinclair (1987), in a classic study of older women, found one woman reported an enhanced quality of life when a group of young women lived next to her and offered her considerable companionship. The older woman's life changed: 'For a while my life was so different… We helped each other quite a lot' (Ford & Sinclair, 1987, p. 9). Old age does not have to be a time of communicative isolation from younger people despite intergenerational differences. This was evidenced through experiences and stories of community cross-generational support during the COVID-19 pandemic; research showed increased cross-generational communications via phone or virtual media during this time (Nature Ageing, 2021).

Ryan et al. (1995) proposed a model of 'communication predicament' in relation to older people receiving health care from younger carers. They suggested the predicament is linked to the older person's communication skills changing alongside certain barriers, maybe linked to intergenerational issues, associated with their communication partners. The altered skills create barriers that led to compromised communication. Ryan et al. (1995) also suggested a 'communication enhancement' model that focuses on the promotion of health through communication. Both models emphasise the importance of the conversational partners for the older person, suggesting 'problem(s) may not lie with the older person's communication, but rather with the interaction between the two, based on the appropriateness of the accommodation that occurs' between them' (Worrall & Hickson, 2003, p. 36).

Old age can also be a time when illness and age-related functional changes, such as impaired sight, hearing, speech or cognition, present extra challenges to communication and the maintenance of communication skills.

CULTURALLY SENSITIVE COMMUNICATION

As the world's population becomes more diverse and our cultures become multi- rather than monocultural, nurses and other health care professionals need to ensure culturally sensitive, individualised care. One way is to always communicate inclusively, respectfully and effectively with people from different cultures, ethnicities and backgrounds while respecting their individuality and individual needs. To develop culturally sensitive communication, nurses should do the following (Markey et al., 2021; Purnell & Fenkl, 2020; Teal & Street, 2009):

- Reflect on their own cultural views and beliefs, recognising and appreciating cultural differences in work and care environments and between individuals and how differences may impact on care.
- Reflect on their communication styles and how they are influenced by their own culture and the culture of the organisation in which they practice.
- Understand how cultural differences can impact care decisions.
- Avoid making assumptions based on stereotypes.
- Demonstrate knowledge and understanding of an older person's and their family's and carers' cultures.
- Safeguard against monoculturalism or their own cultural views and beliefs unduly influencing the care they provide to people from other cultures.
- Modify care to be congruent with each older person's wishes.

Failure to recognise cultural diversity can negatively impact therapeutic communication between people of all ages (Purnell & Fenkl, 2020). However, in older age, culturally insensitive communication may compound additional communication challenges brought about by ageing. Making sure this doesn't happen is about ensuring respectful, honest, inclusive dialogue and using extra resources to enhance communication whenever necessary. The sorts of resources nurses can use include the following:

- Working with interpreters—and allowing sufficient time when booking them
- Using translation technology; while not always perfect, when trained interpreters are not readily available, technology can help
- Finding out how patients and their families and carers would like to receive information and accommodating their preferences
- Using non-verbal communication skills such as pictures and hand gestures to enhance patients' understanding of what you want to communicate
- Using written materials translated into a patient's language of choice; remember to first assess the person's literacy levels and adjust the use of written materials accordingly
- Involving family, significant others or community members in conversations; remember, not all patients want to discuss sensitive information in front of their family, friends or carers

CHALLENGES TO COMMUNICATION IN OLDER AGE

Worrall and Hickson (2003, p. 93) described five areas of communication in which impairments can occur as a result of the natural course of ageing or illness: language, conversational discourse, speech, voice, and hearing. Deficits in these areas are likely to have the following effects:

- Language: Decreased speed and ability to retrieve words, decreased ability to understand increasingly complicated messages
- Conversational discourse: Difficulty in understanding long and complicated conversations, lessened efficiency and increased ambiguity in conversing, decreased cohesion within conversations
- Speech: Decreased respiratory support for speech output, imprecise articulation, slower rate of speech
- Voice: Increase in pitch for men, decrease in pitch for women, decreased voice quality
- Hearing: Diminished sensitivity to pure tones, difficulty in discriminating speech when it's hard to hear

In addition, deficits in seeing also impact communication, as do alterations in cognition, sensory awareness and behaviour. The main communication challenges associated with these areas are discussed below.

Visual Impairment

Many older people experience some reduction in vision. Visual impairment significantly affects individuals' ability to collect information about their surroundings and therefore can have a marked impact on an older person's ability to communicate.

The most common problems likely to affect visual acuity are as follows:

- Presbyopia—the natural lessening of the ability to focus on nearby things
- Cataracts
- Glaucoma
- Senile macular degeneration
- Diabetic retinopathy
- Regardless of the cause of visual impairment, it is likely to have some effect on communication, leading to
- Reduced orientation to the environment
- Reduced ability to discriminate between non-verbal cues
- Reduced ability to read or write or use information communication technology
- Reduced ability to interact with others

Assessing Vision

Obtaining an accurate history of visual impairment and determining how an older person deals with reduced vision is clearly within the remit of the nurse (see Chapter 17). Nurses should consider, together with the older person and their relatives and friends,

- The nature and duration of the visual impairment
- The cause of the impairment, if known to the older person
- Its impact on daily living
- The anticipated impact on sight of hospitalisation or admission to a residential nursing home
- Mechanisms for reducing the visual impairment

A general assessment helps the nurse recognise signs and symptoms that require referral to a specialist. However, the accuracy of an assessment may be compromised if the older person has memory loss or a mental or physical illness.

Communicating and helping an older person with a visual impairment involves skilled communication using both verbal and non-verbal cues. The following pointers may be useful:

- Ensure spectacles are appropriate, clean and within easy reach.
- If a magnifier is used, ensure it is held close to the eye and the object being magnified is moved closer until it is in focus.
- Ensure appropriate glare-free lighting and that bedside lights work and are within easy reach.
- Avoid glare from windows; draw curtains or blinds accordingly.
- Ensure some lighting at night to avoid disorientation or accidents.
- Facilitate orientation to the environment through colour-coded doors with large clear labels.
- Ensure call bells or alarm systems are within easy reach.
- If writing information down, use a black felt-tip pen after checking the patient can read the size and style of your writing.
- Encourage regular eye tests.
- Stand or sit within the older person's visual field so they are aware of your presence. This is particularly important when visual impairment minimises peripheral vision.
- Suggest the use of large-print books or papers or talking books, and increase the size of print on tablets, computers and phones. Ebersole and Hess (2019) suggested extra strategies to complement those listed above and to enhance communication with older people who have a visual impairment, including:
  - Identify yourself clearly.
  - Make it clear when you are leaving and entering the room.
  - Make sure you have the person's attention before you speak; you may find touch useful in gaining or holding attention.

Since people with a visual impairment find it hard to become oriented to a new environment, particular care is required to help familiarise them to anything unfamiliar. This is particularly acute when older people are admitted to a hospital or a nursing care facility after the familiar surroundings of their own home or other setting. For more information on sight and older people, see Chapter 17, and visit the Royal National Institute of Blind People website to keep up to date with new information and technological advances.

Auditory Impairment

Hearing loss is prevalent in older adults around the world and is often cited as the most common sensory impairment in adults over the age of 65. Hearing loss is considered a public health challenge in the United Kingdom, as 70% of individuals aged 70 and older report problems with hearing (See the RNID website at https://rnid.org.uk/). Deafness in old age can result from blockage of the ear canal by wax or narrowing, closure or hardening due to ageing; infection of the middle ear with subsequent auditory damage; and tinnitus, or ringing in the ears. It is generally categorised into conductive or sensorineural hearing loss, although a combination of the two is possible.

Effects of Auditory Impairment on Communication

Hull (1989) described the frustrations of older people with hearing impairments, emphasising the consequences of not being able to understand the sounds of a previously familiar world. Hearing impairment may be associated with misinterpretation, embarrassment, fear, making inappropriate responses and withdrawal. These are likely to lead to isolation and diminished well-being. Hull suggested hearing loss may also result in an older person

feeling control of the senses is being lost, particularly if confirmed by others.

As long ago as 1996, the Royal National Institute for the Deaf, which campaigns to make life fully inclusive for deaf people and those with hearing loss or tinnitus, starkly described the effects of hearing loss as a series of exclusions: 'exclusion from conversation, exclusion from day to day interaction, exclusion from information, exclusion from leisure activities, exclusion from family and friends [and] exclusion from mainstream life'. This emphasis on exclusion serves as a reminder of the challenges of auditory impairment to an older person's well-being and opportunities for communication.

Deafness has an impact on the sender and receiver of the message in a variety of ways:

- The ability to listen is diminished.
- As hearing levels decrease, the older person may suggest others are not speaking clearly, thereby creating strained relationships.
- Hearing loss may affect the person's speech, as auditory monitoring of speech is compromised.
- Non-verbal communication may also be affected. For example, gaze or eye contact may be minimised as the hearing-impaired person focuses attention on the speaker's lips, trying to lip-read.
- Responses may be slower because of the need to seek clarity through several communication channels rather than through listening alone.

These issues impact the relationship the nurse establishes with a person with compromised hearing and the degree to which the older person feels able to re-establish independence and autonomy (Fig. 15.2).

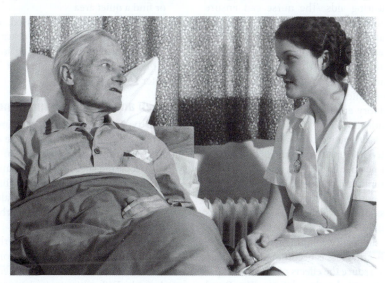

Fig. 15.2 Eye contact. Photo taken of Romilly Ingram Redfern (1902–1991), Professor Sally Redfern's father. Printed with permission.

Assessing Hearing

Assessment plays a vital part in establishing a therapeutic partnership with a person who has an auditory impairment. Nurses need to be able to determine whether hearing difficulties are present in order to provide appropriate care and make rapid referrals for treatment or monitoring by other health care workers. The following steps may be used to guide initial assessments:

- Establish details of the hearing loss, its duration and if any compensatory mechanisms (e.g., hearing aid, lip-reading) are used.
- Establish how the hearing loss affects the person's life.
- Establish when hearing was last checked.
- Check current drug therapy to rule out ototoxicity.
- Discuss the anticipated impact of hospitalisation or moving into an unfamiliar environment.
- Observe the person's behaviour to determine signs of auditory impairment.

Communicating With an Older Person With an Auditory Impairment

Hearing impairment is very common among older people. Age-related hearing loss cannot be reversed as it is caused by a degeneration of sensory cells that occurs during ageing. Although it can significantly affect communication, nurses are well situated to assist older people by using age-appropriate communication skills and auditory devices developed to minimise or avoid problems (Weinreich, 2017). Hull (1989) suggested health-care professionals could help older people with hearing impairments in a number of ways that hold true over 30 years later. First, he proposed amplification using hearing aids. The nurse can ensure a hearing aid is working, set at the appropriate level and worn correctly. The nurse may also be able to monitor the effectiveness of the hearing aid in enhancing communication. Second, Hull drew attention to the environment in which the interaction occurs: nurses should, whenever possible, seek to ensure interactions occur in noise-free environments and auditory enhancement equipment such as hearing or audio-induction loops are activated. Third, he suggested the use of alternative communication strategies such as using written information, ensuring lip-reading is facilitated by careful positioning during interactions and using a variety of communication skills. Andersson et al. (1994) highlighted the positive effects of counselling older people with hearing loss. The use of specialist social workers who can make individual assessments of a person's auditory needs and recommend supportive equipment to help people to adapt and live with hearing loss is becoming increasingly common and is likely to reduce the effects of isolation experienced by older people with hearing deficits. The Royal National Institute for Deaf People (n.d.) produced some tips

for nurses who communicate virtually with older people with a hearing loss, such as using videoconferencing rather than a simple phone if possible and using the typed chat feed. During the COVID-19 pandemic, as more and more people wore masks, it became important to consider using transparent masks or visors to enable people to lip-read and see facial expressions to aid communications (Brown, 2020). These inovations, developed as a response to a quickly developing pandemic, can now be used in everyday practice as a means of providing enhanced person-centred care.

The following list provides useful ways to improve communication techniques when caring for someone with an auditory impairment:

- Make sure your mouth can be seen to facilitate lip-reading.
- Use non-verbal cues, such as facial expressions and gestures, to enhance speech.
- Articulate words carefully.
- Face the person with whom you are interacting, sitting or standing at the same level.
- Make sure there is sufficient light on your face.
- Gain the person's attention before you speak. Touching may be a useful way of doing this.
- Speak at a normal volume; do not shout.
- Pause between sentences and confirm if you have been understood.
- If you are misunderstood, repeat the sentence using different words.
- Supplement spoken information with written information or use information communication technology.
- Reduce background noise such as radios or televisions, or find a quiet area.
- Make sure hearing aids, if used, and audio-conduction loops are switched on and working.

More information on hearing loss is available on the Royal National Institution for Deaf People website and in Chapter 16.

Speech and Language Impairment

Several types of speech disorder are associated with illness-related changes during old age and may in some way impinge on verbal communication. The three most commonly occurring speech disorders are as follows:

- Disorders of reception: Exacerbated by, for example, hearing impairment, anxiety or altered consciousness
- Disorders of perception: Exacerbated by, for example, strokes, dementia or delirium
- Disorders of articulation: Exacerbated by, for example, compromised respiratory function or stroke illness
  These disorders can be categorised into four groups:
- Anomia: Difficulties in retrieving words during conversation

- Aphasia (or dysphasia): Impaired language through disruption in its understanding and expression that can affect listening, speaking, calculating, reading and writing
- Apraxia: Difficulties in carrying out voluntary movements associated with speech
- Dysarthria: Difficulties due to muscle weakness or uncoordinated speech production

For older people, speech impairment is most commonly associated with aphasia and dysarthria.

Aphasia

The most common cause of speech impairment in older people is likely to fall within the category of aphasia and be a consequence of a stroke. The extent of the impairment depends on the severity and location of the stroke. Damage to the right hemisphere of the brain can result in alteration in attention, orientation, perception, retention and integration. Damage to the left hemisphere is likely to result in damage to centres associated with language.

The complexity of aphasia is emphasised by the Stroke Association (n.d.) and Groher (1989), who discussed several types of aphasia and their impact on communication. Grohler categorised them into fluent and non-fluent aphasias due to their impact on speech. Fluent aphasias include the following:

- Wernicke's aphasia: Speech is usually fluent, but the content of the message is impaired. For instance, incorrect words may be used or words mispronounced. Older people with this type of aphasia may find it hard to find the correct word or syllables and often speak in repetitive jargon. Comprehension of the spoken language may also be impaired. Wernicke's aphasia results in compromised speech, reading and writing.
- Conduction aphasia: Typified by difficulties in repeating words despite sound auditory comprehension. Speech may remain intact.
- Anomic aphasia: Difficulties occur in recalling specific words. People with this disorder may learn to substitute alternative words for the intended one, thus keeping the content of the message intact. Speech and understanding remain intact.
- Transcortical sensory aphasia: Less common than the other forms of fluent aphasia. The symptoms are similar to those found in Wernicke's aphasia but more severe. Speech may still be fluent but incomprehensible, and words may be replaced by sounds that mimic the intended word but have no meaning. People with this aphasia may accurately echo sounds that they hear.

Non-fluent aphasias include the following:

- Broca's aphasia: Characterised by problems of verbal production. Grammatical structure goes awry, and increased length of time is taken to produce words, result-

ing in slow speech that uses a minimum of words. In Broca's aphasia comprehension may remain intact.
- Transcortical motor aphasia: People with this disorder exhibit problems finding words during conversations, and their auditory abilities range from poor to good. As with transcortical sensory aphasia, people with this disorder are able to echo sounds they hear, although initiation may be difficult.
- Global aphasia is characterised by severe problems with language, reception and expression, linked with unintelligible speech and compromised understanding.

These communication-linked disorders have far-reaching effects, ranging from an inability to speak coherently to difficulties interpreting and comprehending messages conveyed orally or in writing. Clearly any of these disorders has a profound effect on an older person's social and psychological well-being and may ultimately impinge on physical status as well.

Communicating With an Older Person With Aphasia

Each edition of the Ebersole and Hess (2019) textbook provides a series of pointers nurses may use when communicating with older people with aphasia:

- Explain interventions in an accessible way.
- Avoid childlike or patronising language.
- Keep calm and patient, and allow enough time for responses.
- Speak slowly and clearly.
- Ask one question at a time, and wait for an answer before moving on to the next.
- Speak about things that interest the person.
- Augment verbal communication with visual cues (e.g., pictures, objects) and non-verbal cues.
- Encourage speech, even if it is hard to understand.
- Show interest in the person.

Groher (1989, p. 35) noted the importance of standing on the unaffected side of the person with stroke illness, thereby maximising the likelihood of non-verbal cues being seen. He offered useful advice in relation to word-finding problems, suggesting if you know the word being searched for, you could consider helping with sentence completion by saying, for instance, 'I want a drink of…', then pausing. The patient may then find it easier to fill in the missing word.

Aphasia often has an isolating effect on older people. Several clubs and groups help people with aphasia to communicate more effectively. Rayner and Marshall (2003) trained six volunteers from one such group as conversation partners for other people with aphasia. The training aimed to extend the volunteers' knowledge of aphasia and provide them with a selection of communication strategies that would help them to talk with people with aphasia and also enhance their own communication skills. The initiative was evaluated positively and high-lights the benefits of innovations designed specifically to address older people's communication needs for their well-being. Thompson and McKeever (2014, p. 18) noted an older person's health can be 'improved when nurses use communication to express concern and commitment and, in return, invite trust and human connection'.

Case Study 15.1 illustrates a nurse's awareness of how to communicate with an older person with stroke.

Dysarthria

Dysarthria is another common disorder related to speech impairment that can affect older people. Dysarthria com-promises the intelligibility of speech by poor muscle coor-dination and can be associated with respiratory function, difficulties in articulation, phonation (i.e., the ability to pro-duce sounds) and resonance (i.e., the quality of the sounds, such as loudness, depth) (Groher, 1989). These problems can cause distortions of all sounds, making speech tremu-lous or robotic, too slow or fast, slurred or softer, and hard to understand. Dysarthria is linked with several different illnesses and conditions of older age such as stroke or other brain injuries, tumours and Parkinson's disease. Sensitive communication that uses the tips below from the NHS website (https://www.nhs.uk/conditions/dysarthria/) and takes into account the treatment prescribed by a speech and language therapist is necessary to establish therapeutic communication.

- Reduce distractions and background noise when you're having a conversation.
- Look at the person as they talk.
- After speaking, allow them plenty of time to respond. If they feel rushed or pressured to speak, they may become anxious, which can affect their ability to communicate.
- Be careful about finishing their sentences or correcting errors in their language, as this may cause resentment and frustration.
- If you do not understand what they're trying to com-municate, do not pretend you understand, as they may find this patronising and upsetting. It's always best to be honest about your lack of understanding.
- If necessary, seek clarification by asking yes/no ques-tions or paraphrasing. For example, say, 'Did you ask me if I'd done the shopping?'

In addition the NHS gives tips for people who have dys-arthria (https://www.nhs.uk/conditions/dysarthria/) that might be useful to pass on to them or their carers:

- Take a deep breath before you start speaking.
- Put extra effort into saying key words.
- Speak slowly, saying one word at a time if necessary.
- Leave a clear space between each word.

CASE STUDY 15.1   Communicating With a Stroke Patient: A Nurse's Story

Mr Jenkins lay motionless in bed. He had just been ad-mitted to my ward from the Medical Assessment Unit after having a stroke. Although he was unable to talk or move, his eyes followed every movement I made as I tried to make him comfortable and adjust his intravenous infusion. I was to work with him for the rest of the shift.

After about 10 minutes, I realised it felt rather eerie be-ing watched so closely; I wasn't used to that. I went to fetch another pillow and thought about it and then I re-alised this was his way of communicating with me that I'd been so busy adjusting the intravenous infusion and trying to make him comfortable I'd said very little. Recog-nising this absence of verbal communication took me by surprise. I was usually aware of the importance of talking with people even when they weren't able to respond in words. After that I started to talk more about what I was doing. His eyes continued to follow me and my conversa-tion more attentively, as if they were listening themselves to what I was saying. He began to relax as I continued to talk about what was going to happen to him during the rest of the shift, who I was and who the rest of the team were who would be looking after him, and how long he might expect to have the intravenous infusion.

Recognising his need for explanation and the degree of normality conferred by my talking was an important way to settle Mr Jenkins into the ward and reassure him about his care.

- Make sure you're in the same room as the person you're talking to and face them.
- Attract the listener's attention—for example, by touch or calling their name before you begin talking to them.
- Keep sentences short, and avoid long conversations if you're feeling tired.
- Reduce background noise—for example, switch off the TV or radio.
- Repeat yourself if needed.

Assessment

Nurses may be among the first people to identify a speech impairment, which should be accurately noted and referred for specialist intervention early on to facilitate an appropri-ate plan of action. Assessment may be facilitated through the use of skilled communication and enhanced, in the case of aphasia, by using the shortened, non-specialist Frenchay Aphasia Screening Test (FAST) (Enderby et al., 2013), which focuses largely on comprehension and verbal expression and takes less than 10 minutes to complete.

Coping with a speech impairment may be an all-consuming task for an older person, taking up a large amount of energy and concentration. For many people speech impairment causes considerable frustration, as speech is generally regarded as the mainstay of communication, and effective alternatives are hard to find. Nurses who care for people with a speech disorder need to be aware of the far-reaching effects of this impairment on an older person's social, psychological, emotional and physical well-being.

Communication and Dementia

Over the past few decades knowledge of dementia has considerably increased, including its impact on the person living with dementia, their family and relatives and their formal and informal carers. (Visit the Alzheimer's Society website for more information.) Treatments and approaches to care have altered and progressed, but sensitive, skilled communication remains central to person-centred, high-quality care, and nurses are in key positions to provide it. Regardless of diagnostic category or the stage of a person's illness, each person with dementia and their families and friends may be bewildered and frustrated as their illness progresses. These challenges are more prominent as a person struggles to make sense of slipping between cognitive clarity and opaqueness, watches and feels relationships and independence change without understanding why, and becomes confused as to why the rules of everyday life no longer make sense. It becomes hard to maintain past levels of communication, so nurses need to be creative and clear in the ways they communicate and ensure communication is altered to suit each person with dementia.

Effects of Dementia on Communication

Dementia can have a far-reaching impact on the ways people communicate. When alterations to communication are combined with other behaviours linked to dementia, such as wandering or forgetfulness, or the safety precautions needed in a pandemic, they may result in frustration, anger and further isolation for both the person with dementia and the people who provide care. Some of the most common effects of dementia on communication are outlined below.

- Speech and language disruption vary with the stage of dementia but are likely to include, during the course of the disease, poor comprehension, reduced vocabulary that results in the need to search for appropriate words, difficulty in naming objects, fragmentation of sentences, digression from the topic of conversation, echoing sounds, or, in the extreme, the older person may become mute. As the dementia progresses, the person's insight diminishes, and it becomes harder to cover up speech and language deficits. These changes have a significant effect on the older person's communication skills and the quality of their interactions.

- Written skills and the ability to use different technologies also deteriorate, with difficulty in choosing correct words or constructing sentences.
- Difficulty in following conversations results from poor comprehension and diminished attention span. Conversations may be easier when long-term memory is used.

Assessing Communication Impairments Associated With Dementia

Assessment is a complicated process in which all members of the multidisciplinary team have a role. Nurses may find it useful to consider Jacques's (1992) advice that listening to the older person speak provides important information on the use of the right words, appropriate sentence structures, difficulties in articulation and naming objects. Consideration of these factors helps the nurse determine the effects of dementia on communicative abilities and how they impact the care planned for the person. Assessment at an early stage helps nurses recognise progressive deterioration in communication skills and alerts them to the need to modify their own skills to suit the older person's needs. (See Chapter 29 for more information on assessment in dementia.)

Communicating With an Older Person With Dementia

As the disease progresses, it is unlikely significant improvements can be made in the older person's communicative ability. Therefore, efforts need to be directed toward modifying the communication skills of all others who interact with the person, which is naturally time-consuming, as the abilities and needs of the person with dementia vary from day to day and person to person. The goal of successful communication, in this instance, is to create an environment that facilitates flexible communication by all carers, both lay and professional, and is guided by the older person's changing needs. Carers need to adapt their communication styles to suit how the older person experiences dementia. Goldsmith (1996) suggested some useful general strategies for communicating with someone who has dementia:
- Make the environment conducive to communication. For instance, make sure the TV or radio is switched off.
- Leave enough time for the interaction.
- Approach the older person slowly and within his or her line of vision.
- Reinforce your verbal communication with touch if appropriate.
- Listen.
- Use short sentences.
- Allow enough time for responses, and do not immediately decide the older person hasn't understood the conversation if they don't respond.
- Try to illustrate what you are saying with photos or objects.

- Don't feel it is necessary to correct mistakes in conversation.
- Do not be embarrassed by the expression of emotions in the interaction.

In addition to these strategies, many experts now emphasise the importance of non-verbal behaviours in improving communication. For instance, Daily Caring (https://daily-caring.com/dementia-communication-techniques-calm-positive-body-language/) highlights a series of non-verbal behaviours carers could use that focus on voice, gesture, touch, eye contact, body movements and posture, and space. They are similar to some suggested earlier by Tanner and Daniels (1990), based on their observations of interactions between eight carers and their relatives with dementia, that may be useful for nurses to consider in relation to their own practice or to give as advice to relatives of people with dementia. Also remember a person with dementia may have other age-related communcation difficulties to be taken into consideration.

Since Tanner and Daniels's (1990) work, many researchers and pracitioners have investigated the best ways to communicate with older people who have dementia. One of the most common conclusions from this body of knowledge is the importance of fostering trust and respect. However, the ways through which trust and respect are created depends very much on the people concerned and nurses' understandings of each older person. This includes making, sharing and recording assessments of each person's wishes, life stories and interests; observing how the person and the nurse behave in particular situations; having discussions with their family and friends; and evaluating how well (or not) communication strategies work in practice and altering them as needed to create the best environment of care for each person.

Communicating with a person with dementia may be a time-consuming and complex undertaking but one that, if done successfully, has the potential to increase physical, social, emotional and psychological well-being (see Chapter 29).

The management of the COVID-19 pandemic resulted in intense social isolation for many older people, especially those who live alone in the community and people in long-term care facilities who live with dementia. Limitations to family and friend visits and in some cases limited physical contact with staff or other patients or residents, along with the use of personal protective equipment by nurses, other permanent or visiting staff and volunteers, often negatively affected communication. It is difficult to read lips when someone is wearing a mask, and it is also challenging to hear each other or read sign language when maintaining a safe distance. Nurses who care for older adults in these situations need to be aware and alert that safety measures are depersonalising and frightening, particularly to individuals with underlying cognitive impairments or dementia, and as such adapt their care to ensure patients and residents are safeguarded against potential negative outcomes (O'Hanlon & Inouye, 2020).

Sensory Deprivation

Sensory deprivation may be associated with any of the communication challenges discussed above. It may also occur as a result of diminished social contact, isolation or living in an unstimulating environment. In care settings nurses have a key role to play in keeping sensory deprivation to a minimum and ensuring social distancing does not lead to social isolation. Skilled communication, using the full range of verbal, written, graphic and non-verbal cues, is particularly valuable in overcoming sensory deprivation, whether it is associated with environment-, age- or illness-related changes to communication. The information provided in this chapter will help nurses minimise the likelihood of older people experiencing sensory deprivation.

Sensory deprivation can have far-reaching effects on older people that could lead to the following:

- Exaggerated personality traits
- Emotional changes such as boredom, restlessness, irritability and anxiety
- Perceptual disorganisation, including alterations in perceptions of colour, shapes and movements
- An inability to think and solve problems
- In extreme cases, hallucinations
- Increased somatic complaints
- Fluctuating emotional states
- Disturbance to usual routines such as sleeping
- Disorientation due to an unusual environment

These affects may be exacerbated when combined with illness.

Nurses need to create a stimulating environment for individuals who are not acutely ill by working with other health care professionals, particularly occupational therapists, activity specialists and dementia champions. The nurse's communication skills and knowledge of the older person are central to establishing a partnership so each person feels involved in decisions regarding activities designed to meet individual interests. The net result of partnership is to offer a choice of activities that minimise boredom and restlessness. Increasingly, long-term care facilities are creating sensory rooms where the five senses are stimulated to promote relaxation or stimulation and interest as well as to spark conversation.

Sensory deprivation may be minimised by helping older people maintain their own identity by bringing special items from their homes when they need to move into long-term care settings or their hospital stay becomes lengthy. For people who require acute care, a stay in hospital detaches them from the pace of life outside the hospital, so they may feel deprived of their everyday routines or fearful of returning to their previous lifestyle. Nurses should discuss this issue with patients, their friends or relatives as well as other members of the multidisciplinary care team so readjustment following discharge can be optimised.

Challenging Behaviour

Sometimes older people exhibit what is referred to as challenging behaviour, either physically or through their style of communication. Challenging communication behaviours include the following:

- Expressions of frustration with physical, social, emotional or psychological status
- Expressions of anger
- Misunderstandings
- Having insufficient information on which to base decisions
Such behaviours may be linked to a person's illness experience or be part of their natural character. Nurses find it useful to determine the source of the problem and discuss how the problem can be resolved, potentially using the following strategies:

- Keeping calm
- Allowing the person to express strong feelings
- Acknowledging their feelings have been heard
- Using assertive statements (i.e., clear, honest and direct) or assertive techniques in reply, such as the 'broken-record technique'—repeating, in a relaxed way, what you think is important or what you want from the situation with the aim of getting the other person to begin negotiating the way forward
- Listening to what is being said
- Negotiating a way forward
- If the interaction becomes too heated, leaving and returning later
- It's always useful to document what works or doesn't work in certain situations so everyone knows how best challenging behaviours can be managed.

THE THERAPEUTIC VALUE OF COMMUNICATION BETWEEN OLDER PEOPLE AND NURSES

Nursing is an interactive, relational process where the quality of the relationship between nurse and patient has marked effects on the physical, social, emotional and psychological well-being of patients and their quality of life. For many years nursing has been described as therapeutic through its ability to help people make positive movements toward health (Ersser, 1997). The use of highly developed communication skills that allow nurses to 'see and hear the individual behind the label or diagnosis, taking into account the increasing diversity of older people as a demographic group' (Blood, 2013, p. 13) is one way of facilitating this movement.

An interpersonal relationship may start with the negotiation of partnerships between nurses and patients, which involves attending, enabling, interpreting, responding and anticipating. For patients, negotiation means managing themselves, affiliating with experts and interpreting the experience. Each activity is intrinsically associated with communication and thus provides a link between the notion of therapeutic nursing and communication with the nurse during the process of care and becoming 'a companion through the ordeal' (Christensen, 1993, p. 34). Once the partnership is negotiated, the work of the nurse and patient centres on maintaining the therapeutic nature of the partnership, relying on the use of sensitive communication skills to ensure care is person-centred. The emphasis on partnership development during care in hospital and community-based settings has been explored in the nursing literature—for example, in the work of Brendan McCormack on person-centred health care practice (Lieshout et al., 2015). There is growing consensus in nursing that patients know what sets the 'good' nurse apart—for example, being calm, professional, intuitive, acknowledging and respectful of the patient's preferences and values. Dewar and Nolan (2013) explored therapeutic communication through appreciative caring conversations, emphasising who people are and what matters to them, and how people feel about their experience, to provide better relationship-centred care on acute wards for older people. They advocated a model of communication that focuses on the 7 Cs, which encourage nurses to be **c**ourageous, **c**onnect emotionally, be **c**urious, **c**onsider other perspectives, **c**ollaborate, **c**ompromise and **c**elebrate (My Home Life Scotland, n.d.).

Good quality communication is affected by the underpinning values of the nurse or the unit where the nurse works and also by the professional and personal characteristics of the nurse, patient and family or friends who accompany the older person during the interaction (Cook et al., 1990). The interplay between this triad can complicate interactions or facilitate them, as the nurse in a hard-pressed health-care system (i.e., with workforce shortages, high turnover or excess use of agency staff) may find the older person and their family and friends have conflicting opinions. Organisational factors could compromise how nurses want to give their best and be compassionate, as the system is more interested in ticking boxes (Sims et al., 2020). Careful negotiation between all involved is required to retain the focus of the interaction and enhance its therapeutic nature.

In summary, the use of skilled communication allows nurses to gather information from older people and their carers that facilitates sensitive assessment, planning, delivery and evaluation of person-centred care. Coupled with the potential to develop a rapport between the nurse and the older person, skilled communication builds trust, support and understanding, enabling a partnership to be established that facilitates collaborative decision-making.

SUCCESSFUL COMMUNICATION

Although there is no foolproof recipe for successful communication, the following general pointers and those in Box 15.1, help nurses consider how to enhance their communication skills when working with older people:

- Create an open atmosphere between interactors.
- Be available.
- Listen.
- Watch.
- Consider alternative forms of communication such as signing, simple preset movements like 'Nod your head if the answer is yes', word boards or talking mats and other assistive technologies.
- Acknowledge an older person's reality. Nussbaum et al.'s (1989) seminal text warned nurses against the use of disconfirming statements that do not acknowledge the older person's reality (e.g., ignoring comments or using childlike language in response to comments). Disconfirming statements can make people doubt themselves and their understanding of their own situation. Acknowleging an older person's reality is particularly important as many older people fear disconfirming statements in their fear of dementia and confusion. Older people may be seen as disconfirming to young people too—for example, through forgetfulness.
- Avoid oversimplified language and thinking older people lack intelligence if they do not understand. Childlike or patronising language is never appropriate.
- Check out interpretations.
- Avoid ritualistic or unrewarding conversations.
- Consider alternative communication media such as YouTube videos, music, art or literature.
- Create an environment conducive to communication or one that facilitates welcome solitude.

Augment these approaches by following Holden's (1988) authoritative guidelines for helping older people with verbal and non-verbal deficits. For verbal challenges, she proposed the following strategies. First, recognise communication impairments do not go hand-in-hand with older age. Second, talk with and do not ignore the person. If the patient is unable to speak to you, try alternatives such as writing notes or using gestures. Talk normally using simple language. Keep to one topic to avoid confusion, and choose a topic that is relevant. Do not fill in the blanks and complete sentences for the other person. Remember to check for communication aids: correct dentures, working hearing aids, clean spectacles. Always retain your patience and understanding.

Holden (1988) also addressed non-verbal challenges related to memory loss and movement disorder. For memory loss, she advised certain games (e.g., Scrabble, I Spy, Monopoly) and quizzes together with reminder notes, lists,

BOX 15.1   Behaviours That Enhance and Inhibit Communication (Tanner & Daniels, 1990)

To gain attention:
- Using non-verbal cues such as touch, eye contact and gesture
- Being in close proximity during the interaction
- Turning to face the older person
- Saying the person's preferred name
- Using a focus such as an object or photograph

During the conversation:
- Using a warm and encouraging tone of voice
- Speaking slightly louder
- Saying the person's name
- Making the content clear and simple by using short sentences
- Repeating and rephrasing statements
- Checking understanding by asking for clarification
- Using non-verbal cues such as eye contact, gesture and facial expression
- Using an object as a focus
- Interpreting the older person's behaviour or communication

In response to communication from the older person:
- Using non-verbal communication such as touch, eye contact, gesture, facial expression or laughter
- Using an appropriate tone of voice
- Using short sentences with simple content
- Giving confirmation
- Asking for clarification.

Behaviours that inhibit communication (Tanner & Daniels, 1990):
- Addressing older people while they are doing something else and not getting their attention
- Speaking too quickly and too quietly
- Not checking understanding
- Using a frustrated or exasperated tone of voice
- Using complicated sentences
- Having unrealistic expectations
- Giving insufficient explanation
- Using patronising language
- Excluding the older person from communication
- Not listening
- Using minimal non-verbal communication

written directions, and large-face clocks and calendars to facilitate everyday activities. Increasingly, computerised versions of games and reminder systems are available, as are various vitual assistant applications such Alexa-like technologies that promote easier engagement between older people and their environments. Movement disorders are likely to affect communication through clumsiness, inappropriate use of gestures or difficulty with daily living activities such as dressing, which alter appearance and affect interactors' perceptions. Holden suggested hand exercises to increase dexterity and formal relearning of other movements. Where older people have difficulty recognising objects through one channel (e.g., sight), Holden advised the use of other channels—touch, smell or sound—to enhance information and therefore provide a more complete picture of the object.

Enhance your approach with the use of reminiscence or story-telling to promote intergenerational understanding by

- Sharing attitudes, histories, backgrounds and experiences
- Increasing your awareness of life events
- Assessing psychological and social feelings of well-being
- Gathering information about the older person's physical, psychological and social function
- Identifying deficits in communication skills
- Facilitating rapport

Successful communication between nurses and older people can be enhanced and evaluated through an assessment of the older person's communication ability, ranging from language comprehension and expression to non-verbal skills. One useful tool to establish good communications knowledge is the FAST (Enderby et al., 2013), which can be used to identify language deficits such as language comprehension, expression, reading and writing and problems associated with articulation. The FAST is particularly useful because it was designed for use by non-specialists and can be used with other tests of sight, hearing and cognition to provide a useful starting point for formal assessment of communication skills, although the informal collection of information through everyday interactions should not be overlooked. Nurses must be able to highlight problems with communication so their care can be sensitively tailored to meet individual needs and they can make prompt referrals for specialist help when needed. Case Study 15.2 demonstrates a nurse's awareness of how to improve her communication with a patient with Parkinson's disease who had a history of falling.

CASE STUDY 15.2 Communicating With a Patient With Parkinson's Disease and a History of Falls: A Nurse's Reflections

For once I was early. I walked slowly into the day hospital. It was my first day back from holiday, and I felt refreshed and ready to tackle some of the challenges I'd left behind. I was thinking about how to solve some of those problems when, as I walked past the sitting room, my attention was drawn to a new patient. She was sitting by herself next to the window. She was smartly dressed and didn't seem distressed, but she had a distant look, her face strangely stiff and masklike. I carried on walking, thinking I would find out more about her at the handover report, especially as I was the primary nurse for that half of the unit.

Mrs Jackson had just been referred to the day hospital. Her general practitioner had been worried by the increased number of falls Mrs Jackson had experienced over the past fortnight and referred her for assessment by the rehabilitation team. She'd had Parkinson's disease for the past 10 years. She lived on her own and until recently had been very independent. Now, however, she was becoming more and more depressed because of her increased immobility and fear of falling.

The handover report ended, and I went straight to talk to Mrs Jackson. We spoke generally about her falls and tried to identify reasons for them. We thought about the layout of her home and the sort of activities she liked to do and tried to work out a plan of how she might do things she could talk through with the occupational therapist when he visited her later that morning. All the time

we were together I was aware of how slowly and carefully Mrs Jackson spoke to me; conversation took a lot of effort, and I was aware I was constantly thinking of finishing her sentences to hurry things along. I didn't, though, because that wouldn't really have helped.

When I handed over my patients at lunchtime to the afternoon staff, I talked through my concerns about communicating with Mrs Jackson—how I'd listened very carefully to her because she spoke slowly and quietly, how I was careful not to finish her sentences for her because I wanted to get on and how when she wrote down some of the things she needed to talk about with the occupational therapist, I noticed her hand had a slight tremor. I realised as I passed this information on how important it was for other people to know so they would encourage her to talk rather than leave her in isolation at her next visit and also recognise although her speech seemed slow and laborious, she was able to direct what was going on around her and was very enthusiastic about reducing the falls she had been experiencing.

As I went home I thought more about Mrs Jackson. I reflected on how some chronic illnesses affect the ways people communicate and how, although the person with the illness is used to these changes, sometimes carers find the effects difficult to deal with. I was pleased I'd had time to spend talking with Mrs Jackson, and I hadn't felt rushed in the ways I communicated with her.

CONCLUSION AND LEARNING POINTS

Many older people who require nursing care in the community or in hospital have problems associated with communication. This chapter focuses on the most common challenges to communication presented in older age and highlights how nurses can enhance their communication skills to help older people and their friends and relatives cope. Each challenge requires skilled therapeutic intervention to maintain or enhance every older person's physical, social and psychological well-being and quality of life.

All nurses, regardless of their speciality, need to be constantly aware of the changes associated with ageing and illness that might affect communication. It's also important to be aware of intergenerational differences between nurses and older people. Together with the development of a sensitive style of communication, nurses can facilitate therapeutic communication that provides information, support and social interaction to older people and their carers.

KEY LEARNING POINTS

- Communication is important throughout life but may be more complex in older age because of age-related and environmental challenges to communication.
- Although good individualised communication can be therapeutic, poor communication can impede care and negatively influence a person's quality of life.
- Today's multicultural societies comprise of culturally and linguistically diverse people. Older people and their families and carers need nurses to be culturally competent in their communications.

- Challenges to communication in older age include the natural course of ageing (e.g, altered hearing and seeing), illness (e.g., stroke or dementia), sensory deprivation (e.g., living in different care environments or in isolating situations such as during the COVID-19 pandemic) and challenging behaviours.
- Communication strategies need to be individualised, respectful and inclusive of everyone involved with the older person, including informal carers, volunteers, relatives and friends.

REFERENCES

Andersson, G., Melin, L., Scott, B., & Lindberg, P. (1994). Behavioural counselling for subjects with acquired hearing loss: A new approach to hearing tactics. *Scandinavian Audiology, 23*, 249–256.

Andrews, N., Gabbay, J., le May, A., Miller, M., O'Neill, M., & Petch, A. (2015). *Developing evidence-enriched practice in health and social care*. Joseph Rowntree Foundation.

Andrews, N., Gabbay, J., le May, A., Miller, M., Petch, A., & O'Neill, M. (2020). Story, dialogue and caring about what matters to people: Progress towards evidence-enriched policy and practice. *Evidence & Policy, 16*(4).

Argyle, M. (1994). *The psychology of interpersonal behaviour* (5th ed.). Penguin.

Armstrong, L., & McKechnie, K. (2003). Intergenerational communication: Fundamental but under-exploited theory for speech and language therapy with older people. *International Journal of Language and Communication Disorders, 38*, 13–29.

Batt-Rawden, K. B., & Stedje, K. (2020). Singing as a health-promoting activity in elderly care: A qualitative, longitudinal study in Norway. *Journal of Research in Nursing, 25*(5), 404–418.

Biggs, S. (1993). *Understanding ageing*. Open University Press.

Blood, I. (2013). *A better life: Valuing our later years*. Joseph Rowntree Foundation.

Brown, A. (2020). Will COVID-19 affect the delivery of compassionate nursing care? *Nursing Times, 116*(10), 32–35.

Christensen, J. (1993). *Nursing partnership. A model for nursing practice*. Churchill Livingstone.

Cook, M., Coe, R., & Hanson, K. (1990). Physician–elderly patient communication: Processes and outcomes of medical encounters. In S. Stahl (Ed.), *The legacy of longevity* (pp. 291–309). Sage.

DailyCaring. (n.d.). How to talk to someone with dementia: calm, positive body language. https://dailycaring.com/dementia-communication-techniques-calm-positive-body-language.

Dewar, B., & Nolan, M. (2013). Caring about caring: Developing a model to implement compassionate relationship centred care in an older people care setting. *International Journal of Nursing Studies, 50*(9), 1247–1258.

Dorgo, S., King, G. A., Bader, J. O., & Limon, J. S. (2013). Outcomes of a peer mentor implemented fitness program in older adults: A quasi-randomized controlled trial. *International Journal of Nursing Studies, 50*(9), 1156–1165.

Dowd, J. (1986). The old person as stranger. In V. Marshall (Ed.), *Later life: The social psychology of aging* (pp. 147–189). Sage.

Ebersole, P., & Hess, P. (2019). *Toward healthy aging: human needs and nursing response* (10th ed.). Mosby.

Enderby, P., Wood, V., & Wade, D. (2013). *Frenchay Aphasia Screening Test (FAST)* (3rd ed.). Stass Publications.

Ersser, S. (1997). *Nursing as a therapeutic activity: An ethnography*. Avebury.

Ford, J., & Sinclair, R. (1987). *Sixty years on: Women talk about old age*. Women's Press.

Giles, H., & Coupland, N. (1991). *Language: contexts and consequences*. Open University Press.

Goldsmith, M. (1996). *Hearing the voice of people with dementia: Opportunities and obstacles.* Jessica Kingsley.

Groher, M. (1989). Neurologically based disorders of speech and language among older adults. In R. Hull, & K. Griffin (Eds.), *Communication disorders in aging* (pp. 23–37). Sage.

Hargie, O. (2018). Communication as skilled behaviour. In O. Hargie (Ed.), *A handbook of communication skills* (6th ed., pp. 7–21). Routledge.

Hargie, O., & Marshall, P. (1993). Interpersonal communication: A theoretical framework. In O. Hargie (Ed.), *A handbook of communication skills* (pp. 22–56). Routledge.

Holden, U. (1988). Recognizing the problems. In U. Holden (Ed.), *Neuropsychology and ageing* (pp. 1–22). Croom Helm.

Hull, R. (1989). The hearing-impaired older adult. In R. Hull, & K. Griffin (Eds.), *Communication disorders in aging* (pp. 91–102). Sage.

Jacques, A. (1992). *Understanding dementia*: Churchill Livingstone.

Lieshout, F., Titchen, A., McCormack, B., & McCance, T. (2015). Compassion in facilitating the development of person-centred health care practice. *Journal of Compassionate Health Care, 2*, 5.

Markey, K., O'Brien, B., O'Donnell, C., Martin, C., & Murphy, J. (2021). Enhancing undergraduate nursing curricula to cultivate person-centred care for culturally and linguistically diverse older people. *Nurse Education in Practice, 50*, Article 102936. https://doi.org/10.1016/j.nepr.2020.102936.

Monaghan, A. (1995). Communication. In H. Heath (Ed.), *Foundations in nursing theory and practice* (pp. 275–298). Mosby.

My Home Life Scotland. (n.d.). Caring conversations. http://myhomelife.uws.ac.uk/scotland/caring-conversations

Nature Aging. (2021). Editorial: Stengthening intergenerational connections. *Nature Aging*(323), 1.

NHS. (n.d.). Dysarthria (difficulty speaking). https://www.nhs.uk/conditions/dysarthria/.

Nussbaum, J., Thompson, T., & Robinson, J. (1989). *Communication and aging.* Harper & Row.

O'Hanlon, S., & Inouye, S. K. (2020). Delirium: A missing piece in the COVID-19 pandemic puzzle. *Age and Ageing, 49*(4), 497–498. https://doi.org/10.1093/ageing/afaa094.

Purnell, L., & Fenkl, E. (2020). *Textbook for transcultural health care: A population approach.* Springer Nature.

Rayner, H., & Marshall, J. (2003). Training volunteers as conversation partners for people with aphasia. *International Journal of Language and Communication Disorders, 38*, 149–164.

Royal National Institue for Deaf People (n.d.). Communication tips for health and social care professionals. https://RNID.org.uk/information-and-support/support-for-health-and-social-care-professionals/communication-tips-for-healthcare-professionals

Ryan, E., Meredith, S., MacLean, M., & Orange, J. (1995). Changing the way we talk with elders: Promoting health using the communication enhancement model. *International Journal of Aging and Human Development, 41*, 89–107.

Sims, S., Leamy, M., Levenson, R., Brearley, S., Ross, F., & Harris, R. (2020). The delivery of compassionate nursing care in a tick-box culture: Qualitative perspectives from a realist evaluation of intentional rounding. *International Journal of Nursing Studies* https://doi.10.1016/j.ijnurstu.2020.103580.

Stroke Association. (n.d.). Types of aphasia. https://www.stroke.org.uk/what-is-aphasia/types-of-aphasia

Tanner, B., & Daniels, K. (1990). An observation study of communication between carers and their relatives with dementia. *Care of the Elderly, 2*, 247–250.

Teal, C. R., & Street, R. L. (2009). Critical elements of culturally competent communication in the medical encounter: A review and model. *Social Science & Medicine, 68*(3), 533–543.

Thompson, J., & McKeever, M. (2014). Improving support for patients with aphasia. *Nursing Times, 110*(25), 18–20.

van der Roest, H., Prins, M., van der Velden, C., Steinmetz, S., Stolte, E., van Tilburg, T. G., & de Vries, D. H. (2020). The impact of COVID-19 measures on well-being of older long-term care facility residents in the Netherlands. *Journal of the American Medical Directors Association.* https://doi.org/10.1016/j.jamda.2020.09.007.

Vogelpoel, N., & Jarrold, K. (2014). Social prescription and the role of participatory arts programmes for older people with sensory impairments. *Journal of Integrated Care, 22*(2), 39–50.

Weinreich, H. M. (2017). Hearing loss and patient-physician communication: The role of an otolaryngologist. *JAMA Otolaryngology—Head & Neck Surgery, 143*(10), 1055–1057.

Worrall, L., & Hickson, L. (2003). *Communication disability in aging: From prevention to intervention.* Thomson.

Yuan, S., Hussain, S. A., Hales, K. D., & Cotton, S. R. (2016). What do they like? Communication preferences and patterns of older adults in the United States: The role of technology. *Educational Gerontology, 42*(3). https://doi.org/10.1080/03601277.2015.1083392.

16

Older People and Hearing

Helen Pryce, Nisha Dhanda

CHAPTER OUTLINE

Communication is an important part of social life; hearing difficulties in all age groups can present many challenges for individuals, their families and their contacts. Difficulty with hearing is a common consequence of growing old (Yamasoba et al., 2013). Hearing impairment in older people may cause greater disability than in younger people because of the impact of other disabilities, especially visual impairments, on their everyday life. There is enormous potential for nurses to support people who are affected by age-related hearing problems provided they know how to recognise problems and understand how to support individuals and their families. This chapter explores the evidence that should inform the practice of nurses who work with older people across all care settings.

We start with an overview of the function of the ear and hearing mechanisms and move on to the activities of hearing and listening. We discuss prevalence and aetiology of hearing impairment as well as ear wax and the concepts of function, activity and participation. From this foundation we focus on the knowledge essential to understanding and caring for older people with hearing impairment and those who choose to use hearing aids. The chapter provides advice on ways nurses can contribute to enabling care for both individuals and their regular communication partners. We explore the relationship between hearing loss and

dementia and how communication adjustments and management strategies can reduce the effects of social isolation. Finally we look at tinnitus to complete our exploration of common problems older people experience with their auditory functioning.

THE FUNCTION OF THE EAR

The function of the ear is to convert sound waves in the air to electrical impulses in the auditory nerve. The ear is divided into the external, middle and inner ears. The external ear comprises the pinna and the external auditory canal, which collect sound and direct it to the tympanic membrane that divides the external and middle ears. The middle ear is an air-filled cavity that contains the ossicular chain: the malleus, incus and stapes. This chain of tiny bones converts sound waves in the air to sound waves in the fluid that fills the inner ear, or cochlea. The sound waves in the fluid of the inner ear bend the hairs on the hair cells. As the hairs bend, chemicals are released that generate an electrical impulse in the auditory nerve.

A foundational understanding of how the normal ear works enables nurses to appreciate normal function and the principles of auditory rehabilitation. It also facilitates information-giving to older people and in particular helps nurses make sense of hearing aids and other assistive listening devices. A useful overview of age-related changes in the auditory system is provided by Wang and Puel (2020).

Abnormalities of the external or middle ear, such as impacted wax or a perforation of the tympanic membrane, cause a conductive hearing impairment. The conduction of sound to the inner ear is impaired, so loudness is reduced, similar to turning down the volume on a TV or radio. A sensorineural hearing impairment is due to pathology in the inner ear or the auditory nerve, most commonly loss of hair cells in the cochlea. In addition to reduced loudness, there is commonly loss of frequency and temporal resolution, so even though sounds may be heard, discrimination of individual sounds is poor. Thus, in addition to the reduced perception of sound, the way sounds of different pitches or frequencies are heard is affected. This is similar to a radio where the volume is too low and not tuned properly. Although some sounds may be audible, they are distorted and difficult to recognise, and word recognition becomes difficult.

HEARING AND LISTENING

Hearing and listening are integral to communication that involves speech or other sounds. Hearing is a passive activity in that an individual's ability to hear is a given; listening, on the other hand, is an active and dynamic process. A person's capacity to listen and motivation to engage in the act of listening depend on a number of factors. To begin with, the listener needs to be alert to sounds and, in effect, tune in and focus on interesting ones. Lack of interest in the topic, tiredness, distractions

and low mood make people disinclined to listen. Similarly, if a conversation does not include the listener, while they may be aware people are talking, they may to some extent ignore them and exercise a degree of choice over intentional listening. Difficult listening circumstances, such as in the presence of background noise or when hearing ability is poor, require a greater effort to understand what is being said, and the work of listening becomes harder. A common complaint of older people is sometimes others, including nurses, exclude them from conversations or expect them to communicate in a disabling listening environment (Mamo et al., 2019). It is important for nurses to recognise and make distinctions between hearing and listening and consider interventions that enable older people to maximise their communication potential.

PREVALENCE OF HEARING IMPAIRMENT

Hearing impairment is defined as a mean hearing level of 25 decibels (dB) or greater (see Fig. 16.1). It is common. About 20% of the United Kingdom's adult population have a hearing impairment in their better hearing ear (Akeroyd, 2014), a prevalence that is expected to rise (World Heath Organization, 2018). The proportion of the population with hearing impairment rises significantly in older people (Table 16.1). Individuals with thresholds of 25 decibels hearing level (dBHL) or worse have at least a mild hearing impairment. Those with thresholds of 45 dBHL or more have at least a moderate impairment and should have audiological rehabilitation. Of individuals in the United Kingdom with a hearing impairment in their better hearing ear, about three-quarters are over 60, and one-quarter are over 80. In the great majority of cases it is a sensorineural hearing impairment.

AETIOLOGY OF HEARING IMPAIRMENT

Sensorineural hearing impairment becomes increasingly common with advancing years. This does not mean it is

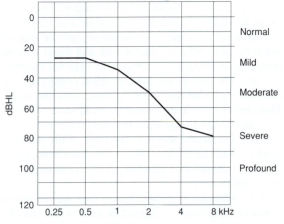

Fig. 16.1 Typical pure-tone audiogram of sensorineural hearing impairment with normal descriptors for hearing thresholds.

Age Group (years)	Hearing ≥ 25 dBHL (%)	Hearing ≥ 45 dBHL (%)
61–70	36.8	7.4
71	60.3	17.6
81	93.4	63.6

TABLE 16.1   **Prevalence of Hearing Impairment in the Better-Hearing Ear in Age Bands**

dBHL = Decibel hearing level.

caused by age, and it is unfair to older people to attribute it to their age. The only significant cause of sensorineural hearing loss that can be readily identified is noise exposure, most commonly industrial noise. People who worked in shipyards, steelworks and similar heavy industries commonly have sensorineural hearing impairment; hence old terms such as 'boilermaker's deafness'. However, the majority of older patients with hearing impairment did not work in noisy occupations. There are probably many factors involved, some related to lifestyle and some to environment. In the great majority of people, no specific causes can be identified.

Sensorineural hearing impairment is usually more marked at high frequencies (Moore, 2016). These are the frequencies at which vocal sounds such as 'd', 't', 's', 'sh' and 'f' occur. This is part of the reason why older people often say they can hear people speaking but have difficulty making out what is said. They can hear vowels and laryngeal tones—commonly the middle of words—but not the beginning or end. Shouting at such a person usually does not help and may make things more difficult.

Older people can also have a conductive hearing impairment, although it affects only a small proportion of the hearing impaired in this age group. It can be caused by simple obstruction of the external auditory canal by wax or diseases of the middle ear. The most easily identified is chronic otitis media, where there is usually a perforation of the tympanic membrane, sometimes with discharge. The ossicles may be damaged, either eroded by infection or fixed by scar tissue.

EAR WAX

Ear wax is produced in the lateral third of the external auditory canal. It keeps the lining of the ear canal moist and serves a protective function. Ear wax or cerumen is continuously moved outward by the natural migration of the skin in the ear canal and can be removed by normal washing with soapy water and a flannel. Repeated use of cotton buds is not recommended, as it can push the ear wax into a compact clump deep in the canal and if used with force can cause damage to the delicate lining of the canal (Somerville, 2002). Ear wax tends be less copious but harder in older adults due to increased amounts of keratin.

Where wax is impacted, there are three options. The most desirable is to use softening ear drops that can be purchased over the counter or prescribed by a physician or nurse prescriber. It is preferable to use gentle preparations such as docusate sodium or simple oil-based solutions rather than solvents, which, if used incorrectly, can lead to irritation and inflammation. An informative review of the evidence is offered in National Institute for Health and Care Excellence guidance (2019). If ear drops fail, ear syringing or manual extraction can be performed by a skilled nurse or doctor; however, the evidence base for mechanical methods of removing ear wax is limited (Radford, 2020). In the community, practice nurses or general practitioners undertake ear syringing; in hospital services physicians and nurses working in specialist services or who have demonstrated competence may undertake ear syringing. Although a relatively safe procedure in skilled hands (Radford, 2020), some patients dislike it, particularly if they experience the unpleasant sensation of vertigo but more usually due to the water being too cold or too hot. A more common method of wax removal is microsuction, where a small vacuum is placed inside the ear canal to dislodge and suck out the wax. This method is the more recent preferred choice for health professionals who carry out the procedure. Details on these methods are provided by the British Society of Audiology guidelines (2021).

It has been estimated one-third of older adults experience cerumen impaction (Gabriel, 2015). If wax is impacted against the tympanic membrane or if it totally occludes the ear canal, it may cause a conductive hearing impairment. Where impaction has occurred, removal can improve a person's perception of ability to hear. However, many older people incorrectly assume wax removal will significantly improve their hearing and are left disappointed. Wax obstruction can feel uncomfortable and interfere with hearing-aid fitting; for these reasons its removal is often indicated (Somerville, 2002). It is important older people understand they are unlikely to notice a marked improvement in their ability to hear given the high prevalence of acquired sensorineural hearing impairment.

HEARING FUNCTION, ACTIVITY AND PARTICIPATION

A useful way to begin thinking about the scope for nursing interventions is to reflect on the international classifications of impairment, activity and participation (World Health Organization, 1999). Hearing loss reduces ability to hear a range of important sounds, from the phone ringing to speech and conversation.

Impairment is the abnormal function of the hearing mechanism that can be measured, for example by audiometry. Activity changes are influenced by an individual's circumstances, for example hearing in a noisy place. Participation is the consequent restriction in social engagement that might follow. There are a number of ways to assess levels of activity and participation, but the easiest is often simply to ask if there's anything a person would like to be able to hear better and if there are things they have stopped doing as a result of changes to their hearing. It is also useful to learn how confident people feel in addressing their hearing loss and how important it is for them to take action. This varies according to individual values and preferences.

The most effective models of rehabilitation embrace the physical and social environment as well as an understanding of cognitive and psychological aspects (Edwards, 2016).

ASSESSMENT OF HEARING

Self-Report

Optimal understanding of the nature of a person's hearing problem and the benefits or limitations they might anticipate from interventions require an appreciation of the individual's perception of the problem and others in the immediate environment. Studies have shown older people tend to underreport hearing difficulties and often ask for help by saying a member of their family thinks they have a problem (Gopinath et al., 2012). The usual admission query 'Do you have problems with your hearing?' is totally inadequate, as most people say no. More useful questions to ask include whether they need the television or radio volume louder than others do and to explore their experience and ability to participate in conversation in noisy situations such as social gatherings in shops and church.

Audiometry

Pure-tone audiometry is the basic test that assesses hearing thresholds over a range of frequencies for each ear (see Fig. 16.1). The approved methodology for testing was written by the British Society of Audiology (2018). Testing is carried out in soundproofed rooms or booths. Tones through a range of frequencies are played into each ear, and the patient reports when they hear them. The scale is designed so normal hearing thresholds are between 0 and 20 dBHL, and it is displayed on an audiogram. Rather than reporting audiometry as numerical thresholds that mean relatively little to the non-specialist, it is usually reported in terms that convey the hearing disability an individual with those thresholds is likely to suffer. The terms in Figure 16.1 are widely used. Although audiometry remains the gold standard of assessing hearing sensitivity, it does not provide information on how a person processes speech (Musiek et al., 2017). Instead it provides a baseline of how well a person can detect tones at various pitches, which can be used to prescribe hearing aids. The

audiogram should be a starting point for hearing assessment and management options.

Shared Decision Making With Hearing Loss

A hearing loss creates substantial work for the affected individual. Straining to hear conversation and worrying about missing phone calls and doorbells are sources of stress and effort (Ramsdell, 1978). The help available for hearing loss also creates work. The practicalities of attending appointments are difficult for people with comorbidities. Hearing aids may help with some sounds but not all, and the tradeoff between using hearing aids and getting benefit varies from individual to individual (Pryce & Hall, 2014). For some people, changing a phone to an amplified one or using a TV aid to hear TV may be a better choice than using hearing aids all the time. There has been a move across health care toward shared decision making to determine the best treatment for each individual set of ciurcumstances. Only an individual can determine where the tradeoffs in the work required to manage hearing loss are. Decision aids such as the hearing loss option grid can help weigh up the pros and cons of different options (Pryce & Hall, 2014).

For nurses who support older people over an extended period of time, such as community nurses and those in long-term care settings, it is important to review progress at agreed on intervals to ensure the older person's preferences continue to be met. Being alert to increasing changes in hearing and facilitating early referral are crucially important.

THE EXPERIENCE OF AGE-RELATED HEARING IMPAIRMENT

A significant consequence of unaddressed age-related hearing impairment is communication is incomplete and frustrating. When communication breakdown becomes a regular occurrence, it is often easier for people to withdraw from social situations rather than undergo the listening effort to engage in conversation. Evidence suggests when hearing loss is not appropriately managed in older adults, there is a greater risk of becoming socially isolated (Shukla et al., 2020). We refer to social isolation as 'the objective state of having few social relationships or infrequent social contact with others' (National Academies of Sciences, Engineering, and Medicine, 2020). *Social isolation* is often used interchangably with *loneliness*, and while they both refer to a sense of withdrawal, social isolation can be thought of as the absence of connectedness, which may or may not lead to loneliness and dementia (Sundström et al., 2019).

Both hearing loss and social isolation have been identified as modifiable risk factors for dementia, and the associations between the three are very much intertwined. A deterioration in communication is the common denominator that can lead to reduced quality of life and well-being in older adults who live with these conditions. This has been especially noted in residential care facilities where there is much irony placed in the focus of communal spaces and activities, yet residents describe isolation and missing social contact (Pryce & Gooberman-Hill, 2012). The introduction of water clubs in residential care facilities not only improved hydration but also created an environment for conversation and social interaction between care home residents who would otherwise not engage (Gleibs et al., 2011). This simple strategy helped improve communication and well-being and could be used as an example for other social initiatves.

A wealth of research in recent years suggests a relationship between hearing loss and cognitive impairment or dementia based on observational studies that analysed the number of people within a study group who naturally developed cognitive impairment or dementia over time and whether having hearing loss earlier in life predicted the risk of developing dementia (Lin et al., 2011; Gallacher et al., 2012). The nature of observational studies makes it difficult to determine a cause-and-effect relationship between hearing loss and dementia because of the many factors that could influence the development of a disease that cannot be predicted or controlled for. Similarly, appropriate measures of social isolation have not been included in observational studies or used interchangeably with loneliness, frequency of contact with family and friends, or marital status. This makes it difficult to quantify or measure social isolation, especially in the context of a causal pathway.

Hearing loss in midlife has been identified as the biggest modifiable risk factor for dementia in later life (Livingston et al., 2020). However, there is no evidence hearing aids reduce the risks of developing dementia. Hearing aids need to be prescribed appropriately as part of a shared decision-making process. What's more common is hearing loss and dementia co-occurring without adequate consideration of a person's communication needs. Both conditions involve a decline in communication to some extent. With hearing impairment, receptive language skills are often affected. This refers to abilities such as listening, hearing, remembering and understanding words and sentences. As dementia progresses, both receptive and expressive language skills are affected. This refers to articulating and expressing speech sounds in a coherent manner. Strategies to enhance the communication opportunities for people living with hearing loss and dementia include providing an optimal acoustic environment that is conducive to conversation (i.e., carpeted floors, soft furnishings, minimal noise sources, natural daylight without glare), understanding disordered

language and 'reading between the lines' of what a person is trying to communicate, making people feel heard and understood through positive body language and empathy, and encouraging and maintaining social connectedness by understanding a person's social identity and asking how many people they feel connected to. On a more practical level, learning the basic functions of hearing aids and assistive listening devices allows immediate relief for individuals who rely on these devices to aid communication and require assistance.

The impact of hearing loss on a person's life varies but can include threats to self-esteem, a reduced sense of security and loneliness (Shukla et al., 2020). Reduced feelings of well-being can contribute to the risk of depression and an increased dependence on others. The consensus view in the literature is hearing difficulties reduce the quality of life of older people by interfering with communication and the social and emotional domains of their lives. Successive studies have shown this to be true for people who live independently and those classified as dependent, such as residents in care homes (Pryce & Gooberman-Hill, 2012).

Understanding the impact on an individual's life is an essential step in audiological rehabilitation. Some studies suggest the restrictions people experience in their ability to participate (i.e., their hearing handicap) influence their decision to seek help (Pryce et al., 2016). Environmental factors that impact an individual's experience include physical and non-physical attributes of their worlds such as the communication skills of their immediate family members and their ability to create an enabling listening environment within the home. Although personal factors are specific to an individual, common experiences are frustration, embarrassment, irritability, anxiety and feeling upset, which culminate in a developing sense of isolation, becoming unsociable and feeling awkward in company. There is evidence older people with a hearing impairment show more symptoms of depression than their counterparts with good hearing (Lawrence et al., 2020).

Age-related hearing impairment tends to develop slowly, and people may be unaware until it restricts their daily lives. In one of the few phenomenological studies of older individuals' experience of hearing problems, Karlsson Espmark and Scherman (2003) highlighted individuals may consider it is other people's fault they can't hear, blaming others for mumbling or talking too quietly. Such complaints are usually indicative of impaired hearing. Importantly, Karlsson Espmark and Scherman's study illuminated a dilemma: on one hand being with others is desirable, but on the other it brings hearing difficulty to the fore, thus creating distress. In terms of personal identity, their work also explored the association of hearing problems with the state of being old and the discomfort of realising you must be old because you have a problem hearing and yet otherwise do not feel old.

This issue of spoiled identity affects how people cope with the problem. For example, they might mask difficulties by guessing and using a range of techniques to give the impression they can hear. Wallhagen (2010) linked the threat to social identity and associated stigma with shame and argued these feelings interfere with an individual's search for the most effective solutions. It often manifests as a reluctance to acknowledge the problem and in part explains why hearing aids may sit hidden in drawers as an unwelcome symbol of personal failure.

The existential value of hearing (Karlsson Espmark & Scherman, 2003)—in other words, the sense of hearing promoting a feeling of existing and being alive—provides a compelling reason to maximise a person's opportunity to hear. To effectively support older people who are living with hearing difficulties, the nurse needs to understand the role of hearing in personal identity, its contribution to well-being and the day-to-day experience. In addition, for nurses who have the opportunity to support families, it is important to consider the impact of the hearing problem on significant others. The influence of cultural factors on how an older person manages living with a hearing impairment should also be considered in the language and approach nurses use to provide care and management options. Stigma associated with hearing loss is highly prevalent in some cultures and should be taken into account when exploring management options (Wallhagen, 2018).

THE IMPACT OF HEARING LOSS ON FAMILIES AND FRIENDS

Family-centred care is increasingly part of audiology and hearing therapy (Scarinci et al., 2013). As communication is a shared experience, it is inevitable hearing loss has an impact on the people around the older individual. For some it results in restricting conversations to the essential, and for others the distress reduces their own health and fuels family tension. Scarinci et al. (2013) referred to this effect as third-party disability. Several studies suggest the impact on spouses and significant others is a reflection of the experience of the person with the impaired hearing (Scarinci et al., 2013). There is mutual frustration at having to repeat things and annoyance at the different volumes desired for comfortable television and radio listening. For partners, intimate interactions are restricted, and there is a tendency for tension to build in relationships (Donaldson et al., 2004). As a result it is critical family and friends are considered in planning how to manage hearing loss. Providing family with information on options for hearing loss, including environmental aids, hearing tactics and ways to support hearing aid use, are key.

Caring families are also affected, and in particular the well-being of the main carer is threatened due to increasing levels of stress (Donaldson et al., 2004). Nurses concerned with the alleviation of caregiver stress may find unmanaged hearing disability adds an intolerable burden that can be alleviated with appropriate audiological management and nursing interventions, whereas solutions to other problems can be more elusive. The provision of a hearing aid, information about communication and environmental aids—also known as assistive listening devices—significantly reduce the main family carer's perception of the hassles associated with the hearing problem (Donaldson et al., 2004; Sawyer et al., 2019).

MANAGEMENT OF HEARING LOSS

Some cases of conductive hearing impairment can be managed surgically. However, the principal management of sensorineural hearing impairment is provision of a hearing aid or aids. It is estimated only about one-third of the United Kingdom population who would potentially benefit from a hearing aid has one (Sawyer et al., 2019). There are probably many reasons for the low take-up, but one of the main ones is hearing impairment is often seen as a sign of ageing, and people therefore do not wish to be seen with an aid. Anyone with a hearing disability and who is motivated has the potential to benefit from a hearing aid. Motivation is essential because it takes some time and effort on the part of the patient to learn how to use it. Patients who are persuaded by relatives to get a hearing aid often do not use it.

Hearing aids are chosen and appropriately adjusted so the amount of amplification varies across frequencies to match the hearing thresholds of the individual ear. They are like spectacles; a hearing aid probably will not suit another person and may not even suit the opposite ear of its owner.

People who have a hearing aid but still have significant hearing disability should be reassessed as they probably require their hearing-aid prescription to be updated. Individuals with a more severe hearing impairment often benefit significantly by using hearing aids in both ears.

Provision of hearing aids is only one part of audiological rehabilitation. Patients require instruction in operating their hearing aid and advice on its use in different listening situations. A hearing aid should be reviewed a few weeks after fitting to confirm it provides adequate reduction in disability and users understand how to use it. Advice should also be given on hearing tactics and environmental aids.

What Happens in the Hearing-Aid Clinic?

People who visit a hearing-aid clinic for the first time will be reassured if they know what to expect (Oh & Lee, 2016) and may find it easier to attend with the support of a companion or a social carer or nurse. Prior to the visit it is desirable obstructive wax is removed as it interferes with hearing-aid fitting. The visit to the audiology clinic normally starts with seeing the audiologist, who takes a brief history and then examines the ears to check for obstructive wax or middle-ear disease. Tests for hearing often begin with voice tests followed by pure-tone audiometry and an assessment of disability. Further tests may also be undertaken.

Pure-tone audiometry is carried out by an audiologist in a room with special sound deadening to keep ambient noise levels low. The patient wears earphones so tones can be presented to one ear at a time. The hearing assessment takes 10–15 min and is used to determine how powerful a hearing aid is required and what sort of specific adjustments are needed to maximise benefit.

Patients prescribed with behind-the-ear (BTE) or in-the-ear (ITE) aids require a tailor-made transparent acrylic ear mould to connect the aid to the ear. An impression is taken of the ear using soft silicon. This is not a difficult or painful procedure, although it may feel a little strange, and the silicon feels warm. It is similar to the experience of getting dentures or teeth crowns fitted. When the patient returns to have the hearing aid fitted at the next appointment, the fit of the mould is checked to ensure it fits snugly so amplified sound from the aid is kept in the ear canal.

Ill-fitting moulds allow escaping amplified sound to re-enter the microphone, and a whistle is heard due to acoustic feedback.

Types of Hearing Aids

There are many types of hearing aid (Fig. 16.2). The first hearing aids were large body-worn devices attached to clothing and connected by wire to an ear mould. These devices are rarely used nowadays except for individuals with profound hearing impairment or those who require aids with large controls. These aids have largely been replaced by BTE hearing aids: a small aid is placed behind the ear, and sound is transmitted to a custom ear mould or generic domepiece via tubing. These are comonly prescribed through the NHS. There are also hearing aids that fit inside the concha (ITE) or ear canal (ITC) and house all the electronics within a single unit. There are also even smaller aids that fit completely inside the ear canal (i.e., completely in canal, or CIC): the power of CIC aids is limited so they are of use only for people with a relatively mild impairment.

Basically all hearing aids consist of a microphone, an amplifier and a loudspeaker, powered by a battery. They have an on/off switch, a volume control and a battery compartment. Everyone dealing with patients, particularly those who are older, should be able to manipulate a hearing aid, as some people have difficulty doing it themselves. In body-worn and BTE aids, the on/off switch is usually operated by opening/closing the battery compartment. The battery compartment is obvious on inspection. The batteries

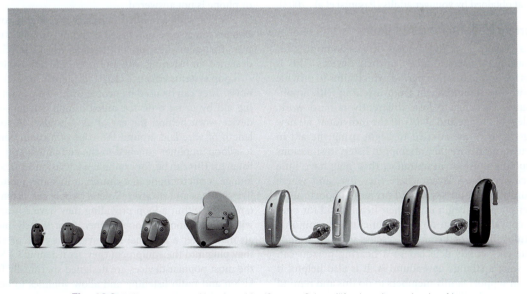

Fig. 16.2 Different types of hearing aids. (Source: Oticon [life-changing technology].)

are similar to those used in other small electronic devices such as watches and cameras.

Hearing aids should not usually whistle. This is acoustic feedback where sound coming out of the speaker re-enters the microphone. If a hand is placed over the ear when the aid is worn, some feedback is to be expected, for example when brushing hair. If hearing aids whistle at other times, a common reason is the mould is not inserted properly in the ear. Other causes are a poorly fitting ear mould, broken tubing and the mould being blocked by wax.

A simple and effective way to tell if a hearing aid is working—that it has a charged battery—is to hold it in your hand, switch it on, turn up the volume and listen for the whistle when you put your other hand over it.

Factors other than hearing also influence the choice of hearing aid. A reasonable degree of manual dexterity is required, so very small hearing aids may not be practical. In addition, the smaller the aid, the easier it is to lose; it may be inadvertently sent to the laundry or dropped unseen into pockets or down the side of chairs.

Some people with a profound hearing impairment do not benefit from hearing aids because they have little residual hearing. They can sometimes be helped by a cochlear implant. A cochlear implant is a speech processor connected to a row of electrodes fed directly into the cochlea. The device sends an electrical signal that stimulates the auditory nerve directly. Inserting a cochlear implant is a straightforward surgical procedure, but the patient requires a lot of training over a period of many months to learn how to use the implant. Several studies have shown people over 65 obtain significant benefit from cochlear implantation, similar to that obtained by younger adults (Pasanisi et al., 2003).

Supporting New Hearing-Aid Users

There is usually a varying period of weeks-months for new hearing-aid users to adapt to their devices. This is know as the acclimatisation period, which aims to provide users with maximum benefit from listening with amplified sound. Learning to hear differently is hard work. Regardless of the age and ability of the individual, all new hearing-aid users are advised to begin using the aid in quiet situations before they attempt to listen in situations of competing noise or near traffic. They may have little influence over noise levels where they live, and where opportunity exists, nurses should promote opportunities for older people to begin using their hearing aid for one-to-one conversations in an environment with minimal distractions. It can be helpful to discuss the new sounds and different sounds detected so a hearing person can explain what a strange new sound is. It is also helpful if nurses can support family members to do this and remind the family sound will be strange at first.

Hearing aids are designed to amplify speech, but they do not restore normal hearing, so patients are sometimes disappointed at first by their new hearing aid. A period of acclimatisation is needed for hearing sound differently that takes at least 3 months (Oh & Lee, 2016). The brain is used to hearing sounds at low volume, particularly at frequencies where the impairment is most marked. Hearing aids, if well fitted to the patient's impairment, amplify differently across different frequencies, so everyday sounds, particularly speech, sound different. Many patients at first describe the sound as 'tinny', because it is different to the sound they are used to.

Nurses can also support older people by reinforcing information about how hearing aids work, how to insert the aid and use the controls, and maintenance, including battery replacement and cleaning. An equally important role is to develop the skills of communication partners who are unfamiliar with talking to people who use hearing aids.

Assistive Listening Devices

Assistive listening devices, also known as environmental aids, are designed to promote independence and safety. Older people with hearing impairment may have difficulty hearing the doorbell or the phone ring, leading to increased isolation as carers have difficulty making contact. Simple measures such as moving the doorbell and phone to a more appropriate area of the house can be helpful. Doorbells and phone bells can be amplified or, for the more severely hearing impaired, linked to a light. Simple measures can have a significant effect on the person's quality of life and reduce stress levels in relatives who are concerned when the door or phone is not answered.

Phones with amplified handsets are readily available. Phones can also be purchased with built-in inductive couplers that allow hearing-aid users to select the 'T' setting designed for listening with any loop-induction system.

Loop systems enhance clarity as there is no background noise. They can be used by people without a personal hearing aid by using a device called a loop listener—a small device worn behind the ear or as a headset. A loop is a length of wire laid around the edge of a room connected to a loop amplifier attached to the equipment you wish to listen to. This can be, for example, a television set in a shared lounge, a microphone in a church or in some public places like cinemas and theatres. Several people can listen simultaneously within a loop providing they have a hearing aid with 'T' function or a loop listener. Alternatively, individuals may prefer a personal loop system, a neck or ear loop they plug into the equipment they are listening to. Some of the most popular devices are designed specifically for television and radio listening and allow volumes to be raised for people with hearing disability without disturbing others.

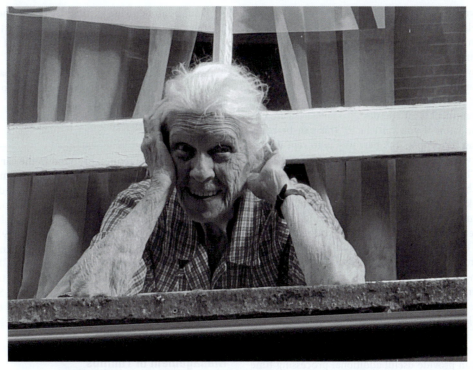

Fig. 16.3 Communication cues. (Photograph courtesy of Ruth Harris.)

Communicators are devices that amplify sound and are designed to assist with one-to-one conversation (Fig. 16.3). There are several designs on the market with the basic features of a microphone for the speaker and an earpiece for the listener. Unlike personal hearing aids, there is no scope for fine adjustments, simply a choice of volume setting. The earpiece is standard, and provided it is wiped clean between users, the communicator can be used as required by anyone. Although communicators can be very useful, they have a tendency to be forgotten resources rather than pieces of enabling equipment that should be readily available to older people (Harkins & Tucker, 2007). Assistive listening devices transform people's experienece of hearing every day sounds (Harkins & Tucker, 2007) and can overcome many common problems with reverberations and distance (Lesner, 2003).

It is important older people and their families and carers are made aware of the choices available to them; a good source of information is the Royal National Institute for Deaf People helpline. Local social service departments, social workers, occupational therapists and, where available, hearing therapists and specialist sensory impairment nurses can provide advice and referral and assist in the selection and provision of appropriate environmental aids.

Strategies to Help Communication

The behaviours that help people hear better are often deceptively simple and easy to use (see Fig. 16.4). All people with hearing loss, whether or not they use hearing aids, benefit from simple changes in behaviour.

- Look at someone's face when speaking: This is an obvious help in terms of lip-reading and gathering clues from facial expressions to make sense of speech sounds. It is very easy to start a conversation and, while speaking, look away or even walk out of the room. Avoid doing this.
- Take cues from facial expression and gestures: Most speech cues are difficult to read unless you can see a person's face. It gives so much important contextual information.
- Keep background noise to a minimum: This might mean turing off TV or music in a room. When out and about, it might mean asking to turn down music in restaurants or similar settings. Alternatively it means moving to a quieter spot.
- Position as close to the speaker as possible: Sitting closer to someone who has hearing difficulties helps. Optimum distance is 3-6 feet away, so the speaker's face can be clearly seen.

- Slow down speech: The easiest way to make speech more intelligible is to slow down delivery. It also helps to shorten sentences. But this is a balance; the person with hearing loss needs enough contextual cues to make sense of what the conversation is about. For example, rather than shortening to 'It's on Tuesday', say something like 'We were talking about your appointment. Your appointment is on Tuesday'.
- Let people know if you can't hear: This can be really challenging for people. The best way is to repeat back whatever was heard, even if it doesn't make sense. For example: 'I heard you say something about an appointment?' It helps the speaker fill in the specific gaps and lets them know the listener was trying to follow them.
- Don't shout: Shouting distorts the sound and the face of the speaker, making it harder to follow rather than easier. It also quickly communicates frustration or anger.
- Be a helpful conduit: If you're in a social situation with someone who is struggling to hear, try cueing them into the conversation so they don't get left behind. Simple cues to the topic or background can help a great deal. For example, 'Jo was telling me she's going away next week'.
- Rephrase rather than repeat: It is natural for people to simply say a message again when someone has not heard. It can provide useful additional processing time for the message, but if little of it was heard, it is unlikely to make sense second time around. It is nearly always better to rephrase the message to provide more lip shapes and sounds to go on.

- Don't be afraid to use writing: There are times when writing something down is the best way to get the message across. Don't forget to use reading glasses if necessary.

Case Study 16.1 demonstrates successful management by a nurse of an older man who was reluctant to admit to his hearing loss.

TINNITUS

Tinnitus is the perception of sound in the ear or head that does not arise from the external environment. Sounds such as vascular bruits are not tinnitus, and neither are auditory hallucinations such as hearing voices. Sounds are most often described as ringing, buzzing like a cricket, hissing, whistling and humming (Chan, 2009). The nature of the perceived sound is of little relevance in management. Around 20% of older people have tinnitus (Chan, 2009).

For a small proportion of people with tinnitus, it is severe enough to affect their everyday life. Some people find it very distressing. Many people with tinnitus also have depression, although it is unclear which comes first (Cederroth et al., 2019).

Management of Tinnitus

The most important aspect of tinnitus management is reassurance. It is important to teach patients tinnitus is a symptom, not a disease. Patients with tinnitus are often worried they have some serious condition, most often a brain

---

CASE STUDY 16.1   **Harry Donaldson's Experience**

Mr Donaldson attended his local health centre for a routine health check, accompanied by his daughter. The assessment results were similar to the previous year. Mr Donaldson considered himself fit for a man his age. His daughter mentioned he seemed a bit low. The practice nurse noticed his daughter occasionally answered for him, and he tended to joke and tease, avoiding direct answers to some of her questions.

Although he stated his hearing was fine, the practice nurse was not convinced. The nurse purposely spoke in a quiet voice with her back turned to Mr Donaldson to check whether he could answer mundane questions about the weather. He could not and explained this was due to wax and said he did not want a hearing aid. At this point his daughter argued with him, complaining bitterly about how bad his hearing had become and how difficult it was for everyone else. He denied any problem with his hearing. The nurse gently encouraged him to allow her to look in his ears for wax.

When he returned to the health centre, his daughter was asked to wait outside while microsuction was completed. The practice nurse took the opportunity to spend time discussing how hearing may change with age and the impact it can have on people's lives. She also persuaded him to try a communicator to see if it helped him follow what she was saying. His relief was visible. He told her how he had become known by family and friends as the 'really man', as he often said 'really' in an attempt to answer appropriately when he did not follow what others were saying. He agreed to be referred for a proper hearing test (i.e., audiometry) and was reassured if prescribed a hearing aid, he could decide when, where and how often he used it.

Recognition of the hearing problem and the provision of reassuring information were crucial steps for both Mr Donaldson and his daughter. Mr Donaldson's daughter can now help her father learn how to use his hearing aid and maximise the benefit from it.

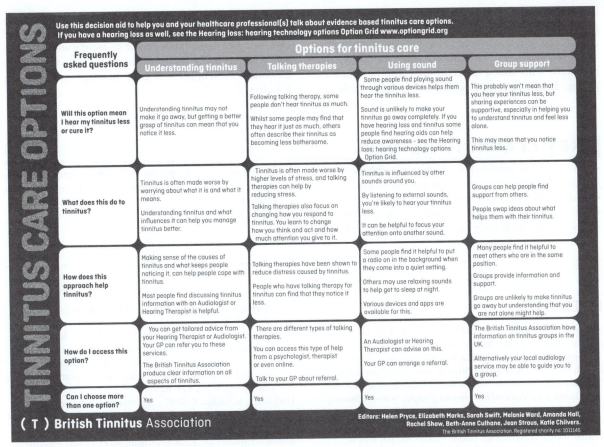

TINNITUS CARE OPTIONS

Use this decision aid to help you and your healthcare professional(s) talk about evidence based tinnitus care options.
If you have a hearing loss as well, see the Hearing loss: hearing technology options Option Grid www.optiongrid.org

Frequently asked questions	Options for tinnitus care			
	Understanding tinnitus	Talking therapies	Using sound	Group support
Will this option mean I hear my tinnitus less or cure it?	Understanding tinnitus may not make it go away, but getting a better grasp of tinnitus can mean that you notice it less.	Following talking therapy, some people don't hear tinnitus as much. Whilst some people may find that they hear it just as much, others often describe their tinnitus as becoming less bothersome.	Some people find playing sound through various devices helps them hear the tinnitus less. Sound is unlikely to make your tinnitus go away completely. If you have hearing loss and tinnitus some people find hearing aids can help reduce awareness - see the Hearing loss: hearing technology options Option Grid.	This probably won't mean that you hear your tinnitus less, but sharing experiences can be supportive, especially in helping you to understand tinnitus and feel less alone. This may mean that you notice tinnitus less.
What does this do to tinnitus?	Tinnitus is often made worse by worrying about what it is and what it means. Understanding tinnitus and what influences it can help you manage tinnitus better.	Tinnitus is often made worse by higher levels of stress, and talking therapies can help by reducing stress. Talking therapies also focus on changing how you respond to tinnitus. You learn to change how you think and act and how much attention you give to it.	Tinnitus is influenced by other sounds around you. By listening to external sounds, you're likely to hear your tinnitus less. It can be helpful to focus your attention onto another sound.	Groups can help people find support from others. People swap ideas about what helps them with their tinnitus.
How does this approach help tinnitus?	Making sense of the causes of tinnitus and what keeps people noticing it, can help people cope with tinnitus. Most people find discussing tinnitus information with an Audiologist or Hearing Therapist is helpful.	Talking therapies have been shown to reduce distress caused by tinnitus. People who have talking therapy for tinnitus can find that they notice it less.	Some people find it helpful to put a radio on in the background when they come into a quiet setting. Others may use relaxing sounds to help get to sleep at night. Various devices and apps are available for this.	Many people find it helpful to meet others who are in the same position. Groups provide information and support. Groups are unlikely to make tinnitus go away but understanding that you are not alone might help.
How do I access this option?	You can get tailored advice from your Hearing Therapist or Audiologist. Your GP can refer you to these services. The British Tinnitus Association produce clear information on all aspects of tinnitus.	There are different types of talking therapies. You can access this type of help from a psychologist, therapist or even online. Talk to your GP about referral.	An Audiologist or Hearing Therapist can advise on this. Your GP can arrange a referral.	The British Tinnitus Association have information on tinnitus groups in the UK. Alternatively your local audiology service may be able to guide you to a group.
Can I choose more than one option?	Yes	Yes	Yes	Yes

(T) **British Tinnitus** Association

Editors: Helen Pryce, Elizabeth Marks, Sarah Swift, Melanie Ward, Amanda Hall, Rachel Shaw, Beth-Anne Culhane, Jean Straus, Katie Chilvers.
The British Tinnitus Association. Registered charity no: 1011145

Fig. 16.4 Tinnitus care decision aid. (Source: British Tinnitus Association.)

tumour. They need reassurance this is not likely to be the case. Tinnitus is usually associated with hearing impairment and is uncommon in people with normal hearing. Most people with significant tinnitus should have their hearing tested. Other investigations are rarely indicated.

Tinnitus seems worse in quiet surroundings. People often say it is louder when they go to bed at night; the world is quieter. They need an explanation of the helpful role of background noise; radio or television provides other noise that masks the tinnitus. People who have significant hearing impairment should be fitted with a hearing aid to help their hearing and increase the level of background noise, making the tinnitus less obvious. Individuals with tinnitus should be given information about local self-help groups and national organisations that provide advice.

Many medications have been tried for tinnitus, but none has been shown to be effective (McFerran et al., 2019). People who also have depression should have appropriate antidepressant treatment. A number of possible interventions can help tinnitus, including psychological therapies such a mindfulness-based cognitive behavioural therapy (McKenna et al., 2017), psychotherapy from hearing therapists, hearing aids and sound generators, and tinnitus groups (Pryce et al., 2019). The tinnitus care decision aid in Figure 16.4 can help summarise the options for treatment and help shared decision making (Pryce et al., 2021).

An increase in reports of the distress associated with the experience of tinnitus may be indicative of an underlying problem. Nurses should be alert for other signs of low mood and take steps to detect and prevent depression.

CONCLUSION

Nurses are ideally placed to contribute to selected aspects of auditory rehabilitation and help the large number of older people who acquire hearing disability. As people grow older, other opportunities for self-actualisation may diminish, and the importance of promoting communication increases. Hearing disability is an example of a chronic problem that may limit individuals' opportunities to communicate and participate as they would like, but thankfully with skilled intervention, it can be effectively managed, and the negative impact on individuals and those around them can be reduced. Unfortunately, many nurses have limited knowledge and skills in this aspect of care, and like many other people in society who are well-meaning but badly informed, many do little to promote communication opportunities for hearing-impaired older listeners.

KEY LEARNING POINTS

- Nurses can do much to help older people with their hearing. Improving communication often takes simple tactics.
- Hearing loss need not be a barrier to participation.
- By knowing about the options to support hearing, nurses can enable their patients to maximise their communication and interactions.

- By knowing what options there are to help with tinnitus, nurses can support their patients to reduce its impact.

REFERENCES

Akeroyd, M. A., Foreman, K., & Holman, J. A. (2014). Estimates of the number of adults in England, Wales, and Scotland with a hearing loss. *International Journal of Audiology, 53*(1), 60–61.

British Society of Audiology. (2018). *Recommended procedure: Pure-tone air-conduction and bone conduction threshold audiometry with and without masking.*https://www.thebsa.org.uk/wp-content/uploads/2018/11/OD104-32-Recommended-Procedure-Pure-Tone-Audiometry-August-2018-FINAL.pdf

British Society of Audiology. (2021). Aural care: Ear wax removal. https://www.thebsa.org.uk/resources

Cederroth, C. R., Gallus, S., Hall, D. A., Kleinjung, T., Langguth, B., Maruotti, A., Meyer, M., Norena, A., Probst, T., Pryss, R., & Searchfield, G. (2019). Towards an understanding of tinnitus heterogeneity. *Frontiers in Aging Neuroscience, 11*, 53.

Chan, Y. (2009). Tinnitus: Etiology, classification, characteristics, and treatment. *Discovery Medicine, 8*(42), 133–136.

Donaldson, N., Worrall, L., & Hickson, L. (2004). Older people with hearing impairment: A literature review of the spouse's perspective. *Australian and New Zealand Journal of Audiology, 26*(1), 30–39.

Edwards, B. (2016). A model of auditory-cognitive processing and relevance to clinical applicability. *Ear and Hearing, 37*(1), 85s–91s.

Gabriel, O. T. (2015). Cerumen impaction: Challenges and management profile in a rural health facility. *Nigerian Medical Journal: Journal of the Nigeria Medical Association, 56*, 390–393.

Gallacher, J., Ilubaera, V., Ben-Shlomo, Y., Bayer, A., Fish, M., Babisch, W., & Elwood, P. (2012). Auditory threshold, phonologic demand, and incident dementia. *Neurology, 79*(15), 1583–1590.

Gleibs, I. H., Haslam, C., Haslam, S. A., & Jones, J. M. (2011). Water clubs in residential care: Is it the water or the club that enhances health and well-being? *Psychology & Health, 26*, 1361–1377.

Gopinath, B., Hickson, L., Schneider, J., McMahon, C. M., Burlutsky, G., Leeder, S. R., & Mitchell, P. (2012). Hearing-impaired adults are at increased risk of experiencing emotional distress and social engagement restrictions five years later. *Age and Ageing, 41*(5), 618–623.

Harkins, J., & Tucker, P. (2007). An internet survey of individuals with hearing loss regarding assistive listening devices. *Trends in Amplification, 11*(2), 91–100.

Karlsson Espmark, A. K., & Scherman, M. H. (2003). Hearing confirms existence and identity—Experiences from persons with presbyacusis. *International Journal of Audiology, 42*, 106–115.

Lawrence, B. J., Jayakody, D. M. P., Bennett, R. J., Eikelboom, R. H., Gasson, N., & Friedland, P. L. (2020). Hearing loss and depression in older adults: A systematic review and meta-analysis. *Gerontologist, 60*(3), e137–e154.

Lesner, S. A. (2003). Candidacy and management of assistive listening devices: Special needs of the elderly. *International Journal of Audiology, 42*, 2S68–2S76.

Lin, F. R., Metter, E. J., O'Brien, R. J., Resnick, S. M., Zonderman, A. B., & Ferrucci, L. (2011). Hearing loss and incident dementia. *Archives of Neurology, 68*(2), 214–220.

Livingston, G., Huntley, J., Sommerlad, A., Ames, D., Ballard, C., Banerjee, S., Brayne, C., Burns, A., Cohen-Mansfield, J., Cooper, C., Costafreda, S. G., Dias, A., Fox, N., Gitlin, L. N., Howard, R., Kales, H. C., Kivimäki, M., Larson, E. B., Ogunniyi, A., … Mukadam, N. (2020). Dementia prevention, intervention, and care: 2020 report of the Lancet Commission. *The Lancet, 396*(10248), 413–446.

Mamo, S. K., Reed, N. S., Mcnabney, M. K., Rund, J., Oh, E. S., & Lin, F. R. (2019). Age-related hearing loss and the listening environment: Communication challenges in a group care setting for older adults. *The Annals of Long-Term Care: The*

Official Journal of the American Medical Directors Association, 27, e8–e13.

McFerran, D. J., Stockdale, D., Holme, R., Large, C. H., & Baguley, D. M. (2019). Why is there no cure for tinnitus? *Frontiers in Neuroscience, 13*.

McKenna, L., Marks, E. M., Hallsworth, C. A., & Schaette, R. (2017). Mindfulness-based cognitive therapy as a treatment for chronic tinnitus: a randomized controlled trial. *Psychotherapy and Psychosomatics, 86*(6), 351–361.

Moore, B. C. J. (2016). A review of the perceptual effects of hearing loss for frequencies above 3 kHz. *International Journal of Audiology, 55*(12), 707–714.

Musiek, F. E., Shinn, J., Chermak, G. D., & Bamiou, D. E. (2017). Perspectives on the pure-tone audiogram. *Journal of the American Academy of Audiology, 28*(7), 655–671.

National Academies of Sciences, Engineering, and Medicine. (2020). *Social isolation and loneliness in older adults: Opportunities for the health care system.* The National Academies Press.

National Institute for Heatlh and Care Excellence. (2019). Hearing loss in adults: Quality standard earwax removal. https://www.nice.org.uk/guidance/ng98/chapter/Recommendations#removing-earwax

Oh, S. H., & Lee, J. (2016). General framework of hearing aid fitting management. *Journal of Audiology & Otology, 20*(1), 1.

Pasanisi, E., Bacciu, A., Vincenti, V., Guida, M., Barbot, A., Berghenti, M. T., & Bacciu, S. (2003). Speech recognition in elderly cochlear implant recipients. *Clinical Otolaryngology, 28*(2), 154–157.

Pryce, H., & Gooberman-Hill, R. (2012). 'There's a hell of a noise': Living with a hearing loss in residential care. *Age and Ageing, 41*(1), 40–46.

Pryce, H., & Hall, A. (2014). The role of shared decision-making in audiologic rehabilitation. *Perspectives on Aural Rehabilitation and Its Instrumentation, 21*(1), 15–23.

Pryce, H., Hall, A., Laplante-Lévesque, A., & Clark, E. (2016). A qualitative investigation of decision making during help-seeking for adult hearing loss. *International Journal of Audiology, 55*(11), 658–665.

Pryce, H., Moutela, T., Bunker, C., & Shaw, R. (2019). Tinnitus groups: A model of social support and social connectedness from peer interaction. *British Journal of Health Psychology, 24*(4), 913–930.

Pryce, H., Ward, M., Turton, L., Stanley, J., & Goss, J. (2021). A multi-site service evaluation of the tinnitus care decision aid. *International Journal of Audiology, 61*(1), 1–4.

Radford, J. C. (2020). Treatment of impacted ear wax: A case for increased community-based microsuction. *BJGP Open, 4*(2), Article bjgpopen20X101064.

Ramsdell, D. A. (1978). The psychology of the hard of hearing and deafened adult. In H. Davis, & R. Silverman (Eds.), *Hearing and deafness* (4th ed., pp. 499–510). Holt, Rinhart and Winston.

Sawyer, C. S., Armitage, C. J., Munro, K. J., Singh, G., & Dawes, P. D. (2019). Correlates of hearing aid use in UK adults: Self-reported hearing difficulties, social participation, living situation, health, and demographics. *Ear and Hearing, 40*(5), 1061–1068.

Scarinci, N., Meyer, C., Ekberg, K., & Hickson, L. (2013). Using a family-centred care approach in audiologic rehabilitation for adults with hearing impairment. *Perspectives on Aural Rehabilitation and Its Instrumentation, 20*(3), 83–90.

Shukla, A., Harper, M., Pedersen, E., Goman, A., Auen, J. J., Price, C., Applebaum, J., Hoyer, M., Lin, F. R., & Reed, N. S. (2020). Hearing loss, loneliness, and social isolation: A systematic review. *Otolaryngology—Head and Neck Surgery, 162*, 622–633.

Somerville, G. (2002). The most effective products available to facilitate ear syringing. *British Journal of Community Nursing, 7*, 94–101.

Sundström, A., Adolfsson, A. N., Nordin, M., & Adolfsson, R. (2019). Loneliness increases the risk of all-cause dementia and Alzheimer's disease. *The Journals of Gerontology: Series B, 75*, 919–926.

Wallhagen, M. (2018). Stigma: What does the literature say? *The Hearing Journal, 71*(9), 14–16.

Wallhagen, M. I. (2010). The stigma of hearing loss. *Gerontologist, 50*(1), 66–75.

Wang, J., & Puel, J. L. (2020). Presbycusis: an update on cochlear mechanisms and therapies. *Journal of Clinical Medicine, 9*(1), 218.

World Health Organization. (1999). *International classification of impairments, disabilities and handicap.* World Health Organization.

World Health Organization. (2018). *Addressing the rising prevalence of hearing loss.* World Health Organization. https://apps.who.int/iris/bitstream/handle/10665/260336/9789241550260-eng.pdf.

Yamasoba, T., Lin, F. R., Someya, S., Kashio, A., Sakamoto, T., & Kondo, K. (2013). Current concepts in age-related hearing loss: Epidemiology and mechanistic pathways. *Hearing Research, 303*, 30–38.

17

Older People's Eye Health

Penelope Stanford

CHAPTER OUTLINE

Vision is often taken for granted. Until it's impaired, its impact on well-being may not be appreciated or understood. For example, a visual impairment or ocular condition is not always obvious. It's important for nurses and health care professionals to understand the nature of vision and eye health as part of the holistic care of an older person.

The ageing profile of the global population is a well-known predictor of public health and a useful forecast for eye health care planning. The World Health Organization (WHO, 2019, p. 8) states 'ageing is the primary risk factor for many eye conditions'. A person's vision is relevant to every area of nursing care and is fundamental to a holistic approach. This chapter sets out to explain the concept of vision for older people by discussing normal and altered anatomy and physiology, some common major and minor ocular conditions, and the impact of vision on an older person's social world.

VISION: AN OVERVIEW

Globally, visual impairment is defined as an eye condition that affects the visual system and visual function (WHO, 2019, including people who need a refractive correction, such as spectacles and contact lenses, to see. Importantly, the WHO (2019) recognises vision impairment as a disability, as it can have a negative impact on a person's life. Older people are susceptible to adverse effects on their physical, psychological and social well-being. The WHO (2019) exemplifies these negative impacts as limited mobility, risk of falls, bone fractures from falls, social isolation and cognitive deterioration. The WHO also suggests older people with a visual impairment are more likely to need support in a care or nursing home environment when compared to their non-visually impaired peers (WHO, 2019).

As with other aspects of the body, the ageing process affects the eyes, with conditions of the visual system transcending the age continuum. Current world population estimations by the United Nations (UN, 2019) suggest by 2050, 16% of people will be over 65, compared to 9% in 2019. As people age, existing eye conditions may deteriorate, and age-related eye conditions can develop. With this in mind, predictions of an upsurge in the population of older people and the fact visual impairment is common in people over 50 (WHO, 2019) means there are likely consequences for health care resources (Burton et al., 2021) and potentially for the well-being of individuals.

Of the five senses, evidence suggests eyesight is the most valuable (WHO, 2019; Enoch et al., 2020). Losing vision has a significant impact on the physical, psychological and social well-being of an older person. For individuals with an existing ocular condition, the ageing process may add another dimension to independence and coping mechanisms as they navigate the way they live. Challenges include self-care, communication, social interaction, mobility and consequently general well-being. Not all eye conditions cause permanent vision loss, but they may cause discomfort and pain and therefore can have a substantial impact on the person, their lifestyle and their overall well-being.

Older people living with dementia and a visual impairment face specific challenges. The Thomas Pocklington Trust (2016) explained an older person living with dementia and visual impairment may limit their involvement in meaningful activities, which are behaviours valued by the person, such as hobbies, walking and engaging with others. It is understood that without meaningful activities in their life, an older person living with a visual impairment and dementia can lose self-confidence and feel they are not contributing to family or community (Thomas Pocklington Trust, 2016). Visual impairment can be associated with negative lifestyle changes and result in a loss of sense of purpose for the older person. Specifically, there are mental health implications for an older person living with a visual impairment, such as anxiety and depression (Evans et al., 2007; GBD 2019 Blindness and Vision Impairment Collaborators, 2021).

IMPACTS OF VISUAL IMPAIRMENT ON OLDER PEOPLE

Vision is very much an individual experience. Different eye conditions, surroundings and individual resilience impact a person's experience with visual loss. The key message is assumptions should not be made; avoid stereotypical perceptions of the blind person with dark glasses and a white stick, which are reflective of the widely used phrase 'not all disabilities are visible'. In the care environment particularly, always ask a person about their vision, what they can see, how their vision and visual impairment affect them and what help they may or may not need. This is essential to a person-centred approach. Visual impairment impacts daily living and has many implications for a person's physical, social and psychological well-being.

The most prevalent conditions that affect the vision of older adults are discussed later in this chapter. Significantly, some visual impairments can be corrected, such as refractive errors and cataracts. Bourne et al. (2017) cited these two common causes of visual impairment in people over 50. Both can be managed with prescription glasses and cataract surgery, respectively, but it is a public health issue to ensure older people are aware treatment is available and how to access it in a health care system with finite resources.

ANATOMY OF THE EYE

It is important to understand the basic anatomy of the eye, also known as the globe, to inform knowledge and understanding of an older person's vision, the impact of eye conditions and their implications for nursing practice. The structure of the eye is shown in Figure 17.1. The eye is a

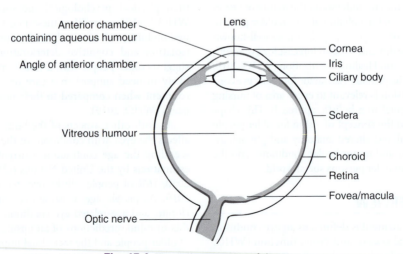

Fig. 17.1 The main structures of the eye.

fascinating and complex structure that enables a person to see and carry out activities of daily living. Understanding normal and abnormal physiology is integral to the nursing care of all older people regardless of the health care context. Usually, two eyes are present to support the breadth and depth of vision. Vision, or normal refraction known as emmetropia, is enabled by light from an object focusing on the retina (Batterbury & Murphy, 2018). The visual process is facilitated by the clarity of the refractive elements of the eye: the tear film, cornea, aqueous humour, vitreous and retina.

The anatomy and physiology of the eye are detailed in several ophthalmic textbooks, including Bowling (2016) and Batterbury & Murphy (2018). To summarise, the eye globe, or bulbus oculi, consists of three layers from the outside to the inside: the sclera, choroid and retina (Fig. 17.1).

- Sclera: The white outside layer helps maintains the shape of the eye. The extraocular muscles are attached to the sclera and control the movement of the eye.
- Choroid: The middle layer of the eye is rich in blood vessels that nourish the retina. The choroid also deflects light rays.
- Retina: A layer of photosensitive cells that receive and process light transfer the information via the optic nerve to the visual cortex in the brain.

The globe is protected by the bony structure of the orbit and structures such as the skull and orbital fat pads in the orbital space. The movable skin folds of the eyelids cover the globe and close to protect the eye.

The cornea is a clear, avascular, oval-shaped structure at the front of the eye. It comprises of five layers and provides two-thirds of the refractive element of the eye. The anterior chamber lies beneath the cornea and in front of the iris. It contains the clear aqueous humour that helps maintain the shape of the eye; the fluid provides nourishment to the posterior cornea and lens.

TEARS

Tears are multifunctional and essential for the optical function and health of the eye. Water and mucus content produce a tear film that nourishes the outside layer of the cornea, and lipids prevent the evaporation of tears (Batterbury & Murphy, 2018). Tears are produced in the lacrimal gland. The eyelids and blink reflex distribute tear film over the ocular surface. Tear film provides oxygen to the outside surface of the eye, including the conjunctiva and cornea. Tear film production decreases as people age, particularly in women post menopause. In conjunction with an increase in evaporation of tears, older people have a predisposition for dry eyes.

NORMAL VISION

The anatomical and physiological structures of the eye promote normal vision, often referred to as emmetropia. Emmetropia is enabled by a number of factors, including normal functioning of the anatomical elements and clarity of the refractive structures: the tear film, cornea, aqueous humour, crystalline lens and vitreous. Light passes through the cornea, pupil and lens to the rods and cones in the retina through the optic nerve to the occipital lobe in the brain, where it is interpreted as sight.

ASSESSING VISION IN AN OLDER ADULT

Assessing an older person's vision is important to identify potential imbalance in the refractive parts of the eye, determine the presence of ocular disease and identify visual problems. Many people are familiar with having their vision tested. The aim of eyesight tests is to determine the need for spectacles and assess a person's eye health, which may establish the presence of sight-threatening eye diseases such as chronic glaucoma—insidious raised intraocular pressure caused by inadequate drainage of the aqueous humour from the anterior chamber.

Vision is an objective and subjective entity, meaning it can be measured by vision tests and according to an individual's perception of the world around them. A vision test provides a baseline measurement for understanding a person's eyesight. An awareness of how vision is tested facilitates an understanding of a person's visual ability.

Shaw and Lee (2017) noted clinical standard distance vision testing means testing visual acuity and is performed by asking a person to read either a Snellen chart or a Log Mar (i.e., minimum angle of resolution) chart. If a person cannot read or recognise the alphabet, alternative tests are the Kay's picture test and the tumbling E test, where the person is asked to identify the 'E' shape on a chart. Each type of chart shows figures in decreasing size. An example of a normal visual acuity, according to the Snellen measurement, is recorded as 6/6; the LogMar equivalent is 0.0 (Shaw & Lee, 2017). The type of chart used for visual acuity is dependent on patient need and clinical area protocol. People who can't read the English alphabet or who are limited by a learning disability, cognitive impairment or dementia may find the tumbling E test or Kay's picture chart acceptable. A functional vision assessment based on how the person interacts with their environment is a suitable alternative assessment to objective measurement for older people unable to read vision charts.

Objective testing of vision provides a measurement of visual status. However, nurses are accustomed to also considering an individual's subjective experience, an approach that lends to understanding the broader context of a person's vision. Self-reporting of vision, or asking the older person about what they can see and how they function in their daily life, offers a valuable perspective. Ehrlich et al. (2019) suggested visual problems are often self-reported and described as difficulty reading printed material and/ or being unable to recognise someone they know from a distance such as from across the road despite wearing spectacles. The real experience of visual problems can aid an understanding of how visual difficulties impact a person's life.

NEAR-VISION TESTING

Near-vision testing is performed at a routine eye test. Bowling (2016) advised near vision is tested using a near-vision chart; a person is asked to hold the chart at a distance they would normally read. The test begins with each eye tested separately, with the other eye covered. The person is then asked to read the chart using both eyes. The near-vison test is particularly useful for assessing the presence of presbyopia, the loss of ability to focus due to the reduced flexibility of the crystalline lens. Signs and symptoms of presbyopia present from the age of 40 (Marsden, 2017).

CONTRAST SENSITIVITY

Contrast sensitivity refers to how the visual system differentiates an object from its background (Bowling, 2016). For example, a visually impaired person may have difficulty identifying food on their plate if the plate is a similar colour to the food, such as green peas on a green plate. This is a good example of how objects, in this case peas, are distinguished and therefore considered an aspect of functional vision assessment. Specific detail about the degree of contrast sensitivity can be tested by a Pellei-Robson contrast sensitivity letter chart (Bowling, 2016).

VISUAL FIELD

Vision is promoted by a person using their peripheral vision—when looking straight ahead, the ability to see objects at the side (Marsden, 2017). Some ophthalmic conditions in older people like glaucoma and systemic illness such as stroke may result in restricted peripheral vision. Commonly, people do not notice limitations in their peripheral vision. They may be observed bumping into things and ignoring objects outside their central line of vision. This can be particularly hazardous in situations such as crossing the road. The person may be startled if objects appear suddenly. It is therefore useful for nurses and the health care team to have a basic

understanding of visual-field testing. Visual field can be manually tested by a confrontation test. The nurse sits in front of the older person, then asks them to close one eye and look at the nurse, who then moves their hand around different sections of the person's visual field (Seewoodhary, 2009). A sophisticated visual-field test for people with suspected field loss is a computer analysis of the perimeter of vision known as a Humphrey field analyser (Bowling, 2016).

CERTIFICATE OF VISUAL IMPAIRMENT

The certificate of visual impairment (CVI) is an official recognition of visual impairment. As advised by the Royal National Institute of Blind People, a CVI facilitates social care referral. Rahman et al. (2020) reported during 2017–2018, 22 844 new certifications were recorded in England. The CVI enables people to access individual support and informs public health planning for people with visual impairments.

A CVI generates connections with the person's local council and assessment for sight loss support (Department of Health, 2017). The registration process is usually initiated by an ophthalmologist. Eye clinic liaison officers (ECLO), available in some eye departments, or charities such as the Royal National Institute of Blind People offer valuable support to help with the CVI process. Tables 17.1 and 17.2 set out the Department of Health (2017) CVI classifications for severe visual impairment and sight impairment.

There are many consequences of visual impairment, including falls and Charles Bonnet syndrome.

TABLE 17.1 Severe Vision Impairment: Certificate of Visual Impairment	
Impairment Group	**Classification**
Group 1	People who have visual acuity worse than 3/60 Snellen (or equivalent)
Group 2	People who are 3/60 Snellen or better (or equivalent) but worse than 6/60 Snellen (or equivalent) who also have contraction of their visual field
Group 3	People who are 6/60 Snellen or better (or equivalent) who have a clinically significant contracted field of vision that functionally impairs them (e.g., significant field loss

Source: Department of Health (2017).

TABLE 17.2 Sight-Impaired: Certificate of Visual Impairment

Impairment Group	Classification
Group 1	People who are 3/60 to 6/60 Snellen (or equivalent) with full field.
Group 2	People between 6/60 and 6/24 Snellen (or equivalent) with moderate contraction of the field (e.g., superior or patchy loss, media opacities or aphakia)
Group 3	People who are 6/18 Snellen (or equivalent) or better if they have a marked field defect

Source: Department of Health (2017).

FALLS

The ageing process may mean people are susceptible to falls. Age combined with visual impairment increases that risk. The causes of falls in older people with a visual impairment are multifactorial. Ocular conditions have the potential to cause a person to fall due to the nature of associated vision loss. For example, chronic glaucoma destroys peripheral vision, and people affected do not have a broad view of potential hazards. Imbalance and exposure to hazards inside and outside the home are common in all types of visual impairment (Lord, 2006). A number of vision-related predisposing factors are associated with older people who fall, including uncorrected refractive error, incorrect spectacle prescription, ill-fitting spectacles and poor contrast sensitivity. Multifocal spectacles may affect distance and depth perception (Lord, 2006), and therefore although the refractive error is corrected, the different lens prescriptions are difficult to become accustomed to and may occasionally affect balance, for example when using an escalator.

An injurious fall may result in a hospital admission, a concern for the individual and their family with implications for health and social care resources. Citing glaucoma as a visual impairment–related risk factor for falls, McGinley et al. (2020) established that over a 6-year period, 11.7% of people admitted to hospital following a fall had glaucoma. The study established each fall per person cost one hospital National Health Service (NHS) trust £2,487, and the total cost of falls over the 6-year period was £200,568. The authors estimated that when generalised to the United Kingdom population, people with glaucoma who fall add

further costs to the NHS of £28.6 million due to hospital admissions, and people with glaucoma are more likely to require a fall-related hospital admission. Age was not specified in the study, but chronic glaucoma commonly affects older adults.

When in hospital following an injurious fall, a holistic assessment of the older person is essential to prevent further events. Vision is an integral part of that assessment, but there are indications that once in hospital, a simple eyesight assessment is not prioritised as part of a patient's care plan. A national audit of inpatient falls (Royal College of Physicians, 2015) of patients over 65 found less than half of individuals hospitalised following a fall had a vision assessment conducted at any point in the hospital episode. In response, the Royal College of Physicians (2015) published guidance on testing vision in hospital. Titled *Look Out! Bedside Vision Check for Falls Prevention*, the guide offered a number of basic visual tests using pictures and text that can be used by nurses and other members of the health care team at the bedside to provide a baseline understanding of a patient's vision. Assessment of vision as a key performance indicator was not met in the 2021 national audit of inpatient falls (Royal College of Physicians, 2021), suggesting there was no improvement in the frequency of hospital vision tests in patients over 65 following a fall.

The home environment may be hazardous to people with a vision impairment as they navigate familiar surroundings with deteriorating eyesight. Home hazards include poor lighting and loose carpets; despite supporting evidence, these issues are common denominators in falls (Valipoor et al., 2020). Waterman et al. (2016) illustrated the potential of home interventions such as home safety, exercise or social home visits to prevent falls in a three-arm randomised controlled trial ($n = 49$) of people over 65 with a visual impairment. Findings indicated the participants found the interventions helpful in maintaining their visual independence and well-being. The authors concluded programmes should be further researched to explore the potential of home safety and home exercise interventions to prevent falls in older people with a visual impairment.

The nature of visual impairment means older people are at risk of falls; prevention is not only person-centred but also a public health issue. Raising awareness of falls and fall-prevention interventions can be addressed by information, education and fall-risk assessment—not only for falls but particularly the vulnerability of older adults with a visual impairment.

Ms Cole's fictional story in Case Study 17.1 will help you to make critical links between the theoretical aspects of this chapter and the lived experience of an older person with a vision impairment.

CASE STUDY 17.1

Ms Cole is 75 years old, is single and lives alone in the two-story terraced house where she was born. She is proud of her house and its decor. She explains she feels 'down' and has no interest in anything.

Ms Cole was diagnosed with chronic glaucoma 20 years ago, managed by eye drops she instils herself. Her vision acuity is 6/18 (Snellen) in both eyes. Ms Cole has bruising on her arms and lower limbs. The stairwell is quite dark, and the carpet appears loose. Ms Cole has slipped a few times on the bottom stair.

She seems to have low mood and says she has lost her confidence going out and meeting people. The bruising prompted a community nurse home visit as she does not feel able to travel to the medical centre alone.

Care issues to consider:

- Ms Cole's visual acuity suggests she has impaired vision. When did she last have her eyes tested by the optician?
- Peripheral vision can be reduced in people with chronic glaucoma, suggesting her vision is restricted and she cannot see obstacles around her. This could account for the bruising.
- Although Ms Cole has instilled glaucoma drops for many years, it is recommended her ability is reassessed as it may have changed over time.
- The dark stairwell and loose carpet are likely to increase the risk of a fall.
- Ms Cole is proud of her home and may not want to consider home adaptations to enhance her well-being.
- As she has already slipped, she may worry about falling outside the home and therefore not want to go out independently.
- As Ms Cole's vision deteriorates, she may lose interest or not have adequate vision to continue to enjoy hobbies, watching television or going out independently, leading to social isolation.

CHARLES BONNET SYNDROME

Charles Bonnet syndrome (CBS) is a little-known condition that widely affects older people living with visual impairment. CBS was discovered in 1760 by Charles Bonnet, who observed his grandfather's predisposition to hallucinations as his vision deteriorated (Best et al., 2019). It took until 2020 to be recognised and listed in the WHO International Classification of Diseases. The WHO (2020) defined CBS as 'visual release hallucinations'. Progress with its recognition is due to the campaigning of Judith Potts from the charity Esme's Umbrella to increase public awareness. CBS is common in older adults; most recent estimates of mean age range are between 74.9 and 83.8 years (Menon et al., 2003). The hallucinations are often temporary and not related to cognitive disorders. While noted to be more prevalent in people with age-related macular degeneration, Menon et al. (2003) suggested CBS is associated with any acquired visual impairment pathology.

The actual cause of CBS is unclear; it is theorised to be due to damage along the visual pathway (Pang, 2016) that causes hyperexcitability in the visual cortex (Best et al., 2019). People have reported temporary visions and hallucinations consisting of animals, fairies, pools of water and so forth. It is also possible the hallucinations could contribute to falls as people attempt to step over objects that appear in their path. Best et al. (2019) found an apparent reticence to admit to hallucinations due to concerns of appearing to have psychological problems. Increasing public awareness

of CBS would encourage people to talk about their experiences, understand the cause of their hallucinations and possibly provide some reassurance.

There is no known cure for CBS, although several pharmaceutical interventions have been explored. Best et al. (2019, p. 1) devised the interventions in Table 17.3 to help people manage hallucinations.

Older people may find these interventions helpful, according to Best et al. (2019), as they allow people to take control of their hallucinations. However, this advice does not take into account mobility issues and fall risks for people with ocular and physical comorbidities. Therefore advice about managing hallucinations should take an individualised approach.

TABLE 17.3   Managing Visual Hallucinations

- When the hallucinations start, look from right to left once every 15 seconds without moving your head.
- Try to touch the hallucination.
- Stare straight at the hallucination.
- Turn your head to alternate sides, then move the head toward each shoulder in turn.
- Walk around the room or to another room.
- Shine a torch from below your chin in front of (not into) your eyes.
- Change the light level in your room or the activity you are doing.

CBS is a consequence of visual impairment that is not widely known. It is essential knowledge and advice are provided and disseminated to older people, health care professionals, families and the wider population so individuals with the condition can be appropriately supported.

EYE CONDITIONS

Awareness of common age-related eye conditions is essential for health care professionals who care for older people across all settings to understand the impact on vision and well-being. The following section discusses several age-related eye conditions, selected based on evidence of commonality among older adults. Some systemic diseases common in older people are connected to eye conditions. Examples taken from Shaw and Lee (2017) are cited in Table 17.4.

REFRACTIVE ERROR

Emmetropia is facilitated by light entering the eye and focusing on the retina. When this is impeded, a person may be diagnosed with a refractive error. Uncorrected refractive error is the most common cause of avoidable visual impairment in older people (Naidoo et al., 2016). The incidence of refractive error was illustrated in a review of population studies by Wolffsohn and Davies (2019), who established presbyopia as the cause of refractive error in 50% of people over 50. Therefore, access to eye tests is an area of a public health concern, and health education is needed to direct people to the importance of eye tests (Scott et al., 2016). However, the cost of eye tests, even with NHS subsidies,

TABLE 17.4 Age-Related Eye Conditions

Systemic Disease	Ocular Manifestation
Hypertension	Retinal oedema, retinal haemorrhages
Giant cell arteritis (arterial disease)	Infarctions, oedema optic disc
Diabetes	Diabetic retinopathy, cataract, glaucoma, uveitis
Thyroid disease	Exophthalmos (i.e., protrusion of the eye ball), leading to lid retraction and corneal exposure decompression of the optic nerve
Herpes zoster	Inflammation of the conjunctiva, inflammation of the cornea, uveitis, glaucoma, cataract
Cerebrovascular accident	Peripheral field defects, scotoma

may be prohibitive for individuals on low budgets (Stanford, 2020). In the course of a general nursing assessment, nurses assess patients from a holistic perspective and can ask patients about their vision and, in the scope of health education, suggest eye tests and referral to an optometrist. A person's eyesight is part of their general well-being; nurses should be aware of the importance of regular eye tests every 2 years if there is no ocular comorbidity. In addition, regular cleaning and repairs to glasses contribute to optimal vision.

Ocular structures are susceptible to many changes across the life span, such as the result of a systemic disease like diabetes. Age itself can alter the eye and vision or exacerbate existing ophthalmic conditions. The next section discusses age-related changes to the eye and how the changes to ophthalmic physiology may impact an older person's well-being. Buchan et al. (2019) identified several specific eye conditions as a public health concern, citing older age as a major risk factor. Ethnicity is also a significant risk factor that underpins some eye diseases and subsequent visual loss; therefore, awareness is essential in caring for older people from specific ethnic backgrounds.

A report by Public Health England (PHE, 2021) called Atlas of Variation reviewed disparities in eye care across the United Kingdom. Specific risk factors were highlighted in ethnic groups such as East Asian people for cataracts and acute glaucoma; people of Black, African Caribbean and South Asian origin are more likely to have a predisposition to chronic glaucoma. People with Asian ethnicity are also known to be susceptible to earlier-onset cataracts. Diabetic retinopathy is prevalent in people from Black, Afro Caribbean and South Asian backgrounds. Atlas of Variation compared these risk factors against the general United Kingdom population to establish eye diseases by ethnicity. It was also noted there is a greater threat to vision from diabetic retinopathy in people in specific ethnic groups when compared to the White population in the United Kingdom. Cultural awareness of eye health and beliefs about treatment are essential for culturally competent eye care (Stanford et al., 2014) and applicable for making links between eye diseases and people from a range of ethnic backgrounds (PHE, 2021).

EYELID DISORDERS

Older adults may experience changes to their eyelids and associated structures that are age-related or due to existing eyelid conditions exacerbated by age. The changes may involve the structure of the eyelids (e.g., ptosis) and eyelid margins (e.g., ectropion and ectropion), instability of the tear film and an inflammatory disease known as blepharitis.

PTOSIS

Ptosis is the drooping of the upper eyelid. Although ptosis is not limited to older adults, changes in the structure of the eyelid are linked to the ageing process. Ageing causes aponeurotic or ageing ptosis, which is the result of thinning and laxity of the eyelid muscles, nerves and muscle damage (Lee et al., 2020).

Aponeurotic ptosis may be unilateral or bilateral and varies in extent. A drooping eyelid can mean the older person's vision is partially or fully obscured. If a person has an existing visual impairment, ptosis may impact negatively their independence and general well-being. Depending on advice from the ophthalmologist, surgical correction is required to return the eyelid to its optimal position (Lee et al., 2020).

DRY EYE DISEASE

Dry eye disease is a complex and uncomfortable condition that predisposes ocular complications in older adults. The Definition and Classification Subcommittee of the International Dry Eye WorkShop (2007) provided the official classification of eye disease. First, lacrimal gland (i.e., where tears are produced) dysfunction results in tear deficiency and a reduction in secretion of tears and tear volume. Second, extreme loss of water causes dry eyes; oil from the Meibomian glands prevents evaporation or the ocular surface becomes exposed. Preservatives in eye drops, particularly glaucoma eye drops, are known to cause dry eyes and irritation (Definition and Classification Subcommittee of the International Dry Eye WorkShop, 2007).

BLEPHARITIS

Blepharitis is inflammation of the eyelid margins, and although it can affect people of any age, it is most common in adults over 50 (Eberhardt & Rammohan, 2019). The condition is classified according to the part of the eyelid affected—anterior or posterior—and both types may occur simultaneously (Eberhardt & Rammohan, 2019).

Blepharitis is caused by dysfunction of the Meibomian glands and/or staphylococcus infection; symptoms include redness of the eyelids, watery eyes and irritation combined with crusting around the eyelids (Batterbury & Murphy, 2018). A person with blepharitis may find it distressing due to the discomfort and body image caused by the symptoms.

Blepharitis can also be associated with a bacterial infection caused by Demodex mites (Zhu et al., 2018). Found in the hair follicles and sebaceous glands in the eyelid, the mites carry bacteria in situ (Zhu et al., 2018). Blepharitis can put patients at risk of postoperative ophthalmic complications. As a result, a common reason for the cancellation of cataract surgery is the risk of postoperative infection (Hosseini et al., 2018).

Following diagnosis, health education is an important factor in prevention and treatment of blepharitis. Eye hygiene is essential. For example, warm compresses aid comfort and also soften crusting. Cleansing and massaging eyelid margins, warm compresses and topical or systemic antibiotics and topical anti-inflammatory treatments may alleviate but not cure the condition (Amescua et al., 2018). Tea tree oil helps resolve Demodex mites (Eberhardt & Rammohan, 2019).

EYELID MALPOSITION: ENTROPION AND ECTROPION

Entropion and ectropion are two malformations of the eyelid margins. Correct positioning of the eyelids is essential for eye health. If the eyelids do not close completely, the front of the person's eye is exposed, putting them at risk of discomfort and infections such as watery eyes (i.e., epiphora) and conjunctivitis. If the cornea is exposed because the eyelid does not close, the cornea and subsequently the rest of the eye are susceptible to infections that affect vision and ultimately can lead to the loss of the eye. There are a number of causes of eyelid malposition, such as scarring from infection, injury and facial palsy, but as people age, eyelid muscles can become lax, resulting in acquired lid abnormalities like entropion and ectropion (Batterbury & Murphy, 2018).

ENTROPION

Entropion is a malformation of the lower eyelid that results from the inward turning of the eyelid muscles (Bowling, 2016). Muscle thinning and loss of elasticity associated with the ageing process cause the lower eyelid to move inward toward the eyeball (Bowling, 2016). Symptoms are reported as a feeling there is something in the eye and general eye discomfort. Eyelashes inevitably turn toward the globe, causing irritation and potential ocular damage (Bowling, 2016). Surgical and non-surgical interventions are available to manage the eyelid defect.

ECTROPION

Ectropion is a malformation of the eyelid that causes it to turn outward due to scarring, infection or slack muscles that are the result of ageing (Batterbury & Murphy, 2018). A person with ectropion cannot close their eye completely, exposing the front of the eye and making it vulnerable to corneal damage and infection (Shaw & Lee, 2017). Frequent applications of eye ointment promote comfort; ectropion may be corrected by a surgical intervention (Batterbury & Murphy, 2018).

CATARACTS

Cataracts are a disorder of the crystalline lens that result in opacity and subsequently disordered vision (Batterbury & Murphy, 2018). Cataracts can affect people across the age spectrum but are more common in older adults. As well as ageing, other risk factors that affect both the wider and older populations include diabetes, exposure to ultraviolet light, smoking and certain medications such as oral steroids (Batterbury & Murphy, 2018). Age-related cataracts develop slowly, are often unilateral and may take some time for the person to notice. Cataracts can affect a person's vision to such an extent their quality of life is significantly impacted, including the ability to complete daily living activities, hobbies, caring responsibilities and driving. It is estimated in England and Wales, 2.5 million people aged 65 and older have some degree of visual impairment caused by cataracts (MacEwan et al., 2019). However, they can be surgically removed to improve vision. Cataracts are named according to their appearance on a slit lamp (i.e., microscopic) eye examination (Table 17.5).

CATARACT SURGERY

Cataracts can be removed only by a surgical procedure. The Royal College of Ophthalmologists (2020) cited cataract extraction as the most common NHS surgical procedure: during 2018–2019, 452,000 cataract surgery operations were undertaken in England and 20,000 in Wales, with an average patient age of 76. The demand for surgery in older adults is expected to increase by 25% in the next 10 years (Royal College of Ophthalmologists, 2015). Visual impairment as a result of cataracts is a global concern across the population of older people, reflecting a worldwide impetus for cataract surgery to facilitate vision and improve quality of life (WHO, 2019).

Spectacle correction can facilitate eyesight in a person who has cataracts, but once meaningful sight is no longer achievable, according to the National Institute for Health and Care Excellence (NICE) guidance Cataracts in Adults, a referral to an ophthalmic cataract service should be made by an optometrist or general practitioner (National Institute for Health and Care Excellence [NICE], 2017a). NICE, in 2018, added further advice regarding patient access to cataract surgery. In the publication 'Serious Eye Disorders', NICE cited the impact of cataracts on a person's quality of life, not only their visual acuity, as a predominant for surgical intervention (NICE, 2018a). Quality of life, loss of colour vision, glare and difficulty reading are advised as mitigating factors for surgery (NICE, 2018a). Nonetheless, health services have finite resources, and many patients may find themselves on a long cataract waiting list. The NHS standard for elective surgery is 18 weeks from referral to operation (NHS, 2019), but there are variances in access to cataract surgery in the United Kingdom that suggest inequalities (PHE, 2021). The COVID-19 pandemic increased pressure on ophthalmic services; in May 2021 PHE reported 125,000 people in the United Kingdom had been waiting more than 6 months for treatment (PHE, 2021). Applying these statistics, the negative impact of visual impairment on an older adult and their family and the value of cataract removal to enhanced quality of life becomes compromised (Burton et al., 2021).

Advances in cataract surgical techniques, anaesthesia and day surgery mean recovery is fast, which allows people to carry on with their everyday lives. This is evident across the older age group; as Toyama et al. (2018) noted, cataract surgery is as safe and effective for people older than 90 as it is for younger people. Age is therefore no limit to the visual and life outcomes afforded by cataract surgery.

GLAUCOMA

Glaucoma is estimated to affect 64 million people in the world population (WHO, 2019). There are several types of glaucoma; the most common that affect older adults are primary angle closure glaucoma (PACG) and chronic open angle glaucoma (COAG) (WHO, 2019). Both types irreversibly affect vision and consequently can negatively affect mental health. Research revealed depression is 10 times

TABLE 17.5 Classification of Cataracts	
Type of Cataract	Appearance on the Slit Lamp
Nuclear cataract	• The opacity is situated in the central aspect of the crystalline lens. • Visual symptoms include loss of clarity of vision, glare and double vision. • Visual symptoms may change according to pupil dilatation in response to light.
Subcapsular cataract	• The crystalline lens is encased in a capsule. • The opacity starts to form directly under the lens capsule.
Cortical cataract	• The opacity extends in a snowflake effect toward the centre of the lens.

Source: Batterbury & Murphy (2018).

higher in people with glaucoma when compared to the general population (Gamiochipi-Arjona et al., 2021).

PRIMARY ANGLE CLOSURE GLAUCOMA

Also known as acute glaucoma, PACG is a sudden closure of the trabecular meshwork or drainage system by the outside edge of the iris (Bowling, 2016), characterised by a sudden onset of symptoms that include blurred vision, halos around lights, significant reduction in vision, a hazy cornea and red eye (Wormald & Shah, 2008). The person is likely to experience severe pain accompanied by vomiting and possibly abdominal pain (Bowling, 2016). The intraocular pressure of the eye can rise to 50–100 millimeters of mercury from the normal range of 15–21 millimeters of mercury. PACG has the potential to cause irreversible damage to eyesight. Although it is a difficult condition to treat—the NICE guidance relates to COAG only (Wormald & Shah, 2008)—Bowling (2016) advised medical and/or surgical treatment and a laser procedure known as an iridotomy. Nursing interventions include assessment and management of the person's pain, nausea, vomiting and the distress of the visual disturbance. However, treatment does not restore eyesight, which is likely to have negative psychological and social impacts for the individual and their family (Gamiochipi-Arjona et al., 2021).

PRIMARY OPEN ANGLE GLAUCOMA

Commonly known as chronic glaucoma, primary open angle glaucoma (POAG) is prevalent in people over 40, those with a family history (Batterbury & Murphy, 2018) and people with African heritage (Tham et al., 2014). POAG is a painless condition characterised by a chronic gradual increase in intraocular pressure that eventually causes optic neuropathy (Wormald & Shah, 2008). Vision deteriorates from the periphery, and its slow progression means the person often does not notice the ensuing visual impairment (WHO, 2019).

In parallel with a predicted growth in the older population, projections suggest by 2035 there will be a 44% increase in people with chronic glaucoma in the United Kingdom (Royal College of Ophthalmologists, 2017). This statistic accentuates the significance of public health messages to people across the age spectrum, including older people, individuals over 40 and first-degree relatives of people with chronic glaucoma. Eye health education, vision testing and interventions are vital for quality-of-life outcomes (Burton et al., 2021). Chronic glaucoma is often initially identified at a routine eye test, thus indicating the importance of eye health promotion (Burton et al., 2021; NICE, 2022; 2017b).

Chronic glaucoma may be difficult to treat. Initially the aim is to decrease intraocular pressure in the eye (Wormald & Shah, 2008). The NICE (2022) recommends selective laser trabeculoplasty, a minimally invasive intervention, as the first line of treatment for people with newly diagnosed chronic glaucoma. For individuals who are unsuitable for selective laser trabeculoplasty, prostaglandin analogue eye drops are prescribed (NICE, 2022). The NICE (2022) recommends glaucoma surgery for people with advanced disease. Even so, the NICE (2022) acknowledged in both groups of people, long-term eye drop therapy may be required.

A pharmaceutical approach to treatment may be necessary for people who are unsuitable for or unresponsive to surgical intervention. Adherence to prescribed eye drops for chronic glaucoma is essential not as a cure but to prevent further damage to vision (Stanford, 2020). Health education about instillation and adherence to eye drop regimes is therefore inherent to patient care. Instilling eye drops can be a challenge for some older people due to issues with manual dexterity, cognitive function in remembering to instil eye drops safely and at the correct time, and general illness. An individualised approach is vital to appropriate interventions to promote eye drop adherence and subsequently ambitions to achieve optimum intraocular pressure. A systematic review by Waterman et al. (2013) set out to identify best practices for promoting eye drop adherence in people with chronic glaucoma. No age groups were specified in the review, but the condition affects adults over 40 and therefore is pertinent to older people's experiences. The review concluded glaucoma education, teaching eye drop instillation, promoting eye drop adherence and ongoing support were essential factors in adherence to eye drop regimes. Glaucoma education continues to be central to patient care in the NICE (2022) guidelines.

DIABETIC RETINOPATHY

Diabetes and its ocular complications affect people in the older age group; Sinclair et al. (2020) reported 19.3% of people aged 65–99 years have diabetes, with type 2 the most common form and particularly prevalent in people with Afro Caribbean and South Asian heritage (PHE, 2021). All parts of the eye are susceptible to damage from diabetes (Khan et al., 2017). One specific eye condition that affects the retina is diabetic retinopathy. The WHO (2019) noted diabetes can cause the formation of abnormal retinal blood vessels that become blocked or leak into the retina, causing scarring and visual loss. The risk of diabetic retinopathy is thought to be associated with the duration of the disease, glycaemic control and presence of hypertension (WHO, 2019). Furthermore, Bowling (2016) explained evidence

TABLE 17.6 **Stages of Diabetic Retinopathy**	
Stage of Diabetic Retinopathy	**Characteristics**
Background	Early stage retinopathy: Retinal micro aneurysms, dots and blot-type haemorrhages.
Preproliferative	Appearance of cotton wool spots on the retina; severe retinal haemorrhages can result in retinal ischaemia.
Proliferative	Neovasculation progression: New vessels move toward the optic disc with potential far-reaching visual consequences.

Source: Bowling (2016).

to suggest risks of diabetic retinopathy are commensurate with the age of onset of type 1 diabetes, notably before 30. After 10 years, the consequences of type 1 diabetes are associated with a 50% risk of diabetic retinopathy (Bowling, 2016). The visual disturbances reported by people with diabetic retinopathy include interference with colour vision, focus, glare, contrast sensitivity and changes in the refractive ability of the eye (Khan et al., 2017).

The four stages of diabetic retinopathy are mild nonproliferative, moderate nonproliferative, severe nonproliferative and proliferative (see Table 17.6). Each stage has the potential to cause irreparable damage and severely affect vision. Diabetic retinopathy responds to a variety of treatments, depending on the extent of the disease and access to health care. Leley et al. (2021) described therapies such as laser photocoagulation, corticosteroid via intravitreal injections and anti-growth factor to reduce swelling of the macula and stimulate new growth of vessels. Vitreous haemorrhages occur as a result of neovascularisation and can cause retinal detachments that require surgical intervention.

Diabetes is also a causative factor in other ocular abnormal physiology. Neovascularisation and haemorrhages in the advanced stage of diabetic retinopathy progress to other parts of the eye such as the trabecular meshwork, resulting in raised intraocular pressure—classified as secondary or rubeotic glaucoma. The increasing prevalence of diabetes in the population and subsequently in older adults means an increase in the occurrence of diabetes-associated eye disorders such as cataracts, glaucoma and diabetic retinopathy (Konstantinidis et al., 2017). It is therefore inevitable people will carry vision-impacting comorbidities into older age or begin to develop the long-term effects of diabetes in their eyes.

Regular eye screening of older people with diabetes can pre-empt the ocular complications caused by the disease, facilitating early intervention to prevent loss of vision (Pearce & Sivaprasad, 2020). Older people's access to screening is essential and pivotal to health promotion. People with diabetes and those who are at risk require preventative and targeted health education that is sensitive to racial differences and health beliefs and translated into appropriate languages. Education should focus on diabetes management and health protection such as access to national diabetic screening programmes for annual monitoring and to trigger treatment of diabetic retinopathy (Pearce & Sivaprasad, 2020; Sinclair et al., 2020). Given the physical and psychological consequences of impaired vision, for older people living with type 1 diabetes or newly diagnosed with type 2, screening for diabetic retinopathy should part of a long-term personalised health care plan.

AGE-RELATED MACULAR DEGENERATION

The ageing process is evident in the macula, a part of the retina that facilitates central vision. Bowling (2016) described age-related macular degeneration (AMD) as a degenerative disorder of the macula. AMD is the main cause of visual impairment in Europe in people over the age of 50, with a predicted increase from 67 million to around 77 million people by the year 2050 (Li et al., 2020). People can experience loss of fine vision and impairment of colour perception, but peripheral vision can remain, and consequences include not being able to read, drive or do simple tasks like prepare vegetables (Holekamp, 2019). Risk factors include smoking, raised blood pressure, age and familial risk from a first-degree relative with the condition (Bowling, 2016). The NICE (2018b) classified AMD in six stages: normal eyes, early AMD, late AMD indeterminable, late AMD wet active, late AMD dry and late AMD wet inactive. These categories provide an indication for treatment according to retinal changes, risk of progression and threat to vision.

The pathology of AMD is determined by ischaemia of the choroidal blood vessels that serve the retina. In wet macular degeneration, choroidal bold vessels leak blood and fluid under the retina, resulting in damage to the macula. Small yellow deposits known as drusen occur on the macula as a consequence of the changes associated with AMD and can further compromise retinal health (Batterbury & Murphy, 2018).

Dry AMD progresses slowly. Currently there is no treatment to arrest the retinal damage and subsequent visual impairment (Narayanan & Kuppermann, 2017). People with dry AMD should be referred for social assistance so they can access vision support such as low-vision aids, home adaptations and financial assistance to help them continue their daily living activities. Support from an eye care liaison officer or social worker for the visually impaired helps the person navigate the certificate of visual impairment application process.

The NICE (2018b) advised prompt treatment for people with AMD and, following diagnosis of wet AMD by an optometrist or ophthalmologist, referral to a macular treatment centre in secondary care. The NICE (2018b) recommends referral within 1 working day following diagnosis, with treatment commencing within 14 days.

Evidence from the NICE (2018b) indicated late wet AMD responds to monthly antivascular endothelial growth factor treatment injected into the vitreous to block endothelial growth. The treatment halts the development of abnormal blood vessels over a 3-month course of monthly injections (NICE, 2018b). However, individualised AMD treatments are also effective (Holekamp, 2019). The prognosis following antivascular endothelial growth factor injections is positive, with people maintaining functional vision for at least 10 years following treatment (Garweg et al., 2018).

CONCLUSION AND LEARNING POINTS

The natural process of ageing and the advancing age of the world population inevitably align to the likelihood most people will develop an eye condition at some stage in later life. Physiological changes have the potential to impact the physical and psychological health of an older person's eyes and ultimately their vision. Treatments and interventions are available to improve vision in some age-related conditions. For example, a cataract can be removed by surgery, and anti-vascular endothelial growth factor injections are effective for AMD. However, for other conditions, such as chronic glaucoma, preservation of rather than improvement of vision is the aim of treatment. Access to eye tests and appropriate treatment and support are essential to promote the health and well-being of older adults. Nurses and other health care professionals have a responsibility to understand the normal and altered anatomy and physiology of the eye and vision so they can comprehend patients' lived experience and assess, plan and evaluate appropriate interventions for holistic patient care. Nurses and other health care professionals can use the information in this chapter to inform their knowledge and practice to understand ocular anatomy and physiology, common eye conditions and the impact of visual impairment on the well-being of older people in any health care context.

KEY LEARNING POINTS

- An understanding of the normal and altered anatomy and physiology of the eye and how age-related changes affect the eye and its surrounding structures.
- An awareness of some major and minor ocular conditions that affect older people and how they affect vision.

- An appreciation of how eye health influences other health issues such as the prevention of falls.
- An understanding of the importance of eye tests and eye health for older people.

REFERENCES

Amescua, G., Akpek, E. K., Fafid, M., Garcia-Ferrer, F. J., Lin, A., Rhee, M. K., Varu, D. M., Musch, D. C., Dunn, S. P., & Mah, F. S. American Academoy of Opthalmology Preferred Practice Pattern Cornea and External Disease Panel. (2018). Blepharitis preferred practice patter. *Opthalmology, 126*(1), 56–93.

Batterbury, M., & Murphy, C. (2018). *Ophthalmology: An illustrated colour text* (4th ed.). Elsevier.

Best, J., Lui, P., Ffytche, D., Potts, J., & Moosajee, M. (2019). Think sight loss, think Charles Bonnet syndrome. *Therapeutic Advances in Ophthalmology, 11*, 1–2.

Bourne, R. R. A., Flaxman, S. R., Braithwaite, T., Cicinelli, M. V., Das, A., Jonas, J. B., Keeffe, J., Kempen, J. H., Leasher, J., Limburg, H., Naidoo, K., Pesudovs, K., Resnikoff, S., Silvester, A., Stevens, G. A., Tahhan, N., Wong, T. Y., Taylor, H. R. & Vision Loss Expert Group. (2017). Magnitude, temporal trends, and projections of the global prevalence of blindness and distance and near vision impairment: A systematic review and meta-analysis. *Lancet Global Health, 5*(9), e888–e897.

Bowling, B. (2016). *Kanski's clinical ophthalmology: A systematic approach*. Elsevier.

Buchan, J. C., Norman, P., Shickle, D., Cassels-Brown, A., & MacEwan, C. (2019). Failing to plan and planning to fail. Can we predict the future growth of demand on UK Eye Care Services? *Eye, 33*, 1029–1031. https://doi.org/10.1038/s41433-019-0383-5.

Burton, M. J., Ramke, J., Marques, A. P., Bourne, R. R. A., Congdon, N., Jones, I., Ah Ton, B. A. M., Arunga, S., Bachani, D., Bascaran, C., Bastawrous, A., Blanchet, K., Braithwaite, T., Buchan, J. C., Cairns, J., Cama, A., Chagunda, M., Chuluunkhuu, C., Cooper, A., … Faal, H. B. (2021). The *Lancet Global Health* Commission on Global Eye Health: Vision beyond 2020. *Lancet Global Health, 9*(4), e489–e551.

Definition and Classification Subcommittee of the International Dry Eye WorkShop. (2007). The definition and classification of dry eye disease: Report of the Definition and Classification Subcommittee of the International Dry Eye WorkShop (2007). *Ocular Surface, 5*(2), 65–204.

Department of Health. (2017). Certificate of visual impairment. http://www.gov.uk/dh

Eberhardt, M., & Rammohan, G. (2019). *Blepharitis*. StatPearls Publishing.

Ehrlich, J. R., Hassan, S. E., & Stagg, B. C. (2019). Prevalence of falls and fall-related outcomes in older adults with self-reported vision impairment. *Journal of the American Geriatrics Society, 67*(2), 239–245. doi:10.1111/jgs.15628.

Enoch, J., Jones, L., & McDonald, L. (2020). Thinking about sight as a sense. *Optometry in Practice, 21*(3), 2–9.

Evans, J. R., Fletcher, A. E., & Wormald, R. P. L. (2007). Depression and anxiety in visually impaired older people. *Ophthalmology, 114*(2), 283–288.

Gamiochipi-Arjona, et al. (2021). Depression and medical adherence in Mexican patients with glaucoma. *Journal of Glaucoma. 30*(3), 251–256.

Garweg, J. G., Zirpel, J. J., Gerhardt, C., & Pfister, I. B. (2018). The fate of eyes with wet AMD beyond four years of anti-VEGF therapy. *Graefe's Archive for Clinical and Experimental Ophthalmology, 256*, 823–831. https://doi.org/10.1007/s00417-018-3907-y.

GBD 2019 Blindness and Vision Impairment Collaborators. (2021). Trends in prevalence of blindness and distance and near vision impairment over 30 years: An analysis for the Global Burden of Disease Study. *Lancet Global Health, 9*(2), e130–e143.

Holekamp, N. M. (2019). Review of age-related macular degeneration. *American Journal of Managing Care, 25*(10), S172–S181.

Hosseini, K., Bourque, L. B., & Hays, R. D. (2018). Development and evaluation of a measure of patient-reported symptoms of Blepharitis. *Health and Quality of Life Outcomes, 16*(11). https://doi.org/10.1186/s12955-018-0839-5.

Khan, A., Petropoulos, I. N., Ponirakis, G., & Malik, R. A. (2017). Visual complications in diabetes mellitus: Beyond retinopathy. *Diabetic Medicine, 34*(4), 478–484.

Konstantinidis, L., Carron, T., de Ancos, E., Chinet, L., Hagon-Traub, I., Zuercher, A., & Peytremann-Bridevaux, I. (2017). Awareness and practices regarding eye diseases among patients with diabetes: A cross sectional analysis of the CoDiab-VD cohort. *BMC Endocrine Disorders, 17*(56). https://doi.org/10.1186/s12902-017-0206-2.

Lee, T.-Y., Shin, Y. H., & Lee, J. G. (2020). Strategies of upper blepharoplasty in aging patients with involutional ptosis. *Archives of Plastic Surgery, 47*(4), 290–296.

Leley, S. P., Ciulla, T. A., & Bhatwadekar, A. D. (2021). Diabetic retinopathy in the aging population: A perspective of pathogenesis and treatment. *Clinical Interventions in Aging, 16*, 1367–1378.

Li, J. Q., Welchowski, T., Schmid, M., Mauschitz, M. M., Holz, F. G., & Finger, R. P. (2020). Prevalence and incidence of age-related macular degeneration in Europe: A systematic review and meta-analysis. *British Journal of Ophthalmology, 104*(8), 1077–1084.

Lord, S. (2006). Visual risk factors for falls in older people. *Age and Ageing, 35*(2), ii42–ii45.

MacEwen, C., Davis, A., & Chang, L. (2019) Ophthalmology GIRFT programme national specialty report. https://gettingitrightfirsttime.co.uk/wp-content/uploads/2019/12/OphthalmologyReportGIRFT19P-FINAL.pdf

Marsden, J. (2017). *Ophthalmic care*. M&K Publishing.

McGinley, P., Ansari, E., Sandhu, H., & Dixon, T. (2020). The cost burden of falls in people with glaucoma in National Health Service Hospital Trusts in the UK. *Journal of Medical Economics, 23*(1), 106–112.

Menon, G., Rahman, I., Sharmila, J., Menon, S., & Dutton, G. (2003). Complex visual hallucinations in the visually impaired: The Charles Bonnet syndrome. *Survey of Ophthalmology, 48*(1), 58–72.

Naidoo, S., Leasher, J., Bourne, R., Flaxman, S., Jonas, B., Keeffe, J., Limburg, H., Pesudovs, K., Price, H., White, R., Wong, T., Taylor, H. R., & Resnikoff, S. (2016). Global vision impairment and blindness due to uncorrected refractive error, 1990–2010. *Optometry and Vision Science, 93*(3), 227–234.

Narayanan, R., & Kuppermann, D. (2017). Hot topics in dry AMD. *Current Pharmaceutical Design, 23*(4), 542–546.

National Health Service (NHS). (2019). Guide to NHS waiting times in England. https://www.nhs.uk/nhs-services/hospitals/guide-to-nhs-waiting-times-in-england

National Institute for Health and Care Excellence (NICE). (2017a). Cataracts in adults: Management. https://www.nice.org.uk/guidance/ng77/resources/cataracts-in-adults-management-pdf-1837639266757

NICE. (2017b). Glaucoma diagnosis and management. https://www.nice.org.uk/guidance/ng81

NICE. (2018a). Serious eye disorders. https://www.nice.org.uk/guidance/qs180/resources/serious-eye-disorders-pdf-75545714654917

NICE. (2018b). Age-related macular degeneration. https://www.nice.org.uk/guidance/ng82/resources/agerelated-macular-degeneration-pdf-1837691334853

NICE. (2022). Glaucoma: Diagnosis and management. https://www.nice.org.uk/guidance/ng81

Pang, L. (2016). Hallucinations experienced by visually impaired: Charles Bonnet syndrome. *Optometry and Vision Science, 93*(12), 1466–1478.

Pearce, E., & Sivaprasad, S. (2020). A review of advancements and evidence gaps in Diabetic retinopathy screening models. *Clinical Ophthalmology, 14*, 3285–3296. doi:10.2147/OPTH.S267521.

Public Health England (PHE). (2021). Atlas of variation in risk factors and healthcare for vision in England. https://fingertips.phe.org.uk/profile/atlas-of-variation

Rahman, F., Zekite, A., Bunce, C., Jayaram, H., & Flanagan, D. (2020). Recent trends in vision impairment certifications in England and Wales. *Eye, 34*, 1271–1278.

Royal College of Ophthalmologists. (2015). The way forward: Cataracts. https://www.rcophth.ac.uk/wp-content/uploads/2015/10/RCOphth-The-Way-Forward-Cataract-300117.pdf

Royal College of Ophthalmologists. (2017). The way forward. https://www.rcophth.ac.uk/wp-content/uploads/2015/10/RCOphth-The-Way-Forward-Glaucoma-Summary-300117.pdf

Royal College of Ophthalmologists. (2020). National ophthalmic database audit. https://www.nodaudit.org.uk/u/docs/20/hqs-rgmurnv/NOD%20Audit%20Full%20Annual%20Report%202020.pdf

Royal College of Physicians. (2015). National falls audit. https://www.rcplondon.ac.uk/projects/national-audit-inpatient-falls-naif

Royal College of Physicians. (2021). National audit of inpatient falls audit report. *Royal College of Physicians*.

Royal College of Ophthalmologists. (2017). Look out! Bedside vision check for falls prevention. http://www.rcplondon.ac.uk/fffap

Scott, A., Bressler, N., Ffolkes, S., Wittenborn, J., & Jorkasky, J. (2016). Public attitudes about eye and vision health. *JAMA Opthalmology, 134*(10), 1111–1118.

Seewoodhary, R. (2009). Managing common eye disorders in the outpatient department. In S. Watkinson (Ed.), *Issues in ophthalmic practice: Current and future challenges*. M&K Publishing.

Shaw, M., & Lee, A. (2017). *Ophthalmic nursing* (5th ed.). CRC Press.

Sinclair, A., Saeedi, P., Kaundal, A., Karuranga, S., Malanda, B., & Williams, R. (2020). Diabetes and global ageing among 65–99-year-old adults: Findings from the International Diabetes Federation Diabetes Atlas, 9th edition. *Diabetes Research and Clinical Practice, 162*(108078). doi:10.1016/j.diabres.2020.108078.

Stanford, P., Olleveant, N., & Wu, L. (2014). Traditional Chinese medicine, health beliefs and glaucoma awareness: Implications for UK practice. *International Journal of Ophthalmic Practice, 5*(4), 134–138.

Stanford, P. (2020). Chronic open-angle glaucoma guidelines: A UK perspective. *Asorn Insight, fall,* 5–10.

Tham, Y., Xiang, L., Wong, T., Quigley, H., Aung, T., & Cheng, C. (2014). Global prevalence of glaucoma and projections of glaucoma burden through 2040: A systematic review and meta-analysis. *Ophthalmology, 121*(11), 2081–2090. https://doi.org/10.1016/j.ophtha.2014.05.013.

Thomas Pocklington Trust. (2016). Sight loss, dementia and meaningful activity. https://www.pocklington-trust.org.uk/sector-resources/research-archive/sight-loss-dementia-and-meaningful-activity

Toyama, T., Ueta, T., Yoshitani, M., Sakata, R., & Numaga, J. (2018). Visual acuity improvement after phacoemulsification cataract surgery in patients aged ≥90 years. *BMC Ophthalmology, 18*, 280. https://doi.org/10.1186/s12886-018-0950-8.

United Nations (UN). (2015). World population aging. https://www.un.org/en/development/desa/population/publications/pdf/ageing/WPA2015_Report.pdf

UN. (2019). Department of Economic and Social Affairs population division highlights. https://population.un.org/wpp

Valipoor, S., Pati, D., Kazem-Zadeh, M., Mihandoust, S., & Mahammadigorji, S. (2020). Falls in older adults: A systematic review of literature on interior-scale elements of the built environment. *Journal of Aging and Environment, 34*(4), 351–374. doi:10.1080/02763893.2019.1683672.

Waterman, H., Ballinger, C., Brundle, C., Chastin, S., Gage, H., Harper, R., Henson, D., Laventure, B., McEvoy, L., Pilling, M., Olleveant, N., Skelton, D. A., Stanford, P., & Todd, C. (2016). A feasibility study to prevent falls in older people who are sight impaired: The VIP2UK randomised controlled trial. *Trials, 17*, 464. https://doi.org/10.1186/s13063-016-1565-0.

Waterman, H., Evans, J. R., Gray, T. A., Henson, D., & Harper, R. (2013). Interventions for improving adherence to ocular hypotensive therapy. *Cochrane Database of Systematic Reviews, 2*(4). doi:10.1002/14651858.CD006132.pub3.

Wolffsohn, J., & Davies, L. (2019). Presbyopia: Effectiveness of correction strategies. *Progress in Retinal and Eye Research, 68*, 124–143.

World Health Organization (WHO). (2019). World report on vision. https://www.who.int/publications/i/item/world-report-on-vision

WHO. (2020). ICD-11 for mortality and morbidity statistics. https://icd.who.int/browse11/l-m/en

Wormald, R., & Shah, R. (2008). Acute and chronic angle glaucoma. In R. Wormald, K. Henshaw, & L. Smeeth (Eds.), *Evidence-based ophthalmology*. BMJ Books.

Wykoff, C. C. (2019). Diabetic retinopathy and its management. In H. Beaver, & A. Lee (Eds.), *Geriatric ophthalmology*. Springer.

Zhu, M., Chao, C., Haisu, Y., Liping, L., & Kaili, W. (2018). Quantitative analysis of the bacteria in blepharitis with Demodex infestation. *Frontiers in Microbiology, 9*, 1–7. https://doi.org/10.3389/fmicb.2018.01719.

18

Promoting Safe Mobility for Older People

Julie Whitney

IMPORTANCE OF MOBILITY

Before embarking on a chapter on how to promote safe mobility, it's important to define it. For this chapter, mobility is 'the ability to move oneself (e.g., by walking, by using assistive devices, or by using transportation) within community environments that expand from one's home, to the neighbourhood, and to regions beyond' (Webber et al., 2010, p. 444).

Many mobility tasks are required for everyday functioning, from simple activities of daily living like getting out of bed, getting up from a chair, walking and stair climbing to more complex mobility requirements like professional sports, leisure activities and certain jobs.

Mobility is essential to the well-being of older people. Webber et al. (2010) suggested it is considered in different life spaces, extending outward from a room to the home, immediate outdoor space, neighbourhood and world. They argued professionals involved in rehabilitation often neglect mobility in the wider spheres of the life space, leaving older people potentially housebound or restricted in their activity (Webber et al., 2010).

WHAT IS NEEDED FOR EFFECTIVE MOBILITY?

Several domains contribute to a person's ability to effectively participate in society in a way that allows them to be economically active, active in occupations such as caring for others and able to serve their well-being through leisure, sport, and education. Webber et al. (2010) proposed five key determinants of mobility—cognitive, psychological, physical, environmental and financial—as well as influences from culture, gender and biography. Although this chapter concentrates on the physical with reference to the cognitive and psychological domains, it is important not to forget other influences on mobility (see Fig. 18.1).

In the presence of disease or injury, mobility may be maintained through compensatory mechanisms within or between domains. For example, someone with visual impairment may be able to compensate using joint position sense, or proprioception. In the same way, impairments in different domains may have a cumulative effect; for example, dementia, muscle weakness and peripheral neuropathy may combine to have a greater impact on mobility than the sum of their parts.

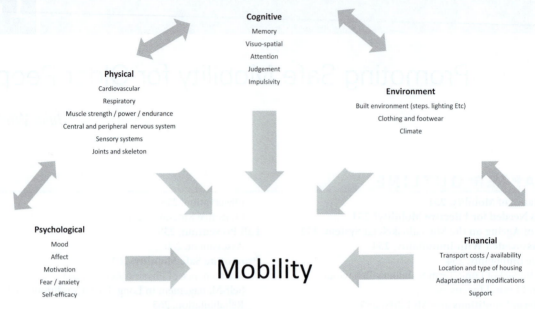

Fig. 18.1 Different domains associated with mobility.

The World Health Organization's (WHO) International Classification of Functioning, Disability and Health (ICF) is a useful method by which to understand mobility in terms of assessment, goal setting and intervention programmes (WHO, 2001).

The ICF uses a holistic approach, ensuring interventions do not merely attempt to diagnose, treat and/or manage a structural or physiological impairment but also consider the effects of a condition on a person's ability to undertake daily activities and participate in the social sphere. Figure 18.2 illustrates how an older person's mobility might be considered using the ICF.

EFFECTS OF AGEING ON THE MUSCULOSKELETAL SYSTEM

Ageing has an effect on muscles, bones and joints. However, some effects are exacerbated by long-term conditions and sedentary behaviour, both of which are more prevalent in older populations.

Muscles reach their peak in terms of mass and strength around age 30. After that there is a steady decline, with reductions in strength of 1%–2% and in power of 3.5% per year after age 65 (Keller & Engelhardt, 2014). Muscle mass is reduced due to a predominant loss of type II fibres. Type II, or fast-twitch, muscle fibres are responsible for explosive contractions that generate large forces over a short duration, such as that required for a stepping strategy to prevent a trip or slip becoming a fall. Severe muscle atrophy and weakness associated with ageing is termed *sarcopenia*. Sarcopenia is diagnosed in older people who have loss of muscle mass accompanied by either muscle weakness or functional impairment (Cruz-Jentoft et al., 2018).

Rather than there being a linear relationship between muscle strength and function, where function declines proportionally to losses in muscle strength, a threshold of muscle strength under which specific functions are negatively impacted has been observed. For example, once quadriceps muscle strength drops below a specific level, getting up from a chair becomes difficult or impossible. Figure 18.3 illustrates the decline in muscle strength over the life course and how the variance in this decline increases with age. This variance supports the idea that deterioration in strength and mass is not merely age related but influenced by genetics and lifestyle. The key aim of health promotion is to prevent older people developing weakness and keeping away from the disability threshold by promoting ongoing physical activity. Rehabilitation aims to address muscle weakness to enable people to cross over the disability threshold to become more functionally independent.

Ageing is also associated with a gradual reduction in bone mineral density, with 80-year-olds losing approximately half

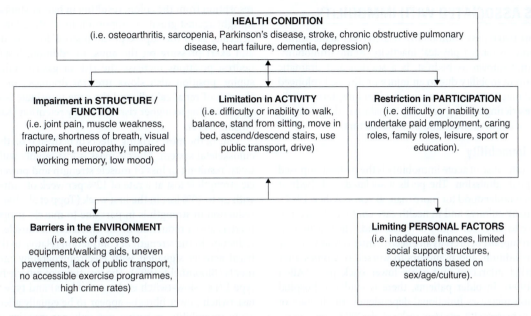

HEALTH CONDITION
(i.e. osteoarthritis, sarcopenia, Parkinson's disease, stroke, chronic obstructive pulmonary disease, heart failure, dementia, depression)

Impairment in STRUCTURE / FUNCTION
(i.e. joint pain, muscle weakness, fracture, shortness of breath, visual impairment, neuropathy, impaired working memory, low mood)

Limitation in ACTIVITY
(i.e. difficulty or inability to walk, balance, stand from sitting, move in bed, ascend/descend stairs, use public transport, drive)

Restriction in PARTICIPATION
(i.e. difficulty or inability to undertake paid employment, caring roles, family roles, leisure, sport or education).

Barriers in the ENVIRONMENT
(i.e. lack of access to equipment/walking aids, uneven pavements, lack of public transport, no accessible exercise programmes, high crime rates)

Limiting PERSONAL FACTORS
(i.e. inadequate finances, limited social support structures, expectations based on sex/age/culture).

Fig. 18.2 How mobility maps onto the WHO's International Classification of Functioning, Disability and Health.

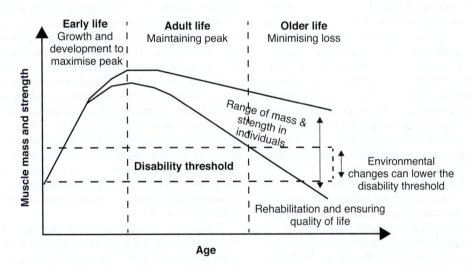

Modified WHO/HPS, Geneva 2000

Fig. 18.3 Life course of muscle mass and strength.

their peak bone mass. This occurs due to hormonal changes in post-menopausal women and a reduction in the activity of bone-building cells, or osteoblasts. These changes are compounded by a reduction in the time spent on weight-bearing activities. Severe reduction in bone mineral density leads to osteoporosis and an increased risk of fracture.

Finally, ageing affects the joints, with increased likelihood of damage to the articular cartilage on joint surfaces and loss of extensibility in ligaments, tendons and joint capsules. Osteoarthritis, which results from joint degeneration and leads to pain and stiffness, is one of the most common long-term conditions that affects older people worldwide.

RISKS ASSOCIATED WITH IMMOBILITY

There are two types of immobility-related risks: acute immobility and prolonged physical inactivity. Acute immobility, sometimes known as bedrest, is a sudden and dramatic reduction in mobility due to an injury or illness. Prolonged physical inactivity may occur as a result of long-term conditions, restricting activity, or it may be habitual, derived from a range of cultural, social and personal factors.

Acute Immobility

A common cause of acute immobility is the bedrest imposed by hospital admission. The perils associated with bedrest have been understood for more than 50 years (Asher, 1947), yet in many cultures and in health care contexts, bedrest in response to illness or injury is widespread. There is no evidence to support bedrest as an effective intervention for any health condition, and it appears to worsen outcomes after myocardial infarction and acute lower back pain (Allen et al., 1999). In older patients, there is evidence hospital admission increases functional dependency, the impact of which increases with age (Covinsky et al., 2003).

Prolonged time spent in bed adversely affects virtually every body system. Notable effects include a reduction in aerobic capacity. Supine lying causes blood to pool in the thorax and abdomen, increasing atrial pressure and the secretion of atrial natriuretic peptide (ANP) as well as aortic arch pressure causing a reduction in antidiuretic hormone (ADH) secretion. These changes result in diuresis, which leads to hypovolaemia. Low circulating blood volume in conjunction with increased venous compliance in the lower limbs increases risk of orthostatic hypotension when sitting or standing up after bedrest. The risk of orthostatic hypotension develops quickly and has been noted after less than 24 hours of bedrest.

The supine position exerts pressure on the chest, decreasing lung tidal volume, while the increased blood volume in the chest reduces residual volume. This position also compromises the mucociliary escalator and cough efficacy. The result is pooling of secretions in the lower parts of the lungs, causing alveolar atelectasis and impaired gas exchange. All these changes elevate the risk of developing lower respiratory tract infections.

Bedrest also has haematological consequences. The risk of thromboembolism is increased in three ways, described as Virchow's triad. Venous stasis, hypercoagulability and endothelial damage to vessel walls in the legs combine to lead to deep vein thrombosis. Emboli from the deep vein thrombosis can travel to the brain and cause stroke, to the coronary arteries to cause myocardial infarction or to the lungs to cause pulmonary infarction (Knight et al., 2018).

The principal gastrointestinal complication of immobility is constipation. Slower gut transit time increases water resorption from the colon, resulting in harder stools. Being upright against gravity is important in eliciting the urge to defecate, as in the supine position stool does not descend and exert pressure on the anus. In addition, head-down bedrest positions increase the risk of gastric reflux. The supine position also slows ureteral drainage, increasing the risk of renal calculi, and the urge to urinate is diminished, leading to higher risk of urinary retention (Knight & Nigam, 2019).

One of the most striking effects of bedrest is on the musculoskeletal system. Muscle mass is lost rapidly with inactivity, resulting in loss of muscle strength and power. Muscle strength is lost at a rate of 12% per week of immobility, with up to 40% lost in the first week (Topp et al., 2002). This reduction in strength is in part due to muscle atrophy, but there is also a reduction in the efficiency of muscle, with a reduction in the strength of contraction relative to the electrical activity signalled with electromyography measurements (Bloomfield, 1997). The two types of muscle fibres—type I (i.e., slow-twitch endurance fibres) and type II (i.e., fast-twitch power fibres)—appear to be equally affected by acute immobility, meaning not only are muscles weaker, but also they fatigue more quickly. The muscle groups most adversely affected are the large antigravity muscles in the lower limbs such as the knee and hip extensor muscles. The muscle atrophy that occurs with immobility leads to several other physiological changes. With reduced muscle activity, oxygen requirements are lower, leading to erythropoiesis and, in the longer term, hypoxaemia and increased risk of skin damage or cerebral hypoxia, resulting in delirium (Knight et al., 2018). With less use, muscle fibres become less sensitive to insulin, impacting the ability of muscle to use circulating glucose to power contractions, which in turn may increase blood glucose levels and heighten the risk of developing type II diabetes mellitus. Severe illness compounds these changes, accelerating the muscle protein breakdown that already occurs as a result of bedrest (Parry & Puthucheary, 2015).

Without the stimulus of weight-bearing, reductions in bone mineral density, particularly in lower limb bones, is noted (Bloomfield, 1997). There are also changes to the structure of tendons and ligaments and the articular surface of the joints, resulting in increased joint stiffness and contractures.

All the effects described above and the resulting sensory deprivation means prolonged bedrest often negatively impacts mental health, resulting in depression or anxiety, or has a deleterious effect on cognitive function.

Older people may be at higher risk of complications due to the compounding effect of ageing on all systems, further exacerbated because older people with long-term conditions also appear to spend more time in bed (Fox et al., 2009).

The Impact of Long-Term Sedentary Behaviour or Physical Inactivity

Sedentary behaviour, defined as time sitting, is associated with poor health outcomes. A sedentary lifestyle over the life course increases the risk of developing cardiovascular disease (de Rezende et al., 2014), diabetes mellitus and cancer and predicts all-cause mortality (Biswas et al., 2015; Stamatakis et al., 2019). Evidence suggests these effects can be counteracted in sedentary individuals by participation in moderate-vigorous exercise (Stamatakis et al., 2019). Older people are more likely to be sedentary and less likely to participate in vigorous exercise. Sedentary behaviour in older people is also predictive of cardiac disease and mortality (de Rezende et al., 2014).

On the other hand, engagement in regular physical activity is associated with better health, fewer long-term health conditions and lower mortality. Physical activity is defined as 'any bodily movement produced by skeletal muscles that requires energy expenditure' (WHO, 2022). Regular moderate-vigorous physical activity reduces the risk of cardiovascular disease, some cancers, obesity, diabetes and dementia (Lear et al., 2017).

LONG-TERM CONDITIONS AND MOBILITY

Most long-term conditions have a higher prevalence and incidence among older adults, many of which are associated with specific mobility impairments. The conditions described below are not comprehensive but provide an overview of the mobility disorders present in common age-related conditions.

Dementia

Dementia involves a deterioration in memory, thinking, behaviours and the ability to perform activities of daily living. However, evidence indicates it is also associated with specific mobility impairments. People living with dementia, when compared to older people who are cognitively intact, have worse static and dynamic balance (Szczepanska-Gieracha et al., 2016). Gait is also affected; people with dementia often have slower walking speeds, shorter step length, more gait variability and impaired coordination. Some of these changes are observed prior to the onset of memory difficulties and clinical diagnosis, which suggests balance and gait impairments are important primary symptoms of dementia (Beauchet et al., 2016). The effects on gait and balance may explain why people living with dementia are two to three times more likely to fall each year (Allan et al., 2009) and three to four times more likely to sustain a hip fracture than individuals without dementia (Harvey et al., 2016). Care of the older person living with dementia is discussed in more depth in Chapter 29.

Stroke

Stroke is the most common cause of disability in the developed world. Walking and balance impairments are common after stroke. Stroke survivors demonstrate a consistent pattern where less weight is taken through the affected leg, and body weight excursions are smaller in that direction, causing difficulties with all activities of daily living that require effective walking and balance. Walking and balance impairments increase the risk of falls and hip fracture (Zheng et al., 2017).

Parkinson's Disease

Parkinson's disease is a progressive neurodegenerative disorder clinically defined by signs of bradykinesia (i.e., slowness of movement) in conjunction with either resting tremor or rigidity. Postural instability is also a common feature. Unlike the other motor features of Parkinson's disease, it does not improve with anti-Parkinsonian medication (Palakurthi & Burugupally, 2019). Bradykinesia results in symptoms such as freezing and festination. Freezing of gait, or an inability to start effective stepping, is particularly noticeable when initiating walking and turning and is exacerbated by encountering obstacles, doorways, stress and distraction. Festination is a pattern of walking where step length gets progressively shorter and walking speed increases. Freezing, festination and postural instability increase the risk of falls and fall-related injuries (Genever et al., 2005).

Osteoarthritis

Osteoarthritis is the most common form of arthropathy, with more than 10% of the population over 60 experiencing symptoms of joint pain and stiffness. It is an important precursor to disability and considered to be the fourth-highest cause of years lived with disability in the world. Osteoarthritis is caused by degeneration of the articular cartilage and surrounding joint structures and is closely associated with ageing. It commonly affects lower-limb joints, impacting standing, walking and stair climbing tasks (Hunter & Bierma-Zeinstra, 2019). Gait patterns are altered to reduce weight transfer through the painful joint, and muscle weakness and deformity lead to impaired balance. For these reasons, there is some evidence osteoarthritis is a risk factor for falls in older adults.

Frailty

Frailty, a susceptibility to incomplete recovery following a stressor event such as illness or injury, increases in prevalence with age, affecting <7% of people between 60 and 69 rising to 65% of individuals over 90 (Gale et al., 2014). Although the term *frailty* covers a wider concept than immobility, it is characterised by symptoms such as muscle weakness, fatigue, weight loss and slow walking speed

(Fried et al., 2001). Therefore, older people living with frailty almost universally experience mobility-related disability and have an increased risk of falls and fractures. See Chapter 6 for more discussion of frailty.

ASSESSMENT OF MOBILITY

Before assessing mobility, it is important to consider the purpose of the assessment. If an older person has sustained an injury or had a period of illness, an assessment may be required to ascertain whether there has been a significant change in their mobility and function. It is important to understand any changes in mobility to ensure the person's safety. For example, when an older person arrives on a hospital ward, it is important to check they are able to walk safely, and walking aid requirements have not changed. Another example is on hospital discharge, when adaptations to the home environment and care provision may be needed as a result of a change in mobility status.

Other reasons for assessment of mobility are to respond to specific problems such as pain or reduced function, where an assessment may be required to identify the underlying cause to ensure the most appropriate treatment, management or rehabilitation plan. Finally, assessment of mobility and related functions is often carried out to ensure appropriately tailored prevention programmes such as those aimed at reducing the risk of falls. Screening and assessment for fall risk is covered in a separate section.

There are three components to assessment: asking the right questions, observation and objective assessment.

Questions

The purpose of questioning for a mobility assessment is to identify the difficulties the person experiences with their mobility, explore the underlying reasons and the duration and degree of the problem. Examples of questions are provided in Figure 18.4.

Observation

One of the most important parts of the mobility assessment is observation. Careful observation of expression, sitting posture, walking, balance and transfers provides vital information about specific mobility impairments and activity limitations.

Observing Balance

Maintaining balance is a complex process that requires the coordination of multiple sensorimotor systems. To maintain balance, the centre of mass (i.e., a hypothetical point in the body around which its mass is equally distributed) must remain within the base of support (i.e., the area covering all points of contact with the ground). As the centre of mass gets closer to the edge of the base of support, balance becomes more perilous (see Fig. 18.5). The visual, somatosensory and vestibular systems provide positional information to the central nervous system, which responds with appropriately timed and scaled muscle contractions, mostly in the lower limbs and trunk, to control stability. It is possible to observe the effects of different sensory systems on balance by reviewing the effect of removing vision by closing eyes or removing adequate somatic sensation by standing on a foam cushion.

Mobility assessment questions

Tell me about your walking, are you having any difficulties?
What can you not do since you've had this difficulty walking?
Do you use a walking aid?
Do you walk outdoors?
What do you think is the cause (of pain, weakness, shortness of breath, lack of confidence, fatigue)?
How long has this been a problem (did it start suddenly, or has it gradually got worse)?
Have you tried anything to help improve your walking?
Do you have difficulties getting up from a chair, getting in and out of bed or using stairs?
Do have any difficulties keeping your balance?
Have you had any falls?

Fig. 18.4 Mobility assessment questions.

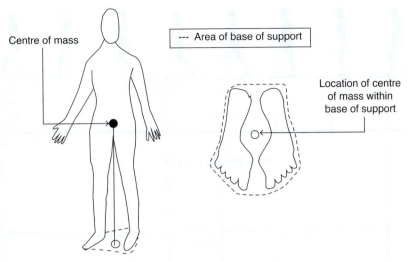

Fig. 18.5 Centre of mass and base of support.

All humans sway both backward and forward and side to side when standing still. This is a necessary function to maintain standing balance as a small degree of movement ensures the sensory systems can provide continuous feedback. Sway may be observed to be decreased or increased.

Although static balance provides some information about stability, it is important to also observe dynamic balance when the person is moving. Dynamic balance requires appropriately timed and scaled muscle responses to perturbations (i.e., a movement of the body). There are two types of perturbation: internal and external. Internal perturbations occur as a result of the forces produced by a movement of the body such as lifting an arm above the head. When postural mechanisms work effectively, before a limb movement, a series of muscle contractions in the legs and trunk serve to withstand the destabilising movement before it begins. This is called an anticipatory muscle contraction. These are observable only through electromyography measurement, but if anticipatory muscle activity is reduced or absent, an observer will notice bodily movement causes significant instability. External perturbations are forces outside the person that may cause instability. External forces may come from contact with an object (e.g., being pushed or pulled) or an unstable support surface (e.g., standing on a moving vehicle). Postural muscle responses to external perturbations are reactive.

Observing Gait

Observing a person walking, or a gait assessment, is a vital part of any assessment of mobility. This can be done during the walk to a clinic room, as the person returns from answering the door to a community visit or while a person moves around on a hospital ward. Effective analysis of walking complements a clinical assessment and provides clues as to why a person is experiencing mobility difficulties. Some key elements to look out for when observing gait include the following:
- Speed: Can be tested formally
- Walking aid use
- Symmetry between right and left legs in:
  - Step and stride distance
  - Support phase duration
  - Arm swing
- Base of support
- Noticeable abnormalities at different points in the cycle (e.g., absent heel strike at start of stance phase or poor foot clearance in midswing)
- Proportion of the cycle in double vs single support phase

Using the stages of the gait cycle as illustrated in Figure 18.6 helps with describing abnormalities.

Table 18.1 provides examples of gait observations and what condition they may indicate. Any hypotheses made while observing gait needs to be followed up with an appropriate examination.

Objective Measurement

A number of objective tests can be used to assess and measure mobility function. The tool chosen depends on the purpose of the measurement. There are two main reasons to conduct objective measurement:
- To use in a screening or assessment schedule to identify impairments, activity limitations or participation restriction that might be addressed with interventions.

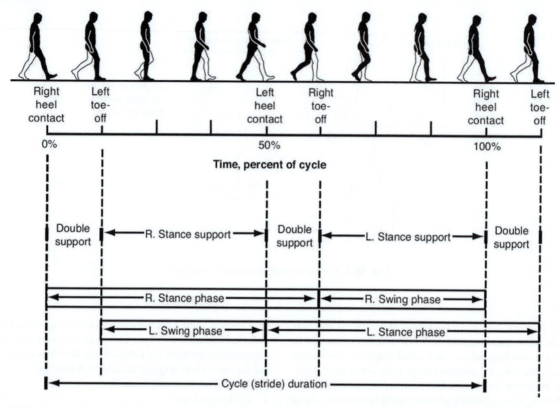

Fig. 18.6 Gait cycle. (Reproduced with permission from Rose, J., & Gamble, J. G., Eds. [2005]. *Human Walking* [pp.26]: Lippincott Williams and Wilkins.)

TABLE 18.1	Gait Observations
Gait Observation	**Possible Indication**
Narrow base of support, short step length, increased double support time, loss of arm swing and flexed posture	Parkinsonian gait
Reduced duration of stance phase with depression of the weight-bearing hip (Trendelenburg gait)	Pain and weakness associated with osteoarthritis of the hip
Reduced duration of left stance phase with absent heel strike; reduced foot clearance in left swing phase due to lack of adequate knee flexion and ankle dorsiflexion.	Left hemiparesis following right sided stroke
Increased knee flexion but reduced ankle dorsiflexion in swing phase	Foot drop due to peripheral neuropathy

- To use as an outcome measure to evaluate the efficacy of an intervention or management plan. Data on minimally clinically important difference, specific to each measure, are required to do this.

Table 18.2 provides details of commonly used objective measures of mobility.

FALL PREVENTION

Falls among all age groups are the second-leading cause of death due to accidental injury in the world. People over 65 have the greatest number of fatal falls (WHO, 2018). A fall is 'an unexpected event in which the participant comes to rest on the ground, floor or lower level' (Lamb et al., 2005, p. 1619).

TABLE 18.2 Objective Measures of Mobility

Name of Measure	What Does It Measure?	Screening or Assessment?	Outcome Measure?
Grip strength	Muscle strength—grip strength is correlated with leg strength	Yes—predictive of morbidity and mortality	No—no consensus on a minimal clinically important difference (MCID) (Bohannon, 2019)
Four-step balance scale (Rossiter-Fornoff et al., 1995)	Standing balance in increasingly more challenging positions	Yes—CDC (https://www.cdc.gov/steadi/pdf/STEADI-Assessment-4Stage-508.pdf) suggests inability to tandem stand (one component of the balance measure) for 10 seconds is associated with increased risk of falls.	Yes—in theory is sensitive to small improvements in balance. No agreed MCID.
Timed unsupported steady stand (Proceedings of SRR, 1996)	Standing balance in one position	Useful as a basic screen for assessing ability to stand unsupported	No—there are issues with ceiling effects; not very challenging for individuals with better balance function
Berg balance scale	Functional balance—static and dynamic	Yes—predicts falling and functional balance	Yes—is sensitive to change and there are published MCIDs dependent on initial balance score (Donoghue & Stokes, 2009).
Gait speed	Walking speed	Yes—predicts disability, mortality, hospitalisation, cognitive decline and care home admission.	Yes—there are numerous studies with suggested MCIDs (Hornyak et al., 2012).
Timed Up & Go	Composite measure of sit-to-stand, walking, turning and stand-to-sit	Yes—predicts fall risk and functional impairment (Shumway-Cook et al., 2000)	Yes—data for MCIDs are available for specific conditions such as Parkinson's disease
Short physical performance battery	A combination of 4 metre (8 foot) walking speed, time taken for five times sit-to-stand and balance test (similar to four-step balance test)	Yes—predicts disability, falls, hospitalisation and mortality	Yes—some evidence for MCIDs (Kwon et al., 2009).
Elderly mobility scale	Assessment of bed mobility, sit-to-stand, walking and functional reach; intended for hospital inpatients	No—limited evidence for predicting care home placement (Yu et al., 2007)	Yes—but limited evidence for responsiveness to change
Barthel Index (Mahoney & Barthel, 1965)	Self-reported/observed measure of basic function; personal activities of daily living and mobility	Yes, used in stroke and can be used as an assessment of basic function	No—limited evidence it is responsive to change, especially for individuals with higher functional levels
Nottingham Extended Activities of Daily Living index	Scale validated in stroke; includes instrumental activities of daily living	Yes—but primary use is as an outcome measure	Yes—data available on MCIDs (Wu et al., 2011)

Continued

TABLE 18.2	Objective Measures of Mobility—cont'd		
Name of Measure	**What Does It Measure?**	**Screening or Assessment?**	**Outcome Measure?**
Fall efficacy scale	Measures concern about falling in a range of activities	Yes—there are cut points for low, medium and high levels of concern (Delbaere, Close et al., 2010)	Yes—has been used to evaluate interventions but limited evidence of MCIDs
IPEQ for older people	Measures physical activity levels in older people	Yes—able to discriminate between low, moderate and high levels of activity (Delbaere, Hauer et al., 2010).	No—limited evidence of use in measuring change in activity

Humans, due to our bipedal posture, are inherently unstable and at high risk of falling. The factors that increase fall risk are multiple, but all relate in some way to the body's ability to maintain an upright posture. Many factors are influenced directly by the ageing process or indirectly as a result of age-related long-term conditions or physical inactivity. As a result, around 30% of people over 65, rising to half of individuals over 80, fall each year. Falls pose a problem for older people; first, because concern over falling may result in a reduction in physical activity with the consequent deconditioning increasing fall risk, and second, fall-related injuries are costly, both to the person's quality of life and their impact on health and social care costs.

There are several ways to prevent falls. A public health approach seeks to change fall risk at a population level using interventions such as education, regulation or environmental changes. The evidence to support such interventions is limited to a small number of studies.

The more common approach is to identify fall-risk factors in each individual older person and apply interventions to manage or minimise these factors. National Institute for Health and Care Excellence (NICE, 2013) guidelines recommend a three-stage process for older people living in the community:

- Screen all older people for increased risk of falls.
- Undertake a multifactorial fall-risk assessment in individuals at high risk.
- Identify modifiable risk factors and provide tailored interventions aimed at them (NICE, 2013).

Screening

It is recommended community-dwelling older people (i.e., people aged 65 and over) are asked in any health care contact about whether they have fallen in the past year (NICE, 2013). This simple question acts as a screening tool; a previous fall is one of the strongest predictors of future falls. For the same reason, any older person who presents to health care as a result of a fall should automatically be considered high-risk.

Guidance also suggests using gait or balance-screening tools to identify individuals who have not fallen but may be at risk (NICE, 2013). Screening tools such as the Timed Up & Go Test can be used for this purpose, but there needs to be an established cut point to identify impairments. A number of studies have investigated this area, and a Time Up & Go Test result of >14 seconds is considered to be predictive of high fall risk (Shumway-Cook et al., 2000). The test measures the time taken to stand from a chair without arms, walk 3 metres, turn around and return to sit on the same chair.

Screening on its own does not prevent falls. The purpose of screening is to identify older adults at higher risk who require a more detailed assessment of fall-risk factors. People who are considered high risk after screening should have a multifactorial fall-risk assessment. Figure 18.7 illustrates a theoretical model that underlies fall-prevention practices.

Since there is no effective method by which to accurately screen hospital inpatients at risk of falls, NICE (2013) recommends all inpatients over 65, or individuals between 50 and 64 with fall-risk factors, have a multifactorial fall risk assessment.

Assessment

The purpose of assessment in fall prevention is to identify relevant risk factors that are amenable to modification, thereby reducing the risk of falls.

Falls are not random events but are predictable based on the presence of a range of risk factors related to different body systems. Table 18.3 provides an overview of some of the common fall-risk factors.

To identify modifiable risk factors, NICE (2013) recommended a multifactorial assessment that includes the following assessments:

- Cardiovascular examination
- Cognition
- Fall history
- Fear related to falling

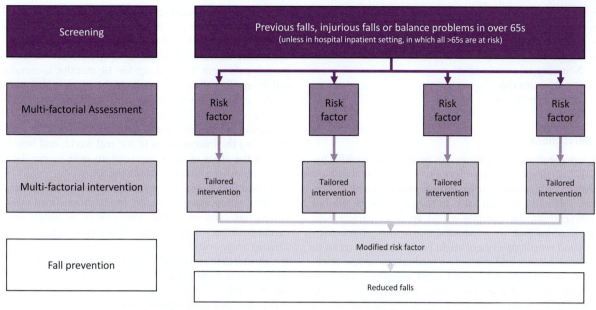

Fig. 18.7 Rationale for fall-prevention screening, assessment and intervention.

TABLE 18.3 Fall Risk Factors

Sociodemographic	Increased age	Medical conditions	Stroke
	Previous falls		Dementia/delirium
	Female		Parkinson's disease
	Inactivity		Depression
			Incontinence
			Arthritis
			Foot problems
			Dizziness
Environment	Poor footwear	Gait and balance	Difficulty with sit-to-stand
	Incorrect glasses		Slow walking speed
	Use of walking aids		Unsteady gait
			Unsteady when standing still
			Difficulty leaning or reaching
Medication	Multiple medications	Psychological	Fear of falling
	Hypnotics/anxiolytics		Difficulty with divided/selective attention
	Antidepressants		(dual tasks)
	Antipsychotics		
	Antihypertensives		
Sensorimotor	Proprioception		Visual impairment
	Vibration sense		Depth perception
	Tactile sense		Contrast sensitivity
	Muscle weakness		Sensory impairment
	Slow reaction time		

- Functional ability
- Gait, balance and mobility, and muscle weakness
- Home hazards
- Medication review
- Neurological examination
- Osteoporosis risk
- Urinary continence
- Vision

Interventions

Fall prevention interventions can be split into multifactorial or single interventions. Multifactorial interventions are centred on a comprehensive assessment of fall-risk factors (see Table 18.3), which leads to the provision of tailored interventions. An example is that an older person with impaired balance, weak muscles, a psychotropic prescription and visual impairment might be directed to exercise to improve balance and strength, a medication review, referral to an optician and home hazard assessment (in relation to vision and impaired balance risk factors). A single intervention addresses one fall risk factor. An example of a single intervention is a home hazard assessment with no complementary interventions.

Fall prevention interventions are generally considered to work differently in different settings. There are important differences between community-dwelling older people, those who live in residential care and hospital inpatient populations.

Fall prevention in community-dwelling older people. Multifactorial fall prevention interventions were examined in a Cochrane review, published in 2018 (Hopewell et al., 2018). Forty-three trials were included in the meta-analysis, which found interventions significantly reduced the rate of falls by 23%, but there was no significant reduction in the likelihood of having a fall, recurrent falls or fall-related hospital admissions.

Exercise is the single intervention most widely tested in community-dwelling populations and was evaluated in a separate Cochrane review (Sherrington et al., 2019). The rationale for exercise as a fall-prevention intervention is based on the high prevalence of fall-risk factors, such as muscle weakness, slow walking and balance impairment, which are potentially modifiable using exercise. Meta-analysis in this review found exercise in general was associated with significant reductions in rates of falls (by 23%) and risk of falling (by 15%). Another review found exercise that challenges balance—that is, makes the person 'wobbly'—carried out for more than 3 hours per week is associated with the largest reductions in falls (Sherrington et al., 2017).

Subsequent to these reviews, Lamb et al. (2020) published a large multicentre randomised controlled trial investigating the effect of both multifactorial and exercise

interventions compared to screening alone. Neither intervention reduced the risk of falls or fractures compared to screening alone. This trial was pragmatic, in that interventions were delivered through existing NHS services, and participants were followed up for 18 months. Generally, follow-ups for fall studies are limited to 1 year, and many of the effective interventions were delivered by highly motivated experts. The findings from Lamb et al. suggest recreating the motivation and interest of "experts" in those delivering the interventions in the real world, and how to sustain the effect of such interventions over longer durations still poses a considerable challenge.

In addition to exercise as a single intervention, evidence suggests home assessment and modification, medication review, insertion of cardiac pacemakers in people with cardio-inhibitory carotid sinus hypersensitivity, first eye cataract surgery and a podiatry intervention may be effective measures to reduce fall rates. These findings come from an older systematic review that has not yet been updated; a current review in this area is likely to identify more comprehensive and contemporary evidence on effective single interventions.

Fall-prevention interventions for older people in hospital and care home settings. The reason why hospital inpatients and care home dwellers are considered separately to community-dwelling older people in the context of fall prevention reflects the different nature of fall risk in these groups. Older people who live in care homes are by the nature of their need to be in 24-hour care a frail population. Frailty is likely to manifest in difficulties with function, gait and balance as well as fall risk factors including, impaired muscle strength, sensory function and coordination. Cognitive impairment, including dementia, is highly prevalent in the care home population.

Similar to care homes, hospitals tend to include a population who are more likely to exhibit fall-risk factors than individuals who live in the community. Older people in hospital frequently have comorbidities on which the effects of acute illness or injury superimpose an increased risk of falls. Common factors associated with acute illness or injury that may increase the risk of falls include dehydration, orthostatic hypotension, delirium and the impact of muscle atrophy due to disuse/bedrest and acute illness.

A Cochrane review published in 2018 found uncertainty in the effects of multifactorial interventions for hospital inpatients, although these interventions appeared to be more effective in sub-acute rehabilitation settings (Cameron et al., 2018). The same review found no convincing evidence to support the use of bed alarms or additional physiotherapy to prevent falls. The findings in care home studies were similar, with uncertainty based on low-quality evidence that exercise, multifactorial interventions or medication review effectively reduce falls. There was some evidence that where care home residents are vitamin D deficient, replacement may reduce the rate but not the risk of falling. Since this review was published, a large multisite study in care homes in the United Kingdom found introducing a 'guide to action' tool to care home support staff who undertake multifactorial risk assessments and interventions led to a 43% (IRR 0.57) (95% confidence interval 0.45 to 0.71, P<0.001) reduction in the rate of falls between 91 and 180 days follow-up (Logan et al., 2021).

The Role of Regulators in Monitoring Falls

The Care Quality Commission regulates all health and social care providers in England. Providers are expected to meet requirements for safe care by assessing for risk of injury or harm and implementing necessary mitigations. There is also a duty to report incidents that affect the health, safety or welfare of an individual in receipt of care from an organisation. With respect to falls, this reinforces the need to undertake regular multifactorial fall-risk assessments and address modifiable risk factors as well as report all fall incidents that occur in hospitals and care homes, including accurately indicating the resultant level of harm. It is important to ensure efforts to reduce the risk of falls do not have the unintended consequence of limiting physical activity. Exposure to falls is higher when standing or walking compared with sitting or lying down. However, as described above, there are significant risks associated with physical inactivity. The key to safe mobility is to enable a person to be as active as possible while implementing fall-prevention measures to optimise safety.

PROMOTING SAFE MOBILITY

When promoting safe mobility, the primary aim is to ensure an older person can optimise and maintain their functional abilities and independence in line with their expectations and goals. Activity restriction—that is, any action that aims to restrict movement—should be avoided. Being active and upright increases exposure to falling. However, the beneficial effects on overall health and well-being far outweigh this risk. In fact, as described in the preceding section, improving strength and balance through exercise is known to reduce risk of falls.

Maintenance of Physical Activity

The early parts of this chapter detailed the short- and long-term impacts of physical inactivity on health and well-being. It is vital all health care professionals discuss reducing sedentary behaviour and increasing physical activity as part of the 'making every contact count' initiative. Physical activity is something that should be encouraged and promoted in all groups, including those living with long-term conditions

and disability. Recommendations for weekly physical activity levels for people over 65 include the following (Department of Health and Social Care, 2019):

- At least 150 minutes (2.5 hours) of moderate intensity aerobic activity, building up gradually from current levels. Moderate intensity activity includes brisk walking or cycling that passes the 'talk test'—the ability to continue to talk in sentences while undertaking the activity.
- Activities to improve/maintain muscle strength, balance and flexibility at least twice a week.
- Avoiding prolonged periods of sitting, breaking it up with regular activity such as standing up.

Older people with specific long-term conditions may benefit from more individualised interventions to ensure they can take part in physical activity safely and it is tailored to their needs. Examples of such programmes include pulmonary rehabilitation for people with long-term respiratory conditions, cardiac rehabilitation for individuals recovering from myocardial infarction and/or associated interventions such as coronary stenting or bypass grafting, and programmes for people with stroke, osteoporosis and falls. It is important older people who have little experience of exercise and have a long-term condition seek programmes suitable for their condition led by appropriately qualified instructors. Older people should be encouraged to see a physiotherapist or check their fitness instructor is registered and qualified to manage their condition.

Self-Management in Long-Term Conditions

As described above, maintaining physical activity and reducing sedentary behaviour are key to self-management for older people with long-term conditions. Other aspects of self-management likely to be helpful include adopting healthy behaviours such as improved nutrition, stopping smoking and cutting down alcohol intake. Self-management involves learning how to anticipate and manage exacerbations to reduce the risk of hospital admission and can also include advice on how to optimise management of symptoms and adherence to medication.

Rehabilitation

The WHO defines rehabilitation as 'a set of interventions designed to optimise functioning and reduce disability in individuals with health conditions in interaction with their environment' (WHO, 2020).

Rehabilitation works most effectively when it is person-centred, adheres to a biopsychosocial model and includes input from the multidisciplinary team. See Table 18.4 for more details of the multidisciplinary team members involved in rehabilitation.

Rehabilitation begins with a detailed, personalised, holistic assessment of a person that covers physical, psychological and social domains. The culmination of an assessment involves developing a problem list, ideally in partnership with or coproduced with the patient, with identified problems relating to impairment of function or structure, activity limitation and/or participation restriction. Problem lists help direct the goal-setting process, which is seen as a vital component of the rehabilitation process. Goal setting focuses rehabilitation activities, encourages involvement of the person receiving rehabilitation and enhances motivation to participate in the activities required to achieve goals.

Rehabilitation can be thought of as a combination of restoration, adaptation and modification. Restoration involves restoring the bodily structures and functions impacted by illness, injury or disability. An example is recovery of range of movement and muscle strength following a fracture. Adaptation involves learning and cementing new ways in which skills, activities or functions can be undertaken when it is not possible to fully restore normal structures or physiological function. An example is functional training after a stroke, when a task is completed using new combinations of muscle groups and/or sensory inputs to compensate for damaged pathways. Modification of the environment can be used to enable functional independence. An example is using a walking aid to provide additional stability or raising the height of a chair to allow independence in standing up.

Rehabilitation is a complex intervention but is usually achieved through exercise, education, self-management and psychosocial support. Exercise involves task-specific training programmes, where functional activities are practised in full or broken into manageable sections with the aim of improving skill in the particular task. General exercise can help to improve overall fitness, strength, endurance and flexibility.

Optimising Uptake and Adherence to Physical Activity Interventions and Exercise

Rehabilitation relies on the active participation of the older person. It is important to account for factors that influence the motivation to start a programme and the behaviour change required to continue with it. The COM-B behaviour change wheel describes three essential conditions that must be met for behaviour to change: capability, opportunity and motivation (Michie et al., 2011). Health care professionals should consider how these conditions might be optimised when designing rehabilitation interventions.

The way information is framed influences perceptions of interventions. Older people at risk of falls sometimes perceive fall-prevention advice as patronising or distressing as it threatens their autonomy and identity. Emphasising the positive effects of exercise on balance and independence rather than the more negative approach of risk avoidance is thought to be more helpful (Yardley et al., 2006).

Recent analysis suggests physical activity reduces with increasing age in all groups, but individuals from Asian and Black ethnicities are less likely than average to be physically active (Gov.UK, 2020). Reasons include language barriers, cultural and religious expectations about physical activity—including access to single-sex spaces for exercise—and competing pressures on time such as caring responsibilities

TABLE 18.4   Members of the Multidisciplinary Team Involved in Rehabilitation

Dietician	Ensures nutrition is optimised to support people in their recovery and rehabilitation.
Geriatrician	A medical speciality concerned with the health care of older people.
Nurse	Provides support to optimise a person's health and ability to participate in a rehabilitation programme.
Occupational therapist	Provides assessment and interventions to support people regaining independence in activities that are important to them.
Orthotist	Creates and fits a range of aids to support people with deformities in nerves, muscles and/or bones.
Physical medicine and rehabilitation physician	A medical speciality concerned with optimising functional ability and quality of life after injury or illness that causes disability.
Physiotherapist	Provides assessment and interventions to support the restoration of movement and function.
Podiatrist	Provides assessment and interventions for a range of lower leg and foot conditions.
Prosthetist	Creates and fits an artificial replacement for a missing limb.
Psychologist	Provides assessment and interventions for cognitive, emotional and functional difficulties.
Rehabilitation support worker	Supports people with rehabilitation programmes such as exercise or practising tasks involved in daily activity.
Social worker	Provides support with short- and long-term care needs.
Speech and language therapist	Provides assessment and interventions to support people with difficulties with communication, eating, drinking and swallowing.

(Ige-Elegbede et al., 2019). Involving patients and members of the public in the coproduction of fall-prevention and rehabilitation services is one way to ensure services can be tailored to meet the needs of local populations more effectively.

Walking Aids

A walking aid might be considered to support mobility for several reasons. It may be necessary to decrease loading on a limb. This might be simply to take some of the body weight through the upper limb by using a stick to ease pain on weight-bearing through an arthritic joint. On the other hand, where recovery from a lower-limb fracture precludes weight-bearing, a frame or crutches might be required to enable the person to move without taking weight through the injured limb. Other reasons for using a walking aid include to improve stability and reduce the risk of falls, provide additional proprioceptive/sensory feedback or increase exercise tolerance. For example, using a rollator frame may reduce the work of breathing associated with walking for a person with a severe respiratory condition.

Walking aids should be prescribed with caution as they are frequently associated with falls and fall-related injuries. Persistent use of a walking aid may result in disuse of the normal postural mechanisms required to maintain balance. This means an older person who starts using a walking aid may become more dependent on it, and as postural stability worsens due to disuse,

they may need to progress to using more supportive walking aids. Prescriptions of walking aids should always be carefully considered by weighing up the benefits of improved safe mobility against the risk of long-term worsening of postural stability and the increased risk of falls and injuries. The aim is usually to use the lowest level of aid that can support safe mobility.

Different types of walking aids are described in Table 18.5. Walking sticks, crutches and frames should be fitted to the height of the intended user. The correct height can be ascertained by measuring the distance from the crease of the wrist to the floor when a person is standing upright with their arms by their sides and their elbows very slightly flexed.

Safe Moving and Handling Regulations: Applying the Law and Using Patient-Handling Systems

Supporting older people to move safely sometimes requires health and social care professionals to provide physical support and assistance. If this includes lifting, moving or handling, it is important to consider the safety of both the older person and members of staff involved in the handling process. Legislation and guidelines to support safe moving and handling should be understood and adhered to. Before carrying out any activity that requires moving or handling, a TILE risk assessment should be undertaken (Health and Safety Executive, 2016):

TABLE 18.5	**Different Types of Walking Aid (Least to Most Supportive)**
Walking aid	**Indication and Considerations**
Walking stick	Pain, postural instability, reduced exercise tolerance, reduced sensation/proprioception in the legs.
Walking stick with shaped handle	As above but where there is pain or deformity in the hand or wrist.
Crutches	When non- or partial weight-bearing is required, usually for short-term recovery from an injury; more difficult to use than sticks so a patient may need to learn how to use them safely.
Walking frame without wheels (i.e. 'zimmer frame')	When crutches do not provide sufficient support to enable non- or partial weight-bearing.
Walking frame with two front wheels (i.e. 'rollator frame')	When a stick or sticks don't provide sufficient support to minimise pain on weight-bearing, to support safe and steady mobility or, to optimise exercise tolerance. The front wheels allow the user to push the frame forward for a more 'normal' physiological gait pattern. Wheels also mean the frame does not need to be lifted—a point in the gait cycle at which the aid provides no support, increasing the risk of falls.
Three-/four-wheeled walker	Can be used by people who have the same needs as a rollator frame user but can control a wheeled walker using brakes. Allows a person to walk outdoors, as zimmer and rollator frames are not designed for outdoor terrain.
Gutter frame	Used in rehabilitation when ability to bear weight through the lower limbs, balance or exercise is very limited and the person cannot manage to stand or walk with the standard rollator frame. May be required as a temporary measure in an accustomed frame user who sustains a hand or wrist injury and cannot use their usual frame.

- Task: The transfer or mobility activity to be undertaken
- Individual: The staff member who will support the older person with an activity (Do they have any injuries, illnesses or increased susceptibility to injury?)
- Load: Information about the older person, their condition, their ability to participate, weight and attachments such as lines
- Environment: Lighting, space, clutter, spillages

The TILE risk assessment can help determine which technique should be used to support an older person with an activity and whether the use of equipment is indicated. Where possible, the older person should be encouraged to be as active as possible in any manoeuvres, but the amount of support required should be individually assessed for each situation. Table 18.6 describes equipment that might be used for specific tasks and which are the most active from the patient perspective.

TABLE 18.6	Equipment to Support Moving and Handling		
Mobility Task	**Most Active for the Patient**		**Least Active for the Patient**
Bed mobility	Use of bed levers, handles		Slide sheets
Sit-to-stand	Raised chair or toilet seat, toilet surround, grab rails	Riser chair, handling belt	Sit-to-stand aid (i.e., Sara Steady)
Transfers	Raised seat, riser chair, handling belt	Standing hoist	Full body hoist
Walking	Supervision, use of simple walking aids or grab rails	Walking frames, handling belts	Wheelchair for longer distances
Getting up after fall without injury	Guidance to patient to get up independently		Floor-level hoist

CONCLUSION AND LEARNING POINTS

The ability to move around safely and effectively is fundamental to independence and well-being. Mobility requires the complex coordination of a range of physiological and bio-mechanical processes spanning across nearly all structures that make up the human body. This means that there are many situations in which mobility can be disrupted, with consequences such as disability and falls. Interventions addressing mobility include avoidance of bedrest, promotion of physical activity as well as focused exercise programmes to address specific impairments or limitations.

KEY LEARNING POINTS

- Safe, effective mobility is an essential requirement for functional independence and social participation.
- Ageing, inactivity and long-term conditions impact the bodily structures and functions required for safe and effective mobility.
  - The impact of acute immobility associated with bedrest is profound and should be avoided whenever possible.
  - Lifelong inactivity increases morbidity and mortality. People of all ages should be encouraged to be less sedentary and engage in regular physical activity.
- Mobility can be assessed through questions, observation and objective measurement. Mobility assessment forms part of a multifactorial fall-risk assessment, which can support interventions to prevent falls in older adults in the community, care homes and hospitals.
- Exercise is the fall prevention intervention most widely tested. Programmes that challenge balance and are undertaken for more than 3 hours a week are most effective.
- Rehabilitation is frequently required for reduced mobility.
  - Rehabilitation works best when delivered through a multidisciplinary, person centred approach using goal setting.
  - Rehabilitation uses exercise, self-management and psychosocial support to achieve goals.
- Supporting older people with safe mobility requires an understanding of the indication for different walking aids and methods by which to optimise safe moving and handling.
- It is not inevitable that all older people are destined to be limited by mobility disability. Safe mobility should be promoted for all older people, from hospital inpatients to those living independently in the community.

REFERENCES

Allan, L. M., Ballard, C. G., Rowan, E. N., & Kenny, R. A. (2009). Incidence and prediction of falls in dementia: A prospective study in older people. *PloS One, 4*, e5521.

Allen, C., Glasziou, P., & Mar, C. D. (1999). Bed rest: A potentially harmful treatment needing more careful evaluation. *The Lancet, 354*, 1229–1233.

Asher, R. A. J. (1947). Dangers of going to bed. *British Medical Journal, 2*, 967–968.

Beauchet, O., Annweiler, C., Callisaya, M. L., De Cock, A. M., Helbostad, J. L., Kressig, R. W. et al., (2016). Poor gait performance and prediction of dementia: Results from a meta-analysis. *Journal of the American Medical Directors Association, 17*, 482–490.

Biswas, A., Oh, P. I., Faulkner, G. E., Bajaj, R. R., Silver, M. A., Mitchell, M. S. et al., (2015). Sedentary time and its association with risk for disease incidence, mortality, and hospitalization in adults: A systematic review and meta-analysis. *Annals of Internal Medicine, 162*(2), 123–132.

Bloomfield, S. A. (1997). Changes in musculoskeletal structure and function with prolonged bed rest. *Medicine & Science in Sports & Exercise, 29*, 197–206.

Bohannon, R. W. (2019). Minimal clinically important difference for grip strength: A systematic review. *Journal of Physical Therapy Science, 31*, 75–78.

Cameron, I. D., Dyer, S. M., Panagoda, C. E., Murray, G. R., Hill, K. D., Cumming, R. G. et al., (2018). Interventions for preventing falls in older people in care facilities and hospitals. *Cochrane Database of Systematic Reviews, 9*(9), CD005465.

Covinsky, K. E., Palmer, R. M., Fortinsky, R. H., Counsell, S. R., Stewart, A. L., Kresevic, D. et al., (2003). Loss of independence in activities of daily living in older adults hospitalized with medical illnesses: Increased vulnerability with age. *Journal of the American Geriatrics Society, 51*(4), 451–458.

Cruz-Jentoft, A. J., Bahat, G., Bauer, J., Boirie, Y., Bruyère, O., Cederholm, T. et al., Writing Group For The European Working Group On Sarcopenia In Older People 2 (EWGSOP2), & the Extended Group for EWGSOP2. (2018). Sarcopenia: Revised European consensus on definition and diagnosis. *Age and Ageing, 48*(1), 16–31.

De Rezende, L. F., Rey-López, J. P., Matsudo, V. K., & Do Carmo Luiz, O. (2014). Sedentary behavior and health outcomes among older adults: A systematic review. *BMC Public Health, 14*, 333.

Delbaere, K., Close, J. C. T., Mikolaizak, A. S., Sachdev, P. S., Brodaty, H., & Lord, S. R. (2010). The Falls Efficacy Scale International (FES-I): A comprehensive longitudinal validation study. *Age and Ageing, 39*, 210–216.

Delbaere, K., Hauer, K., & Lord, S. R. (2010). Evaluation of the incidental and planned activity questionnaire for older people. *British Journal of Sports Medicine, 44*, 1029–1034.

Department of Health and Social Care. (2019). UK Chief Medical Officers' Physical Activity Guidelines. https://assets.publishing.service.gov.uk/government/uploads/system/uploads/attachment_data/file/832868/uk-chief-medical-officers-physical-activity-guidelines.pdf

Donoghue, D., & Stokes, E. K. (2009). How much change is true change? The minimum detectable change of the Berg Balance Scale in elderly people. *Journal of Rehabilitation Medicine, 41*(5), 343–346.

Fox, M. T., Sidani, S., & Brooks, D. (2009). Perceptions of bed days for individuals with chronic illness in extended care facilities. *Research in Nursing & Health, 32*(3), 335–344.

Fried, L. P., Tangen, C. M., Walston, J., Newman, A. B., Hirsch, C., Gottdiener, J. et al., (2001). Frailty in older adults: Evidence for a phenotype. *Journals of Gerontology. Series A, Biological Sciences and Medical Sciences, 56*(3), M146–M156.

Gale, C. R., Cooper, C., & Aihie Sayer, A. (2014). Prevalence of frailty and disability: Findings from the English Longitudinal Study of Ageing. *Age and Ageing, 44*, 162–165.

Genever, R. W., Downes, T. W., & Medcalf, P. (2005). Fracture rates in Parkinson's disease compared with age- and gender-matched controls: A retrospective cohort study. *Age and Ageing, 34*, 21–24.

Harvey, L., Mitchell, R., Brodaty, H., Draper, B., & Close, J. (2016). Differing trends in fall-related fracture and non-fracture injuries in older people with and without dementia. *Archives of Gerontology and Geriatrics, 67*, 61–67.

Health and Safety Executive. (2016). Manual Handling Operations Regulations 1992. https://www.hse.gov.uk/pubns/books/l23.htm

Gov.UK. (2020). Physical activity. https://www.ethnicity-facts-figures.service.gov.uk/health/diet-and-exercise/physical-activity/latest

Hopewell, S., Adedire, O., Copsey, B. J., Boniface, G. J., Sherrington, C., Clemson, L. et al., (2018). Multifactorial and multiple component interventions for preventing falls in older people living in the community. *Cochrane Database of Systematic Reviews, 7*(7), CD012221.

Hornyak, V., Vanswearingen, J. M., & Brach, J. S. (2012). Measurement of gait speed. *Topics in Geriatric Rehabilitation, 28*.

Hunter, D. J., & Bierma-Zeinstra, S. (2019). Osteoarthritis. *The Lancet, 393*, 1745–1759.

Ige-Elegbede, J., Pilkington, P., Gray, S., & Powell, J. (2019). Barriers and facilitators of physical activity among adults and older adults from Black and Minority Ethnic groups in the UK: A systematic review of qualitative studies. *Preventive Medicine Reports, 15*, 100952.

Keller, K., & Engelhardt, M. (2014). Strength and muscle mass loss with aging process. Age and strength loss. *Muscles, Ligaments and Tendons Journal, 3*(4), 346–350.

Khan, T., Grenholm, P., & Nyholm, D. (2013). Computer vision methods for Parkinsonian gait analysis: A review on patents. *Recent Patents on Biomedical Engineering, 6*, 97–108.

Knight, J. N., Nigam, Y., & Jones, A. (2018). Effects of bedrest 2: Respiratory and haematological systems. *Nursing Times, 115*(1), 44–47.

Knight, J., & Nigam, Y. (2019). Effects of bedrest 4: Renal, reproductive and immune systems. *Nursing Times, 115*(3), 51–54.

Kwon, S., Perera, S., Pahor, M., Katula, J. A., King, A. C., Groessl, E. J. et al., (2009). What is a meaningful change in physical performance? Findings from a clinical trial in older adults (the LIFE-P study). *The Journal of Nutrition, Health and Aging, 13*, 538–544.

Lamb, S. E., Bruce, J., Hossain, A., Ji, C., Longo, R., Lall, R. et al., Prevention Of Fall Injury Trial Study Group. (2020). Screening and intervention to prevent falls and fractures in older people. *New England Journal of Medicine, 383*(19), 1848–1859.

Lamb, S. E., Jørstad-Stein, E. C., Hauer, K., & Becker, C. Prevention of Falls Network Europe and Outcomes Consensus Group. (2005). Development of a common outcome data set for fall injury prevention trials: The Prevention of Falls Network Europe consensus. *Journal of the American Geriatrics Society, 53*(9), 1618–1622.

Lear, S. A., Hu, W., Rangarajan, S., Gasevic, D., Leong, D., Iqbal, R. et al., (2017). The effect of physical activity on mortality and cardiovascular disease in 130 000 people from 17 high-income, middle-income, and low-income countries: The PURE study. *The Lancet, 390*, 2643–2654.

Logan, P. A., Horne, J. C., Gladman, J. R. F., Gordon, A. L., Sach, T., Clark, A. et al., (2021). Multifactorial falls prevention programme compared with usual care in UK care homes for older people: Multicentre cluster randomised controlled trial with economic evaluation. *BMJ, 375*, Article e066991.

Mahoney, F. I., & Barthel, D. W. (1965). Functional evaluation: The Barthel index. *Maryland State Medical Journal, 14*, 61–65.

Michie, S., Van Stralen, M. M., & West, R. (2011). The behaviour change wheel: A new method for characterising and designing behaviour change interventions. *Implementation Science, 6*(42).

National Institute for Health and Care Excellence (NICE). (2013). Falls in older people: Assessing risk and prevention. *Clinical Guideline, 161.* https://www.nice.org.uk/guidance/cg161/chapter/1-Recommendations

Palakurthi, B., & Burugupally, S. P. (2019). Postural instability in Parkinson's disease: A review. *Brain sciences, 9*, 239.

Parry, S. M., & Puthucheary, Z. A. (2015). The impact of extended bed rest on the musculoskeletal system in the critical care environment. *Extreme Physiology & Medicine, 4*, 16.

Proceedings of SRR. (1996). *Clinical Rehabilitation, 10*, 352–357. https://journals.sagepub.com/doi/abs/10.1177/026921559601000416?journalCode=crea

Rossiter-Fornoff, J. E., Wolf, S. L., Wolfson, L. I., & Buchner, D. M. (1995). A cross-sectional validation study of the FICSIT common data base static balance measures. Frailty and Injuries: Cooperative Studies of Intervention Techniques. *Journals of Gerontology. Series A, Biological Sciences and Medical Sciences, 50*(6), M291–M297.

Sherrington, C., Fairhall, N. J., Wallbank, G. K., Tiedemann, A., Michaleff, Z. A., Howard, K. et al., (2019). Exercise for preventing falls in older people living in the community. *Cochrane Database of Systematic Reviews, 1*(1), Article CD012424.

Sherrington, C., Michaleff, Z. A., Fairhall, N., Paul, S. S., Tiedemann, A., Whitney, J. et al., (2017). Exercise to prevent falls in older adults: An updated systematic review and meta-analysis. *British Journal of Sports Medicine, 51*, 1750–1758.

Shumway-Cook, A., Brauer, S., & Woollacott, M. (2000). Predicting the probability for falls in community-dwelling older adults using the Timed Up & Go Test. *Physical Therapy, 80*(9), 896–903.

Stamatakis, E., Gale, J., Bauman, A., Ekelund, U., Hamer, M., & Ding, D. (2019). Sitting time, physical activity, and risk of mortality in adults. *Journal of the American College of Cardiology, 73*, 2062–2072.

Szczepanska-Gieracha, J., Cieslik, B., Chamela-Bilinska, D., & Kuczynski, M. (2016). Postural stability of elderly people with cognitive impairments. *American Journal of Alzheimer's Disease and Other Dementias, 31*, 241–246.

Topp, R., Ditmyer, M., King, K., Doherty, K., & Hornyak J. 3rd, (2002). The effect of bed rest and potential of prehabilitation on patients in the intensive care unit. *AACN Clinical Issues, 13*(2), 263–276.

Webber, S. C., Porter, M. M., & Menec, V. H. (2010). Mobility in older adults: A comprehensive framework. *The Gerontologist, 50*, 443–450.

World Health Organization (WHO). (2001). International Classification of Functioning, Disability and Health (ICF). https://www.who.int/standards/classifications/international-classification-of-functioning-disability-and-health

WHO. (2018). Falls. https://www.who.int/news-room/fact-sheets/detail/falls#:~:text=Falls%20are%20the%20second%20leading,greatest%20number%20of%20fatal%20falls

WHO. (2020). Rehabilitation.https://www.who.int/news-room/fact-sheets/detail/rehabilitation

WHO. (2022). Physical Activity. https://www.who.int/news-room/fact-sheets/detail/physical-activity

Wu, C.-Y., Chuang, L.-L., Lin, K.-C., Lee, S.-D., & Hong, W.-H. (2011). Responsiveness, minimal detectable change, and minimal clinically important difference of the Nottingham Extended Activities of Daily Living scale in patients with improved performance after stroke rehabilitation. *Archives of Physical Medicine and Rehabilitation, 92*, 1281–1287.

Yardley, L., Donovan-Hall, M., Francis, K., & Todd, C. (2006). Older people's views of advice about falls prevention: A qualitative study. *Health Education Research, 21*, 508–517.

Yu, M. S. W., Chan, C. C. H., & Tsim, R. K. M. (2007). Usefulness of the elderly mobility scale for classifying residential placements. *Clinical Rehabilitation, 21*, 1114–1120.

Zheng, J.-Q., Lai, H.-J., Zheng, C.-M., Yen, Y.-C., Lu, K.-C., Hu, C.-J. et al., (2017). Association of stroke subtypes with risk of hip fracture: A population-based study in Taiwan. *Archives of Osteoporosis, 12*, 104.

Care of the Foot

Joanne Paton

The suffering and burden of living with painful feet is well recognised. As a consequence of foot pain, people become irritable and unable to concentrate and lose the desire to be mobile.

Foot problems are common in older people. The effect of foot problems, particularly foot pain and deformity, is significant, contributing to poor balance, falls, injury, disability, reduced mobility, social isolation and reduced quality of life (López-López et al., 2018). Many foot problems can be avoided by taking care of the feet. This can be done by an individual, a family member or informal carer, or a health care professional who is not a foot specialist such as a health care assistant or nurse. The role of the nurse in relation to feet involves

- Health education
- Assessment
- Non-specialist foot care
- Referral to a foot-care specialist (i.e., podiatrist)

The incidence of foot problems is increasing as a consequence of increased life expectancy (Rodríguez-Sanz et al., 2018). Benvenuti et al. (1995) found 86% of a sample of 459 'community dwelling older people' (p. 479) had 'at least one foot symptom or sign', (p. 481) many of which could result in reduced mobility. Decreased mobility can leave older adults unable to participate in their regular normal activities. Consequences range from loss of independence to falls, fall-related injury and severe alterations in lifestyle.

The feet consist of skin, bones, muscles, tendons, ligaments, nerves and blood vessels. Healthy feet enable people to stay physically active by balancing the body effectively in walking, running, dancing and many other daily activities. Feet are vulnerable to repetitive mechanical stress and skin irritation due to heavy daily use, but like the rest of the body, feet succumb to changes that occur with age. Older patients with foot problems exhibit normal degenerative changes in the bone and soft tissues of the foot and lower limb, often in combination with one or more age-related chronic conditions that impact foot health such as arthritis, cardiovascular disease and diabetes.

Feet may be misused and abused throughout life as a person follows shoe fashion, ignorant of the problems being established for the future. Consider the ancient cultural tradition of binding feet in China and the effect on women of wearing high-heeled shoes or shoes with pointed toes. Most shoes are not the shape of a healthy foot. Not surprisingly, women have statistically more problems with their feet than men do as they get older (Dawson et al., 2002; Gates et al., 2019; Munro & Steele, 1998).

COMMON FOOT CHANGES WITH AGE

Advancing age is a risk factor for foot problems. Ageing causes thinning of the epithelial and subcutaneous fatty layers in the skin. (See Chapter 5 for more information on the biology of ageing.) The number of fibroblasts, which are responsible for synthesising protein and collagen, are reduced. The resulting reduction in collagen and elastic fibres in connective tissue causes the tissue to become more dense. Joint range of motion and flexibility are reduced such that the foot becomes more rigid. Skin loses elasticity and resilience to become more fragile and prone to injury (Edelstein, 1988). There is a decrease in both active sweat glands and sebaceous glands, leaving the skin at risk of becoming dry, flaky and scaly. Older skin, which is easily damaged, repairs at a slower rate than in younger individuals and is at greater risk of infection. The fat pads under the feet (i.e., plantar surface) are important as shock absorbers. Atrophy of the fat pads as a result of ageing reduces the foot's ability to absorb shock and increases risk of injury.

Toenails grow more slowly with age, due to decreased vascular supply to the nail beds, and nail plates thickens, resulting in brittle, thick and dull nails prone to fungal infection. Improper-fitting shoes can cause persistent trauma to the nail matrix and lead to thickening. Osteoporosis can affect the bones of the feet, predisposing them to fractures even during normal everyday activities. A reduction in muscle fibre in old age leads to decreased arch integrity. There is often reduced blood supply to the feet with age, as arteriosclerosis increases peripheral resistance to blood flow. Delivery of oxygen and nutrients is reduced, resulting in an increased healing time after injury.

With ageing, sensory acuity diminishes, which may be exacerbated by pathological conditions such as diabetes. A reduced sensory perception threshold may mean older adults are less aware of uncomfortable shoes. Foreign objects can, for example, get into shoes and cause significant tissue damage to individuals with diminished sensory perception. In addition, a decrease in temperature sensitivity may increase susceptibility to thermal trauma, so people should guard against burns from hot-water bottles or when sitting near a fire.

As people get older, loss of visual acuity, muscle strength, joint suppleness and sensory perception can have major implications on postural control, leading to balance deficits and increased fall risk. In combination, the effects of ageing can interfere with a person's ability to care for their feet, which increases pain and further reduces mobility. Loss of mobility can lead to loss of contact with family and friends who used to help with foot care. Lack of interest and neglect may ensue.

PREVALENCE OF FOOT PROBLEMS

Foot pain and deformity are common problems for older people and have a serious impact on quality of life and mobility. When these problems are successfully managed, relief from pain facilitates an older person's rehabilitation from chronic disorders and other disabilities (Bruno & Helfand, 1990).

Several studies found a high prevalence of foot disorders in the older population. Around half of older people report having from a foot problem. This estimate is believed to be higher in older adults who live in care homes or receive foot health assessment from a podiatrist. Harvey et al. (1997) conducted a large ($n = 792$) community-based study in Wales to find 53% of people in a population aged 60 and over had three or more foot problems. Another study found more than half of individuals aged 75 years or older obtained care from podiatry services. Difficulty cutting toenails was reported by participants as the most common problem (Crawford et al., 1996). Another study indicated the most prevalent problems that affect older people are toenails that are difficult to cut, pain from corns and calluses, and toe deformities (White & Mulley, 1989). Although it is difficult to predict who will develop foot problems, other factors can increase the risk of foot symptoms. Older women display a higher incidence of foot disorders, with an increased likelihood of corns, calluses and bunion deformity when compared to men (Munro & Steele, 1998). Some studies cite a causal relationship between obesity and foot pain. And people with foot pain are more likely to present with multiple chronic diseases (e.g., diabetes, stroke, rheumatoid arthritis) or chronic pain in other areas of the body (e.g., hands, back, hips, knees).

Podiatry care improves foot pain and mobility for older people through a wide range of foot-related interventions, from debridement of calluses to the provision of insoles. A systematic review of the literature found when podiatry was integrated into an interprofessional fall-prevention intervention, the fall rate significantly decreased (Wylie et al., 2019). Despite the preventable nature of many consequences of foot pain and pathology, a number of studies suggest a proportion of people who need treatment for foot ailments do not receive it (Pushpangadan & Burns, 1996). It was estimated 40% of people over 65 need podiatry treatment, but only half receive podiatry care (Pushpangadan & Burns, 1996). This was supported by Harvey et al. (1997), who found 20% of people whose feet had been assessed had sufficient pathology to be in need of care from a podiatrist, but they had not received it. The group least likely to receive treatment for foot conditions were older people who lived alone (Harvey et al., 1997). Podiatry services may not be targeted toward individuals with greatest need, and where podiatric services are available, not all older people with painful feet consult practitioners for treatment or guidance (Munro & Steele, 1998).

COMMON FOOT PROBLEMS

Common foot problems in older people include dry skin (i.e., anhydrosis), calluses, corns, toenail pathologies, fungal infections and chilblains, and musculosketal pain. These problems are often a result of normal changes of ageing in combination with the effects of inadequate foot care, mechanical overuse and increased suseptibility to infection. The foot health of older adults is often compromised by complications from coexisting systemic diseases such as diabetes, vascular disease and arthritis.

Corns and Calluses

Corns and calluses are common skin pathologies that develop as the body's protective response to excessive mechanical stresses. These hyperkeratotic lesions are produced when the outermost layer of the skin, the stratum corneum, becomes thickened as a result of the epidermis being stimulated by stress to produce more cells. A callus is a diffuse area of hyperkeratosis of a regular depth, formed by the body in response to friction. A corn is a much denser focal area of hyperkeratosis, organised to form a nucleus. Corns are formed by the body in response to pressure or friction over a joint. These lesions are typically found on the plantar surface of the foot and the apex and dorsum of the prominent joints of the toes. They are not always painful and serve to protect underlying tissues from excessive stresses. However, corns and calluses may produce pain on walking.

Podiatric treatment of corns and calluses usually consists of debridement with a scalpel followed by pressure relief using a cushioning insole or sometimes an orthotic. Insoles can be bought over the counter or custom-made by a podiatrist or orthotist to better target and relieve pressure.

Cracks and Fissures

Cracks and fissures are breaks or tears in the skin. Two types of fissures commonly occur in the feet. Fissures between the toes (i.e., interdigital) are usually a result of the skin continuously being too moist. This type of fissure is often associated with fungal infections. Refer to the section on fungal infections for further information. The second type of skin fissure occurs because the skin becomes too dry (i.e., anhydrosis). In this situation the skin around the base of the heel appears dry, flaky and cracked. Heel fissures can be painful to walk on and, if left untreated, leave the skin open to infection. Heel fissures are more common in people who wear open sandals without socks, where the skin becomes stripped of its natural oils.

Open fissures should be managed by a podiatrist. Self-management advice can be given to help prevent dry, hard skin from cracking. Weekly gentle rubbing with a wet pumice stone after bathing, along with the daily application of moisturiser, improve the skin's integrity and reduce the risk of fissures. Always warn against removing too much skin.

Bunions

Bunion is a lay term associated with a deformity of the hallux (i.e., first or big toe)—*hallux abducto valgus*—and is a common forefoot deformity, especially in women (Fig. 19.1). Hallux abducto valgus is a lateral deviation of the hallux and a splaying of the first metatarsal medially. A bunion is a prominence on the inside of the foot around the big toe joint. If exposed to repetitive friction from poor-fitting footwear, a chronically inflamed adventitious bursa—a fluid-filled sac—can develop in response to constant rubbing or friction. The bursa is commonly situated on the medial side of the head of the first metatarsal. It serves to protect the deeper tissues from injury when the area is traumatised by shoe pressure.

Symptoms of bunions include inflammation, redness, swelling and sometimes acute pain in the affected area. The discomfort may affect the patient's gait. A similar deformity can arise on the outside (i.e., lateral) side of the foot over the joint at the base of the little toe, sometimes known as a 'tailor's bunion'; in times gone by, tailors sat cross-legged, so this area was susceptible to constant trauma. Both genetic and lifestyle factors are likely to contribute to hallux abducto valgus development. However, once developed, ill-fitting footwear can exacerbate symptoms. It's important for the patient to wear shoes that accommodate the extra width of the foot caused by the deformity and to avoid trauma to the exposed bony prominences.

Toenails

Many older people are particularly affected by nail deformities. Patients may present with very long, thickened and neglected nails. This often painful and potentially problematic condition may be exacerbated by an inability to bend easily to reach the feet as a consequence of ageing, obesity or arthritis in the knees or hips. Difficulty manipulating nail clippers or scissors because of stiffness in the hands and fingers or visual impairment also makes the simple task of nail cutting seemingly impossible for many older people.

Onychogryphosis usually occurs as a result of trauma to the nail bed or matrix and results in a deformity referred to as a 'ram's horn nail'. The nail plate is much distorted and deviates to one side as it grows. When neglected, the nail can curve under or over the adjacent toes, causing painful lesions and ulceration.

Onychomycosis and onychauxis appear similar, but differentiation between the two conditions is relevant to inform treatment. Onychauxis is simple thickening of the nail plate without any associated deformity. The nail may become yellow or white in appearance. Onychauxis is often caused by chronic trauma from footwear but may be related to psoriasis or impaired nutrition to the nail bed and matrix due to insufficient arterial supply.

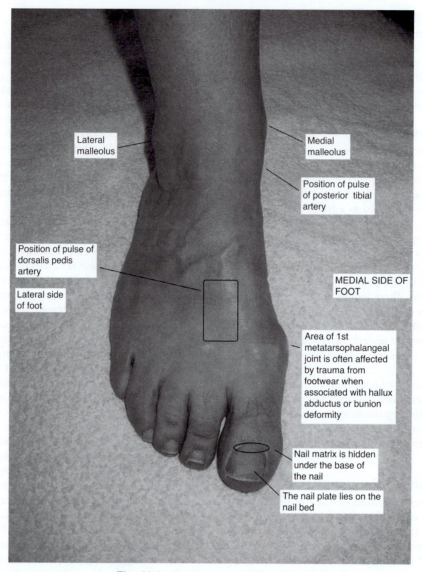

Lateral malleolus

Medial malleolus

Position of pulse of posterior tibial artery

Position of pulse of dorsalis pedis artery

MEDIAL SIDE OF FOOT

Lateral side of foot

Area of 1st metatarsophalangeal joint is often affected by trauma from footwear when associated with hallux abductus or bunion deformity

Nail matrix is hidden under the base of the nail

The nail plate lies on the nail bed

Fig. 19.1 Surface anatomy of the foot.

Onychomycosis is the term given to a nail infected by fungal organisms. The nail appears thickened, discoloured and, in severe cases, crumbly with a characteristic odour. Occasionally in mild cases, the nail plate is only partially affected, and the infection may be evident by a small amount of white discolouration at the free edge of the nail. Approximately 90% of onychomycosis cases in toenails are caused by dermatophytes—trichophyton metagrohytes and tichophyton rubrum (Leung et al., 2020).

Oral antifungal therapies are much more effective in treating onychomycosis than topical medicaments.

Terbinafine is the recommended oral antifungal therapy and can be prescribed by a GP after diagnosis is confirmed through a fungal culture (Leung et al., 2020). However, many older people are resistant to taking additional tablets, and terbinafine has contraindications for older people. Terbinafine should be used with caution in people who have psoriasis, depression or liver or kidney problems (National Institute for Health and Care Excellence, 2020). A topical antifungal nail preparation should be considered first in the treatment of mild cases of onychomycosis in older adults.

Skin Fungal Infections

Skin fungal (i.e., mycotic) infections are a relatively common, often reoccuring foot problem in older people. Over time fungal infections can spread to the nail bed to become onychomycosis. The condition is referred to as tinea pedis; the lay term is 'athlete's foot'. *Tinea* refers to the dermatophyte organism that causes the infection (i.e., tinea interdigitale tinea rubrum and tinea mentagrophytes). *Pedis* refers to the foot. There are three clinical presentations of tinea pedis. The most common form occurs interdigitally and is characterised by moist inflamed skin usually between the fourth and fifth toes. Fissuring, or splitting, of the skin may occur, which can be very painful. The patient should be encouraged to dry carefully and gently between their toes and then apply an antifungal preparation as described below. The second type of tinea pedis is recognised by excessive scaling and desquamation of the skin on the soles of the feet. This type is called a mocasin infection and is generally more difficult to treat with topical preparations because skin on the soles is thicker. The final clinical presentation is less common in older adults and presents as vesicles and itching around the arch of the foot.

To identify the fungal organism, a scraping of the affected skin is sent to a local microbiology laboratory for microscopy and culture. Ninety percent of tinea pedis is treated within a week or two using topical over-the-counter antifungal preparations (Otani, 2017). Topical preparations of terbinafine 1%, clotrimazole 1%, or miconazole nitrate 2% are effective against most organisms. Topical creams or ointments are a better choice than lotions or sprays for older adults because they tend to be less astringent and less likely to cause irritation (Otani, 2017). Occasionally a more widespread or particularly persistent infection requires tablets. Terbinafine tablets can be obtained with a prescription from a GP.

Nurses play a useful role in managing tinea pedis. It is sensible to encourage prompt treatment of these infections to prevent a skin fissure or secondary bacterial infection. These problems can lead to more serious complications, especially if the patient has impaired arterial flow to the feet or a disorder such as diabetes, when ulceration may result. To prevent reinfection, the patient's socks, towels and bed linen should be washed at 60°C to destroy any fungal elements, and shoes and slippers should be sprayed with any of the above preparations available in aerosol form. The patient should be encouraged to wear different shoes on alternate days and then leave them to dry out, preferably in sunshine, which helps eradicate remaining fungal spores.

Chilblains

Chilblains of ideopathic origin are unusual in older people. The occurrence of chilblains or chilblain-like lesions is more likely to be a marker of another systemic (e.g., lupus erythematosus) or vascular (e.g., Raynaud's) condition worthy of further investigation (Nyssen et al., 2020). Ideopathic chilblains develop in older people who experience an abnormal localised response to cold in the skin's blood vessels in their extremities. The susceptible individual can avoid chilblains by wearing warm hosiery and footwear and taking care to avoid exposing the feet to direct heat after coming in from the cold. Smoking cessation should be encouraged. Current chilblain treatments are unsatisfactory and should not be recommended. Calcium channel blockers, in particular nifedipine, and topical betamethasone, a corticosteriod cream, are sometimes used to manage chilblains, but their effect has not been confirmed by randomised clinical trials (Nyssen et al., 2020; Souwer et al., 2017). Ideopathic chilblains usually resolve spontaneously within a couple of weeks (Nyssen et al., 2020). Common sites for chilblains are the apices of toes, over the exposed medial border of the foot associated with hallux abducto valgus and at the back of the heel. The lesions can also affect hands and appear as small red or cynosed ichy swellings. Emerging research showed chilblain-like lesions on the hands and feet of 19% of people with COVID-19 (Recalcati, 2020) but less frequently in older patients with the virus.

Metatarsalgia

Metatarsalgia is a general term that denotes pain in the ball of the foot or forefoot. In older adults, metatarsalgia is often a symptom of a musculoskelal condition such as capsulitis, synovitis or mortons neuroma. Capuslitis or synovitis of the metatarsal phalangeal joint capsule, often associated with plantar plate disruption, commonly affects the second or third metatarsal heads. Mortons neuroma is nerve entrapment usually sited between the third and fourth metatarsal heads. Typically, patients describe their symptoms as aggravated by weight-bearing and increasing with activity. The pathology of metatarsalgia is usually associated with poor foot biomechanics in combination with a loss of subcutaneous fat and thinning skin, resulting in a loss of shock absorption and pain, particularly over the plantar metatarsal heads. Typical biomechanical foot deformities associated with metatarsalgia include a pronated foot type, recognised as a foot with a low medial long arch and the appearance of being rolled inward, or a foot with an abnormal metatarsal parabola, or a particularly long second or third toe.

Most cases of metatarsalgia respond well to conservative measures, including rest, over-the-counter pain relief and properly fitting footwear. A change in footwear is often an effective first approach to reducing biomechanical stress on the foot. Patients should be encouraged to choose wide shoes with fastenings and cushioned soles. Narrow court or

CASE STUDY 19.1

Mrs Dunn, a fit and active 85-year-old woman, lives with her husband in a flat in an area of town that is being gentrified. They are hoping to be rehoused in the near future. Mrs Dunn is visiting the practice nurse, Michelle, at her GP's office for her annual flu vaccination. The weather is unusually cold, and she has to remove layers of clothing, which takes some time, during which she chats with Michelle. Mrs Dunn sits down with relief and complains about how sore her feet have been recently, so Michelle takes the opportunity to examine them. She finds small, dark cyanosed patches on Mrs Dunn's toes and on the balls of her feet, and her feet feel very cold. Michelle suspects these lesions are typical of the congestive stage of chilblains and advises Mrs Dunn to buy a proprietary preparation to treat them, which acts as a vasodilator and may help relieve the symptoms. She also advises her to

keep her feet warm by wearing a thin pair of socks over her stockings and to find some insulating insoles for her boots. Michelle also says it's a good idea to keep outdoor shoes on when she returns home until her feet warm up. Rubbing the feet gently with a towel after washing them in warm water may also help improve blood flow, and avoiding standing in the cold is also sensible advice. Mrs Dunn reveals her flat is very cold and draughty, and she admits to toasting her feet in front of the electric fire, which Michelle warns against. She reassures Mrs Dunn when she and her husband move into their new, well-insulated, centrally heated home, her chilblains will probably be less of a problem. Keeping warm and preventing chilblains from forming is the best form of management in susceptible people.

high-heeled shoes should be avoided. If symptoms persist, the GP can refer to a podiatrist for insoles.

Heel Pain

The most common cause of heel pain in older adults is plantar fasciitis. Typically, patients complain of pain under the medial anterior aspect of the heel at the insertion of the plantar fascia into the calcaneum, which feels worse on rising from bed or after a period of rest. Current thinking supports the theory the aetiology of the condition is more likely to be degenerative than inflammatory; plantar fasciitis would be better defined as plantar fasciosis. Plantar fasciitis is an overuse injury associated with a poor foot biomechanics. Feet with either very high or low arches can generate excessive mechanical stress during prolonged periods of standing or walking, causing injury to the plantar fascia. Other causes of heel pain include tarsal tunnel syndrome, fat pad atrophy, sciatica and calcaneal stress fracture.

In most cases, plantar fasciitis is self-limiting and resolves within a year. Conservative therapy can help patients with heel pain maintain the activities of daily living. Patient-directed treatments include nonsteroidal anti-inflammatory drugs, weight loss, activity modification, calf stretches, over-the-counter insoles, heel cushions or arch supports. In the minority of cases that fail to respond to conservative therapy and remain symptomatic for more than 6 months, custom-made insoles, corticosteroid injections and extracorporeal shock wave therapy can provide relief.

Osteoarthritis

Pain and stiffness in the joints of the foot or feet is the key symptom of osteoarthritis that drives people to seek medical attention. At first, the pain tends to occur only with activity, but as the osteoarthritis progresses, the frequency of pain increases to periods of rest and at night. Although osteoarthritis is not part of the ageing process, age is a strong risk factor (Shelton, 2013). Osteoarthritis can occur in multiple joints of the body. In feet, however, it is most commonly seen at the first metatarsophalangeal joint and affects one in 40 people over the age of 50 (Gould et al., 1980). Early in the disease, patients typically present with palpable osteophytes and tenderness along the dorsal joint margin of the first metatarsophalangeal joint. This presentation usually occurs in combination with reduced joint range of dorsiflexion motion (<60 degrees) and discomfort when the joint is pushed to end range. At this stage, the condition is termed hallux limitus. In severe cases with advanced joint degeneration and significant osteophyte formation, the joint becomes fixed. Defined as hallux rigidus, by this point in the disease progression, because of the lack of joint motion, the joint is often pain free.

Bilateral hallux limitus is associated with repetitive wear and tear generated in the joint during the thousands of steps taken a day, particularly in a foot that functions with poor biomechanics. With a unilateral presentation of osteoarthritis, the underlying cause is likely to be a past major traumatic incident such as dropping a heavy weight or a stubbed toe. Conservative treatment is usually targeted toward pain

TABLE 19.1 SINBAD System of Wound Classification

Category	Definition	Score
Site	Forefoot	0
	Midfoot and hindfoot	1
Ischemia	Pedal blood flow intact: at least one palpable pulse	0
	Clinical evidence of reduced pedal flow	1
Neuropathy	Protective sensation intact	0
	Protective sensation lost	1
Bacterial infection	None	0
	Present	1
Area	Ulcer <1 cm^2	0
	Ulcer ≥1 cm^2	1
Depth	Ulcer confined to skin and subcutaneous tissue	0
	Ulcer reaching muscle, tendon or deeper	1
Total possible score		6

relief. Nonsteroidal anti-inflammatory drugs are the first treatment in managing periods of acute pain. Other interventions aimed at reducing joint dorsiflexion, such as low-heeled, stiff-bottomed shoes or shoes with rocker-shaped sole units, may be beneficial in controlling symptoms.

Ulceration

It is important to assess and document the severity of any foot wound or ulcer. The site, ischeamia, neuropathy, bacterial infection, area and depth (SINBAD) wound classification and score is a simple, validated tool for documenting important wound characteristics and predicting ulcer healing rates (Table 19.1) (Ince et al., 2008).

Ischaemic Ulcers

Ischaemic ulcers are often shallow and located over bony prominences on the margins of feet. The ulcer may have a 'punched out' appearance and well-demarcated borders. This sort of ulcer often causes a great deal of pain. Ischaemic ulcers are caused by insufficient arterial supply to the area of the lesion, resulting in skin tissues becoming devitalised and necrosed. Patients who have an ischaemic foot ulcer present with signs and symptoms characteristic of peripheral arterial disease, which affects up to 15% of adults over 70 (Selvin & Erlinger, 2004). Nurses play a key role in the baseline vascular assessment of older people. Non-palpable foot pulses, either dorsalis pedis or posterior tibial (see Fig. 19.1), in the presence of skin breakdown or

in combination with other observable signs of peripheral arterial disease, should be referred to vascular services for further assessment. Other observable signs include monophasic doppler wave forms, intermittent claudication, atrophic skin and nail changes, slow capillary refill time and pale, cold feet with a temperature gradient increasing proximally—where the leg is warmer than the foot when tested with the back of the hand.

Typical intermittent claudication symptoms include pain in the calf on walking that disappears when the person rests for a few minutes. The Edinburgh Claudication Questionnaire is a useful aid in the clinical diagnosis of intermittent claudication (Bendermacher et al., 2006). A handheld Doppler is now widely used by nurses to assist in screening for peripheral arterial disease. A monophasic Doppler signal is one in which only one sound can be heard, indicating reduced flow in the diseased artery. A normal arterial Doppler signal has three sounds (i.e., triphasic) that indicate a healthy elastic artery and therefore a good blood flow to the area it supplies.

Edinburgh Claudication Questionnaire

- Do you get a pain or discomfort in either leg on walking?
- Does this pain ever begin when you are standing still or sitting?
- Does this pain occur if you walk uphill or hurry?
- Does this pain occur if you walk at an ordinary pace on the level?
- What happens if you stand still?
- In what part of your leg do you feel the pain?

Absent pulses accompanied by gangrene or resting pain—described as unremitting, severe, cramp-like pain in the toes or forefoot—can be a sign of critical limb ischaemia. The pain is often worse at night when the feet get hot. Typically, patients describe having to hang their leg over the edge of the bed to get relief. Critical limb ischaemia requires urgent referral to a vascular team. The dorsalis pedis and posterior pulses may not be palpable, and if they are audible when using Doppler ultrasound, they are monophasic.

Venous Ulcers

Venous ulcers are commonly present in the area of the medial malleolus or occasionally the lateral malleolus (Fig. 19.1). Varicosities are probably evident, and other clinical findings include oedema and venous dermatitis. Venous stasis ulcers vary in size from a few centimetres to many centimetres in diameter, and they occasionally extend around the circumference of the leg above the ankle.

Neuropathic Ulcers

Neuropathic ulcers are most frequently a complication of diabetes but can be associated with other neurological disorders in which a sensory deficit exists, such as spina bifida and leprosy, or a result of injury to the peripheral nerves. Neuropathic ulcers are often deep and complicated by infection. Neuropathic ulceration occurs during the process of walking, when tissue damage is caused by increased plantar loads and tissue stress in the absence of protective sensory pain feedback. The development of claw toe deformity and prominent metatarsal heads is associated with elevation in forefoot pressure in the diabetic neuropathic foot. This alteration in foot structure and pressure distribution, in combination with neuropathy, predisposes the foot to ulceration. Connective tissue abnormalities in the diabetic population are common and affect the skeleton, joints and peri-articular tissues. Connective tissue complications stem from a substantial increase in levels of non–enzymatic glycation that occur in collagen, stimulated by poor glycaemic control. Increased non-enzymatic glycation alters collagen metabolism, increasing the formation of intermolecular cross-links. This process results in collagen becoming stiffer. Although considered part of the normal ageing process, progressive stiffening of collagen is substantially accelerated for people with diabetes.

The clinical presentation of stiffening collagen is thick, tight, waxy skin in combination with joint contracture; because of its similarities to scleroderma, this manifestation is sometimes termed *pseudo-scleroderma*. It usually affects the small joints of the hands and feet. The screening test for this condition is the prayer sign: the patient is asked to place their hands together as if praying and then to fan and extend their fingers. In the presence of limited joint mobility, the patient is unable to place their palms flat together.

Previously considered of little consequence, diabetic pseudo-scleroderma has often been ignored as part of a diabetic patient's management plan. However, limited joint mobility in feet is associated with both increased peak pressure and neuropathic ulceration. This link is believed to reflect the profound effect of limited joint mobility on lower limb function combined with an inability for patients with sensory neuropathy to modify dysfunction to prevent injury by protective sensory feedback (Birke et al., 1995). Possible biomechanical risk factors for increased plantar loads and subsequent diabetic foot ulceration include limited range of motion at the first metatarsal phalangeal joint, ankle and subtalar joint; lesser toe deformity; reduced fibro fatty padding over the metatarsal heads; and tibialis anterior muscle weakness.

Development and healing of neuropathic foot ulceration is associated with the magnitude of plantar pressure. Neuropathic ulceration usually occurs over the areas of the foot that receive the greatest pressure, such as the metatarsal heads at the plantar aspect of the first toe. In a patient with neuropathy, callosity further increases plantar load and the likelihood of ulceration. Ulceration risk is reduced through callus debridement.

A person with neuropathic ulceration should be encouraged to rest to relieve pressure and facilitate healing. A gold-standard total-contact cast, diabetic air-cast walker boot, or similar offloading device relieves pressure on the lesion while keeping the patient mobile.

Pressure Ulcers

Pressure ulcers occur over bony prominences, most often the malleola bones or the posterior surface of the calcaneum in patients with reduced mobility. Tissue necrosis is caused by prolonged tissue pressure, capillary occlusion and subsequent local necrosis of tissue. See Chapter 24 for information on the causes and treatment of pressure ulcers.

Neuroischaemic Ulcers

The etiology of diabetic foot ulcers is often multifactorial. Complications of diabetes mellitus can involve peripheral neuropathy, as discussed above, in combination with microangiopathy (i.e., abnormality of small blood vessels) and peripheral arterial disease, making diabetic feet particularly vulnerable to ulceration. Enabling patients to maintain their blood glucose levels as close as possible to normal can delay the onset of diabetic foot complications that increase the risk of foot ulceration.

Because of the mixed aetiology, neuroishaemic ulcers (see Case Study 14.2) are more difficult to manage.

Foot ulcers in people with diabetes are prone to infection and can deteriorate very rapidly to become limb or life threatening. It is crucial that any new foot ulcer in a patient with diabetes is urgently referred to a multidisciplinary diabetic foot care team. The team usually consists of an endocrinologist, vascular surgeon, orthopaedic surgeon, podiatrist and orthotist who together take a holistic approach to diabetic foot wound management. Multidisciplinary teams are common in the UK as the approach is aligned to current National Institute for Health and Care Excellence guidance. However, service provision varies in different health care organisations because of inconsistencies in team membership (Paisey et al., 2017).

MANAGEMENT OF FOOT PROBLEMS

Diabetic Foot Screening

Diabetic foot screening is the cornerstone of diabetic foot care. Every person with diabetes should undergo an annual standardised diabetic foot screening. Diabetic foot screening is also recommended on admission to hospital or with the onset of a new foot problem. Nurses and other health care professionals involved in the management of older adults with diabetes can conduct the screening.

The procedure combines simple, evidence-based vascular and neurological assessments. The purpose is to stratify the diabetic foot in terms of ulcer risk and identify individuals at greatest risk for targeted foot care, ulcer prevention and education. Once the risk status is determined, the patient should be informed and a management plan targeted to their level of risk.

As part of the diabetic foot screening procedure, the nurse should observe for factors known to increase ulcer risk, including structural foot deformities, significant calluses, a previous or current foot ulcer, previous amputation and inability to self-care for the feet. The vascular assessment is based on the clinical signs of peripheral arterial disease and non-palpable foot pulses, either tibialis posterior and dorsalis pedis. If either pulse on each foot is palpable, the vascular supply is sufficient. If the pulse on either foot isn't palpable in a patient with diabetes, a more in-depth vascular assessment is required. Referral to a podiatrist for vascular investigation is appropriate. A neurological assessment is conducted using a 10 g Semmes-Weinstein monofilament that tests sensory perception loss alongside clinical symptoms of neuropathy (Diabetes Foot Screening, n.d.). Depending on the number of risk factors for ulceration, the patient is classified as low, moderate or high risk of foot disease or active foot disease (Fig. 19.2).

The Semmes-Weinstein monofilament test was developed to detect patients at risk of neuropathic ulceration. Sensory perception testing in combination with a clinical examination to determine if the patient has any foot deformity (e.g., claw toes, bunions) is the most sensitive method of identifying patients at risk (Schaper et al., 2016).

CASE STUDY 19.2

Mr White is a retired farm worker who lives alone in an isolated cottage in a rural area. He has type 2 diabetes, which was diagnosed 10 years ago by routine screening of his blood chemistry before he underwent a minor surgical procedure at the local hospital. His diabetes is controlled by diet and metformin, an oral medication that helps lower blood glucose levels. He finds it difficult to maintain his blood glucose at a low level, and it varies between 190–300 mg/dl (10–18 mmol/l) (normal fasting blood glucose levels are (70–100 mg/dl, or 3.0–5.5 mmol/l). World Health Organization (1999) guidelines for diagnosing diabetes mellitus specify a fasting blood glucose level of more than 100–125 mg/dl; 5.6–6.9 mmol/l is considered prediabetes. He is overweight and has a body mass index of 30 (normal range is 18.5–25).

The district nurse, Julie, visits Mr White to chat about how he can improve his blood glucose levels. He shows her a blister on his big toe, which has been present for about a week but does not cause him pain. Julie examines the lesion and discovers he has a 2-cm-diameter ulcer on the dorsum of the hallux on his left foot. She uses a 10 g Semmes-Weinstein monofilament to detect the presence of neuropathy and finds he is unable to feel the filament at all on that foot and can't feel the pain of the ulcer. These findings indicate he has peripheral neuropathy. Julie is concerned, and after applying a dry dressing, she arranges an urgent appointment (i.e., within 24 hours) with the local diabetes specialist podiatrist.

The podiatrist finds only one pulse is palpable in Mr White's left foot, indicating the ulcer is neuroischaemic in origin. A referral is made to the diabetic multidisciplinary foot team at the hospital. An endocrinologist reviews Mr White's glucose self-management. The dose of metformin is increased, and after reviewing a lipid sample, Mr White is offered 20 mg simvastatin daily. He is encouraged to make some lifestyle changes, including being more active and adopting a healthier diet. Mrs White cooks for Mr White, so to support the couple to make the dietary changes, they are referred to a dietitian. The vascular team conducts and reviews an arterial duplex scan. The orthotist assesses Mr White's footwear; the toe boxes on his shoes are pressing on the area and considered to be the underlying cause of the ulcer. Mr White agrees to wear open-toe sandals to accommodate dressings and relieve pressure. The podiatrist cleans the wound and applies an appropriate dressing and some protective padding. He advises Mr White to keep the dressing dry, arranges for it to be changed, provides Mr White with an emergency contact number and explains when to seek urgent medical help. The team and Mr White discuss a plan of care to facilitate ulcer healing.

Mr White's blood glucose levels come down to 155–160 mg/dl (8–9 mmol/l) and, with suitable dressings and the change in footwear, the ulcer heals in 6 weeks. He is now waiting for vascular reconstruction in the affected leg. Once completed, the likelihood of further tissue loss in that limb may be avoided. The orthotist measured Mr White for therapeutic footwear with a deep toe box. Mr White is waiting for the shoes to be made and fitted. In future, the podiatrist will monitor Mr White's condition regularly, and the district nurse will visit him to keep an eye on his medication and diabetes.

Diabetic foot risk stratification and triage

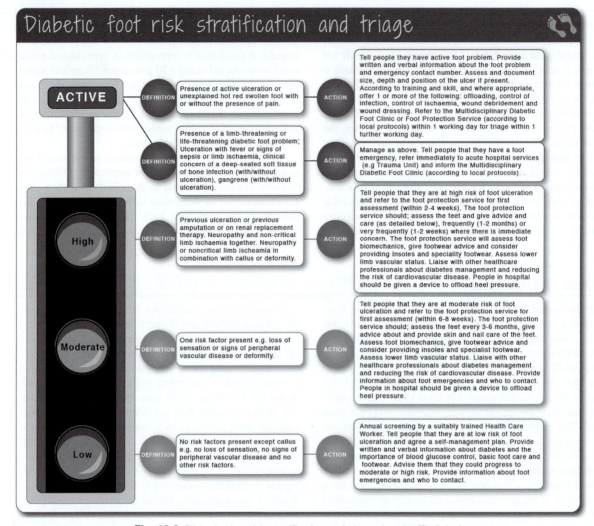

ACTIVE

DEFINITION Presence of active ulceration or unexplained hot red swollen foot with or without the presence of pain.

ACTION Tell people they have active foot problem. Provide written and verbal information about the foot problem and emergency contact number. Assess and document size, depth and position of the ulcer if present. According to training and skill, and where appropriate, offer 1 or more of the following: offloading, control of infection, control of ischaemia, wound debridement and wound dressing. Refer to the Multidisciplinary Diabetic Foot Clinic or Foot Protection Service (according to local protocols) within 1 working day for triage within 1 further working day.

DEFINITION Presence of a limb-threatening or life-threatening diabetic foot problem; Ulceration with fever or signs of sepsis or limb ischaemia, clinical concern of a deep-seated soft tissue of bone infection (with/without ulceration), gangrene (with/without ulceration).

ACTION Manage as above. Tell people that they have a foot emergency, refer immediately to acute hospital services (e.g Trauma Unit) and inform the Multidisciplinary Diabetic Foot Clinic (according to local protocols). .

High

DEFINITION Previous ulceration or previous amputation or on renal replacement therapy. Neuropathy and non-critical limb ischaemia together. Neuropathy or noncritical limb ischeamia in combination with callus or deformity.

ACTION Tell people that they are at high risk of foot ulceration and refer to the foot protection service for first assessment (within 2-4 weeks). The foot protection service should; assess the feet and give advice and care (as detailed below), frequently (1-2 months) or very frequently (1-2 weeks) where there is immediate concern. The foot protection service will assess foot biomechanics, give footwear advice and consider providing insoles and speciality footwear. Assess lower limb vascular status. Liaise with other healthcare professionals about diabetes management and reducing the risk of cardiovascular disease. People in hospital should be given a device to offload heel pressure.

Moderate

DEFINITION One risk factor present e.g. loss of sensation or signs of peripheral vascular disease or deformity.

ACTION Tell people that they are at moderate risk of foot ulceration and refer to the foot protection service for first assessment (within 6-8 weeks). The foot protection service should; assess the feet every 3-6 months, give advice about and provide skin and nail care of the feet. Assess foot biomechanics, give footwear advice and consider providing insoles and specialist footwear. Assess lower limb vascular status. Liaise with other healthcare professionals about diabetes management and reducing the risk of cardiovascular disease. Provide information about foot emergencies and who to contact. People in hospital should be given a device to offload heel pressure.

Low

DEFINITION No risk factors present except callus e.g. no loss of sensation, no signs of peripheral vascular disease and no other risk factors.

ACTION Annual screening by a suitably trained Health Care Worker. Tell people that they are at low risk of foot ulceration and agree a self-management plan. Provide written and verbal information about diabetes and the importance of blood glucose control, basic foot care and footwear. Advise them that they could progress to moderate or high risk. Provide information about foot emergencies and who to contact.

Fig. 19.2 Diabetic ulcer risk stratification and triage chart (traffic lights).

There are many different methods for using monofilaments described in the literature but no universally accepted guidelines. The method outlined below is modified from guidance produced by the International Working Group for the Diabetic Foot (Schaper et al., 2016). Sensory examination should be carried out in a quiet and relaxed setting.

1. Apply the monofilament on the patient's hands, elbow or forehead so they know what to expect.
2. The patient must not be able to see whether or where the examiner applies the monofilament. Three sites to be tested on both feet are indicated: the first and fifth metatarsal heads and the plantar surface of the distal hallux.

3. Apply the monofilament perpendicular to the skin surface.
4. Apply sufficient force to cause the filament to bend or buckle. The total duration of the approach—skin contact and removal of the filament—should be approximately 2 seconds.
5. Apply the filament along the perimeter of, not on, an ulcer site, callus, scar or necrotic tissue. Do not allow the filament to slide across the skin or make repetitive contact at the test site.
6. Press the filament to the skin and ask the patient whether they feel the pressure applied and where.

7. Repeat this application twice at the same site, but alternate it with at least one mock application in which no filament is applied for a total three questions per site. Protective sensation is present at each site if the patient correctly answers two out of three applications. Protective sensation is absent with two out of three incorrect answers, and the patient is considered to be at risk of ulceration.

8. Encourage the patient during testing by giving positive feedback.

The health care provider should be aware of the possible loss of buckling force if the filament is used for too long a period.

The plantar aspects of the foot's metatarsal heads are used as test areas; these sites are particularly prone to high pressure and most likely to develop ulceration. Any area with calluses should be avoided because sensation is impaired by the presence of hard, thickened skin, which could lead to a false diagnosis of neuropathy.

Wound Care

Although local wound management is important, the underlying cause of the wound or ulcer should be addressed before healing can occur. For an ischaemic ulcer, this might involve surgical vascular reconstruction; for a diabetic ulcer, improved blood glucose control may be the priority. As such, wound management involves working with the wider multidisciplinary team. See Chapter 24 for more on skin care.

The treatment aim of local wound management is to create an optimum environment for reepithelialisation and healing. This begins with cleansing the wound to remove excess exudate and decrease the bacterial burden in the presence of local infection. Studies show using tap water in place of saline does not affect rates of infection or healing (Beam, 2006). Wound debridement to remove devitalised tissue can be achieved using autolytic-promoting dressings, including alginates, hydrocolloids and hydrogels. Regular sharp debridement of surrounding calluses by a podiatrist or specialist nurse is effective for tissue-damaging plantar pressures. In some cases biological debridement or laval therapy can be effective in reducing the time of debridement (Dumville et al., 2009). It is important to note debridement of a foot wound is contraindicated if the wound presents with a dry intact eschar, as is sometimes seen overlying the heel. In this scenario, the dry eschar provides a biological covering or barrier.

Once the wound bed is prepared, apply a dressing. The choice of dressing is often difficult but should consider factors such as wound classification, amount and type of exudate, site of the wound and practicalities of accommodating the dressing in footwear or an offloading device. Further patient-centred considerations are pain avoidance at dressing changes (i.e., choosing a dressing that is easy to remove) and maintenance of quality of life. When assessing the suitability of a dressing, check it has remained intact and in place, leakage has been prevented even under pressure and the skin has not become macerated (Harding et al., 2019).

When you apply a dressing to a foot wound, take special care to avoid bandaging individual toes and creating a tourniquet effect. Bandages are often appropriate and useful secondary dressings particularly because their application removes the need for adhesive strapping and taping on fragile older skin. However, when you apply bandages to a foot wound, avoid creases and bumps under the weight-bearing plantar surface.

In patients with plantar wounds, particularly those with diabetic neuropathy and elevated plantar pressures, it is crucial to offload or redistribute pressure away from the ulcer site. The magnitude of plantar pressure under the foot is associated with the development and healing of neuropathic foot ulceration. The gold standard is a total-contact cast (Bus et al., 2020). Where total-contact casts are contraindicated, other removable devices such as a diabetic walker or forefoot offloader should be applied (Bus et al., 2020). A multidisciplinary team oversees application and management of total-contact casts.

Self-Care

It's easy to neglect your feet until discomfort draws attention to a problem. It is not unusaul for people to prioritise routine self-care of their hands and fingernails over and above caring for their feet and toenails. Yet the feet are arguably in greater need of care and attention, being more prone to pain and injury through wear and tear. Nurses can assist in preventing foot problems by promoting and educating older people about the importance of preventive self-foot care and supporting and enabling them to take responsibility for their own foot care self-management. In order to prevent foot problems, a regular regime of foot care and surveillance should be established. Older people, especially those with diabetic neuropathy, should be encouraged to inspect their feet regularly, looking for unusual swelling, reddness or rubs, cracks or cuts in the skin and taking care to check areas that are less easy to get at—for example, the plantar aspect of the feet or between the toes. Older people should be advised any new lesion could be an early warning sign of a potential foot problem and to seek advice from a medical professional. Many older people find it difficult to see the bottoms of their feet. If a family member is not available to undertake regular foot checks, a strategically placed mirror may provide a solution.

Much preventative foot self-care consists of simple tasks like routine foot care and general hygiene. For example, feet should be washed regularly and dried carefully, especially between the toes. Older people should be advised to soak their feet for no more than 5–10 minutes and then, after drying carefully, especially between the toes, to apply a moisturising cream—not a specialty foot cream, which can be expensive, but any moisturising cream. A thin layer of petroleum jelly can be applied to the most painful areas after bathing and before bed, with a sock to protect bed linen. This prevents moisture from escaping any area of callosity and helps soften the skin, making it less painful. As many older patients have trouble reaching their feet, a partner, relative or friend may be willing to help them. Moisturising cream applied to the feet daily helps keep the skin in good condition but should be avoided interdigitally. Excess moisture between toes can be managed with antiperspirant spray several times a week, or surgical spirits can be applied with a cotton wool bud. If the skin in this area is allowed to become too wet, it can split or fissure. Toenails should be cut straight across and not too short, and sharp corners or edges should be smoothed with a nail file. Cutting down the sides of the nails is inadvisable as it can lead to ingrown toenails.

Raising awareness in older adults about the need to reduce risky behaviours has an important role in preventing foot problems. It's always advisable for older adults not to walk barefoot, even at home, as it increases the risk of injury from standing on foreign objects or inadvertently kicking furniture. Footwear provides protection.

Home remedies for foot pain are best avoided. The use of corn cures, which often contain acids, can cause skin damage. It may be tempting, but it is unwise to treat your own painful corns or calluses using a razor blade or pair of scissors. The most helpful advice is to wear adequate, well-fitting footwear, as described below. A change in footwear often brings comfort and a tremendous improvement in pressure lesions, enabling the older person to enjoy walking.

Footwear

Choice of footwear is important to prevent or exacerbate existing foot problems and reduce the risk of falls (Menz et al., 2018). Nurses are in a good position to advise patients and their carers on their choice of footwear. Style is commonly seen as more important than comfort in every age group, but older adults, particularly with foot pain, should choose shoes for comfort, support, function and safety rather than fashion. Women in particular may find it challenging to follow footwear recommendations around style and fit. Women's footwear styles, particularly court or heeled shoes, are considered by some to be symbols of social normality and youth, forming an important aspect of personal image. When talking with patients about shoe choices, practitioners should be sensitive to the psychological impact of footwear choice. Investing time to listen and understand the thoughts and feelings of the patient without judgement, then empowering them to make the right shoe choice, is more likely to influence behaviour than lecturing an individual on what they should wear on their feet. Drawing around the patient's feet with them standing on a piece of paper, then comparing this to a similar drawing made around their shoes, can reveal a mismatch that may persuade them to discard ill-fitting shoes. This technique is a particularly helpful method of introducing the concept of age-related changes in foot size and shape in individuals who have not had their feet measured for many years.

A recent systematic review of the literature concluded over 60% of people wear incorrectly fitted footwear (Buldt & Menz, 2018). With age, it's not uncommon for the forefoot to spread. Forefeet of older adults tend to be comparatively broader, often leading to particular difficulties finding shoes with the correct width (Ansuategui Echeita et al., 2016) A correct fit is important, and the length of the shoes may be inadequate. Width and depth of toe boxes should be roomy enough to allow you to naturally spread your toes. It can be difficult to find well-fitting shoes when there is gross toe deformity. Ideally shoes have a fastening—laces, a bar or a Velcro strap—that enables them to be tightened snugly to the foot while the person moves through the gait cycle and adapts to uneven walking surfaces. A thick or cushioned sole to absorb the stresses that pass through the foot during walking is also desirable. If shoe uppers are made of leather, they conform more easily to foot shape, but sometimes cheaper shoes with synthetic uppers are acceptable. Shopping for shoes late in the day when feet tend to be at their largest is a good idea to ensure a good fit and avoid wasting money on inadequate, unsuitable, uncomfortable shoes.

Some people have such difficult foot deformities or gross oedema around their feet and ankles it is almost impossible to buy shoes they can wear. They can be referred to a local orthotist for tailor-made footwear. People with mobility difficulties can use equipment to assist with fastening shoes (see Resources list). Replacing ordinary shoelaces with elastic ones or finding shoes with a zip fastener may be easier to manage. Long-handled shoehorns assist people who cannot bend to put on their shoes. If slippers are worn indoors, they should provide support and fit properly, with firm, non-slip soles so there is no need to shuffle to keep them on, which increases the risk of falls. Menz et al. (2006) found indoor fallers were more likely to go without shoes or slippers. Loose-fitting socks and stockings avoid restricting superficial circulation over the toes and heels. Cotton socks, which absorb sweat, are useful for people who are prone to developing fungal infections where the skin is moist.

Surgery

Once a patient has exhausted or considered all conservative treatment options, foot surgery may be indicated. Foot surgery is not without possible complications; it's important to try conservative treatment options before surgery is considered as the last resort. Even then, patients must be given a clear understanding of the risks involved before consenting to surgery. In some cases surgery is an excellent option to relieve foot pain, improve function and enable a return to normal activity. However, benefits need to be weighed against possible risks, including surgical complications, social isolation, long rehabilitation and the chance the surgery makes the condition worse. Forefoot surgery is often performed using local anaesthesia. Conditions of the forefoot amenable to surgical invervention include deformed lesser toes (i.e., hammer toe, claw toe), hallux valgus (i.e., bunion) and mortons neuroma. Deformed lesser toes can rub against shoes during walking and cause dorsal or apical corns and calluses. Surgical interventions for lesser toe deformities such as digital arthroplasty, which restores function in an abnormal joint or replaces it with a prosthetic joint, or arthrodesis, which is correction of the joint with fusion so no movement occurs, straighten toes and prevent further trauma from shoes. If a lesser toe is excessively dorsiflexed (i.e., pushed upward and out of normal alignment), it may be simpler to amputate it and keep a cosmetically acceptable result. Extreme dorsiflexion can occur in the second toe from pressure from a medially deviated first toe (i.e., hallux abductus), which comes to lie under the second toe and forces the second toe into this position.

Mid and rear-foot procedures are less common and more complex. Midfoot surgery may be indicated in the presence of a particularly severe bunion. The surgical management of an acquired flat foot involves a combination of midfoot and rear-foot surgery. Flatfoot reconstruction involves tendon transfer (i.e., distal section of a tendon transferred to an additional site), calcaneal displacement osteotomy (i.e., cutting and realignment of the heel bone) and double or triple arthrodesis (i.e., surgical fusion between the calacaneum, talus and cuboid). Whether these procedures are used in isolation or in combination depends on the individual case. The rehabilitation period for this type of procedure is prolonged.

CONCLUSION AND LEARNING POINTS

Foot problems are reported by at least one in three community-dwelling older people, with higher prevalence rates observed in institutional and clinical settings. The most common foot conditions in older people are nail disorders, corns and calluses, toe deformities (i.e., hallux valgus and lesser toe deformities), musculoskeletal disorders (i.e., metatarsagia, plantar fasciitis) and ulceration.

Risk factors for foot problems include age, being a woman, obesity and multiple chronic diseases, particularly diabetes. Foot problems have a significant detrimental effect on mobility and quality of life for older people. Nurses have an extremely important role to play in the assessment, evaluation and examination of foot pathology in older adults. Advising older adults about self-care and carrying out practical interventions can improve their quality of life. Nurses and podiatrists working together can do much to optimise treatment, lessen discomfort from foot problems and contribute to the well-being of older people and their ability to carry out day-to-day activities.

KEY LEARNING POINTS

- Foot problems are common in older people.
- Age related change increases the risk of foot problems.
- Nurses play an important role in the assessment and diagnosis of foot problems in the older person.
- Common dermatological problems to affect older people include corns, callus and nail deformity.
- Poor lower limb biomechanics in combination with the repetitive wear and tear of walking can lead to common musculoskeletal conditions such as metatarsalgia, plantar fasciitis and osteoarthritis.
- Foot ulceration is serious. Assessment should consider the immediate referral to the appropriate team

(multidisciplinary diabetic foot care team or vascular team). If left untreated ulceration can lead to loss of limb or life.
- When caring for older people particularly those known to have diabetes it is important to take time to remove the patient's shoes and socks and check the feet for ulceration.
- Nurses have the skills and knowledge to foot screen, triage, educate and refer older people with diabetes.
- Nurses are well placed to offer preventative advice on routine foot care and hygiene as well as choice and fit of footwear.

RESOURCES

Diabetes UK: https://www.diabetes.org.uk
Royal College of Podiatry: https://cop.org.uk
British Footwear Association: https://britishfootwearas-
   sociation.co.uk
Disabled Living Foundation: https://www.whereyoustand.org/
   groups-and-organisations/item/disabled-living-foundation

Disabled Living: https://www.disabledliving.co.uk
Society of Shoe Fitters: https://www.facebook.com/
   Society-of-Shoefitters-121804411325196

REFERENCES

Ansuategui Echeita, j, Hijmans, J. M., Smits, S., Van der Woude, L. H. V., & Postema, K. (2016). Age-related differences in women's foot shape. *Maturitas, 94*, 64–69.

Birke, J. A., Franks, B. D., & Foto, J. G. (1995). First ray joint limitation, pressure, and ulceration of the first metatarsal head in diabetes mellitus. *Foot & Ankle International, 16*(5), 277–284. doi:10.1177/107110079501600506.

Beam, J. W. (2006). Wound cleansing: Water or saline? *Journal of Athletic Training, 41*(2), 196–197.

Bendermacher, B. L., Teijink, J. A., Willigendael, E. M., Bartelink, M. L., Büller, H. R. et al., (2006). Symptomatic peripheral arterial disease: The value of a validated questionnaire and a clinical decision rule. *British Journal of General Practice, 56*(533), 932–937.

Benvenuti, F., Ferrucci, L., Guralnik, J. M., Gangemi, S., & Baroni, A. (1995). Foot pain and disability in older persons: An epidemiologic survey. *Journal of the American Geriatrics Society, 43*(5), 479–484.

Bruno, J., & Helfand, A. E. (1990). Physical medicine considerations in managing the older patient. *Journal of the American Podiatric Medical Association, 80*(7), 364–369.

Buldt, A. K., & Menz, M. B. (2018). Incorrectly fitted footwear, foot pain and foot disorders: A systematic search and narrative review of the literature. *Journal of Foot and Ankle Research, 11*(1), 43.

Bus, S. A., Armstrong, D. G., Gooday, C., Jarl, G., Caravaggi, C., Viswanathan, V., et al., (2020). Guidelines on offloading foot ulcers in persons with diabetes (IWGDF 2019 update). *Diabetes/Metabolism Research and Reviews, 36*(1), e3274.

Crawford, V. L. S., Ashford, R. L., McPeake, B., & Stout, R. W. (1996). Palliative podiatric care: Service provision and treatment in an elderly population. *The Foot, 6*(1), 10–12.

Dawson, J., Thorogood, M., Marks, S.-A., Juszczak, E., Dodd, C., Lavis, G., et al., (2002). The prevalence of foot problems in older women: A cause for concern. *Journal of Public Health Medicine, 24*(2), 77–84.

Diabetes Foot Screening. (n.d.). Diabetic foot risk stratification and triage.https://www.diabetesframe.org/wp-content/up-loads/2021/03/traffic_light_NHS_England.pdf

Dumville, J. C., Worthy, G., Bland, J. M., Cullum, N., Dowson, C., Inglesias, C., et al., (2009). Larval therapy for leg ulcers (VenUS II): Randomised controlled trial. *BMJ, 338*, b773.

Edelstein, J. E. (1988). Foot care for the aging. *Physical Therapy, 68*(12), 1882–1886.

Gates, L. S., Arden, N. K., Hannan, M. T., Roddy, E., Gill, T. K., Hill, C. L., et al., (2019). Prevalence of foot pain across an international consortium of population-based cohorts. *Arthritis Care & Research, 71*(5), 661–670.

Gould, N., Schneider, W., & Ashikaga, T. (1980). Epidemiological survey of foot problems in the continental United States: 1978–1979. *Foot & Ankle, 1*(1), 8–10.

Harvey, I., Frankel, S., Marks, R., Shalom, D., & Morgan, M. (1997). Foot morbidity and exposure to chiropody: Population based study. *BMJ, 315*(7115), 1054–1055.

Harding, K., Carville, K., Chadwick, P., Moore, Z., Nicodème, M., Percival, S., et al., (2019). WUWHS Consensus Document: Wound Exudate, effective assessment and management.https://www.woundsinternational.com/resources/details/wuwhs-consensus-document-wound-exudate-effective-assessment-and-management

Ince, P., Abbas, Z. G., Lutale, J. K., Basit, A., Ali, S. M., Chohan, F., et al., (2008). Use of the SINBAD classification system and score in comparing outcomes of foot ulcer management on three continents. *Diabetes Care, 31*(5), 964–967.

Leung, A. K. C., Lam, J. M., Leong, K. F., Hon, K. L., Barankin, B., Leung, A. A. M., et al., (2020). Onychomycosis: An updated review. *Recent Patents on Inflammation and Allergy Drug Discovery, 14*(1), 32–45.

López-López, D., Becerro-de-Bengoa-Vallejo, R., Losa-Iglesias, M. E., Palomo-López, P., Rodríguez-Sanz, D., Brandariz-Pereira, J. M., et al., (2018). Evaluation of foot health related quality of life in individuals with foot problems by gender: A cross-sectional comparative analysis study. *BMJ Open, 8*(10), Article e023980 –e023980.

Menz, H., Morris, M., & Lord, S. (2006). Footwear characteristics and risk of indoor and outdoor falls in older people. *Gerontology, 53*(3), 174–180.

Menz, H. B., Auhl, M., & Spink, M. J. (2018). Foot problems as a risk factor for falls in community-dwelling older people: A systematic review and meta-analysis. *Maturitas, 118*, 7–14.

Munro, B. J., & Steele, J. R. (1998). Foot-care awareness: A survey of persons aged 65 years and older. *Journal of the American Podiatric Medical Association, 88*(5), 242–248.

National Institute for Health and Care Excellence. (2020). BNF Terdinafine. https://www.nice.org.uk/bnf-uk-only

Nyssen, A., Benhadou, F., Magnée, M., André, J., Koopmansch, C., & Wautrecht, J.-C. (2020). Chilblains. *VASA, 49*(2), 133–140.

Otani, M. (2017). Treatment of tinea pedis in elderly patients using external preparations. *Medical Mycology, 58*(2), j35–j41.

Paisey, R. B., Abbott, A., Levenson, R., Harrington, A., Browne, D., Moore, J., Bamford, M., & Roe, M. (2017). Diabetes related major lower limb amputation incidence is strongly related to diabetic foot service provision and improves with enhancement of services: Peer review of the South-West of England. *Diabetic Medicine,* 35(1): 53–62. doi:10.1111/dme.13512.

Pushpangadan, M., & Burns, E. (1996). Caring for older people. Community services: Health. *BMJ, 313*(7060), 805–808.

Recalcati, S. (2020). Cutaneous manifestations in COVID-19: A first perspective. *Journal of the European Academy of Dermatology and Venereology, 34*(5), e212–e213.

Rodríguez-Sanz, D., Tovaruela-Carrión, N., López-López, D., Palomo-López, P., Romero-Morales, C., Navarro-Flores, E., et al., (2018). Foot disorders in the elderly: A mini-review. *Disease-a-Month, 64*(3), 64–91.

Schaper, N. C., Van Netten, J. J., Apelqvist, J., Lipsky, B. A., & Bakker, K. International Working Group on the Diabetic Foot. (2016). Prevention and management of foot problems in diabetes: A Summary Guidance for Daily Practice 2015, based on the IWGDF Guidance Documents. *Diabetes/Metabolism Research and Reviews, 32*(1), 7–15.

Selvin, E., & Erlinger, T. P. (2004). Prevalence of and risk factors for peripheral arterial disease in the United States: Results from the National Health and Nutrition Examination Survey, 1999–2000. *Circulation, 110*(6), 738–743.

Shelton, L. R. (2013). A closer look at osteoarthritis. *The Nurse Practitioner, 7,* 38.

Souwer, I. H., Bor, J. H., Smits, P., & Lagro-Janssen, A. L. (2017). Assessing the effectiveness of topical betamethasone to treat chronic chilblains: A randomised clinical trial in primary care. *British Journal of General Practice, 67*(656), e187–e193.

White, E. G., & Mulley, G. P. (1989). Footcare for very elderly people: A community survey. *Age and Ageing, 18*(4), 276–278.

World Health Organization. (1999). Mean fasting blood glucose. https://www.who.int/data/gho/indicator-metadata-registry/imr-details/2380

Wylie, G., Torrens, C., Campbell, P., Frost, H., Gordon, A. L., Menz, H. B., et al., (2019). Podiatry interventions to prevent falls in older people: A systematic review and meta-analysis. *Age and Ageing, 48*(3), 327–336.

Breathing

Janelle Yorke

This chapter focuses on aspects of breathing in older adults. There are well-documented physiological changes associated with ageing. Respiratory conditions can be debilitating and impact physical and emotional well-being, resulting in feelings of helplessness and depression. The chapter builds on issues raised in Chapter 5, emphasises the importance of thorough respiratory assessments and explores a range of therapeutic interventions intended to maximise breathing in older adults. See Table 20.1 for a useful list of abbreviations.

OVERVIEW OF THE RESPIRATORY SYSTEM

The main function of the respiratory system is gas exchange. Oxygen is required at cellular level for the production of energy, which the cells use for metabolism. If oxygen is not readily available to the tissues, the cells cease to function and ultimately die. Elimination of carbon dioxide occurs by an elegant transport mechanism that begins when atmospheric oxygen is drawn into the lungs via the respiratory tract and comes into contact with the alveolar membrane. Oxygenation occurs through three main processes: ventilation, external respiration and internal respiration.

Ventilation refers to the mechanism by which atmospheric gases are delivered to the alveolar membrane and alveolar gases are expelled. This is a mechanical process that is dependent on volume changes within the thoracic cavity. When there is a change in volume, there is a corresponding change in pressure, which leads to an increased flow of gases to equalise the pressure. This is explained by Boyle's law, which forms the basis of inspiration and expiration (Waugh & Grant, 2022). Ventilation is affected by the action of thorax muscles and controlled by the respiratory centre in the brainstem via the phrenic and intercostal nerves. The respiratory centre is mainly stimulated by raised levels of arterial carbon dioxide and low levels of oxygen. Breathing is not normally under conscious control, although it can be stopped for a few seconds at will.

A number of gases make up the atmosphere, including oxygen, carbon dioxide, nitrogen and water. Each has its own molecular weight and is pulled to earth by gravitational forces. The term used for the collective pressure of these gases is *atmospheric pressure*, which equates to 760 mmHg (101 kPa) at sea level (Waugh & Grant, 2022). Inspiration occurs when atmospheric pressure is greater than the pressure within the lungs, and expiration occurs when pressure inside the lungs exceeds the atmospheric pressure. However, each gas also exerts its own pressure independently, according to Dalton's and Henry's laws. These are

TABLE 20.1	Abbreviations Used in Chapter 20
Abbreviation	**Definition**
ABG	Arterial blood-gas analysis
BiPAP	Biphasic positive-pressure ventilation
COPD	Chronic obstructive pulmonary disease
CPAP	Continuous positive airway pressure
EPAP	Expiratory positive airway pressure
FEV_1	Forced expiratory volume in 1 second
FRC	Functional residual capacity
FVC	Forced vital capacity
GOLD	Global Initiative on Chronic Obstructive Lung Disease
Hb	Haemoglobin
HbO_2	Oxyhaemoglobin
IPAP	Inspiratory positive airway pressure
LTOT	Long-term oxygen therapy
MDI	Metered-dose inhaler
NIPPV	Non-invasive positive-pressure ventilation
NIV	Non-invasive ventilation
$PaCO_2$	Partial pressure of carbon dioxide in arterial blood
PaO_2	Partial pressure of oxygen in arterial blood
RV	Residual volume
SpO_2	Saturation of peripheral haemoglobin
TLC	Total lung capacity

referred to as partial pressures and are measured in clinical practice by arterial blood-gas (ABG) analysis.

Once inspiration is complete, oxygen moves from the alveoli to the pulmonary blood capillary by a process of diffusion. Similarly, carbon dioxide diffuses from the pulmonary blood capillary to the alveolus for elimination during expiration in a process is called external respiration. Once oxygen has moved across the alveolar membrane, 97% combines with haemoglobin (Hb) to form oxyhaemoglobin (HbO_2). The remaining 3% is dissolved in the plasma. Each molecule of Hb can carry four molecules of oxygen.

The final stage of respiration involves the exchange of gases at the tissue level between the capillaries and tissue cells, known as internal respiration. Gas exchange occurs as a result of changes in pressure gradients by the same process of diffusion. Carbon dioxide is then carried as a waste product of metabolism. The majority (70%) of carbon dioxide is carried as bicarbonate via the carbonic acid bicarbonate buffer system. The remaining carbon dioxide is carried as either carbaminohaemoglobin (23%) or dissolved in the plasma (3%). Carbon dioxide is then expelled from the lungs during expiration. In health, the amount of carbon dioxide produced should equal the amount exhaled; this forms the acid–base balance. For a more detailed discussion, please refer to Waugh and Grant (2022) or any general physiology text.

ACUTE AND CHRONIC BREATHING PROBLEMS ASSOCIATED WITH OLDER ADULTS

Many acute or chronic respiratory conditions affect older adults. Chronic respiratory problems develop throughout life, many of which are associated with smoking or environmental factors. The disabling effects tend to increase with age, leaving some individuals housebound. Chronic obstructive pulmonary disease (COPD) is a term used to encompass conditions such as chronic bronchitis, emphysema and asthma. The 2021 guidelines from the Global Initiative on Chronic Obstructive Lung Disease (GOLD) state deranged inflammatory processes are associated with noxious particles or gases in the lungs of a patient with COPD (GOLD, 2021). COPD is a major cause of global morbidity and mortality. An estimated 328 million people have COPD worldwide; by 2030, it is expected to become the leading cause of death (GOLD, 2021).

Patients with emphysema have enlarged air sacs distal to the terminal bronchioles, accompanied by destruction of the alveolar walls. Symptoms of emphysema, namely breathlessness, stem from structural changes that lead to progressive airflow limitation, hyperinflation, air-trapping and reduced gas transfer at the alveolar-capillary interface. A diagnosis of chronic bronchitis is usually made by the presence of a productive cough for most days of the week for a minimum of 3 months over a 2-year period. Asthma is associated with symptoms of wheezing and breathlessness rather than sputum production. Each COPD condition has acute exacerbations, defined by GOLD (2021) as 'an acute event characterised by worsening of symptoms that is beyond day-to-day variations and leads to a change in medication'. Exacerbations of COPD accelerate decline in lung function, resulting in increased breathlessness, reduced physical activity, reduced health-related quality of life, increased hospital admissions and decreased survival (Case Study 20.1).

Immune systems decline with age, making older adults at higher risk of influenza and complications like pneumonia (see Chapter 23). Flu is a highly contagious viral infection and one of the most severe winter illnesses. It spreads easily from person to person, usually when an infected person coughs or sneezes. Pneumonia is a serious infection that leads to inflammation in the lungs. The air sacs fill with pus and other liquid, blocking oxygen from reaching the bloodstream (American Lung Association, 2020). It is

CASE STUDY 20.1

Mrs Smith, a retired 82-year-old cotton mill worker, was diagnosed with COPD more than 10 years ago. She lives at home with her husband, who smokes around 20 cigarettes per day; Mrs Smith stopped smoking a few years ago. She was admitted to hospital following an acute exacerbation of COPD, general deterioration of her activity levels and increasing breathlessness. During the hospital admission Mrs Smith's saturations remained <92%, and a referral for assessment for LTOT was made. An arterial blood gas assessment was performed—LTOT is indicated in patients with an arterial partial pressure of oxygen (PaO_2) when stable of <7.3kPa. Mrs Smith's results confirmed hypoxaemia with a PaO_2 7kPa, and she was prepared for discharge with LTOT.

A risk assessment was conducted to prepare Mrs Smith and her husband for discharge that included the following:

- Fire safety in the home
- Current smokers who resided in or visited the home
- Space for the equipment
- Inability of patient to use complex equipment
- Compliance with oxygen prescription—evidence shows LTOT needs to be used for at least 15 hours per day for maximal clinical benefit
- Risk of falls
- Risk of pressure sores from use of a nasal canulae
- Presence of pets and children

An education package was developed that included the following:

- Written safety instructions and alert of fire risk for patients and relatives
- Written information of the dangers of using home oxygen within the vicinity of an open flame such as pilot lights, cookers, gas fires and candles
- Dangers of people smoking in the house
- Advice and information on smoking cessation to avoid the patient relapsing
- Importance of the person receiving LTOT to not smoke due to increased fire risk and reduced clinical benefit
- Responsibility of the person receiving LTOT to use oxygen safely
- Education on self-care and prevention of pressure sores around nasal area, including use of water-based lubricants
- Importance of maintaining a nutritional diet and hydration
- Support for social and mental health well-being
- Requirement for portable oxygen to enable Mrs Smith to leave the house for outings

Further assessment and advice were provided by the field engineer from the oxygen supply company.

more likely to be fatal or cause more profound and longer illness in older people compared with younger people because of the increased incidence of comorbidities such as COPD and because older adults tend to be less well nourished and active. Diagnosis and management of pneumonia may be complicated by these factors, and there is often a dilemma of whether home or hospital treatment is best for the patient.

The World Health Organization declared a global pandemic on March 11, 2020, caused by the acute respiratory syndrome coronavirus 2 (COVID-19). There were over 83 million confirmed cases and more than 1.8 million deaths globally in the first year. In a systematic review of studies published between December 2019 and May 2020, older adults were found to be particularly susceptible to COVID-19, with mortality reported to be as high as 10% in adults aged 70 years and above compared to <1% in younger adults. One in five elderly people were critically ill (Singhal et al., 2021). Although these rates may change with increased understanding about the disease and vaccination, older people are likely to remain particularly vulnerable to COVID-19, which is an important consideration for nurses and health care professionals. For survivors, long-term functional decline and a decrease in health-related quality of life has been reported 6 months following hospitalisation due to COVID-19 (Hodgson et al., 2021). Older adults and people who live with, visit or provide care for them can take steps to protect themselves against COVID-19 that include vaccination and biosecurity measures such as handwashing, mask wearing and social distancing.

During the peak of the pandemic, severe COVID-19 that necessitated intensive care management affected around 5% of people with a diagnosis and more likely to occur in older and frail people (Singhal et al., 2021). Intensive care intervention, including mechanical ventilation, requires careful consideration and shared decision making between the patient, family and clinicians. Anticipatory care for an older person with access to palliative care is essential. However, further pandemic waves with different viral variants and the success of vaccination programmes in many developed countries has resulted in a decline in intensive care admissions (Vasileiou et al., 2021).

Consider the following when caring for an older person with COVID-19:

- Good hydration
- Breathing techniques
- Proning: Current evidence indicates benefit in some patients in hospital; community patients may benefit from changing positions (Koeckerling et al., 2020)
- Cooling using wet facecloths; however, avoid fans due to increased infection risk

It is also important to consider psychological support and the importance of explaining the use of personal protective equipment. If visiting is restricted due to biosecurity measures, maintaining connections with family through regular contact using digital techniques is essential to mental well-being.

Oxygen therapy is a key consideration in the acute management of COVID-19. The primary aim of oxygen is to correct hypoxaemia. For a person with suspected COVID-19–related breathlessness, SpO_2 <94% in room air, then oxygen therapy, should be considered (Voshaar et al., 2021). If the person is at home, an assessment of the situation for safe and timely delivery of home oxygen is required; consideration of hospital admission must be a shared decision.

The RECOVERY trial found the use of dexamethasone reduced mortality in hospitalised patients with COVID-19 who required respiratory support through mechanical ventilation or oxygen therapy (RECOVERY Collaborative Group, 2021). A significant number of trial participants were in the same age category as nursing home residents; care home residents with COVID-19 infection and increasing oxygen requirements may benefit from dexamethasone administration.

FACTORS THAT AFFECT BREATHING IN OLDER ADULTS

Factors that affect breathing in older adults can be physiological, psychosocial and/or environmental. It is difficult to assess physiological ageing processes, as few lungs are free from some pathophysiological or environmental changes. However, older lungs have lost much of the protein elastin, which is necessary for maintaining airway patency. As a consequence, lungs become less compliant, which increases airway resistance. Loss of elasticity can result in alveolar hypoventilation and lead to a ventilation–perfusion mismatch (Lumb & Thomas, 2021).

Changes also occur in the composition of collagen. Cross-links form between the subunits of the collagen, resulting in increased rigidity, which is thought to be responsible for the alterations of respiratory mechanics (Waugh & Grant, 2022). General musculoskeletal changes associated with ageing also affect the mechanics of breathing. For example, osteoporosis in the rib cage and vertebra can lead to kyphosis, which is observed as stooped posture that compromises respiratory effort and impairs inspiration.

Epithelial mucus production is increased, and macrophages become less efficient, impairing the immunological processes that protect an individual against infection. Loss of muscle tone and strength in the diaphragm, intercostal and accessory muscles, together with an increase in sensitivity of the upper respiratory tract, lead to a reduced and less effective cough reflex. In younger people, the respiratory system is able to respond to challenges such as an infection or heavy exercise by compensatory mechanisms (e.g., increased respiratory rate and depth and a strong cough reflex). However, where changes have occurred due to age, that option is reduced. Weak respiratory muscles contribute to reduced lung volumes. These effects are confounded by inactivity and lack of stamina. Environmental conditions, both at home and work, also affect overall respiratory status. The seminal work by Dunn et al. (1995) established clear links between factory emissions and cases of asthma. An older person may have had a longer period of exposure to unfavourable conditions. Some have been exposed without protection to environmental pollutants, including asbestos dust or mustard gas, conditions that would not be tolerated today. Housing conditions also contribute to respiratory problems. A cold, damp home environment results in reduced resistance to infection, thus predisposing the occupant to bronchitis and tuberculosis. Dietary deficiencies also have an adverse effect; for example, iron deficiency anaemia reduces the oxygen-carrying capacity of the blood, leading to breathlessness and lethargy.

Although maintaining a healthy lifestyle from an early age gives the best chance later on, few individuals reach old age without some compromise to health. However, it is never too late to benefit from positive changes to lifestyle and environment. Cigarette smoking is the chief initiating agent in the development of COPD. It causes hypertrophy of the mucus-secreting glands and increases the risk of infection by reducing the number and efficiency of epithelial cilia. Tobacco plays a major role in the development of emphysema due to an imbalance between protease and antiprotease activity in the lungs. Excess protease activity damages and dissolves alveolar walls and the small airways. Cigarette smoke induces the proliferation of alveolar macrophages, which contain protease. On the death of the macrophages, the protease released exceeds the neutralising capacity of the antiprotease system (Lumb & Thomas, 2021). This allows tissue damage to occur. Cigarette smoke is also carcinogenic.

The most important intervention in modifying the course of COPD and many other respiratory disorders is smoking cessation (Lumb & Thomas, 2021). However, alternative strategies must be considered, as nicotine dependency is a relapsing condition that sometimes requires multiple interventions (National Institute for Health and Care Excellence, 2021). A person-centred assessment is required and for some people referral to specialist smoking cessation services.

Physiological and social/environmental factors impact an older adult's psychological status. Chronic respiratory conditions can be debilitating, which may affect psychological well-being and cause feelings of helplessness and depression that restrict socialisation outside the home.

Community nurses and general practitioners are ideally placed to note these factors and assist in obtaining appropriate help and advice. There is good quality evidence that increased levels of physical activity, psychological support and nutritional support, as part of a multiprofessional pulmonary rehabilitation programme, provide survival and quality of life benefits (GOLD, 2021).

RESPIRATORY ASSESSMENT

A thorough respiratory assessment is key to planning effective care to prevent, manage and treat respiratory conditions. This process is not very different for an older person than it is for a younger person, but it may be complicated by difficulties such as unreliable historians and complex multiple pathologies and therapeutic regimes that affect the clinical symptoms (Lumb & Thomas, 2021).

An accurate patient history is vitally important, although memory and concentration loss may be apparent. Older adults may have sensory deficits such as hearing or vision loss that impede the process. Other sources of information should be used to validate information where necessary, including family and significant others and previous medical or nursing documentation, although retrospective documentation has the potential for inaccuracy. When considering history, enquire about social circumstances and support. A number of older people live alone and are financially less secure following retirement. This has repercussions on their lifestyle and diet and contributes to respiratory problems. Ask questions about smoking habits, physical activity, allergies, occupational history, living arrangements, quality of housing (e.g., presence of damp or mould, adequacy of heating) and pastimes in a sensitive manner.

All clinical assessments should follow a logical systematic approach. This involves using the skills of inspection, palpation, percussion and auscultation to obtain primary data, then supporting these findings using secondary data such as chest X-rays. Table 20.2 outlines and discusses the primary data that might be ascertained during a clinical respiratory assessment. Assessment is best performed with the person sitting upright and forward. However, this is difficult for some older clients; support may be required. Adapt the assessment technique depending on individual needs.

A number of older clients rely on long-term therapies for chronic respiratory conditions. Assessment of their respiratory status must be undertaken in relation to these therapies. The amount of respiratory support the person is receiving at the time of assessment should be noted, including treatments such as oxygen, medications and fluids. It is important to understand the effects of these therapies; for example, increased fluid input may lead to cardiac failure and subsequent pulmonary oedema that presents as dyspnoea. It is

good practice to provide ongoing education to patients and ask them to demonstrate their use of inhalers—in particular metered-dose inhalers (MDI)—and discuss competence issues related to equipment being used such as home oxygen therapy. Exercise tolerance should also be noted so it can be used to evaluate any improvement or deterioration in the patient's condition over time.

Secondary Data

Pulmonary Function Tests

As described in Lumb and Thomas (2021), pulmonary function testing is a useful adjunct to clinical assessment. Static lung volumes such as total lung capacity (TLC), residual volume (RV) and functional residual capacity (FRC), and dynamic lung volumes such as forced vital capacity (FVC) and forced expiratory volume in 1 second (FEV_1), can be measured. These tests require specialist equipment that is not always readily available in acute settings. Changes in an older adult's pulmonary function are related to musculoskeletal changes in the chest wall and in elastic recoil. Baseline assessment of these data is useful to determine changes in chronic conditions over time. Although TLC remains essentially unchanged in older adults, some of its components alter; for example, FRC increases as elastic recoil decreases. They may also present with increased RV, particularly in the presence emphysema and/or chronic bronchitis. In both restrictive and obstructive diseases, FVC and FEV_1 are reduced, the difference lying in the amount of RV and the ratio between FVC and FEV_1, described as $FEV_1\%$.

Peak Expiratory Flow Rate

The measurement of peak flow is a useful guide to dynamic lung function in acute settings, and serial measurements are used to diagnose and monitor asthma and evaluate the effect of therapies such as nebulized salbutamol. Peak expiratory flow rate, or peak flow, as it is commonly termed, is the flow generated in the first 0.1 second of a forced expiration; the resulting figure is extrapolated over a minute. Results indicate the degree of airway resistance, with reducing volumes achieved as the condition deteriorates. The best of three readings should be recorded, with the patient standing or sitting upright where possible to increase inspiratory capacity. The same device should be used for successive readings, as different peak flow meters give different readings (British Thoracic Society & SIGN, 2016). Peak flow assessments are commonly carried out in the community by practice and community nurses and general practitioners.

Pulse Oximetry

The pulse oximeter in clinical practice is now a well-established, non-invasive tool to estimate peripheral oxygen

TABLE 20.2 Clinical Respiratory Assessment: Primary Data (Lumb & Thomas, 2021)

Assessment	Data Obtained	Assessment Issues
Inspection	Respiratory rate, pattern and depth	Inspection may increase respiratory rate
	Signs of dyspnoea (e.g., sitting forward, use of accessory muscles)	Older adults have increased respiratory rate (16–25 beats/minute)
	Conscious level/mental acuity	Trend of respiratory rate most sensitive indicator of deterioration
	Signs of pain	Rate should be accurately counted and documented
	Colour	Change in mental status is the most sensitive indicator of hypoxia and hypercapnia in older adults
	Chest movement/structure/spinal deformities	
	Patient position	
	Ability to speak/move	Older people have a larger anterior posterior chest diameter, especially in the presence of COPD
	Finger-clubbing/nicotine staining/ evidence of tremor	
	Jugular venous pressure	Barrel chest can indicate chronic airflow limitation
	Presence of cough	Abnormal spinal curvatures may impede adequate ventilation
	Colour, consistency and culture of sputum	Decreased chest expansion may be caused by pain, poor position and reduced mobility
		Older adults have decreased effectiveness of cough mechanism and reduced ciliary action
		Alterations in sputum colour and consistency may indicate tuberculosis, malignancy or infection
Palpation	Pulse	Environmental factors may alter findings (e.g., fan therapy, blankets)
	Blood pressure	
	Skin temperature/skin turgor	Systemic oedema may indicate cardiac or hepatic dysfunction, causing secondary respiratory difficulties
	Tracheal position	
	Chest wall tenderness/movement	May reveal presence of masses
	Abnormal lesions	Older person expected to have reduced skin turgor
	Presence of systemic oedema	Vibrations over chest wall during expiration may indicate retained secretions
	Presence of lymph nodes	
	Tactile fremitus	
Percussion	Areas of density/consolidation	Percussion not often performed by nurses
	Presence of air	COPD patients may have hyper-resonant chest, whereas adults with pneumonia, consolidation or fluid-filled areas have areas of dullness
Auscultation	Normal bilateral air entry to all zones	Should be performed from the back over each lobe of lung
	Added breath sounds (e.g., crackles, wheeze, stridor)	Commence auscultation at bases as most pathologic conditions occur here in older adults
		Do not to continue for too long as patient may become dizzy and exhausted
		Older person may have decreased basal breath sounds due to spinal changes, poor position, reduced mobility and decreased ability to take deep breaths
		Crackles can indicate fluid or secretions
		Older adults can have increased retention of mucus due to age-related decreased pulmonary function
		Wheeze can indicate airflow restriction

delivery. The COVID-19 pandemic meant community pulse oximetry, where patients are provided with a portable machine to use at home, was expedited in an effort to keep people out of hospital. Normal readings are cited by most authors to be >95% (Hogsten & Switzer, 2001). Patients with chronic respiratory conditions such as COPD may have a lower normal baseline due to changes in chemoreceptor activity. Cyanosis is not normally visible unless oxygen saturation drops below 75%. The main function of the pulse oximeter is to facilitate the early detection of hypoxaemia before it can be seen clinically. The pulse oximeter estimates oxygen delivery by measuring the saturation of peripheral Hb with oxygen and expressing it as a percentage (SpO_2). It is important to ensure the person has an adequate Hb before accepting the result as valid. Apply the probe to a warm, well-perfused digit or the nose or earlobe. The area should not be under direct sunlight, as it can affect readings. Heavy nail varnish obscures the light penetrating through the nail bed (Hinkelbein et al., 2007). It is sensible to avoid using the patient's dominant hand, which they are more likely to move; motion has been shown to affect readings. Roffe et al. (2021) provided reassurance in their study that oximeters can be applied to either side in a patient with hemiparetic stroke. However, a hand with a tremor affects readings, and so patients with problems such as Parkinson's disease or muscle tremor may be better with the probe placed on the earlobe, which is less likely to be affected by motion artefact or vasoconstrictive effects.

The pulse oximeter is a useful adjunct to clinical respiratory assessment when used properly. Kaye et al. (2002), for example, performed a case-control study in a group of nursing-home residents that found a decrease in oxygen saturation of >3% from the baseline or a saturation of <94% suggested the presence of pneumonia in this population. The SpO_2 should always be interpreted in light of the clinical picture and degree of oxygen therapy being received. The British Thoracic Society recommends ABG analysis be performed for patients with a resting SpO_2 <92% to determine the presence of hypoxemia and the need for oxygen therapy (British Thoracic Society, 2015).

The most important thing to remember about pulse oximeters is they do not measure the adequacy of ventilation or lung performance, only peripheral oxygenation. It is not possible to assess carbon dioxide elimination with a pulse oximeter. An increase in carbon dioxide may be present in a patient with a chest infection, for example, when the metabolic rate and thus production of carbon dioxide are increased, but the patient is unable to increase the rate and depth of breathing to exhale the increased production. In this case capnography or an ABG would be necessary to fully evaluate the patient's condition.

Arterial Blood Gases

ABG analysis is the gold standard for evaluating gas exchange, and its use is indicated in any patient with severely deteriorating respiratory or haemodynamic function. It is also used to obtain a baseline for patients prior to surgery where a chronic condition might indicate potentially varied values from normal. ABG analysis provides information regarding the partial pressure of oxygen (PaO_2) and carbon dioxide ($PaCO_2$) and the presence of acid–base disturbances by evaluating the blood pH (normal range 7.36–7.44). A normal PaO_2 is >12 kPa, and $PaCO_2$ 4.7–6.0 kPa on room air (Lumb & Thomas, 2021). Patients with chronic conditions such as COPD may need to have ABG analysis performed frequently to evaluate their condition, and thus the use of capillary sampling from the earlobe is an acceptable and common practice (Lumb & Thomas, 2021). As with any investigations, it is important to evaluate results in light of therapy, such as oxygen, being received by the patient and the patient's normal baseline.

Radiography

Many older patients need to have a chest X-ray taken at some point, perhaps as part of a preoperative respiratory assessment or to evaluate the progress of an ongoing or acute condition. A chest X-ray provides information regarding both local and diffuse problems—for example, local consolidation due to a tumour or infection or diffuse shadowing due to the presence of fluid in the lungs (i.e., pulmonary oedema). A chest X-ray can also provide information regarding rib fractures, position of the diaphragm, size of the thoracic cage and the amount of functioning lung present (Lumb & Thomas, 2021). In most cases patients have chest X-rays in the radiography department of a hospital, but in some circumstances mobile equipment can be used. All chest X-rays should be reviewed and reported on by a radiologist with specialist training in the technique. Some patients also have other radiographic investigations (e.g., ventilation–perfusion scans, ultrasounds) for certain conditions that require specific preparation and aftercare. It is always important to fully explain to the patient what to expect and to be aware of any particular side effects, such as allergic reactions to dyes, that need to be looked for following the procedure.

INTERVENTIONS FOR OLDER ADULTS WITH BREATHING DIFFICULTIES

Acute Airway Management

In some cases breathing difficulties are due to a partial or complete obstruction of the airway. This could be caused by unconsciousness due to a cerebrovascular accident, post-anaesthetic or airway obstruction from foreign objects, or the presence of a tumour. In such circumstances airway manoeuvres or adjuncts may be required.

The most basic method of opening the airway is to ensure proper positioning of the head and neck. Often, a simple chin lift is adequate to remove signs of obstruction such as snoring and ease dyspnoea. Patients should be placed in a lateral position to prevent the tongue from falling back and protect the airway from aspiration in the case of vomiting.

Positioning needs to be combined with the use of an oropharyngeal airway in patients where no gag reflex is present to maintain an open airway and provide a route for oropharyngeal suction. This device, sometimes referred to as a Guedel airway, prevents the tongue from falling back and obstructing the airway but does not protect from gastric aspiration; again the patient should be positioned laterally. Oropharyngeal airways come in sizes 2, 3, and 4 and before insertion should be sized to correspond to the vertical distance between the patient's incisors and the angle of the jaw. Care should be undertaken to avoid damage to the hard palate, and the airway should be inserted in an upside-down position before rotating it 180° when the soft palate is reached. It should then be further inserted until it lies in the oropharynx. This reduces the risk of the tongue being pushed back, causing further obstruction. The flat portion of the airway should fit snugly against the patient's teeth (or gums if edentulous), and following insertion, patency of the airway should be rechecked (Resuscitation Council UK, 2021).

Nasopharyngeal airways can be used to facilitate the removal of secretions from a patient with an inadequate cough; they are better tolerated by a semiconscious or awake patient. They are also useful as an airway adjunct for patients with trismus (i.e., lock jaw) or maxillofacial injuries, although they are contraindicated in any patient with a suspected basal skull fracture (Resuscitation Council UK, 2021) and should be used with caution in a patient with a history of bleeding or epistaxis (i.e., nose bleeds). Adult sizes are 6–7 mm in diameter and are often measured by the diameter of the patient's little finger. Before insertion the tube should be lubricated, and the right nostril should be checked for patency; this is the nostril recommended by the Resuscitation Council UK (2021). Some brands have a safety pin that needs to be placed at the flange end before insertion to prevent the airway disappearing beyond the nasal flares. The airway should be directed toward the patient's feet, with the beveled end inserted first using a slight twisting action. If it is not possible to pass the airway through the right nostril, the left nostril can be used. As with the oropharyngeal airway, patency should be checked following insertion. In addition, consideration needs to be given to the discomfort that might be experienced by an awake patient.

A tracheostomy is an opening in the wall of the trachea below the cricoid cartilage. With the increase in critical care facilities and the growing population of older people, many older patients have permanent or temporary tracheostomy tubes in place in the hospital or community environment. Most tracheostomies are temporary following respiratory failure and weaning from mechanical ventilation or following trauma when there has been a potential risk to the airway. Nursing a patient with a tracheostomy requires vigilance and a good level of knowledge and skill to prevent complications such as obstruction, which could lead to a respiratory arrest. The key aspects of management are the maintenance of adequate tube patency with the use of humidification, suctioning and cleaning of the inner tube on a regular basis. Vigilance for signs of respiratory distress is required, and they should be reported immediately. Any patient with a tracheostomy should have emergency equipment available nearby, including spare tracheostomy tubes, tracheal dilators, and equipment for manual ventilation (i.e., ambu-bag) and suctioning. It should also be remembered patients may be highly anxious about the presence of a tracheostomy tube, which can hinder their ability to speak, so psychological support and reassurance are vital parts of care.

In an emergency situation (e.g., cardiac arrest), the use of an endotracheal tube provides a secure airway for ventilation. Patients can usually be transferred to a critical care unit. Insertion of endotracheal tubes is the responsibility of a competent, trained clinician. Familiarity with the equipment required is important to facilitate a smooth intubation process. Nurses should check the equipment on the emergency trolley with this in mind. Following extubation, close monitoring of respiratory status is required.

Removal of Secretions

In older adults the cough reflex may not be very effective, making the removal of secretions difficult. Older people with COPD may have copious secretions that are difficult to expectorate. Nurses should work with the physiotherapist, assisting the older person with coughing and deep breathing. They should be shown how to inspire deeply, pause, then cough forcibly to expel secretions. This manoeuvre may be too exhausting, in which case the older person is encouraged to take deep breaths on inspiration and long exhalations. This could move secretions sufficiently to stimulate a cough reflex. They can also be taught how to breathe through pursed lips, which increases pressure in the lungs during expiration and prolongs the period for gas exchange and intrinsic positive end-expiratory pressure and arterial oxygen tension (PaO_2).

Expectoration is sometimes perceived as an antisocial activity. The older person can be given sputum pots and tissues and supported to recognise the importance of clearing secretions. An upright posture, either in bed or a chair, can be achieved by careful positioning of pillows to allow support and full chest expansion, thus permitting maximum ventilation. Positioning is especially important when osteoporosis has resulted in kyphosis. The older person may find it easier to manage lung expansion by leaning over a cushioned table (i.e., the orthopnoeic position). Careful attention should be paid to the patient's hydration status, as dehydration makes secretions more sticky, tenacious and difficult to expectorate. Caution should also be taken to prevent cross-infection through expectoration in view of the increasing incidence of respiratory pathogens.

If secretions cannot be expectorated, it may be necessary to use oropharyngeal or nasopharyngeal suction. Nasopharyngeal suction is an invasive and potentially traumatic procedure that should be used only following a thorough assessment by a competent practitioner and where less invasive techniques are not possible. Associated adverse events include hypoxaemia, cardiac dysrhythmias, trauma and cardiac arrest (Moore, 2003). There is a dearth of research evidence related to suctioning, and practitioners are advised to consult policies and protocols within their organisation. Further research is required in this area to inform guidelines in the future.

Individuals with COPD may suffer recurrent exacerbations with an increase in volume and purulence of sputum. Mucolytics are oral medicines believed to increase expectoration of sputum by reducing its viscosity, thus making it easier to cough up. Improved expectoration of sputum may lead to a reduction in exacerbations of COPD. There is evidence that treatment with mucolytics leads to a small reduction in the likelihood of having an acute exacerbation and hospitalisation, and it is not associated with an increase in adverse events (Poole et al., 2019).

Administration of Nebulizers

Prevention and relief of symptoms are central to managing the patient with breathlessness, and bronchodilators are the key agents. The major benefit of bronchodilator therapy is to alleviate bronchial obstruction and airflow limitation, reduce hyperinflation and improve emptying of the lung and exercise performance (Cazzola & Page, 2014). Bronchodilators can be administered using a metred-dose inhaler (MDI) or nebulization.

For older adults, nebulizers may be used both in hospital and at home. A nebulizer converts a drug in solution to a fine mist for inhalation and can be driven by either air or oxygen via a mask or mouthpiece. The choice of beta-agonists, anticholinergic drugs, theophylline or combination therapy depends on individual response. However, improvements are often found by combining agents (GOLD, 2021). There is good-quality evidence that longer-acting inhaled beta-agonists such as salmeterol and formoterol are of particular benefit to older adults as they have a duration of action of up to 12 hours and can significantly improve symptoms, exercise capacity and health status (Cazzola & Page, 2014). Corticosteroid therapy may be given through nebulizers as an anti-inflammatory agent, although their effects on asthma and COPD remain controversial. The bronchodilator should always be given first and time allowed for it to take effect (e.g., 5–10 minutes) so when the corticosteroid is inhaled, it is delivered to the bronchioles, where its anti-inflammatory effects are required. After using the nebulizer, wash the patient's face to prevent skin irritation. It is also advisable to rinse the patient's mouth after steroid inhalation to avoid the risk of oral candidiasis.

If patients are going to be discharged home with a nebulizer, it is essential they are given specific information regarding the number of inhalations per day, instructions on how to prepare the nebulizer and how to clean and care for the equipment. Written instructions should also be provided, and help should be available through community nurses and general practitioners, who are ideally placed to provide appropriate advice and assistance.

The use of MDI therapies is commonly prescribed, and patients are usually discharged home with an MDI. Their use requires the person to have good coordination. Chronic respiratory weakness or arthritis may make MDIs impossible to use. Time should be taken to teach a patient how to use the inhaler. For some, a device attached to the MDI that allows the medication to be held in the chamber long enough for inhalation over a number of breaths (i.e., spacer device) is more appropriate. This eliminates the need to coordinate triggering the MDI with inspiration (National Institute for Health and Care Excellence, 2017).

RESPIRATORY THERAPIES

Oxygen Therapy

Oxygen is one of the most common drugs given to patients in both hospital and community settings. Indications for its use are to treat or prevent hypoxaemia. Although oxygen administration may be lifesaving, it is not without risks, which should be considered at all times (British Thoracic Society, 2015).

Guidance is available on the administration of oxygen for adults in the community, with separate guidance for its use in hospital (British Thoracic Society, 2015) or emergency situations (O'Driscoll et al., 2017). Particular attention should be paid to the risks associated with smoking and the amount of oxygen therapy to be prescribed. See Case Study 20.2 for details of a patient with COPD. Patients who have COPD with carbon dioxide retention should not normally be administered

---

CASE STUDY 20.2

Mr Patrick O'Reilly, a retired 87-year-old builder, is admitted from a residential home with an acute onset of respiratory distress. He was diagnosed with COPD 15 years ago and continues to smoke 30 cigarettes a day. He is normally unable to walk more than 20 minutes without becoming breathless and has required hospital admission three times over the past year. He is prescribed 24% oxygen, 4-hourly salbutamol and atrovent nebulizers, and steroid therapy. A sputum pot is provided, and a specimen is collected for microbiological assay. He is also referred for chest physiotherapy. Following nursing assessment, the following priorities are identified:

- Psychological support and reassurance to alleviate fears regarding his condition and inability to breathe, and an awareness of the effects of a change in environment.
- Positioning to enhance chest expansion and the ability to cough and clear secretions.
- Assistance with activities of daily living (e.g., hygiene, mobilisation, nutrition, sleep), taking account of his level of dyspnoea and oxygen therapy.
- Ensuring nebulizers and oxygen therapy are delivered according to the prescription, assembled correctly and

appropriately humidified. Mr O'Reilly must be informed of the dangers of smoking while receiving oxygen, and steps should be taken to ensure the therapy is tolerable (e.g., mouth and eye care).
- Ongoing assessment and monitoring of clinical observations, noting the importance of an increase in respiratory rate over time and ensuring data are interpreted according to Mr O'Reilly's normal parameters.

Two weeks later, Mr O'Reilly's condition has improved sufficiently for him to be discharged back to the residential home. Before this, the following issues are considered:

- Rehabilitation programme to increase respiratory muscle strength and level of mobility
- Assessment of most appropriate inhaler device for Mr O'Reilly and teaching him how to use it correctly
- Follow-up appointment at chest clinic and associated transport arrangements
- Future medical management of Mr O'Reilly's condition
- Discussion of potential lifestyle changes to reduce recurrence of acute illness (e.g., nutritional advice to enhance immune function and smoking reduction)

---

high percentages of oxygen (i.e., >24–28%) as it can affect their respiratory drive. Oxygen at higher concentrations given over prolonged periods can be toxic to the cells of the respiratory tract and alveoli, possibly causing irreversible damage. Thus, the smallest amount of oxygen necessary to maintain an adequate PaO_2 should be given for the shortest period of time possible. This means a patient on oxygen therapy needs to be regularly evaluated using clinical assessment, SpO_2, ABG analysis and other available tools.

Oxygen may be administered using a variety of devices of both fixed and variable rates. Nasal cannulae are suitable for low-flow oxygen rates (i.e., up to approximately 6 l/min) or for short-term use to enable a dyspnoeic patient to remove their face mask while eating or talking. A nasal cannulae is useful for a confused patient who is unable to tolerate a face mask. However, caution should be applied if the patient breathes through their mouth; in this case the nasal cannulae is of limited benefit. Simple face masks are more useful in acute settings. Both a nasal cannulae and simple face masks are low-flow devices or variable-performance devices; the amount of oxygen delivered to the patient is variable because it is affected by the patient's breathing depth and rate. Documentation should state the flow in litres per minute, but the percentage of oxygen cannot be accurately calculated. Fixed performance systems such as the Venturi system or high-humidity devices are not dependent on the minute volume of the patient, which

means the percentage of oxygen delivered to the patient can be determined accurately as long as the correct flow of oxygen is set at the oxygen flowmeter. Some devices allow up to 100% oxygen to be delivered by a system of rebreathing expired gas that is housed in a reservoir bag beneath the mask. These systems are commonly referred to as 100% masks or reservoir masks and are useful in acute settings.

A patient who receives oxygen therapy for long periods of time may find masks claustrophobic. Alternatively, feeling unable to breathe makes some patients highly anxious and dependent on the mask, then unwilling to remove it for any reason. Pay close attention to good psychological care, ensuring effective communication between the nurse and patient and the development of a trusting and supportive relationship. Negotiation may be necessary to achieve an optimal outcome.

Oxygen is a dry gas that is likely to dry the mucous membranes of the oro- and nasopharynx. Provide adequate humidification and frequent oral hygiene or drinks. Eyes are also at risk of drying, particularly if masks are not fitted correctly, so attention should be given to ophthalmic care. Oxygen equipment should be changed regularly, labelled with the patient's details, and kept clean and dry to prevent infection and discomfort. This may be a particular problem with humidification systems fitted into the circuit, which can cause accumulation of water in the tubing, making it more difficult for the patient to breathe.

Long-Term Oxygen Therapy

Long-term oxygen therapy (LTOT) improves pulmonary function in patients with COPD and lengthens survival in patients with COPD and other chronic respiratory conditions.

It is advisable for all patients to be assessed by a respiratory physician prior to LTOT. Guidelines from the British Thoracic Society (2015) suggest patients with COPD who have a PaO_2 of <7.3kPa, with or without hypercapnia, and an FEV_1 of <1.5l should receive LTOT, and it should be administered for at least 15 hours per day to achieve maximum benefit. When home oxygen is arranged, the type of facility (e.g., concentrator and/or portable oxygen) and the recommended flow rate should be recorded. Three systems are currently available: gas cylinders, liquid oxygen systems and oxygen concentrators (Kacmarek, 2000). A concentrator with nasal prongs is recommended as the best method of delivery, with the flow rate set at 2–4 litres per minute (British Thoracic Society, 2015). With these systems air is drawn into the unit through a filter and compressed. Room air is then separated into oxygen and nitrogen plus trace gases. The concentrated oxygen is stored in a small cylinder for delivery to a flow meter. Oxygen concentrators deliver oxygen concentrations of up to 95% depending on the flow rate (Kacmarek, 2000).

LTOT can be very restricting for patients, which in turn can affect their physiological and psychological states. Portable systems may be considered for some patients. Development of technology that allows systems that are lightweight, compact and capable of providing oxygen for extended periods is ongoing (Kacmarek, 2000). Some patients use extension tubing to increase mobility. Nursing considerations for LTOT are similar to those for in-hospital oxygen administration. Humidification is generally unnecessary with a nasal cannulae if the flow rate is <5l/min. If humidifiers are used, they should be washed in soapy water and dried twice weekly. A cannulae may cause soreness around the nasal cavity. Patients should be advised to use water-based lubricants. Education regarding fire hazards when using oxygen at home is important, and smoking must cease before LTOT is offered. Patients must understand why they are having the therapy, how the equipment functions, how to care for it and what to do if there are problems. Follow-up and reassessment for all patients on LTOT at regular periods are vital, as studies have highlighted a number of problems associated with its use (British Thoracic Society, 2017). Assessment should involve regular ABG analysis. However, if a patient is receiving nocturnal therapy, daytime ABGs have been shown not to correlate with nighttime gas exchange (Tarrega et al., 2002). ABG analysis should be performed at 07:00 a.m. in order to determine appropriate settings for nighttime therapy (Tarrega et al., 2002).

Non-Invasive Ventilation

Non-invasive ventilation (NIV) is an important treatment option for patients with severe breathing difficulties (British Thoracic Society, 2017). For an older person with COPD not previously considered suitable for invasive ventilation, NIV has been shown to significantly improve survival. NIV is a global term that encompasses a number of respiratory therapies, including continuous positive airway pressure (CPAP) and non-invasive positive pressure ventilation (NIPPV).

Continuous Positive Airway Pressure

For some patients, oxygenation is not improved through oxygen therapy alone, and the use of CPAP is of great benefit. CPAP increases the volume of gas in the lungs at the end of quiet respiration (i.e., the FRC). CPAP increases compliance and helps correct ventilation–perfusion mismatch (Lumb & Thomas, 2021). The indications for CPAP are outlined in Table 20.3.

The application of CPAP involves a tightly fitting mask, which some patients find claustrophobic and uncomfortable (Fig. 20.1). In addition, the constant high-flow gas can be difficult to tolerate; CPAP is suitable only for patients who are alert and able to maintain their own airway and clear their own secretions. Setting up CPAP requires skill and expertise. It can be delivered by continuous or demand flow systems:

- Continuous flow systems use a continuous flow of gas throughout the respiratory cycle and are very noisy, which can interfere with the sleep and rest of all people in close proximity.
- Demand flow systems are triggered only at the start of inspiration. Although demand-flow systems are quieter and more economical, they create additional respiratory effort and are unsuitable for many patients.

The type of valve attached determines the amount of CPAP delivered. Many patients are started on a fairly low level of CPAP, such as 2.5 or 5.0 cm H_2O. A low level is

TABLE 20.3 Continuous Positive Airway Pressure (CPAP)

Indications for CPAP	Possible Applications
Hypoxic respiratory failure (type 1)	Acute left ventricular failure
Atelectasis/low lung volumes	*Pneumocystis carinii* pneumonia
Increased work of breathing	Acute lung injury
	Pulmonary oedema
	Asthma
	Obstructive sleep apnoea

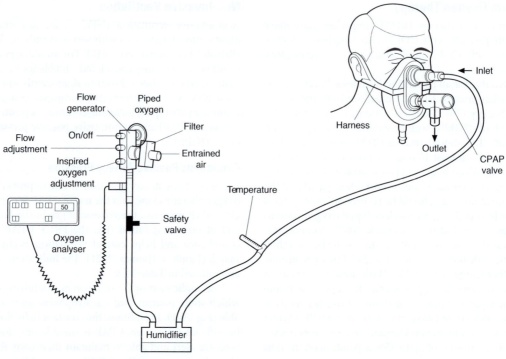

Fig. 20.1 Patient with continuous positive airway pressure (CPAP) circuit.

easier to tolerate but may not increase the FRC sufficiently to improve oxygenation. Higher levels of CPAP can be used, such as 7.5 or 10.0 cm H_2O, although they can cause problems and increase the risk of barotrauma (i.e., pressure damage). Attention needs to be paid to the risks of circuit blockage, recognised by an increase in airway pressure and obvious patient distress. Circuit blockage should be rectified immediately to prevent the occurrence of barotrauma.

Non-Invasive Positive-Pressure Ventilation

NIPPV can be used as an alternative to intubation and mechanical ventilation in patients with type 2 (i.e., ventilatory) respiratory failure (Lumb & Thomas, 2021). NIPPV augments alveolar ventilation by positive-pressure ventilation without the need for an endotracheal tube. Biphasic positive-pressure ventilation (BiPAP) is one type of NIPPV so widely used it is the main mode of NIV in acute-care settings. BiPAP is similar to two alternating pressures of CPAP: a higher one is set during inspiration (i.e., inspiratory positive airway pressure, IPAP) and a lower pressure during expiration (i.e., expired positive airway pressure, EPAP). Levels of IPAP and EPAP should be set according to prescribed parameters based on the patient's condition and assessment data. The indications for NIPPV/BiPAP

as identified by the British Thoracic Society and Intensive Care Society (2017) are outlined in Box 20.1.

The British Thoracic Society (2017) also recommends NIPPV be used as a holding measure, with a view to intubation if unsuccessful, and as a maximum level of treatment for patients who are not candidates for intubation and invasive ventilation. The latter may apply for older adults, as it is not always appropriate to admit a patient to an intensive care unit.

Setting up NIPPV requires skill and expertise, and there are potential problems. Physiotherapists or respiratory nurse specialists are the experts in this field and commonly initiate treatment in hospital and community settings. Nasal or full face masks can be used. A nasal

---

BOX 20.1   Indications for Non-Invasive Positive-Pressure Ventilation and Biphasic Positive-Pressure Ventilation

Patients with chronic obstructive pulmonary disease
Hypercapnoea: $PaCO_2$ >6.5 kPa
Hypoxaemia: PaO_2 <8 kPa
Respiratory acidosis: pH <7.30

mask may be more comfortable and easier to tolerate and facilitates communication. However, nasal masks cannot be used if the patient is mouth-breathing. Another advantage of NIPPV is the ventilator delivers additional predetermined breaths should the patient become hypoxic or apnoeic. Because of the system backup and comfortable mask, this method of treatment is well tolerated for relatively long periods of time. Patients can be discharged home with NIPPV as long as there is appropriate support in the community.

Both CPAP and NIPPV can be extremely frightening for the patient, and many patients are confused as a result of the associated hypoxia. It can take up to 20 or 30 minutes for the physiological effects of CPAP and NIPPV to take place at an alveolar level. It is important that treatment, once started, is not stopped abruptly, and care is grouped together to accommodate these factors. An ABG should be taken 1 hour after starting treatment to assess and monitor the effects on oxygenation and acid–base balance.

In view of the complex issues associated with caring for an older person receiving NIV, it is essential nurses have a good understanding of the key issues and nursing interventions required. Frequently, it is appropriate for the patient to be nursed in a high-dependency unit for close assessment and monitoring.

Monitoring and Evaluating the Effectiveness of Respiratory Therapies

The success of CPAP can be assessed by observing improvements in oxygenation (i.e., through ABG analysis or pulse oximetry), a reduction in respiratory rate, an increase in tidal volume and reduced work of breathing. The same applies to patients receiving oxygen therapy and NIV. The need for high levels of vigilance when caring for patients cannot be overemphasised, as deterioration can be rapid, particularly in an older person who has less compensatory capacity. Patients receiving high levels of oxygen (i.e., greater than 50%) or NIV should not be left unattended. Observations of respiratory rate, depth and rhythm, level of consciousness and vital signs should be documented at frequent intervals, and any deterioration should be reported immediately.

ASSOCIATED CARE ISSUES

Chronic Breathlessness

The term breathlessness is generally used to describe the subjective experience of breathing discomfort. As a subjective experience, like pain and other nociception stimuli, breathlessness is influenced by psychological and emotional processes (American Thoracic Society, 2012). Breathlessness is the key presenting symptom of many cardiac and respiratory conditions common in older adults such as COPD, respiratory viruses such as influenza and COVID-19, heart disease or neuromuscular disease. Breathlessness is a distressing symptom for individuals and their carers. When it becomes a chronic condition, people may restrict their activities to avoid feeling it. Unfortunately, this leads to a downward spiral of deconditioning and worsening breathlessness (Johnson et al., 2014). Epidemiological studies underscore the high prevalence of breathlessness in older adults, with rates as high as one in four adults aged 70 and older experiencing breathlessness (Smith et al., 2016).

Breathlessness that persists despite optimal treatment of the underlying condition is sometimes referred to as refractory breathlessness, more recently described as chronic breathlessness syndrome (Johnson & Currow, 2015). Chronic breathlessness can be challenging to manage, but strong evidence has developed over the past decade for non-pharmacological interventions (Booth et al., 2011). Therapies are aimed at modulating the perception of breathlessness and the individual's response. They are typically delivered within a self-management framework in which people learn skills to reduce the impact on functioning and improve emotional well-being (Spathis et al., 2017).

The breathlessness service has emerged as a new model of care for chronic breathlessness in which expert multidisciplinary teams educate and train patients to self-manage using a range of non-pharmacological therapies, including breathing techniques, exercise and physical activity, planning and pacing, a handheld fan and relaxation strategies (Booth et al., 2011). However, it takes time and persistence to learn and practice non-pharmacological techniques; this requires thoughtful consideration for older adults.

Nutrition

Breathing difficulties can lead to insufficient intake of fluid or nutrition due to oxygen administration, open-mouth breathing, an increased insensible loss due to pyrexia and the inability to eat and drink due to the level of dyspnoea experienced. All these factors lead to secretions becoming more tenacious and difficult to expectorate, exacerbating difficulties that might already be present. Adequate systemic hydration is a priority, and nurses should be vigilant in monitoring input and output. However, with conditions such as pulmonary oedema, fluid restriction may be required. Some patients, for example those with a tracheostomy in place, may also be nil by mouth, so strict attention should be given to ensuring the mouth remains moist with mouthwashes and toothbrushing. Patients who have an irritating cough or unpleasant-tasting mouth may get relief from sipping warm drinks or sucking ice cubes, sweets or lozenges if appropriate. Referral or discussion with a speech and language therapist may be required before starting oral intake for patients with a recent history of swallowing or eating difficulties.

Nutritional requirements of older adults are different from those of younger people, with specific requirements for increased protein, some vitamins and calcium (Clegg & Williams, 2018). These requirements are further altered in the presence of breathing difficulties, thus requiring an appreciation of the patient's special needs. For example, medical conditions and drug therapies can affect the absorption of nutrients. Malnutrition can increase the risk of pulmonary infection due to a decrease in respiratory muscle function, compounded by the presence of foul-tasting sputum and hypoxia, which can lead to anorexia and a disinclination to eat or drink. Weight loss has been shown to be a particularly important predictor of poor prognosis in COPD, so attention should be given to its avoidance (Chapman-Novakofski, 2001). Supplementary nutrition via the enteral or parenteral route may be necessary as part of acute-care requirements; the importance of ensuring the mouth, teeth and dentures are in good condition cannot be overemphasised if malnutrition is to be avoided, thus helping prevent the occurrence of chest infections that cause breathing difficulties. Small meals are often better tolerated by patients with dyspnoea and help prevent abdominal distension, which could impede adequate lung expansion. Similarly, obesity increases the work of breathing and makes breathing difficulties worse. Therefore, health promotion plays an important part in the ongoing plan of care. See Chapter 21 for more information on eating and drinking.

Sleep, Rest and Activity

An older adult with breathing problems may find it increasingly difficult to maintain a balance between activity and rest. Lack of energy to perform even the simplest activity is often experienced. Rest is disturbed by dyspnoea, which is aggravated if the patient falls into an unsuitable position. Coughing disrupts sleep and rest. Regular position changes to aid ventilation prevent consolidation in the dependent areas of the lung. Pressure area care if needed also disturbs sleep.

There is little doubt being unable to breathe, or fighting for breath, is one of the most frightening experiences for people of all ages. For an older person with chronic breathing difficulties, the fear of falling asleep and not waking is very real. This anxiety can turn a restful night into a time of terror. Hypnotics should rarely be used, as they may cause respiratory depression. Alternative strategies need to be considered to aid patient comfort and provide reassurance. In the hospital setting, consideration should be given to the position of the patient in the ward. Some patients find reassurance by being placed close to the nurses' station. Others prefer a quieter place to allow them to sleep without disturbance. If sleep during the night is broken, patients can be encouraged to sleep and rest during the day. See Chapter 25 for more on sleep and rest in older adults.

In addition to ensuring sufficient sleep and rest, it is essential to consider the importance of activity. The patient's position is important, as a recumbent position reduces the capacity for gas exchange and exacerbates hypoxia, which could result in an acute confusional state and increase patient risks. It is important early mobilisation is achieved. Movement and exercise should be planned and increased each day.

There is a clear association between physical activity levels and hospital admission rates (Garcia-Aymerich et al., 2003). Progression to a more comprehensive rehabilitation programme is beneficial for older patients with COPD and cardiac disease (Dalal et al., 2010; GOLD, 2021).

SUMMARY AND LEARNING POINTS

This chapter highlights the normal pathophysiological changes associated with breathing in older adults and discusses the process of respiratory assessment and management. The importance of treating each person individually and holistically is emphasised. To meet the needs of this patient group, health care practitioners should ensure they develop the knowledge and skills necessary to work with patients to achieve their optimal goals.

KEY LEARNING POINTS

- Older adults are at increased risk of breathing problems as a result of disease such as COPD, COVID-19 or pneumonia, and the ageing process includes a declining immune system.

- Pneumonia is a serious and often fatal infection in older adults because they are less well nourished and active than younger people and have a higher incidence of comorbidities such as COPD.

- Older people are more susceptible to COVID-19, with a high mortality rate (as high as 10%) in adults aged 70 years and above.
- Immunisations and good infection prevention and control measures are important to reduce the risk of respiratory illnesses to an older person.
- Respiratory assessment of older adults may be complicated by multiple pathologies and therapeutic regimes as well as the person's limitations in providing a reliable history.
- Oxygen therapy is used to treat hypoxaemia and may be lifesaving, but is not without risks and requires careful assessment and management.
- Chronic breathlessness, or chronic breathlessness syndrome, is a common distressing symptom in older adults that limits activity and quality of life.
- There is good evidence non-pharmacological interventions reduce the perception of breathlessness and improve physical functioning and emotional well-being.

REFERENCES

American Thoracic Society. (2012). An official American Thoracic Society statement Update on the Mechanisms, Assessment, and Management of Dyspnea. *American Journal of Respiratory and Critical Care Medicine, 185*(4), 435–452.

American Lung Association. (2020). What is the connection between influenza and pneumonia? https://www.lung.org/lung-health-diseases/lung-disease-lookup/pneumonia/what-is-the-connection

Booth, S., Moffat, C., Burkin, J., Galbraith, S., & Bausewein, C. (2011). Nonpharmacological interventions for breathlessness. *Current Opinion Support Palliative Care, 5*, 77–86.

British Thoracic Society. (2015). BTS Guidelines for home oxygen use in adults. *Thorax, 70*(1).

British Thoracic Society & SIGN. (2016). British guideline for the management of asthma. https://www./BTS_SIGN%20Asthma%20Guideline%202016.pdf

British Thoracic Society & Intensive Care Society. (2017). Guideline for the ventilatory management of acute hypercapnic respiratory failure in adults. *Thoracic, 12*, 72–76.

Cazzola, M., & Page, C. (2014). Long-acting bronchodilators in COPD: Where are we now and where are we going? *Breathe, 10*(2), 110–120.

Chapman-Novakofski, K. (2001). Nutrition management in long-term care and home health: Nutrition management of chronic obstructive pulmonary disease in older adults. *Journal of Nutrition for the Elderly, 20*, 45–46.

Clegg, M. E., & Williams, E. A. (2018). Optimising nutrition in older people. *Maturitas, 112*, 34–38.

Dalal, H. M., Zawada, A., Jolly, K., Moxham, T., & Taylor, R. S. (2010). Home based versus centre based cardia rehabilitation. Cochrane stematic review and meta-analysis. *British Medical Journal, 340*, B5631.

Dunn, C. E., Woodhouse, J., Bhopal, R. S., & Acquilla, S. D. (1995). Asthma and factory emissions in northern England: Addressing public concern by combining geographical and epidemiological methods. *Journal of Epidemiology and Community Health, 49*, 395–400.

Garcia-Aymerich, J., Farrero, E., & Felez, M. A. (2003). Risk factors of readmission to hospital for a COPD exacerbation: a prospective study. *Thorax, 58*, 100–105.

Global Initiative for Chronic Obstructive Lung Disease (GOLD). (2021). Global strategy for the diagnosis, management, and prevention of chronic obstructive pulmonary disease.https://goldcopd.org

Hinkelbein, J., Koehler, H., Genzwuerker, H. V., & Fiedler, F. (2007). Artificial acrylic finger nails may alter pulse oximetry measurement. *Resuscitation, 74*, 75–82.

Hodgson, C. L., Higgins, A. M., Bailey, M. J., Mather, A. M., Beach, L., Bellomo, R., et al., (2021). The impact of COVID-19 critical illness on new disability, functional outcomes and return to work at 6 months: A prospective cohort study. *Critical Care, 25*, 382.

Hogsten, P., & Switzer, M. (2001). Hemodynamic monitoring. In P. S Kidd, & K. D. Wagner (Eds.), *High acuity nursing* (3rd ed.). Prentice Hall p. 315.

Johnson, M. J., & Currow, D.C. (2015). Chronic refractory breathlessness is a distinct clinical syndrome. *Current Opinion in Supportive and Palliative Care, 9*, 203–205. doi:10.1097/SPC.0000000000000150

Johnson, M. J., Currow, D. C., & Both, S. (2014). Prevalence and assessment of breathlessness in the clinical setting. *Expert Review Respiratory Medicine, 8*, 151–161.

Kacmarek, R. (2000). Delivery systems for long-term oxygen therapy. *Respiratory Care, 45*, 84–92.

Kaye, K. S., Stalam, M., Shershen, W., & Kaye, D. (2002). Utility of pulse oximetry in diagnosing pneumonia in nursing home residents. *American Journal of Medical Science, 324*(5), 237–242.

Koeckerling, D., Barker, J., Mudalige, N. L., Oyefeso, O., Pan, D., Pareek, M., et al., (2020). Awake prone positioning in COVID-19. *Thorax, 75*(10).

Lumb, A. B., & Thomas, C. R. (2021). *Nunn and Lumb's applied respiratory physiology* (9th ed.). Elsevier.

Moore, T. (2003). Suctioning techniques for the removal of respiratory secretions. *Nursing Standard, 18*(9), 47–53.

National Institute for Health and Care Excellence. (2017). *Asthma: diagnosis, monitoring, and chronic asthma management.* https://www.nice.org.uk/guidance/ng80

National Institute for Health and Care Excellence. (2021). *Smoking cessation.* https://cks.nice.org.uk/topics/smoking-cessation.

O'Driscoll, B. R., Howard, L. S., & Earis, J. (2017). BTS guideline for oxygen use in adults in healthcare and emergency settings. *Thorax, 72* ii1–ii90.

Poole, P., Sathananthan, K., & Fortescue, R. (2019). Mucolytic agents versus placebo for chronic bronchitis or chronic obstructive pulmonary disease. *Cochrane Database of Systematic Reviews, 5,* Article CD001287. doi:10.1002/14651858. CD001287.pub6.

RECOVERY Collaborative Group. (2021). Dexamethosone in hospitalized patients with COVID-19. *New England Journal of Medicine, 384*(8), 693–704.

Resuscitation Council UK. (2021). *Advanced life support course: Provided manual.* https://www.resus.org.uk.

Roffe, C., Sills, S., Wilde, K., & Crome, P. (2001). Effect of hemiparetic stroke on pulse oximetry readings on the affected side. *Stroke, 32*(8):1808–1810.

Singhal, S., Kumar, P., Singh, S., Saha, S., & Dey, A. B. (2021). Clinical features and outcomes of COVID-19 in older adults: A systematic review and meta-analysis. *BMC Geriatrics, 21,* 321.

Smith, A. K., Currow, D. C., Abernethy, A. P., Johnson, M. J., Miao, Y., Boscardin, W. J., et al., (2016). Prevalence and outcomes of breathlessness in older adults: A national population study. *JAGS, 64,* 2035–2041.

Spathis, A., Booth, S., Moffat, C., Hurst, R., Ryan, R., Chin, C., et al., (2017). The Breathing, Thinking, Functioning clinical model: A proposal to facilitate evidence-based breathlessness management in chronic respiratory disease. *NPJ Primary Care Respiratory Medicine, 27*(1), 27. doi:10.1038/s41533-017-0024-z.

Tárrega, J., Güell, R., Antón, A., Mayos, M., Farré, A., Jerez, F. R., et al., (2002). Are daytime arterial blood gases a good reflection of nighttime gas exchange in patients on long term oxygen therapy? *Respiratory Care, 47*(8), 882–886.

Vasileiou, E., Simpson, C. R., Shi, T., Kerr, S., Agrawal, U., Akbari, A., et al., (2021). Interim findings from first-dose mass COVID-19 vaccination roll-out and COVID-19 hospital admissions in Scotland: A national prospective cohort study. *Lancet, 397*(10285), 1646–1657.

Voshaar, T., Stais, P., Köhler, D., & Dellweg, D. (2021). Conservative management of COVID-19 associated hypoxemia. *ERJ Open Research, 7.* doi:10.1183/23120541.00026-2021.

Waugh, A., & Grant, A. (2022). *Ross & Wilson: Anatomy and physiology in health and illness* (13th ed.). Elsevier.

Eating and Drinking

Sue M. Green

Eating and drinking are fundamental activities that enable us to meet biological, social, psychological and cultural needs. Diet and fluid intake exert a positive or negative effect on health and recovery from illness. An understanding of physical and psychological changes experienced through older adulthood that affect food and fluid intake enables comprehensive nursing assessment and care planning. Supporting older adults to change or modify dietary habits promotes health and prevents disease and is an important component of health promotion activity undertaken by nurses. Nurses also play an important role in delivering nutritional interventions that promote recovery or comfort. For nurses to provide good nutritional care, screening and assessment of nutritional status, care planning with the multidisciplinary team and safe, effective delivery of nutritional interventions are crucial. The first section in this chapter presents an overview of factors that influence food and fluid intake in older adults. The second section discusses malnutrition, dehydration, promotion of a healthy diet and provides an overview of nutritional interventions for older adults.

FACTORS THAT INFLUENCE FOOD AND FLUID INTAKE IN OLDER ADULTS

During the normal process of ageing, food and fluid consumption may be affected by physiological changes, including changes in metabolic rate, appetite, the gastrointestinal system, functional ability and dietary intake. Changes associated with ageing occur at different rates and intensity in older adults. A person in their tenth decade may have a very good appetite, while a person in their seventh decade with a long-term condition may experience significant gustatory changes that affect appetite.

Metabolic Rate and Appetite

Slowing of metabolic rate is caused by reduced activity and muscle mass and results in lower energy and nutrient requirements. Although activity reduction is not inevitable in older people, it is often a consequence of changed lifestyle with retirement from working life, medical conditions and reduced energy levels. Muscle mass and function diminish as part of the ageing process and may progress to sarcopenia—accelerated, progressive and generalised loss of skeletal muscle and function (Cruz-Jentoft & Sayer, 2019). The rate of muscle mass loss is influenced by lifestyle factors such as habitual diet and activity levels.

Appetite initiates and sustains oral nutritional intake in terms of both the amount and range of food eaten. Nurses who work with older people are familiar with older adults describing a loss of appetite. Physiological regulation of appetite is complex, and its loss is not solely attributable to disease or treatment. Loss of appetite in older adults, or anorexia of ageing, is well described and occurs when homeostatic regulation of energy intake is altered, leading to a reduction in food intake. Anorexia of ageing plays a role in the development of sarcopenia and cachexia (Morley, 2017) and is associated with risk of frailty (Cox et al., 2020). Contributing factors to anorexia of ageing include increased feelings of fullness at meals caused by changed stomach capacity and slower gastric emptying generating early satiety signals to the central nervous system. Hormonal changes associated with ageing include reductions in oestrogen and testosterone, which are associated with appetite.

Reductions in the taste and smell threshold (i.e., the ability to detect taste or smell) and acuity (i.e., the intensity of taste or smell) are commonly reported in older age and illness and can cause changes in the amount and type of food eaten (Doty, 2018). This sometimes results in flavour preference changes, with a preference for saltier, spicier and more sugary foods and drinks. Thirst sensation also tends to decline with age, resulting in reduced drive to drink.

Appetite is also influenced by psychosocial factors. Preparing food and eating alone often results in lower food intake, giving poorer dietary quality and variety over time. Depression sometimes causes reduced appetite and ability to shop and prepare food. Side effects of a number of drugs diminish appetite in older people—for example, quinagolide, amphotericin, donepezil and amiloride.

Gastrointestinal System

The processes associated with ingesting, digesting and eliminating waste change as we grow older. Mastication of food in the mouth requires good dentition; jaw, lip and tongue musculature; and volumes of saliva. The complex process of swallowing requires good sensory capacity and musculature of the pharyngeal region. Key components of the gastrointestinal system are the olfactory and gustatory systems, which influence appetite. They also modulate saliva production and swallowing, so changes can influence food intake. Gastric emptying and gut motility also slow as part of the ageing process, causing prolonged feelings of fullness and constipation. Reduced function and sensation in the upper gastrointestinal tract can increase reflux and risk of aspiration. Secretion of products involved in digestion, such as gastrointestinal enzymes, gastric acid secretion and hormones involved in digestion, may diminish, affecting absorption of nutrients. Decreased immune function results in increased susceptibility to foodborne and other gastrointestinal infections. Age-related changes in the ancillary organs of digestion (i.e., liver, gall bladder and pancreas) also influence nutrient digestion and absorption. As with other changes associated with ageing, gastrointestinal changes are variable, with different effects on eating and drinking. More time to enjoy meals at a leisurely pace often comes with age, which can mitigate some of these effects.

Functional Ability

Reduced muscle mass, diminished sight and hearing, cognitive decline and the effects of long-term conditions reduce functional ability. The ability to perform activities of daily living such as shopping and housework significantly influence food and drink intake. Loss of functional ability is described in detail in Chapter 19, but in relation to nutrition, it affects the ability to acquire, prepare and eat food independently. Independent food acquisition requires the ability to travel to a shop or market, purchase food and drinks, and transport them home or the ability to access the internet and use online shopping resources. Food preparation requires the ability to store food and prepare it safely and appropriately. The process of eating and drinking itself (i.e., moving food from a vessel to the mouth) requires the ability to wash hands and achieve a good eating position as well as cognition and good hand and arm function. At completion of a meal or snack, disposal of waste and effective cleaning are important to remove bacteria from kitchen utensils and surfaces. Loss of functional ability as a result of ageing influences all these processes. A risk factor for a poor-quality diet in older adults is functional limitation (Nazri et al., 2021), suggesting decline in functional ability as a process of ageing is a significant factor that influences food and fluid intake.

Dietary Intake

The term *dietary intake* considers both the amount and quality of the food we eat and our food consumption pattern. Dietary intake depends on a variety of factors, including socioeconomic status, health status, functional ability and wider societal effects. The dietary intake of many older people is good and follows national healthy eating guidelines. Dietary intake may be in excess of nutritional requirements, leading to obesity.

Energy and nutrient requirements are lower in older people, particularly those over 75 (Public Health England, 2016). Associated with this is the tendency for food intake to decline gradually with age with an accompanying decline in nutrient intake. This gives rise to low levels of micronutrients such as iron and calcium. Vitamin D intake in older people requires particular consideration because exposure to sunlight plays a key role in maintaining adequate levels in the body. It is difficult to obtain sufficient vitamin D from food and drinks alone (Public Health England, 2016). Adults over 65 in many European countries are advised to take daily vitamin D supplements of about 10 micrograms every day to compensate for lack of exposure to sunlight.

Very old adults are most at risk of poor dietary intake due to low energy requirements and physical factors associated with old age, leading to protein and micronutrient deficiencies. A recent review summarised the epidemiological evidence from European studies of ageing that investigated diet and nutritional status in very old adults (Granic et al., 2018). Cereals, cereal products and bread were shown to be the main source of carbohydrates and contributed to intake of other macronutrients, folate and iron. Meat and milk were identified as the main source of protein and B12. Low dietary intakes of vitamin D, calcium and magnesium were highlighted. Adequate protein intake, particularly in combination with physical activity, may delay functional and mental decline in very old adults (Mendonça et al., 2020).

In terms of the societal effects, the older age group spans over 40 years, from people born at the time of World War I to people born in the 1950s. Over the past 100 years, there has been a huge change in dietary patterns and food availability. Food common in the early part of 21st century, such as offal and suet-based products, are seldom eaten by younger age groups, and the advent of convenience foods and rapid growth in opportunities to eat away from home have led to less home cooking. However, although we can consider changes in dietary patterns over several decades, generalising about an individual's food intake based on their age would be incorrect. We adapt to societal changes as we grow older, and individual social circumstances and health status vary, so it's important to assess each person's preferences and diet.

Despite the general changes in factors that influence food and fluid intake in older age, many older people eat well and are able to maintain health or even eat more energy than their body requires and gain weight. However, a period of ill health or the development of a long-term condition, both of which become increasingly common with age, can lead to reduced food and fluid intake and cause dehydration, loss of body weight and nutritional deficiency.

Malnutrition

Malnutrition is a common issue in older adults (Volkert et al., 2019). Malnutrition is a change in body composition and physiology as a result of nutrient intake in excess of or less than the body requires. Water is as an essential nutrient required to maintain life. Water insufficiency is defined as *dehydration*. Malnutrition encompasses over- and undernutrition but in the context of this chapter refers to a deficiency of nutrients, particularly protein and energy. Overnutrition, or energy intake in excess of energy requirements, is discussed using the term *obesity*.

Dehydration

Dehydration due to insufficient fluid intake is not an uncommon issue in older people and is associated with higher morbidity and mortality (Hooper et al., 2015). Risk factors for dehydration are multifactorial and associated with changes experienced during ageing, environmental factors and functional ability (Masot et al., 2018). Risk factors may be modifiable (e.g., lack of availability of fluids) or unmodifiable (e.g., reduced thirst due to ageing). Older people who live nursing homes often become dehydrated (Masot et al., 2018), so it is particularly important to review institutional factors related to detection of dehydration and provision of fluids.

Obesity

Obesity is an increasing problem in older adults (Volkert et al., 2019). For example, the 2018 Health Survey for England indicated a high percentage of people aged 65–74 who were overweight or obese (men 78%, women 73%) (Conolly & Craig, 2019). After 74, the proportion of overweight and obese adults decreased (Conolly & Craig, 2019). The causes of obesity are multifactorial in all age groups, but older adults may be particularly susceptible to weight gain due to reduced activity levels, side effects of medication and long-term conditions.

The association between obesity status and ageing well is complex. Conditions associated with obesity include type II diabetes mellitus, hypertension, coronary heart disease, some cancers and joint disorders. Increased amounts of adipose tissue are often accompanied by sarcopenia (Roh & Choi, 2020). As with younger people, obesity can reduce physical activity levels and functional ability. However, the term *obesity* encompasses a broad body mass index (BMI) range, and the degree of obesity and age of the person need to be considered. In older adults body fat can provide a buffer for illness when appetite is reduced and weight is lost, preventing the person from becoming underweight. Body fat also protects bony prominences, reducing risk of fracture or pressure injury by absorbing the energy of an impact or pressure. Weight reduction is sometimes associated with a reduction of muscle mass and bone mineral density (Goisser et al., 2020). While it is unclear what level of obesity, if any, might be beneficial for older adults and whether it changes as people move toward very old age, weight loss in obesity reduces weight-related health problems and the risk of developing obesity-related conditions. It can also improve functional ability and mobility.

Undernutrition

Protein energy malnutrition refers to a deficiency of protein and energy (i.e., calories), giving rise to weight loss. Other types of malnutrition include iron deficiency anaemia and deficiencies caused by low intake of vitamins D and B12. Protein energy malnutrition may be accompanied by micronutrient deficiency but can occur alone. Similarly, specific micronutrient deficiencies can occur in isolation or with other micronutrient deficiencies.

A substantial proportion of individuals cared for by health care professionals experience malnutrition (British Association for Parenteral and Enteral Nutrition, 2020), with the prevalence varying across care settings (O'Keefe et al., 2019). Malnutrition is associated with poorer clinical outcomes, increased health care costs and longer recovery from illness and surgery (British Association for Parenteral and Enteral Nutrition, 2020).

As stated by O'Keeffe and colleagues (2019), malnutrition is a complex multidimensional problem. A wide variety of interrelating factors are associated with malnutrition that impact individuals in different ways, including socioeconomic, psychological, pathological and drug-related factors.

Socioeconomic Factors

Low socioeconomic status is associated with poorer quality diet and nutritional status in older adults (Nazri et al., 2020). Dietary intake relies on a person's ability to acquire and prepare food. Income determines the quality and quantity of food bought, as do the availability of shops or the ability to order food online and the capacity to transport food home. At home food needs to be stored and prepared. Low income may drive an older person to reduce fuel costs, leading to compromised cold storage and cooking facilities. Poor living conditions often reduce storage and cooking options and increase risk of foodborne illnesses. Social support to undertake obtain and prepare food, whether in the form of family and friends or paid carers, can enhance food availability. Poor diet quality is also associated with smoking habit in all age groups (Nazri et al., 2020).

Psychological Factors

In all age groups, psychological factors sometimes result in low food and fluid intake, leading to malnutrition and dehydration. There is some evidence poor cognitive function and depression are associated with malnutrition in older adults (O'Keefe et al., 2019). Changes in life circumstances

that lead to a loss of independence, such as a move to residential care or hospital admission, can precipitate changes in mood with the potential to affect dietary intake. The devastating effect of receiving a life-changing diagnosis or a significant bereavement can also result in low mood and potentially affect dietary intake.

Medical Condition–Related Factors

Many medical conditions contribute to the development of malnutrition as a consequence of the condition or its treatment and management. In older adults the presence of some conditions limits their ability to acquire and prepare food. Limited mobility is a consequence of a variety of conditions due to muscular skeletal issues, fatigue, breathlessness and reduced dexterity and can affect a person's ability to shop and prepare meals. Conditions that result in cognitive deficits, such as dementia, can disrupt normal shopping and food-preparation habits and lead to poor dietary intake.

Conditions that affect the gastrointestinal tract are frequently associated with poor dietary intake. In the older population, anorexia is commonly experienced as a result of disease or medication. For example, loss of appetite is common in older people with COVID-19 (Lechien et al., 2020).

The process of eating and drinking in terms of transferring food from the plate to the mouth and chewing is affected by many conditions. Examples include stroke, Parkinson's disease and neurodegenerative diseases. Once food has been transferred to the mouth and prepared for swallowing by forming a bolus, it needs to be safely and effectively moved from the mouth to the stomach by swallowing. Conditions that cause changes in the form and function of the pharyngeal, laryngeal or oesophageal regions involved in swallowing, such as head and neck cancer, stroke and altered consciousness, influence dietary intake. Difficulty swallowing, or dysphagia, is a key factor in the development of malnutrition, which must be managed to ensure adequate nutritional intake.

Poor diet quality has also been associated with poor oral health (Nazri et al., 2020). Poor dentition and other oral problems significantly affect food and drink intake by restricting the type and amount of food and drink consumed.

Conditions that affect the stomach, small and large intestine, and ancillary organs of digestion also influence dietary intake. The movement of nutrients and other products of digestion through the gastrointestinal tract is changed by some conditions, either by obstructing or reducing movement or by speeding up its normal rate. For example, stomach cancer may block or slow the movement of chyme into the small intestine, and bacterial infection such as *Clostridium difficile* can cause diarrhoea. Nausea and vomiting are extremely unpleasant symptoms that result in dehydration and malnutrition if not managed. Both are caused by a wide range of conditions and reduce the drive to eat, sometimes resulting in fluid and electrolyte imbalance. Conditions that reduce absorption of nutrients from the gastrointestinal tract also predispose to malnutrition. Examples include pernicious anaemia caused by declining production of intrinsic factor to aid absorption of vitamin B12 and coeliac disease, which results in villous atrophy.

Conditions that cause changes in the metabolic rate are associated with malnutrition. For example, cancer cachexia, a multifactorial syndrome characterised by weight loss, leads to malnutrition (Zhang & Edwards, 2019). In all age groups, conditions that result in a higher nutrient use due to increased demand increase the risk of malnutrition. Conditions more prevalent in older age that increase nutrient demand are dementia as a result of wandering and longstanding Parkinson's disease.

Frailty is associated with malnutrition and discussed in depth in Chapter 6. Poor diet quality has been associated with risk of frailty in community-dwelling older adults (Hengeveld et al., 2019); being frail can lead to poor dietary intake.

Medication

Medication use and polypharmacy are more common in older people (see Chapter 31) and in some studies have been associated with malnutrition (O'Keefe et al., 2019). This is sometimes due to the effect of the conditions for which the medication is prescribed or is a side effect of the medication. Some medications cause drug-nutrient interactions that affect nutritional status by reducing or increasing bioavailability of nutrients. One example is the pharmacodynamic and pharmacokinetic interactions between drugs and fruit juices. Orange juice enhances iron absorption but also enhances aluminium absorption from some antacids.

Use of herbal medicines and over-the-counter dietary supplements can give rise to potential herb–drug or supplement–drug interactions (Agbabiaka et al., 2018). Commonly used herbal medicines that interact with prescribed medications include flaxseed, evening primrose oil, St John's wort and peppermint (Agbabiaka et al., 2018). The assessment process should include herbal and supplement use to determine potential risk.

Admission to Health Care Institutions

Following admission to residential care or hospital, older people experience a loss of independence with a huge impact on their lifestyle and normal living routines. Although food acquisition is easier because food and drinks are provided, the psychological effects of the lifestyle change may reduce or precipitate poor intake. People admitted to institutional care environments usually have medical conditions that require management or an inability to cope that contributes to the development of malnutrition.

Organisational and environmental issues limit the availability of food for some people for a variety of reasons. Ethnic identity may be expressed by a habitual dietary pattern that can be disrupted on admission to health care institutions. Food and drinks provided may not be culturally appropriate or meet religious requirements. Provision of a range of diets to support ethnic, cultural and religious requirements is crucial. Likewise, therapeutic and modified texture diets need to be provided to ensure people can manage their conditions. People who are reliant on enteral nutrition by tube frequently experience problems with nutrition and hydration delivery either because the tube cannot be replaced or used or the formulation that provides nutrients is not available (Green et al., 2019).

NUTRITIONAL CARE

The United Nations General Health Assembly in 1948 outlined everyone has the right to food intake adequate for health and well-being. People who use health care services should have adequate nutrition and hydration to sustain life and good health and reduce the risks of malnutrition and dehydration while they receive care and treatment. The exception to this is when meeting nutritional or hydration needs is not in the service user's best interests or is done without their consent.

Regulation 14 of the UK Health and Social Care Act 2008 (Regulated Activities) Regulations of 2014 outlines that 'providers, where it is their role, must make sure that people have enough to eat and drink to meet their nutrition and hydration needs and receive the support they need to do so'. This is reinforced by the Care Quality Commission (2022) the independent care regulator of health and adult social care in England, which indicates the nutritional needs of people should be assessed and food provided to meet those needs. Other nations, for example Scotland have similar standards (Healthcare Improvement Scotland, 2014). Nurses play a central role in ensuring older adults receive appropriate nutritional care.

Nutritional care should be considered a process (Fig. 21.1) with screening and assessment as the first stage. People identified with or at risk of malnutrition or obesity or with specific dietary needs should have a plan of care developed and implemented. The next stage of the process involves the implementation of the plan followed by evaluation as time progresses. Organisational audit and service evaluation and development can be built around

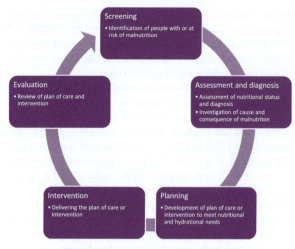

Fig. 21.1 Process of nutritional care.

this process. Although it is helpful to consider each stage of the process separately, in practice they connect, interrelate, and may occur simultaneously; for example, components of screening overlap with assessment and evaluation, and planning and intervention may be an iterative process informed by resource availability and an older person's wishes.

Each aspect of the process of care is reviewed to systematically support the nutrition and hydration care of older adults.

Malnutrition Risk Screening and Nutritional Assessment

Providing good nursing care for older adults requires careful consideration of their nutrition and hydration status to ensure appropriate nutritional support is planned and provided. The first stage of the nutritional care process is screening and assessment. These two terms are often used interchangeably and sometimes involve the same methods. Screening is the process of identifying individuals at risk of malnutrition; assessment is a thorough investigation of nutritional status, identifying cause and consequence. As with all aspects of care, it's important to work with a multidisciplinary team to provide individualised care.

Screening for Malnutrition Risk

On admission to care or shortly after, older people should be screened for risk of malnutrition using a valid and reliable tool, except in groups and individuals where this is not deemed appropriate. Screening can be done during a routine health check or as part of an outpatient department or community visit. Screening for nutritional risk may not be appropriate for some people or groups of people—for

example, those receiving palliative or end-of-life care. In this situation the reason for not screening for malnutrition should be recorded in the person's health care records or stated in unit policy. Health care professionals should still assess dietary needs and preferences.

Screening for malnutrition risk is a rapid and easy process that can be done in both institutional and community settings. Regional legislation and health care provider policies about nutritional care usually make reference to a screening tool or other simple measure such as weight. Screening tools comprise of a number of items usually focused on anthropometric measures (i.e., measurement of physical properties of the body) and other items related to nutritional intake that, when scored, give an indication of overall risk.

Numerous screening tools have been developed over the past 30 years. Some are generic, and others focus on screening older adults. Few tools have undergone rigorous validity and reliability testing (Power et al., 2018). Tools that have been tested extensively include the Malnutrition Universal Screening Tool (MUST) (British Association for Parenteral and Enteral Nutrition, 2020), which is widely used in adult populations. The MUST relies on weight and height measurement to calculate BMI and weight loss. Proxy measures of height and weight can be calculated if they can't be measured. The Mini Nutritional Assessment Tool (MNA) is another widely used nutrition screening and assessment tool that has undergone extensive validity and reliability testing (Nestlé Nutrition Institute, 2020). It is designed to identify people over 64 who are malnourished or at risk of malnutrition. Both the MUST and MNA offer self-screening versions older people and their carers can use directly.

Many screening tools do not directly measure anorexia and inadequate intake, which are early markers of malnutrition risk in older adults. Tools that do, such as the Simplified Nutritional Appetite Questionnaire, can be used with healthy community-dwelling older adults to create opportunity for early intervention (Lau et al., 2020).

The choice of tool in a health care setting should consider its ease and acceptability of use and its validity and reliability. Barriers to the use of malnutrition screening tools are present in some health care settings, including organisational culture, time and resources to screen and intervene as well ease and acceptability of the screening tool (Green et al., 2014). The consistent use of one malnutrition screening tool in a health care setting enables easy detection of differences over time, training and auditing to identify issues.

Self-screening for malnutrition and screening by social care workers is increasingly promoted. For example, the British Association for Parenteral and Enteral Nutrition (2020) designed a web-based tool using MUST components

TABLE 21.1 Basic Dietary Assessment Questions

Eating Patterns/Habits
Do you eat a particular type of diet, for example, for religious reasons?
What type of food and drinks do you like?
Could you tell me what you normally eat in a day?
Has your appetite changed recently?
Have you been prescribed nutritional supplement drinks by your dietitian or doctor? If you have, do you drink them?

Socioeconomic Factors
Where do you normally live?
Does someone help you with shopping and cooking?
Does anything stop you from buying and cooking what you like to eat?
Has anything changed recently that makes shopping and eating more difficult?

Symptoms That Affect Eating and Drinking
Does anything stop you from eating and drinking well, such as feeling sick or not being able to swallow properly?
If something is stopping you from eating and drinking well, what effect does it have, and how long have you had it?
Does your mouth feel comfortable when you eat and drink?
Do you think you have lost or gained weight recently?

Multidisciplinary Team Work
Have you spoken to a dietitian or speech and language therapist about your eating?
Has your doctor advised you what you should eat and drink?

to support community-dwelling adults to identify their own risk of malnutrition. People who identify as being at risk of malnutrition can download a dietary advice sheet. Self-screening supports older people and their relatives and carers to identify risk of malnutrition and encourages increased dietary intake and GP consultation. It relies on the cognitive ability and inclination, so it does not replace screening by health care professionals. Specific tools to assess eating difficulties exist, such as the self-rating Eating Assessment Tool (Möller et al., 2020) and the Edinburgh Feeding Evaluation in Dementia (EdFED) scale, designed to measure feeding difficulty in people with dementia (Spencer et al., 2020).

Nutritional Assessment

Nutritional assessment enables identification of specific nutritional needs to determine dietary intake and nutritional status and inform the development of a care plan. It comprises of a range of questions and measures that consider psychosocial and physiological aspects related to nutrition. A simple nutritional assessment may be included as part of an initial assessment. On admission to care it is important to ask each person about their dietary needs and preferences, including belief-based or religious dietary requirements, and identify risk factors associated with eating and drinking such as choking. Assessment of appetite, dietary habits and recent food and drink consumption helps identify symptoms that affect nutritional

status. Table 21.1 gives examples of questions used during this process. Older adults should also be assessed for risk of refeeding syndrome (National Institute for Health and Care Excellence [NICE], 2006), which occurs when a person who has adapted to a very low dietary intake is given carbohydrates, causing electrolyte and metabolic changes as the body copes with the nutrient influx. Serious consequences include hypophosphatemia and hypokalaemia, resulting in cardiac arrhythmias and respiratory muscle dysfunction. Criteria for determining people at high risk of developing refeeding problems have been published by several national organisations, including the National Institute for Health and Care Excellence (2006). These include identifying if the person has a BMI that indicates they are underweight; unintentional weight loss; little nutritional intake for a period of days; low potassium, phosphate or magnesium blood levels; a history of alcohol use; or prescribed medications associated with risk of refeeding such as chemotherapy.

As part of the assessment process, identification of symptoms that influence food and drink intake is made. Symptoms such as nausea and constipation can often be treated promptly, resolving poor dietary intake. Oral health can also influence nutritional intake and may be done with a tool, although evidence to support tools in assessing older people's oral health is limited (Everaars et al, 2020).

At this stage referral to another health care professional to undertake a more thorough assessment may be required. For example, if assessment reveals difficulty in swallowing or increased risk of choking, refer to a speech and language therapist, or if manual dexterity affects food intake, refer to an occupational therapist. Dietitians are the experts in nutritional assessment, and a person who requires assessment beyond simple nutritional assessment should be referred for dietetic review. People identified as at risk of refeeding syndrome should be referred to a doctor and dietitian as a priority before nutritional support.

A recent Cochrane review (Culp et al., 2015) indicated limited evidence to support the use of an individual clinical symptom, sign or test to indicate water-loss dehydration (i.e., drinking too little fluid). A combination of approaches should be used as part of the clinical assessment process.

The nutritional assessment enables information to be recorded for future reference and should be used to develop a care plan.

Planning Care

Each person with an identified nutritional need should have an effective and individualised nutritional care plan (British Association for Parenteral and Enteral Nutrition, 2020). This could be a written document or contained within the electronic patient record. Planning nutritional care, as with planning of all care, requires a nursing need,

goal and actions along with evaluation to ensure it meets the person's needs. For older adults with long-term nutritional needs, a care plan that is transferable across settings supports clinical and social care teams to work together. It is important to state people with long-term conditions who require nutritional support are often experts by experience and used to managing their own nutritional care plan. Any new plans of nutritional care must be informed by the existing plan and agreed on with the person where possible. The nutritional care plan identifies planned interventions.

Interventions

Nutritional intervention is an umbrella term for a wide range of approaches aimed at supporting appropriate diet and nutrient intake. Interventions range from dietary counselling to complex therapies such as parenteral nutrition. They are considered in terms of policy development at international, national and local levels; public health and individual dietary education at provider and patient or resident levels; enhancement of eating environments; mealtime activities; products and procedures to assist a person to eat and drink; oral nutritional supplementation; enteral nutrition by tube; and parenteral nutrition. Table 21.2 shows examples of these approaches.

TABLE 21.2 **Nutritional Intervention Approaches**	
Nutritional Intervention Approach	**Examples of Interventions**
Policy development at international, national and local levels	• Policy development and action by international organisations to support health in older people (e.g., Age International, United Nations Human Rights) • Policy development and action by national organisations focussed on supporting health in older people (e.g., Age UK, Caroline Walker Trust) • Health care provider nutrition and hydration policy • Policy development by people with expertise in nutritional care (e.g., dietitians, nutrition nurses, gastroenterologists) • Clear requirement that diets that meet cultural and religious needs are available to order and deliver • Clear requirement for plan of care focusing on nutrition and hydration needs if required • Audit cycle includes focus on nutrition and hydration care • Service improvement on nutrition and hydration care follows audit
Public health and individual dietary education at provider and patient or resident levels	• International and national campaigns • Health care worker education (online or in person) • Online or in-person education for older people
Third-sector and commercial organisations	• Focused campaigns to improve food availability (e.g., lunch clubs) • Services to support mealtime activity and dietary intake (e.g., Food Train, Eat Well Age Well)
Eating environment	• Designated eating areas in acute and community settings • Eating areas clean, quiet, set for eating • Seating arrangements suitable to facilitate eating and consistency • Food waste and plates removed following completion of meals

Nutritional Intervention Approach	Examples of Interventions

TABLE 21.2 Nutritional Intervention Approaches—cont'd

Nutritional Intervention Approach	Examples of Interventions
Mealtime activities	• Ability to toilet and wash hands before and after eating • Focus on mealtime activity (i.e., protected mealtimes) • Menu completion on day food served • Mealtime supervised by registered nurse • Meal choice reminder when meal served • Alternative foods available • Mealtime volunteers • Relatives or carers invited to mealtimes • Intentional rounding • Food kept hot until person available to assist with eating
Products and procedures to support mealtime intake	• Provision of aids for posture and eating • Occupational and physiotherapy input as required • Speech and language therapist input as required • Mealtime assistants • Provide snacks in the evening • Ensure drinks are always available • Texture-modified foods • Finger-food menu • Coloured plates and glasses • Intentional rounding as mealtimes • Family carers assisting at mealtimes • Meal delivery service
Oral nutritional supplements, enteral nutrition by tube and parenteral nutrition	• Strategy, guidance or policy on oral nutritional supplement prescription • Dietetic service provision to ensure appropriate prescription and delivery of enteral nutrition • Energy-dense food and protein-supplemented food and drinks • Nutrition support team in acute care settings to ensure appropriate prescription and delivery of parenteral nutrition and enteral nutrition • Home enteral nutrition teams to support delivery of enteral nutrition by tube in the community • Dedicated parenteral nutrition service to support parenteral nutrition delivery in the community

Policy focused on good nutrition and hydration care is important as it sets the standard governments and organisations should strive to achieve and drives improvements. A clear policy supports local guidelines and initiatives to improve nutrition and hydration provision. At a local level, an NHS trust or health care provider policy focused on nutrition and hydration lays out specific expectations for staff and informs nutritional care strategies.

Key to supporting good nutrition and hydration in older adults are public health and individual dietary education. Adherence to a healthy diet rich in nutrient-dense foods is important at all stages of life but especially in later life, when age-related diseases are more prevalent (Granic et al., 2018). Preventive measures that seek to improve nutritional status by modifying risk factors in conjunction with dietary health promotion strategies are essential.

Education programmes can be delivered to older people and their informal carers and to health and social care staff. Nutrition education should be embedded within the curriculum of all prequalifying health care programmes; focused sessions on care for older adults must include nutrition and hydration. There is opportunity for dietitians and other health care professionals with expertise in aspects of nutrition and hydration care to provide education to support continuing professional development. Supporting education and learning about nutrition and hydration for older people is an important part of nursing, as is facilitating older adults to support their peers to develop their knowledge and understanding. Dietary counselling has a positive effect on energy intake and body weight in older adults (Reinders et al., 2018).

One of the roles of nurses and carers who work in institutional and residential settings is to ensure eating environments and mealtime activities are conducive to good dietary and fluid intake. Nurses also need to ensure support aids that facilitate eating and drinking are used appropriately, and procedures to assist a person to eat and drink are safe and effective.

Interventions that enhance the eating environment aim to produce a calm, sociable, clean setting with good seating and lighting. Eating with others promotes dietary intake (i.e., social facilitation of eating) compared to eating alone (Ruddock et al., 2019). Creating a dining area or room with tables and chairs can provide dining companions. If an older adult lives alone or prefers to eat alone, ensuring space for a chair and table enables they can sit upright with a meal in from of them. Noisy and dirty rooms reduce appetite for eating and drinking, as does not removing food waste. In residential care, asking older adults if they would like to participate in preparing rooms for eating helps provide a sense of purpose and enhances their cognitive ability to recognise mealtime. Sitting in the same place in the dining room at each meal promotes familiarity and association of the space with eating.

Assisting older people with eating and drinking is a fundamental aspect of nursing care that requires knowledge and skills to identify a range of physical, psychological and social issues that impair eating and to plan appropriate interventions. A simple intervention can be delegated to a volunteer, such as supporting a visually impaired person to choose from a menu or providing skilled assistance to move food from the plate to the mouth. However, although this is part of the nurse's role, it requires a team approach that involves therapists, catering and service staff. Referral to occupational therapy and physiotherapy supports the identification of appropriate equipment and positions. A speech and language therapist can advise on dietary modifications to ensure safe eating and drinking. Equipment includes eating aids such as plates guards and adapted cutlery and, in the future robot assisted eating. Mealtime assistants can help with simple tasks such as unwrapping food and providing drinks; family carers can be invited to assist their family member to eat. Nursing assistance often uses intentional rounding, a structured approach where nurses check and prompt people to eat. The use of coloured plates and glasses can improve intake as it makes food easier to see and prompts drinking (McLaren-Hedwards et al., 2022). Texture-modified and finger foods promote independence in eating because they can be easily transferred to the mouth. For example, thick soup is easier to spoon than

thin consommé, and a small new potato is easier to pick up than mashed potato. Providing snacks during the day and particularly before bed improves energy by encouraging frequent food intake. Drinks should be available at all times to ensure frequent fluids are taken. In the community, meal delivery services can support older people to eat a two-course meal each day.

Management of Obesity

Obesity can be managed through lifestyle interventions (i.e., incorporating behavioural, physical activity and dietary changes), pharmacological interventions and surgery (NICE, 2014). A review of interventions for obesity management in people over 60 concluded older age should not be a contradiction to lifestyle or surgical management of obesity (Haywood & Sumithran, 2019). The review showed lifestyle interventions had positive effects on outcomes such as physical function and cardiovascular measures; bariatric surgery gave comparable weight loss with similar or slightly increased complication rates. The review identified little evidence concerning pharmacological management of obesity in older people (Haywood & Sumithran, 2019).

As with younger adults, behaviours that increase physical activity and reduce dietary intake should be determined at an individual level. Dietary changes that result in a low-energy diet when combined with increased physical activity promote fat loss while retaining lean mass (Haywood & Sumithran, 2019). Dietary change alone may result in slower weight loss and loss of muscle mass. Physical activity is also associated with improved mood. Depending on the ability of the older adult, low-intensity activities such as walking and swimming are more appropriate to support weight loss and lean muscle gain.

Oral Nutritional Supplements, Enteral Nutrition by Tube and Parenteral Nutrition

Oral nutritional supplements, enteral nutrition by tube and parenteral nutrition are used to promote and maintain dietary intake. Oral nutritional supplements include milk-based drinks, juices, puddings and soups. Less often used to enhance intake are fortified biscuits and other products. Oral nutritional supplements can positively affect energy intake and body weight in older adults (Reinders et al., 2018) but only if actually consumed. Waste is a common issue in institutional and community settings where supplements are opened but only a portion or none at all is consumed. For effective and efficient use of oral nutritional supplements, their use should be monitored and plans changed accordingly. Oral nutritional supplement drinks can be served frozen, cold or hot to increase palatability. They may be used as part of a meal—for example, added to porridge or used instead of soup. Serving in a glass or bowl is sometimes preferable to serving in the container.

The delivery of nutrients and fluid via tube to the gastrointestinal tract is indicated for people who are unable to take food or fluid by mouth or cannot maintain adequate oral intake. If the upper gastrointestinal tract is accessible and functional, nasogastric or nasojejunal supplementation is usually given in the short-term. For longer-term feeding, a gastrostomy or jejunostomy tube can be inserted. Jejunal feeding is preferred when the stomach is not functional or the risk of pulmonary aspiration is high.

The management of enteral nutrition is similar for all age groups. However, support of an older adult with an enteral tube at home requires specific consideration. Older people discharged home with a gastrostomy or jejunostomy tube require support to adapt to this complex nutritional intervention. Frequently spouses are placed in a position where they are required to support their partner, which sometimes causes anxiety and apprehension about how they will cope. Home enteral nutrition teams and commercial home care services can provide significant support while older people adapt to their new way of living.

Parenteral nutrition is delivery of nutrition and hydration directly into the venous system via a catheter. It is indicated in gastrointestinal failure and several conditions where bowel rest is mandatory. Intravenous nutrition is costly and carries appreciable risks of infective, metabolic and mechanical complications. The management of parenteral nutrition is similar across all age groups.

Third-Sector Interventions

Third-sector organisations provide many services that support nutritional intake in older people, including resources both in and outside the home. In each region a number of non-governmental and non-profit organisations provide food and meals along with opportunities for socialisation that enhance the enjoyment of eating and drinking. Examples include Age UK–run cafés and restaurants that serve fresh, home-cooked food. A meal is provided at low cost, and it is sometimes possible to provide transport to and from the venue. Some organisations do daily deliveries of hot or frozen and ready-to-cook two-course meals. Food banks provide opportunities to obtain dietary products and may deliver boxes to older adults. Evidence suggests daily meals from a non-profit provider improve nutritional status in the short-term (O'Leary et al., 2020). However, third-sector services are not always accessed equally by all groups; race, ethnicity, and socioeconomic status have been shown to affect service use (Meyer, 2019). Nurses are in a position to support older adults and their carers to identify needs and signpost to local third-sector or social services.

Mouth Care

Mouth care is an important nursing intervention that should be considered with nutrition and hydration assessments. People who consume little or nothing orally are at risk of poor mouth condition because the release of saliva to rinse and lubricate the mouth and the mechanical action of swallowing to remove debris is reduced. This can lead to a dry mouth, coated tongue and risk of gum infection and tooth decay. Poor mouth condition has also been associated with increased risk of respiratory infection (Everaars, 2020). Regular mouth and lip care using a safe and effective procedure must be given. Guidelines and resources to support oral health care in adults in care homes (NICE, 2020) and hospital patients (Health Education England, n.d.) are available to guide practice.

Evaluation

Evaluation is an important stage in nutritional care at both group and individual levels. Evaluation is done using nutritional screening and assessment to determine differences following planning and intervention. Organisational processes used to evaluate nutrition and hydration care include an audit cycle, strategy evaluation and other quality processes such as Plan Do Study Act. Barriers and facilitators to good nutrition and hydration are considered as part of the evaluative process, such as investigation of why malnutrition screening tools are not used (Green et al., 2014) and barriers to screen-and-treat approaches to malnutrition in primary care (Harris et al., 2019).

Ethical Issues

A chapter on eating and drinking in older adults cannot conclude without consideration of ethical issues associated with the provision of nutrition and hydration. At the end of life, people may voluntarily choose to stop eating and drinking or request the cessation of nutritional support. As a nurse this can present conflicting emotions due to the need to advocate for the older person and deliver care to support nutrition and hydration intake. Discussion to inform decisions about nutrition and hydration care should involve a multidisciplinary team, the older adult and their family and carers. The European Society for Clinical Nutrition and Metabolism published guidelines on ethical aspects of artificial nutrition and hydration, which are focused on adult care and provide a summary of ethical issues around nutrition and hydration for physicians and other health care professionals (Druml et al., 2016).

CONCLUSION AND LEARNING POINTS

This chapter provides an overview of factors that influence nutritional intake in older adults and interventions to support good nutritional status. The nurse's role is to provide

CASE STUDY 21.1

June Pia, an 89-year-old woman, experienced a stroke that resulted in oropharyngeal dysphagia. She initially had a nasogastric tube, but prior to discharge from hospital, she received a percutaneous endoscopic gastrostomy (PEG) tube. She was transferred to a nursing home following discharge and a needs assessment, as she was unable to live independently. June was registered as sight impaired and had limited mobility due to decreased strength in her left leg as a result of the stroke. She considered her cognitive abilities unaffected by the stroke and enjoyed conversation and listening to the radio.

On admission to the nursing home, her MUST score was zero with a BMI of 23. June's height was 1.5 metres. She described herself as being a size 16 before she lost some weight in her 80s when her partner of many years died and she had an episode of ill health. Her oral health assessment indicated good oral health with some natural teeth. She was prescribed a feed regime by the dietitian to be administered via the PEG and received her medication via this route too. June had started drinking fluids in hospital, and the speech and language therapist had recommended slightly thick drinks and soft, bite-size foods.

Over the course of 12 months, with regular review by the home enteral nutrition speech and language therapist and dietitian, June was able to improve her swallowing ability and safely consume regular food and thin fluids to meet her nutrition and hydration needs orally. She really enjoyed her meals and snacks and felt the nursing home chef provided high-quality food. Her prescribed medication was reviewed and reduced by her general practitioner, and she was now able to take it orally.

June always expressed she did not like the PEG tube. She described it as a nuisance and felt it affected how she was able to dress and sleep at night. The home enteral nutrition team were keen to advocate for June and recommended removal of the tube when she had maintained her nutrition and hydration status orally for several months. Her GP was initially reluctant to refer her to endoscopy as he felt it was an unnecessary potentially traumatic procedure, but he referred her when it was clear this was her wish. June had an uneventful tube removal and returned to the nursing home, where she continued to enjoy eating and drinking and maintained good nutritional status.

---

dietary advice and ensure nursing care provides sufficient nutrients to meet nutritional requirements. Within the scope of professional practice, nurses need to work collaboratively with other health professionals to ensure high-quality nutritional standards for screening, assessment and support. Nutritional intake is more than the nutrients and water required to meet cellular needs; for most people it's one of life's great pleasures. This is especially important to recognise in older adults and near the end of life when freedom from adhering to dietary restrictions and societal norms may be welcome. As Jenny Joseph (1992) writes of getting older,

> You can wear terrible shirts and grow more fat
> And eat three pounds of sausages at a go
> Or only bread and pickle for a week

The Registered Nurses role is also to support older people to enjoy eating and drinking where possible and to maintain nutrition and hydrational status to enhance their quality of life.

KEY LEARNING POINTS

- Many factors influence food and fluid intake in older adults as a result of the aging process and the development of long-term conditions.
- Malnutrition (i.e., undernutrition and obesity) and dehydration are common in older adults and caused by a variety of factors.
- Nutritional care is a fundamental nursing activity that involves screening, assessment, planning, intervention and evaluation.

- A variety of interventions promote nutritional and fluid intake that meets group and individual needs.
- Ensuring good nutritional care requires a whole-team approach and working with dietitians, speech and language therapists, catering services and other health care staff.
- Ethical issues associated with the provision of nutrition and hydration may necessitate discussion with a multidisciplinary team, older adults and their carers to inform decisions.

REFERENCES

Agbabiaka, T. B., Spencer, N. H., Khanom, S., & Goodman, C. (2018). Prevalence of drug-herb and drug-supplement interactions in older adults: A cross-sectional survey. *British Journal of General Practice, 68*(675), e711.

British Association for Parenteral and Enteral Nutrition. (2020). Malnutrition/undernutrition. https://www.bapen.org.uk

Care Quality Commission. (2022). Regulation 14: Meeting nutrition and hydration needs. https://www.cqc.org.uk/guidance-providers/regulations-enforcement/regulation-14-meeting-nutritional-hydration-needs

Conolly, A., & Craig, S. (2019). *Health Survey for England 2018: Overweight and obesity in adults and children.* NHS Digital.

Cox, N. J., Morrison, L., Ibrahim, K., Robinson, S. M., Sayer, A. A., & Roberts, H. C. (2020). New horizons in appetite and the anorexia of ageing. *Age and Ageing, 49*(4), 526–534.

Cruz-Jentoft, A. J., & Sayer, A. A. (2019). *Sarcopenia. Lancet, 393*(10191), 2636–2646.

Doty, R. L. (2018). Age-related deficits in taste and smell. *Otolaryngologic Clinics of North America, 51*(4), 815–825.

Druml, C., Ballmer, P. E., Druml, W., Oehmichen, F., Shenkin, A., Singer, P., Soeters, P., Weimann, A., & Bischoff, S. C. (2016). ESPEN guideline on ethical aspects of artificial nutrition and hydration. *Clinical Nutrition, 35*(3), 545–556.

Everaars, B., Weening-Verbree, L. F., Jerković-Ćosić, K., Schoonmade, L., Bleijenberg, N., de Wit, N. J., & van der Heijd, G. J. (2020). Measurement properties of oral health assessments for non-dental healthcare professionals in older people: A systematic review. *BMC Geriatrics, 20*(1), 1–18.

Goisser, S., Kiesswetter, E., Schoene, D., Torbahn, G., & Bauer, J. M. (2020). Dietary weight-loss interventions for the management of obesity in older adults. *Reviews in Endocrine & Metabolic Disorders, 21*(3), 355–368.

Granic, A., Mendonça, N., Hill, T. R., Jagger, C., Stevenson, E. J., Mathers, J. C., & Sayer, A. A. (2018). Nutrition in the very old. *Nutrients, 10*(3), 269.

Green, S. M., James, E. P., Latter, S., Sutcliffe, M., & Fader, M. (2014). Barriers and facilitators to screening for malnutrition by community nurses: A qualitative study. *Journal of Human Nutrition and Dietetics, 27*(1), 88–95.

Green, S. M., Townsend, K., Jarrett, N., & Fader, M. (2019). The experiences and support needs of people living at home with an enteral tube: A qualitative interview study. *Journal of Human Nutrition and Dietetics, 32*, 646–658.

Harris, P. S., Payne, L., Morrison, L., Green, S., Ghio, D., Hallett, C., Parsons, E. L., Aveyard, P., Roberts, H. C., Sutcliffe, M., Robinson, S., Slodkowska-Barabasz, J., Little, P. S., Stroud, M. A., & Yardley, L. (2019). Barriers and facilitators to screening and treating malnutrition in older adults living in the community: A mixed-methods synthesis. *BMC Family Practice, 20*(1), 100.

Haywood, C., & Sumithran, P. (2019). Treatment of obesity in older persons: A systematic review. *Obesity Reviews, 20*(4), 588–598.

Health Education England. (n.d.). Mouth care matters. https://mouthcarematters.hee.nhs.uk/links-resources/mouth-care-matters-resources-2

Healthcare Improvement Scotland. (2014). Standards for food, fluid and nutritional care. https://www.healthcareimprovementscotland.org/our_work/standards_and_guidelines/stnds/nutritional_care_standards.aspx

Hengeveld, L. M., Wijnhoven, H. A., Olthof, M., Brouwer, I. A., Simonsick, E. M., Kritchevsky, S. B., Houston, D. K., Newman, A. B., & Visser, M. (2019). Prospective associations of diet quality with incident frailty in older adults: The Health, Aging, and Body Composition Study. *Journal of the American Geriatrics Society, 67*(9), 1835–1842.

Hooper, L., Abdelhamid, A., Attreed, N. J., Campbell, W. W., Channell, A. M., Chassagne, P., Culp, K. R., Fletcher, S. J., Fortes, M. B., Fuller, N., Gaspar, P. M., Gilbert, D. J., Heathcote, A. C., Kafri, M. W., Kajii, F., Lindner, G., Mach, G. W., Mentes, J. C., Merlani, P., & Hunter, P (2015). Clinical symptoms, signs and tests for identification of impending and current water-loss dehydration in older people. *Cochrane Database of Systematic Reviews.* https://www.cochranelibrary.com/cdsr/doi/10.1002/14651858.CD009647.pub2/full.

Joseph, J. (1992). *Selected poems.* Bloodaxe Books Ltd.

Lau, S., Pek, K., Chew, J., Lim, J. P., Ismail, N. H., Ding, Y. Y., Cesari, M., & Lim, W. S. (2020). The Simplified Nutritional Appetite Questionnaire (SNAQ) as a screening tool for risk of malnutrition: Optimal cutoff, factor structure, and validation in healthy community-dwelling older adults. *Nutrients, 12*(9), 2885.

Lechien, J. R., Chiesa, E. C., Place, S., Van Laethem, Y., Cabaraux, P., Mat, Q., Huet, K., Plzak, J., Horoi, M., Hans, S., Rosaria Barillari, M, Cammaroto, G., Fakhry, N., Martiny, D., Ayad, T., Jouffe, L., Hopkins, C., Saussez, S., Blecic, S., & De Siati, D. R (2020). Clinical and epidemiological characteristics of 1420 European patients with mild-to-moderate coronavirus disease. *Journal of Internal Medicine, 288*(3), 335–344.

Masot, O., Lavedán, A., Nuin, C., Escobar-Bravo, M. A., Miranda, J., & Botigué, T. (2018). Risk factors associated with dehydration in older people living in nursing homes: Scoping review. *International Journal of Nursing Studies, 82*, 90–98.

McLaren-Hedwards, T., D'cunha, K., Elder-Robinson, E., Smith, C., Jennings, C., Marsh, A., & Young, A. (2022). Effect of communal dining and dining room enhancement interventions on nutritional, clinical and functional outcomes of patients in acute and sub-acute hospital, rehabilitation and aged-care settings: A systematic review. *Nutrition and Dietetics, 79*(1),140–168.

Mendonça, N., Kingston, A., Granic, A., Hill, T. R., Mathers, J. C., & Jagger, C. (2020). Contribution of protein intake and its interaction with physical activity to transitions between disability states and to death in very old adults: The Newcastle 85+ Study. *European Journal of Nutrition, 59*(5), 1909–1918.

Meyer, S. J. The use of social services by older males. *Journal of Social Work, 19*(4), 450.

Möller, R., Safa, S., & Östberg, P. (2020). A prospective study for evaluation of structural and clinical validity of the Eating Assessment Tool. *BMC Geriatrics, 20*(1), 269.

Morley, J. E. (2017). Anorexia of ageing: A key component in the pathogenesis of both sarcopenia and cachexia. *Journal of Cachexia, Sarcopenia and Muscle, 8*(4), 523–526.

National Institute for Health and Care Excellence (NICE). (2006). Nutrition support for adults: oral nutrition support, enteral tube feeding and parenteral nutrition. https://www.nice.org.uk/guidance/cg32/chapter/1-guidance

NICE. (2014). Obesity: identification, assessment and management. https://www.nice.org.uk/guidance/cg189/chapter/About-this-guideline#copyright

NICE. (2020). Oral health for adults in care homes overview. https://pathways.nice.org.uk/pathways/oral-health-for-adults-in-care-homes

Nazri, N. S., Vanoh, D., & Kah Leng, S. (2021). Malnutrition, low diet quality and its risk factors among older adults with low socio-economic status: A scoping review. *Nutrition Research Reviews, 34*(1), 107–116.

Nestlé Nutrition Institute. (2020). MNA mini nutritional assessment. https://www.mna-elderly.com/mna_forms.html

O'Keeffe, M., Kelly, M., O'Herlihy, E., O'Toole, P. W., Kearney, P. M., Timmons, S., O'Shea, E., Stanton, C., Hickson, M., Rolland, Y., Sulmont Rossé, C., Issanchou, S., Maitre, I., Stelmach-Mardas, M., Nagel, G., Flechtner-Mors, M., Wolters, M., Hebestreit, A., De Groot, L., & O'Connor, E. M (2019). Potentially modifiable determinants of malnutrition in older adults: A systematic review. *Clinical Nutrition, 38*(6), 2477–2498.

O'Leary, M. F., Barreto, M., & Bowtell, J. L. Evaluating the effect of a home-delivered meals service on the physical and psychological wellbeing of a UK population of older adults: A pilot and feasibility study. *Journal of Nutrition in Gerontology & Geriatrics, 39*(1), 1.

Power, L., Mullally, D., Gibney, E. R., Clarke, M., Visser, M., Volkert, D., Bardon, L., de van der Schueren, A. E., & Corish, C. A. (2018). A review of the validity of malnutrition screening tools used in older adults in community and healthcare settings: A MaNuEL study. *Clinical Nutrition, 24,* 1–13.

Public Health England. (2016). *Government dietary recommendations*. Public Health England.

Reinders, I., Volkert, D., de Groot, L., Beck, A., Feldblum, I., Jobse, I., Neelemaat, F., de van der Schueren, M., Shahar, D., Smeets, E., Tieland, M., Twisk, J., Wijnhoven, H., & Visser, M. (2018). Effectiveness of nutritional interventions in older adults at risk of malnutrition across different health care settings: Pooled analyses of individual participant data from nine randomized controlled trials. *Clinical Nutrition, 38*(4), 1797–1806.

Roh, E., & Choi, K. M. (2020). Health consequences of sarcopenic obesity: A narrative review. *Frontiers in Endocrinology, 11*, 332.

Ruddock, H. K., Brunstrom, J. M., Vartanian, L. R., & Higgs, S. (2019). A systematic review and meta-analysis of the social facilitation of eating. *The American Journal of Clinical Nutrition*, 110(4), 842–861.

Spencer, J. C., Damanik, R., Ho, M. H., Montayre, J., Traynor, V., Chang, C. C., & Chang, H. C. (2020). *Review of food intake difficulty assessment tools for people with dementia*. Western Journal of Nursing Research.

Volkert, D., Beck, A., Cederholm, T., Cruz-Jentoft, A., Goisser, S., Hooper, L., Kiesswetter, E., Maggio, M., Raynaud-Simon, A., Sieber, C., Sobotka, L., van Asselt, D., Wirth, R., & Bischoff, S. (2019). ESPEN guideline on clinical nutrition and hydration in geriatrics. *Clinical Nutrition, 38*(1), 10–47.

Zhang, X., & Edwards, B. J. (2019). Malnutrition in older adults with cancer. *Current Oncology Reports, 21*(9), 80.

Bladder and Bowel Health

Sue Woodward

The passage of urine and faeces is, for most people in Western society, a very personal and private function, which many people are able to take for granted. Continence is one of children's first socialisations in childhood and in adult life is a largely subconscious, if still voluntary, function. Considerable control over micturition and defecation is necessary to meet the commonly accepted criteria of continence. This involves complex neuromuscular coordination in conjunction with an awareness of societal norms.

Especially at times of illness or disease, control may become vulnerable for older adults who are dependent on the care of others to access toilet facilities at home or in residential or hospital care. The nurse has a key role in both hospital and community settings in identifying older adults

at risk of elimination problems. With a thorough assessment of individual needs, appropriate care can be planned to maintain normal function and prevent problems or to remedy problems already apparent.

Traditionally, nurses approached elimination care in a routinised manner. Most nurses were familiar with bedpan rounds, bottle rounds, bowel books and 4-hourly toileting regimens. Care of the bowel and bladder tended to be seen as a low-status task that required little knowledge or expertise and was often left to the most junior or non-registered staff. Working with older adults was often identified as synonymous with an endless routine of changing incontinent patients and wet beds. This may be partly responsible for the unfavourable image held by some nurses of working with older adults. Yet care for elimination needs is one of the fundamentals of nursing care and an aspect nurses have responsibility for.

The majority of older people manage to maintain normal elimination function to the end of their life. Problems are not a necessary or inevitable concomitant of ageing and should never be passively accepted. Bladder and bowel symptoms do not 'just happen'; there is always a cause or reason for them. If it can be discovered, it can often be remedied or at least its effects on the individual minimised.

ATTITUDES AND EFFECTS

The Person

Elimination is a challenging subject for most older people to talk about. Elimination difficulties are a cause for shame, embarrassment and guilt and are typically kept hidden. Consequently, many people who have problems do not seek help. For example, only a minority of incontinent people seek health care, and many delay seeking help for incontinence, often for years. Lack of health-seeking behaviour has also been reported among carers of older people with dementia (Drennan et al., 2011) who may be seeking to protect the dignity and personhood of the person cared for. Active case finding is therefore needed, especially in high-risk groups such as older adults (National Institute for Health and Care Excellence [NICE], 2018).

It is easy to assume frail older people are passive recipients of nursing care with little input to the process. However, Robinson (2000), in a study of nursing-home residents with incontinence using grounded theory methodology, found people engage in a process she called 'managing urinary incontinence', with a range of strategies used with varying success. Many older adults believe urinary incontinence is an inevitable part of ageing and within that context seek to protect their own physical, psychological and social integrity. Residents invest much more in protecting themselves from the consequences of leakage than in seeking treatment for incontinence, with most expressing the feeling 'you manage', for example, by accepting pads instead of toilet use to reduce the risk of falls, cognitive efforts to preserve dignity and avoiding alienating staff. Robinson (2000) identified six common strategies (Table 22.1). For many residents they enabled 'making the best of it' (p. 74) and getting on with other aspects of life. For individuals who did not employ successful strategies, incontinence caused suffering and physical and/or mental anguish.

Low rates of older people seeking help with bladder and bowel symptoms have been noted in particular populations. Women, for example, may attribute symptoms of urinary incontinence to the effects of ageing (Rashidi Fakari et al., 2021) and therefore put up with symptoms for many

TABLE 22.1 Nursing-Home Residents' Strategies for Managing Urinary Incontinence (Robinson, 2000)

Strategy	Examples
Limiting	Self-imposed restriction on activities Avoid taking diuretics Restrict fluid intake Use pad instead of calling for night staff Stay near a toilet, avoid travel
Improvising	Methods to accomplish voiding (e.g., receptacles) Travel and transfer to the toilet Aesthetic and hygienic methods
Learning	Learning how to access toilets in the facility Learning how to transfer Importance of controlling fluid intake
Monitoring	Environment: routine and other residents Checking for evidence of leakage Observing staff behaviour
Speaking up	Communicate needs, opinions and ideas Express preferences
Letting it go	Accidental, deliberate or negotiated urination outside usual receptacle Wait until morning to tell staff when wet at night

years, perhaps encouraged by advertisments for female urinary incontinence pads on commercial television that reinforce self-management. The perception of loss of control can be associated with self-esteem and shame, which may explain why many people fail to seek professional help for incontinence and why others do not take up offers of assistance, even when easily accessible in their locality.

Many older incontinent women restrict their social activities and go only to places where they know the toilet facilities. The degree of incontinence is not always directly related to the degree of restriction. Many avoid social contact, and urinary incontinence has been associated with loneliness and mental health problems such as anxiety and depression (Stickley et al., 2017). Generally, urge incontinence has more impact than stress leakage, probably because of the unpredictable nature of the symptom.

The presence of urinary incontinence may determine where somebody lives, may even rob an individual of the ability to live independently and has been cited as a precipitating factor for admission to a nursing home, while faecal incontinence was not (Schluter et al., 2017). Most studies, however, have shown urinary incontinence is not an independent predictor of admission to long-term care (Musa et al., 2019). One year after a stroke, people with urinary incontinence are four times more likely to be institutionalised than those who are continent (Williams et al., 2012). Even allowing for the consideration some people with incontinence are more disabled than individuals who are not incontinent, this is a major influence on placement. The same is likely to be true for other conditions.

Unlike urinary incontinence, very little research has been conducted on the effects of faecal incontinence on the individual, although common sense suggests the impact would be even greater. Even less is known about the impact of incontinence on long-term care preferences of older people, although one study suggests urinary and faecal incontinence may influence their decisions about placement in long-term care (Carvalho et al., 2020).

Elimination problems cause misery and discomfort and can be a burden to carers (Gotoh et al., 2009). Nighttime problems, faecal incontinence and the need to have intimate contact with a partner or family member to provide care are particularly difficult for relatives to cope with. These problems merit a serious nursing effort to provide a remedy when possible or optimum management to control symptoms. Timely early nursing support can mean an older person is able to remain in their own familiar surroundings for longer (Carvalho et al., 2020).

Although most older people think nothing can be done to cure or improve incontinence, attitudes can be changed by health education. A systematic review of continence promotion programmes advocates the need for ongoing health promotion programmes that include health-seeking behaviour (Newman et al., 2020); the long-term effectiveness of these programmes is beginning to emerge (Tannenbaum et al., 2019).

The Nurse

A nurse needs to approach the subject of elimination difficulties with the utmost sensitivity and tact if a good rapport and trust are to be established and take the time to find a mutually understood vocabulary. Nurses have unique and privileged access to intimate information. Using this position of privilege, nurses can be alert to the possibility of problems with every patient, not just those with overt difficulties. However, nurses may be reluctant to bring the subject into the open, either accepting problems as irremediable or pretending nothing is wrong in order to spare the patient's embarrassment. The use of trigger questions and active case finding is therefore encouraged (Yates, 2018) to enable incontinence to be assessed and treated in the best way possible.

Elimination has long been identified as a major problem for nursing older people. Problems such as incontinence occupy a high proportion of nursing time and energy. The amount of time spent promoting continence is inversely related to the amount of incontinence on a ward or in a care home.

Nurses' knowledge and attitudes toward incontinence have been explored in different nursing populations, including among nurses who work in care homes (Saxer et al., 2009), advanced nurse practitioners (Keilman & Dunn, 2010) and nursing students (Luo et al., 2016). Attitudes are found to be different among different grades of nursing staff and in different settings, but negative attitudes and inadequate knowledge seem to be becoming less common. One study found, in general, nursing assistants are more positive than registered nurses, and nurses in acute units may be more negative than those working in longer-stay care (Vinsnes, 2001). Various continence programmes have been found to reduce incontinence (see below), but compliance with such programmes is often low, even in research settings once the formal study phase is over.

There have been calls to improve education about incontinence for nurses, but education alone does not seem to change attitudes. A recent systematic review indicated studies of educational interventions for nurses led to improvement in knowledge, but this does not always translate into improved outcomes for patients and change in clinical practice (Ostaszkiewicz et al., 2020). There is a rapidly growing literature on promoting continence (see Roe et al., 2015, and Edwards et al., 2021, for comprehensive reviews), and today the motivated nurse has considerable scope for positive management of elimination. However, change in established practice is not always easy to achieve, perhaps due to clinical inertia in which nurses fail to follow protocols, guidelines and preventative measures (Artero-López et al., 2018).

DELIVERY OF CONTINENCE SERVICES

It is easy for service providers to make assumptions about the individuals they are supposed to serve. It is only recently we have seriously asked what people want or need, and with an embarrassing problem like incontinence, the majority of people affected have been reluctant to tell us or complain when things were not good. Most do not seek help and expect little when they do. Simple screening questions can be used to screen effectively for incontinence in primary care, but in routine practice such questions are rarely asked. Clear guidance is now available for commissioners of continence services to co-produce high-quality community services that reduce harms for older people as a result of incontinence (NHS England, 2018).

TABLE 22.2	Incontinence and the Multidisciplinary Team (Norton, 1996)
Community	**Hospital**
District nurse	Physician
Continence adviser	Urologist
General practitioner	Gynaecologist
Physiotherapist	Geriatrician
Occupational therapist	Neurologist
Social worker	Nurse
	Physiotherapist

Multidisciplinary Team

For many years incontinence has been seen as solely a nursing problem, with little interest or input from other members of the multidisciplinary team in either hospital or community settings. It is not uncommon for an older person who presents with incontinence to a general practitioner to be told, 'It's your age,' and referred directly to a district nurse for supply of pads and pants, with no physical examination or further investigation (Orrell et al., 2013). This therapeutic nihilism is a recognised barrier to older people being able to access good continence care.

In fact, incontinence is often a complex and multifaceted problem that may need input from a wide variety of disciplines (Table 22.2). Although it is obviously not practical for all specialties to physically work together, there needs to be careful consideration of who does what, preferably with protocols to guide appropriate referral (NHS England, 2018) and ensure good liaison. It is important to ensure there are neither gaps nor too many overlaps in the service. It is often a community nurse, trained in continence care, who is responsible for initiating assessment and coordinating services around the older person (NHS England, 2018). For people with more complex needs, referral to specialist services, including urology, colorectal services or a geriatrician, may be required. It is also clear the collaborative effort of the entire nursing team is required to improve the assessment and management of care for older people with incontinence (McDaniel et al., 2020).

Role of the Nurse Specialist Continence Adviser

With the recognition of the very positive role of the nurse in managing incontinence, the concept of the nurse specialist has grown. In 2009 there were 624 practicing continence specialists in a database maintained by the Bladder and Bowel Community (https://www.bladderandbowel.org) with a recommended average annual caseload of 458 patients per member of full-time staff (UK Continence Society, 2014). These nurses have a very diverse role, from clinical casework and running incontinence and urodynamics clinics to teaching, researching, acting as a resource, developing products, appraising, and acting as supplies liaison. An informal friendly approach by nurses with good communication skills relieves patients' embarrassment and anxiety, giving them confidence and trust in the nurse, thus facilitating information exchange and effective effectiveness. A recent systematic review of the values of wound ostomy and continence nurses found them to be improved quality of life for patients, teaching and mentoring, cost reduction, improved efficiency, improved wound outcomes, improved incontinence outcomes, advanced treatments, research and leadership (Corey & Duff, 2021).

With an ageing population, the role of the continence specialist nurse is increasingly important (Franken et al., 2018). International service specifications for continence care that move toward community-delivered, nurse-led services are echoed in the UK guidance (NHS England, 2018). Continence nurse specialists are expert clinicians and can ensure clinical and cost effective prescribing and use of resources (Kumah & McGlashan, 2019) that improve symptoms with high levels of patient satisfaction.

ELIMINATION NEEDS

For people who are older or have a disability, the ability to remain continent often depends on a complex interplay of their physical bladder and bowel control and a host of other factors. Incontinence may be transient, for example during an acute illness or a urinary tract infection (UTI), which may be the case for one-third of older people who are incontinent in the community and half of hospital inpatients. Transient incontinence has a reversible underlying cause, normally has a sudden onset and lasts for less than 6 months.

Certain basic needs are common to both micturition and defecation if these functions are to be achieved. The individual must be able to identify an acceptable place for elimination; get to that place; hold excreta until that place is reached; empty the bowel or bladder easily, completely and in private once there; and perform a number of toilet-related skills. This may sound obvious, but failure in any one of these abilities makes the individual vulnerable to incontinence and is so common each is considered in turn, along with possible measures to solve problems.

Identifying an Acceptable Place

An older person's ability to identify correctly an acceptable place for elimination may be impaired in several ways. Most people expect to use a lavatory behind a locked door. In unfamiliar surroundings, this presumes an ability to follow signposts and read and correctly interpret labels on doors. Impaired vision, dim lighting or unclear or absent signs create difficulties. Sometimes gender symbols are difficult to distinguish. The problem is often compounded by a reluctance or embarrassment to ask for help. In some instances of cerebrovascular disease, an individual loses the ability to recognise the function of common objects such as a lavatory by vision alone (i.e., agnosia). A person who is confused or has dementia may likewise experience difficulty in correctly identifying right and wrong receptacles and may, for instance, use a wastebin or washbasin in error.

In institutional care, expectations are often different from those in general society, and people are expected to void into bedpans, bottles, commodes or behind curtains or doors without locks or any privacy, often in close proximity to their peers in shared rooms. It is easy to see how a lifetime's conditioned response only to excrete in private is disrupted and how a disoriented person may not be able to identify the 'acceptable' place. The very confused person may lose all socially acceptable behaviour, and the concept of continence or incontinence may become irrelevant.

Correct identification can be aided by providing clear explanations of what is expected; ensuring good lighting and clear signage and labelling of facilities at an appropriate height for older people and using pictures rather than words if patients have lost the ability to read; and, if necessary, improving vision by provision of spectacles (Murphy et al., 2021).

Ability to Get There

It is no good knowing there is a correct place for elimination unless that place can be reached. The problem may be an unsuitable environment or an individual's physical disabilities. At home, some older people have a lavatory that involves climbing stairs or, rarely, is outside. If shared with others, it may be occupied when needed. Public lavatories are often difficult for anyone with even a slight disability to use and are usually in sparse supply. They may be closed or vandalised and not repaired, or older people may not have a radar key to open a locked door. Many older women have a horror of public lavatories, believing they risk catching diseases, and would rather avoid their use. Some older-care wards were built in the days when all patients were nursed in bed, and some nursing homes have been adapted from private residences. Lavatories have been built on as an afterthought, often at the opposite end of the ward to the day room and down a corridor or around a corner. Sometimes toilets are too small to close the door if using a wheelchair. Patients have reported opening a toilet door when it was in use by another person, not being able to summon help when needed and having to wait up to 30 minutes for a commode.

Mobility is essential in getting to the lavatory. Degree of incontinence is closely related to degree of immobility, especially in institutional settings. This is helped by ensuring that beds and chairs are of the correct height and design to aid rising, that routes to the toilet are uncluttered with obstacles (e.g., loose mats) and that individuals have the optimum mobility aids for their needs. A physiotherapist should be involved in ensuring maximum mobility and in advising carers on safe transfer techniques. Good foot care and well-fitting shoes make a great difference.

Opening the lavatory door and getting into the compartment may present problems if design is poor. The height of the lavatory and availability of handrails often determines whether sitting and rising are possible independently. Manual dexterity is crucial in removal of clothing, positioning and cleansing. Appropriate clothing, a raised seat or a dressing aid help facilitate independent toileting.

When physical disabilities are severe, an alternative such as a hand-held urinal (male or female) or a commode may be more appropriate if privacy in their use can be ensured. However, many commodes are supplied without adequate consideration for privacy. Design improvements can improve comfort and safety in the future with toilet adaptations and alternatives to suit an individual's disabilities.

Sometimes depression or apathy results in lack of motivation to attempt to reach the lavatory. A person with an impoverished social environment may simply cease to try. We are all subject to peer pressure and a wish to conform. If staff have an attitude that incontinence does not matter, and it can be quicker to change a pad than to toilet someone, they can actively promote incontinence. This is particularly a problem in long-stay care if incontinence is the norm and no expectation is put on the individual to attempt to be continent. The Francis Inquiry (Her Majesty's Stationery Office, 2013) into care provided by the Mid Staffordshire NHS Foundation Trust identified many reports of poor and undignified care of people for their continence needs. Dignity should always be a guiding principle when providing care to older people with bladder and bowel care needs (Ostaszkiewicz et al., 2020). Occasionally, incontinence is a protest or sign of despair from an individual in an unacceptable personal situation.

Ability to Hold Excreta

An individual needs to be able to control bladder and bowel contents reliably while getting to the lavatory. This requires competent urethral and anal sphincters and the ability to inhibit detrusor (i.e., bladder muscle) and rectal contractions. Any of these functions can be impaired by disease or ageing (see below). With increasing age, sensation tends to diminish, and the individual gets little warning and often experiences increased urgency of micturition or defecation. It is a cruel fact this urgency sometimes coincides with decreased ability to hurry.

Ability to Empty

Constipation and bladder-voiding difficulties are common in old age and have many possible causes (see below). Privacy is an important component in enabling complete evacuation.

Toilet-Related Skills

Sitting or standing in the correct position for long enough, using lavatory paper, flushing the lavatory, handwashing and many other incidental skills are all part of independence in toileting. The nurse's assessment determines which, if any, of these prerequisites for successful elimination are lacking for each individual. Care should be planned that aims to maximise each individual's potential for independent continence.

Drugs

Many drugs influence continence. The most obvious are diuretics, which exacerbate urgency and frequency and may contribute to constipation. Sedation in any form lessens awareness of a full bladder or bowel. Both are overused for older people, with a recent study identifying the continuing problem of excessive polypharmacy and potentially inappropriate prescribing in care homes (MacRae et al., 2021). The most commonly reported adverse drug events in MacRae et al.'s study were in drugs predisposing to constipation (35.8%), sedation (27.7%) and renal injury (18.0%).

Many drugs have unintended side effects, such as constipation (e.g., many analgesics) or difficulty emptying the bladder (e.g., Parkinson's drugs, some antipsychotics and antidepressants). Polypharmacy is common in old age; it

is essential all incontinent people have their drug regimens reviewed to determine if medication influences continence (see Chapter 31).

Emotions

Many incontinent people appear anxious or depressed. It is difficult to say whether this is a cause or effect of their problem. Most of us can identify with needing to use the toilet more often when under stress. Unfortunately, worrying about leakage can become a self-fulfilling prophecy, especially for individuals who experience urgency.

DEFECATION

Many older people seem obsessed by their bowels. Having lived through an era when the medical profession extolled the virtue of at least one bowel motion per day and weekly purgation, many become distressed if they do not achieve this. In fact, the range of normality is wide and lies between three motions per day and one every 3 days, with little if any variation due to age or gender.

Normal Defecation

Figure 22.1 shows the normal anatomy of the colon and rectum. The colon receives about 600 ml of faecal matter from the small bowel per day. Normal colonic activity includes propulsion of the faecal matter and absorption of fluid, so 150–200 ml of faeces finally reach the rectum each day. Normal defecation usually follows a mass movement of bowel contents, often stimulated by eating or physical activity. They usually deliver a substantial proportion of colonic contents to the rectum.

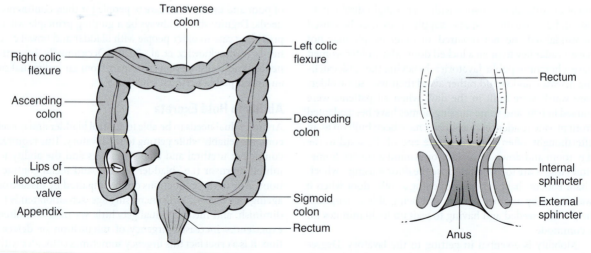

Fig. 22.1 Normal anatomy of the colon and rectum.

Rectal filling leads to a sensation of needing to defecate and automatic reflex relaxation of the smooth-muscle internal anal sphincter (i.e., rectoanal inhibitory reflex). This enables the stool to move into the upper anal canal, where sensitive nerve receptors distinguish different rectal contents (e.g., gas, liquid or solid). The external anal sphincter is voluntary skeletal muscle. If passage of stool or flatus is inconvenient at this moment, the person can contract the external sphincter to retain rectal contents. This contraction is maintained for long enough for the internal sphincter to recover its resting tone automatically and the rectum to relax. The stool is propelled backward into the rectum, and usually the feeling of needing to empty the bowels becomes less acute.

Once at the toilet, the external sphincter and puborectalis muscle are relaxed. This, sometimes coupled with a slight voluntary rise in abdominal pressure, stimulates a coordinated rectal contraction, and the rectum should empty with minimal effort. If the call to stool is ignored, defecation can be delayed for considerable periods. An increasing amount of fluid is absorbed from the stool, so the longer the delay, the harder the stool tends to become.

CONSTIPATION

Each of us knows what someone means when they say they are constipated; however, in fact different people mean very different things, depending on past experience and expectations. The most common use of the term refers to difficult and/or infrequent defecation.

Constipation is associated with a variety of symptoms besides difficulty in evacuating rectal contents. Stools may be hard or pellet-size, and there may be a feeling of incomplete evacuation. Some people can evacuate only by using a finger in the rectum to help. Many constipated people complain of abdominal pain or cramps, bloating and general malaise or fatigue. In extreme cases, nausea, headaches and halitosis are present.

By itself, constipation seldom has serious or life-threatening consequences. Minor anorectal conditions such as haemorrhoids, fissures or rectal mucosal prolapse may be precipitated or exacerbated, and, in immobile older people, faecal incontinence may result. It may be a precipitating factor for confusion in vulnerable individuals. Old wives' tales such as poisoning of the blood have little factual basis, although this does not stop many people from believing in the imperative of a daily bowel motion for inner cleanliness. Constipation does, however, cause chronic discomfort and distress. If faecal impaction results, overflow faecal incontinence may occur; very rarely, bowel perforation from a faecaloma occurs in older people.

A large-scale prospective population survey (Verkuijl et al., 2020) found women were twice as likely to develop constipation as men and that constipation was much more prevalent in women of childbearing age than older women. Ageing does not, of itself, decrease colonic motility or transit time or decrease rectal sensation or bowel frequency. It may be the image of constipation increasing with age has more to do with expectations and attitudes, immobility, frailty and other concomitant conditions rather than age itself, as there is no evidence ageing is a cause of constipation. Many more older people take regular laxatives than younger people. Older people may report fear of constipation and feel the need to use laxatives on a daily basis, often self-medicating with over-the-counter medication and reporting symptoms such as bloating, urges, excessive flatus, nausea and cramps as a result. They often have a preference for a particular type of laxative and continue with it even after seeking help for constipation symptoms (Mihaylov et al., 2008).

Constipation results from a failure of colonic propulsion (i.e., slow transit), a failure to evacuate the rectum or a combination of both (McCrea et al., 2008). Box 22.1 lists the most common underlying causes of each. It is possible to have more than one of these problems contributing to symptoms of constipation, and often there is a complex interaction of causes.

Stool consistency affects both transit and evacuation and is to some extent regulated by diet. Dietary fibre is indigestible carbohydrates (i.e., non-starch polysaccharides) that are not digested in the small bowel. When it reaches the colon, it provides an ideal nutritional medium for the normal commensal colonic bacteria. Bacterial cell bodies form 40%–55% of the bulk of material in the colon and in addition help retain fluid in the gut lumen as bacteria contain 80% water. Normally stool weight varies considerably despite a constant fibre intake. Although it is commonly believed low dietary fibre is associated with constipation, and it is known an increase in fibre improves colonic transit time and increases stool weight, there is little evidence chronically constipated people eat a different diet from non-constipated people or that an increase in fibre intake controls the problem if it is severe. Constipated people seem to respond less well to fibre than others (Ho et al., 2012).

People who are unwell or generally weak may be unable to generate enough abdominal effort to stimulate a defecation reflex. Poor toilet facilities or lack of privacy can exacerbate this. Confused people sometimes fail to realise what social behaviour is required for toileting and ignore the urge to defecate.

The physical environment plays a role in constipation for some older people. As physical height declines, a toilet may be too high for the feet to touch the floor with ease.

BOX 22.1 Common Causes of Constipation

Delay in Colonic Transit

- Inadequate dietary fibre
- Inadequate fluid intake (i.e., dehydration)
- Immobility
- Neuropathy: Gut wall (i.e., myenteric plexus) or peripheral or central nervous system (e.g., Parkinson's disease, diabetic neuropathy)
- Myopathy
- Megacolon or megarectum
- Hormonal or endocrine disorder (e.g., hypothyroidism)
- Drug-induced (e.g., opiate analgesia, anticholinergics, iron)
- Bowel disorders (e.g., irritable bowel syndrome, diverticular disease, carcinoma)
- Psychiatric disorders (e.g., anorexia nervosa, depression)

Evacuation Difficulties

- Hard stools
- Secondarily to painful anorectal conditions (e.g., haemorrhoids, fissure, solitary rectal ulcer)
- Descending perineum or rectocoele
- Paradoxical pelvic floor contraction (i.e., anismus)
- General debility and ineffective abdominal effort
- Poor toilet facilities (e.g., lack of access, privacy or poor posture on toilet)
- Hirschsprung's disease
- Neuropathy
- Confusion or intellectual impairment
- Rectal mucosal prolapse or solitary rectal ulcer syndrome

This inhibits effective use of abdominal muscles to aid defecation. Provision of a footstool can enable a better defecation posture. In institutional settings, attention to adequate privacy is important.

Each constipated person needs a thorough individual assessment to discover the cause. Rectal examination for stool presence and consistency is an important component of a nursing assessment (Royal College of Nursing, 2019), although digital rectal examination provides an unreliable indicator of colonic loading, particularly when stools are soft and putty-like rather than hard. Plain abdominal radiography may not be helpful, but a transit study using radiopaque markers gives an accurate picture of the speed of colonic transit and is particularly useful in laxative-refractory constipation (Sharma et al., 2021).

Treating Constipation

Mild constipation sometimes respond to simple dietary manipulation, which is probably useful in prophylaxis, although the effectiveness of only increasing fibre for someone whose constipation is bad enough to seek medical attention is doubtful. Increased bulk should improve transit time, thus decreasing the opportunity for water absorption and breakdown of bacterial cell bodies, and improve peristalsis, delivering a softer stool to the rectum and probably protecting against diverticular disease. However, although fibre increases stool bulk and has many health benefits (Gill et al., 2021), it does not improve stool consistency or treatment outcomes (Yang et al., 2012).

The average adult daily intake of fibre for adults in the United Kingdom is 18 g (British Dietetic Association, 2021), around 60% of the recommended amount. However, as noted above, constipated people often derive less benefit from fibre than non-constipated people as the non-starch polysaccharides tend to be broken down more with slow transit. Raw bran may upset mineral balance in vulnerable individuals. Fibre often needs to be combined with minor lifestyle changes, such as allowing adequate time for defecation and not ignoring the call to defecate. Great care should be taken to increase fibre intake gradually as a sudden increase can cause bloating and abdominal discomfort. Fibre supplements should be avoided in immobile older people as it is likely to add to the problem and even result in faecal incontinence. A systematic review did not identified strong or consistent evidence for the benefit of fibre in an institutionalised population (Kenny & Skelly, 2001). As there are many types of non-starch polysaccharides, and its content in individual foods varies, it is difficult to estimate intake and predict response.

The most widely used treatment for constipation is laxatives. Considering how widely used both prescribed and over-the-counter laxatives are, there have been remarkably few comparative trials (Petticrew et al., 1997). It is often a case of trial and error to find a laxative that works for an individual with minimal side effects. Older people are at risk of increased adverse effects of laxative use, such as electrolyte disturbances, due to age-related changes (Pont et al., 2019).

Bulking agents can help individuals who find dietary fibre supplements unpalatable; however, they should always be introduced gradually, after clearance of any impacted faeces and with adequate fluid intake; otherwise there is a danger of intestinal obstruction or merely adding to the impacted mass. Bulk-forming laxatives are not always appropriate for use with older people due to the associated need to increase fluid intake (Emmanuel et al., 2017). There is no evidence increasing fluid intake to abnormally high levels helps constipation. Although clinically dehydrated individuals may benefit, normal gut secretions far exceed the daily fluid intake, and excess intake is voided by the urinary not the digestive system.

Stimulant laxatives should be used with extreme caution if it is suspected the patient is faecally impacted, especially with concurrent disease such as diverticulitis. Osmotic laxatives such as lactulose and polyethylene glycols act by retaining fluid in the stool and thereby softening it. Polyethylene glocols such as Movicol and Laxido are licenced for use in disimpaction (NICE, 2022). There is a need for many more placebo-controlled studies before it is possible to make general recommendations on laxative use, however, recruitment to such studies may be challenging. One major funded study into the comparative effectiveness of laxative use vs. laxatives plus lifestyle advice ended early due to low recruitment (Speed et al., 2010).

Individuals who are resistant to fibre or oral laxatives may find a rectal stimulant in the form of a suppository or enema has better results. The results are often more predictable and easier to manage.

As lack of exercise and mobility are widely cited as causes of constipation in old age, it seems logical exercise might improve constipation. The mode of action might be to stimulate colonic motility and mass movements or that the mobile individual has more opportunity to use the toilet. In reality increasing exercise for many older people is challenging to achieve. Although some studies have suggested exercise may improve outcomes for people with constipation, most studies are methodologically flawed, and evidence is therefore inconclusive (Gao et al., 2019). Nurses should be mindful older people may feel preached at to eat more fibre, drink more fluid and exercise more, but the evidence to support these interventions is limited, and there is no proven link between exercise and alleviation of constipation (Annells & Koch, 2003).

FAECAL INCONTINENCE

Studies have found widely varying prevalence rates of faecal incontinence, depending on the definition of incontinence used and the population. Prevalence increases with advancing age in both sexes. A recent systematic review of the prevalence of faecal incontinence among older people living in care homes found medians of included studies of faecal incontinence alone, double incontinence and all faecal incontinence to be 3.5% (interquartile range [IQR] 2.8%), 47.1% (IQR 32.1%), and 42.8% (IQR 21.1%), respectively) (Musa et al., 2019). Faecal incontinence was most commonly associated with cognitive impairment, limited functional capacity, urinary incontinence, reduced mobility, advanced age and diarrhoea. Faecal incontinence has a prevalence in a hospital population of 11%, increasing with age to >21% in older people over 85.

There are many causes of faecal incontinence (Norton & Chelvanayagam, 2004) (see Table 22.3). Childbirth, with consequent sphincter damage, is probably the most common, but chronic diarrhoea, local anorectal pathology and neurological disease are also common. Treatment depends on accurate diagnosis and remedy for the underlying cause and is the same in old age as for younger folks (Norton & Chelvanayagam, 2004). Dependent older people may be incontinent of faeces secondarily to impaction (see below).

Constipation, Impaction and Faecal Incontinence in Old Age

There is a well-recognised association between severe constipation with faecal impaction and incontinence of solid or liquid stool, often referred to as spurious diarrhoea or overflow, particularly among frail older adults in institutional care. However, the mechanism for this incontinence remains somewhat obscure. It has often been suggested impaction of the rectum causes anal relaxation, but anal resting and squeeze pressures have been found to be similar in impacted individuals compared with pressures in age-matched non-impacted controls. There is, however, a reduction in sensation and in the volume of rectal distension needed to elicit internal sphincter relaxation via the rectoanal inhibitory reflex and some loss of the anorectal angle in incontinent individuals. It is unclear which of these mechanisms is the cause or effect of impaction or subsequent incontinence. It may be that once impaction is present—possibly caused by a combination of immobility, low fluid and fibre intake, drug side effects, confusion, lack of privacy and many other factors—lack of sensation makes it difficult to contract the external sphincter appropriately

TABLE 22.3 Common Causes of Faecal Incontinence (Norton & Chelvanayagam, 2004)

Primary Problem	Common Causes
Anal sphincter or pelvic floor damage	Obstetric trauma
	Iatrogenic (e.g., haemorrhoidectomy, anal stretch, lateral sphincterotomy)
	Idiopathic degeneration
	Direct trauma or injury (e.g., impalement)
	Congenital anomaly
Gut motility/stool consistency	Infection
	Inflammatory bowel disease
	Irritable bowel syndrome
	Pelvic irradiation
	Diet
	Emotions/anxiety
Anorectal pathology	Rectal prolapse
	Anal or rectovaginal fistula
	Haemorrhoids or skin tags
Neurological disease	Spinal cord injury
	Multiple sclerosis
	Spina bifida, sacral agenesis
Secondary to degenerative neurological disease	Alzheimer's disease, or environmental (see below)
Impaction with overflow 'spurious diarrhoea'	Institutionalised or immobile older people
Lifestyle and environmental	Poor toilet facilities
	Inadequate care/non-available assistance
	Drugs with gut side-effects
	Frailty and dependence
Idiopathic	Unknown cause

to prevent leakage when the internal sphincter relaxes in response to rectal distension.

Older people with hard faeces in the rectum may have diminished rectal sensation and not experience a normal urge to defaecate. However, not all faecal impaction is in the presence of hard stool; many older people with impaction develop massive faecal loading with soft stool. Laxatives and excess fibre intake are responsible for most of this soft impaction. Treatment of constipation has been found to resolve faecal incontinence in a nursing-home population (Chassagne et al., 2000). Careful assessment is vital to diagnose faecal impaction, a common cause of intestinal obstruction in older adults. If misdiagnosed,

anti-diarrhoeal medication may be administered, which can exacerbate the constipation (De Giorgio et al., 2015).

Patients who are generally frail and dependent on others for help with daily activities of living need to have their bowel care actively planned to pre-empt problems, particularly impaction with overflow. With meticulous attention to routine, diet, fluid intake, maximising mobility with passive movement if necessary, motivation, staff/carer attitudes, defecation posture, drug regimens and the many other factors that can contribute to the issue, many problems can be kept in check. However, the emphasis is often on management rather than prevention, and increased workforce training to prevent and manage faecal incontinence may be needed. Figure 22.2 gives expert-consensus-derived algorithms for the management of faecal incontinence in old age (Abrams et al., 2017).

MICTURITION

Disorders of micturition become increasingly common with age. However, ageing per se does not lead to incontinence. It is usually a combination of impairment of bladder function and a variety of precipitating factors that upset an often delicate balance and produce incontinence. Bladder capacity decreases with age, thereby increasing frequency of micturition. Urethral outlet pressure decreases in women. A meta-analysis identified a global prevalence of 37% of urinary incontinence in older women aged 55 and over, with some important contributory factors being obesity, diabetes, educational level, childbirth and presence of UTIs (Batmani et al., 2021).

Nocturia (i.e., rising at night to pass urine) affects most older people, with nocturia one or two times at night considered normal. Over the age of 80, 70% to 90% of people get up at night to pass urine. There is evidence many older people experience a disturbed diurnal rhythm of urine production. Instead of producing most urine during waking hours, older people often produce urine evenly throughout the 24 hours or even more at night. This is probably due to changes in the production of antidiuretic hormone and exacerbated by renal or heart disease, worsened if sleep is disturbed for other reasons. Frail older people may additionally spend more hours in bed, increasing the likelihood of needing to empty the bladder while in bed. Simple measures such as elevating the feet or using compression stockings toward the end of the day to encourage venous return, reducing fluid intake for a few hours before bedtime and changing timing of diuretics can be helpful to people with troublesome nocturia (Fonda et al., 2002).

Many people experience diurnal frequency and urgency, and, in community-dwelling adults, about 20% have some degree of urinary incontinence, which affects upward of 50%

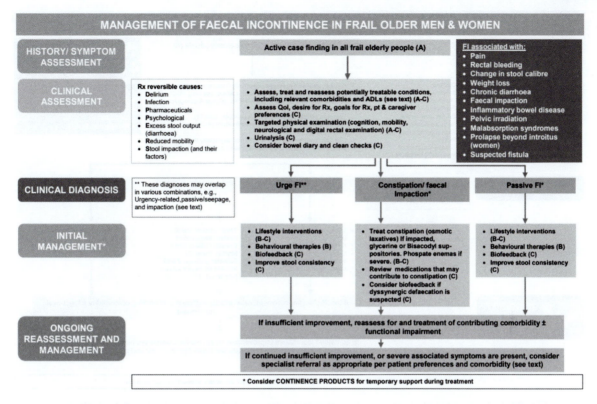

MANAGEMENT OF FAECAL INCONTINENCE IN FRAIL OLDER MEN & WOMEN

Fig. 22.2 Management of faecal incontinence in frail older men and women. *UTI*, Urinary tract infection; *CNS*, central nervous system; *MSU*, midstream urine; *LUT*, lower urinary tract. (Reproduced from Abrams et al. [2017] with permission of International Continence Society.)

in nursing homes (NHS England, 2018). As age advances, men, who have lower prevalence rates than women in younger age groups, also report increased levels of incontinence. In men aged 70 to 80 years the prevalence rates are about half those in women. Severity of incontinence also increases with advancing age (Nitti, 2001). However, it is important not to assume everyone who reports incontinence is bothered by it. For some individuals it is a minor nuisance, but bother is more commonly reported in women, and how bothersome people find symptoms influences health care–seeking behaviour.

UTIs are present in over 10% of older people and up to 50% of individuals in institutional care. One in two men is likely to experience symptoms attributable to prostatic hypertrophy by the 8th decade of life. Urge urinary incontinence is associated with a 26% increased risk of falls and a 34% increased risk of fractures. A recent meta-analysis confirmed urinary incontinence is a risk factor for falls in both older men and women and is associated with recurrent falls (Moon et al., 2021).

Control over bladder function, as with bowels, is likely to face many other insults in addition to physiological dysfunction with increasing age, including other diseases, multiple medications, difficulties with mobility and mental agility. Incontinence is often precipitated by these extrabladder factors. Resnick (1984) coined the mnemonic DIAPPERS:

- D Delirium (e.g., confusion)
- I Infection (e.g., symptomatic UTI)
- A Atrophic urethritis or vaginitis in women
- P Psychological (e.g., severe depression, neurosis)
- P Pharmacologic
- E Excessive fluid intake or output
- R Restricted mobility and environmental
- S Stool impaction (e.g, constipation)

It is usually necessary to treat both the bladder and these other factors to achieve continence.

Complete urinary continence may not be achievable for all older people. This does not mean care has failed. A state of dependent continence or social continence may enable an

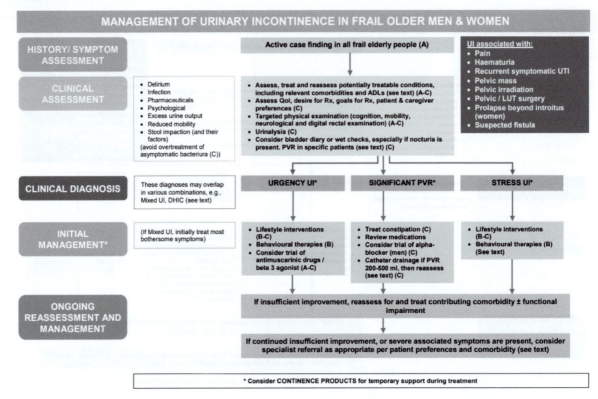

Fig. 22.3 Management of urinary incontinence in frail older men and women. *UTI*, Urinary tract infection; *CNS*, central nervous system; *MSU*, midstream urine; *LUT*, lower urinary tract. (Reproduced from Abrams et al. (2017) with permission of International Continence Society.)

individual to maintain dignity and continue desired activities despite imperfect bladder control (Fonda et al., 2002).

Bladder Dysfunction in Old Age

Most people with urinary symptoms have an underlying bladder dysfunction. In old age, two or even three separate problems may be present in combination. It is important to obtain an accurate diagnosis, as the treatments are different. Usually a careful history and examination indicates the cause, but if in doubt, urodynamic studies are necessary to distinguish bladder dysfunctions (Abrams et al., 2017). Figure 22.3 gives expert consensus–derived algorithms for the management of urinary incontinence in old age (Abrams et al., 2017). Assessment should be multidisciplinary and approached in a stepwise logical order, first to identify and treat reversible causes and subsequently to determine the best management option for individuals with established incontinence (Karim & Rantell, 2021). A fit older person should be treated for incontinence in exactly the same manner as younger people, with the full range of options, including surgery, considered.

Lifestyle Alteration and Education

Box 22.2 gives suggested components of assessment in frail older adults (Lekan-Rutledge & Colling, 2003). Most patients can be managed with non-pharmacologic treatments and lifestyle changes nurses can initiate. Treatment often involves addressing mobility and toilet access, diet to avoid constipation, adequate but not excessive fluid intake, caffeine reduction and advice on increasing exercise and reducing obesity. As would be expected, increased fluid intake increases the volume and frequency of voiding. However, increased fluid intake probably does not actually cause frequency or incontinence in the absence of other problems such as an overactive bladder. Ensuring adequate fluid intake does not increase incontinence and helps protect against UTI and bladder cancer. Excessive fluid intake (over 3 litres in 24 hours) may increase incontinence, and restricting fluids for 2 hours before bed may improve nocturnal voiding (Gray & Krissovich, 2003).

Although the evidence base for many suggested lifestyle changes is not strong, clinically and in combination, they are often found to be useful. Several systematic reviews explored

BOX 22.2 Components of Assessment in Frail Older Adults

History and Symptoms
- Symptoms of stress, urge, mixed or functional incontinence
- Voiding and incontinence pattern
- Fluid intake and type
- Bowel habits
- Smoking
- Functional assessment
  - Activities of daily living, mobility and exercise
  - Cognition and affect
- Other medical conditions and medication
- Impact of incontinence, quality of life and motivation
- Environment and carers
- Patient's preferences for treatment

Clinical and Physical Assessment
- Assess for reversible causes and treat if present (e.g., DIAPPERS)
- Physical examination (e.g., abdominal, rectal, vaginal, prostate)
- Bladder diary for 3–5 days for voids, volumes and incontinence
- Urinalysis
- Postvoid residual urine volume

Environmental Assessment
- Distance to toilet
- Accessibility of toilet or alternative (e.g., commode or urinal)
- Carer's availability and willingness to help
- Walking aids
- Dexterity and clothing

Formulate Diagnosis
- Based on the assessment determine, and where possible address, all factors that may be relevant to each individual patient.
- Consider need for specialist referral

(Adapted from Fantl, et al., 1990; Resnick, et al., 1988; Yu, et al., 1990.)

conservative management of urinary incontinence in older people in a variety of populations and settings, which included interventions directed at education for older adults (Flanagan et al., 2012; Roe et al., 2015; Stenzelius et al., 2015). All these reviews concluded more robust studies are needed.

Overactive Bladder

Although stress urinary incontinence (see below) is common among the general population, especially among women, an unstable or overactive bladder—also known as urge urinary incontinence—is the most common bladder dysfunction in old age. The person loses the ability to inhibit detrusor contractions reliably and experiences urgency and frequency. If this is severe, or the person is immobile or asleep or no lavatory is at hand, incontinence may result.

Behavioural interventions are the mainstay of treatment for an overactive bladder. Table 22.4 outlines the various programmes described in the literature (Wyman et al., 2009). However, many variations and combinations of therapy are described. Bladder training, with or without the help of medication, should be the first option in treatment for cognitively intact individuals. There is good evidence bladder retraining reduces urge, stress and mixed urge and stress incontinence in older women (Wyman et al., 2009). Although there is no nursing consensus as to what is meant by bladder training, most programmes involve keeping a baseline chart for 3 to 7 days and then working out an individualised pattern of target toilet visits gradually to extend the time between voidings. With plenty of support and encouragement, many patients learn to overcome their urgency and establish a normal pattern without urgency. There is evidence of an incremental benefit from advice on lifestyle and diet (e.g., caffeine reduction), bladder training and pelvic muscle exercise, with a decrease in severity of incontinence of 61% 2 years after behavioural management, compared with an increase of 184% in severity of incontinence in controls (Dougherty et al., 2002). Timed voiding may also be of benefit; family caregivers may be able to implement an individualised toileting programme that leads to a significant reduction in incontinent episodes, especially if the patient is mobile and has only mild to moderate cognitive impairment.

Urge incontinence can also be controlled pharmacologically by inhibiting unstable detrusor muscle contractions. Adding an antimuscarinic drug alongside behavioural treatment is well tolerated in older people, but side effects such as constipation may become problematic. The antimuscarinics oxybutynin chloride and tolterodine are probably the most widely used drugs available at present as they are off patent and therefore the least expensive options. Current guidelines (NICE, 2019a) recommend prescribing the drug with the lowest acquisition cost. However, many prescribers opt for a newer, more expensive drug such as trospium or solifenacin as they have a lower side-effect profile and are therefore better tolerated. Some drugs that were previously used, such as propantheline and imipramine, should not be prescribed for overactive bladder, and oxybutinin should not be prescribed for people at risk of deterioration in their physical or mental health (NICE, 2019a). Side effects of anti-muscarinic

TABLE 22.4   Behavioural Interventions for Managing Urinary Symptoms and Promoting Bladder Health (Wyman et al., 2009)

Technique	Description	SYMPTOM			
		Frequency	Urgency	UUI	MUI
Habit Changes (Managing Symptoms and Promoting Bladder Health)					
Lifestyle modification	Diet, fluid, bowel and weight management; smoking cessation	X	X	X	X
Timed voiding*	Urination at a fixed interval that avoids the symptom (useful for urgency and UI not associated with frequency)		X	X	X
Training Techniques (Managing Symptoms)					
Urgency control techniques	Deep breathing and using complex mental tasks (reciting poetry, counting backward from 100 by 7 s etc.) to ignore urgency	X	X	X	X
Bladder training	Progressively increasing interval between voidings; utilises distraction and relaxation techniques to gradually increase the time between urinations	X	X	X	X
Multicomponent behavioural training*	Teaching to not rush to bathroom in response to urgency and use of PFM contractions to supress bladder contraction and delay voiding, with use of pelvic floor muscle exercises	X	X	X	X
Pelvic floor muscle training	Daily regimen of pelvic floor muscle contractions to maintain or build strength and endurance			X	X
Delayed voiding*	Progressively increasing interval between onset of urgency and voiding	X	X	X	X

*Using a bladder diary. *UUI*, Urgency urinary incontinence; *MUI*, mixed urinary incontinence; *PFM*, pelvic floor muscle.

drugs, such as a dry mouth, disturbed vision and constipation, are very common with therapeutically effective doses. Postural hypotension is also a possibility in frail older adults. Prescribers should be mindful of the potential for anticholinergic burden when adding an antimuscarinic drug alongside other drugs with similar effects and the potential impact it may have for cognitive decline for older people (Bell & Avery, 2021).

Mirabegron is a relatively new β3-adrenoreceptor agonist for treatment of overactive bladder with urge urinary incontinence and has similar efficacy to anticholinergic drugs but without the risk of anticholinergic effects. Mirabegron has been recommended since 2013 for the treament of overactive bladder but only for people in whom antimuscarinic drugs are contraindicated, not clinically effective or have unacceptable side effects (NICE, 2013). Initially data from use in trials with older people were lacking, but it has been shown to be safe in older people (Makhani et al.,

2020) and does not appear to impair cognitive function (Griebling et al., 2020).

Electrical stimulation, usually administered via vaginal or skin electrodes at home or in a clinic setting, has shown promise compared to no active treatment or placebo in early studies (Stewart et al., 2016), although there is insufficient evidence and therefore current guidelines recommend this intervention is used (NICE, 2019a).

Stress Urinary Incontinence

Stress urinary incontinence is most common in parous women and may be associated with atrophic changes in the vagina and urethra or vaginal prolapse. The symptom of stress incontinence is leakage on physical exertion such as cough. If severe, even minimal rises in abdominal pressure such as during walking or the act of standing from a chair, provoke leakage. If incontinence is slight to moderate, there is strong evidence relief is gained from pelvic muscle exercises. Women who undergo pelvic floor muscle training for stress incontinence are eight times more likely to report being cured and having improved symptoms (Dumoulin et al., 2018). Pelvic floor exercises may also help someone with urgency to hang on a little more effectively and avoid urge incontinence.

Simple teaching of techniques such as the knack (i.e., intentionally contracting the pelvic floor muscles before and during a cough or other rise in intra-abdominal pressure) can dramatically reduce urine loss within 1 week.

The success of pelvic muscle exercises depends on

- Patient motivation: There is no doubt these exercises are boring, and it is difficult to remember to do them as often as needed. Regular follow-up has an important role in keeping a patient motivated and giving feedback on progress.
- Correct teaching: Most people are unaware of the pelvic floor and do not perform the exercises correctly unless properly taught and reassessed at intervals. A digital vaginal or rectal examination is the best way to teach pelvic floor exercises. Many patients practise them incorrectly, and even counterproductively, without this teaching.
- Correct initial diagnosis: Pelvic floor exercises are not a panacea for all types of incontinence.

Sometimes vaginal cones or electrotherapy are a useful adjunct to pelvic floor exercises.

Long-term adherence to exercises is sometimes a problem, and long-term benefit probably depends on at least some exercises being performed on an ongoing basis. Various health education techniques have been tried to enhance long-term compliance with exercises, but none has been found more advantageous than good physiotherapy teaching alone (Alewijnse et al., 2003), with women with the highest urine loss initially being the most likely to keep performing the exercises.

Drugs have a limited role in stress incontinence. Oestrogen replacement may help if oestrogens are administered topically; a Cochrane review found significantly more women report improvement in symptoms than those given a placebo (Cody et al., 2012). There was no benefit from systemic osetrogen, however, with some women reporting worsening symptoms. Current guidelines recommend systemic oestrogen treatment is not used (NICE, 2019a).

Urinary incontinence in men following prostatectomy has been found to be less severe and to resolve more quickly if men practise pelvic muscle exercises (Van Kampen, 2000), but long-term results seem to be similar whether or not exercises are performed, suggesting perhaps it is most cost-effective to reserve intensive exercise programmes for individuals who are most symptomatic (Dumoulin et al., 2017).

More severe stress incontinence, particularly if associated with prolapse, usually requires surgical correction, for which advanced age is no contraindication. Older women may achieve better results from surgery than younger ones as they are less likely to undertake vigorous exercise that may disrupt the repair. Traditionally, a suprapubic rather than vaginal approach to surgery gives the best results. However, a technique for insertion under local or brief general anaesthetic of tension-free vaginal tape is now in widespread use as a minimally invasive technique, usually performed as a day-case without open surgery. The National Institute for Health and Care Excellence recommends three types of surgery for stress incontinence in women in the United Kingdom—colposuspension, rectus fascial sling and the retropublic sling—and has produced a patient decision aid (NICE, 2019b). Recently the safety of mesh surgery has been called into question and there have been legal cases worldwide against the manufacturers, sparking debate about the utility of this surgery (Glazener, 2015). Complications associated with mesh procedures for stress urinary incontinence include haemorrhage, organ perforation, mesh erosion, infection, sexual dysfunction, bowel problems and pain (Keltie et al., 2017), which may require further surgery that may or may not be successful. There is little data about longer-term rates of complications and concerns rates seen in everyday practice may be higher than previously thought, with many women feeling their concerns and complaints were not taken seriously. A pause in mesh surgery was implemented in 2017 and called for in 2020 (Independent Medicines and Medical Devices Safety Review, 2020). If mesh surgery is considered, it should always be a last resort.

Another minimally invasive approach is to inject collagen or similar synthetic material around the bladder neck to give added support, which can be done under local anaesthetic as an outpatient. Success rates of 43% have been found in older women injected, which are maintained in the long-term (Plotti et al., 2018). Sometimes a vaginal ring pessary produces symptomatic relief.

Incomplete Voiding

In both sexes, postvoid residual urine volume increases with age, often due to a combination of urethral outflow obstruction and impaired detrusor muscle contractility, with 50–100 ml considered normal and volumes above that as potentially significant. Prostatic enlargement in men is the most common cause of outflow obstruction, which can occur in either gender because of faecal impaction or a pelvic mass. The patient usually experiences frequency and difficulty voiding. Residual urine may accumulate in the bladder, and overflow incontinence usually presents as continuous non-specific dribbling. Treatment involves relief of the obstruction. Simple mechanical methods such as an intravaginal pessary to support genital prolapse are often overlooked but can provide ongoing help to many older women who do not wish for surgical solutions for prolapse.

If the detrusor muscle fails to contract for micturition, or if the contraction is not sustained until the bladder is empty, a chronic residual collection of urine may be present. This can become infected and lead to overflow incontinence. It is now recognised many frail older people have both an overactive unstable bladder, causing frequency, and impaired contractility on micturition and therefore incomplete emptying. This can be a drug side effect of antimuscarinic drugs used to treat overactive bladder, but previous spinal injury, back surgery or pelvic surgery have been identified as independent risk factors (Park & Palmer, 2015). An important element of patient assessment is an estimation of postvoid residual urine volume, either using portable ultrasonography or an in–out catheter; this is very often missed as a cause of incontinence in older people of both genders (Abrams et al., 2017).

The use of intermittent (i.e., in–out) catheterisation to drain this residual urine is widespread. Some people can be taught to self-catheterise, in which case a clean, non-sterile technique is taught; for others, a relative or nurse must do the catheterisation. Some patients regain detrusor tone with this management and resume voiding; for others, the intermittent catheterisation must become long-term management. Age is not associated with failure to learn the technique, but mobility issues, difficulty reaching the perineum and cognitive impairment are (Hentzen et al., 2018).

Urinary Tract Infection (UTI)

Older people with a UTI may not present with the same symptoms as younger people. Probably the most useful way to treat a UTI is to distinguish between acute infection and asymptomatic bacteriuria. An older adult with a sudden onset of the symptoms and cystitis—dysuria, pain, frequency, pyrexia and possibly confusion—should receive the appropriate antibiotic therapy, but it should be noted symptoms are often a lot less acute than in younger patients. As many as 80% of older women with urinary incontinence who live in care homes have an asymptomatic bacteriuria (Biggel et al., 2019). Avoiding routine treatment of asymptomatic bacteriuria has been recommended practice, and clinicians were previously encouraged not to treat asymptomatic UTIs to reduce antibiotic prescribing. However, a recent retrospective audit of over 1 million GP records showed reduced or deferred prescribing in older people resulted in increased morbidity and mortality from sepsis, especially from *Escherichia coli* bacteraemia; early prescribing is advocated (Gharbi et al., 2019). Early recognition and treatment is important, especially as symptoms may be less severe in older people.

It is wise to remember symptoms of atrophic urethritis mimic cystitis in older women. Inspection of the vulva reveals if atrophic changes, such as dry, inflamed mucosa, are present. Women with recurrent UTIs may benefit from low-dose topical oestrogen therapy (Leckie, 2010).

INCONTINENCE IN INSTITUTIONAL CARE

Prevalence of incontinence in nursing homes varies from 40% to 70%, depending on case mix; an average of over 50% is accepted as usual (NHS England, 2018). It is associated with immobility, reduced ability to perform activities of daily living, use of restraints and cognitive impairment (Leung & Schnelle, 2008), with dementia and immobility the two factors most strongly associated. It is possible to improve mobility by a structured exercise programme in this group, but the benefits for continence status are unclear, as few who are dependent are capable of becoming independent. Pads are the most commonly used method of management, often in excess of 77%, and have been associated with increased incidence of urinary tract infections (Omli et al., 2010). Residents in nursing homes believe incontinence is inevitable and spend more time and energy hiding the problem than seeking treatment (Robinson, 2000). Continence in this patient group is characterised by four categories (Fig. 22.4) (Wagg, 2017).

Incontinence in residents in homes or hospitals is often associated with multiple undiagnosed and untreated problems, which, if remedied, leads to restoration of continence for some. It cannot be overemphasised an individual assessment is the crucial first step in any nursing intervention. Transient causes may be reversible (e.g., treating an acute UTI or changing medications). However, appropriate assessment of residents is often not carried out.

Toileting Programmes

Most toileting programmes reported for frail older people achieve an average reduction of one or two incontinent episodes per day (Lekan-Rutledge & Colling, 2003; Wagg, 2017). Mobility and unimpaired cognition are likely to be predictors of success.

Prompted Voiding

Prompted voiding provides an opportunity to be assisted to the toilet at regular intervals. Most studies have used a 2-hourly schedule of asking the patient discreetly, up to three times, if they would like help to go to the toilet and taking them if requested. Social interaction and positive verbal feedback are given when the request is appropriate and the toilet used. Twenty percent to 40% of frail

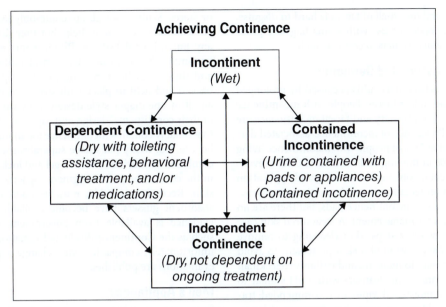

Achieving Continence

Incontinent
(Wet)

Dependent Continence
(Dry with toileting assistance, behavioral treatment, and/or medications)

Contained Incontinence
(Urine contained with pads or appliances)
(Contained incotinence)

Independent Continence
(Dry, not dependent on ongoing treatment)

Fig. 22.4 A paradigm for continence. (Reproduced from Wagg et al. [2017] with permission of International Continence Society.)

nursing-home residents respond well, with severity of incontinence reduced by approximately half. There is some suggestion prompted voiding produces short-term benefits, but there is no evidence of long-term effectiveness or whether the effects continue when prompted voiding is stopped (Eustice et al., 2000). A 3-day trial of prompted voiding is usually sufficient to tell if an individual patient will respond, suggesting this is not a learning response but a positive response to being provided with the opportunity to be continent. It does not help at night. Various regimes, including both 2-hourly and 3-hourly prompts, have been shown to be effective in the short term, but studies of longer term effects are lacking.

The results of many studies are statistically significant, but the clinical significance of results is less clear as few patients become completely continent. Addition of antimuscarinic medication to a prompted voiding programme may yield results that are statistically significant but probably not large enough to be clinically useful in the nursing-home setting except in occasional individual cases.

Habit Training

Habit training is the most complex toileting programme devised for frail older people in nursing homes. It attempts to identify each individual's own natural habit or voiding pattern, then to implement an individualised prompted voiding schedule. An individualised toileting programme may be most difficult to implement in an institutional

setting using largely untrained staff, and caregivers often find it difficult to adhere to protocols (Ostaszkiewicz et al., 2004). The difficulties of introducing innovative programmes and getting staff to comply should not be underestimated. Given the paucity of evidence underpinning this intervention, it is questionable whether habit training is worthwhile.

MANAGEMENT OF INTRACTABLE INCONTINENCE

Even with the best available management and care, some patients remain incontinent. It is important this is recognised as inevitable and nurses do not feel guilty about it. An individual can usually be helped to maintain dignity and comfort in some way. The nurse should teach the patient, or the family, the most suitable management techniques and has an important supportive role in care.

Persistent incontinence can cause other problems; the odour and sore skin caused by leakage of faeces are particularly difficult to cope with. Smell is an understandable concern of many people with incontinence. Freshly voided urine should not smell unpleasant—and if it does, it may be infected. It is contact with air that leads to breakdown of the constituents of urine and the consequent smell. Prompt changing of soiled pads or clothes and storage of soiled materials in an airtight container, along with the hygiene measures outlined below, are the best option. But this is not always possible, and the smell of faeces is hard to disguise. Deodorants developed for use with stoma bags are probably the most useful products to combat smell.

Incontinence-Associated Dermatitis

Incontinence associated dermatitis is caused by prolonged exposure to urine and/or faeces. People with incontinence of liquid stool or both urinary and faceal incontinence are at greatest risk. Prevalence of incontinence-associated dermatitis is upward of 51% of people with incontinence living at home and 30% in nursing and residential care. Prevention and treatment involves skin cleansing and application of leave-on skin protectants alongside continence promotion and correct use of incontinence pads, but there are no specific guidelines for management. A structured skin care regime includes two key steps: skin cleansing to remove urine/faeces and application of a skin protectant to avoid or minimise exposure to moisture and irritants (Beeckman et al., 2016). No-rinse skin cleansers with a pH similar to normal skin or premoistened wipes are recommended; traditional soap should not be used. A wide range of leave-on products are available with different formulations that contain petrolatum, dimethicone, zinc oxide or liquid film-forming acrylate, but there is little evidence of the comparative effectiveness of products for preventing and treating incontinence-associated dermatitis in adults (Beeckman et al., 2016); it is often a case of trial and error to find a product that works for an individual. A funded study to develop and assess the feasibility of a manualised package of care to prevent and treat incontinence-associated dermatitis in care homes is underway (see https://fundingawards.nihr.ac.uk/award/NIHR128865).

Incontinence Products

A good incontinence aid enables an incontinent person to be socially accepted and to lead a relatively normal life. A large range of products for containment are available. The Continence Product Advisor website (https://www.continenceproductadvisor.org) is designed to help people with incontinence and their carers navigate their way to a product suitable for them. An aid must be carefully selected with regard to the individual's degree, type and pattern of incontinence, local anatomy, physical and mental abilities, personal preference, washing or disposal facilities and cost. No one aid suits everyone, and a range should be provided. The nurse must be the patient's advocate in this and be prepared to make a case for the supply of the most appropriate items.

Body-Worn Pads and Pants

Most incontinent women, and some men, use a disposable absorbent pad held in place by pants to collect urine or faeces. Sanitary towels are commonly used by individuals who have not sought help, but they do not cope with any but minimal leakage. Plastic pants are undignified, uncomfortable and can cause considerable skin problems and should not be in routine use. Most pads are plastic-backed and held in place with stretch pants. Others have an all-in-one diaper-style design. They vary in the quality of their constituents, design and capacity. The smallest pad that reliably contains incontinence for an individual should be selected. Many pads have superabsorbent powder that combines with urine to form a gel and lock the urine away in the core of the pad to augment capacity and protect the skin. Recently, washable, reusable pads and pants with absorbent gussets have become available. Good-quality evidence is available from government-funded sources such as the Continence Products Evaluation Network, but unfortunately, companies often change a product before evaluations are published.

Men's Appliances

Some men are able to use a penile sheath or appliance in preference to a pad. A retracted penis or poor manual dexterity make their use difficult. A penile sheath should be carefully selected for appropriate size and is most satisfactory if a self-adhesive variety is used or if held in position with double-sided adhesive tape. It should be connected to a leg bag. Appliances such as pubic pressure urinals should always be fitted by an experienced appliance fitter.

Bed and Chair Protection

Washable bed sheets with a stay-dry surface are comfortable, popular and cost-effective, but in some instances laundry provision is inadequate to cope with them. However, these products offer little protection for a person's skin, and nurses should consider carefully the use of bed and chair protection, refocusing care from protection of the environment to protection of the patient and using body worn pads.

INDWELLING CATHETERS AND OLDER PEOPLE

Generally, the use of an indwelling catheter should be seen very much as a last resort when all other methods of managing micturition have been tried and failed. Widespread, indiscriminate use of catheters has fallen into disrepute, as has their use solely for nursing convenience. A move away from catheters can benefit even severely incontinent patients in many instances.

The decision to use a catheter should be made only for clear and valid reasons, with a definite goal that can be evaluated and in full consultation with all concerned, especially the patient. The individual's quality of life should be the prime consideration. Will the use of a catheter significantly improve independence, comfort and dignity? For some patients (e.g., someone with severe incontinence that is poorly controlled by an aid) a catheter is a great benefit, even enabling community rather than institutional care. Catheters may be indicated for wound healing if incontinence-associated dermatitis is severe, but each decision should be made on an individual basis and re-evaluated at planned intervals.

Managing a Catheter

Many long-term catheters are poorly managed. If a patient has to live with a catheter, drainage must be made convenient and dignified. For day use, a leg bag inside trousers or under a skirt hides the urine from public view. A link system should be used with connection of single-use night bags at the bottom of leg bags without breaking the closed system on a daily basis. The outlet tap should be simple to use and understand, but many fail to meet these criteria. Leg bags should be changed weekly.

Patient teaching and individualised care overcome many problems. The importance of diet, exercise, fluid intake, personal hygiene and avoiding constipation should be emphasised. Sexual function should be discussed, and if the patient is sexually active an alternative to a urethral catheter considered. Sometimes a patient or a partner may be taught to remove and replace the catheter, thus increasing independence, or a catheter can be inserted into the bladder suprapubically via the abdominal wall.

Leakage may be caused by too large a catheter or balloon or by an overactive bladder, which may respond to anticholinergic medication. Catheter blockage is a recurrent problem in 40% to 50% of long-term catheters (Getliffe, 2003) and is most likely in the presence of alkaline urine, often caused when the bladder is colonised by bacteria that produce the enzyme urease, which breaks down urea to release the alkaline ammonia. Preventive administration of acidic catheter maintenance solutions of 50 ml volume should be used only when all other options have been explored (Royal College of Nursing, 2021), but pre-emptive changing may be a better answer. There is no evidence drinking acidic drinks such as cranberry juice prevents bacteriuria or infections. Infections are inevitable with long-term catheter drainage and should be treated only if the patient is symptomatic. If a catheter causes repeated problems, its use should be questioned, since the patient may be better off without it.

SEXUAL FUNCTION

Ageing is not synonymous with becoming asexual. People are often sexually active well into old age (see Chapter 26). Many residents in long-term care facilities remain interested in sex, and some remain sexually active in their care homes. Incontinence can negatively impact sexual functioning yet is rarely discussed or assessed. A recent survey of women over 55 identified 68% of those with a partner were sexually active, and of these only 5% avoided sexual activity because of their incontinence (Visser et al., 2014). Erectile dysfunction in men also impacts sexual relationships. Nurses must not shy away from discussing this topic as impairment of sexual functioning often goes hand in hand with bladder and bowel problems (Rantell, 2021).

CONCLUSION AND LEARNING POINTS

Many older people are at risk of less-than-perfect control over their elimination. It is a nursing responsibility to assess each individual and to plan care in collaboration with other members of the multidisciplinary team. Care should attempt to remedy any bladder or bowel problem and maximise the individual's ability to cope with elimination in a continent manner. In this area nurses can make a significant contribution to the comfort, dignity and well-being of individuals who come into their care.

KEY LEARNING POINTS

- Incontinence is not an inevitable consequence of ageing.
- Bladder and bowel problems among older people are common and frequently hidden, so active case finding is essential.
- Detailed assessment is vital to understand the underlying causes of symptoms and determine the best treatment options.

- The least invasive option should be considered first, including behavioural and conservative interventions, and pharmacological interventions should be prescribed according to current guidelines.
- Bladder and bowel problems are often associated with psychological harm, and nurses should be alert to the risk of anxiety and depression and potential impact on relationships.

REFERENCES

Abrams, P., Cardozo, L., Wagg, A., & Wein, A. (2017). *Incontinence* (6th ed.). International Continence Society.

Alewijnse, D., Metsemakers, J. F. M., Mesters, I. E., & van den Borne, B. (2003). Effectiveness of pelvic floor muscle exercise therapy supplemented with a health education programme to promote long-term adherence among women with urinary incontinence. *Neurourology and Urodynamics, 22*, 284–295.

Annells, M., & Koch, T. (2003). Constipation and the preached trio: Diet, fluid intake, exercise. *International Journal of Nursing Studies, 40*(8), 843–852.

Artero-López, C., Márquez-Hernández, V. V., Estevez-Morales, M. T., & Granados-Gámez, G. (2018). Inertia in nursing care of hospitalised patients with urinary incontinence. *Journal of Clinical Nursing, 27*, 1488–1496.

Batmani, S., Jalali, R., Mohammadi, M., & Bokaee, S. (2021). Prevalence and factors related to urinary incontinence in older adults women worldwide: A comprehensive systematic review and meta-analysis of observational studies. *BMC Geriatrics, 21*, 212.

Beeckman, D., Van Damme, N., Schoonhoven, L., Van Lancker, A., Kottner, J., Beele, H., Gray, M., Woodward, S., Fader, M., Van den Bussche, K., Van Hecke, A., De Meyer, D., & Verhaeghe, S. (2016). Interventions for preventing and treating incontinence-associated dermatitis in adults. *Cochrane Database of Systematic Reviews, 11*, Article CD011627. https://doi.org//10.1002/14651858.CD011627.pub2.

Bell, B., & Avery, A. (2021). Identifying anticholinergic burden in clinical practice. *Prescriber, 32*, 20–23. https://doi.org//10.1002/psb.1901.

Biggel, M., Heytens, S., Latour, K., Bruyndonckx, R., Goossens, H., & Moons, P. (2019). Asymptomatic bacteriuria in older adults: The most fragile women are prone to long-term colonization. *BMC Geriatrics, 19*, 170.

British Dietetic Association. (2021). Fibre: Food fact sheet. https://www.bda.uk.com/resource/fibre.html#:~:text=How%20much%20fibre%20should%20I,aim%20for%2015g%20per%20day

Carvalho, N., Fustinoni, S., Abolhassani, N., Blanco, J. M., Meylan, L., & Santos-Eggimann, B. (2020). Impact of urine and mixed incontinence on long-term care preference: A vignette-survey study of community-dwelling older adults. *BMC Geriatrics, 20*(1), 69.

Chassagne, P., Jego, A., Gloc, P., Capet, C., Trivvale, C., Doucet, J., Denis, P. & Bercoff, E. (2000). Does treatment of constipation improve faecal incontinence in institutionalized elderly patients? *Age and Ageing, 29*, 159–164.

Cody, J. D., Jacobs, M. L., Richardson, K., Moehrer, B., & Hextall, A. (2012). Oestrogen therapy for urinary incontinence in post-menopausal women. *Cochrane Database Syst Rev., 10*(10), CD001405. Doi:10.1002/14651858.CD001405.pub3. https://10.1002/14651858.CD001405.pub3.

Corey, H., & Duff, V. (2021). The value of nurses specialized in wound, ostomy, and continence: A systematic review. *Advances in Skin & Wound Care, 34*(10), 551–559.

De Giorgio, R., Ruggeri, E., Stanghellini, V., Eusebi, L. H., Bazzoli, F., & Chiarioni, G. (2015). Chronic constipation in the elderly: a primer for the gastroenterologist. *BMC Gastroenterology, 15*, 130.

Dougherty, M. C., Dwyer, J. W., Pendergast, J. F., Boyington, A. R., Tomlinson, B. U., Coward, R. T., Duncan, R. P., Vogel, B., & Rooks, L. G. (2002). A randomized trial of behavioral management for continence in older rural women. *Research into Nursing Health, 25*, 3–13.

Drennan, V. M., Cole, L., & Iliffe, S. (2011). A taboo within a stigma? A qualitative study of managing incontinence with people with dementia living at home. *BMC Geriatrics, 11*, 75.

Dumoulin, C., Adewuyi, T., Booth, J., Bradley, C., Burgio, K., Hagen, S., Hunter, K., Imamura, M., Morin, M., Morkved, S., Thakar, R., Wallace, S., & Williams, K. (2017). Adult conservative management. In P. Abrams, L. Cardozo, A. Wagg, & A Wein (Eds.), *Incontinence* (6th ed., pp. 1443–1628): International Continence Society.

Dumoulin, C., Cacciari, L., & Hay-Smith, E. C. (2018). Pelvic floor muscle training versus no treatment, or inactive control treatments, for urinary incontinence in women. *Cochrane Database of Systematic Reviews, 10*, CD005654. https://doi.org/10.1002/14651858.CD005654.pub4

Edwards, D., Harden, J., Jones, A., & Featherstone, K. (2021). Understanding how to facilitate continence for people with dementia in acute hospital settings: A mixed methods systematic review and thematic synthesis. *Systematic Reviews, 10*(1), 1–22.

Emmanuel, A., Mattace-Raso, F., Neri, M. C., Petersen, K.-U., Rey, E., & Rogers, J. (2017). Constipation in older people: A consensus statement. *International Journal of Clinical Practice, 71*, e12920. https://doi.org/10.1111/ijcp.12920.

Eustice, S., Roe, B., & Paterson, J. (2000). Prompted voiding for the management of urinary incontinence in adults. *Cochrane Database of Systematic Reviews, 2*, Article CD002113. https://doi.org/10.1002/14651858.CD002113.

Fantl, J. A., Newman, D. K., Colling, J., DeLancey, J. O. L., Keeys, C., Loughery, R., et al. (1996). *Urinary incontinence in adults: acute and chronic management. Clinical practice guideline 2, 1996 update*. Rockville, MD: Agency for Health Care Policy and Research.

Flanagan, L., Roe, B., Jack, B., Barrett, J., Chung, A., Shaw, C., & Williams, K. S. (2012). Systematic review of care intervention studies for the management of incontinence and promotion of continence in older people in care homes with urinary incontinence as the primary focus (1966–2010). *Geriatrics Gerontology International, 12*(4), 600–611.

Fonda, D., Benvenuti, F., Cottenden, A. et al. (2002). Urinary incontinence and bladder dysfunction in older persons. In: Abrams P., Khoury S., Wein A., Cardozo L. (eds) Incontinence. *Health Books, Plymouth*, 625–695.

Franken, M. G., Corro Ramos, I., Los, J, & Al, M. J. (2018). The increasing importance of a continence nurse specialist to improve outcomes and save costs of urinary incontinence care: an analysis of future policy scenarios. *BMC Family Practice, 19*(1), 31.

Gao, R., Tao, Y., Zhou, C., Li, J., Wang, X., Chen, L., Li, F., & Guo, L. (2019). Exercise therapy in patients with constipation: A systematic review and meta-analysis of randomized controlled trials. *Scandinavian Journal of Gastroenterology, 54*(2), 169–177.

Getliffe, K. (2003). Managing recurrent urinary catheter blockage: Problems, promises and practicalities. *Journal of Wound Ostomy and Continence Nursing, 30*, 146–151.

Gharbi, M., Drysdale, J. H., Lishman, H., Goudie, R., Molokhia, M., Johnson, A. P., Holmes, A. H., & Aylin, P. (2019). Antibiotic management of urinary tract infection in elderly patients in primary care and its association with bloodstream infections and all cause mortality: Population based cohort study. *British Medical Journal, 364*, l525. doi:10.1136/bmj.l525.

Gill, S. K., Rossi, M., Bajka, B., & Whelan, K. (2021). Dietary fibre in gastrointestinal health and disease. *Nature Reviews Gastroenterology and Hepatology, 18*, 101–116.

Glazener, C. M. (2015). What is the role of mid-urethral slings in the management of stress incontinence in women? *Cochrane Database of Systemic Reviews, 1*(7), Article ED000101. doi:10.1002/14651858.ED000101.

Gray, M., & Krissovich, M. (2003). Does fluid intake influence the risk for urinary incontinence, urinary tract infection and bladder cancer? *Journal of Wound Ostomy and Continence Nursing, 30*, 126–131.

Gotoh, M., Matsukawa, Y., Yoshikawa, Y., Funahashi, Y., Kato, M., & Hattori, R. (2009). Impact of urinary incontinence on the psychological burden of family caregivers. *Neurourology and Urodynamics, 28*(6), 492–496.

Griebling, T. L., Campbell, N. L., Mangel, J., Staskin, D., Herschorn, S., Elsouda, D., & Schermer, C. R. (2020). Effect of mirabegron on cognitive function in elderly patients with overactive bladder: MoCA results from a phase 4 randomized, placebo-controlled study (PILLAR). *BMC Geriatrics, 20*, 109.

Hentzen, C., Haddad, R., Ismael, S. S., Peyronnet, B., Gamé, X., Denys, P., Robain, G., & Amarenco, G. GRAPPPA (Clinical Research Group of Perineal Dysfunctions in Older Adults). (2018). Intermittent self-catheterization in older adults: Predictors of success for technique learning. *International Neurourology Journal, 22*(1), 65–71.

Her Majesty's Stationery Office. (2013). *Report of the Mid Staffordshire NHS Foundation Trust public inquiry.* The Stationery Office.

Ho, K. S., Tan, C. Y., Mohd Daud, M. A., & Seow-Choen, F. (2012). *Stopping or reducing dietary fiber intake reduces constipation and its associated symptoms. World Journal of Gastroenterology, 18*(33), 4593–4596.

Independent Medicines and Medical Devices Safety Review. (2020), First do no harm: The report of the independent medicines and medical devices safety review. https://www.immdsreview.org.uk/downloads/IMMDSReview_Web.pdf

Karim, F., & Rantell, A. (2021). Understanding the basic assessment and treatment of lower urinary tract symptoms in older women. *Nursing Older People, 33*(5), 33–41.

Keilman, L. J., & Dunn, K. S. (2010). Knowledge, attitudes, and perceptions of advanced practice nurses regarding urinary incontinence in older adult women. *Research and Theory for Nursing Practice, 24*(4), 260–279.

Keltie, K., Elneil, S., Monga, A., Patrick, H., Powell, J., Campbell, B., & Sims, A. J. (2017). Complications following vaginal mesh procedures for stress urinary incontinence: An 8 year study of 92,246 women. *Scientific Reports, 7*(1), 12015.

Kenny, K. A., & Skelly, J. (2001). Dietary fiber for constipation in older adults: A systematic review. *Clinical Effectiveness in Nursing, 5*, 120–128.

Kumah, C., & McGlashan, D. (2019). Benefits of nurse-led continence prescription services for effective stock management and streamlined prescribing. *British Journal of Community Nursing, 24*(9), 424–431. https://doi.org/10.12968/bjcn.2019.24.9.424.

Leckie, K. J. (2010). What is the evidence for the role of oestrogen in the prevention of recurrent urinary tract infections in postmenopausal women? An evidence-based review. *Journal of Clinical Gerontology and Geriatrics, 1*(2), 31–35.

Lekan-Rutledge, D., & Colling, J. (2003). Urinary incontinence in the frail elderly. *American Journal of Nursing, 3*(Suppl), 36–46.

Leung, F. W., & Schnelle, J. F. (2008). Urinary and fecal incontinence in nursing home residents. *Gastroenterology Clinics of North America, 37*(3), 69–707.

Luo, Y., Parry, M., Huang, Y.-J., Wang, X.-H., & He, G.-P. (2016). Nursing students' knowledge and attitudes toward urinary incontinence: a cross-sectional survey. *Nurse Education Today.* 40,134–139, https://doi.org/10.1016/j.nedt.2016.02.020

Makhani, A., Thake, M., & Gibson, W. (2020). Mirabegron in the treatment of overactive bladder: Safety and efficacy in the very elderly patient. *Clinical Interventions in Aging, 15*, 575–581.

MacRae, C., Henderson, D. A., Mercer, S. W., Burton, J., De Souza, N., Grill, P., Marwick, C., & Guthrie, B. (2021). Excessive polypharmacy and potentially inappropriate prescribing in 147 care homes: a cross-sectional study. *British Journal of General Practice Open, 5*(6). BJGPO.2021.0167 doi:10.3399/BJGPO.2021.0167.

McCrea, G. L., Miaskowski, C., Stotts, N. A., Macera, L., & Varma, M. G. (2008). Pathophysiology of constipation in the older adult. *World Journal of Gastroenterology, 14*(17) 2631–2368.

McDaniel, C., Ratnani, I., Fatima, S., Abid, M. H., & Surani, S. (2020). Urinary incontinence in older adults takes collaborative nursing efforts to improve. *Cureus, 12*(7), e9161. doi:10.7759/cureus.9161.

Mihaylov, S., Stark, C., McColl, E., Steen, N., Vanoli, A., Rubin, G., Curless, R., Barton, R., & Bond, J. (2008). Stepped treatment of older adults on laxatives. The STOOL trial. *Health Technology Assessment, 13*, iii-iv, ix–139. doi:10.3310/hta12130.

Moon, S., Chung, H. S., Kim, Y. J., Kim, S. J., Kwon, O., Lee, Y. G., Yu, J. M., & Cho, S. T. (2021). The impact of urinary incontinence on falls: A systematic review and meta-analysis. *PloS One, 16*(5), e0251711. doi:10.1371/journal.pone.0251711.

Musa, M. K., Saga, S., Blekken, L. E., Harris, R., Goodman, C., & Norton, C. (2019). The prevalence, incidence, and correlates of fecal incontinence among older people residing in care homes: A systematic review. *Journal of the American Medical Directors Association*, e193–e198.

Murphy, C., De Laine, C., Macaulay, M., Hislop Lennie, K., & Fader, M. (2021). Problems faced by people living at home with dementia and incontinence: Causes, consequences and potential solutions. *Age and Ageing, 50*(3), 944–954.

National Institute for Health and Care Excellence (NICE). 2013. Mirabegron for treating symptoms of overactive bladder. https://www.nice.org.uk/guidance/ta290/chapter/1-Guidance

NICE. (2018). Faecal incontinence in adults: management. https://www.nice.org.uk/guidance/cg49

NICE. (2019a). Urinary incontinence and pelvic organ prolapse in women: management. https://www.nice.org.uk/guidance/ng123

NICE. (2019b). Surgery for stress urinary incontinence. https://www.nice.org.uk/guidance/ng123/resources/surgery-for-stress-urinary-incontinence-patient-decision-aid-pdf-6725286110

NICE. (2022). British national formulary. https://bnf.nice.org.uk/drug/macrogol-3350-with-potassium-chloride-sodium-bicarbonate-and-sodium-chloride.html#indicationsAndDoses.

Newman, D. K., Ee, C. H., Gordon, D., Srini, S., Williams, K., Cahill, B., Gordon, B., Griebling, T., Nishimura, K., & Norton, N. (2020). Continence promotion, education & primary prevention. https://www.ics.org/publications/ici_4/files-book/comite-21.pdf

NHS England. (2018). Excellence in continence care: Practical guidance for commissioners, and leaders in health and social care. https://www.england.nhs.uk/wp-content/uploads/2018/07/excellence-in-continence-care.pdf

Nitti, V. W. (2001). The prevalence of urinary incontinence. *Reviews in Urology, 3*(Suppl 1), S2–S6.

Norton, C. (1996). *Nursing for continence* (2nd ed.). Beaconsfield Publishers.

Norton, C., & Chelvanayagam, S. (2004). *Bowel continence nursing*. Beaconsfield Publishers.

Omli, R., Skotnes, L. H., Romild, U., Bakke, A., Mykletun, A., & Kuhr, E. (2010). Pad per day usage, urinary incontinence and urinary tract infections in nursing home residents. *Age and Ageing, 39*, 549–554.

Orrell, A., McKee, K., Dahlberg, L., Gilhooly, M., & Parker, K. (2013). Improving continence services for older people from the service-providers' perspective: A qualitative interview study. *BMJ Open, 3*(7), Article e002926. http://dx.doi.org/10.1136/bmjopen-2013-002926.

Ostaszkiewicz, J., Chestney, T., & Roe, B. (2004). Habit retraining for the management of urinary incontinence in adults. *Cochrane Database of Systematic Reviews, 2*, Article CD002801. https://doi.org/10.1002/14651858.CD002801.pub2.

Ostaszkiewicz, J., Dickson-Swift, V., Hutchinson, A., & Wagg, A. (2020). A concept analysis of dignity-protective continence care for care dependent older people in long-term care settings. *BMC Geriatrics, 20*, 266.

Park, J., & Palmer, M. H. (2015). Factors associated with incomplete bladder emptying in older women with overactive bladder symptoms. *Journal of the American Geriatric Society, 63*(7), 1426–1431.

Petticrew, M., Watt, I., & Sheldon, T. (1997). Systematic review of the effectiveness of laxatives in the elderly. *Health Technology Assessment, 1*(13), 1–52.

Plotti, F., Montera, R., Terranova, C., Luvero, D., Marrocco, F., Miranda, A., Gatti, A., De Cicco Nardone, C., Angioli, R., & Scaletta, G. (2018). Long-term follow-up of bulking agents for stress urinary incontinence in older patients. *Menopause, 25*(6), 663–667.

Pont, L. G., Fisher, M., & Williams, K. (2019). Appropriate use of laxatives in the older person. *Drugs & Aging, 36*(11), 999–1005.

Rantell, A. (2021). *Sexual function and pelvic floor dysfunction: A guide for nurses and allied health professionals.* Springer Nature.

Rashidi Fakari, F., Hajian, S., Darvish, S., & Alavi Majd, H. (2021). Explaining factors affecting help-seeking behaviors in women with urinary incontinence: A qualitative study. *BMC Health Services Research, 21*(60).

Resnick, N. M. (1984). Urinary incontinence in the elderly. *Medical Grand Rounds, 3*, 281–290.

Resnick, N. M., Baumann, M., Scott, M., Laurino, E., & Yalla, S. V. (1988). Risk factors for incontinence in the nursing home: a multivariate approach. *Neurourology & Urodynamics, 7*, 274–276.

Robinson, J. (2000). Managing urinary incontinence in the nursing home: Residents' perspectives. *Journal of Advanced Nursing, 31*, 68–77.

Roe, B., Flanagan, L., & Maden, M. (2015). Systematic review of systematic reviews for the management of urinary incontinence and promotion of continence using conservative behavioural approaches in older people in care homes. *Journal of Advanced Nursing, 71*(7), 1464–1483.

Royal College of Nursing. (2019). *Bowel care.* Royal College of Nursing.

Royal College of Nursing. (2021). *Catheter care.* Royal College of Nursing.

Saxer, S., de Bie, R. A., Dassen, T., & Halfens, R. J. G. (2009). Knowledge, beliefs, attitudes, and self-reported practice concerning urinary incontinence in nursing home care. *Journal of Wound, Ostomy and Continence Nursing, 36*(5), 539–544.

Schluter, P. J., Ward, C., Arnold, E. P., Scrase, R., & Jamieson, H. A. (2017). Urinary incontinence, but not fecal incontinence, is a risk factor for admission to aged residential care of older persons in New Zealand. *Neurourology and Urodynamics, 36*(6), 1588–1595.

Sharma, A., Rao, S. S. C., Kearns, K., Orleck, K. D., & Waldman, S. A. (2021). Review article: Diagnosis, management and patient perspectives of the spectrum of constipation disorders. *Alimentary Pharmacology and Therapeutics, 53*, 1250–1267.

Speed, C., Heaven, B., Adamson, A., Bond, J., Corbett, S., Lake, A. A., May, C., Vanoli, A., McMeekin, P., Moynihan, P., Rubin, G., Steen, I. N., & McColl, E. (2010). LIFELAX—diet and LIFEstyle versus LAXatives in the management of chronic constipation in older people: randomised controlled trial. *Health Technology Assessment, 14*(52), 1–251. doi: 10.3310/hta14520. https://www.journalslibrary.nihr.ac.uk/hta/hta14520/#/abstract.

Stenzelius, K., Molander, U., Odeberg, J., Hammarström, M., Franzen, K., Midlöv, P., Samuelsson, E., & Andersson, G. (2015). The effect of conservative treatment of urinary incontinence among older and frail older people: a systematic review. *Age and Ageing, 44*(5), 736–744.

Stewart, F., Gameiro, L. F., El Dib, R., Gameiro, M. O., Kapoor, A., & Amaro, J. L. (2016). Electrical stimulation with non-implanted electrodes for overactive bladder in adults. *Cochrane Database of Systematic Reviews, 12*, Article CD010098. doi:10.1002/14651858.CD010098.pub4.

Stickley, A., Santini, Z. I., & Koyanagi, A. (2017). Urinary incontinence, mental health and loneliness among community-dwelling older adults in Ireland. *BMC Urology, 17*, 29.

Tannenbaum, C., Fritel, X., Halme, A., van den Heuvel, E., Jutai, J., & Wagg, A. (2019). Long-term effect of community-based continence promotion on urinary symptoms, falls and healthy active life expectancy among older women: Cluster randomised trial. *Age and Ageing, 48*(4), 526–532.

UK Continence Society. (2014). Minimum standards for continence care in the United Kingdom. https://ukcs.uk.net/resources/Documents/15091716_Revised_Min_Standards_for_CC_in_UK.pdf

Van Kampen, M. (2000). Effect of pelvic floor re-education on duration and degree of incontinence after radical prostatectomy: A randomised controlled trial. *Lancet, 355*, 98–102.

Verkuijl, S. J., Meinds, R. J., Trzpis, M., & Broens, P. M. A. (2020). The influence of demographic characteristics on constipation symptoms: A detailed overview. *BMC Gastroenterology, 20*, 168.

Vinsnes, A. G. (2001). Healthcare per Vinssonnel's attitudes towards patients with urinary incontinence. *Journal of Clinical Nursing, 10*, 455–462.

Visser, E., de Bock, G. H., Berger, M. Y., & Dekker, J. H. (2014). Impact of urinary incontinence on sexual functioning in community-dwelling older women. *Journal of Sexual Medicine, 11*(7), 1757–1765.

Wagg, A. (2017). Incontinence in frail older persons. In P. Abrams, L. Cardozo, A. Wagg, & A. Wein (Eds.), *Incontinence* (6th ed, pp. 1309–1441). International Continence Society.

Williams, M. P., Srikanth, V., Bird, M., & Thrift, A. G. (2012). Urinary symptoms and natural history of urinary continence after first-ever stroke—a longitudinal population-based study. *Age and Ageing, 41*(3), 371–376.

Wyman, J. F., Burgio, K. L., & Newman, D. K. (2009). Practical aspects of lifestyle modifications and behavioural interventions in the treatment of overactive bladder and urgency urinary incontinence. *International Journal of Clinical Practice, 63*(8), 1177–1191.

Yang, J., Wang, H. P., Zhou, L., & Xu, C. F. (2012). Effect of dietary fiber on constipation: a meta analysis. *World Journal of Gastroenterology, 18*(48), 7378–7383.

Yates, A. (2018). How to perform a comprehensive baseline continence assessment. *Nursing Times, 114*(5), 26–29.

Yu, L. C., Rohner, T. J., Kaltreider, D. L., Hu, T. W., Igou, J. F., & Dennis, P. J. (1990). Profile of urinary incontinent elderly in long-term care institutions. *Journal of the American Geriatrics Society, 38*(4),433–439.

23

Infection Prevention and Control and Thermoregulation in Older People

Edward Purssell, Dinah Gould

CHAPTER OUTLINE

Susceptibility to infection increases in older people because of the physiological changes that accompany ageing, especially in the immune system. A second important problem is presented by changes in thermoregulatory control that place older people at increased risk of hypothermia and hyperthermia. These risks can be further compounded by the living conditions and behavioural changes often adopted with increasing age. For example, older people frequently live alone, may become lonely, suffer from depression and become less inclined to prepare well-balanced meals. This situation can be exacerbated by reduced mobility and dental problems (e.g., ill-fitting dentures, gum disease). The resulting malnutrition in turn disrupts metabolism and increases susceptibility to infection. Malnutrition

339

contributes to dysfunction of the immune system in older people, resulting in increased susceptibility to infection. It is a significant predictor of mortality (Chakhtoura et al., 2017).

Traditionally a great deal of attention was given to the prevention and control of infection in acute-care settings. It has been estimated in England alone 300,000 inpatients annually develop a health care–associated infection (HCAI), contributing directly to morbidity and mortality and inflating the costs of health care (National Institute for Health and Care Excellence [NICE], 2018). A high proportion of these infections are caused by methicillin-resistant *Staphylococcus aureus* (MRSA) and *Clostridioides difficile*. In epidemiological studies, increasing age is an important risk factor. The majority of hospital inpatients are over 65 and are very often subjected to invasive procedures that increase susceptibility to infection. Overuse of antimicrobial drugs has generated the emergence of antibiotic-resistant micro-organisms. Antimicrobial resistance is now recognised as a global problem and one of the greatest threats to human health (World Health Organization [WHO], 2016). In recent years the vulnerability of people outside acute-care settings has also become increasingly apparent. Frequent use of health services places older people at high risk of HCAIs. Clusters of other infections, notably influenza (Pop-Vicas et al., 2015) and norovirus (Rajagopalan & Yoshikawa, 2016), and outbreaks of scabies infestations (Gould, 2010) are frequently reported in nursing and care homes.

This chapter describes the chain of infection common to all pathogens (i.e., micro-organisms able to cause infection) and outlines the risks of infection, the principles of infection prevention applied to older people and thermoregulation and thermoregulatory challenges.

AGEING, IMMUNITY AND THE TRANSMISSION OF INFECTION

The chain of infection is an epidemiological model applicable to all types of pathogenic organisms (van Seventer & Hochberg, 2017). It consists of a series of events that must occur to allow pathogens to spread and describes the interaction between the micro-organism, its host and the environment. Each part of the chain can be conceptualised as a link, and there are six links in the chain. The model provides the basis for recognising and implementing infection prevention and control measures at each stage. The six links in the chain of infection are

1. The reservoir of infection
2. The portal of exit from the reservoir
3. The mode of transmission of the pathogen
4. Its portal of entry into a new host
5. The means by which the pathogen gains access to the new host and invades a susceptible site

6. The interaction between the pathogen and the host, resulting in the signs and symptoms of infection (National Infection Prevention and Control Manual, 2012)

Each step is discussed in greater depth below.

The Reservoir of Infection

The reservoir is where pathogens live and multiply. Four types of reservoir exist. Other people are an important source: patients or residents in care and nursing homes and people living in the community operate as reservoirs for influenza, norovirus, COVID-19, coughs and colds. The index case (i.e., the first documented patient when a cluster of infections occurs) may show signs of infection or may be asymptomatic, either because the infection is mild and never becomes symptomatic—because the infection is in the very early stages when symptoms are not yet evident—or because they are already recovering. Inanimate contaminated surfaces and objects (i.e., fomites) can operate as major reservoirs of infection. Examples include frequently handled objects such as bedpans and urinals and bedside curtains. HCAIs (e.g., *Staphylococcus aureus*, *Pseudomonas* spp., *Klebsiella* spp.) are frequently spread via inanimate surfaces. At one time it was thought cross-infection occurred from surfaces and objects predominantly in the close patient environment, but it is now apparent transfer can occur from distant locations (Weber et al., 2013). Cross-infection by this route occurs because the hands of staff become contaminated, and hand hygiene is either omitted or not conducted thoroughly enough to remove all the pathogens they are carrying (Pittet et al., 2006). The environment can operate as a reservoir for some pathogens. Water is the reservoir for the organisms responsible for Legionnaire's disease (*Legionella pneumophila*), typhoid and cholera. The bacteria that cause tetanus (*Clostridium tetani*) originate in soil. Finally, animals can be the source of some infections. Examples include rabies and exotic and emergent infections (e.g., Ebola, Middle East respiratory syndrome, avian influenza). Infections that originate in animal hosts and are transferred to humans are called zoonoses.

The Portal of Exit From the Reservoir

Micro-organisms can escape from their reservoir by direct contact between surfaces (e.g., via hands); in coughs, sneezes and spluttered speech; in vomit and faeces; on skin scales; and in body fluids.

Mode of Transmission

The classical view is pathogens are spread by direct contact, in droplet nuclei, via contaminated food and water or by insect vectors. Direct contact occurs via hands and fomites and is the route taken by HCAIs. Spread by droplet nuclei occurs in two ways. Large droplet nuclei (>5 microns) escape into the atmosphere but rapidly settle on surrounding surfaces. The pathogens they contain are then transferred to a new host by direct contact, often by hands. This is the route thought to be taken by viruses responsible for the common cold. Smaller droplet nuclei (<5 microns) escape as tiny aerosols. They dry out, and the pathogens they are carrying are inhaled. This route is thought to be important for influenza. Bacteria that cause food poisoning are spread in contaminated food (e.g., *Salmonella enteritidis*); some of the classic communicable diseases (e.g., typhoid, cholera) are waterborne. Insect vectors spread infection mechanically (e.g., on the feet of houseflies), or transmission is biological, meaning the pathogen survives and multiples within the insect before it is transferred to the new host. Malaria (*Plasmodium* spp.) is spread from mosquitos through biological transmission. In reality many pathogens are probably spread by more than one route. Norovirus can be spread in droplet nuclei from contaminated bodily excretions, via hands and other fomites and from bivalve shellfish (Rajagopalan & Yoshikawa, 2016). It is also likely that coughs, colds and COVID-19 are spread in both large and small droplet nuclei via aerosols and direct and indirect contact (Graham et al., 2020). *Salmonella* survives on environmental surfaces and can be spread via hands and fomites as well as in food. Major outbreaks of salmonella have been reported among frail older people in communal accommodation.

Portals of Entry

Pathogens gain access to the new host by inhalation (e.g., influenza, colds), ingestion, via the urogenital tract (e.g., urinary pathogens, sexually transmitted infections), inoculation via skin and mucous membranes (e.g., surgical site and needlestick injuries) and vertical transmission from mother to foetus.

The Interaction Between Pathogen and Host

The ability of the pathogen to establish infection depends on the immunity of the host (see page 343), the size of the infective dose and virulence. It is axiomatic that the greater the number of pathogens to which the prospective host is exposed, the more chance the pathogens have of overwhelming the immune system and establishing infection. Exposure may be the result of a single event such as receiving a large infective dose (e.g., eating a food that is heavily contaminated) or may arise through frequent risky behaviour. At the time of writing, the public health bodies in the United Kingdom reported the greatest rate of increase in sexually transmitted infections is among people over 60. The high rate of newly single people in this age group and increased use of online introductory platforms are considered to be important contributory factors, especially in a population that has no need to use

contraception and thus lacks the protection of barrier methods. Where another person is the reservoir of infection, the release of large numbers of pathogens is likely to result in large numbers of others becoming infected. The way they behave can also be influential: a heavily colonised health worker whose work is peripatetic (e.g., physiotherapist going from ward to ward or domiciliary nurse going from home to home) can act as a 'super-spreader'. An individual heavily colonised or infected with a respiratory pathogen who becomes disinhibited through alcohol use can spread large numbers of infectious particles in a crowded space such as a bar.

Virulence

Virulence is the ability of the pathogen to cause infection and can be taken as a measure of the severity of the resulting disease. The severity of the infection is increased if the pathogen is highly virulent and the new host receives a large infective dose. The ability of the pathogen to invade the host's tissues and generate harm is sometimes described as aggressiveness. Many of the bacteria notorious for their ability to cause HCAI are not highly aggressive and are often described as opportunists. *Escherichia coli*, *Klebsiella* spp. and *Pseudomonas* spp. are all opportunists that cause infection only in patients with low resistance or if the micro-organisms gain access to an anatomical site usually free of such bacteria (e.g., transfer of *E. coli* from the heavily contaminated bowel into the urinary tract). The human immunodeficiency virus (HIV) is sometimes described as a 'pathogenic weakling' because it survives poorly outside the tissues and relies on spread by sexual and parenteral routes.

A virulence factor is a property of a potential pathogen that increases its ability to establish infection. It is often enhanced by cellular structure. For example, the thick coat that surrounds *Mycobacterium tuberculosis* protects it from host defence mechanisms in lung tissue. Strains of *E. coli* protected with a thick mucus coat are more likely to set up urinary infections. *Neisseria gonorrhoeae* attaches itself to the female cervical epithelium by minute hair-like projections (i.e., pili) on the surface of its cells. Mutant strains that lack pili are not pathogenic. Many organisms, including *Staphylococcus aureus*, evade the host response because surface toxins on their cells confer protection against phagocytes.

Risk of Infection

The risk of infection varies from one person to another, is altered by changes that affect general health and the ageing process, and is influenced by numerous other factors. Throughout the life cycle but especially in middle age and beyond, men are more likely to succumb to infection than women.

Twin studies have demonstrated genetic factors play a role determining susceptibility to infection. Identical twins share all their genetic material and are useful when studying the influence of genetic vs. environmental factors on susceptibility to disease. Identical twins who live apart are not exposed to the same environmental risk factors, but if one of the pair develops tuberculosis, the other is more likely to do so than non-identical twins, who are no more genetically alike than ordinary siblings. This does not suggest tuberculosis is a genetic condition, but it does indicate a genetic component plays a role in susceptibility to tuberculosis. Sickle disease and thalassaemia are genetically inherited conditions that increase an individual's resistance to malaria. Chronic diseases such as diabetes and malignancy increase susceptibility to infection, as do many immunosuppressive treatments and chemotherapy. As chronic diseases are more common in older people, risk of infection is correspondingly increased.

Good general health, optimal nutrition and hydration all contribute to ability to avoid infection. Intact skin, anatomical adaptations, the normal flora of the body and naturally produced antimicrobial substances such as hydrochloric acid and lysozyme are important contributors to innate immunity. If any of these mechanisms fail, pathogens are more likely to gain access to the tissues. Invasive devices that bypass the body's natural defences increase susceptibility, as does frailty in older people (Chakhtoura et al., 2017).

Intact Skin and Mucous Membranes

The anatomical arrangement of the tissues, the secretion of fluids that wash foreign materials from the body and the presence of normal flora covering the skin and lining the gastrointestinal tract reduce the risks of pathogenic invasion. Intact skin and mucous membranes are the body's chief defences against infection. The skin has a low pH because sebaceous secretion is acidic (i.e., the 'acid mantle'), supporting a population of commensal bacteria that keep pathogens out. Infection supervenes when the skin is broken or becomes excessively moist, especially if hygiene is poor.

Gastrointestinal Tract

Powerful acid and alkaline secretions protect the gastrointestinal system from infection. The pH of gastric acid (2) destroys most bacteria ingested with food. In the small intestine, the high pH (8–9) destroys most pathogens. The bacteria responsible for typhoid and cholera have adapted to survive and multiply at this pH, however.

Respiratory Tract

Coughing and sneezing reflexes are protective. In the nose, the nasal conchae increase the surface area of the mucosal surface and cause air to eddy, trapping small particles as inspired air travels over them. Lymphoid tissue in the pharyngeal, palatine and lingual tonsils traps remaining pathogens. The entire respiratory tree, except for the alveoli, is lined with specialised mucus-secreting epithelium (i.e., muco-ciliary escalator). The mucus traps foreign substances and is carried upward to the pharynx by the action of the cilia, swallowed and removed from the body by the gastrointestinal tract.

Female Reproductive Tract

Throughout the reproductive years the vagina contains a population of lactobacilli that metabolise glycogen in cervical secretions, forming lactic acid. The pH of the healthy adult vagina is low (4.5), inhibiting the growth of other micro-organisms. Before menarche and after menopause, the cervical secretions are scant because oestrogen production is low. Vaginal pH is correspondingly higher and infection is more common in older women.

Urinary Tract

The bladder has little protection against invading pathogens, and urinary infections are common, especially during pregnancy and among older women. Regular and complete emptying of the bladder tends to militate against infection by flushing micro-organisms out of the bladder and urethra.

Secretions With Natural Antimicrobial Properties

Lysozyme is an enzyme secreted by macrophages present in many body fluids, including tears and saliva. It destroys bacteria by attacking their cell walls.

The Immune System

The immune system is diverse and complex and can be thought of as consisting of three 'layers' of protection. The first is the skin, mucous membranes and associated substances such as stomach acid, and secreted substances such as lysozyme that break down proteins and lactoferrin, which removes iron necessary for bacterial growth. Beyond this, most of the immediate immune response is provided by the innate immune system, which provides a non-specific response. Finally, there is the most flexible and complex part of the immune response: the adaptive, acquired or specific immune system, which provides a specific response for each antigen. The immune system is incredibly complex, and not all aspects are well understood, so here only the general principles are discussed. It has been said anyone who claims to fully understand the immune system really does not understand the immune system!

Natural Barriers to Infection

One of the most important ways of protecting the body from infection is to maintain these natural barriers and protective mechanisms. In older people, these may be damaged through natural processes or as a result of treatments. For example, wounds and ulcers breach skin integrity, and use of antacid drugs might reduce the effectiveness of stomach acid in protecting the gastrointestinal tract. This is particularly important in areas of the body such as the eyes that are said to be immunologically privileged, which means antigens are tolerated without significant local inflammatory responses. If you think of the possible effects of inflammation in the eyes, it is easy to see why this has evolved, but the limitation is they are an important portal for infection.

Innate Immune System

Although it is complex, some of the parts of the immune system have fairly descriptive names. The innate immune system, for example, is known thus because you are born with it; it is innate. The important feature of the innate immune system is the cells that comprise it are able to recognise particular molecules widely found on microorganisms. These molecules are known as pathogen-associated molecular patterns and are recognised by complementary pattern-recognition receptors on the cell. Cells of the innate immune system include dendritic cells, Langerhans cells, macrophages, monocytes, neutrophils and natural killer cells. Some of these cells, such as monocytes, macrophages, neutrophils, directly remove pathogens through phagocytosis; others, such as dendritic and Langerhans cells, do not primarily remove pathogens but enhance the immune response by stimulating adaptive immunity. Important features of innate immunity are that although it is rapid, it not specific to a particular microorganism and lacks the immunological memory found in the adaptive immune system.

Adaptive Immune System

The adaptive immune system comprises two main branches, often referred to as humoral or antibody-related immunity and cell-mediated immunity. Unlike innate immunity, adaptive immunity is antigen specific. An antigen is a substance able to stimulate a specific immune response, and an individual bacterium and virus will contain many antigens, some of which are better at stimulating an immune response than others. This is particularly important for vaccination, as vaccines need to contain antigens that do not mutate or vary too much and stimulate a good immune response. The influenza vaccine, for example, contains two important antigens, hemagglutinin (H) and neuraminidase (N), which do change over time, hence the need for annual vaccination (Centers for Disease Control and Prevention, 2015).

Some antigens, such as polysaccharides, which are found on some bacteria such as Pneumococci, are able to stimulate an immune response, but due to the lack of T-cell involvement in this response, it is relatively weak and does not result in robust immunological memory. For example, the pneumococcal conjugate vaccine provides a more robust response than the polysaccharide vaccine. If you consider the number and variety of different antigens an individual meets throughout their lives, the enormous diversity of adaptive immune responses becomes apparent. As this number is far greater than the ability of the genome to produce different receptors for these antigens, an increase in diversity occurs over an individual's lifespan through somatic mutation.

Antibody Responses

Antibodies are produced in largest amounts by differentiated B cells known as plasma cells. There are five broad classes of antibodies, also referred to as immunoglobulins or Ig:

- IgA: Main antibody in external secretions and on mucous membranes
- IgD: Exact function is not known
- IgG: Main circulating antibody, important in secondary response
- IgE: Triggers allergic reaction
- IgM: Main primary response antibody (Moser & Leo, 2010)

The process of producing an antibody response is that most antigens are taken up by a variety of cells that together are known as antigen presenting cells (APC). Important APCs include monocytes and dendritic cells. These cells take up antigens and process them within the cell. They are then 'presented' to B cells by molecules known as MHC Class II on the antigen-presenting cell, which interact with B cell receptors. The important feature of this interaction is that although APCs are not antigen specific, B cells are antigen-specific; that is, the antigen has to be presented to a B cell specific for the antigen, which can then produce antibodies for that specific antigen.

The first antibody produced in the immediate or primary response is IgM. After a period of a few days, many B cells go through a process known as class or isotype switching; that is, they change the class of antibody they produce. As it is the main antibody, most class-switch to produce IgG. At the same time, the specificity of the antibody being produced increases, producing antibodies with better affinity, which is a measure of the strength of the interaction between antibody and antigen, and avidity, which is a measure of the overall strength of this interaction. They also mature to become high level antibody producing cells known as plasma cells. During the first (i.e., primary) response to an antigen, this process takes 10 to 14 days;

during subsequent (i.e., secondary) exposures, it is much quicker, and due to the existence of memory cells, IgG and the other antibody types can be produced immediately. This occurs because of one of the cardinal features of the adaptive immune system: immunological memory. On subsequent exposure to the same antigen, the immune response is more rapid and more robust. This is one of the main rationales for vaccination. The vaccine provides the primary response by presenting an antigen in a form that does not cause disease. The result is when the vaccinated person meets the pathogen for the first time, even though they have not been exposed to the organism before, immunologically the immune system *has* seen the antigen before, and a secondary immune response results. Cells that have not been exposed to antigen before are referred to as naive cells.

Cell-Mediated Responses

Antibodies are very important in the immune response to organisms that live outside host cells but are not able to reach those that have an intracellular lifestyle, most importantly viruses. For this, cell-mediated immunity is important. This response is undertaken by cells known as cytotoxic T cells. All nucleated cells in the body express molecules known as MHC Class I on their surface. These molecules present fragments of proteins known as peptides that are being produced by the cell, on the outside of the cell. A non-infected cell expresses normal human proteins that are recognised as such by cytotoxic T cells, and the cell is ignored. If the cell is infected by a virus, it eventually produces viral proteins, so the MHC Class I molecules express foreign viral proteins. These are recognised as such by cytotoxic T cells, which then kill the infected cell. Again, as part of the adaptive immune system, this is antigen specific, and immunological memory results.

Immune-System Coordination

These processes are complex and require a high degree of coordination. Although for clarity different parts of the immune system are discussed separately, this is an oversimplification, because it is really a highly coordinated and interlinked system. In order for it to function, each part must work and be able to communicate with the others. For example, viruses have intra- and extra-cellular stages, making them susceptible to the innate immune system and antibodies during the extra-cellular stage and to cytotoxic cells in their intracellular state.

Communication may occur through direct contact, such as that between APC and T-helper cells, or through the production of chemical messengers known as cytokines and other soluble substances such as the many inflammatory mediators. The main cells responsible for coordinating and regulating the immune system are helper T-cells. You may hear T-helper cells referred to as CD4 cells, and cytotoxic T-cells as CD8 cells, with CD standing for cluster of differentiation. They are cellular molecules used for identifying different cells. T-helper cells come in different populations that stimulate different types of immune response. Some lead to primarily antibody (or humoral) responses, others cell-mediated responses, while still others downregulate the responses. It is a lack of these cells that causes AIDS in people with end-stage HIV disease, as the virus infects cells that carry CD4 molecules. This leads to immunological dysregulation and results in the infections and malignancies seen in these patients. T-cell 'help' is essential for a robust immune response.

It is important to remember the immune response varies between individuals, and an adaptive immune response takes time, typically 10 to 14 days. In older people this may be longer still. A person does not have robust immunity the day after a vaccination.

Conditions of the Immune System

The three main problems with the immune response are insufficient immunity, exaggerated immunity and autoimmunity. Autoimmunity, an immune response to self-antigens, is the cause of a number of conditions, such as type 1 diabetes and rheumatoid arthritis. The main problems associated with exaggerated immunity are allergy, which is due to an overproduction of IgE, and sepsis, which results from a dysregulated host response and leads to systemic inflammation and organ dysfunction (Gyawali et al., 2019).

The Ageing Immune System

One of the main problems with the ageing immune system is there is a relative decline of some cell types. Although neutrophil and macrophage populations do not seem to be affected by age, some changes occur in their function, including changes in cytokine production, a reduction in their phagocytic and bactericidal ability, and increased production of inflammatory reactive oxygen species. T-cells mature in the thymus, an organ that involutes (i.e., shrinks) with age, although the total number may remain stable as the population of mature T cells is not affected. A similar phenomenon of reduced production and a relative increase in longer-lived memory cells may also occur in B cells (Keenan & Allan, 2019). However, there may be age-related changes in function, with reduced ability to switch the type of antibody being produced (i.e., isotype switching) and reduction in antibody affinity, making the antibody response less robust (Weiskopf et al., 2009). The overall result of these changes in the T- and B-cell populations is immune response to new acute and latent viral infections and vaccinations is reduced (Simon et al., 2015).

This reduction in the production of new cells and changes in antibody production may reduce the ability to respond to new antigens, as memory cells that seem less affected by age can respond only to antigens to which the individual has already been exposed. Thinking of the different sources of potential pathogens, when cared for at home by individuals who they will have had frequent contact with, people are likely to be exposed to organisms to which they have existing immunity. In hospitals or care facilities there is a greater chance of exposure to new organisms or those with increased pathogenicity.

One of the main issues associated with the immune response is although it is beneficial overall, a robust immune response often has negative aspects as well. One is inflammation, which can be painful and cause local or systemic pathogenesis. The accumulation of inflammatory mediators in older people can lead to chronic inflammation, sometimes referred to as inflammaging (Montecino-Rodriguez et al., 2013).

Another condition that may at least partly result from changes in the immune response is cancer. It is likely this is primarily due to cellular and genetic damage that accumulates throughout an individual's lifetime, but the decline in the immune response and increase in inflammation may also play a role (Simon et al., 2015).

Physiological Changes Associated With Ageing

Physiological changes in older people affect every organ system in the body in addition to any disease process the individual may develop. These physiological changes result from molecular and cellular damage that accrues over the lifespan, resulting in decreased ability to repair damage and reduced homeostatic control (Chakhtoura et al., 2017).

Urinary System

In older people, susceptibility to infection is increased by reduction in bladder capacity, bladder spasms, decreased urinary flow rate and residual urine after voiding. In men it is exacerbated by prostate disease and in women through prolapse of the bladder and decreased oestrogen production. Changes in the epithelium that lines the urinary tract increase the ability of invading pathogens to attach themselves (i.e., enhanced virulence factor).

Respiratory System

The cough reflex is blunted, mucociliary clearance of the lower airways. In older adults, elasticity of the lungs and respiratory muscle strength are reduced and respiratory

secretions contain less immunoglobulin, placing them at increased risk of pneumonia.

Skin and Soft Tissues

There is general decrease in integrity and increased risk of mechanical damage through loss of subcutaneous tissue and loss of collagen from the dermis with ageing, leading to slower wound repair. The blood vessels become smaller, impairing the delivery of immune cells able to mount the protective inflammatory response. The skin becomes drier through reduced ability of the stratum corneum to bind water molecules. It has been estimated that by age 70, nearly three quarters of the population has at least one underlying skin problem that contributes to a thinner, more fragile integument (Sinikumpu et al., 2020).

Gastrointestinal System

With age, salivary production decreases, chewing and swallowing are slowed through reduced muscular strength of the tongue, gastric acidity and intestinal mobility are decreased and the resident intestinal flora are modified, allowing easier access by invading pathogens. Dehydration is also a common problem in older people and is often multifactorial: poor oral intake and impaired endocrine response manifest as decreased thirst.

Central Nervous System

The structure and function of immune cells in the central nervous system changes with age. Cognitive decline and chronic infection and inflammation are frequently linked.

Endocrine System

There is gradual increase in cortisol release with age and increased catabolism as a result. The net effect is reduced appetite, weight loss, reduced energy expenditure and decreased muscle mass. These changes are important contributory factors to frailty.

Musculoskeletal System

Loss of skeletal muscle mass leads to decreased strength and functionality. The effect is increased following catabolism induced by trauma (e.g., accident, major surgery).

Special Senses

Reduced sense of smell and taste may result in anorexia, reduced dietary intake and malnutrition.

INFECTION PREVENTION AND CONTROL

The chain of infection can be broken at three different levels: through interventions targeted at the individual, through policies and procedures intended to reduce the risks of infection for particular groups of people and by public health measures aimed at entire communities and populations.

Interventions Targeted at Individuals

Individual strategies involve identifying factors that increase individual susceptibility to infection or constitute a specific infection risk and delivering the appropriate care or advice tailored to meet individual need. Placing a patient at high risk of infection in protective isolation or giving individualised advice to somebody at high risk of developing COVID-19 are examples of this approach.

Policies and Procedures

Policies and procedures are designed to protect all patients or residents and staff in a hospital, community health care setting or nursing home. Examples are policies for cleaning, antibiotic stewardship and screening patients for MRSA before hospital admission. Between 1999 and 2010, the government in the United Kingdom delivered a range of strategic drivers to increase the status of infection control (Health Foundation, 2015), and the focus on community health care settings increased (NICE, 2018). In the past emphasis was placed on preventing infection in inpatient settings. Although this remains of key importance, there is a clear need to reduce health care–associated infection and other infections in primary care and community settings, in line with the move of health care beyond traditional hospital boundaries. In the United Kingdom, the NICE responded by issuing guidelines for infection prevention and control in and outside hospital (NICE, 2018).

Public Health Measures

Public health measures are policies to promote the health of an entire community, for example through notification of infectious diseases to statutory bodies, immunisation and inspection of premises where food is produced and sold. In the United Kingdom and many other countries, the immunisation schedule offered to older people includes the pneumococcal vaccine, an annual vaccine against influenza and vaccination for herpes zoster.

Risk Factors Associated With Hospital Admission and Communal Living

People in hospital and those living in closed and semi-closed environments (e.g., nursing/care homes, prisons, cruise ships) are at increased risk of infection irrespective of age because they share facilities, consume mass-produced food and have contact with other people who can operate as reservoirs. In premises where health care is delivered, infection risk is increased through frequent patient/resident contact with staff and exposure to the risks of antimicrobial-resistant micro-organisms. Very sick patients in hospital are handled more often and by larger numbers of people, undergo more invasive procedures (e.g., mechanical ventilation, urethral catheterisation) and are more likely to receive antibiotics. Long-stay patients have correspondingly greater exposure to hospital flora and are more likely to succumb to infection and operate as reservoirs of antimicrobial-resistant hospital strains, presenting an infection risk to others. Frail older people with chronic conditions are frequently discharged from acute hospitals to nursing homes and may import antimicrobial-resistant micro-organisms that can then be spread to other residents (Barr et al., 2007).

Health Care–Associated Infections

Health care–associated infections (HCAIs) are infections contracted through treatment or contact with a health or social care setting or health care delivered in a community setting (NICE, 2018). HCAIs can originate outside health care settings and be brought into hospital by patients, visitors or staff and transmitted to patients (NICE, 2018). Norovirus is a good example of an infection that can readily be imported into hospital and spread rapidly (Rajagopalan & Yoshikawa, 2016). Estimates of HCAIs vary. Epidemiological studies are expensive and challenging to undertake, so the most recent accurate figures are now somewhat dated. They suggest in England, 6.4% inpatients had at least one HCAI at the time of the prevalence survey, compared with 5% to 10% estimates elsewhere. Frequency was 23.4% in intensive care units (Health Protection Agency, 2012). The most commonly reported HCAIs were pneumonia and other respiratory infections (22.8%), urinary tract infections (17.2%), surgical site infections (15.7%), gastrointestinal infections (8.8%) and bloodstream infections (7.3%). Collectively these infections accounted for over 80% of all HCAIs.

The consequences of HCAIs are considerable. They are the most frequently occurring untoward events reported in health care. They increase avoidable morbidity and mortality, delay recovery, inflate the costs of health care (e.g., by prolonging stay, prompting re-admission, increasing use of antibiotics and consumables) and reduce patient satisfaction and public confidence in the health service. Cost estimates for HCAIs vary. According to the O'Neill Report (2016), HCAIs cost the NHS £1 billion annually, accounting for almost 1% of the total budget spent on health care. Individually, bloodstream infections are the most expensive, but surgical site infections add most to the overall costs of health care because they occur more often. The impact of HCAIs on patients is profound. They cost the NHS three times as much as patients who do not become infected; stay in hospital three times longer; are more likely to suffer pain, disability and need the attention of their family doctor or the domiciliary nursing services; consume more antibiotics; and are slower to resume their former activities and responsibilities (Plowman et al., 2001). HCAIs also contribute to the global problem of antimicrobial resistance, which is particularly challenging to treat (WHO, 2016).

Over the years opinions on HCAIs have changed. The traditional view was they were an inevitable consequence of receiving health care. Today it is thought HCAIs are avoidable and represent poor-quality care. Prevention hinges on the implementation of good fundamental infection-prevention precautions and educating staff, patients and the public about their contribution to infection prevention (WHO, 2016).

Infection Prevention Policies and Precautions

In all settings where health care is delivered, infection prevention and control policies need to address levels of risk. The following are important:

- Hand hygiene
- Policies for the use of cleaning agents, disinfection and sterilisation
- Disposal of clinical waste
- Disposal of soiled laundry
- Isolation of infectious patients and potentially infectious patients/residents
- Standard precautions/principles (e.g., environmental cleaning, use of personal protective equipment, safe handling and disposal of sharps and procedures to be followed in the case of needlestick injury and exposure to blood/body fluids)

The same principles apply in all settings, but modification is necessary according to where people live. In nursing homes the aim is to promote comfort and relaxation while still maintaining clinical standards when undertaking specific procedures such as dressing changes and giving injections. The fabric of the environment in this type of setting and the equipment available are key issues. Providing the requisite training and updating for staff responsible for frontline care can be challenging because they are often unregistered and supervised by only a small number of registered nurses. A vast body of research has been undertaken to assess and tackle the risks of infection in acute-care settings. Far less work has been undertaken in settings dedicated to the care of older people despite the increasing complexity of care delivered and the very high vulnerability of older people to infection. To complicate matters further, care and nursing homes vary considerably in the numbers and types of residents admitted, staff and amenities. Risk assessment and ability to adapt guidelines safely to meet local need is of paramount importance. See Chapter 11 for more on care homes.

Risk Management

Risk management is an important part of any infection prevention and control infection strategy. It is a systematic process in which potential risks are identified, analysed, prioritised and evaluated (Rausand, 2013). The objectives are to minimise the number of risks, enhance quality of care and contain costs.

Environmental Risks

For many years the health care environment was not considered to contribute much to the development of infection, but opinion has now changed. It is apparent microorganisms in the inanimate environment are able to reach vulnerable people, resulting in colonisation and infection (Weber et al., 2013). When identifying risk in different settings, it is important to bear in mind the health care environment consists of everything on the premises: all fixtures, fittings, equipment, patients and staff. It is also necessary to differentiate between risk in different settings: those where the risk of infection is very high and stringent precautions are necessary (e.g., theatres and critical care units), other health care settings (e.g., general hospital wards, clinics) and settings where people live and may also receive health care (e.g., nursing homes). The same principles of infection prevention apply everywhere, however, and encompass cleaning regimens, use of equipment, hand hygiene, personal and protective equipment and isolation for patients/residents who are contagious.

Cleaning

High standards of cleaning are essential to maintain the appearance, structure and efficient functioning of any environment where people live and receive care. Cleaning requires skill and training. Managers need sufficient knowledge to monitor whether the correct practices are being adopted. Key questions to ask are how soon recontamination is likely to occur after cleaning has been undertaken, whether the approach required to clean or disinfect equipment is likely to result in damage and practicality. Some items (e.g., floors, sluice hoppers and toilets) become recontaminated very rapidly, and the need for disinfection must be carefully evaluated. In lower-risk environments, cleaning rather than routine disinfection is often recommended. Disinfectants require time to exert effect, and the length of time varies between different agents, both of which affect choice in a given setting.

Equipment

In hospital, nurses or technicians are responsible for looking after equipment that is too delicate or expensive for domestic staff to handle and for items directly involved in patient care that need regular cleaning to avoid heavy contamination. In many community settings (e.g., health centres), nurses take responsibility for the routine cleaning and decontamination of all clinical equipment.

Items in the close patient environment (i.e., patient zone) are very likely to be contaminated and can operate as fomites (Lindberg et al., 2017). The obvious solution is to use disposables and otherwise ensure as far as possible that items are reserved for individual use. Inevitably some are shared (e.g., equipment used to monitor vital signs); others used by health workers (e.g., pens, scissors) are carried between the close environment of one patient and the next. The practicality of decontaminating such items every time they enter and leave a patient zone or finding alternatives is beginning to receive attention from health preventionists (Lindberg et al., 2017).

Hand Hygiene

HCAIs are spread predominantly by direct contact via hands (Pittet et al., 2006). Hand hygiene has traditionally been regarded as the most important means of prevention and continues to be the topic of considerable research, especially as potentially highly virulent community-acquired pathogens can be spread via hands (Bloomfield et al., 2007). Cross-infection is possible if a health worker moves from one patient/resident to another, for example travelling between different homes in the community, or handles different sites on the same person (e.g., giving an injection after bed-bathing). The hands of visitors as well as staff can be heavily contaminated with pathogens that cause HCAIs (Birnbach et al., 2015). Visitors who enter premises where health care is delivered should be encouraged to cleanse hands; hand hygiene is essential if they deliver direct care.

The WHO (2009) issued comprehensive hand hygiene guidelines and promotes the Five Moments for Hand Hygiene (Sax et al., 2007), which stipulate hands should be cleansed

1. Before touching a patient
2. Before undertaking clean/aseptic procedures
3. After exposure to blood/body fluids
4. After touching a patient
5. After touching the immediate patient environment

The Five Moments have been modified for use in care/nursing homes where patients are not restricted to an immediate bedspace (NICE, 2018). Some modification may also be necessary in hospitals as patients frequently move between locations in the same ward and from one department to another (e.g., physiotherapy and occupational therapy departments). Although the WHO (2009) guidelines are disseminated globally, overcrowding in hospitals in low-income countries challenges adherence to the Five Moments because bedspaces are so close together. Modification may also be necessary in very low-risk environments (e.g., outpatient radiology departments) where slavish adherence has the potential to reduce productivity and in emergencies (e.g., cardiac arrest).

Personal Protective Equipment

Personal protective equipment (PPE) has an established place protecting health workers when there is a known risk of exposure to blood or other body fluids and possible contact with transmissible pathogens.

Gloves are important as part of contact precautions to protect patients and whenever invasive procedures are undertaken. The evidence base underpinning the use of PPE is problematic, however. Most comes from expert panels and consensus groups. Relatively few empirical studies have been undertaken. Most studies explore how effectively items of PPE prevent transmission in laboratory or simulated settings rather than in trials under in-use conditions. Most of the research concerning the effectiveness of gloves has been undertaken in relation to MRSA, and recommendations are pragmatic. The consensus is they should be changed between patients/residents to prevent cross-infection and changed between different procedures involving the same patient/resident to prevent endogenous (i.e., self-infection) infection. Hands must still be cleansed after gloves have been worn as they are not impermeable to virus particles, and recontamination frequently occurs when they are removed. In recent years there have been concerns overuse of gloves is wasteful and challenges sustainability, and they are often worn unnecessarily, sometimes resulting in distress to patients (e.g., if used during routine bed-bathing). In the United Kingdom there is a move to reduce unnecessary use.

Face Masks

Masks were originally used in the operating theatre to protect patients. They are now used throughout other clinical settings to protect staff from respiratory viruses and splashing with body fluids. Uptake increased since the COVID-19 pandemic in 2020, and there is some controversy concerning effectiveness. Most studies to evaluate effectiveness of surgical masks have been performed either by analysing postoperative infection rates or by laboratory studies and simulation tests rather than prospectively in clinical settings. Even if they incorporate filters, the efficiency of masks is imperfect because virus-laden particles can escape around the sides. Simple paper and cloth masks are unlikely to be very effective because they are not sufficiently close-fitting and become damp and contaminated rapidly. They may increase the risks of transmission if they are handled frequently and not properly disposed of. Mask-wearing by the general public was encouraged during the COVID-19 pandemic largely to increase confidence when people were obliged to leave home. Advice about mask-wearing to prevent infection needs to present a balanced view, pointing out the limitations. Older people may find it difficult to hear when masks are worn, and wearing masks that loop around the ears is difficult for individuals who use hearing aids. Ability to hear and communicate is recognised as one of the main factors that helps reduce risks of dementia.

Respirators (e.g., N95) are designed to protect the wearer from very small particles, including viruses. Interest and use increased in the Far East in response to the SARS pandemic and in other countries as a consequence of COVID-19. Respirators filter out 95% of particles with a diameter of 0.3 micrometres and are fluid-resistant, but to remain effective, they must be tightly fitting. They are expensive, hot, uncomfortable and not practical except for use in high-risk settings.

Eye Protection

Eye and face protection that confirms to British Standards Institution standards is required when splashing or aerosols of blood, body fluids, secretions or excretions are possible. This is unusual in care home situations but a risk in theatre or dentistry where high-speed drills are used. Eye protection (e.g., goggles or visors) may not be disposable and must be disinfected after use by washing in a liquid detergent solution, followed by thorough drying.

Clothing

Research from the 1960s evaluated the contamination of uniforms worn in high-risk settings (e.g., burns units, operating theatres). It became apparent uniforms can transfer micro-organisms, especially if they become damp. More recent studies confirmed clothing becomes contaminated on general wards, especially during prolonged patient care episodes. Modern close-weave textiles have been developed that are splash-proof and have antibacterial properties, but they are expensive. When considering their purchase, thought needs to be given to laundering. The advantages of this type of clothing are lost if health workers are responsible for their own laundering, as most domestic washing machines employ eco-friendly cycles that do not destroy potential pathogens. In industrial laundries, risk of transferring infection still exists, because cross-contamination can occur, especially if staff work in both 'clean' and 'dirty' areas.

Aprons

Disposable plastic aprons are worn if clothing is likely to be exposed to blood, body fluids, secretions or excretions and where there is a risk of skin being contaminated from extensive splashing, such as in the operating theatre or accident department. Plastic aprons are more suitable than cotton gowns as the weave is permeable. Plastic carries fewer bacteria than cotton because bacteria cannot adhere readily to cold, slippery surfaces, and plastic dries out quickly. Plastic aprons are cheap and should be used as intended by the manufacturers—discarded between patients/residents or after an activity that results in heavy soiling.

Need for PPE differs according to clinical setting and patient risk and is heavily influenced by the activities undertaken by health workers. When considering choice of PPE, it is important to determine cost, amount of travel undertaken by staff (e.g., between different organisations or types of organisations), who is responsible for laundry and comfort if use is likely to be prolonged and disposal, especially for staff in community settings. It is easier to ensure PPE is used and disposed of correctly in institutions, but this creates significant challenges for domiciliary care.

Isolation

Isolation is an established part of any infection prevention programme. The aim is to prevent the transmission of antibiotic-resistant pathogens—those that are highly contagious or cause serious infection. The effectiveness of isolation has been questioned, and it can be difficult to undertake, especially if patients do not understand why it is necessary and become confused, lonely, bored, anxious and possibly uncooperative. A recent survey exploring the care of patients isolated for infectious conditions suggested in clinical practice the main issues are identifying which patients need to isolate quickly and prioritising who should be segregated when isolation accommodation is in short supply (Gould et al., 2018). There is some evidence patients become anxious and depressed during isolation (Purssell et al., 2020). Reducing contact with family members resulted in mental deterioration and dementia in older people in nursing homes during the COVID-19 pandemic in 2020 (Suárez-González et al., 2021). Understanding the effectiveness and impact of social distancing and isolation strategies in care homes for older people is important to consider as we prepare for further outbreaks (Williams et al., 2021).

THERMOREGULATION

Normal Body Temperature

Although it is common to talk about body temperature as if there is one value, in reality the body contains different areas, each with its own normal temperature. At its most simple, this can be thought of as consisting of a core temperature, which is that of the internal organs, and the shell, which is that of the skin, subcutaneous tissues and limbs. The temperature of the core is normally relatively stable, but the shell temperature varies widely according to factors such as ambient conditions, activity and time of day. Although it is tempting to provide normal temperature values, they vary according to the individual, their circumstances and measurement site. On average, however, there is approximately 0.4°C difference between healthy adults below 65 and those above (Blatteis, 2012).

The regulation of body temperature is achieved through a complex system that involves most bodily systems, so changes to these systems with advancing age impacts an individual's ability to control their temperature. For example, heat is distributed around the body primarily by the blood through the cardiovascular system, which is also important for regulating body temperature through vasoconstriction for saving hat and vasodilation for losing it. Although body temperature does not need to be as tightly controlled as some physiological parameters, heat extremes can cause significant damage or lead to death.

The body is naturally hot and usually produces far more heat than it needs through the action of metabolic, muscular and other functions. This heat is transferred around the body primarily through the bloodstream and lost to the environment through conduction, convection, radiation and evaporation. If more heat needs to be lost, vasodilation and sweating may occur. Because the normal requirement is to lose heat, heat-conserving mechanisms such as the action of brown adipose tissue, vasoconstriction and shivering are inhibited. As we will see later, fever results from the disinhibition of these mechanisms. Another important method of temperature regulation is behavioural changes—for example, changing position or adding or removing clothing.

Fever and Hyperthermia

It is most important to differentiate fever, which is a regulated rise in temperature, from hyperthermia, which is an unregulated rise. Substances that cause a regulated rise in temperature are known as pyrogens, which may be endogenous or exogenous in origin. Fever is normally caused by endogenous pyrogens, or substances produced within the body. These are collectively known as pyrogenic cytokines and include IL-1α, IL-1β, TNF-α, TNF-β, IL-6 and ciliary neurotrophic factor, produced during infection as part of the immune response (Dinarello, 2004). Further downstream, cellular cyclooxygenases convert phospholipases into prostaglandin E2, which causes disinhibition of nerves that usually prevent heat-generating responses, resulting in responses such as activation of brown adipose tissue, vasoconstriction and shivering thermogenesis to raise body temperature. Although there is no single temperature that indicates normality or fever, that the consensus is a tympanic temperature ≥37.2°C or a change of ≥1.3°C from baseline indicates fever in older people (Chung et al., 2014).

Commonly used antipyretic drugs that lower febrile temperatures, such as aspirin, paracetamol and ibuprofen work differently, but all have the effect of inhibiting the action of the cyclooxygenase enzymes. As fever is a regulated rise in temperature, it will be defended by the body as long as the pyrogenic cytokines are present, unless treated with antipyretic drugs. Use of physical methods to reduce fever are not therefore be effective and may cause shivering as the body attempts to maintain the temperature at its increased level. If shivering occurs in the presence of a high temperature, it may be the person is being cooled too quickly and are, paradoxically, cold. This is known as a rigor, and it should be avoided as it can be distressing and unpleasant.

The most important task when faced with a febrile patient is to quickly identify the cause. In many cases it is a self-limiting viral infection, for which no treatment apart from symptomatic care is required. However, more serious infections should not be discounted without appropriate consultation. For example, people over 75 or people who are very frail are at an increased risk of sepsis (NICE, 2017). However, the absence of fever does not necessarily mean the patient does not have an infection, as the normal clinical signs and symptoms of infection may be atypical or absent in older people (Székely & Garai, 2018). Diagnosing sepsis in older people is particularly challenging. Some symptoms that would suggest infection of the nervous system in younger people, such as altered mental state or delirium, may a less specific sign of infection in older adults or the result of other conditions. Urinary tract infections may cause confusion rather than more classic signs, and pneumonia may present with weakness, falls and hypoxia. Biological markers of infection such as C-reactive protein and raised blood counts may be abnormal as the result of other and multiple morbidities and infection (Clifford et al., 2016).

The regulated rise in temperature associated with fever is quite different from hyperthermia, which is an unregulated rise. Unlike fever, which is not in itself dangerous, both hypothermia and hyperthermia can be harmful. A number of age-related changes predispose older people to altered temperature, including difficulties in adapting to changing environmental temperature, changes in sensory perception (e.g., hearing, vision), decreased thermal sensitivity, decreased sweating responses, reduced cardiac output making vasodilation more difficult and reduced or altered physical activity (Székely & Garai, 2018). The loss of physical abilities may also mean it is difficult for older people to make important behavioural changes. Both heat and cold defence may be inhibited, predisposing to hypo- and hyperthermia.

Hypothermia

Hypothermia is generally defined as a core body temperature <35°C, although a more patient-focused approach would define it as a decrease in temperature that results in signs of physiologic dysfunction (Cheshire, 2016). Hypothermia may be classified as being mild if the core temperature is 32.3°C to 35°C, moderate if it is 28°C to 32.2°C, or severe if it is <28°C. The clinical features associated with mild hypothermia include shivering, vasoconstriction, tachycardia and tachypnoea but in addition may include apathy, ataxia, diuresis and impaired judgement. As the body temperature falls and consciousness decreases, blood pressure, heart rate and respiratory rate fall, pupils may dilate, the gag reflex may be lost and shivering and body tone decrease. If the person is on cardiac monitoring, abnormalities such as atrial dysrhythmias and other changes may be seen. In severe hypothermia, apnoea, coma and ventricular dysrhythmias and cardiac arrest may result.

The main focus in a hypothermic patient should be to safely rewarm them; the exact method by which this is achieved depends on the degree of hypothermia and the available resources. In general, rewarming techniques are either passive, where the natural heat-producing properties of the body are used to achieve a rise in temperature, or active, where the patient is warmed either externally or internally. Passive rewarming normally consists of removing any wet clothing, moving to a warmer environment and wrapping up the person to insulate them. This strategy clearly requires the individual is able to generate sufficient heat, and it may take a considerable amount of time, so it is suitable only for mild hypothermia in individuals who are able to produce sufficient heat for rewarming to occur (McCullough & Arora, 2004).

If this is not sufficient, active external rewarming is the next step. It is relatively easy to undertake by applying heat to the skin. Remembering the main way heat is distributed around the body is through circulation, this method requires a functioning cardiovascular system. Furthermore, caution needs to be taken to avoid complications such as a sudden drop in core temperature as cold blood suddenly returns to the heart, acidosis as lactic acid from the periphery circulates centrally, and shock due to sudden peripheral vasodilation. Internal core rewarming can be highly invasive and includes interventions such as forced-air rewarming, warmed intravenous fluids and extracorporeal blood warming (McCullough & Arora, 2004).

Hyperthermia

Hyperthermia is an unregulated rise in temperature, in contrast to fever, which is a regulated rise. Fever has a 'glass ceiling' above which temperature does not appear to rise, and it certainly does not achieve temperatures of >42°C, at which physical damage might occur. This is the result of multiple mechanisms to prevent these sorts of temperatures. However, there are no such preventative defences against external warming and other causes of hyperthermia, which depend on physiological responses to lose heat and behavioural changes to remove the source of the heat. Hyperthermia can therefore be defined as a core temperature of >40.5°C (Cheshire, 2016), although changes may be seen at temperatures far lower than this, and as with hypothermia, a more patient-focused definition describes it as an increase in temperature that results in signs of physiologic dysfunction.

Hyperthemia can be passive in origin—for example, through exposure to heat sources such as the sun—or the result of activity such as exercise. The former is more common in older adults, and the risk of it occurring is increased by impairments in thermoregulatory physiology and heat dissipation mechanisms or if the person is unable to remove themselves from the source of the heat.

There are three levels of hyperthermia: heat cramps and oedema, heat exhaustion, and heat stroke. Heat cramps are more common following exercise. In older adults, heat oedema in the feet and ankles may be more common. Prickly heat or heat rash is a minor condition caused by sweat glands becoming plugged. Heat exhaustion is characterised by fatigue, thirst and irritability with nausea and vomiting. The individual may appear flushed with sweating, and they may be tachycardic, with weakness, cramps, headache, dizziness and paraesthesia. Heat stroke presents with delirium, confusion, hallucinations, seizures and coma; the individual may appear flushed but may have a loss of sweating that can progress to heart failure, hypotension, myocardial and hepatic injury and ultimately thrombocytopenia and disseminated intravascular coagulation (Cheshire, 2016).

Treatment is to remove the source of heat. Active cooling may be applied, remembering this is different to fever, where active cooling is not recommended. Other treatments are to manage symptoms or physiological abnormalities, such as by correcting dehydration or electrolyte imbalance.

SUMMARY AND KEY POINTS

This chapter describes the chain of infection common to all pathogens and outlines the risks of infection, the principles of infection prevention applied to older people and challenges to thermoregulation and how to manage them. In the wake of the COVID-19 pandemic, it is likely in future greater attention will be paid to the prevention of infection, especially for high-risk groups such as older people.

KEY LEARNING POINTS

- The chain of infection comprises six links: the reservoir of infection, the means of exit, the method of transmission, entry into a new host, invasion of a susceptible site and the interaction that results in infection. Each offers the opportunity to reduce or prevent infection.
- Older people have an increased risk of infection due to changes in the immune system, comorbidities and social factors.
- Diagnosing infection in older people is complicated by these same factors, making specialist involvement important.
- It is important to remember the social aspects of infection such as isolation and loneliness.
- Older people are at increased risk of hypo- and hyperthermia. It is important to differentiate hyperthermia from fever.

REFERENCES

Barr, B., Wilcox, M. H., Brady, A., Parnell, P., Darby, B., & Tompkins, D. (2007). Prevalence of methicillin-resistant *Staphylococcus aureus* colonization among older residents of care homes in the United Kingdom. *Infection Control and Hospital Epidemiology, 28*, 853–859.

Birnbach, D., Rosen, L., Fitzpatrick, M., Arheart, L., & Munoz-Price, S. (2015). An evaluation of hand hygiene in an intensive care unit: Are visitors a potential vector for pathogens? *Journal of Infection and Public Health, 8*, 570–574.

Blatteis, C. M. (2012). Age-dependent changes in temperature regulation—A mini review. *Gerontology, 58*(4), 289–295. https://doi.org/10.1159/000333148.

Bloomfield, S., Aiello, A. E., Cookson, B., O'Boyle, C., & Larson, L. (2007). The effectiveness of hand hygiene procedures in reducing risks of infections in home and community settings including handwashing and alcohol-based hand santizers. *American Journal of Infection Control, 35*(Supp 1), S27–S64. https://doi.org/10.1016/j.ajic.2007.07.001.

Centers for Disease Control and Prevention (2015). In J Hamborsky, A Kroger, & S Wolfe (Eds.), *Epidemiology and prevention of vaccine-preventable diseases* (13th ed.). Public Health Foundation.

Chakhtoura, N. G., Banomo, R. A., & Jump, R. L. P. (2017). Influence of aging and environmental presentation of infection in older adults. *Infectious Disease Clinics, 31*(4), 593–608.

Cheshire, W. P. (2016). Thermoregulatory disorders and illness related to heat and cold stress. *Autonomic Neuroscience, 196*, 91–104. https://doi.org/10.1016/j.autneu.2016.01.001.

Chung, M.-H., Huang, C.-C., Vong, S.-C., Yang, T.-M., Chen, K.-T., Lin, H.-J., Chen, J.-H., Su, S.-B., Guo, H.-R., & Hsu, C.-C. (2014). Geriatric Fever Score: A new decision rule for geriatric care. *PloS One, 9*(10), e110927. https://doi.org/10.1371/journal.pone.0110927.

Clifford, K. M., Dy-Boarman, E. A., Haase, K. K., Maxvill, K., Pass, S. E., & Alvarez, C. A. (2016). Challenges with diagnosing and managing sepsis in older adults. *Expert Review of Anti-infective Therapy, 14*(2), 231–241. https://doi.org/10.1586/14787210.2016.1135052.

Dinarello, C. A. (2004). Review: Infection, fever, and exogenous and endogenous pyrogens: some concepts have changed. *Journal of Endotoxin Research, 10*(4), 201–222. https://doi.org/10.1177/09680519040100040301.

Gould, D. J. (2010). Scabies. *Nursing Standard, 25*(9), 42–46.

Gould, D. J., Drey, N. S., Chudleigh, J., King, M. F., Wigglesworth, N., & Purssell, E. (2018). Isolating infectious patients: organizational, clinical, and ethical issues. *The American Journal of Infection Control, 46*(8), e65–e69. https://doi.org/10.1016/j.ajic.2018.05.024.

Graham, N. S. N., Junghans, C., Downes, R., Sendall, C., Lai, H., McKirdy, A., Elliott, P., Howard, R., Wingfield, D., Priestman, M., Ciechonska, M., Cameron, L., Storch, M., Crone, M. A., Freemont, P. S., Randell, P., McLaren, R., Lang, N., Ladhani, S., … Sharp, D. J. (2020). SARS-CoV-2 infection, clinical features and outcome of COVID-19 in United Kingdom nursing homes. *Journal of Infection, 81*(3), 411–419. https://doi.org/10.1016/j.ajic.2018.05.024.

Gyawali, B., Ramakrishna, K., & Dhamoon, A. S. (2019). Sepsis: The evolution in definition, pathophysiology, and management. *SAGE Open Medicine, 7*. 2050312119835043. https://doi.org/10.1177/2050312119835043.

Health Foundation. (2015). *Infection prevention and control: Lessons from acute care in England. Towards a whole health economy approach. Health Foundation Learning Report.* Health Foundation.

Health Protection Agency. (2012). *English national point prevalence survey on healthcare-associated infections and antimicrobial use, 2011: Preliminary data.* London: Health Protection Agency.

Keenan, C. R., & Allan, R. S. (2019). Epigenomic drivers of immune dysfunction in aging. *Aging Cell, 18*(1), e12878. https://doi.org/10.1111/acel.12878.

McCullough, L., & Arora, S. (2004). Diagnosis and treatment of hypothermia. *American Family Physician, 70*(12), 2325–2332.

Lindberg, M., Lindberg, M., & Skytt, B. (2017). Risk behaviours for organism transmission in health care delivery: A two month unstructured observational study. *International Journal of Nursing Studies, 70*, 38–45.

Moser, M., & Leo, O. (2010). Key concepts in immunology. *Vaccine, 28*, C2–C13. https://doi.org/10.1016/j.vaccine.2010.07.022.

Montecino-Rodriguez, E., Berent-Maoz, B., & Dorshkind, K. (2013). Causes, consequences, and reversal of immune system aging. *Journal of Clinical Investigation, 123*(3), 958–965. https://doi.org/10.1172/JCI64096.

National Infection Prevention and Control Manual. (2012). Chain of infection. https://www.nipcm.hps.scot.nhs.uk/infection-prevention-and-control-manual-for-older-people-and-adult-care-homes/print?section=2820

National Institute for Health and Care Excellence (NICE). (2017). Sepsis: Recognition, diagnosis and early management—Guidance. https://www.nice.org.uk/guidance/ng51/chapter/recommendations#risk-factors-for-sepsis

NICE. (2018). Healthcare associated infections: Prevention and control in primary and community care. National Institute for Health and Care Excellence. https://www.nice.org.uk/guidance/cg139

O'Neill Report. (2016). *Tackling drug-resistant infections globally. Infection prevention, control and surveillance: Limiting the spread and development of drug resistance.* http://amr-review.org/sites/default/files/Health%20infrastructure%20and%20surveillance%20final%20version_LR_NO%20CROPS.pdf

Pittet, D., Allegranzi, B., Sax, H., Dharan, S., Pessoa-Silva, C. L., Donaldson, L., & Boyce, J. (2006). Evidence-based model for hand transmission during patient care and the role of improved practices. *Lancet Infectious Diseases, 6*, 641–652.

Plowman, R., Graves, N., Griffin, M. A. S., Swan, A. V., Cookson, B., & Taylor, L. (2001). The rate and cost of hospital-acquired infections occurring in patients admitted to selected specialties of a district general hospital in England and the national burden imposed. *Journal of Hospital Infection, 47*, 198–209.

Pop-Vicas, A., Rahman, M., Gonzlo, P. L., Gravenstein, S., & Mor, V. (2015). Estimating the effect of influenza vaccination on nursing home residents' morbidity and mortality. *Journal of the American Geriatric Society, 63*, 1798–1804.

Purssell, E., Gould, D., Chudleigh, J. Impact of isolation on hospitalised patients who are infectious: systematic review with meta-analysis *BMJ Open* 2020;10:e030371. https://doi.org/10.1136/bmjopen-2019-030371.

Rajagopalan, S., & Yoshikawa, T. T. (2016). Norovirus infections in long-term care facilities. *Journal of the American Geriatrics Society*. https://doi.org/10.1111/jgs.14085.

Rausand, M. (2013). *Risk assessment, theory, methods and applications*. John Wiley.

Sax, H., Allegranzi, B., Uçkay, I., Larson, E., Boyce, J., & Pittet, D. (2007). 'My five moments for hand hygiene': A user-centred design approach to understand, train, monitor and report hand hygiene. *Infection Control Hospital Epidemiology, 67,* 9–21.

Simon, A. K., Hollander, G. A., & McMichael, A. (2015). Evolution of the immune system in humans from infancy to old age. *Proceedings of the Royal Society B: Biological Sciences, 282*(1821), 20143085. https://doi.org/10.1098/rspb.2014.3085.

Sinikumpu, S. P., Jokelainen, J., Haarala, A. K., Keränen, M. H., Keinänen-Kiukaanniemi, S., & Huilaja, L. (2020). The high prevalence of skin diseases in adults aged 70 and older. *Journal of the American Geriatrics Society, 68*(11), 2565–2571. https://doi.org/10.1111/jgs.16706.

Suárez-González, A., Rajagopalan, J., Livingston, G., & Alladi, S. (2021). The effect of COVID-19 isolation measures on the cognition and mental health of people living with dementia: A rapid systematic review of one year of quantitative evidence. *eClinicalMedicine, 39*, 101047. https://doi.org/10.1016/j.eclinm.2021.101047.

Székely, M., & Garai, J. (2018). Thermoregulation and age. In *Handbook of clinical neurology* (pp. 377–395). Elsevier. https://doi.org/10.1016/B978-0-444-63912-7.00023-0.

van Seventer, J. M., & Hochberg, N. S. (2017). Principles of infectious diseases: Transmission, diagnosis, and control. *International Encyclopedia of Public Health*, 22–39. https://doi.org/10.1016/B978-0-12-803678-5.00516-6

Weber, D., Anderson, D., & Rutala, W. A. (2013). The role of the surface environment in healthcare-associated infections. *Current Opinions in Infectious Diseases, 26*, 338–344.

Weiskopf, D., Weinberger, B., & Grubeck-Loebenstein, B. (2009). The aging of the immune system. *Transplant International, 22*(11), 1041–1050. https://doi.org/10.1111/j.1432-2277.2009.00927.x.

Williams, C. Y. K., Townson, A. T., Kapur, M., Ferreira, A. F., Nunn, R., Galante, J., Phillips, V., Gentry, S., & Usher-Smith, J. A. (2021). Interventions to reduce social isolation and loneliness during COVID-19 physical distancing measures: A rapid systematic review. *PLoS One, 16*(2), e0247139. https://doi.org/10.1371/journal.pone.0247139.

World Health Organization (WHO). (2009). *WHO guidelines on hand hygiene in health care*. Geneva: World Health Organization. https://www.who.int/publications/i/item/9789241597906.

WHO. (2016). Global action plan on antimicrobial resistance. Geneva: World Health Organization. https://www.who.int/publications/i/item/9789241509763.

24

Maintaining Healthy Skin

Gillian Elizabeth Pedley

CHAPTER OUTLINE

This chapter provides an overview of general skin assessment in older adults. The causes of pressure injury, predisposing risk factors and risk assessment are discussed, along with the principles of pressure ulcer prevention. The final section provides an overview of wound healing and principles of wound management.

The skin is the part of the human body visible to others, and it reflects our emotions, well-being and state of health. It performs essential homeostatic, sensory and protective roles. Skin assessment provides a visible summary of internal functioning and requires an understanding of normal age-related changes in the skin and the ability to distinguish them from abnormal skin lesions and signs of systemic disease. It also provides an indicator of a person's ability to attend to personal care needs and indirectly reveals clues about the person's level of functional ability. General skin assessment should include past and present skin history, skin changes, medication and a visual assessment (Box 24.1). For an account of the anatomy and physiology of the skin, age-related changes and skin assessment, see Nigam and Knight (2017).

Skin lesions are common in older people, and observation should be made of their location, structural characteristics, size, colour and grouping. Skin lesions may be triggered by long-term sun exposure. New lesions or lesions that have undergone changes, are asymmetrical, have irregular borders, variable pigmentation, a mottled appearance or are 6 mm or more in diameter require further investigation to rule out malignency. Age-related changes and higher levels of morbidity in later life make older adults' skin more vulnerable to injury from unrelieved pressure. For this reason skin assessment in older adults must include an inspection for early signs of pressure ulcers.

PRESSURE ULCERS: CAUSES, RISK FACTORS AND RISK ASSESSMENT

Pressure ulcers are localised soft-tissue injuries caused by unrelieved pressure, shear or friction, or a combination of these. If prolonged, mechanical stressors impair local microcirculation and result in ischaemic changes or necrosis in the tissues served by the affected vessels. Visible skin changes occur, ranging from redness to localised tissue death and ulceration of the skin, subcutaneous fat and muscle. Pressure ulcers occur most frequently on areas of the body where soft tissues are vulnerable to compression between two hard surfaces, usually the bony prominences or 'pressure points', where there is little opportunity for pressure to dissipate through fatty tissues and another firm surface such as a mattress, chair or medical device (e.g., urinary catheter or endotracheal tube). The three

BOX 24.1   Framework for the Visual Assessment of Skin: Key Assessment Areas, Common Findings and Their Possible Significance

Colour and Altered Pigmentation
- Bruising/petechiae: Vitamin deficiency, bleeding disorder, trauma
- Cyanosis: Cardiovascular and/or pulmonary insufficiency
- Jaundice: Gastrointestinal disease
- Pallor: Anaemia, reduced vascularity, arterial insufficiency of limb
- Erythema: Inflammation/infection, pressure-induced ischaemia
- Ankle flare, staining of lower limbs and varicosities: Chronic venous hypertension/venous insufficiency

Texture
- Smooth, atrophic skin: Arterial insufficiency
- Coarse skin: Hypothyroidism
- Dry skin: Reduced sebum and water content of skin

Turgor/Oedema
- Reduced elasticity and resilience: Reduced collagen, reduced hydration
- Taut, shiny and reduced skin mobility: Oedema

Temperature
- Difference between trunk and extremities: Maintenance of core and peripheral temperature

- Difference between lower limbs: Vascular insufficiency
- Elevated temperature: Inflammation, hyperthyroidism
- Low temperature: Low core temperature, hypothyroidism

Lesions/Rashes/Scars/Areas of Discontinuity
- New growths: Normal age-related changes, abnormal lesions
- Eczema: Arthritis, chronic venous insufficiency
- Infection: Bacterial, viral, fungal
- Cuts and abrasions
- Pressure ulcers and blisters
- Leg ulcers: Venous/arterial insufficiency
- Rashes

Hygiene
- Odour: Poor hygiene, poor self-care ability, loss of continence, infection
- Condition of skinfolds, feet, nails, genitalia and perianal area: Self-care ability
- Infestation: Head lice, body lice, scabies

most common sites for pressure ulcer development are, in descending order of prevalence, the sacrum (37%), heels (25%) and buttocks (12%) (Moore et al., 2019).

Aetiology: Anatomical Structures

The structures of the dermis are supported in a matrix of collagen and elastin that protects blood and lymph vessels, nerves, glands and hair follicles against mechanical damage. Collagen has little extensibility but has high strength and resists deformation. Elastin has elastic properties and enables tissues to recover their shape after being stretched. Together, collagen and elastin protect the tissues from the effects of pressure. The loose connective tissue underlying the dermis is composed primarily of fat cells. It is compressible, provides padding over bony prominences and permits the movement of the dermis over deeper structures. It contains little collagen and therefore lacks tensile strength and is vulnerable to mechanical stressors. Underlying the subcutaneous layer and surrounding the muscle is the fascia. Its high collagen content provides resistance to distortion

and protects the soft muscle layer. The ageing process affects these protective mechanisms and makes the tissues less resistant to mechanical forces. For example, collagen synthesis gradually declines between the ages of 20 and 60, with a marked decline thereafter. As collagen levels fall, more load is transmitted to the cells and interstitial fluid. Elastin content of the tissues also declines. These changes help explain the rise in pressure ulceration associated with advancing age.

Aetiology: Maintaining Tissue Perfusion

Effective tissue perfusion requires an intact microcirculation and is fundamental in maintaining tissue integrity and preventing pressure ulcers. The following section reviews the physiology of microcirculation and its response to pressure.

Microcirculation

The microcirculation comprises arterioles, venules, metarterioles (i.e., shunting vessels) and capillaries. The capillary walls are one cell thick and formed from endothelial cells. Their thin structure facilitates the diffusion of gases, nutrients and metabolites. This exchange of nutrients and waste products between the blood and tissues is achieved by an intermittent flow and stasis of blood through the capillaries and is controlled by the precapillary sphincters, their action mediated by the chemical composition of the capillary blood. When the sphincters are closed, blood flow ceases, and an exchange of nutrients, oxygen, carbon dioxide and metabolites occurs. This accumulation of metabolites and carbon dioxide and a fall in oxygen triggers relaxation of the precapillary sphincters, and oxygenated blood flows into the capillary, flushing out the deoxygenated blood and waste products. The microcirculation system is interwoven with a network of lymph vessels that drains extravascular fluid back into the blood.

Capillary blood pressure ranges from 32 mm Hg at the arteriolar end of the capillary to 12 mm Hg at the venous end. These values vary according to systolic blood pressure and other factors that influence blood pressure. Compression of microcirculation by external forces in excess of capillary pressure in theory impedes blood flow, but the soft tissues and microcirculation contained within are exposed to external pressures in excess of capillary pressure on a daily basis. Two inbuilt circulatory mechanisms, autoregulation and reactive hyperaemia, enable the soft tissues to resist the effects of pressure without incurring lasting ischaemic changes and cell damage.

Autoregulation. In response to external forces, a process of autoregulation enables capillary pressure to rise and stabilise 10 mm Hg above the external pressure, up to the pressure of the diastolic blood pressure. This protective response may be less dramatic in hypotensive clients and may be absent in those who develop ulcers (Schubert, 1991).

Reactive Hyperaemia. External pressure sufficient to occlude capillary blood flow results in ischaemia, and the accumulation of carbon dioxide, hydrogen ions and metabolites produces local arteriolar dilatation. Removal of the external occluding pressure causes a sudden increased blood flow through the dilated capillaries, known as reactive hyperaemia, and is visible on lightly pigmented skin as a clearly demarcated pink/red 'flush'. The patency of the capillaries in the hyperaemic area can be assessed by the application of light finger pressure. Application of pressure occludes the capillaries, which can be observed as a whitening of the area when the pressure is removed, called blanching hyperaemia. The white area rapidly turns deep pink as the capillaries refill with blood, demonstrating they are patent. Failure of a reddened area to turn white under light finger pressure indicates the capillaries may no longer

be patent. This is termed non-blanching hyperaemia (i.e., non-blanchable erythema) and is considered an early sign of pressure injury.

Ischaemic-Reperfusion Injury

Ischaemic-reperfusion injury may cause or exacerbate pressure ulcer formation and contribute to deep tissue injury (DTI). Reperfusion of tissues after extended periods of ischaemia produces high levels of intracellular reactive oxygen species (i.e., free radicals) (Swan, 2017). These unstable molecules react readily with others, damaging cell proteins, DNA and RNA, which may result in cell death. In vitro studies have shown cell damage to increase with repeated cycles of ischaemic reperfusion. Tissue damage also appears more severe with repeated ischaemic reperfusion compared to tissue injury caused by sustained ischaemia.

Aetiology: The Role of Pressure, Shear and Friction

Intact sensation and the ability to carry out spontaneous changes in position to alleviate pressure and redistribute weight are important protective mechanisms. Spontaneous body movements are triggered by the sensation of discomfort and pain from compressed ischaemic tissues. This continuous cycle of spontaneous movement relieves pressure and permits reperfusion of the affected area, preventing permanent damage. Excessive body loading, either as a perpendicular force or as shear, is the primary cause of pressure ulcers. The role of pressure, shear and friction in the causation of pressure ulcers is outlined below.

Pressure

At levels that exceed capillary pressure, a load or force applied at right angles to the body acts to compress and occlude the blood supply, causing ischaemia. Local accumulation of toxic metabolic by-products increases the rate of cell death. The surviving cells are compromised and more susceptible to damage by mechanical forces. Pressure may also cause angulation and distortion of the arterioles sufficient to disrupt the endothelial cells and trigger the clotting process: platelets accumulate in the damaged vessels, causing occlusion and necrosis of the cells supplied by the vessel. Accumulated metabolites and hypoxia act on the precapillary sphincters, causing a marked hyperaemic response on removal of the occluding pressure. This increases the blood flow and amount of fluid that filters through the capillary wall into the interstitial space. Excess interstitial fluid is normally removed by lymph vessels, but under hypoxic conditions, lymphatic smooth muscle may be damaged, leading to loss of lymph motility and impaired lymph flow. The excess fluid that separates capillaries from cells makes it more difficult for capillary oxygen to reach the tissues. Compression of tissues may cause interstitial fluid to be squeezed from between the cells, resulting in cell-to-cell contact pressure of sufficient magnitude to cause cell rupture. A sudden reduction in interstitial pressure associated with removal of the external force, coupled with the rise in capillary pressure from the hyperaemic response, may result in capillary bursting. Impaired lymph function hinders removal of the products of capillary bursting from the interstitial space, which is thought to contribute to cell necrosis. A reduction in the amount of collagen fibres in the tissues, as occurs with ageing, reduces the resistance to compression and squeeze.

Shear

Shear occurs when lateral forces are applied to the tissues, in conjunction with pressure, to create an opposite parallel sliding movement. As soft tissues are dragged over the rigid skeleton, they are stretched and distorted. This commonly occurs when gravity causes a patient to slide down the bed or chair; the frictional forces of the skin against the chair surface cause the outer layers of tissues to remain static while the skeleton and deeper tissues slide forward. The extent to which the tissues are subject to shearing depends on their consistency and structure. For example, the subcutaneous layer, which contains adipose tissue, provides padding and dissipates pressure, but its mobility makes it particularly prone to shear. In contrast, the high collagen content of the underlying tough, firm fascia and to a lesser extent the dermis enables these structures to resist mechanical deformation. Although pressure is the primary cause of occlusion, animal studies have shown the presence of shear reduces the amount of pressure required to cause tissue damage, which has important clinical implications for the moving and positioning of patients and the choice of seating.

Friction

Friction may injure the epidermis and dermis, making these structures less resistant to pressure, or it may act in conjunction with shear and/or pressure as described above.

Summary

Age-related changes reduce soft-tissue tolerance to pressure, shear and friction. Conditions that impair sensation or movement, including anaesthesia, sedation and mental ill health, also negatively impact protective mechanisms.

Diagnosis and Classification of Pressure Ulcers

Pressure ulcer diagnosis requires the clinician to distinguish pressure-induced soft-tissue injury from other forms of tissue destruction and from the body's normal hyperaemic response to pressure. Numerous pressure ulcer classification systems exist (also called categorisation or staging). For pressure ulcers with tissue loss, rather than measuring the depth of the ulcer in millimetres, classification requires the practitioner to identify the deepest layer of damaged tissue. This approach is used because of diversity among individuals in the amounts of muscle and fat and the variations in muscle and fat distribution on different parts of the body. For example, a shallow ulcer on a heel may reach the bone, while an ulcer of similar depth located on the buttock may reach only the adipose layer. Classification requires not only visualisation of the wound bed—often masked by slough and necrotic tissue—but also that the clinician has sufficient knowledge to distinguish between the different tissues.

The International NPUAP-EPUAP Pressure Ulcer Classification System (National Pressure Ulcer Advisory Panel, European Pressure Ulcer Advisory Panel and Pan Pacific Pressure Injury Alliance, 2014) (Table 24.1) is one of the most widely used classification systems. Its development was driven by the need for a standardised approach to pressure ulcer definition and classification in order to enhance the quality and consistency of clinical practice and allow comparisons between research findings. The classification draws on earlier published systems and has been refined through expert panel consensus meetings and improved understanding of pressure ulcer aetiology. It is not intended to represent sequential stages in the severity of tissue damage. The classification considers intact skin with a localised area of non-blanchable erythema or redness over a pressure point to be an established indicator of early or impending pressure ulceration.

The early identification of pressure injury in people with heavily pigmented skin using traditional diagnostic indicators presents challenges as the higher levels of melanin may mask the pink/red hue of the hyperaemic response and non-blanchable erythema, with the risk of delayed identification and intervention. This applies to both stage 1 ulcers and suspected DTI. Evidence of delayed identification in people with darker skin tones is evident in pressure ulcer incidence and prevalence data where this is reported by skin tone. For example, VanGuilder et al. (2008) reported a 37% stage 1 pressure ulcer prevalence in patients with light skin tones, 31% in patients with medium skin tones and 12% in patients with dark skin tones. Conversely, stage 4 pressure ulcer prevalence was 5%, 6% and 12%, respectively. To ensure early recognition in all patients, practitioners need to be aware of, and able to recognise, the signs of pressure injury across the full spectrum of skin tones. In patients with a skin tone too dark

TABLE 24.1   International NPUAP-EPUAP Pressure Ulcer Classification System

Category/Stage	Description
Category/Stage I pressure ulcer: Non-blanchable erythema	Intact skin with non-blanchable redness of a localised area usually over a bony prominence. Darkly pigmented skin may not have visible blanching; its colour may differ from the surrounding area. The area may be painful, firm, soft, warmer or cooler as compared to adjacent tissue. Category/Stage I may be difficult to detect in individuals with dark skin tones. May indicate at-risk individuals (a heralding sign of risk).
Category/Stage II pressure ulcer: Partial thickness skin loss	Partial thickness loss of dermis presenting as a shallow open ulcer with a red-pink wound bed, without slough. May also present as an intact or open/ruptured serum filled blister. Presents as a shiny or dry shallow ulcer without slough or bruising*. This category/stage should not be used to describe skin tears, tape burns, perineal dermatitis, maceration or excoriation.
Category/Stage III pressure ulcer: Full-thickness skin loss	Full-thickness tissue loss. Subcutaneous fat may be visible, but bone, tendon or muscle are not exposed. Slough may be present but does not obscure the depth of tissue loss. May include undermining and tunnelling. The depth of a Category/Stage III pressure ulcer varies by anatomical location. The bridge of the nose, ear, occiput and malleolus do not have subcutaneous tissue and Category/Stage III ulcers can be shallow. In contrast, areas of significant adiposity can develop extremely deep Category/Stage III pressure ulcers. Bone/tendon is not visible or directly palpable.
Category/Stage IV pressure ulcer: Full-thickness tissue loss	Full-thickness tissue loss with exposed bone, tendon or muscle. Slough or eschar may be present on some parts of the wound bed. Often includes undermining and tunnelling. The depth of a Category/Stage IV pressure ulcer varies by anatomical location. The bridge of the nose, ear, occiput and malleolus do not have subcutaneous tissue, and these ulcers can be shallow. Category/Stage IV ulcers can extend into muscle and/or supporting structures (e.g., fascia, tendon or joint capsule), making osteomyelitis possible. Exposed bone/tendon is visible or directly palpable.
Unstageable: Depth unknown	Full-thickness tissue loss in which the base of the ulcer is covered by slough (yellow, tan, grey, green or brown) and/or eschar (tan, brown or black) in the wound bed. Until enough slough and/or eschar is removed to expose the base of the wound, the true depth, and therefore the category/stage, cannot be determined. Stable (i.e., dry, adherent, intact without erythema or fluctuance) eschar on the heels serves as the body's natural (i.e., biological) cover and should not be removed.
Suspected deep tissue injury: Depth unknown	Purple or maroon localised area of discoloured intact skin or blood-filled blister due to damage of underlying soft tissue from pressure and/or shear. The area may be preceded by tissue that is painful, firm, mushy, boggy, warmer or cooler as compared to adjacent tissue. Deep tissue injury may be difficult to detect in individuals with dark skin tones. Evolution may include a thin blister over a dark wound bed. The wound may further evolve and become covered by thin eschar. Evolution may be rapid, exposing additional layers of tissue even with optimal treatment.

*Bruising indicates suspected deep tissue injury.

Source: National Pressure Ulcer Advisory Panel, European Pressure Ulcer Advisory Panel and Pan Pacific Pressure Injury Alliance (2014).

to detect non-blanchable erythema, the skin over bony prominences should be examined for demarcated areas of persistent discolouration (i.e., hyperpigmentation or hypopigmentation), comparing opposite sides of the body to aid assessment. Where DTI is present, discolouration may have a purple hue (Sullivan, 2014). (See next paragraph for explanation of DTI.) Palpation of the area may reveal localised hardness (i.e., induration). Where there is established tissue damage, heat due to the inflammatory process or coolness due to reduced perfusion may also be noted. Bogginess may be felt, particularly over the calcaneus (i.e., heel). Patient reports of pain over pressure points can be an important early indicator of tissue injury and should be acted on promptly. Unlike most earlier classifications, this system provides specific indicators within the descriptors to assist with identification in patients with darker skin tones. For a visual respresentation of pressure injury classification in people with darker skin tones, see

Talley Group Limited (2020). For further discussion on this topic, see Oozageer Gunowa et al. (2018).

Some pressure ulcers form deep within the tissues, where areas of necrosis can occur with little initial outward sign other than discolouration of the overlying skin, referred to as deep tissue injury (DTI). Eventual skin breakdown may reveal a substantial area of necrotic tissue. DTI may present as a localised, clearly defined area of non-blanchable dark-red, purple or purple-tinged discolouration of intact skin overlying a pressure point or as a blood-filled blister. The area may also feel different, as described in the paragraph above. The EPUAP-NPUAP classification includes a separate category for suspected DTI and for unstageable pressure ulcers, where the base of the ulcer is obscured by slough or necrotic tissue such that the extent of tissue injury cannot be confirmed. Evidence pertaining to the inter-rater reliability of the classification system is limited.

Incidence and Prevalence

Two approaches are used to measure the occurrence of pressure ulcers: prevalence and incidence. Prevalence is the proportion of people in the population who, at a specific time, have pressure ulcers. The term *point prevalence* is used to distinguish the number of people with pressure ulcers at a specific point in time from *period prevalence*, which describes the number of patients with ulcers over a specified period of time. Prevalence is the most commonly reported measure in the literature. Published rates across all specialty ranges show wide variations: a systematic review of European data reported a mean prevalence of 10.8% (range 4.6%–27.2%) (Moore et al., 2019). Prevalence rates were highest in acute care, followed by acute and long-term care combined, long-term care, and community care, respectively.

Incidence is the rate at which new ulcers develop within the *at-risk* population. When evaluating the effectiveness of prevention strategies, it is necessary to distinguish between the overall number of existing ulcers (i.e., prevalence) and the number of new ulcers (i.e., incidence) that have occurred since the introduction of a new policy or preventive intervention. Incidence rates vary by specialty, and care settings within specialties, and are influenced by both the vulnerability of patients and the effectiveness of preventive care. Differences in dependency and frailty levels between similar groups of patients with apparently similar risk may be sufficient to affect rates and cause variations across settings within the same specialty. For this reason rates specific to each ward or team, rather than global specialty, hospital or community rates, provide a more informative measure with which to target resources to areas of need.

Wide variations in incidence and prevalence rates are evident in published literature and reflect inconsistencies in approaches used. Comparison of rates requires a standardised approach to the identification and categorisation of pressure ulcers and in the methods used to record and calculate these statistics. For incidence rates this also includes consistency in defining the at-risk population denominator used for calculations. In the United Kingdom, NHS Improvement (2018) introduced definitions and measurement guidance for defining, measuring and reporting pressure ulcers in order to promote consistency in data.

Pressure Ulcer Risk Factors

Risk factors are intrinsic or extrinsic characteristics that increase susceptibility to the effects of pressure, shear and friction. Many risk factors are cited in the literature, but their exact role and significance in pressure ulcer formation is not fully understood. Some commonly cited risk factors include the following.

Age. The prevalence of pressure ulcers increases with age. Statistically significant differences are reported between the age of individuals who develop pressure ulcers and those who don't. The normal physiological processes of ageing and the increased likelihood of disease and disability with advancing age make the occurrence of pressure ulcers more common among older people.

Drugs. Any drug that decreases sensation or mobility—for example, sedatives, opiates and alcohol—may contribute to pressure ulcer development. Steroids have been shown to mimic and exacerbate the ageing process by reducing the collagen content of the dermis Hall et. al., 1974, which may make the tissues less tolerant to pressure.

Mobility and Activity Levels, Patient Handling and Positioning. Reduced mobility and activity levels are significant predisposing risk factors. Medical conditions, interventions and situations that reduce mobility or sensation of pain can interfere with the spontaneous movements normally made in response to ischaemic discomfort. Examples include long waits on hospital trolleys, surgery, anaesthesia and sedation. Medical conditions such as stroke, advanced cognitive impairment and Parkinson's disease impact mobility and activity levels. The moving, handling and positioning of patients can cause injury from pressure, friction and shear if undertaken incorrectly. The combination of these three forces poses particular risks when patients are positioned in a sitting or semisitting position in bed or an ill-fitting chair. Tightly tucked-in bedding can restrict the movement of a debilitated patient and exert pressure on vulnerable areas such as the toes.

Skin Factors. Dry skin is common in later life due to reduced sebum production and reduced water content. The skin becomes more fragile and vulnerable to the effects of pressure, shear, friction and moisture. Chemical irritation from prolonged contact with urine and faeces and prolonged exposure to moisture may result in skin maceration, making the tissues less tolerant to mechanical stressors. Equally, overzealous use of soap and poor rinsing of the skin after washing aggravates dry skin problems and can be harmful because protective oils are lost, the skin pH is altered and dehydration occurs, making the skin less resistant to friction. A systematic review of risk factors found out of 27 studies that included moisture-related variables in their statistical modelling, 13 (48%) identified moisture-related variables to be statistitcally significant predictors for pressure ulcers (Coleman et al., 2013). Research findings indicate that having a category 1 ulcer is associated with a subsequent development of a category 2 or greater pressure ulcer (Shi et al., 2020), but practitioners should be mindful that not all forms of pressure injury are preceeded by non-blanching erythema indicative of a category 1 ulcer (Kottner, 2020).

Body Weight and Nutritional Status. Nutrients are necessary for maintaining body repair processes and body weight. Malnutrition may be more common in institutionalised older patients than is generally recognised, and associations between pressure ulcers and poor nutritional status are reported in the literature (Coleman et al., 2013). For example, low serum albumin, low body weight and a nutritional intake below the recommended daily allowance for protein, calories and zinc have been cited as significant predictors of pressure ulceration. Factors that influence food intake, such as requiring assistance with eating, particularly where cognitive impairment is present, have also been reported to increased the likelihood of developing a pressure ulcer. See Chapter 21 for further reading on eating, drinking and nutrition.

Perfusion-Related Factors. Conditions that decrease the quality or quantity of blood that reaches the tissues increase the likelihood of pressure ulcers. Cardiac disorders, anaemia, peripheral vascular disease, arteriosclerotic disease and low blood pressure are thought to be predisposing factors in pressure ulcer development due to their impact on tissue perfusion. A review of studies that investigated perfusion-related variables showed over 70% confirmed perfusion to be a risk factor for pressure ulcers, with diabetes showing strong evidence (Coleman et al., 2013).

Psychological Factors. The emotional stress of severe illness and disability stimulates the adrenal glands to increase production of glucocorticoids. This leads to an inhibition of collagen formation and an increased risk of tissue breakdown. A small number of studies have shown an association between psychosocial factors and pressure ulcer development (Anderson & Andberg, 1979), but the effects of an individual's emotional state on tissue breakdown is not fully understood.

Conceptual frameworks aim to describe the complex interrelationships and causal pathways between pressure ulcer risk factors. One of the earliest, a schema for the aetiology of pressure ulcer formation, identifies two groups of critical causative factors: a) the intensity and duration of pressure, and b) the ability of the skin and soft tissues to tolerate pressure (Braden & Bergstrom, 1987). These in turn are influenced by risk factors. The three risk factors—reduced mobility, reduced activity and reduced sensory perception—increase the risk of prolonged, intense pressure. Tissue tolerance is influenced by the intrinsic factors nutrition, age and arteriolar pressure, and by the extrinsic variables moisture, friction and shear. The framework proposes these factors alter the structures of the skin and soft tissues and their ability to withstand pressure. This framework forms the theoretical basis for the Braden scale risk assessment tool.

A more recent framework (Coleman et al., 2014) proposed the direct and indirect causes of pressure ulceration (Fig. 24.1) based on a review of biomedical, physiological and epidemiological research evidence by Coleman et al. (2013). Immobility, skin condition/pressure ulcer status and poor perfusion are identified as direct causal or primary risk factors, which are influenced by five indirect causal factors: poor sensory perception and response, diabetes, moisture, poor nutrition and low albumin. The framework recognises other indirect causal factors thought to impact on pressure ulcer development for which the research evidence remains limited: older age, medication, pitting oedema, chronic wounds, infection, acute illness and raised body temperature. Informed by Coleman's framework, the International Guideline for Prevention and Treatment of Pressure Ulcers/Injuries (European Pressure Ulcer Advisory Panel, National Pressure Injury Advisory Panel and Pan Pacific Pressure Injury Alliance, 2019) lists 15 risk factors to consider when assessing pressure ulcer risk:

- Skin status over pressure points, including existing or previous pressure ulcer
- Pain over pressure points
- Perfusion, circulatory and oxygen deficits
- Poor nutritional status
- Increased skin moisture
- Increased body temperature

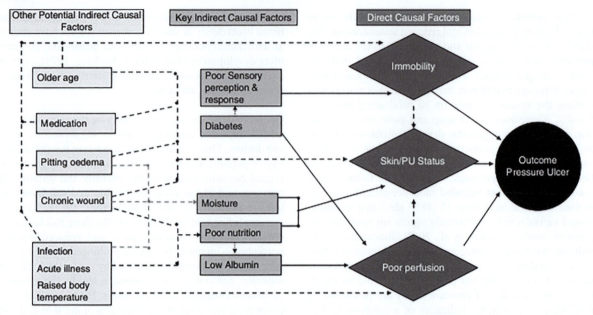

Fig. 24.1 Proposed causal pathway for pressure ulcer development. (Source: Coleman et al. [2014].)

- Increased age
- Impaired sensory perception
- Diabetes mellitus
- Laboratory blood results
- General health and mental health status
- Mobility and activity limitations
- Friction and shear
- Time spent immobilised before and during surgery
- Factors specific to critical illness (e.g., time spent in ICU, mechanical ventilation, APACHE II score, use of vasopressors)

Identifying Patients at Risk

The nursing assessment of any older patient should include an assessment of their risk of pressure ulcers. The assessment, and any required preventive actions, must be implemented promptly to avoid skin deterioration. The United Kingdom's pressure ulcer quality standard sets the benchmark for initial assessment within 6 hours of admission or, for community care services, at the first referral visit (National Institute for Health and Care Excellence [NICE], 2015). For professional and legal reasons, the assessment must be documented, and because the patient's condition may change, regular reassessment is necessary. The frequency of reassessment is determined by the patient's condition.

Risk Assessment Tools

Assessment of pressure ulcer risk requires a systematic approach, using clinical judgement supported by a recognised pressure ulcer risk assessment tool to standardise the assessment and identify the patient's level of risk (NICE, 2014). The three published risk assessment scales most commonly used worldwide are the Norton, Waterlow and Braden scales. Risk factors form the basis of these scales. They require the clinician to attribute a score to each risk factor, then sum the scores to obtain an overall indication of risk. All published scales identify a threshold or cut-off score that delineates individuals with elevated risk from lower-risk groups. In some scales a high score indicates elevated risk, while in others elevated risk is represented by a low score.

Norton Scale. The Norton scale (Norton et al., 1975) was the first published pressure ulcer risk assessment tool (Table 24.2). It was originally designed as a data collection tool in an investigation into the role of skin products and skin care for preventing pressure ulcers in older people. It has five components: physical condition, mental state, activity, mobility, and incontinence. The physical condition of the patient is assumed to reflect nutritional status. Each category has four items, each weighted from 1 to 4, giving a minimum possible score of 5 and maximum score of 20. A score of 16 or less indicates elevated risk. Many of the later risk assessment tools are based on the Norton scale.

TABLE 24.2 Pressure Ulcer Risk Assessment Scales: Norton Scale

Physical Condition		Mental Condition		Activity		Mobility		Incontinent	
Good	4	Alert	4	Ambulant	4	Full	4	Not	4
Fair	3	Apathetic	3	Walk with help	3	Slightly limited	3	Occasionally	3
Poor	2	Confused	2	Chair-bound	2	Very limited	2	Usually of urine	2
Very bad	1	Stuporous	1	Bedfast	1	Immobile	1	Doubly	1

Instructions for use:
1. Score the patient 1–4 under each heading (A–E) and total the scores.
2. A score of 14 or less was formerly taken to indicate the patient was at risk and in need of preventive care. A score of 16 or less is now used.
3. When sacral oedema is present, the patient might be at risk, even with a high score.
4. Assess the patient regularly.
Source: Norton et al. (1975).

Waterlow Scale. The Waterlow scale (Waterlow, 1985) is widely used in the United Kingdom and has undergone several revisions, most recently 2005 (http://www.judy-waterlow.co.uk/the-waterlow-score-card.htm). The scale contains nine risk factor categories, each with between four and seven weighted items. Scores for each category are summed, and the total is used to identify whether the patient has a medium, high or very high risk; a high score indicates a high risk. It is intended for use on a wide range of patient groups, including older people, but it lacks discriminatory power when used to predict risk in this client group—most older inpatients are identified as high or very high risk. Appraisal of the scale's reliability when used in care settings for older people has shown interrater reliability to be low (Cook et al , 1999; Kottner & Dassen, 2010).

Braden Scale. The Braden scale (Table 24.3) is based on Braden and Bergstrom's (1987) conceptual framework. It assesses mobility, activity, sensory perception, skin moisture, friction, shear and nutritional status (Bergstrom et al., 1987; Braden & Bergstrom, 1989). Unlike the previous scales, a definition of each subscale category is provided, which helps remove ambiguity and increases the likelihood of interrater agreement. Each dimension is rated from 1 (least favourable) to 3 or 4 (most favourable); the total score range is from 16 to 23. A score of 16 or less indicates pressure ulcer risk, although the authors recommended each clinical area should determine its own cut-off point. The scale has been subjected to well-designed validation studies in acute and long-term older care settings, including nursing homes, as well as medical-surgical and intensive care settings. A systematic review and meta-analysis concluded the scale performs best when used with Caucasian inpatients over 60 (Huang et al., 2021). The meta-analysis results suggested a cut-off score of 18 may provide the greatest accuracy, but the authors noted this required further investigation due to the differing cut-off thresholds used in the studies reviewed.

Effectiveness of Risk Assessment Tools

The effectiveness of pressure ulcer risk assessment scales in preventing pressure ulcers remains unclear. One reason is a historical lack of standardisation in the design of validation studies such that comparison of results is difficult. Study design weaknesses are also a factor and include inadequate definitions of measures, particularly skin assessment, pressure ulcer classification and a lack of blinding of assessors. Appraising effectiveness of scales to predict pressure ulcers while simultaneously providing preventative care is a further source of difficulty; the ideal study design would require withholding preventative interventions, which would be unethical. In addition, the majority of the published risk scales contain a fundamental design weakness in that they are constructed from assumed risk factors rather than using statistical techniques to identify key indicators of risk and their relative significance for predicting pressure ulcers. The numerical weightings assigned to risk factors are largely based on assumed importance rather than being statistically derived. A recent systematic review identifed just two studies of sufficient quality to meet the inclusion criteria and concluded there is little robust evidence that risk assessment scales are more effective in identifying patients with elevated risk than the professional judgement of experienced practitioners or that the use of asessment tools reduces the incidence of pressure ulcers (Moore & Patton, 2019). In consequence, risk assessment tools should not be used to replace or override clinical judgement. International clinical guidance issued jointly by three expert groups advocates a structured approach to risk assessment, and if used, a risk assessment tool should be part of a broader comprehensive assessment, with clinical judgement used to interpret assessment findings (European Pressure Ulcer Advisory Panel, National Pressure Injury Advisory Panel and Pan Pacific Pressure Injury Alliance, 2019).

PRESSURE ULCER PREVENTION STRATEGIES

Prevention strategies are based on a full risk assessment and the identified patient-specific risk factors. In general, prevention strategies aim to reduce interface pressure and improve soft tissue ability to withstand compressive forces. They include reduction of mechanical forces (e.g., pressure, friction and shear) and other external risk factors and the alleviation of internal risk factors where possible. Successful prevention strategies require collaborative, interprofessional working and ongoing education and training of clinicians, carers and patients.

Reducing Interface Pressure

Relief of pressure is the principal aim of prevention. It applies as much to chair-bound patients as to those who are bed-bound.

Relief of pressure is achieved through regular repositioning, through the selection of an appropriate pressure-reducing support surface that spreads pressure over a wide surface area, or by using a support surface that alternates the amount of pressure exerted on the patient's soft tissues.

Repositioning

Risk-reduction strategies for the vulnerable person should encompass a 24-hour repositioning plan constructed around the patient's daily routine and lifestyle and agreed with the patient and carers. The plan and repositioning frequency should be based on individual assessment of need and aim to offload bony pressure points and spread body weight over a wide surface area.

Where the patient's condition allows, promoting mobility should be one of the primary interventions to alleviate

TABLE 24.3	Pressure Ulcer Risk Assessment Scales: The Braden Scale for Predicting Pressure Sore Risk			
Patient's Name		**Evaluator's Name**		**Date of Assessment**
Sensory perception Ability to respond meaningfully to pressure-related discomfort	**1. Completely limited** Unresponsive (does not moan, flinch or gasp) to painful stimuli, due to diminished level of consciousness or sedation or limited ability to feel pain over most of body surface	**2. Very limited** Responds only to painful stimuli. Cannot communicate discomfort except by moaning or restlessness or has a sensory impairment which limits the ability to feel pain or discomfort over half of the body	**3. Slightly limited** Responds to verbal commands, but cannot always communicate discomfort or need to be turned or has some sensory impairment which limits ability to feel pain or discomfort in one or two extremities	**4. No impairment** Responds to verbal commands. Has no sensory deficit that would limit ability to feel or voice pain or discomfort
Moisture Degree to which skin is exposed to moisture	**1. Constantly moist** Skin is kept moist almost constantly by perspiration and urine. Dampness is detected every time patient is moved or turned	**2. Very moist** Skin is often, but not always, moist. Linen must be changed at least once a shift	**3. Occasionally moist** Skin is occasionally moist, requiring an extra linen change approximately once a day	**4. Rarely moist** Skin is usually dry; linen only requires changing at routine intervals
Activity Degree of physical activity	**1. Bedfast** Confined to bed	**2. Chairfast** Ability to walk severely limited or non-existent. Cannot bear own weight and/or must be assisted into chair or wheelchair	**3. Walks occasionally** Walks occasionally during day, but for very short distances, with or without assistance. Spends majority of each shift in bed or chair	**4. Walks frequently** Walks outside the room at least twice a day and inside room at least once every 2 h during waking hours

TABLE 24.3   Pressure Ulcer Risk Assessment Scales: The Braden Scale for Predicting Pressure Sore Risk—cont'd

Patient's Name		Evaluator's Name		Date of Assessment
Mobility Ability to change and control body position	**1. Completely immobile** Does not make even slight changes in body or extremity position without assistance	**2. Very limited** Makes occasional slight changes in body or extremity position but unable to make frequent or significant changes independently	**3. Slightly limited** Makes frequent though slight changes in body or extremity position independently	**4. No limitations** Makes major and frequent changes in position without assistance
Nutrition Usual food intake pattern	**1. Very poor** Never eats a complete meal. Rarely eats more than one-third of any food offered. Eats two servings or fewer of protein (meat or dairy products) per day. Takes fluids poorly. Does not take a liquid supplement or is nil-by-mouth and/or maintained on clear liquids or intravenous fluids for more than 5 days	**2. Probably inadequate** Rarely eats a complete meal and generally eats only about one-half of any food offered. Protein intake includes only three servings of meat or dairy products per day. Occasionally will take a dietary supplement or receives less than optimum amount of liquid diet or tube feeding	**3. Adequate** Eats over half of most meals. Eats a total of four servings of protein (meat, dairy products) each day. Occasionally will refuse a meal, but will usually take a supplement if offered or is on a tube-feeding or total parenteral nutrition regimen which probably meets most of nutritional needs	**4. Excellent** Eats most of every meal. Never refuses a meal. Usually eats a total of four or more servings of meat and dairy products. Occasionally eats between meals. Does not require supplementation
Friction and shear	**1. Problem** Requires moderate to maximum assistance in moving. Complete lifting without sliding against sheets is impossible. Frequently slides down in bed or chair, requiring frequent repositioning with maximum assistance. Spasticity, contractures or agitation lead to almost constant friction	**2. Potential problem** Moves feebly or requires minimum assistance. During a move skin probably slides to some extent against sheets, chair, restraints or other devices. Maintains relatively good position in chair or bed most of the time but occasionally slides down	**3. No apparent problem** Moves in bed and in chair independently and has sufficient muscle strength to lift up completely during move. Maintains good position in bed or chair at all times	
				Total score

Source: Braden & Bergstrom (1989).

pressure. In seated patients, regular sit-to-stand exercises are beneficial. Standing aids such as the Sara Stedy™ can be used for less able patients to relieve pressure on the sacral area and for standing practice to build strength and stamina in the lower limbs. For individuals nursed in bed, the effects of pressure, friction and shear can be minimised by limiting the extent to which the head of the bed is elevated, limiting the length of time the patient is nursed in a semi-recumbent position, and appropriate use of positioning techniques, profiling beds and pillows to counter the effects of gravity and pressure. This includes careful limb positioning to prevent contractures and pressure injury where bony prominences touch each other. To protect the vulnerable pressure points of the trochanter, a 30-degree lateral side lying position (30-degree tilt) rather than a lateral 90-degree turn is advocated. High interface pressures and low transcutaneous oxygen tensions have been recorded when patients lie directly on the trochanter (Seiler et al., 1986). At an angle of 30 degrees, direct pressure on the trochanter is avoided and instead is dissipated through the gluteal muscle, increasing the time the tissues can withstand pressure. In this position, Seiler et al. (1986) found neither the sacral nor the trochanteric skin became hypoxic. The extent to which 30-degree side lying is effective in an older person with reduced muscle bulk and collagen content is not extensively discussed in the literature, but from a theoretical perspective, it is conceivable the age-related changes in the tissues may make them less able to dissipate pressure.

Constant Low Pressure Static Support Systems

Pressure is inversely proportional to the area of contact and can be reduced by increasing the area of contact between the body and the support surface. This can be achieved by using mattresses and cushions designed to yield and achieve good immersion of the body, thereby spreading the pressure over the widest area possible. Examples of static support systems include foam support surfaces and low air loss devices.

High-Specification Foam. For many patients pressure redistribution can be achieved successfully using high-specification foam mattresses in place of a standard mattress or mattress overlay (McInness et al., 2015). Overlays must be of sufficient depth to allow good immersion of the body and spread of weight, which may be difficult to achieve with heavier patients. The quality and effectiveness of foam products is influenced by the type and density of the foam and the foam depth. A high specification should be used as a minimum for patients with elevated risk. Some support surfaces are made from laminated foam; these combine layers of foam of differing densities—for example, a high-density, firm foam core for durability covered

by softer, low-density outer layers of foam that give easily under areas of high pressure such as the bony prominences, increasing the contact surface area and redistributing the pressure to surrounding areas. Some manufacturers also cube-cut, score or profile the surface of the foam to improve immersion. Viscoelastic foam is temperature-sensitive and may be used as the outer layer on a laminated support surface; when warmed by body heat, it becomes softer, moulding around the patient.

The correct choice of mattress or cushion cover is of equal importance in order to avoid interference with the performance of the support surface. A water-vapour permeable, low-friction, two-way stretch cover should be used. Covers need regular inspection for tears and abrasions that make them permeable to fluid ingress. The foam insert needs inspection for signs of staining. Foam retains humidity and should be used on an open-mesh bed base to promote air circulation and prevent mould formation. Some mattresses require regular turning to prolong their life expectancy. Without proper care, both the mattress and cover can deteriorate. To prevent this, manufacturers' instructions should be carefully followed. All foam products have a limited life expectancy, after which a permanent compression-set occurs along with loss of the pressure-reducing support properties (i.e., 'grounding' or 'bottoming out'), consequently foam support surfaces need regular testing for bottoming out.

Low Air Loss Devices. A low air loss support surface is electrically operated and comprises a series of air sacs that lie edgeways across the width of the bed. Air within the sacs is constantly lost and replaced such that they are always slightly underinflated. This process enables them to contour around the patient, giving good immersion and pressure distribution. The constant flow of air from the small perforations in the upper surface of low air loss mattresses assists with reducing the skin microclimate temperature and humidity and, in turn, the surface humidity and heat of the skin surface. This is advantageous since a dry skin surface has a lower friction coefficient, causing less distortion of tissues (Kottner et al., 2018).

Alternating Pressure Devices

Electrically operated, an alternating pressure device is made as a mattress overlay, replacement mattress, replacement bed or cushion. The device consists of a series of air sacs, or cells, that inflate and deflate in a series of two- or three-phase timed cycles, each of which includes a period of low or zero interface pressure. The size of the air cells, the weight of the patient and the robustness of the design influence the effectiveness of these devices. The amount of inflation is governed by the patient's weight. Underinflation causes grounding, a particular consideration for obese/

bariatric patients, and overinflation produces high interface pressures. Designs vary in their degree of sophistication: some automatically adjust to the weight of the patient; others must be set manually. The air cells must be large enough to lift the patient sufficiently clear off the bed. The manufacturer's instructions should always be consulted in order to select the most appropriate device and the correct settings for the patient's body weight.

Selecting Support Surfaces

Choice of equipment is guided by evidence of effectiveness and the individual needs of the patient. Degree of risk, treatment objectives and body weight are among the initial considerations. Good quality research evidence on the performance of support surfaces is limited. Best practice guidance advocates the use of of high-specification (i.e., specialist) foam mattresses or overlays for individuals at risk. It also advises the relative benefits of using alternating air mattresses or overlays should also be considered (European Pressure Ulcer Advisory Panel, National Pressure Injury Advisory Panel and Pan Pacific Pressure Injury Alliance, 2019). A systematic review of support surfaces for pressure ulcer prevention (McInness et al., 2015) concluded the use of low-tech high-specification foam mattresses reduces the incidence of pressure ulcers in individuals at risk when compared with standard foam support surfaces, but there was insufficient evidence on the performance between types of high-specification foam support surfaces to guide choice. Reviewers reported some evidence in favour of alternating devices compared with standard mattresses, but studies comparing the effectiveness of alternating pressure and constant low-pressure systems gave conflicting results, and no clear difference was found between the relative benefits of high-tech (i.e., mechanical) constant low pressure devices and alternating pressure devices. Also noted was the insufficient clinical trials addressing the value of seat cushions.

Patient acceptance and ability to tolerate the proposed support surface are central to a successful preventive plan. Patients may reject pressure-relieving equipment because they find it uncomfortable, because the noise from the motor is disturbing or because the equipment hinders their ability to move independently. The movement of alternating-pressure mattresses can be sufficiently disconcerting to interfere with a patient's ability to rest. In some cases, the selection of a less-sophisticated option that provides better comfort and rest but affords lower levels of pressure relief may be necessary to achieve patient acceptance. Additional considerations include ease of transportation, size and weight of the equipment in relation to the room it is to be used in, and the ease of operation, maintenance and cost. The impact of the proposed equipment on rehabilitation,

mobility, general independence and safety also requires assessment. Replacement mattresses, overlays and cushions alter the overall dimensions of the support surface. The extent to which this affects the patient's ability to maintain good posture and independent mobility requires careful consideration. Unless well secured, overlays can slide against the underlying mattress as the patient gets into and out of bed, increasing the risk of a fall. This is an important consideration, particularly if the overlay is being used in the patient's own home. Most replacement mattresses are deeper than a standard mattress, increasing the overall height of the bed. Similarly, the addition of a cushion alters the seat height. Adjustable-height beds minimise this, but where a fixed-height bed is being used, as in the patient's own home, or the range of chair sizes is limited, the increased height may impair patient mobility.

Seating and Cushions

Sitting presents a higher risk to patients because the body's weight is concentrated over a small surface area, the buttocks (i.e., ischial tuberosities, trochanters, sacrum) and thighs, and to a lesser extent the arms and feet. Patients who are unable to reposition their trunk in response to pressure-induced discomfort are at particular risk of pressure ulcers. Ill-fitting seating may not only increase the risk of pressure damage but also place excess stress on body structures, encourage poor posture, contribute to fatigue and ultimately make it more difficult for individuals with limited movement to readjust their posture and body weight. For these reasons, care should be given to the assessment and choice of seating and cushions and to the length of time spent sitting.

Seating assessment should consider comfort, body size, rehabilitation needs, mobility and occupational/recreational needs, the effect of contractures or deformity on posture, and weight distribution. Seating selection aims to promote good posture; minimise pressure, friction and shear; and facilitate independent access in and out of the chair. Seat depth should allow for a 2-cm gap behind the knees. A seat base that is too deep places pressure on the popliteal fossa, impairing circulation to the extremities. To overcome the discomfort, the user slides forward, increasing the risk of shear and pressure on the sacral area. Armchairs with deeply angled backs should be avoided as they push the buttocks forward, encouraging forward sliding. Chairs with a tilt-in-space function allow the whole chair to be tilted backwards 20 to 45 degrees on its frame while maintaining the angle of the chair seat and back. They can be used to prevent buttocks sliding forward and for pressure reduction by shifting weight off the ischial tuberosities and increasing blood flow to the area. Seat width should allow for a 2-cm clearance on either side of the buttocks.

If too wide, the seat encourages the user to loll to one side, placing undue pressure on one side of the body. If the seat base, inclusive of cushion, is too high, the patient's feet will not rest on the floor and pressure that is normally taken through the feet will be transferred to the thighs and buttocks, increasing the risk of injury to these areas. Seating that is too low or too short in depth prevents pressure being taken through the thighs, increasing the risk of injury to the buttocks. The additional muscular effort required to rise from chairs that are too low can result in less mobile and older adults being stranded. As a general guide, the total height of the chair, inclusive of cushion, should not exceed the length of the patient's leg from the popliteal fossa to the floor. Poorly padded chairs backs may lead to pressure on the spinous processes in the thin, kyphotic individual. Any form of seating that causes the person to slide forward or down the chair may result in excessive pressure on the heels and heel ulceration.

Excessively high mean interface pressures have been reported in wheelchairs used without cushions (Rithalia, 1989). A wide range of high-specification foam, gel, air and alternating-pressure cushions are available for use with both wheelchairs and armchairs. Foam cushions may be moulded or cube-cut or include gel inserts to improve immersion and the ability to conform to body contours. The relative effectiveness of pressure-reducing cushions is unclear due to insufficient good quality clinical trials (McInness et al., 2015); nevertheless, their use is advocated in clinical practice guidelines (European Pressure Ulcer Advisory Panel, National Pressure Injury Advisory Panel and Pan Pacific Pressure Injury Alliance, 2019). Cushion covers can impinge on a cushion's effectiveness and should be chosen in line with manfacturers' guidance. All cushions need regular checks for defects such as bottoming-out, gel or air leakage, and covers need checks for wear and tear. Cushions cannot relieve pressure completely and additional pressure relief strategies are required.

Specialist seating exists that can be tailored to high-risk patients with complex needs. Occupational therapists have particular expertise in this area, and advice can be sought through occupational therapy or rehabilitation services. For a more detailed account of seating, see Stockton, Gebhardt, and Clark's (2009) clinical practice guideline.

Heels

Heels are a frequent location for pressure injury. Their small surface area and lack of subcutaneous tissue make pressure redistribution difficult. Correct choice of seating may reduce the risk of heel damage in seated patients. A range of heel protectors are available for use with patients nursed in bed. These devices should lift the heels clear off the bed but, in doing so, should not put undue pressure on the surrounding areas such as the Achilles tendon or calf. The effect of the device on limb position needs consideration in patients who have had recent lower limb surgery; patient comfort and the ability to decontaminate the equipment after use are other essential considerations. In the absence of heel protectors, pillows can be used, but care in their positioning is essential to prevent pressure under the calf or knee. Self-adherent bordered foam dressings, designed to protect heels and the sacrum from friction, may be beneficial in reducing pressure ulcer occurrence, but there is currently insufficient evidence to support their routine use (NICE, 2019). Ring cushions and similar devices have been shown to impede blood and lymph flow in the surrounding area, contributing to tissue breakdown.

Maintaining and Improving Tissue Tolerance to Pressure

Individual assessment will identify specific interventions required to enhance tissue tolerance to pressure. A successful risk-reduction plan requires dialogue between team members, the patient, and the family or carers and draws on the diverse skills and knowledge of the multidisciplinary team. Specialist help beyond the expertise of the team may also be required. Risk-reduction plans include correction or restabilisation of underlying disease processes such as heart failure and management of associated symptoms such as oedema that make tissues more vulnerable to damage. Management of pain is equally important; if present, pain influences the patient's psychological state and desire to move. Adequate sleep and rest promote psychological well-being and support tissue regeneration and repair.

Nutritional Support

Nutritional screening is an integral component in the general health assessment of older adults and is essential where pressure ulcer risk is identified. Malnutrition and dehydration result from many disease processes, and older people are more at risk from malnutrition than many other client groups. Where screening indicates malnutrition, a formal assessment of nutritional status is required (European Pressure Ulcer Advisory Panel, National Pressure Injury Advisory Panel and Pan Pacific Pressure Injury Alliance, 2019). Nutritional interventions to prevent pressure ulcers are largely based on consensus opinion and good practice recommendations due to the low quality of existing research trials (Langer & Fink, 2014). Individuals who do not achieve a nutritional intake that meets the recommended daily requirements for their age and activity level or who show evidence of being nutritionally compromised require a plan of nutritional support under the guidance of a dietician (European Pressure Ulcer Advisory Panel, National Pressure Injury Advisory Panel and Pan Pacific Pressure

Injury Alliance, 2019). Factors that influence eating ability also need consideration, especially when cognitive impairment is present. For a detailed discussion on nutritional assessment and nutritional problems in older adults, see Chapter 21.

Skin Care

Dry skin is a common feature in later life. Dry skin lacks suppleness and can fissure and crack, making the epidermis less resistant to injury. Skin exposed to constant moisture is more susceptible to maceration, particularly if the moisture contains chemical irritants as found in body fluids. The principles of a skin care strategy are to minimise irritation and maceration of the epidermis, maintain natural skin oils and improve skin quality and hydration. Care should include the avoidance of repeated, prolonged exposure to moisture and prompt skin cleansing after soiling to reduce the potential of irritants to damage the epidermis. A mild cleanser rather than soap should be used and a wide range of emollient cleansers are available. Some are pH-balanced and contain a water-repellant barrier that may help maintain skin integrity of incontinent patients. Applying an emollient after showering helps retain the moisture absorbed by the skin during showering and improves its hydration. Skin that has lost its natural oils may also benefit from the application of oil-based creams. Barrier creams that contain silicone or zinc help prevent skin damage from repeated incontinence or diarrhoea, but lanolin-based products should be avoided as some patients are sensitive to them. Cavilon™ barrier film may be used to protect intact or superficially damaged skin from irritation from urine or wound exudate. This is applied as a fluid that rapidly dries to provide a colourless barrier that lasts up to 72 hours. Semipermeable film or hydrocolloid dressings can be useful in protecting vulnerable areas such as heels, elbows and the sacrum from moisture or friction damage.

Promoting Continence

Many incontinence problems are amenable to improvement with support from a continence specialist (see Chapter 22). Incontinence pads can encourage skin maceration through sweating and, if incorrectly fitted, act as a source of pressure in the sedentary patient. Incontinence pads with insufficient absorbancy or that are infrequently changed contribute to incontinence-associated dermatitis (IAD), a form of moisture-related contact dermatitis from prologed contact with urine or faeces. Skin affected by IAD is less able to withstand pressure, friction and shear and is sometimes mistaken for a category 2 pressure ulcer, leading to inappropriate management. Both conditions can co-exist (see Voegeli, 2017, for an in-depth account and differential diagnosis). Interventions include careful cleansing, application of a barrier product, and identification and management of the underlying cause.

Moving and Handling

The principles of skilled handling techniques include the avoidance of friction and shear on the sacrum and heels. Facilitation of normal movement should be the primary strategy for moving patients, supported by standing aids and similar devices where necessary. This promotes self-care and minimises trauma from unskilled handling. Encouraging ambulation via physiotherapy and exercises designed to increase coordination, balance, flexibility and muscle strength increases the patient's ability and confidence to readjust posture, move and mobilise independently. In addition to their lead role in educating the patient toward mobility, physiotherapists can advise on positioning and safe moving and handling techniques. See Chapter 18 for discussion of safe mobility.

Continuity of Care

When patients are transferred or discharged, liaison between service providers is required to ensure continuity of pressure ulcer prevention and to enable ordering of appropriate support surfaces in advance of a patient's arrival. This is particularly relevant when the patient is being transferred into community settings, as sufficient time is needed for delivery and setup of equipment. Within the acute-care sector, emergency, radiology and operating departments are areas where patients may be immobile for long periods and where special consideration should be given to pressure relief. Monitoring the duration of waiting times for ambulance transfer or portering services may also identify points in the patient journey that contribute significantly to pressure ulceration and where greater continuity of care is desirable.

Education and Practice Development

Patients are central to a prevention plan. Their involvement, together with family and carers, in setting and agreeing objectives is essential for success. Motivation to accept and participate in a plan depends on the patient's understanding of the causes and significance of pressure ulcers, risk factors and means of prevention. The prevention plan should incorporate education that takes account of the patient's and family's existing knowledge, cognitive abilities, specific needs and lifestyle, with the aim of motivating them to participate and ultimately take responsibility for preventive care in so far as condition and ability allow. This is particularly true if clients live at home, where they and/or their family may have primary responsibility for implementing the prevention plan. Equally, centralised pressure ulcer education for all health care professionals is integral to quality improvement (European Pressure Ulcer Advisory Panel, National Pressure Injury Advisory Panel and Pan Pacific Pressure Injury Alliance, 2019), covering such areas as risk assessment, skin assessment, prevention measures, repositioning, support surfaces and patient education (NICE, 2014).

Summary

Physiological age-related changes reduce tolerance of soft tissues to pressure, shear and friction, placing older compromised adults at greater risk of pressure ulcers. Despite the large volume of literature, current research on the causes and prevention of pressure ulcers is undermined by weaknesses in research design; there is a need for more methodologically sound empirical investigations to confirm understanding and inform decision-making.

PRESSURE ULCER MANAGEMENT

High-quality preventive care helps avoid the development of pressure ulcers for most patients but may not always prevent their occurrence in significantly compromised patients, particularly those who are at the end of life. When severe, pressure ulcers are life-threatening. Restoring skin integrity in patients with deep wounds presents notable challenges to the multidisciplinary team.

Pressure ulcer management requires knowledge of the wound-healing process and factors that influence healing. Wound healing involves a variety of complex mechanisms interlinked in a continuous process of repair (Singh et al., 2017). The stages and mechanisms of wound healing are briefly summarised in Box 24.2. The speed at which wounds progress through the stages of healing depends on the nature of the wound. Pressure ulcers can have large areas of tissue damage with loss of the skin and subcutaneous layers. These wounds cannot be sutured; the body must replace the lost tissue by the process of granulation, which occurs from the base of the wound. Once the deficit is repaired, epithelialisation takes place.

Wound Assessment

A wound assessment is necessary to select appropriate treatment, judge its effectiveness and the rate of healing or deterioration of the wound. Although pressure ulcer classification systems provide some information on the degree of tissue loss, on their own they do not provide sufficient information on the size of the wound or factors that influence the healing process. To be effective, wound assessment must be holistic and give consideration to the physiological, psychological and social factors that might influence the healing process. Most individuals who develop pressure ulcers do so during times of ill health,

---

BOX 24.2   Stages and Mechanisms of Wound Healing

Inflammation

Damaged tissues release histamine and other substances; the vasodilatation and increased permeability of capillaries that result from this chemical response bring neutrophils and, later, macrophages, which have a major role in clearing bacteria and debris from the wound. Vasodilatation enhances the blood supply to the damaged area and provides the additional nutrients required in the rebuilding process. Patients who have a depressed inflammatory response as a result of disease or drug therapy may experience delay in this phase of healing.

Proliferation

New blood vessels and collagen strands develop to form granulation tissue. Dietary amino acids, vitamins and trace elements are essential in this process.

Maturation

This is an ongoing process of collagen synthesis and degradation that continues for many months after the wound appears visibly healed. Cross-linking, remodelling and realignment of collagen occur to ensure maximum strength.

Contraction

Part of the healing process is achieved by contraction of the wound—an inward centripetal movement of the wound edges initiated by myofibroblasts. Contraction is an important healing mechanism for wounds with tissue loss such as pressure ulcers, as it reduces the deficit to be repaired.

Epithelialisation

Hair follicles and the wound margins provide the main source of epidermal regeneration, and in shallow wounds that contain viable hair follicles, migration of epidermal cells across the wound surface can occur fairly rapidly. For deeper wounds, healing is much slower because the sources of epidermal regeneration other than at the wound margins are lost.

---

and their compromised health status is likely to affect the body's healing ability. Multipathology, polypharmacy and impaired nutritional status are more common among the older population. These influencing factors may contribute to a slowed healing rate. Medical problems that impair oxygen uptake, tissue perfusion, or nutritional or fluid intake undermine the body's ability to repair itself. Medical treatments may also impair the healing process, such as steroid therapy and cancer treatments.

The location of the wound and the patient's activity level influence the choice of wound dressing. Location may also indicate the potential risk for infection, such as wounds on the buttocks and sacrum. Odour may be indicative of infection and can have a distressing effect on the patient and family.

Pain assessment is an integral part of wound assessment and may result from the underlying disease process, the wound itself or the wound management regimen. Pain can limit the patient's ability to tolerate a plan of care and may interfere with sleep. As wound repair proceeds most rapidly during sleep, impaired sleep may, in turn, delay the healing process (see Chapter 25).

Wound Measurement

Regular wound measurement is necessary to monitor changes in wound size and assess progression of healing and effectiveness of the wound management plan. Ruler measurements of wound width and length, combined with photographs and/or tracings of the circumference on transparent film can be used (see Nichols, 2015, for a practial description). Areas of necrosis, slough, granulation and epithelial tissue can be marked on the photograph or tracing to help monitor healing or deterioration. Contraction results in the wound changing shape as it heals. This process, in conjunction with debridement, initially may make the wound appear larger, which should be borne in mind when reviewing the wound.

The depth and amount of tissue loss are important in pressure ulcer wound assessment. Significant tissue destruction can occur without being evident at the wound surface, and the surface diamensions of the wound may be significantly smaller than the underlying cavity. The extent of any undermining should be gently assessed by an experienced practitioner using a sterile disposable probe. Deep pressure ulcers that have penetrated the fascia and muscle can quickly extend along and around bones and joints and present a major risk of systemic infection. For this reason a skilled appraisal of deep cavity ulcers is required, and appropriate specialist help should be sought.

Assessment of the Wound Bed

Inspection of the wound bed and wound margins helps identify the stages of healing and factors that may delay the healing process, such as the presence of devitalised tissue and infection. By their very nature, pressure ulcers frequently contain dead tissue resulting from ischaemia. Skin affected in this way loses the ability to control evaporation of moisture, and dehydration occurs, resulting in a dry, black, leathery area—an eschar. Continued evaporation extends the dehydration process into the subcutaneous layers. Visualisation of the wound bed also identifies specific features that need consideration when preparing the wound bed for healing and selecting an appropriate wound dressing. These include shape and accessibility; the condition of the surrounding skin; the amount and type of exudate; the presence of slough, eschar, or infection; and the presence of granulation tissue or epithelial tissue. These considerations are captured in the TIME systematic approach to chronic wound assessment and wound bed preparation:

- **T**isssue
- **I**nfection/inflammation
- **M**oisture imbalance
- **E**pithelial edge advancement

For a review of wound bed preparation using the TIME framework, see Harries et al. (2016) and Atkin et al. (2019).

Principals of Management

The general principles of wound care are to support the body's own mechanisms for wound cleansing and healing. This includes nutrition supplements if indicated by the nutritional assessment. The cause of the pressure ulcer must also also be addressed to prevent further skin breakdown. Meeting psychosocial needs, maintaining quality of life and ensuring patient participation should feature in the wound care plan.

Pressure ulcers are chronic wounds, and their management focuses on correcting imbalances that occur within the wound microenvironment (Harries et al., 2016). Due to factors such as the recurrence of necrotic tissue, repeated trauma (e.g., unrelieved pressure) and heavy bacterial loading, deep pressure ulcers exhibit prolonged and complex inflammatory processes and produce high levels of exudate. These events cause biochemical and cellular changes within the wound that have a negative effect on healing. To promote healing, preparation of the wound bed aims to debride necrotic tissue, control exudate and correct bacterial imbalance by applying a primary wound dressing that creates an optimal moist healing environment appropriate to the stage of healing, depth of tissue loss and condition of the wound bed. The wound assessment provides the information required to select an appropriate wound dressing and identify the specific factors that affect healing, enabling corrective interventions.

Wound Cleansing

Routine cleansing of wounds is unnecessary and may delay the healing process due to mechanical or chemical trauma or cooling the wound through the application of cold cleansing fluids. Where there is loose, superficial debris or remnants of dressing products to be removed, cleansing is best achieved by irrigation. On occasion mechanical swabbing with gauze may be justified to remove adherent tissue and debris from the wound bed. This method should be avoided where possible due to the risk of mechanical trauma to granulating tissue and risk of introducing gauze fibres into the wound that can act as foci for bacterial growth.

Wound Dressings

Modern wound products aim to create an ideal environment that maximises tissue repair. The properties of the ideal dressing include maintenance of a moist wound-dressing interface, absorption of excess exudate, prevention of bacterial contamination, maintenance of an optimum temperature, promotion of patient comfort, prevention of trauma to the wound and surrounding skin on removal, and being free from toxins, residues and contaminants. Cost, wear time and ease of use are other considerations. Rarely does a single dressing product meet the needs of a wound throughout all the stages of healing, so the dressing prescription will require review as the wound progresses and its specific requirements change. This necessitates regular evaluation and reassessment of the wound, surrounding skin and patient comfort. For an overview of dressing products and their use, see Vowden and Vowden (2017).

Summary

Wound healing is a complex process. Pressure ulcers are wounds that have a complex aetiology and pathology. The combined features of ageing and multipathology present particular considerations in the management of these wounds. As with prevention, the assessment, care and evaluation of pressure ulcers require a holistic, multidisciplinary approach.

CONCLUSION AND KEY POINTS

Skin care has been traditionally viewed as a basic, routine task that can be left to the least skilled staff. The maintenance and restoration of healthy skin require a sophisticated knowledge base and present complex challenges to the multidisciplinary team.

KEY LEARNING POINTS

- Skin lesions are common in older people. New lesions or lesions that have undergone changes require assessment and investigation.
- Pressure ulcers are localised soft-tissue injuries caused by unrelieved pressure, shear or friction. Age-related physiological changes and higher levels of morbidity in later life make older people more susceptible.
- Pressure ulcers can form deep within the tissues, with little initial outward sign other than discolouration of overlying intact skin.
- Assessment of older people should include their pressure ulcer risk using a systematic, structured approach and take account of differences in skin pigmentation.
- Relief of pressure is the principal aim of prevention; interventions include promoting mobility, repositioning and the use of specialist equipment. Good quality research evidence on the effectiveness of preventative equipment is limited.
- A holistic wound assessment identifies the stage of healing and the presence of factors that may delay the healing process, and guides wound bed preparation and the choice of dressing.

REFERENCES

Anderson, T. P., & Andberg, M. M. (1979). Psychosocial factors associated with pressure sores. *Archives of Physical Medicine and Rehabilitation, 60*, 314–346.

Atkin, L., Bućko, Z., Conde Montero, E., Cutting, K., Moffatt, C., Probst, A., Romanelli, M., et al., (2019). Implementing TIMERS: The race against hard-to-heal wounds. *Journal of Wound Care, 28*(3), S1–S49.

Bergstrom, N., Braden, B., Laguzza, A., & Hollman, V. (1987). The Braden scale for predicting pressure sore risk. *Nursing Research, 36*, 205–210.

Braden, B., & Bergstrom, N. (1987). A conceptual schema for the study of the etiology of pressure sores. *Rehabilitation Nursing, 12*(8–12), 16.

Braden, B. J., & Bergstrom, N. (1989). Clinical utility of the Braden scale for predicting pressure sore risk. *Decubitus, 2*(44–46), 50–51.

Coleman, S., Gorecki, C., Nelson, A., Closs, J., Defloor, T., Halfens, R., Farrin, A., et al., (2013). Patient risk factors for pressure ulcer development: Systematic review. *International Journal of Nursing Studies, 50*(7), 974–1003.

Coleman, S., Nixon, J., Keen, J., Wilson, L., McGinnis, E., Dealey, C., Stubbs, N., et al., (2014). A new pressure ulcer conceptual framework. *Journal of Advanced Nursing, 70*(10), 2222–2234.

Cook, M., Hale, C., Watson, B. (1999). Interrater reliability and the assessment of pressure sore risk using an adapted Waterlow scale. *Clinical Effectiveness in Nursing, 3*, 66–74

European Pressure Ulcer Advisory Panel, National Pressure Injury Advisory Panel and Pan Pacific Pressure Injury Alliance.

(2019). *Prevention and treatment of pressure ulcers/injuries: Quick reference guide.* In E. Haesler (Ed.). EPUAP/NPIAP/PPPIA.

Hall, D. A., Reed, F. B., Nuki, G., Vince, J. D. (1974). The relative effects of age and corticosteroid therapy on the collagen profiles of dermis from subjects with rheumatoid arthritis. *Age and Ageing, 3,* 15–22

Harries, R. L., Bosanquet, D. C., & Harding, K. G. (2016). Wound bed preparation: TIME for an update. *International Wound Journal, 13*(Suppl S3), 8–14.

Huang, C., Ma, Y., Wang, C., Jiang, M., Foon, L. Y., Lv, L., & Han, L. (2021). Predictive validity of the braden scale for pressure injury risk assessment in adults: A systematic review and meta-analysis. *Nursing Open, 8,* 2194–2207.

Kottner, J. (2020). Clinical relevance of nonblanchable erythema in pressure ulcer development. (Commentary). *British Journal of Dermatology, 182,* 262–263.

Kottner, J., & Dassen, T. (2010). Pressure ulcer risk assessment in critical care: Interrater reliability and validity studies of the Braden and Waterlow scales and subjective ratings in two intensive care units. *International Journal of Nursing Studies, 47,* 671–677.

Kottner, J., Black, J., Call, E., Gefen, A., & Santamaria, N. (2018). Microclimate: A critical review in the context of pressure ulcer prevention. *Clinical Biomechanics, 59,* 62–70.

Langer, G., & Fink, A. (2014). Nutritional interventions for preventing and treating pressure ulcers. *Cochrane Database of Systematic Reviews,* 6. CD003216 https://doi.org/10.1002/14651858.CD003216.pub2

McInness, E., Jammali-Blasi, A., Bell-Syer, S. E. M., Dumville, J. C., Middleton, V., & Cullum, N. (2015). Support surfaces for pressure ulcer prevention. *Cochrane Database of Systematic Reviews,* 9. CD001735.

Moore, Z., Avsar, P., Conaty, L., Moore, D. H., & O'Connor, T. (2019). The prevalence of pressure ulcers in Europe, what does the European data tell us: A systematic review. *Journal of Wound Care, 28*(11), 710–719.

Moore, Z. E. H., & Patton, D. (2019). Risk assessment tools for the prevention of pressure ulcers. *Cochrane Database of Systematic Reviews, 1* CD006471.

National Institute for Health and Care Excellence (NICE). (2014). *Pressure ulcers: Prevention and management clinical guideline CG179.* NICE.

NICE. (2015). *Pressure ulcers quality standard.* NICE.

NICE. (2019). *Mepilex border heel and sacrum dressings for preventing pressure ulcers.* Medical technologies guidance (MTG 40). https://www.nice.org.uk/guidance/mtg40

National Pressure Ulcer Advisory Panel, European Pressure Ulcer Advisory Panel and Pan Pacific Pressure Injury Alliance (2014). In E. Haesler (Ed.), *Prevention and treatment of pressure Ulcers: Clinical practice guideline*: Cambridge Media.

NHS Improvement. (2018). *Pressure ulcers: Revised definitions and measurement. Summary and recommendations.* NHS Improvement.

Nichols, E. (2015). Wound assessment part 1: How to measure a wound. *Wound Essentials, 10*(2), 51–55.

Nigam, Y., & Knight, J. (2017). Anatomy and physiology of ageing 11: The skin. *Nursing Times, 113*(12), 51–55.

Norton, D., McLaren, R., & Exton-Smith, A. N. (1975). *An investigation of geriatric nursing problems in hospital* (2nd ed.). Churchill Livingstone.

Oozageer Gunowa, N., Hutchinson, M., Brooke, J., & Jackson, D. (2018). Pressure injuries in people with darker skin tones: A literature review. *Journal of Clinical Nursing, 27,* 3266–3275.

Rithalia, S. V. S. (1989). Comparison of pressure distribution in wheelchair seat cushions. *Care Science and Practice, 7,* 87–92.

Schubert, V. (1991). Hypotension as a risk factor for the development of pressure sores in older subjects. *Age and Ageing, 20,* 255–261.

Seiler, W. O., Allen, S., & Stahelin, H. B. (1986). Influence of the 30 degree laterally inclined position and the 'super-soft' 3-piece mattress on skin oxygen tension on areas of maximum pressure: Implications for pressure sore prevention. *Gerontology, 32,* 158–166.

Shi, C., Bonnett, L. J., Dumville, J. C., & Cullum, N. (2020). Nonblanchable erythema for predicting pressure ulcer development: A systematic review with an individual participant data meta-analysis. *British Journal of Dermatology, 182,* 278–286.

Singh, S., Young, A., & McNaught, C.-E. (2017). The physiology of wound healing. *Surgery, 35*(9), 473–477.

Stockton, L., Gebhardt, K. S., & Clark, M. (2009). Seating and pressure ulcers: Clinical practice guideline. *Journal of Tissue Viability, 18,* 98–108.

Sullivan, R. (2014). A 5-year retrospective study of descriptors associated with identification of stage I and suspected deep tissue pressure ulcers in persons with darkly pigmented skin. *Wounds: A Compendium of Clinical Research and Practice, 26*(12), 351–359.

Swan, J. (2017). Development of deep tissue injury: Inside out or outside in? *Wounds UK, 13*(2), 18–24.

Talley Group Limited. (2020). *Pressure ulcers in people with dark skin tones.* https://www.talleygroup.com/medias/documents/PPPIA-Pressure-Ulcers-in-People-with-Dark-Skin-Tones-Poster-A3L-0-1604484440.pdf

VanGuilder, C., MacFarlane, G. D., & Meyer, S. (2008). Results of nine international pressure ulcer prevalence surveys: 1989 to 2005. *Ostomy Wound Management, 54*(2), 40–54.

Voegeli, D. (2017). Prevention and management of incontinence-associated dermatitis. *British Journal of Nursing, 26*(20), 1128–1132.

Vowden, K., & Vowden, P. (2017). Wound dressings: Principles and practice. *Surgery, 35*(9), 489–494.

Waterlow, J. (1985). Pressure sores. A risk assessment card. *Nursing Times, 81,* 49–55.

25

Sleep and Rest

Irene Gilsenan

> *Good sleep doesn't just means lots of sleep: it means the right kind of sleep*
>
> *Colin Espie (2021, p. 5)*

CHAPTER OUTLINE

INTRODUCTION

Sleep is 'a natural temporary state of rest during which an individual becomes physically inactive and unaware of the surrounding environment and many bodily functions (as breathing) slow' (Merriam-Webster, 2021). Considered rationally, it is a curious physiological activity that at a particular time, usually within a 24-hour period, the body closes down and becomes unresponsive to the outside world, and a state of unconsciousness happens. It is perhaps not surprising theories about sleep have been circulating for many centuries, some dating back to ancient Greek philosophers (Horne, 1989). The simple definition above sets out the basic appearance of sleep. A growing body of evidence underpins the stages of sleep, what happens when humans are sleep deprived, what affects sleep, how sleep alters during a person's lifetime and what can be done to improve sleep. Depriving the body of sleep, intentionally or otherwise, has been shown to have a detrimental effect on the health of an individual (Cooke & Ancoli-Isreal, 2011); sleep medicine has emerged as a burgeoning specialty in recent years. Although sleep is a normal human activity, it is of utmost importance to recognise the states of coma and stupor can mimic sleep. Most nurses who care for a sick, older adult have had the experience of being concerned about their unresponsiveness and of deliberating whether the person is actually asleep or their condition or health has deteriorated. In this situation the nurse may need to try and wake the person to assess their well-being, with the risk of irritating them if they were enjoying a lovely sleep!

If nurses consider the baseline that promoting sleep is a core nursing skill, they can help patients function better, recover from illness more effectively and in the longer-term facilitate management and care of older adults at home, in hospital and in long-term care facilities. Nurses have experience looking after patients at night and are acutely aware of the effects on their own personal sleep patterns and functioning while working various shift patterns. In addition, they have long recognised the value of building relationships with patients and their families to assess health and glean personalised knowledge around sleep patterns.

When it comes to the amount of sleep individuals need, it varies a great deal. The old adage of getting 8 hours of sleep is not borne out by people who manage perfectly well on less than 4 hours per night. Others require more than 10 hours nightly to help them feel refreshed and ready for the following day. However, if people feel they have had less sleep than is normal for them, this internalised perception can begin to affect their general health. The structure and pattern of sleep—otherwise known as the architecture of sleep—is complex and personal (Pilkington, 2013). This chapter discusses what normal sleep is, the stages of sleep and changes that come with age, sleep problems in older people, how sleep is assessed and a discussion of sleep therapies.

NORMAL ADULT SLEEP

Studying Sleep

Although sleep studies have been ongoing for many decades examining the activities of the bodily organs and the effects of varying degrees of sleep deprivation, they have mainly been undertaken with younger, healthy adults, and the older population has rarely been included (Bloom et al., 2009).

Equipment used to measure sleep include the electroencephalograph (EEG) to monitor electrical brain activity via electrodes on the scalp; the electro-oculograph (EOG), which monitors the movement of the eyes; and the electromyograph (EMG), which records muscle tone (Morgan & Closs, 1999). These three objective measurements are known as polysomnography and have been used for many decades, although it has been suggested the act of studying sleep influences how subjects behave or react (Bianchi, 2014). More recently subjective sleep diaries and emerging laboratory tests have been used to attempt to measure what happens when we sleep. This means although nurses have a number of investigative tools that can be used to assess sleep type, duration and quality, they perhaps need to consider supporting sleep as part of a holistic approach to care.

Sleep Stages

There are two main types of sleep: non–rapid-eye-movement (non-REM) sleep and rapid-eye-movement (REM) sleep. The classification of the stages of sleep was updated by the American Academy of Sleep Medicine (AASM) in 2005. Before that it was thought there were five sleep stages, but today there is consensus among sleep experts the sleep cycle comprises four stages as defined by the AASM (see Table 25.1). Non-REM sleep is categorised into three stages

TABLE 25.1 What Happens to the Body in the Stages of Sleep

Stage of Sleep	What Is Happening?
N1 (previously known as stage one) (non-REM sleep)	Lightest stage of sleep, a dozing off phase Usually 1–5 minutes in length Can have slow rolling eye movements in this stage Reduced muscle tone and occasional twitching EEG readings of 2 to 7-Hz frequency range EMG levels lower than when awake
N2 (previously known as stage two) (non-REM sleep)	Most time spent in this stage 10–60 minutes in this stage but differs in each cycle Sometimes known as true sleep Body temperature drops and muscles relax EEG readings lower but spike in 12 to 14-Hz frequency range
N3 (previously known as stages three and four) (non-REM sleep)	Sometimes called deep sleep or slow wave sleep Spend most time in this stage in the first part of the night EEG readings of 0.5 to 3-Hz frequency range 20–40 minutes in this stage but varies with cycles
R sleep (previously known as stage five) (REM sleep)	Lots of eye movement Sometimes known as the dreaming stage with increased brain activity Very low muscle tone 10–60 minutes in this stage, getting longer in the cycles as the night wears on Varies with age: 50% of sleep in newborns and 20% of sleep in adults EMG levels at their lowest rate

Sources: Bloom et al. (2009); Sleep Foundation (2020).

(N1 [previously stage 1], N2 [previously stage 2] and N3 [previously stages 3 and 4]. These three stages of non-REM sleep and REM sleep (previously stage 5) sequence over the course of the sleep period, with episodes of REM sleep lengthening until time of waking. The body requires these stages of sleep for different bodily responses. Amlaner and Fuller (2009) suggest the time spent in each stage of sleep varies as people get older.

More detail about the stages of sleep and the differing EEG and EMG recordings are highlighted in Table 25.1.

The International Classification of Sleep Disorders lists 125+ conditions that affect the specific stages of sleep related to issues that include age, pregnancy, medical conditions and medications (Reite et al., 2002).

Purpose of Sleep

Although we spend approximately one-third of our lives asleep (Gilsenan, 2012), the primary function of sleep in humans remains poorly understood. From their studies of animals, Amlaner and Fuller (2009) asserted sleep serves a fundamental function, but there is much we do not understand about it. Horne (1989) linked sleep to health restoration and argued sleep restores us, as we feel so much better when we get enough sleep and so much worse when we don't. Price (2016) built on this idea, suggesting sleep is not only restorative but also helps with energy conservation, learning and memory.

Researchers are currently focused on the role of sleep in replenishing the brain's stores of the carbohydrate energy reserve molecule glycogen. Levels are being related to the concentrations of the compound adenosine, the breakdown product of adenosine triphosphate (ATP), which provides the essential fuel for all cellular metabolism (Lee, 2007). As adenosine accumulates, the brain switches into deeper sleep, during which resynthesis of glycogen and increases in the level of ATP occur. Other chemicals appear to be important in this process, and there is clear evidence a chemical messenger, the cytokine tumour necrosis factor-alpha, promotes longer and deeper non-REM sleep in animals (Horne, 1989). This chemical is released in bacterial and viral infections and causes a febrile response, which explains at least in part why feverish patients are also often sleepy.

The function of REM sleep and its relationship to dreaming have provoked much speculation in published evidence. REM sleep and dreaming may be independent of each other, even though they tend to occur at the same time. Dreaming takes place in the higher centres of the brain, in the cortex, while REM sleep is controlled in the brainstem and midbrain. Repeated selective REM sleep deprivation does not appear to harm individuals who are so deprived, and patients tolerate drugs like tricyclic antidepressants that specifically suppress REM sleep without producing any physical or mental ill health (Tembo & Parker, 2009). REM sleep is at its most plentiful in the foetus and neonate, suggesting it has an important role when rapid growth and development are taking place. It has been suggested there is a lack of external stimulation within the uterus, and REM sleep provides substitute stimulation to aid brain development (Reite et al., 2002).

Although Reite et al. (2002) speculated non-REM sleep, or slow-wave (stage N3) sleep (SWS), is good for restoring the body, and REM stage sleep is good for restoring the brain, other authors dispute this and claim sleep is a 'non-behaviour' to either keep us out of harm's way of predators or to while away the hours of darkness that are usually unproductive (Horne, 1989). This demonstrates a lack of consensus about the functions of sleep and the need for further research, particularly about the impact of sleep on health. The Royal Society for Public Health (2016) determined the potential consequences of poor sleep to public health (see Table 25.2).

SLEEP ARCHITECTURE IN OLDER PEOPLE

We now consider how sleep in older adults differs from sleep in younger people. Research shows age-related changes in depth, continuity and duration of sleep (Bloom et al., 2009). The architecture of sleep in older people is characterised by an increase in the number of sequences of the different stages of sleep, a reduction in the amount of N3 stage SWS, more episodes of intervening wakefulness during the night and more daytime napping . Other authors reiterate disturbances in sleep can occur at any time in a person's life, but as we get older, physical and psychological diseases and conditions play a bigger part in our lives and therefore affect sleep (Bloom et al., 2009; Ersser et al., 1999).

Joshi (2008) confirmed the polypharmacy associated with multiple chronic conditions in later life can lead to altered sleep patterns, but sleep disturbances should not always be seen as inevitable. Amlaner and Fuller (2009) suggested sleep problems are not necessarily age related but more condition related, as participants in studies had mental health issues such as depression, respiratory conditions, moderate-to-poor health generally and a number of physical comorbidities.

Jaussent et al. (2011) examined three sleep complaints: difficulty initiating sleep, difficulty maintaining sleep through the night, and early morning awakening and not being able to go back to sleep. Of nearly 6,000 participants over age 65, 70% reported at least one of these three complaints, with difficulty maintaining sleep being the most common. The study also showed women reported two or

TABLE 25.2	Main Consequences of Poor Sleep to Public Health		
Physical	**Mental**	**Behavioural**	**Performance**
Risk of...	*Risk of...*	*Risk of...*	
Cancer	Depression	Sleepiness	Impaired attention and concentration
Cardiovascular disease and stroke	Psychiatric relapse	Road traffic accidents	Decreased memory
Disorders of the hypothalamic-pituitary-adrenal (HPA) system	Mood fluctuation	Falls and fractures	Reduced multitasking
Metabolic abnormalities	Delirium	Repeat prescribing	Impaired decision making
Weight gain and obesity	Impulsivity	Alcohol and drug dependency	Reduced creativity
Reduced immunity	Anger and frustration	Increased sedative and stimulant use	Reduced communication
Bodily sensations of pain	Higher risk of suicide	Less likely to attend appointments	Reduced socialisation
Thermoregulatory problems	Anxiety and hyperarousal	Longer stay in hospital	Less likely to be employed
Vulnerable seizure threshold	Chronic fatigue	Earlier admission to long-term care	More likely to be on benefits

Source: Royal Society for Public Health (2016).

three complaints, while the men in the study generally reported just one, showing a possible impact of gender and biological sex on sleeping difficulties.

Bianchi (2014) cited sleep studies with a 'young-old' category of individuals between 60 and 74 years old and an 'old-old' category who were between 75 and 87. The young-old group showed fewer differences in quality of sleep, whereas the old-old group exhibited increased wakefulness and issues with getting to sleep. The likelihood of napping was found to increase as people moved from the young-old age range to the old-old age range. Furthermore, there was little evidence of whether and how these trends change as people age beyond the age of 87, which is important as population demographics change.

Sleep studies have been brought up to date with authors such as Shankar et al. (2010) listing aspects of modern-day living that affect sleep, such as electric lights, longer working hours, more time spent commuting to work, shiftwork associated with employment roles in 24-hour services, and the effects of television and the internet. Although these aspects may be regarded as affecting the younger generation more, some older people have developed ingrained sleep behaviours from earlier in life due to previous work patterns, family activities and medical conditions—for example, sleeping in an armchair due to mobility issues.

The amount of sleep older people get has been the subject of many studies. Some older adults sleep for longer periods; others sleep for shorter periods. Horne (1989) suggested napping during the day can be related to boredom and loneliness and not necessarily be health related or due to a lack of sleep at night. Cooke and Ancoli-Israel (2011) implied the hours an older person sleeps must be measured against the ideal daytime functioning for that person; Banks and Dinges (2007) categorically stated between 7 and 8 hours of sleep per night is needed for all physical and psychological functioning.

Horne (1989) also suggested daytime naps up to and beyond 2 hours per day become replacement sleep and should be subtracted from an older adult's expected night-time sleep hours.

Some authors have suggested older people are more likely to go to bed early as they feel sleepy between 7:00 and 9:00 p.m. (Cooke & Ancoli-Israel, 2011), but this may influence the perception of having slept well. For example, Horne (1989) stated if an older person goes to bed at between 9:00 and 10:00 p.m., then they sleep until 3:00 or 4:00 a.m., they may awake feeling refreshed and alert after a good quota of sleep, but because of the time of day, they feel it is wrong to get up, so they stay in bed awake, doubting the quality of the sleep they just had.

Bianchi (2014) reviewed the evidence from sleep studies over a number of years and showed the development of how sleep disturbance conditions are diagnosed. Although there are now more recognised conditions and behaviours that affect sleep, many complex factors influence sleep disturbance, so there is variation in how sleep conditions present, leading Bianchi to suggest each individual experiences sleep disturbance differently. Furthermore, there are concerns about being prescriptive about what is a 'normal' amount of sleep; Bianchi suggests it is more useful to determine how much a person's sleep disturbance deviates from what is normal for them.

The age-related changes in the amount of non-REM and REM sleep stages are summarised in Table 25.3. The relative amount of REM sleep persists until extreme old age, although a decline in the proportion of REM sleep seems to correlate with reduced intellectual functioning and organic brain syndrome (Zisberg et al., 2010). Cooke and Ancoli-Israel (2011) advised the goal in addressing sleep issues for older adults is to promote daytime functioning.

Some studies use a standard measure of sleepiness termed *sleep latency*. This refers to how quickly a person falls asleep as measured by EEG recordings. Sleep latency can be measured at any time of the day or night and is a more valid and reliable measure of sleepiness than naturally occurring naps. Measurement is precise and objective, and the opportunity and environment for sleeping are controlled (Johns, 2000). In a study that compared a group of younger adults aged 19–29 with older adults over 65, the older group reported longer sleep latency with some serious interruptions to their sleep than the younger group. Although the older group did not complain of sleep disturbances, they were more likely to take daytime naps to reduce their sleepiness (Zilli et al., 2009)

CAUSES OF SLEEP PROBLEMS IN OLDER PEOPLE

Nurses need to move beyond the signs and symptoms of poor sleep to identify its various causes to help promote sleep in the older population.

Biological Rhythms, Ageing and Sleep

One view of the ageing process is it is characterised by the disorganisation of biological rhythms. The body's circadian rhythm over a 24-hour period regulates sleep–wake activities and links with patterns of hormonal secretions, blood pressure regulation, immunological responses and body temperature control. These bodily rhythms need to be in tune with one another and can be affected by not only internal events but also external time cues (i.e., zeitgebers), such as the light–dark cycle affecting our perception of rest–activity cycles and eating times (Cooke & Ancoli-Israel, 2011). The regular alternation of sleep–wakefulness and synchronisation of internal rhythms is regarded as a fundamental biological rhythm for humans.

It can be quite tempting when nursing older people to encourage daytime napping, especially if you know the person has had a disturbed night, but Morgan and Gledhill (1991) advised against creating a vicious circle whereby the person sleeps more during the day and less at night, desynchronising their sleep–wake cycle with other rhythms.

A key zeitgeber is daytime light changes—sunrise and sunset—which Pilkington (2013) states are fundamental to maintaining rhythms within the 24 hours of a day. Zisberg et al. (2010) argued these zeitgebers, in association with a daily routine, help older people train their circadian rhythms and avoid behaviours such as daytime napping. Nurses should be wary of imposing regimens of sleep–waking on older people, as their cycles are likely to be less adaptable and more easily disrupted than those of younger people, and they need time to adapt to an unfamiliar routine. Regular daytime activities that include both physical and mental stimulation can help maintain a healthy normal sleep–wake schedule for individuals whose rhythms are in synchrony, but abruptly enforced daytime activity is unlikely to help either the sleep-deprived or the desynchronised older person. The use of bright light therapy and melatonin are discussed later in the chapter.

Sleep Deprivation

Horne (1989) cited the study of a 17-year-old adolescent who deprived himself of sleep for 264 hours to beat the world record. This American schoolboy, Randy Gardner, was studied by an American Navy Sleep Institute to see what effects it had on his body, including visual

TABLE 25.3	Sleep Pattern and Age		
Age	Non-REM Sleep	REM Sleep	Hours Slept
Newborn	50%	50%	16 hours
1–2 years	69%	31%	13 hours
19–30 years	80%	20%	7.5 hours
50–70 years	83%	17%	6 hours
70–85 years	91%	9%	5.5 hours

Source: Adapted from Bianchi (2014).

disturbances, mood changes, difficulty speaking, memory lapses and fragmented speech. When he beat the previous world record by 4 hours and went to sleep, he slept longer for the first few nights as his body attempted to catch up on the lost sleep, then reverted back to his normal sleep patterns.

Dautovich et al. (2010) examined sleeplessness in the older population and found it was problematic to make general assumptions about published studies as they were often undertaken on relatively healthy, medication-free, well-educated adults, which may not be representative of the whole population. Horne (1989) believed sleep deprivation studies in animals or on younger people such as military personnel may not have the wider currency some assume.

Many of the sleep deprivation studies in adults focus on a person's ability to maintain cognitive functions such as memory, alertness and ability to maintain tasks such as driving. Although initially it was thought performance of boring, repetitive tasks deteriorated following sleep deprivation, later studies have shown certain short, interesting tasks such as verbal fluency and non-verbal planning are also sensitive to sleep loss (Horne, 1989). When young adults are sleep-deprived for 36 hours, their ability to perform neuropsychological tests becomes similar to that of a 60-year-old (Harrison & Horne, 2000).

As mentioned earlier, a key function of sleep appears to be cerebral cortex recovery, the area employed in stimulating tasks that involve directing and sustaining attention, inhibiting distraction, aspects of working memory and flexible thinking. Short-term sleep deprivation has been shown to impair these abilities (Harrison & Horne, 2000).

Total sleep deprivation affects not only performance and mood but also the rest–activity and sleep–wake cycles. Subjects tend to become agitated and delirious and have a reduced pain tolerance. Many studies have examined how sleep deprivation occurs in intensive care units, with medications, noise, ventilator settings, light pollution and care activities being highlighted as factors (Parathasarathy & Tobin, 2009; Tembo & Parker, 2009).

Psychosocial and Environmental Context of Sleep

A number of environmental factors may increase sleep disturbance and deprivation in older people.

Hospital or Institutional Admission

Hospital and care environments have long been studied to examine if they are antagonistic or conducive to sleep. Recommendations suggest such places are noisy, have increased light pollution, are places where patients are anxious and in pain, and are where care-giving activity disturbs sleep (Celik et al., 2005; Gilsenan, 2017; Patel et al., 2008; Pilkington, 2013).

Celik et al. (2005) targeted the nursing routines on a critical care unit as events that disturb patients' sleep, citing an average of 51 interventions per patient each night, making it impossible for those patients to obtain a necessary amount of sleep. They cited activities such as bed baths, drug administration, observations and dressings as activities undertaken between the hours of midnight and 5:00 a.m. Although this demonstrates the delivery of 24-hour care, it overrides patients' need for sleep. Many authors suggest nighttime protocols should be implemented, with nurses taking into consideration light, noise and care activities while optimising sleep, protecting the hours overnight and reducing unnecessary interruptions (Humphries, 2008; Lareau et al., 2008; Missildine, 2008).

For older people in long-term care institutions, similar sleep disturbances exist in terms of nighttime activities, but Joshi (2008) suggested modifications to alleviate sleep deprivation that include increasing the amount of daytime physical activity and sunlight the person experiences; limiting naps to just 1 hour in the early afternoon; avoiding stimulating foods; drinks and medications close to bedtime; and managing the light and dark experiences.

Many environmental and psychosocial factors, including boredom, social isolation and physical confinement, are likely to result in excessive sleepiness, whereas heat, cold, light, movement and noise are liable to disturb sleep and encourage wakefulness.

Noise Effects on Sleep

Older people are more likely to be affected by noise-induced sleep disturbances than younger adults, although Basner and McGuire (2018) noted this varies from person to person. The researchers suggested a healthy adult can be aroused briefly from sleep approximately twenty times in an 8-hour sleep period, although the person is unlikely to recall these awakenings. They also noted the auditory system keeps watch while the person slumbers, and specific noises are more likely to wake an individual. For example, if a noise is accompanied by vibration, it can be particularly disturbing. Another factor is where a person is in the cycle of sleep; Morgan and Closs (1999) suggested REM sleep is most affected by exposure to noise.

Many studies over the years have examined sleep disturbances associated with louder noises such as railway lines and major airports (Basner & McGuire, 2018; Morgan & Closs, 1999), but researchers indicated people exhibit a certain amount of adaptation to noise levels and forge regular sleep patterns.

Some authors look at sleep in hospitals or long-term care facilities to examine extraneous noises nurses and care staff should try to reduce, including audible conversations between staff, telephones, televisions and equipment such as waste bins and doors that bang when closed (Gilsenan, 2017; Pilkington, 2013; Robinson et al., 2005). Strange noises in institutional settings also affect sleep. Reid (2001) cited noises from other patients or residents as a potential issue as well as noises made by staff attending patients during the night. There is also frequent use of mobile phones in hospitals and care environments, with relatives using them to contact loved ones at any time. Nurses should encourage contact and support but need to be aware of their contribution to sleep disturbance. Because of the dependency level of patients in hospitals, such as patients with cognitive and sensory impairment, it may be impossible to eliminate all noise interruptions while providing care. Conversely, a study indicated environmental noise was responsible for a maximum of 17% of awakenings from sleep, suggesting although noise is important, other factors are responsible for the majority of disturbances (Freedman et al., 2001).

In terms of managing sleep, increasingly high doses of sedatives are sometimes considered for patients who make a lot of noise or exhibit disruptive behaviours in an attempt to alleviate their distress and help other patients have uninterrupted sleep. However, giving high doses of sedatives is not recommended as a treatment option, and other solutions should be explored:

- Identify the reason why the patient is shouting or exhibiting disruptive behaviour and respond to it.
  - Is the person in pain or anxious about being in hospital?
  - Is there a communication problem that once solved would result in the person becoming more settled?
  - Does the person have a physical condition such as delirium that explains why they are agitated?
- Would a reduction in sedation be more effective than an increase?
- How should the person be supported? Do they need enhanced care and attention from nurses, which may require additional staff?
- Supporting the mental health of older adults, including those with depression, dementia and delirium, should a priority for nurses so patients who exhibit lots of noise and disruptive behaviour can be referred for diagnosis and appropriate treatment.

Dietary Effects on Sleep

Dietary habits appear to have an important influence on sleep patterns. St-Onge et al. (2016) examined the effects of a variety of diets on sleep patterns and found a high-carbohydrate diet reduced stage N3 non-REM SWS and increased REM sleep, whereas higher fat content in a diet reduced REM sleep and increased SWS sleep. However, the effects of diet on sleep are complex. Amino acids such as tryptophan obtained from foods such as nuts, cheese and red meats contribute to the production of the brain transmitter 5-hydroxytryptamine (i.e., serotonin), which affects mood regulation, pain sensitivity and sleep.

Peuhkuri et al. (2012) discussed various foods alleged to have sleep-inducing properties, including milky drinks made with Horlicks powder, a malted barley and wheat additive. They cited studies that concluded milky drinks taken by older people resulted in better sleep quality if the drinks were made with melatonin-rich milk obtained when cows are milked in darkness at nighttime. Timing of foods during the day has also been studied, with recognition that in hospital and long-term care institutions, the last meal of the day may be a long time before bedtime, so providing some nutrition later in the evening such as a milky drink or snack may help sleep overall. Helping older people who are in an unfamiliar environment follow familiar presleep routines, such as having a drink or snack or a warm bath, can aid relaxation and the onset of sleep.

Caffeine has long been considered an antidote to good sleep, but what is not so well known is the levels of caffeine in everyday food and drinks such as tea, coffee, cocoa-based drinks and especially high-energy drinks. Nurses should be aware some over-the-counter analgesics also contain caffeine. Ruxton (2009) set out the range and average levels of caffeine in a number of food and drink items and advocated a safe level of between 38 mg and 400 mg of caffeine per day (see Table 25.4).

According to the European Food Safety Authority (2015), a single dose of 100 mg caffeine taken close to

TABLE 25.4 Caffeine Content of Food and Drinks

Beverage (portion size)	Range (mg/portion)	Average (mg/portion)
Tea (190 ml)	1–90	50
Instant coffee (190 ml)	21–120	75
Ground coffee (190 ml)	15–254	100
Espresso coffee (40 ml)	No data	140
Hot chocolate (150 ml)	1–6	No data*
Dark chocolate (bar)	No data	50
Cola (330 ml)	11–70	40
Energy drink (250 ml)	27–87	80

*Milk chocolate contains approximately half the caffeine levels of dark chocolate.
Source: Ruxton (2009).

bedtime reduces sleep duration in adults. Ruxton (2009) also advocated the benefits of caffeine in the diet and advised against nurses suggesting a total ban on caffeine intake as there is widespread enjoyment of foods that contain caffeine, and they may have other health benefits.

Drugs Associated With Sleep Disorders

As people become older, they experience an increased likelihood of being diagnosed with a medical condition. With diagnosis usually comes a medication regime that can affect sleep patterns. Cooke and Ancoli-Israel (2011) stated polypharmacy is often prescribed without any consideration of how it affects the sleep pattern of the person. Joshi (2008) also raised the possibility of multiple medications causing adverse drug interactions, including sleep disturbances.

Bloom et al. (2009) listed the range of medications with the potential to affect sleep in older adults, including prescription-only items such as 'beta-blockers, bronchodilators, corticosteroids, decongestants and diuretics… cardiovascular, neurological, psychiatric and gastrointestinal medications' (p. 7). Steiger and Pawlowski (2019) stated medications to treat depression can paradoxically also affect sleep by reducing REM sleep cycles. Nurses have to be aware of the range of medications that can be bought over the counter that affect sleep. Medications that contain caffeine are discussed above; treatments for coughs, colds and nasal congestion often contain pseudoephedrine, a stimulant that can inhibit sleep.

Cooke and Ancoli-Israel (2011) found the timing of medications throughout the day should be regulated so medications with a sedative effect are given close to bedtime and medications that stimulate or require activity such as diuretics are administered during the day. Reite et al. (2002) suggested older people may have diminished renal and hepatic function, so care is needed when prescribing any medications, particularly considering the half-life of the drug prescribed as well as potential interactions (see Chapter 31).

Alcohol

The adage that alcohol aids sleep has been studied and found to be untrue. Although evidence supports alcohol promoting drowsiness, therefore helping people fall asleep, increasing research shows alcohol adversely affects sustained and REM sleep. Britton et al. (2020) reported on a 30-year study that examined the health, activities and lifestyles of over 10,000 United Kingdom civil servants and included self-reported sleep patterns and alcohol-related behaviours. They concluded high alcohol consumption may contribute to the incidence of sleep disturbances in older age, and individuals with sleep issues should not use alcohol as a sleep aid.

Nurses should be aware older people can be reluctant to discuss their alcohol consumption, which in some cases increases insidiously for years before coming to the attention of a health care professional (see Chapter 32). Enquiries about alcohol use should always be made in assessing any form of sleep disturbance in older people.

Illness and Sleep Disturbance

The majority of illnesses result in sleep disruption and further confound the sleep problems of older adults. A sleep problem improves only when the underlying medical condition is alleviated or resolved.

Mental Health

Mental health problems associated with sleep disorders include anxiety, depression, dementia, phobias, obsessive-compulsive disorder and other neurotic disorders.

Anxiety and Stress

The Royal Society for Public Health (2016) cited anxiety and stress as key factors in difficulties with sleep. Anxiety and stress are defined as any acute emotional or conflict state caused by a loss or perceived threat such as personal bereavement, sudden changes in lifestyle and unfamiliar circumstances such as illness, hospitalisation or institutional care.

Ganz (2012) and Pilkington (2013) described how when a person is stressed or anxious, the body releases cortisol, which inhibits sleep further, so if someone is anxious and cannot sleep, their body reacts by releasing cortisol, which sets off a vicious cycle of disturbed sleep. Reid (2001) indicated stress and anxiety responses impede falling asleep, increase intermittent waking and affect movement between the stages of sleep. Reid (2001) also suggested older people may have unrealistic expectations of their sleep, and explaining how sleep patterns change with age may reduce some of the anxiety and stress that increase the occurrence of disturbed sleep.

Nurses need to be aware the lives of many older adults include major and minor losses and threats and should not be surprised to see sleep disruption among patients. Nurses should regularly assess sleep patterns and be prepared to support the interventions discussed earlier to improve sleep (Patel et al., 2018).

More persistent periods of sleep disturbance may arise from chronic tension–anxiety states. During these states, older adults may stay in bed longer in an effort to resume sleep and try to nap with little success. High muscle tension may result in complaints of back pain and headache, and pulse rates may rise. They may complain of worried thoughts and anxious dreams, exhibit restless vigilant behaviour and regard tension as normal.

Depression

Many studies have shown an association between poor-quality, unsatisfactory sleep and depression (Cooke & Ancoli-Israel, 2011; Leblanc et al., 2015). According to Steiger and Pawlowski (2019), changes in REM sleep as well as increased arousal during sleep in individuals with depression are seen on EEG recordings. They suggested sleep impairment is both a symptom and a risk factor in individuals with depression, and as many as 80% of people with depression have some form of insomnia.

Depression can be the result of life events such as the death of a loved one or changes in circumstances. Symptoms are similar to the effects of anxiety or stress.

The difference between the reactions of individuals with anxiety or stress and depression, according to Leblanc et al. (2015), is individuals with depression are more likely to fall asleep quickly and remain in bed due to their fatigue and lack of interest, whereas those with anxiety or stress exhibit alertness and hyperactivity, thus affecting their sleep in different ways. Many physical factors impact sleep and depressive symptoms, so assessment and intervention need to be holistic in nature, considering all aspects of the problem and tackling it incrementally (see Chapter 30).

Dementia

Cooke and Ancoli-Israel (2011) stated sleep disturbances in people with a diagnosis of dementia are not surprising as the range of illnesses labelled as dementia often damage the parts of the brain that regulate sleep. Individuals with dementia may be sleepy during the daytime, become agitated and wander during the night—known as sundowning—and have reduced SWS and overall sleep hours. These behaviours create a considerable challenge for individuals who look after these patients—both informal carers in community settings and formal carers in hospital and institutional settings.

Cooke and Ancoli-Israel (2011) found obtaining a reliable history regarding sleep disturbances can be problematic, but nurses should consult with family and carers to ascertain this information.

Bloom et al. (2009) defined the sleep patterns typical of individuals with dementia as irregular sleep–wake disorder and outlined a programme of reducing the amount of time spent in bed during the day alongside increased physical activity, a structured bedtime routine and 30 minutes each day of sunlight exposure as being beneficial, leading to less daytime sleeping and more participation in social events (see Chapter 29).

Other Mental Health Problems

Patients with psychotic depression generally fall asleep readily but have difficulty maintaining sleep and wake early in the morning feeling fatigued, achy and 'washed out'. Patients in the depressed phase of manic-depressive psychosis and those with mild depressive disorders tend to be excessively sleepy by day. Mania or hypomania results in difficulty falling asleep and short sleep time, and people with this condition often wake refreshed after as little as 2 to 4 hours of sleep. It should be noted the older a patient with depression is, the greater the sleep loss in the second half of the night due to the cycles of sleep being affected. Schizophrenia and schizoaffective disorders can result in partial or complete inversion of the day–night sleep cycle, with extreme agitation in the first half of the night. The extent of sleep disruption depends on the severity of the illness (Bloom et al., 2009; Reite et al., 2002).

Physical Pathologies

An anomaly of disturbed sleep is it can be both a symptom and a contributing factor in the development of certain physical pathologies. Cooke and Ancoli-Israel (2011) found as older people have more diagnosed medical conditions, they are likely to suffer from insomnia, affecting the various stages of sleep.

Central nervous system damage or disease may result in pain, abnormal sensations or bodily movements that affect sleep or promote excessive drowsiness. Damage includes raised intracranial pressure from any cause, including tumours, cerebral haemorrhages and stroke (Bianchi, 2014).

Endocrine disorders such as hypothyroidism, diabetes and other conditions associated with changes in body weight are often accompanied by excessive daytime drowsiness and loud snoring. Patients may also have a significant degree of obstructive sleep apnoea (Ancoli-Israel, 2006), which is important to recognize, as appropriate pharmaceutical treatment can improve sleep quality and produce dramatic improvements in daytime and social functioning.

Increasingly, respiratory and cardiac disorders are recognised as producing chronic sleep disruption. Patients with chronic congestive heart failure have evidence of alternating periods of hypo- and hyperventilation during sleep—called Cheyne–Stokes respiration (Ancoli-Israel, 2006). These episodes can be exhausting, and it is not surprising to see a patient with cardiac problems sitting dozing in a chair after a disturbed night's sleep.

Long and Short Sleep

Many authors report a link between long and short sleep duration and the risks for diagnosed medical conditions (Cappuccio et al., 2011; Da Silva et al., 2016; Ganz, 2012; Shankar et al., 2010). Cappuccio et al. (2011) defined short sleep as being equal to or less than 5 or 6 hours per night and long sleep as being over 8 or 9 hours per night. The studies concluded short sleep duration was linked to a higher risk of coronary heart disease, vascular damage, high blood pressure, diabetes mellitus (type 2) and obesity. Long sleep duration was linked to higher levels of depression, unemployment and undiagnosed health conditions as well as coronary heart disease and stroke. There continues to be discussion about whether the health risks of long and short sleep duration affect both genders equally.

Sleep Apnoea

The condition whereby breathing ceases during sleep has long been an area for research and study. That the body has episodes of no airflow (i.e., apnoea) or a partial reduction in airflow (i.e., hypopnoea) is of interest across all age groups. An apnoea may be defined as a total loss of airflow for more than 10 seconds; hypopnoea is defined as a 50% reduction in airflow for at least 10 seconds (Reite et al., 2002). The body continues with respiratory effort during these episodes, and the usual outcome is an arousal or awakening that stimulates breathing to restart. Central apnoeas occur when airflow stops and the patient makes no effort to breathe. Apnoeic events, more common in older people, are obstructive sleep apnoea, when airflow stops while the patient continues to struggle to breathe.

Diagnosis is based on how many episodes of apnoea/hypopnoea occur each hour, resulting in an apnoea/hypopnoea index (AHI) score. The AHI should be less than 5 to 8 per hour for a young adult, although some studies indicate older people can have up to 17 episodes in an hour (Bianchi, 2014; Reite et al. 2002). Bloom et al. (2009) stated 15% of men and 5% of women are affected by apnoea/hypopnea conditions, but this rises to 70% of older men and 56% of older women. The common risk factors are age, obesity, being male and having existing respiratory airway disease (Bianchi, 2014). In their global study of sleep apnoea across 16 countries, Benjafield et al. (2019) estimated up to 425 million adults between 30 and 69 years of age have moderate to severe sleep apnoea.

The observable presentation of this condition is a patient who snores loudly, has reduced oximetry, and perhaps exhibits choking and excess body movements during sleep, although they may be less frequent. During the day the person may have headaches, excessive sleepiness, intellectual deterioration, fatigue and personality changes. The sudden onset of silence after hours of prolonged snoring is particularly alarming for a bed partner or attending nurse or carer, who often wakes up the patient to ensure they are still alive! The snoring itself can be extremely disruptive for everyone around the patient and may lead to much embarrassment and some reluctance to travel away from home. Patients can be treated with nasal continuous positive airway pressure used nightly. This treatment is relatively cumbersome; it requires both motivation and comprehension on the patient's part but is extremely effective in improving

wakefulness and general levels of energy (Morgan & Closs, 1999).

The Royal Society for Public Health (2016) indicates people diagnosed with obstructive sleep apnoea have higher risk of hypertension, stroke and a reduced quality of life.

Alveolar Hypoventilation

In some circumstances the tidal volume (i.e., the volume of air inhaled or exhaled in a single breath) during sleep fails to meet the level needed to maintain the normal elimination of carbon dioxide and replenishment with oxygen of the arterial blood. This problem differs from complete cessation of breathing, as the patient usually does not snore (Reite at al., 2002). It is not clear whether alveolar hypoventilation results from the interaction of normal sleep pathology and coexisting disease, such as in severe chronic obstructive airway disease, or whether there is a more specific defect in ventilatory control such as in obesity–hyperventilation syndrome. Changes of this type occur especially in REM sleep. Other causes include scoliosis, cordotomy, disease of the respiratory control centres, poliomyelitis and myotonic dystrophy.

Sleep-Related Leg Movements

The causes of relatively common leg movements during sleep remain largely unknown. People affected with them are usually middle aged or older, and they (and often their bed partners) complain of nighttime awakenings, unrefreshing sleep and daytime sleepiness. Some notice leg cramps, and in extreme cases they may even fall out of bed. Other symptoms include repetitive leg muscle jerking and uncomfortable feelings in the lower extremities, including tingling and skin-crawling sensations. The symptoms can be felt in one or both legs mainly from the knees downward. These physical activities are accompanied by EEG features of arousal, and the sleepiness is thought to be a consequence of the resulting sleep fragmentation. Nighttime leg movements are not usually accompanied by jerking of the rest of the body. In some cases problems extend into the day, and patients may be unable to sleep at night. Although neurological disorders such as motor neurone disease present in this way, the worst-affected cases often have evidence of chronic renal failure. Before any treatment options are discussed, a full assessment is required to eliminate other symptoms. Treatment options include iron supplements, dopaminergic agents, opioids, physiotherapy and an overhaul of sleep routines (Guo et al., 2017).

Pain

In a study about experiences of sleep in hospital, Grossman et al. (2017) asked staff and patients to list the most disruptive factor to sleep. Patients placed pain at the top of their list, whereas nurses and doctors placed various hospital nighttime noises as their top disturber.

All staff need to be aware a range of both acute and chronic painful physical pathologies disturb sleep, and older people tend to have more ongoing painful conditions than younger people. Tranmer et al. (2003) examined the experiences of both medical and surgical patients in hospitals and found both groups listed pain as a disturber of sleep. Pain may disturb sleep directly or in combination with psychological changes such as anxiety or the inability to undertake a usual routine. Pilkington (2013) surmised sleep disturbances and pain are interrelated in that sleep is disturbed by pain, and pain is made worse by lack of sleep.

Chronic conditions such as low-back pain, peripheral neuropathy, peripheral vascular disease, arthritis and fibromyalgia commonly disturb sleep, mainly by delaying sleep onset and increasing the frequency of awakening. Ancoli-Israel (2006) examined both rheumatoid and osteoarthritis and found both had a link with pain and sleep disturbances; people with these conditions spent more time in stage N1 non-REM sleep, leading to feelings of unrefreshing sleep. For example, individuals who underwent total hip replacement for osteoarthritis had increased sleep satisfaction after the initial postoperative phase, as their overall pain diminished. Some types of chronic pain such as dyspepsia and ulcer pain have a circadian rhythmicity, whereby the pain becomes worse during the night. It appears the interplay between pain and sleep is complex, with pain disrupting sleep quality and architecture, and sleep deprivation reducing pain thresholds.

Other Disorders

A range of parasomnias (i.e., undesirable physical phenomena associated with sleep) are exhibited by all age groups. Sleep-walking in older people is more likely to be due to stress or psychomotor epilepsy than to true somnambulism (i.e., sleepwalking). Nightmares are more prevalent at times of emotional stress and during REM rebound from drug withdrawal. Older adults with sleep-related inadequacy in swallowing saliva are at risk of respiratory aspiration, and sleep-related gastrointestinal reflux may result in oesophageal stricture or aspiration pneumonia. Primary sleep disorders such as narcolepsy and idiopathic central nervous system hypersomnolence persist into old age so may be occasionally seen.

Sleep research has come a long way toward helping us understand sleep problems in older adults. Nurses can use this knowledge to assess, care for, teach and empathise with people. There is now clear evidence much daytime sleepiness is a result of physical problems that disrupt normal sleep, which may be present whether or not the patient complains of insomnia. The subtle and complex interactions of normal ageing, diagnoses of medical conditions, polypharmacy and increasing physical frailty explain much of the disruption to sleep patterns experienced by older people.

Published research shows greater variability in older adults' sleep than in younger people for a number of reasons. That sleep–wake cycles may be more easily disrupted in older people, and the perceived dissatisfaction with sleep is generally supported by objective (i.e., EEG) evidence (Bloom et al., 2009). Many current sleep researchers consider older adults to need the same amount of sleep as younger people, and all seem to agree the potential causes of insomnia increase in old age. Makley et al. (2008) suggested poor sleep in patients who are hospitalised can increase their length of stay, so it is in patients' best interest to ensure staff caring for them have some knowledge and understanding of poor sleep and what can be done to help. Hypnotic medications to aid sleep in older people should be avoided not only to minimise deleterious side effects but also because they fail to address why sleep is disturbed.

The most common causes of sleep disturbance for adults include the following (Ancoli-Israel 2006; Guo et al. 2017; Jaussent et al., 2011):

- Chronic pain, especially due to rheumatism and arthritis
- Nocturnal dyspnoea
- Nocturnal discomfort from pruritus
- Peripheral neuritis
- Enforced uncomfortable positions
- Nocturia
- Dyspepsia
- Cerebral degeneration
- Abnormal movements
- Secondary disturbance of the circadian sleep–wake cycle
- Environmental factors associated with hospitalisation

The most important and consistent finding regarding sleep problems for older adults is the number and length of periods of awakening after sleep has started. However, as in all age groups, there are considerable individual differences. Research findings may reveal statistically significant differences between the sleep of young and old people, but you can never assume an individual in your care conforms to a trend. Detailed assessment of all elements of sleep is essential before care is planned and agreed on.

ASSESSMENT OF SLEEP

In recent years there has been increased awareness of the stages of sleep and more reiteration of what constitutes a good night's sleep. Much has come from technology, such as wearable gadgets that measure heart rate, daily step counts and sleep stages and duration. Although there is a large global market for this technology, the Royal Society for Public Health (2016) has questioned its accuracy in measuring sleep but admits wearables have the effect of raising awareness of sleep.

An initial assessment of sleep or lack of it by medical or nursing staff relies heavily on the subjective report of the sleeper. However, nurses who work in acute hospitals and care homes have the advantage of being present night and day and are in a good position to assess the sleep and wake behaviour of the people in their care, although in acute hospitals, this is likely to be for only a very short period. Nurses in long-term care environments are well placed for detailed ongoing assessment of sleep habits. Nurses work very closely with older adults and their family and carers, which is advantageous in building up a picture of a person's sleep activities. When it comes to scientific measurements of sleep, sleep researchers and medical staff are able to assess sleep using polygraphic recordings of internal events such as neurological and cardiovascular responses.

As with any self-reported symptoms and behaviours, there are challenges in assessing the quantity and quality of patients' sleep. To what extent do the person's subjective complaints and comments about their sleep correspond with objective measurable sleep problems? Some of the research discussed earlier showed some older people have multiple microarousals during the night they are not aware of and spend much time in light stages of sleep, as measured by EEG recordings. Mini awakenings are not generally visible even to the most observant nurse, but the aftermath of daytime sleepiness and complaints of poor sleeping are genuine. On the other hand, some older and younger people who complain of poor sleep do not exhibit EEG abnormalities when monitored in sleep laboratories, reinforcing the ideas discussed earlier that individuals of all ages exhibit a range of sleep habits.

An important distinction should be made between the person who is fatigued but tense and although longing to sleep is rarely able to do so and the person who is tired and suffering from sleep deprivation who, if given the opportunity, is able to make up the sleep by spending a longer time in bed at night and taking daytime naps. Severely sleep-deprived individuals eventually fall asleep whatever the surrounding activities, whereas a fatigued tense person is likely to be vigilant everything happening around them.

It can become difficult if a person's circadian rhythms become out of step with the world they live in so they want to sleep for most of the day and are awake during the nighttime hours. These people require a detailed assessment of their sleep–wake patterns and social responses over the preceding weeks in addition to a 24-hour diary of sleep to be certain of the diagnosis. It is important not to dismiss complaints about poor nighttime sleep. Nurses should accept they may not be able to improve the situation very quickly. It is important

older adults feel listened to and that nurses do everything possible to provide an environment conducive to sleep.

Methods of Assessment

There are a wide range of approaches to the assessment of sleep. Some measure physiological concomitants of sleep (e.g., EEG, EOG, EMG, body movements); others measure psychological aspects of daytime activity affected by the quality of sleep (e.g., reaction times, daytime sleepiness, and mood states). Perhaps most important are subjective reports of sleep from the sleeper.

Although it is unlikely nurses use physiological tests, they can observe and record daytime mood and sleepiness. However, the sleep history recorded on admission or on first assessing them in the community, plus subjective assessments of sleep, provide the most important and useful information. Many validated tools assess the quality of sleep, patterns of sleep and fatigue severity scales (Dautovich et al., 2010; Ersser et al., 1999).

Sleep History

Taking a sleep history allows the nurse to elicit information about the usual sleep patterns, including usual timing and duration of sleep and daytime napping habits. A basic sleep history such as that shown in Box 25.1 can be used as part of an admission process.

Nurses can then dig a little deeper by asking about a person's preferences and pre-sleep activities (Box 25.2) and in this way can assist in altering elements of the environment to encourage and support good sleep patterns.

There may, however, be a need for a more detailed assessment of sleep habits and history. The questionnaire developed by Lacks (1987) in Box 25.3 uses 48 questions that cover seven categories of information about sleep:

1. Description of the symptoms, extent and duration of insomnia (questions 1–7)
2. Psychological contributing factors (questions 8–16)
3. Sleep hygiene (questions 17–27)
4. Psychopathology (questions 28–32)
5. Organic sleep pathology (questions 33–39)
6. Serious medical problems (questions 40–45)
7. Patient's self-help attitudes (questions 46–48)

Using these assessments, the nurse may be able to provide support in terms of encouraging sleep hygiene and recognising contributing psychological factors. For psychopathology, organic sleep pathology or serious medical problems, referral to other specialists may be necessary.

Daily Assessment

Where an older person has an ongoing sleep problem, daily monitoring of sleep may help in the assessment and management of insomnia. Sleep diaries are now widely used

BOX 25.1 Simple Initial Sleep Assessment Questionnaire

1. What time do you normally go to bed at night? What time do you normally wake up in the morning?
2. Do you often have trouble falling asleep at night?
3. About how many times do you wake up at night?
4. If you do wake up during the night, do you usually have trouble falling back asleep?
5. Does your bed partner say (or are you aware) you frequently snore, gasp for air or stop breathing?
6. Does your bed partner say (or are you aware) you kick or thrash about while asleep?
7. Are you aware you ever walk, eat, punch, kick or scream during sleep?
8. Are you sleepy or tired for much of the day?
9. Do you usually take one or more naps during the day?
10. Do you usually doze off without planning during the day?
11. How much sleep do you need to feel alert and function well?
12. Are you currently taking any type of medication or other preparation to help you sleep?

Source: Bloom et al. (2009).

BOX 25.2 Questions to Highlight Routines and Preferences

- How did you sleep last night?
- What time did you go to bed?
- Approximately how long did it take you to get to sleep?
- How many times did you wake up during the night?
- What time did you wake up?
- How long did you sleep for in total?
- What did you consume (if anything) within 4 hours of going to bed (e.g. tea, coffee, milky drink, wine, beer, sleeping pills, dinner)? How long before bed did you consume it?
- What was the temperature outside and in your bedroom?
- What light sources were there when you went to sleep?
- How much noise was there when you went to sleep?
- What activities did you undertake before you went to sleep?
- Any other comments?
- How did you feel throughout the next day (1 = awful, 5 = average, 10 = great)? Include a description if appropriate (e.g., drowsy, grumpy, spaced out).

Source: Espie (2021).

for this purpose and vary according to the type of problem investigated. Sleep diaries or logs focus on sleep quality and quantity, patterns of sleep and wakefulness or how the person feels following sleep. Box 25.4 shows a simple sleep diary that should be used for 2 to 3 weeks alongside history taking to build up a picture of the person's sleep. Completed sleep diaries can be used to calculate estimates of total sleep times, nighttime awakenings and sleep efficiency (Reite at al., 2002). More complicated tools to measure and assess sleep are available. In the past visual analogue scales were used—for example, a 10-cm horizontal line with the anchors 'best sleep ever' and 'no sleep at all' at each end. The sleep was scored by indicating the point on the horizontal line that represented quality.

Patient Objectives Regarding Sleep

After you have made an assessment of sleep, discuss it with your patient to recommend and agree on objectives for sleep. For example,

1. The older person will sleep at their normal time and for their normal duration.
2. The older person will have undisturbed sleep at night.
3. The older person will have rest time during the day.
4. The older person will feel and appear rested.
5. The older person will understand the use of sedatives and analgesics. (Sedatives will be avoided wherever possible unless required to alleviate distress.)
6. The older person will be able to plan a return to a healthy sleep–wake activity pattern.

Nursing Intervention to Promote Sleep

With these objectives in mind, a range of nursing interventions can improve the quality of sleep in hospital and long-term care environments for older adults, including

- Managing the environment in terms of reducing noise from staff, door hinges, waste bins and other equipment and examining the heat, light and ventilation aspects of the area as well as the position of the person's bed
- Examining and planning 24-hour sleep–activity patterns suitable for the individual
- Assisting patients in their pre-sleep routines as near as possible to their normal pattern
- Providing food and drinks at times normal for that patient
- Planning all nursing, medical and other interventions to give patients undisturbed periods of time (e.g., at least 90 min for one complete sleep cycle)
- Providing relief of physical symptoms that interrupt sleep (e.g., pain, urinary frequency, dyspnoea and cough)
- Discussion and relief of psychological distress, including referrals to other health care professionals

BOX 25.3   48-Point Detailed Sleep History Questionnaire

Name _____   Date _____

1. How many nights per week do you usually have difficulty falling asleep?
   _____

2. On nights when you *do* have difficulty falling asleep, how many *minutes* does it usually take you to fall asleep after going to bed?
   _____

3. On nights when you *do not* have difficulty getting to sleep, how many *minutes* does it usually take you to fall asleep after going to bed?
   _____

4. Do you ever wake up in the middle of the night and have difficulty falling back to sleep?   yes   no
   1. If yes, about how many nights does this happen each week?
      _____

   2. On average, how many times do you wake up each night?
      _____

   3. How many minutes does it usually take you to get back to sleep each time you awaken?
      _____

5. How often do you wake up early in the morning, before your scheduled wake time, and are unable to return to sleep?
   _____

6. On nights when you have insomnia, approximately how long do you sleep each night
   _____

7. How long have you had a sleep problem?_____

8. How long would you like to be able to sleep each night? _____

9. Is your sleep problem sometimes worse than other times?   yes   no
   If yes, explain: _____
   _____
   _____

10. Why do you think you have a sleep problem?
    _____
    _____

11. Was the onset of your problem related to any specific event?   yes   no
    If yes, describe: _____
    _____

12. Do you sleep better when you are away from home?   yes   no

13. What do you do when you can't sleep?
    _____
    _____

14. When you try to sleep, is it hard for you to turn off your mind?   yes   no

15. Have you been under stress more than usual recently?   yes   no
    If yes, please explain:_____
    _____

BOX 25.3   48-Point Detailed Sleep History Questionnaire—cont'd

Name _____ Date _____

16. Are you the kind of person who tends to worry a lot?   yes   no

17. How often is your sleep disturbed by environmental factors such as traffic, neighbours or family members?

_____

18. Is your bedroom adequately dark at night?   yes   no

19. On weekends or your days off, do you sleep more than an hour later than your usual wake-up   yes   no
    time?

20. How many times per week do you take naps?

_____

21. Are you on a weight-loss programme?   yes   no

22. Do you engage in some kind of physical exercise?   yes   no
    If yes, describe the time, frequency and time of day:

_____

23. How many cups or glasses of caffeinated beverages (e.g., coffee, tea or cola) do you drink in a day?
    coffee   tea   cola

24. How many days a week do you drink caffeinated beverages after 4:00 p.m.?

_____

25. Do you take any medications that contain caffeine or stimulants (e.g., allergy medication or   yes   no
    painkillers)?
    1. If yes, what medication and dose?

    _____

    2. How often do you usually take it?

    _____

    3. How soon before bed do you take it?

    _____

26. How often do you use alcohol to aid sleep?

_____

27. How many cigarettes a day do you smoke?

_____

28. Does difficulty sleeping ever affect your mood during the day?   yes   no

29. Would you describe yourself as an especially nervous person?   yes   no

30. Estimate how many nightmares you have had in the past year:

_____

31. How often and what amounts of alcohol do you drink?

_____

32. Have you ever been treated or hospitalised for mental, emotional, drug or alcohol problems?   yes   no

33. Does difficulty sleeping affect your functioning during the day?   yes   no
    If yes, describe how it affects your functioning:

    _____

    _____

    _____

Continued

BOX 25.3   48-Point Detailed Sleep History Questionnaire—cont'd

Name _____   Date _____

34. Do you snore?	yes	no
35. Do you ever wake up in the night and feel unable to breathe?	yes	no
36. Do your legs ever jerk repeatedly or feel restless after you go to bed at night?	yes	no
37. Do you ever work the night shift (11:00 p.m. to 7:00 a.m.)?	yes	no
38. Do you work a rotating or split shift?	yes	no

    If yes, please describe:

_____

39. Have you recently taken any prescription or over-the-counter medication for sleeping problems?   yes   no
    (a) If yes, what medication and amount are you taking?

    (b) How many nights a week do you usually take this medication?

    (c) How long have you been taking sleeping medication?

40. Are you currently taking any other medication?   yes   no
    (a) If yes, what medication is it?

    (b) What illness was it prescribed for?

41. Do you have any other physical problems or illnesses?   yes   no
    If yes, please describe:_____

42. Have you ever been hospitalised during the past 10 years?   yes   no
    If yes, please describe:

43. Have you ever had any convulsions or significant head injury?   yes   no
    If yes, please describe:

44. How many times per night do you wake up to use the bathroom?

45. How many nights per week do you have indigestion or heartburn?

46. Have you previously received treatment for sleeping problems?   yes   no
    If yes, please describe

47. Have you tried any self-help remedies for your sleeping problems?   yes   no
    If yes, please describe:

48. Would you be willing to devote 30 minutes per day to a programme of treatment to improve   yes   no
    your sleep?

Source: Lacks (1987).

BOX 25.4 An Example of a Completed Sleep Diary/Log

Sleep Log for ....
- Mark the time you got into bed with a downwards arrow (↓)
- Mark the time you got out of bed with an upwards arrow (↑)
- Shade the areas of sleep (■)

Day	Date	1pm	2pm	3pm	4pm	5pm	6pm	7pm	8pm	9pm	10pm	11pm	Midnight	1am	2am	3am	4am	5am	6am	7am	8am	9am	10am	11am	Noon	Notes
Monday												↓			■	■	■	■	■	↑						
Tuesday												↓			■	■	■	■	■	↑						
Wednesday													↓		■	■	■	■	■	↑						
Thursday													↓		■	■	■	■	■	↑						
Friday												↓			■	■	■	■	■	↑						
Saturday														↓	■	■	■	■	■	■	■	■	■	↑		
Sunday			■	↑										↓	■	■	■	■	■	■	■	■	■	■	■	

Source: Reite et al. (2002).

- With medical and pharmacy colleagues, reviewing medication regimes in terms of dosages, timings, effects of sedatives and stimulants and polypharmacy side effects
- Supporting teaching around good sleep habits
- Treating any underlying medical/surgical conditions

Many authors suggest nursing interventions such as back rubs, ear plugs and headphones, warmed blankets, relaxation tapes, aromatherapy and simple acts like straightening bed linen have a positive effect on patients (Ersser et al., 1999; LaReau et al., 2008; Robinson et al., 2005). The areas of intervention over which nurses have most control are the sleeping environment and nursing interruptions of sleep (Morgan & Closs, 1999) (see Case Study 25.1). However, the total management of factors likely to disrupt sleep patterns requires discussion, decisions and action to be undertaken jointly by nurses and medical, paramedical and administrative staff with help from maintenance engineers and porters. Patel et al. (2008) suggested all health care workers should be aware of sleep and the effects of sleep deprivation. They recommended this fundamental knowledge and skill be taught on every health care course to raise awareness.

Reassessment or Continuing Assessment of Sleep

Interventions, education and support are likely to bring about changes in the way an older person sleeps, but these changes may take time. Nurses may need to revisit and reassess the various factors originally assessed. The primary question asked in reassessment is: 'Have the patient's goals been achieved? If not, why not? Have we or the patient failed to carry out the planned intervention?'

Nurses may also ask if the goals were unrealistic. For example, you may have to accept disturbed nights are inevitable if the patient has an irreversible central nervous system pathology. What else can you do for that person to alleviate the disturbances? A key element is the sleeper's own report of whether they feel refreshed and satisfied with whatever pattern of sleep they have and whether it is considered normal for them (Chaput & Shiau, 2019).

SLEEP THERAPIES

Once the nursing interventions have been tried for optimising the sleep environment, increasing an older adult's understanding of their own sleep, managing expectations of sleep and providing sleep hygiene advice, there may still be difficulties that require further intervention in the form pharmacological and non-pharmacological therapies.

Pharmacological Therapies

Hypnotic drugs such as benzodiazepines and the newer Z-drugs are not recommended to treat chronic insomnia in older people. The British National Formulary (National Institute for Health and Care Excellence, 2021) stipulates using these medications in older adults can cause confusion and poor coordination, leading to falls and injury. In spite of this, a study by Luta et al. (2020) examined prescribed benzodiazepine practices for older adults in Switzerland and found 15%–19% of adults between 65 and 69, 18.4% between 70 and 74, 22.5% between 75 and 80, years and 25.8% over 80 were prescribed these medications.

CASE STUDY 25.1

Esme MacDonald, 89, was admitted to hospital following a fall that resulted in three fractured ribs and a pneumothorax. She is being treated with a chest drain to re-inflate the lung, analgesics and antibiotics. She was widowed 18 months ago and now lives alone. She has two children but they live away in a different city. Esme is usually mobile with a walking stick but is finding it difficult to mobilise while in hospital due to the chest drain.

Nursing assessment: On admission, the nurses assessed Esme's physical, psychological and social conditions and found pain was Esme's foremost symptom. The chest drain was affecting her mobility and the potential for other complications associated with immobility. They noted her comments about 'not sleeping very well' since her husband died and that she often fell asleep in an armchair. She wonders whether she needs a sleeping tablet to help her sleep when she goes home.

Nursing plan: Talk to Esme about her usual nightly routines and try to accommodate those elements for her within the ward area. Explain a number of strategies can be tried to help her sleep such as examining her food and drink intake for elements such as caffeine and her existing medication regime for side effects and interactions. Explain how the nursing staff can help Esme with her sleep—for example, by assisting Esme get into a comfortable position in bed while reassuring her they will attend to her in the night if required. Explain the nursing staff will address her pain using the medications prescribed for her, emphasising sleep is an important element of her recovery, so the pre-bedtime analgesics are important to help her sleep. Reiterate she should inform the staff if she feels the medication regime is not keeping her pain controlled and manageable. Esme should be kept informed of how long the chest drain will stay in situ, when it is likely to be removed and the discharge planning arrangements taking place. When moving around or settling into her bed or chair, the nursing staff should be in attendance to reduce pulling on the chest drain and ensure a safe position for it. A referral to a physiotherapist may be required to encourage deep breathing and mobility.

Key Points

- Sleep is a necessary restorative activity for humans. Although there are changes in sleep patterns and activities as people age, nurses can't make assumptions that all older adults are affected negatively.
- Nurses need to be aware of the various stages to sleep and their importance and benefit.

- Many physical and psychological conditions affect on sleep in older adults, as well as the medications prescribed to treat those conditions.
- Assessment of usual sleep patterns for all patients is useful to assist in promoting good sleep behaviours.
- A number of sleep therapies are available, both pharmacological and lifestyle changes.

Patel et al. (2018) suggested careful evaluation is required for any hypnotic or sedative therapy for older adults and suggested short-term use only. They also advised if such therapy is deemed necessary for an older person, the drugs with the shortest half-lives should be used to reduce any unwanted side effects such as a reduction daytime concentration during tasks.

The use of herbal remedies is increasing in popularity globally, although it is not clear whether older people comprise a significant proportion of current users. Although few of the herbal treatments have extensive research evidence to support their efficacy and safety, Reite et al. (2002) stated valerian, kava and passionflower compounds are easily purchased over the counter as potential remedies for insomnia. The US Food and Drug Administration (2015) advised certain food supplements such as valerian and kava have unwanted effects, and their use should be discussed with a physician. Given older people often take multiple medications, both prescribed and over the counter, the risk of interactions and other adverse effects means more evidence concerning safety is needed before herbal remedies can be recommended for insomnia.

Non-Pharmacological Therapies

Joshi (2008) listed a range of potential cognitive behaviour therapies for insomnia, including relaxation, restricting sleep, stimulus control, light therapy, education around sleep and sleep hygiene, and cognitive approaches. All are well established as safe and effective therapies. The Royal Society for Public Health (2016) advocated their use, citing benefits over sleeping medication and very few if any unwanted side effects.

Psychological Interventions

Stimulus control aims to strengthen and maintain the association between the bedroom and sleep onset and break the link between behaviours that do not help sleep. Joshi (2008, p. 110) listed simple instructions for older patients:

- Go to bed only if you feel sleepy.
- Avoid activities in the bedroom that keep you awake other than sex.

- Sleep only in your bedroom.
- Leave the bedroom when awakening.
- Return to the bedroom only when sleepy.
- Arise at the same time each morning, regardless of the amount of sleep obtained that night.
- Avoid daytime napping.

Relaxation-based treatments include progressive muscle relaxation and tensing, guided imagery, meditation, mindfulness and concentration on breathing techniques (Espie, 2021; Patel et al., 2018). Although these treatments may be less complicated options for nurses and care staff, be aware some people with very painful conditions such as osteoarthritis find the tensing and relaxing of muscles very uncomfortable.

McMillan et al. (2013) cited a study that compared three groups of adults allocated to 6 weeks of cognitive-behavioural therapy (CBT), one of the newer Z-drugs or a placebo. They found CBT reduced the total wake time by over 50%. The study described how the positive effects of CBT continued at the 6-month follow-up. It does need to be stated that for CBT to work well, the cognitive functioning of the individual needs to be intact, and therefore CBT may not benefit older people with degenerative brain conditions and cognitive impairment.

Strengthening Circadian Rhythms

Sleep problems thought to be associated with circadian rhythm disruption are treated with various therapies designed to strengthen and bring the circadian rhythms back into synchronisation. Normally, the hormone melatonin is secreted by the pineal gland and acts as a chemical messenger of the primary circadian pacemaker, stimulating sleep. Melatonin supplements have been trialed at various times of the day to attempt to bring the sleep–wake pattern into some sort or normal order with varying results, but Patel et al. (2018) suggested more research is needed on its wider use in insomnia care and treatment.

Bloom et al. (2009) considered the two prominent circadian rhythm sleep disorders in older adults to be advanced sleep phase disorder and irregular sleep-wake disorder. The treatment for both includes bright light therapy at various times of the day that can delay an irregular sleep–wake cycle and concentrating on good sleep hygiene practices. Further research is needed, but whatever the outcome of studies, nurses should not assume sleep rhythm changes in older people are simply an inevitable consequence of the ageing process.

Exercise and Body Warming

Evidence is available about how physical activity impacts sleep. Not only is physical activity tiring for the body but also it reduces stress and anxiety, helping with sleep (Espie, 2021). Zisberg et al. (2010) found maintaining a good daytime routine helped sleep patterns of older adults living in the community. Therefore, regular physical exercise and a daily routine may promote social wellbeing and relaxation and raise the core body temperature, leading to improved initiation and maintenance of sleep. Espie (2021) suggested exercise needs to be timed earlier in the day as it stimulates the body's adrenaline production. Adrenaline close to bedtime makes sleep more problematic. A little caution should be observed, however, since exercise is not appropriate for everyone, but even simple movement and establishment of a routine can be beneficial.

Some researchers have examined nurse-led approaches to promoting sleep and looked at body warming as a method of improving sleep. Robinson et al. (2005) instigated a programme to help hospital patients in the retiring, resting and rising phases of sleep. One of the interventions was a warmed blanket placed close to the patient with regular bedding placed on top. This snuggling-down-to-sleep approach was rated very highly by patients in the study who had a mean age of 70 years. The authors concluded age-related effects on the thermoregulatory processes in the body can result in older adults feeling cold, which can stop them falling to sleep. With a body-warming intervention, the person feels cosy, and sleep comes more easily.

Although these approaches provide a useful alternative to pharmacological interventions, care is needed in matching therapy with individual needs. Health should be carefully assessed, including circulatory problems and skin condition, cognitive ability and painful conditions.

CONCLUSION AND LEARNING POINTS

This chapter discusses the normal stages of sleep, the changes that come with age, how sleep is assessed, sleep problems in older adults, and potential sleep therapies.

KEY LEARNING POINTS

- Sleep is an activity that needs to be considered on an individual basis with an awareness it affects many aspects of a person's life. Many factors disturb sleep in later life—in particular, circadian decay, physical and mental health, and moving into unfamiliar institutions or environments.

- The complex interactions between day- and nighttime behaviours have a profound influence on the structure and efficacy of sleep.
- Nurses who work a variety of shift patterns are aware of how disrupted sleep affects the way they feel and function. Although you may be aware of and use personal strategies to cope with these aspects of your work, be careful in applying that experience to people in your care to help them sleep better (Gilsenan, 2000).

- As part of the wider health care team, nurses need to identify any primary causes of sleep problems since symptomatic interventions have only limited success.
- Careful assessment, realistic expectations and the provision of advice on day- and nighttime activities, general comfort measures, therapeutic interventions and referrals to other specialists where necessary help.

REFERENCES

Amlaner, C. J., & Fuller, P. M. (Eds.). (2009). *Basics of sleep guide* (2nd ed.). Sleep Research Society.

Ancoli-Israel, S. (2006). The impact and prevalence of chronic insomnia and other sleep disturbances associated with chronic illness. *American Journal of Managed Care, 12*(8), 221–229.

Banks, S., & Dinges, D. F. (2007). Behavioral and physiological consequences of sleep restriction. *Journal of Clinical Sleep Medicine, 3*(5), 519–528.

Basner, M., & McGuire, S. (2018). WHO Environmental Noise Guidelines for the European Region: A systematic review on environmental noise and effects on sleep. *International Journal of Environmental Research and Public Health, 15*(3), 519–564.

Benjafield, A. V., Ayas, N. T., Eastwood, P. R., Heinzen, R., Ip, M. S. M., Morelli, M. J., et al. (2019). Estimation of the global prevalence and burden of obstructive sleep apnoea: A literature-based analysis. *Lancet Respiratory Medicine, 7*(8), 687–698.

Bianchi, M. T. (Ed.). (2014). *Sleep deprivation and disease: Effects on the body, brain and behavior.* Springer.

Bloom, H. G., Ahmed, I., Alessi, C. A., Ancoli-Israel, S., Buyesse, D. J., Kryger, M. H., et al. (2009). Evidence based recommendations for the assessment and management of sleep disorders in older persons. *Journal of the American Geriatric Society, 57*(5), 761–789.

Britton, A., Fat, L. N., & Neligan, A. (2020). The association between alcohol consumption and sleep disorders among older people in the general population. *Scientific Reports, 10,* 5275. doi:10.1038/s41598-020-62227-0.

Cappuccio, F. P., Cooper, D., D'Elia, L., Strazzullo, P., & Miller, M. A (2011). Sleep duration predicts cardiovascular outcomes: a systematic review and meta-analysis of prospective studies. *European Heart Journal, 32,* 1484–1492.

Celik, S., Oztekin, D., Akyolcu, N., & Issever, H. (2005). Sleep disturbances: The patient care activities applied at the night shift in intensive care. *Journal of Clinical Nursing, 14,* 102–106.

Chaput, J. P., & Shiau, J. (2019). Routinely assessing patients sleep health is time well spent. *Preventative Medicine Reports, 14,* Article 100851.

Cooke, J. R., & Ancoli-Israel, S. (2011). Normal and abnormal sleep in the elderly. *Handbook of Clinical Neurology, 98,* 653–655.

Dautovich, N. D., McNamanra, J., Williams, J. M., Cross, N. J., & McCrae, C. S. (2010). Tackling sleeplessness: Psychological treatment options of insomnia. *Nature and Science of Sleep, 2,* 23–27.

Ersser, S., Wiles, A., Taylor, H., Wade, S., Walsh, R., & Bentley, T. (1999). The sleep of older people in hospital. *Journal of Clinical Nursing, 8,* 360–368.

Espie, C. A. (2021). How to sleep better. *Mental Health Foundation.* https://www.mentalhealth.org.uk/publications/how-sleep-better.

European Food Safety Authority. (2015). Scientific opinion on the safety of caffeine. *EFSA Journal, 13*(5), 4102.

Freedman, N. S., Gazendam, J., Levan, L., Pack, A. I., & Schwab, R. J. (2001). Abnormal sleep wake cycles and the effect of environmental noise on sleep disruption in the intensive care unit. *American Journal of Respiratory Critical Care Medicine, 163,* 451–457.

Ganz, F. D. (2012). Sleep and immune function. *Critical Care Nurse, 32*(2), 19–25.

Gilsenan, I. (2000). Caring for staff. In C. Bassett, & L. Makin (Eds.), *Caring for the seriously ill patient* (pp. 216–236). Hodder.

Gilsenan, I. (2012). Nursing interventions to alleviate insomnia. *Nursing Older People, 24*(4), 14–18.

Gilsenan, I. (2017). How to promote patients sleep in hospital. *Nursing Standard, 31*(28), 42–44.

Grossman, M. N., Anderson, S. L., Worku, A., Marsack, W., Desai, N., Tuvilleja, A., et al. (2017). Awakenings? Patient and hospital staff perceptions of nighttime disruptions and their effect on sleep. *Journal of Clinical Sleep Medicine, 13*(2), 301–306.

Guo, S., Huang, J., Jiang, H., Han, C., Li, J., Xu, X., et al. (2017). Restless legs syndrome: From pathophysiology to clinical diagnosis and management. *Frontiers in Aging Neuroscience, 9,* 171.

Harrison, Y., & Horne, J. A. (2000). The impact of sleep loss on decision making: A review. *Journal of Experimental Psychology, 6,* 236–249.

Horne, J. (1989). *Why we sleep: The functions of sleep in humans and other mammals.* Oxford University Press.

Humphries, J. D. (2008). Sleep disturbances in hospitalised adults. *Medical Surgical Nursing, 17*(6), 391–395.

Jaussent, I., Dauvilliers, Y., Ancelin, M. L., Dartigues, J. F., Tavernier, B., Touchon, J., et al. (2011). Insomnia symptoms in older adults: Associated factors and gender differences. *American Journal of Geriatric Psychiatry, 19*(1), 88–97.

Johns, M. W. (2000). Sensitivity and specificity of the multiple sleep latency test (MSLT), the maintenance of wakefulness tests and the Epworth sleepiness scale: Failure of the MSLT as a gold standard. *Sleep Research, 9*, 5–11.

Joshi, S. (2008). Nonpharmacologic therapy for insomnia in the elderly. *Clinics in Geriatric Medicine, 24*, 107–119.

Lacks, P. (1987). *Behavioural treatment for persistent insomnia.* Pergamon.

Lane, T., & East, L. A. (2008). Sleep disruption experienced by surgical patients in an acute hospital. *British Journal of Nursing, 17*(12), 766–771.

Lareau, R., Benson, L., & Watcharotone, K. (2008). Examining the feasibility of implementing specific nursing interventions to promote sleep in hospitalised elderly patents. *Geriatric Nursing, 29*(3), 197–206.

Leblanc, M. F., Desjardins, S., & Desgagne, A. (2015). Sleep problems in anxious and depressive older adults. *Psychology Research and Behavior Management, 8*, 161–169.

Lee, S. (2007). Caring for the patient with a nutritional disorder. In M. Walsh & A. Crumbie (Eds.). *Watson's Clinical Nursing and Related Sciences*, 7th Ed. Bailliere Tindall.

Luta, X., Bagnoud, C., Lambiris, M., Decollogny, A., Eggli, Y., Le Pogam, M. A., et al. (2020). Patterns of benzodiazepine prescription among older adults in Switzerland: A cross-sectional analysis of claims data. *BMJ Open, 10*(1), Article e031156. doi:10.1136/bmjopen-2019-031156.

Makley, M. J., English, J. B., Drubach, D. A., Kreuz, A. J., Celnik, P. A., & Tarwater, P. M. (2008). Prevalence of sleep disturbance in closed head injury patients in a rehabilitation ward. *Neurorehabilitation and Neural Repair, 22*(4), 341–347.

McMillan, J. M., Aitkien, E., & Holroyd-Leduc, J. M. (2013). Management of insomnia and long term use of sedative-hypnotic drugs in older people. *Canadian Medical Association Journal, 185*(17), 1499–1505.

Merriam-Webster. (2021). Sleep: Online dictionary. https://www.merriam-webster.com/medical

Missildine, K. (2008). Sleep and the sleep environment of older adults in acute care settings. *Journal of Gerontological Nursing, 34*(6), 15–21.

Morgan, K., & Closs, S. J. (1999). *Sleep management in nursing practice: An evidence based guide.* Churchill Livingstone.

Morgan, K., & Gledhill, K. (1991). *Managing sleep and insomnia in the older person*: Winslow Press.

National Institute for Health and Care Excellence. (2021). British National Formulary. https://bnf.nice.org.uk

Parthasarathy, S. P., & Tobin, M. J. (2009). Sleep in the intensive care unit. In M. R. Pinsky, L. Brochard, J. Mancebo, & G. Hedenstierna (Eds.), *Applied Physiology in Intensive Care Medicine* (pp. 191–200). Springer.

Patel, D., Steinberg, J., & Patel, P. (2018). Insomnia in the elderly: A review. *Journal of Clinical Sleep Medicine, 14*(6), 1017–1024.

Patel, M., Chipman, J., Carlin, B., & Shade, D. (2008). Sleep in the intensive care unit setting. *Critical Care Nursing, 31*(4), 309–318.

Peuhkuri, K., Sihvola, N., & Korpela, R. (2012). Diet promotes sleep duration and quality. *Nutrition Research, 32*, 309–319.

Pilkington, S. (2013). Causes and consequences of sleep deprivation in hospitalised patients. *Nursing Standard, 27*(49), 35–42.

Price, B. (2016). Promoting healthy sleep. *Nursing Standard, 30*(28), 49–58.

Redeker, N. S. (2000). Sleep in acute care setting: An integrative review. *Journal of Nursing Scholarship, 32*(1), 31–38.

Reid, E. (2001). Factors affecting how patients sleep in the hospital environment. *British Journal of Nursing, 10*(14), 912–915.

Reite, M., Ruddy, J., & Nagel, K. (2002). *Evaluation and management of sleep disorders* (3rd ed.). American Psychiatric Publishing.

Robinson, S., Weitzel, T., & Henderson, L. (2005). The Sh-h-h-h Project: Nonpharmacological interventions. *Holistic Nursing Practice, 19*(6), 263–266.

Roffwarg, H. P., Muzio, J. N., & Dement, W. C. (1966). Ontogenetic development of the human sleep-dream *cycle. Science, 152*(3722), 604–619.

Royal Society for Public Health. (2016). *Waking up the benefits of sleep.* Royal Society for Public Health.

Ruxton, C. (2009). Health aspects of caffeine: Benefits and risks. *Nursing Standard, 24*(9), 4150.

Shankar, A., Syamala, S., & Kalidindi, S. (2010). Insufficient rest or sleep and its relation to cardiovascular disease, diabetes and obesity in a national, multi-ethnic sample. *PLoS ONE, 5*(11), e14189. doi:10.1371/journal.pone.0014189.

Silva, Da, A., A., De Mello, R. G. B., Schaan, C. W., Fuchs, F. D., Redline, S., & Fuchs, S. C (2016). Sleep duration and mortality in the elderly: A systematic review with meta-analysis. *British Medical Journal Open, 6*, Article e008119. doi:10.1136/bmjopen-2015-008119.

Sleep Foundation. (2020). Stages of sleep. https://www.sleepfoundation.org/how-sleep-works/stage-of-sleep

Steiger, A., & Pawlowski, M. (2019). Depression and sleep. *International Journal of Molecular Science, 20*(3), 607–620.

St-Onge, M. P., Mikic, A., & Peitrolungo, E. C. (2016). Effects of diet on sleep quality. *Advanced Nutrition, 7*, 938–949.

Tembo, A. C., & Parker, V. (2009). Factors that impact on sleep in intensive care patients. *Intensive and Critical Care Nursing, 25*, 314–322.

Tranmer, J. E., Minard, J., Fox, L. E., & Rebelo, L. (2003). The sleep experience of medical and surgical patients. *Clinical Nursing Research, 12*(2), 159–173.

U.S. Food and Drug Administration. (2015). FDA 101: Dietary supplements. https://www.fda.gov/consumers/consumer-updates/fda-101-dietary-supplements

Zilli, I., Ficca, G., & Salzarulo, P. (2009). Factors involved in sleep satisfaction in the elderly. *Sleep Medicine, 10*, 233–239.

Zisberg, A., Gur-Yaish, N., & Shochat, T. (2010). Contribution of routine to sleep quality in community elderly. *Sleep, 33*(4), 509–514.

26

Sexuality and Relationships in Later Life

Tommy Dickinson, Roy Litvin, Maria Horne, Christine Brown Wilson,
Paul Simpson, Sharron Hinchliff

CHAPTER OUTLINE

Sexuality and relationships are as important in later years as they are throughout life, and their expression can be positive, joyful, empowering and life-affirming. However, there is a belief that prevails across English-speaking Western societies, in popular culture, in everyday assumptions and throughout health care settings that people become 'post-sexual' or even asexual as they reach advanced ages. This chapter focuses on important aspects of sexuality within the broader context of relationships in later life. We refer to sexuality in its broader sense—encompassing sexual need and expression, identity, intimacy, eroticism, pleasure and reproduction. As such, it is influenced by the interaction of biological, psychological, social, economic, political, cultural, legal, historical, religious and spiritual factors.

Despite sexuality and relationships remaining a central tenet of older people's activities of daily living (Roper et al., 1980), they are often disregarded. The subject of sexuality and older people has until recently largely been ignored by nurses. This chapter discusses the importance of acknowledging that intimacy and sexuality change with ageing, and to deny they exist is detrimental to the holistic care nurses should aim to provide. It focuses on how nurses can enhance their practice in supporting their patients' sexual and intimate expression and offers practical suggestions for broaching sexuality and delivering relationship-centred care for older people and couples.

SEXUALITY AND OLDER PEOPLE IN ECONOMICALLY DEVELOPED SOCIETIES

In light of our definition, this section reflects our expertise concerning later-life sexuality as understood across more economically developed parts of the globe over the past 25 years. Australasia, Britain, North America and parts of Europe have produced the most scholarly output to address ageing sexuality (Simpson, 2015a). Having reviewed the Anglophone literature on the subject, contemporary understandings of later life are premised on a central contradiction. Despite increasing validation of diverse forms of sexual identification and sexual self-expression since about the 1990s, the sexuality of older people remains marked more by constraint than enablement. Even though dating websites have appeared that cater to 'silver singles,' older people generally are encouraged toward a state of 'compulsory non-sexuality' (Simpson, 2021).

But why should constraint be the dominant motif of later-life sexuality? We argue the limitations imposed on older people's intimate and sexual self-expression have much to do with 'ageist erotophobia' (Simpson et al., 2018, p. 1479). This concept refers to fear of older people as sexual and is manifest in failure to imagine them as sexual beings as well as visceral disgust at the thought of older bodies engaged in sexual activity. It has serious ramifications in that it can motivate attempts to deny older people sexual experience. This desexualisation and pathologisation are deeply entrenched and as such indicate the operation of popular thinking that homogenises older people as sexless. Some older people come subconsciously to believe later life is by nature post-sexual (Simpson et al., 2018).

Desexualisation and Difference

For reasons of space, we discuss some key examples of desexualisation rather than offer a comprehensive exegesis of it. Desexualisation and the ageist erotophobia that informs it operate in diverse ways. In effect, later life is age-differentiated. You need only compare the 50-something silver singles who appear on dating websites with the oldest individuals who are regarded as non-sexual. This may simply be by virtue of their stage in the life course and the narrow framing of sexual pleasure around youth-coded, vigorous, penetrative sex (Simpson et al., 2016). Exclusion from sexual status becomes more complex when you consider how the presence of dementia can be automatically framed as risk-laden and thus requiring proscriptive approaches to safeguarding. Gilleard and Higgs (2011) drew attention to the contrast between the less competent, less continent bodies associated with the oldest citizens and the vitality of younger adults. Moore and Reynolds (2016) described a negative aesthetic that ascribes older people as ugly, undesirable and devoid of desire. Such ageism has been attributed to neoliberal, individualist discourses characteristic of consumerist societies that privilege physical vitality and conflate youth with beauty and later life with its opposite (Macia et al., 2015).

Arguably, one of the most discernible forms of difference in later-life sexual and intimate self-expression is that between older men and older women. This could be attributed to the power asymmetry that results from gender ideology that places fewer constraints on older men's ability to claim status as (still) viable sexual beings. Nevertheless, loss of sexual capacity in later life is considered more challenging for men given the fear of loss of masculine status and that men are widely viewed as more reluctant than women to talk through sexual and/or relationship problems. Although older heterosexual women face particular expressions of prejudice and discrimination (see below), it does not follow that older heterosexual men, under the pervasive power of masculinity, escape such problems. Although they are problems of a different kind, they are of equal consequence. Older heterosexual men can find their sexuality limited or even excluded by youth-coded discourses that exert pressure to maintain penetrative sex, especially given the availability of pharma-technologies like Viagra (Lee & Tetley, 2021).

In contrast, older women not only tend to favour the intimacy involved in emotional closeness, sharing, caressing and cuddling (O'Brien et al., 2012), they also face a different set of problems. Older women have reported experiencing desexualisation more intensely because of the harsh, exacting aesthetic standards of consumer societies that equate youth with female beauty (Doll, 2012). Some women might invoke the double-standard that over the life course has encouraged male experimentation while policing women's sexual self-expression and in ways that demand age-appropriate behaviour in later life (Kaklamanidou, 2012). If an older man expressing desire can be stereotyped as a 'chip off the old block' or sometimes a 'dirty old man', sexually assertive older women fear being seen to breach a legitimate ageing femininity that demands decorum and passivity (Kaklamanidou, 2012). Baby boomer women, now middle-aged and older, encounter sex-positive feminist thought, which has helped some articulate a continuing right to sexual enjoyment (Hinchliff & Gott, 2008).

Desexualisation is also seen to work differently in relation to older Black American women. For reasons of space, we focus on older Black women who find their sexuality defined as problematic and more constrained than that of older men. Harley (2021) illuminated how a stereotype of older Black women, informed by a history of colonialism/slavery and racism, serves to limit and regulate their sexuality. Such stereotypes are apparent in the sexless, motherly maid 'Mammie' (beloved of old Hollywood films) and, more recently, in the cautionary figure of the younger 'welfare queen': a woman with a lax lifestyle supported by the state who has children by different fathers. This discourse can be applied to working-class White women but minus the racism. Contemporary British equivalents might be visible in the welfare 'scrounger' like 'Black Dee' in the Channel 4 television programme *Benefits Street*. It is then unsurprising that, historically, many older Black women have felt encouraged to discount themselves as sexual beings and, as Harley concluded, avoided seeking help to achieve or extend pleasurable sexual and intimate lives.

Furthering the theme of the intersectional influences involved in the desexualisation process, Pryzbylo (2021) focused on how ageing femininity is shaped by combined influences of ageism, sexism, heterosexism, racism and ableism. These factors are viewed as central to regulatory narratives of 'successful ageing' that are modelled on and privilege older, able-bodied, White, middle-class heterosexual people. By implication, successful ageing discourse positions older women, and women who make a positive choice in favour of asexuality, as the antithesis of what it means to age 'successfully'.

However, later-life sexuality should not be reduced to a single account of exclusion, which not only obscures diversity of responses but also is grievous to older people who have developed resources of ageing—the knowledge and self-esteem required to challenge and thus avoid compliance with dominant social and cultural expectations (Simpson, 2015b). We should therefore not ignore the agentic capacities of older people to assert themselves as valid sexual beings, though capacities to challenge and defy ageist erotophobia are not equally distributed and are significantly affected by the cross-cutting influences of gender, sexuality, ethnicity and class (Simpson et al., 2017).

LGBTQ+ PEOPLE IN LATER LIFE

The lesbian, gay, bisexual, trans, queer/questioning, with the plus sign signifying a desire to be inclusive (LGBTQ+) community is diverse. See Box 26.1 for a description of common LGBTQ+ identities. Although the L, G, B, T and Q are often grouped together as an acronym that suggests homogeneity, each letter represents a wide range of people of different races, ages, socioeconomic status, ethnicities and identities. Nevertheless, what binds them together as social and gender minorities are their shared experiences of discrimination and stigma, the challenge of living at the intersection of many cultural

---

BOX 26.1 LGBTQ+ Glossary

Asexual/ace: An orientation generally characterised by a lack of stronger sexual attraction for any gender or lower levels of sexual need.

Bisexual/bi: Refers to a person who is sexually and/or romantically attracted to people regardless of the other person's gender identification.

Cisgender/cis: Someone whose gender identity is the same as the sex they were assigned at birth; someone who is not trans. It is good practice to refer to nontrans people as cisgender/cis, rather than with terms like biological man/woman, as it helps to normalise transness and avoid othering trans people.

Closeted/(in the) closet: Keeping secret a part of your identity, usually related to your sexual orientation and/or gender identity.

Coming out: The process of voluntarily sharing your sexual orientation and/or gender identity with others.

Deadnaming: Calling someone by a previous name after they have changed their name. This term is often associated with trans people who have changed their name as part of their transition. Deadnaming can be harmful or can even out trans people to others, so trans people's previous names should not be referred to, even in the past tense, unless they expressly say otherwise.

Gay: Refers to someone who is sexually and/or romantically attracted to the same gender.

Gender expression: How a person expresses their identity through visible features such as clothing, hairstyle and makeup and behaviours.

Gender identity: A person's sense of their own gender, whether male, female or something else (see non-binary), which may or may not correspond to their sex assigned at birth.

Gender-neutral: Refers to something that is not designated as belonging to a particular gender, such as facilities any individual can use regardless of their gender (e.g., gender-neutral bathrooms) or language that does

not carry male/female or masculine/ feminine associations (e.g., they/them pronouns).

Heteronormativity: Attitudes and behaviours that perpetuate the often-harmful assumption that heterosexuality, predicated on the male/female gender binary, is the default or 'normal' mode of sexual orientation.

Homophobia: Systems, beliefs or actions that exclude or oppress lesbian, gay or bi people.

Intersex: Refers to a person with natural variations in sex characteristics that do not fit the typical expectations for male or female bodies.

Lesbian: Refers to a woman who is sexually and/or romantically attracted to other women. Some non-binary people also self-identify as lesbian.

Misgendering: The act of referring to someone as the wrong gender, often by using the wrong pronouns or gendered language that does not match their gender identity.

Non-binary: An umbrella term for people whose gender identity is not, or not fully, described by the binary identities of man and woman. Some people who identify as non-binary use the pronoun they.

Outed/outing: To out someone is to intentionally or unintentionally reveal their LGBTQ+ identity, usually against their will and to someone they had not yet come out to themselves. It's important to treat information about someone's LGBT+ status sensitively, unless you have explicit permission to share that information, in order to avoid outing them. This includes information about their partners, pronouns or deadname.

Pansexual/pan: Refers to a person who experiences sexual and/or romantic attraction to others regardless of gender.

Queer: Traditionally a pejorative term, queer has been reclaimed by some LGBTQ+ people to describe themselves. It is also sometimes used as an umbrella term for the LGBTQ+ community, particularly to denote the rejection of sexual and gender labels. However, some individu-

Continued

BOX 26.1   LGBTQ+ Glossary—cont'd

als still consider the term pejorative, and it should not be used to describe any given person unless they explicitly self-identify that way.

Questioning: The process of exploring your own sexual identification and/or gender identity.

Transgender/trans: An umbrella term to describe people whose gender is not the same as, or not fully defined by, the sex they were assigned at birth. *Trans* is an adjective, so transgender people or trans people are appropriate terminology. Trans itself is a spectrum from self-identification and self-presentation through to full reassignment surgery. Transsexual is an older term that should generally only be used to describe individuals who explicitly self-identify that way.

Transitioning: The changes a trans person makes to their gender expression and to their legal and social life in order to better align with their gender identity. Each person's transition involves different things. For some this involves medical intervention such as hormone therapy and surgeries, but not all trans people want or are able to have this. Transitioning might also involve coming out to friends and family, dressing differently and changing official documents.

Source: Royal Society of Chemistry LGBTQ+ Toolkit (n.d.).

backgrounds and trying to be part of each and, particularly with respect to health care, a long history of discrimination and lack of awareness of health needs by health professionals (see the Fenway Health website). For example, between the 1930s and 1970s, some members of the LGBTQ+ community received aversion therapy: chemical and electrical treatment in psychiatric hospitals in an attempt to 'cure' them of their 'sexual deviations'. Chemical aversion therapy involved using emetics to produce nausea and vomiting in men and woman patients while showing pictures of naked men or women in the hope the two would come to be associated. In electrical aversion therapy, patients were given electrical shocks—sometimes to their genitals—while they viewed pornography or cross-dressed. Men convicted of homosexual offences were given a choice of going to prison or undergoing treatment. Thinking it would be an easier option, many made the calamitous decision to undergo the treatment (Dickinson, 2015; Spandler & Carr, 2022). Sex between men was illegal in England and Wales until the Sexual Offences Act became law in 1967, decriminalising sex between two consenting male adults over the age of 21 in private. Men in Scotland, Northern Ireland, Guernsey, Jersey and the Isle of Man had to wait until 1980, 1982, 1983, 1990 and 1993, respectively.

Older LGBTQ+ people lived through the AIDS crisis of the 1980s and much of the 1990s. The years before effective antiretroviral medication became widely available were filled with profuse suffering, especially within gay communities. Young men in their prime succumbed to this virulent and completely unpredictable pathogen in what has been called as 'the gay holocaust' (Kramer, 1989). The social reaction to AIDS during the first few years of the epidemic was permanently marked by the unique social distribution of the disease. With more than 90% of reported cases coming from intravenous drug users and gay and bisexual men, the community expressed not only its fears about contagion but also its moral judgement. Before the term AIDS was coined in 1982, it was labelled the 'gay cancer' or 'GRID'

(gay-related immune deficiency), and there was a strong sense the condition was associated with sexual identity rather than sexual practice. The power of the medical profession was brought into intimate contact with the gay community, and once again medicine compelled homosexual men to examine their behaviour. The media shaped a lot of public perception regarding the epidemic, and headlines that referred to the 'gay plague' characterised gay men as plague bearers who were highly contagious. There was rhetoric regarding compulsory testing for all gay men and even of quarantine (Dickinson et al., 2022). Nurses need to be mindful of the struggles this minority group may have lived through, ensuring they are non-judgemental and accepting of their patients' sexual orientations and gender identities.

Differences in desexualisation also occur within and between non-normative ageing identity categories—in other words, referring to older lesbian gay, bisexual and trans individuals who also differ along axes of age, class, race and gender identity. The main motif in the literature addressing older gay men draws attention to how experience of desexualisation might be different for them compared to lesbian-identified women and heterosexual men. Mirroring older heterosexual women's experience, older gay men can be subjected to harsh bodily aesthetics that result in judgement of their putative loss of sexual/physical capital (Simpson, 2015b). A perennial feature of this body of literature concerns the idea ageing is accelerated in gay male culture, where a gay man is seen as old and beyond desirability at a relatively young age (40 onward). The concept of accelerated ageing was first articulated in an Australian context (Bennett & Thompson, 1991) and later taken up in North American writing (Hostetler, 2004). Although early exclusion from sexual status is keenly felt by middle-aged and older gay men, the concept has been critiqued for its occlusion of more diverse responses to sexual expression that include celebration and continuity (Simpson, 2015b).

In relation to lesbian-identified women, it has been argued that heteronormative discourse is responsible for an endemic failure to imagine their existence, let alone as sexual beings, given women of a grandmotherly age are presumed to be heterosexual (Treais, 2016). We might also question the idea that ageing is considered much less of a barrier to being valued as a sociosexual being in lesbian cultures that tend to regard attractiveness in a kinder and more holistic way that involves body, personality, mind and so on (Barker, 2004). Lesbian cultures may yield many opportunities for support for older women, but they are not untainted by endemic ageism. Ageism may operate differently and less acutely within lesbian cultures, but recent scholarship has observed younger lesbians are beginning to reject intimacy and friendship with their ageing peers on the aesthetic grounds of age and, mirroring gay male commercialised cultures, whether women have the appropriate toned, youthful look (Slevin & Mowery, 2012).

The themes of invisibility and lack of recognition also apply to older bisexual and trans individuals subject to particular forms of ageist erotophobia. In the case of older bisexual individuals, age-related fear is attributable to a presumed excessive sexuality overlaid with the presumption older people are involved in settled monogamous relationships (Simpson et al., 2018). Along with mononormativity, which reflects the idea a person is either straight or gay, such thinking reinforces the invisibility of older bisexuals, whose identities, when acknowledged, are reduced to stereotypes of promiscuity, unreliability and lack of courage to own their essential gayness while hiding behind heterosexual privilege (Taylor, 2018).

There is very little scholarship on sexuality and older trans individuals, though the transition process appears subject to a range of cultural, psychological, material, legal and health-related constraints and disadvantages, not least of which is access to sexual health support (Donovan, 2002). Older trans individuals especially seem far less legible as sexual subjects than any other. Failure of recognition may have to do with their overassociation with gender rather than sexuality, and when acknowledged, their sexuality can be pathologised as unreal and seen as pathological for being old and trans (Simpson et al., 2016). Arguably their putative abnormality causes trans individuals to be viewed as sexually desperate or indiscriminate or as appealing to a niche market of individuals who fetishise them.

Many older LGBTQ+ people fear the prospect of needing health and social care services (Fenway Health, n.d.). Owing to the heteronormative and gender normative culture of institutionalised regimes in numerous health and residential care settings, many believe their sexual/gender identity and life history will be invisible or that they will experience prejudice from care professionals or their own peers (Knocker, 2012). Nurses should strive to recognise same-sex partners and involve them in the decision-making

process. When caring for older trans people, nurses need to recognise and respond to people's need to express their gender identity, especially during personal care. It is also important to recognise the memories of people living with dementia who are trans and have had gender reassignment surgery, especially in later life, may revert to a point in their past. They may become confused about their appearance and require help knowing how to engage in self-care or express their gender identity, for example by applying cosmetics. Language and the use of correct pronouns are also essential in enabling an older trans person to feel validated. Being misgendered is often distressing and isolating for trans people. After rapport has been established, nurses should ask: 'What is your preferred pronoun?' or 'Which pronouns do you prefer people use for you?' or 'Can you remind me which pronouns you use?' It can feel awkward at first, but asking for a preferred pronoun can avoid hurtful assumptions.

RELATIONSHIPS AND RELATIONSHIP-CENTRED CARE IN LATER LIFE

Relationships are an integral part of our lives as we age and central in the development of intimate relationships. As we journey through key stages in life, our relationships and social networks change. Transitioning through later life, social networks begin to be impacted by age-related losses, such as no longer being able to drive or the death of a spouse along with potentially declining health (Smith, 2012). It is often a combination of these factors that impacts a person's ability to remain engaged in meaningful relationships, leading to loneliness and poorer health outcomes in later life (Courtin & Knapp, 2017). To mitigate such changes, interventions that support older people to maintain meaningful engagement through relationships have been developed that include facilitating social interactions with peers, befriending, animal interventions, leisure/skills development, psychological therapies and service delivery (Gardiner et al., 2018).

As discussed in several chapters, older people are more likely to be in receipt of services as they age due to a range of health and social care needs. Care delivery and how it impacts relationships in later life is a necessary consideration. The Care Act 2014 puts people at the centre of their care, maximising their involvement and integrating social care with health to prevent the need for tertiary care. Adopting a strengths-based approach, the assessment process becomes collaborative, enabling the person to coproduce their care and the services they receive (Social Care Institute for Excellence, 2015). A strengths-based approach focuses on a person's capabilities and considers how they might be maximised. In this sense, the Care

Act 2014 developed the concept of person-centred care in policy from the functional approach of focusing on the needs of the older person to the consideration of the whole person, including their relationships and social networks. Additionally, the NHS Long Term Plan (National Health Service, 2019) champions the importance of what matters to someone as a critical approach to working together to develop and deliver an integrated model of care.

Person-centred care is founded on the value of relationships as staff get to know the person and what is important to them (Brown Wilson & Davies, 2009). Each person has a biography that influences not only how they approach later life but also how they may respond to the care context they find themselves in. This recognition of biography creates a relational dynamic between the person and the people who provide care that personalises the care encounter by finding out what matters (Brown Wilson et al., 2013). Although many health and social care organisations, as part of their remit to deliver person-centred care, often include a section in their assessment such as 'Getting to know you' or, for patients with dementia, 'Who am I?', biographical information is not always considered as part of the care-planning process. Nurses, however, are in a key position to identify what matters to an older person and find ways of delivering care that takes it into account. The move to a strengths-based approach and a focus on co-production provides the impetus for nurses to adopt a biographical approach to care planning. Understanding what is important to an older person and how they wish to be involved in their care enables nurses to engage older people in co-production. Co-production moves beyond partnership working to a recognition the person is an active decision maker in the process of their care (Baim-Lance et al., 2019). This is not without its difficulties, as older people may access services at a time of crisis, where they may have cognitive impairment or speech difficulties that prevent them from being actively involved in their care.

Supporting people with dementia in co-production of their care may pose additional challenges as their ability to communicate verbally decreases as the dementia progresses. Within this context, reminiscence therapy provides a vehicle for people living with dementia to speak about their past, providing insights into what was important to them. Using the senses to prompt memory rather than questions as prompts supports nurses in engaging people living with dementia more effectively in the care-planning process. Furthermore, adopting a strengths-based approach to assessment enables the person with dementia to be seen as having capabilities rather than disability.

Developing relationships between older people and care providers is a key mechanism by which person-centred care

is delivered. However, it may not be enough when considering the intimacy of relationships in an older person's life. Even when older people are engaged in long-term spousal relationships, intimacy or sexual activity is rarely acknowledged. Although it may feel inappropriate to ask highly personal questions in relation to care delivery, and we do not suggest personal relationships should be pathologised, not understanding the nature and importance of intimate relationships may impact the care being delivered and decisions being made. Many care providers feel uncomfortable speaking about intimate or sexual relationships, which then makes it difficult for older people or their partners to initiate such conversations. This is not surprising given our earlier discussion that ageism in society reinforces older people as asexual, also making it difficult for older people to speak about their need for intimate or sexual relationships. Relationship-centred care may be a mechanism to facilitate these conversations.

Relationship-centred care does not seek to replace person-centred care but to extend the philosophy more explicitly to consider relationships between the person and care provider and to understand the context of relationships between the person and the wider community. Adopting a wider community perspective is vital in ensuring older people are supported to age well in place. In the United Kingdom, relationship-centred care has been developed in residential contexts to include everyone in the relationship, such as staff, paid carers and individuals significant to the older person, such as family carers (Nolan et al., 2006). The contributions of older people and family carers are integral to these relationships but not always recognised (Brown Wilson, 2009). The interactions between care providers, family carers and the older person, irrespective of cognitive impairment, influence the type of relationships that develop and so shape the care encounter. For example, sharing personal stories through care routines is a common mechanism that enables personal relationships to develop. For people with dementia, using the senses to introduce ideas similar to reminiscence therapy may prompt discussions and can be used by both carers and family members to strengthen the relationship with the person living with dementia. As staff recognise the contribution older people and families make to the relationship, reciprocal relationships emerge from shared understandings about the community in which the older person is based (Brown Wilson et al., 2013). The ability to see the older person and care delivery in context to the wider community is central to the development of reciprocal relationships in relationship-centred care (Brown Wilson, 2009). Relationship-centred care enables all voices within the relationship to be recognised, with the needs of everyone taken into account.

Case Study 26.1 highlights a common issue experienced by older people and their spouses when being discharged from hospital: the use of hospital equipment and changes to sleeping arrangements.

If you consider Case Study 26.1 in context to person-centred care, knowing what is important and why different routines hold significance was not an area that was considered (i.e., sleeping with a spouse). It was not until the wider context of the marital relationship was considered, including the needs of the wife, that a shared understanding was reached. In adopting a relationship-centred care approach—and considering the needs of everyone in the relationship—care providers were in a better position to enable the conversation about intimate and sexual relationships. Positive and trusting relationships between care providers, older people and their partners are essential for older people to feel comfortable in sharing information about their intimate and sexual relationships.

A number of factors have been associated with relationship-centred care, including leadership. Leadership that encourages staff to work consistently in adopting personal and reciprocal relationships enables staff to move flexibly between person-centred and relationship-centred care (Brown Wilson, 2012). Staff who are able to understand what is significant for the person are more likely to be able to see the wider context and other relationships in the person's life, leading to relationships that enable the older person and the people close to them to feel comfortable in initiating conversations about intimate and sexual relationships. As older people are more likely to require services in later life, we need to consider the value of relationships not only in care delivery but also in how we support older people in maintaining their intimate and sexual relationships. Valuing multiple perspectives is a key feature of co-production, and nurses are in a position to consider all perspectives, ensuring all parties in the relationship feel included and valued.

CASE STUDY 26.1

Bill was discharged from hospital with terminal prostate cancer to spend his final months at home with his wife, Kate, caring for him. The palliative care team arranged for a hospital bed to be installed in the living room as Bill was no longer able to manage the stairs to their bedroom. Kate insisted she did not need a hospital bed and was adamant she could support Bill to bed each evening. The palliative care team felt this was not safe for Bill and considered Bill to be at risk of harm with Kate's actions. Kate was developing a reputation as a pushy wife and someone who did not understand the importance of caring for her husband in this terminal phase. It was not until a nursing student was speaking to Kate during a home visit that Kate confided in the student how important the physical relationship between her and Bill was and that they both wanted to maintain it in whatever form they could until the end of Bill's life. The student adopted a relationship-centred care approach and considered the needs of Kate alongside those of Bill and the palliative care team. For the palliative care team, person-centred care meant for Bill to have his needs met in a safe environment, but no one had asked Bill what he thought of losing the opportunity to sleep in a bed with his wife. For Kate and Bill, maintaining their intimate relationship was of key importance. Once the palliative care team were apprised by the student, other options of ensuring Bill could be supported up the stairs were explored (adapted from Brown Wilson, 2012).

PROMOTING RELATIONSHIPS, INTIMACY AND SEXUALITY FOR OLDER PEOPLE LIVING IN CARE HOMES

Contemporary literature supports the importance of intimacy, the expression of sexuality and relationship needs for people living in residential care environments (Barrett & Hinchliff, 2018). Sexuality, intimacy, and relationship needs remain important for many older people living in care homes; the need for human intimacy for most people lasts until the end of their life (Kuhn, 2002). Promoting positive relationships, intimacy, sexuality and sexual identity (e.g., gay, bisexual, straight) and gender identity (e.g. male, female, transgender) is an important public health issue for older adults in maintaining health and promoting quality of life, well-being and personal identity (World Association for Sexual Health, 2014). Intimate relationships take many different forms, ranging from touching and kissing to masturbation and intercourse, but sex is not important for everyone (Hillman, 2012). Over time, some older adults develop forms of physical intimacy such as touching that might not be what they had previously thought of as sex.

Sexuality is an important issue for many older adults, yet it is a subject health care professionals have an important role in but may do little to meet the needs of older care home residents. Respecting wishes for intimacy, assessing risk and supporting personal freedoms, privacy and choice, especially when there are concerns about mental capacity and sexuality, can be challenging for care professionals (Royal College of Nursing, 2018). It may also challenge their own attitudes, beliefs and values and those of the resident's family and/or friends. However, it is important to keep an open mind and support older care home residents' needs. Having conversations about sexuality, intimacy and relationship needs can be extremely helpful to older people and promotes person-centred care. There is no one-size-fits-all approach to supporting the needs of older care home residents' intimacy, sexuality and relationships needs.

The Care Quality Commission (CQC) guidance document *Relationships and Sexuality in Adult Social Care Services* (CQC, 2020) advises that care professionals should ask care home residents about their sexuality, intimacy and relationship needs. This can be accomplished through needs assessment when care planning. Care professionals can provide opportunities for couples to connect and find private time. The CQC (2020) encourages overnight guests at care homes if possible within the layout of facility, and the guidance covers how care workers can help residents access specialist dating services. However, it is recognised there is sometimes a fine line between person-centered care and managing risk around safeguarding and a need to protect older adults (Age UK, 2021). Risk can be minimised through sensitively approaching sexuality, intimacy and relationship with older adults and ensuring activity is consensual before moving to safeguarding.

Many residents in care homes have cognitive impairment but still express a need to be intimate and/or engage in sexual expression, which may or may not be with their current partner. Although staff and families may accept gestures relating to comfort such as holding hands or cuddling, entering into sexual activity is often frowned on, reflecting society's ageist erotophobia. At this point the dilemma for staff is whose needs are most important: the residents' or the families, which may create tension in the relationships. For example, when confronted with a scenario of residents living with dementia engaging in consensual sexual expression, both families and staff felt it was inappropriate without considering the capacity of the person with dementia to consent. This approach was very much focused on the value of monogamous heterosexual relationships without discussing the developing relationship with the person with dementia (Wiskerke & Manthorpe, 2018). We know people living with dementia are able to consent in the moment; adopting a process-consent approach (Dewing, 2007) enables staff to recognise when the person with dementia is withdrawing their consent and to intervene if sexual activity becomes unwanted. For example, if a person with dementia is seeking out the person and enjoys being in their company, consent may be inferred. Upset, withdrawal or avoidance may be behaviours that signify withdrawal of consent. Sensitivity is required by staff to support

people living with dementia in meeting their intimacy and sexual needs while navigating the emotions and feelings of families who may not understand the change in the older person's behaviour or choices. Having open conversations with families about developing relationships and the positive impact they have on the older person may be a helpful starting point rather than waiting for the relatives to see the intimacy themselves and become upset. There is, however, limited education, training and guidance in care homes for supporting people living with dementia to meet their intimacy and sexual needs (Wiskerke & Manthorpe, 2019), a situation that warrants further attention.

Discussing sexuality, intimacy and relationship needs can be challenging. This is a sensitive discussion area, as it can challenge care staff's attitudes, beliefs, culture and values. Studies highlight that few care professionals are willing or find it difficult to engage in open discussions about intimacy, sexuality and relationship needs with older people, despite growing acknowledgement of and focus on these issues (Simpson et al., 2017; 2018). Nonetheless, having conversations about sexuality, intimacy and relationship needs can be extremely helpful to older people (Ezhova et al., 2020). Care professionals should be aware of and prepared to discuss the intimacy, sexuality and the relationship needs of older adults who reside in care settings in a nonjudgemental way and support them in this area of need. However, although older adults who reside in care settings should expect an open and inclusive approach from care professionals, it must also be acknowledged the rights of individual members of care staff need to be respected, and they should not be required to compromise their religious and/or cultural beliefs. Nevertheless, the religious or cultural beliefs of care staff may compromise the care of older people, a duty under the Nursing and Midwifery Council code of conduct (Nursing and Midwifery Council, 2018), and may be seen as discrimination or denial of the older person's rights. It is important that if older adults wish to discuss such needs, care staff refer them to the care manager, who can undertake or arrange for another member of staff to discuss and assess how best to support their sexuality, intimacy and relationship needs.

From an organisational perspective, registered managers and registered providers should be able to explain how their service supports people to meet their intimacy and sexuality needs, for example by having a relationship and sexuality policy. They include any specific measures put in place to meet people's equality and diversity needs (CQC, 2020). Lack of double rooms, double beds or two-seater sofas in communal areas can prevent intimacy and should be considered when designing care homes. But residents also need privacy to be intimate. Privacy policies need to balance care and protection with resident needs and wishes. Safeguarding policy and practice should be driven by the observable needs and wishes of residents.

Communicating With Older Adults to Assess Needs and Plan Care

When looking at communicating about intimacy, sexuality and relationship needs with older adults who reside in care settings, it is important to build rapport and trust. Explain that sensitive, resident-led discussion about intimacy needs is encouraged when assessing and planning care. The choice of language used to introduce the subject is important. Using the term *intimacy* rather than *sex* as a general way of talking about closeness, which may or may not include sexual experience, is a sensitive way to approach discussions in this area. It is important the care worker lets the resident know they can talk about sexual matters by giving the person permission to raise the topic in any discussion.

SEXUAL HEALTH IN LATER LIFE

Sexual Rights

The sexual rights of older adults are globally acknowledged as the role that sexuality, both as a practice and identity, plays in health and well-being (World Health Organization [WHO], 2006). Sexual rights are rooted in human rights, and as such they are the rights that belong to everyone regardless of age, gender, nationality and race. They are important to healthy sexual ageing: when we live free from discrimination, we tend to live healthier and longer lives (Marmot et al., 2020).

Sexual rights are predominantly associated with young people and discussed with regard to the prevention of sexually transmitted infections (STIs) and unintended pregnancy. It is not widely known that sexual rights apply to older adults. An implication is health care staff may unintentionally breach an older adult's sexual rights by, for example, not advising them of the sexual side effects of a prescribed medication and dismissing the patient's sexual difficulty as age-related and therefore irreparable. Not being proactive when it comes to older adults' sexual health can have a negative impact on well-being and relationships, particularly when sex is important to the person.

It is important that health care practitioners are aware of the sexual rights of older adults and have access to resources that support their work. In recognition of this urgent need, Barrett and Hinchliff (2018) proposed a framework for the sexual rights of older adults to guide health and social care policy, practice, service design and research. Their framework, based on the Declaration of Sexual Rights from the World Association for Sexual Health, aims to ensure that older adults are treated with dignity and respect and are able to influence the direction of their lives through the choices they make. The first sexual right, to equality and non-discrimination, underpins the whole framework (Box 26.2). Nurses are familiar with this as a human right, as it forms a central part of their duty of care (Nursing and Midwifery Council, 2018).

These rights come into sharp focus when we consider that sexual education programs for nurses and allied health professionals infrequently include older age, and older adults are rarely the focus of sexual health campaigns. A sexual rights approach is essential if we are to deliver health care that supports healthy sexual ageing and engenders positive health outcomes. However, as noted, the sexual rights of older adults are not always met, and this is particularly evident in the area of STIs.

SEXUALLY TRANSMITTED INFECTIONS AND HIV

New diagnoses of STIs in people over 50 have increased in many countries over the past 20 years, yet safer sex campaigns and education rarely target older adults. At the time of writing, the highest increases in STIs for older adults living in England were gonorrhoea and syphilis. While the prevalence is lower than that for younger age groups, over a 4-year period the highest increases in gonorrhoea and syphilis were reported in the 65+ age group for men who have sex with men (which includes men who do not identify as gay for cultural, political or personal-experiential reasons), women who have sex with women, and heterosexual women aged 45–54 (see Tables 26.1 and 26.2).

Similar increases were observed in other countries. For example, in China, Tao et al. (2020) reviewed evidence over a 21-year period and found people over 60 had the highest incidence of primary and secondary syphilis. In Australia, the Kirby Institute (James et al., 2020) reported that between 2008 and 2017, gonorrhoea diagnoses increased from 1,202 to 5,451, and syphilis from 506 to 1,483 in the 40+ age group, with the highest number of diagnoses in men. The authors of a US study argued that chlamydia, gonorrhoea and primary and secondary syphilis in the 65+ age group 'more than doubled' from 2007 to 2017 (Smith et al., 2020). And in rural Uganda, self-reported data from women (52%) and men (48%) aged 50+ revealed that 29% had an STI in the past month (Wandera et al., 2020). From a global perspective, a systematic review conducted to estimate the worldwide prevalence of herpes simplex (type 2), which is almost 'entirely sexually transmitted, causing genital herpes', found that 344.5 million people aged 50–99 were infected (James et al., 2020, p. 157). (Note: The sexual orientation and/or gender of participants were not always reported in these studies.)

BOX 26.2   Declaration of the Sexual Rights of Older People

1. **The right to equality and non-discrimination:** Older people have the right to enjoy the sexual rights set out in this declaration without distinction of any kind, particularly related to age.
2. **The right to life, liberty and security:** Older people have the right to life, liberty and security that cannot be arbitrarily threatened, limited or taken away for reasons related to sexuality.
3. **The right to autonomy and bodily integrity:** Older people have the right to control and decide freely on matters related to their sexuality and their body. This includes sexual behaviours, practices, partners and relationships with due regard to the rights of others.
4. **The right to be free from torture and cruel, inhuman or degrading treatment or punishment:** Older people have the right to be free from torture and cruel, inhuman or degrading treatment or punishment related to sexuality.
5. **The right to be free from all forms of violence and coercion:** Older people have the right to be free from sexually related violence and coercion.
6. **The right to privacy:** Older people have the right to privacy related to sexuality, choices regarding their own body and consensual sexual practices without arbitrary interference and intrusion.
7. **The right to the highest attainable standard of health including sexual health:** Older people have the right to the highest attainable level of health and well-being in relation to sexuality, including the possibility of pleasurable, satisfying and safe sexual experiences.
8. **The right to enjoy the benefits of scientific progress and its application:** Older people have the right to enjoy the benefits of scientific progress and its applications in relation to ageing and sexuality.
9. **The right to information:** Older people have the right to access scientifically accurate and understandable information related to sexuality and ageing through diverse sources.**The right to education and to comprehensive sexuality education:** Older people have the right to comprehensive sexuality education that is age appropriate and grounded in a positive approach to sexuality and ageing.
10. **The right to enter, form and dissolve marriage and other similar types of relationships:** Older people have the right to choose whether or not to marry and to enter freely and with full consent into marriage, partnership, or similar relationships.
11. **The right to freedom of thought, opinion and expression:** Older people have the right to freedom of thought, opinion and expression regarding sexuality and the right to express their own sexuality with due respect to the rights of others.
12. **The right to freedom of association and peaceful assembly:** Older people have the right to peacefully organise, associate, assemble, demonstrate and advocate about sexuality and sexual rights.
13. **The right to participation in public and political life:** Older people are entitled to an environment that enables active, free and meaningful participation in, and contribution to, the civil, economic, social and political aspects of life.
14. **The right to access to justice, remedies, and redress:** Older people have the right to access justice, remedies and redress for violations of their sexual rights.

Source: Barrett & Hinchliff (2018).

New diagnoses of HIV are also increasing in the 50+ population: data analysed from 31 countries over a 12-year period showed that they had significantly increased (Tavoschi et al., 2017). Transmission routes were predominantly sex between men, heterosexual sex and injection drug use (Tavoschi et al., 2017). Older adults are more likely to be diagnosed late (Tavoschi et al., 2017), which supports findings from other studies (Schouten et al., 2013; Wilson et al., 2014). Late diagnosis of HIV has serious implications for treatment options and health outcomes and is complicated by pre-existing long-term conditions (Davis et al., 2013).

It is appropriate to ask why new diagnoses of STIs and HIV in people over 50 are increasing. A small but growing body of research sheds light on this although the findings are mixed. A recent study found that adults aged 65–94, recruited from various aged-care facilities in New York, had low levels of STI knowledge (Smith et al., 2020), whereas a national survey of women and men aged 65+ in Australia found that sexually active participants had good general knowledge of STIs but poor knowledge about the protection offered by condoms (Lyons et al., 2017). Knowledge was more accurate in women than men and among people who had sought STI testing (Lyons et al., 2017).

TABLE 26.1 New Gonorrhoea Diagnoses in England

	2014	2018	Increase
Men			
Heterosexual: 45–64	666	1128	69.4%
Heterosexual: 65+	57	104	82.5%
Men who have sex with men (MSM): 45–64	2142	3824	78.5%
MSM: 65+	98	189	92.8%
Women			
Heterosexual: 45–64	244	513	110.2%
Heterosexual: 65+	9	20	122.2%
Women who have sex with women (WSW): 45–64	3	7	133.3%
WSW: 65+	0	0	0

Source: Public Health England (2020).

TABLE 26.2 New Syphilis Diagnoses in England

	2014	2018	Increase
Men			
Heterosexual: 45–64	122	194	59%
Heterosexual: 65+ years	13	21	61.5%
MSM: 45–64	823	1479	79.7%
MSM: 65+	32	80	150%
Women			
Heterosexual: 45–64	31	41	32.3%
Heterosexual: 65+	1	1	0
WSW: 45–64	0	0	0
WSW: 65+	0	0	0

Source: Public Health England (2020).

Evidence suggests that perception of risk of contracting an STI is influenced by psychological factors such as the perceived characteristics of the partner and quality of the relationship which can foster a sense of safety (Lewis et al., 2020). Single middle-aged adults in the United Kingdom viewed themselves as being at low risk from STIs, but their behaviour (e.g., having condomless sex with a new partner) suggested otherwise (Dalrymple et al., 2017; Lewis et al., 2020). Middle-aged heterosexual adults in Scotland did not view themselves as being at risk because they associated risk with casual sex (Dalrymple et al., 2017). Not perceiving themselves to be at risk, plus trusting their partner, reduced the likelihood of condom use in an Australian study of older adults (Fileborn et al., 2018). Interestingly, the perceived STI status of a new partner has been found to be judged on their physical appearance, demeanour and wealth and assumptions about their sexual history, which the authors point out are clearly 'inadequate indicators' (Lewis et al., 2020, p. 160).

Discussion about condom use can be a difficult conversation with a new partner, especially for people recently out of a long-term relationship and those who expect reduced sexual pleasure from condoms (Dalrymple et al., 2017; Fileborn et al., 2018; Lewis et al., 2020). Stigma is a barrier to condom use in older adults who remember the historical negative framing of condoms—for example, the moralisation of sexual activity and the association of condoms with sexual promiscuity in women (Brown et al., 2017).

Talking About Sex in Health Care

The taboo around the sexual health and sexual well-being of older adults has implications for professional practice. There is evidence that health practitioners tend not to ask older people about sexual issues, even if an older adult has had treatment or surgery that can impair their sexual pleasure (Schaller et al., 2020). Sex is a deeply personal topic for many people, which maintains the taboo. Barriers to talking about sex reported by practitioners include lack of

---

BOX 26.3   Three Ps Approach

Privacy

Ensure the conversation takes place in a private setting to avoid being overheard or interrupted. Let the older person know discussions are confidential, and confidentiality will be breached only under certain circumstances in line with the policy of the service you work within.

Permission

Let the older person know it is okay to talk about sexual matters. To start the conversation, practitioners can request permission to ask about the older person's sex life by using generic questions (see Box 26.4). It is important the older person knows the practitioner is comfortable with the subject. Signs of discomfort, such as fidgeting

with a pen or avoiding eye contact, can close down conversations on sensitive topics.

Practice

Helping the older person feel comfortable makes the conversation easier and encourages them to open up. There are various ways to approach this:

- Consider your non-verbal behaviour: Eye contact and active listening are important skills.
- Make the consultation less formal (e.g. do not sit directly behind a desk).
- Use diagrams, magazine articles and leaflets to help communicate about sexual matters.

Source: Hinchliff & Fileborn (2020).

---

knowledge and training, fear of causing offence and assuming older adults are not sexually active (Ezhova et al., 2020; Hinchliff & Gott, 2011).

But research has shown that older adults want their practitioner to ask about sexual health (Sinković and Towler, 2019). Older adults tend to delay seeking help for sexual issues due to embarrassment, waiting to see if the problem gets better on its own, and uncertainty about whether the topic is appropriate for the practitioner (Ezhova et al., 2020; Hinchliff and Gott, 2011). It is important practitioners take a proactive approach, but starting the conversation can be difficult. Included below is guidance that uses the Three Ps (privacy, permission and practice) approach to support sexual communication in health care settings. The Three Ps approach (Box 26.3) provides practical, easy-to-remember advice on talking to older adults about sex, including ways to start the conversation and facilitate comfort for both the older adult and practitioner.

EFFECTS OF ILL HEALTH AND DISABILITY ON SEXUALITY FOR THE OLDER PERSON

Due to changing attitudes regarding sexual activity in older people, many men and women remain sexually active well into later life. In fact, being in good health appears to predict a better quality and interest in sex among older people. Conversely, physical and mental health conditions are associated with sexual inactivity in older men and women. Older people who are diagnosed with a medical condition are more likely to be sexually inactive or to report sexual problems (Traeen et al., 2017). Within this context, some older people appear to accept sexual inactivity as part of the ageing process. These views may shield them from the psychosocial effects of sexual difficulties. Others may view sexual issues as

separate from health, which may prevent them from seeking advice from health care providers. However, for some older people, sexual function is a determinant of a good quality of life, demonstrating the diversity and meaning placed on sexuality in later life (Sinković & Towler, 2019).

Older people encounter age-related physiological changes that can impact on sexual health and function. For example, due to a decline in oestrogen, post-menopausal women develop urogenital atrophy, which is associated

---

BOX 26.4   Examples of Generic Questions

- As part of your care assessment, I can take a sexuality, intimacy and relationship needs history. The questions may be sensitive, but they are important and can help me to provide the best care for you.
- Some residents lose interest in sex. Is this something that has affected you?
- Sexuality is an important part of life for many people. If it's okay, I'd like to ask you some questions about sex as part of your health assessment.
- People who I see in clinic sometimes have sexual problems. Have you noticed anything?
- At this point I normally ask some questions about your sexual health. The questions may be sensitive, but they are important and can help me to provide the best care for you.
- These medications can cause sexual difficulties. Is that something you have experienced?

Source: Courtesy of Sharron Hinchliff.

with dyspareunia (i.e., painful intercourse), vulval pain, itching, burning, dryness, a decline in lubrication and vaginal blood flow. Changes in vaginal pH may increase the risk of vaginal and urinary tract infections, and skin healing may be impaired in atrophied genital tissue (Garrett & Lawton, 2019; Naumova & Castelo-Branco, 2018). Various treatments such as vaginal lubricants and moisturisers, hormone replacement therapy, selective oestrogen receptor modulators and vaginal dehydroepiandrosterone may help with some of these symptoms (Naumova & Castelo-Branco, 2018). In older men, erectile dysfunction (ED) appears to be the most prevalent complaint, which may worsen with age. Hormonal changes such as decreased testosterone associated with andropause (i.e., male menopause) may cause a decline in libido, soft erections and low ejaculatory volume (Morley & Tolson, 2012). A common treatment for ED is phosphodiesterase-5 inhibitors such as sildenafil (commonly known as Viagra), vardenafil and tadalafil. They work by increasing blood flow to the penis. They should be avoided by people on nitrates and alpha-adrenergic blockers, as the combination can cause a dangerous fall in blood pressure. Testosterone therapies may also help with ED and loss of libido. Many physiological changes result from the normal ageing process, but some are caused or exacerbated by ill health.

In Britain, one in six older women and one in four older men consider themselves to have a health condition that affects their sexual activity or enjoyment (Erens et al., 2019). When considering sexual problems in the context of ill health, it is important to bear in mind vasocongestion and myotonia, which are basic physiological processes associated with human sexual physiology. Theoretically, any illness that affects the arteries, central or peripheral nerves, hormones or musculoskeletal function may impact sexual functioning (Bancroft, 2009; Verschuren et al., 2010). As older people are more likely to be diagnosed with a health condition such as cardiovascular disease, a neurological condition, diabetes, arthritis or cancer, they may be vulnerable to the direct, indirect or iatrogenic effects of the illness on their sexual functioning and well-being. We cannot provide a detailed overview of all diseases and their impact on older people's sexuality, but some of the more common ones are briefly considered.

Vascular disease is very common in men with ED, and ED may be an early manifestation of arterial disease. Cardiovascular disease and hypertension are major risk factors for ED. Men who are prescribed diuretics and statins are more likely to report ED (Steptoe et al., 2016). In women, cardiovascular disease is associated with vaginal dryness, dyspareunia, decreased libido, orgasmic difficulties and decrease genital sensation (Morley & Tolson, 2012).

People with cerebrovascular hemisphere strokes may have a decrease in libido. Depression and left hemisphere lesions appear to play a role in post-stroke sexual dysfunction in both men and women (Kimura et al., 2001). Indirectly, a stroke may also impact sexual functioning, for example, with the loss of muscle power, pain, muscle spasms, mobility issues or urinary incontinence. In fact, sexual activity requires some degree of mobility and agility. Pain or mobility issues from any condition may cause sexual problems. For example, hip arthritis or other musculoskeletal deterioration may cause pain and stiffness that interferes with sexual intercourse (Morley & Tolson, 2012).

In diabetes, damage to autonomic and peripheral nerves and degenerative changes to small blood vessels may interfere with sexual function. More than half of men diagnosed with diabetes experience ED (Kouidrat et al., 2017), and diabetic older women are likely to report lower sexual satisfaction, difficulty with lubrication and orgasm (Copeland et al., 2012; Verschuren et al., 2010).

In neurological conditions such as Parkinson's disease, both sexual performance and desire are reduced. Muscle rigidity and slowness of movement may impact the ability to perform sex. L-dopa and dopamine agonists are usually prescribed for Parkinson's disease, and they may increase sexual desire and, in some cases, cause hypersexuality (Verschuren et al., 2010). Epilepsy arising in the temporal lobes may affect sexuality, and the side effects of anti-epileptic medication can further compound the issue. Peripheral neuropathy and spinal cord injuries may also impact on sexual, genital, and sexual response. What appears to be common in most neurological disorders is comorbid depression, which contributes significantly to sexual dysfunction.

Depression in older people can be linked to having a health condition as well as to other psychosocial factors such as loss, loneliness or social isolation. A marked loss of libido is one of the somatic symptoms of depression (WHO, 2004). Although treatment with antidepressants may alleviate some of the symptoms of depression, antidepressants may exacerbate sexual dysfunction. This remains one of the most frequent side effects of these medications, particularly selective serotonin reuptake inhibitors (Clayton & Montejo, 2006), which are frequently prescribed to older people with depression. It is also important to note many drugs, both social or medically prescribed, impact sexual function. Alcohol, narcotics and various anxiolytic drugs have a depressant effect on the central nervous system.

There is always an interplay between the physical and psychosocial aspects of sexual problems, which may be exacerbated by illness. For example, older women with breast cancer may have significant concerns about their body image that may affect them long after treatment (Davis et al., 2020). In men, prostate cancer may not only cause a disruption to sexual function but also have a negative impact on dyadic sexual communication, self-esteem, self-confidence and sexual intimacy (Ussher et al., 2016). Severe incontinence caused by a health condition may mean couples have to sleep in separate beds. Faecal incontinence exerts a particularly adverse effect on sexual intimacy (Morley & Tolson, 2012; Royal College of Nursing, 2018). Following a major life-threatening event like a heart attack or stroke, some older people become fearful of sexual activity. For some single older people, restricted mobility or lack of confidence associated with a health problem may deter them from getting out and meeting other people (Erens et al., 2019). For others, a health condition impacts the quality of a relationship where new roles and dependencies are created that may affect intimacy and sexual activity between partners. This may be particularly visible when a person has dementia, and their partner feels they are not able to pay full attention to their feelings and needs. A person living with dementia may lack the capacity to consent to sexual or intimate activities with their partner, which poses legal, ethical and social considerations with regards to intimacy.

When considering sexuality in older people, it is important to take a holistic view and consider the various physiological changes that come with ageing or are exacerbated by disease directly, indirectly or iatrogenically by the effects of treatments and medications. It is also important to consider the impact of psychosocial ill health on the person's self-image, intimacy within the relationship or difficulty in finding a suitable partner.

ROLES FOR HEALTH CARE WORKERS

Education

In this chapter we discuss the importance of the sexual rights of older people being respected, protected and fulfilled (WHO, 2006) and that sexual health is closely associated with emotional, mental, physical and social well-being in relation to sexuality. In the United Kingdom, the Nursing and Midwifery Council (2018) requires nurses to promote well-being and meet the health and care needs of their patients, including challenging discriminatory attitudes. Addressing sexuality in this context falls within the remit of holistic nursing. Despite this, a study by Saunamäki and Engström (2014) identified some nurses consider sexuality a taboo subject and someone else's responsibility. The topic can be strongly associated with feelings of embarrassment and discomfort for some nurses, and others do not feel confident or well equipped to address sexuality and

intimacy issues with older people (Royal College of Nursing, 2018). Research indicates knowledge is inadequate and negative attitudes are prevalent among health care workers about older people's sexuality (Ezhova et al., 2020; Haesler et al., 2016). Consequently, it can adversely impact care and mean nurses may not be fulfilling their duty of care to address the needs of older people in a holistic manner.

Ezhova et al. (2020) identified some of the barriers to older people seeking sexual health advice and treatment. As indicated earlier, one of them is associated with cultural views toward sex as something controversial or immoral in old age that prevent health providers from initiating conversations about sexual health or offering appropriate advice and treatment. For some nurses, discussing sexuality means confronting an uneasy topic, particularly when sexuality among more diverse groups is considered. A study by Donaldson and Vacha-Haase (2016) highlighted the importance of providing education to help staff develop cultural competence when working with older LGBTQ+ people. Helping care staff work through any ambivalence and understand how experiences of stigma, discrimination and victimisation may have impacted the lives of the older LGBTQ+ population is a key factor. As we discussed, this includes understanding how the historical criminalisation and medicalisation of homosexuality cast a shadow on the lives of older LGBTQ+ people that deterred them from discussing their sexual lives. The issues of stigma and stereotyping older people by health care professionals also exists in the heterosexual community. A study by Youssef et al. (2018) identified heterosexual older people also appeared to be stigmatised when being diagnosed with HIV in old age or when using sexual health services.

Due to their personal or religious beliefs, nurses may have their own views about the appropriateness of certain types of relationships and when people should or should not be sexually active. A study by Mahieu et al. (2016) found age and religious affiliations related to less open attitudes toward sexuality in later life among nursing staff. They may be compounded by what society considers appropriate to talk about. As a consequence, nurses may not address the topic of sexuality with older people, which could be a form of subconsciously protecting the person and themselves from drifting to the edge of what is considered socially or morally acceptable (Magnan et al., 2006). Conversely, when nurses challenge their discomfort and embarrassment, they give permission to their patients to broach the subject of sexuality and not be embarrassed by it (Taylor & Davis, 2006). It's important for nurses to challenge bias, conflicting emotions and beliefs toward older people's sexuality. Creating safe and non-judgemental spaces where staff can explore and question assumptions and stereotypes can help challenge prejudicial attitudes (Hafford-Letchfield et al.,

2018). It is important to add staff rights should be promoted, and they should be allowed to work in ways that feel comfortable and morally acceptable to them, as long as this does not compromise the care of the older person, discriminate or deny their rights in any way (Royal College of Nursing, 2018).

The EX-PLISSIT model (Taylor & Davis, 2006) provides a helpful framework that identifies four levels of interventions when addressing sexuality and sexual health: intervention, permission, limited information, specific suggestions, and intensive therapy, detailed in Box 26.5. This framework helps nurses to address issues of sexuality and meet the sexual health care needs of older people in different care settings. One of the strengths of the EX-PLISSIT model is it encourages self-awareness and reflective practice and asks nurses to challenge their assumptions (Taylor & Davis, 2006). Nurses need to be able to have honest and open conversations with colleagues they trust or with their supervisors to identify areas for development in this important area of practice (Royal College of Nursing, 2018). Likewise, organisational systems should adopt non-discriminatory and non-judgemental approaches, and managers need

to facilitate education and training for staff so practitioners feel safe and adequately trained to address the subject of sexuality with older people (Royal College of Nursing, 2018; Saunamäki & Engström, 2014). What remains apparent in most cases is that knowledge and attitudes can be positively influenced by experience, exposure and the training and education of staff in later-life sexuality (Haesler et al., 2016).

Advocates

Whether in illness or in health, older people continue to have rights and needs in relation to sexuality and intimacy. Nurses are in a good place to advocate for older people by speaking out for them when they are not able to influence a certain situation themselves, by challenging poor practice and discriminatory attitudes toward care or by simply providing dignified person-centred care (National Midwifery Council, 2018). This can be demonstrated by nursing care to assist an older person with their hygiene and grooming needs, dress and physical appearance. Physical presentation, appearance and dress are a visible way of expressing individuality and sexuality and contribute to a person's sense of dignity and self-respect. Nurses can also advocate

---

BOX 26.5 Ex-PLISSIT Model

Permission-giving stage: This stage is about the nurse explicitly giving the older person permission to express any concerns about their sexual health. To create a climate of permission, nurses need to challenge their own values, attitudes and beliefs and have the humility to provide a safe space for the person, listen and hear without judgement. Earlier we provided some generic questions that may help nurses start a conversation about sexuality.

Providing leaflets or posters in the care environment also indicates the organisational culture and care practices consider intimate relationships and sexuality to be integral to well-being.

Limited information stage: In this stage the nurse acts as a source of information—for example, by explaining to the older person the effects of illness or various treatments on sexual functioning. Nurses can clarify misinformation and give correct information in the form of leaflets or signposting to a trusted website. It is essential nurses provide information that is relevant to the older person's specific concerns rather than providing information that is generalised or based on assumptions. This is why listening and hearing the older person's needs is so crucial in the permission-giving stage.

Specific suggestion stage: During this stage the nurse needs to take a problem-solving approach in order to address

the older person's concerns. For example, for an older person who is experiencing pain and stiffness during sex due to an arthritic condition, there may be a need to discuss the option of experimenting with different sexual positions as well as the possibility of taking pain relief before sexual activity. For an older woman who is experiencing vaginal dryness and difficulty with lubrication, it may be appropriate to suggest vaginal lubricants and moisturisers. This stage needs to holistically consider all aspects of sexual health rather than just focus on sexual activity. For example, a person may feel anxious her partner will not find her attractive following a mastectomy or hysterectomy. Suggestions could be varied and focus on addressing the sense of loss following surgery as well as any significant concerns about body image that impact self-esteem.

Intensive therapy stage: This is the most advanced stage of the model, where more intensive therapy may be required. Depending on the nurse's competency, they may or may not have this level of expertise. A referral to specialist services is required if the issues identified are beyond the competency of the nurse—for example, referral for psychosexual or relationship counselling or referral to a mental health service if the sexual health problems are associated with a mental health condition.

Source: Adapted from Taylor, B., & Davis, S. (2006). Using the Extended PLISSIT model to address sexual healthcare needs. *Nursing Standard, 21*(11), 35–40.

for older people by respecting their rights to privacy and confidentiality. For example, an older couple in a care home may want private time to engage in consensual intimate relations, or an older person may wish to withhold certain information about their sexuality or sexual relations from their family members.

There is sometimes tension between supporting older people's human rights and freedoms in relation to sexuality and acting within professional and legal frameworks. According to the Mental Capacity (Amendment) Act 2019, if a person lacks capacity to consent to sexual relations, a decision cannot be made on their behalf with regards to this matter as part of a best-interests decision process. Consequently, this means any sexual relation with a person who lacks capacity to consent to sexual relations constitutes sexual assault. This poses challenges to nurses who, for example, may be supporting an older couple who wish to express intimacy and engage in sexual relations where one partner's capacity begins to deteriorate due to dementia. Another piece of legislation that is important to be aware of in the context of challenging poor attitudes and discriminatory practice is the Equality Act 2010. If a nurse refuses to provide care to an older person based on one of the protected characteristics (i.e., age, disability, gender reassignment, marriage and civil partnership, pregnancy and maternity, race, religion or belief, sex and sexual orientation), it may constitute discriminatory practice and be in breach of their professional code of conduct as well as be unlawful under this act. It's important for nurses to advocate for older people by challenging discriminatory behaviour and for organisational systems and services to promote non-discriminatory approaches.

CONCLUSION AND LEARNING POINTS

Addressing sexuality and relational issues remains a central element of nursing older people and this chapter has offered a range of strategies that nurses can use to do this. Establishing practices that support safe relational, sexual, and intimate expression among older people can enhance their wellbeing. Raising issues of sexuality and intimacy may be difficult for both older people and nurses. However, steps can be taken, before and after a person has been admitted to the care setting, to facilitate such discussions. Acknowledging that older people may still want to be sexually active, or intimate is the first step to addressing the issues and overcoming the barriers. Creating an environment where older people feel comfortable to discuss these issues is paramount.

KEY LEARNING POINTS

- Relationships, sexual expression and intimacy remain important aspects of older people's lives.
- Addressing relationships, sexual expression and intimacy is a central tenet of nursing older people. It is imperative to foster a climate where permission to discuss sexuality and intimacy is implicit in care settings, care processes and practice.
- Nurses should have a high level of self-awareness when working with older LGBTQ+ people to challenge concepts of gender normativity/heteronormativity and promote inclusion. It is essential nurses and all health care professionals develop LGBTQ+-friendly environments that facilitate individuals to disclose and express their identities where they feel it is appropriate, enabling them to feel supported and respected.
- Nurses do not need to be psychosexual therapists to address sexuality and relationship issues with older people in their care. Nurses can open a dialogue on these matters with older people, listen actively, remain congruent and intervene appropriately by teaching or counselling within the limits of their knowledge or by referring to specialists for help.

REFERENCES

Age UK. (2021). Factsheet 78. Safeguarding older people from abuse and neglect. https://www.ageuk.org.uk/globalassets/age-uk/documents/factsheets/fs78_safeguarding_older_people_from_abuse_fcs.pdf

Bancroft, J. (2009). *Human sexuality and its problems* (3rd ed.). Churchill Livingstone.

Baim-Lance, A., Tietz, D., Lever, H., Swart, M., & Agins, B. (2019). Everyday and unavoidable coproduction: Exploring patient participation in the delivery of healthcare services. *Sociology of Health & Illness, 41*(1), 128–142. doi:10.1111/1467-9566.12801.

Barker, J. (2004). Lesbian aging: An agenda for research. In G. Herdt, & B. de Vries (Eds.), *Gay and lesbian aging: Research and future directions* (pp. 29–72). Springer Publishing.

Barrett, C., & Hinchliff, S. (Eds.). (2018). *Addressing the sexual rights of older people: Theory, policy and practice.* Routledge.

Bennett, K., & Thompson, N. (1991). Accelerated ageing and male homosexuality: Australian evidence in a continuing debate. *The Journal of Homosexuality, 20*(3–4), 65–75.

Brown, G., Lyons, A., Hinchliff, S., & Cramer, P. (2017). The challenges in reducing STIs while fulfilling and enhancing the sexual rights of older people. In C. Barrett, & S. Hinchliff (Eds.), *Addressing the sexual rights of older people* (pp. 111–124). Routledge.

Brown Wilson, C. (2009). Developing community in care homes through a relationship-centred approach. Health and Social Care in the. *Community, 17*(2), 177–186. doi:10.1111/j.1365-2524.2008.00815.x.

Brown Wilson, C. (2012). *Caring for older people: A shared approach*. Sage.

Brown Wilson, C., & Davies, S. (2009). Using relationships in care homes to develop relationship centred care- the contribution of staff. *Journal of Clinical Nursing, 18*, 1746–1755. doi:10.1111/j.1365-2702.2008.02748.x.

Brown Wilson, C., Swarbrick, C., Pilling, M., & Keady, J. (2013). The senses in practice: Enhancing the quality of care for residents with dementia in care homes. *Journal of Advanced Nursing, 69*(1), 77–80. doi:10.1111/j.1365-2648.2012.05992.x.

Clayton, A. H., & Montejo, A. L. (2006). Major depressive disorder, antidepressants, and sexual dysfunction. *The Journal of Clinical Psychiatry, 67*(Suppl 6), 33–37.

Copeland, K. L., Brown, J. S., Creasman, J. M., Van Den Eeden, S. K., Subak, L. H., Thom, D. J., et al. (2012). Diabetes mellitus and sexual function in middle-aged and older women. *Obstetrics & Gynecology, 120*(2, Part 1), 331–340.

Courtin, E., & Knapp, M. (2017). Social isolation, loneliness and health in old age: A scoping review. *Health and Social Care in the Community, 25*(3), 799–812. doi:10.1111/hsc.12311.

Dalrymple, J., Booth, J., Flowers, P., & Lorimer, K. (2017). Psychosocial factors influencing risk-taking in middle age for STIs. *Sexually Transmitted Infections, 93*(1), 32–38.

Davis, C., Tami, P., Ramsay, D., Melanson, L., MacLean, L., Nersesian, S., et al. (2020). Body image in older breast cancer survivors: A systematic review. *Psycho-Oncology, 29*(5), 823–832.

Davis, D. H., Smith, R., Brown, A., Rice, B., Yin, Z., & Delpech, V. (2013). Early diagnosis and treatment of HIV infection: magnitude of benefit on short-term mortality is greatest in older adults. *Age and Ageing, 42*(4), 520–526.

Dewing, J. (2007). Participatory research: a method for process consent with persons who have dementia. *Dementia: The International Journal of Social Research and Practice, 6*, 11–25.

Dickinson, T. (2015). 'Curing queers': Mental nurses and their patients, 1935–74. *Nursing History and Humanities MUP*.

Dickinson, T., Appasamy, N., Pritchard, L. P., & Savidge, L (2022). Nursing a plague: Nurses' perspectives on their work during the United Kingdom HIV/AIDS crisis, 1981–96. In J. Western, & H. J. Elizabeth (Eds.), *Histories of HIV/AIDS in Western Europe: New and regional perspectives* (pp. 109–138). Manchester University Press.

Doll, GA (2012). *Sexuality and long-term care: Understanding and supporting the needs of older adults*. Health Professions Press.

Donaldson, W., & Vacha-Haase, T. (2016). Exploring staff clinical knowledge and practice with LGBT residents in long-term care: A grounded theory of cultural competency and training needs. *Clinical Gerontologist, 39*(5), 389–409.

Donovan, T. (2002). Being transgender and older: A first person account. *Journal of Gay and Lesbian Social Services: Issues in Practice, Policy and Research, 13*(4), 19–22.

Erens, B., Mitchell, K. R., Gibson, L., Datta, J., Lewis, R., Field, N., et al. (2019). Health status, sexual activity and satisfaction among older people in Britain: A mixed methods study. *PLoS ONE, 14*(3), Article E0213835.

Ezhova, I., Savidge, L., Bonnett, C., Cassidy, J., Okwuokei, A., & Dickinson, T. (2020). Barriers to older adults seeking sexual health advice and treatment: A scoping review. *International Journal of Nursing Studies, 107*, 1–16.

Fenway Health. (n.d). Pride in Our Health. https://prideinourhealth.libsyn.com/

Fileborn, B., Brown, G., Lyons, A., Hinchliff, S., Heywood, W., Minichiello, V., et al. (2018). Safer sex in later life: Qualitative interviews with older Australians on their understandings and practices of safer sex. *Journal of Sex Research, 55*(2), 164–177.

Gardiner, C., Geldenhuys, G., & Gott, M. (2018). Interventions to reduce social isolation and loneliness among older people: An integrative review. Health and Social Care in the. *Community, 26*(2), 147–157. doi:10.1111/hsc.12367.

Garrett, D., & Lawton, S. (2019). The effects of ageing on female genital and sexual health. *British Journal of Nursing, 28*(18), 1192–1195.

Gilleard, C., & Higgs, P. (2011). Ageing, abjection and embodiment in the fourth age. *Journal of Aging Studies, 25*(2), 135–142.

Haesler, E., Bauer, M., & Fetherstonhaugh, D. (2016). Sexuality, sexual health and older people: A systematic review of research on the knowledge and attitudes of health professionals. *Nurse Education Today, 40*, 57–71.

Hafford-Letchfield, T., Simpson, P., Willis, P., & Almack, K. (2018). Developing inclusive residential care for older lesbian, gay, bisexual and trans (LGBT) people: An evaluation of the Care Home Challenge action research project. *Health & Social Care in the Community, 26*(2), E312–E320.

Harley, D. (2021). Sexual expression and pleasure among Black minority ethnic older women. In P. Hafford-Letchfield, P. Simpson, & P. Reynolds (Eds.), *Sex and diversity in later life: Critical perspectives* (pp. 18–37). Policy Press.

Hillman, J. (2012). *Sexuality and aging: Clinical perspectives*: Springer.

Hinchliff, S., & Fileborn, B. (2020). Sexuality and ageing. In T. Dening, A. Thomas, R. Stewart, & J.-P. Taylor (Eds.), *The Oxford textbook of old age psychiatry* (pp. 785–802). Oxford University Press.

Hinchliff, S., & Gott, M. (2008). Challenging social myths and stereotypes of women and aging: Heterosexual women talk about sex. *Journal of Women & Aging, 20*(1–2), 65–81.

Hinchliff, S., & Gott, M. (2011). Seeking medical help for sexual concerns in mid-and later life: a review of the literature. *Journal of Sex Research, 48*(2–3), 106–117.

Hostetler, A. (2004). Old gay and alone: The ecology of well-being among middle-aged and older single gay men. In B. De Vries, & & G. Herdt (Eds.), *Gay and lesbian aging and research: Future directions* (pp. 143–176). Springer Publishing Co. Inc.

James, C., Harfouche, M., Welton, N. J., Turner, K. M., Abu-Rad-dad, L. J., Gottlieb, S. L., et al. (2020). Herpes simplex virus: Global infection prevalence and incidence estimates, 2016. *Bulletin of the World Health Organization, 98*, 315–329.

Kaklamanidou, B. (2012). Pride and prejudice: Celebrity versus fictional cougars. *Celebrity Studies, 3*(1), 78–89.

Kimura, M., Murata, Y., Shimoda, K., & Robinson, R. (2001). Sexual dysfunction following stroke. *Comprehensive Psychiatry, 42*(3), 217–222.

Kirby Institute. (2018). *HIV, viral hepatitis and sexually transmissible infections in Australia: Annual surveillance report 2018*: Kirby Institute. https://data.kirby.unsw.edu.au/STIs.

Knocker, S. (2012). *Perspectives on ageing: Lesbians, gay men, and bisexuals.* Joseph Rowntree Foundation.

Kouidrat, Y., Pizzol, D., Cosco, T., Thompson, T., Carnaghi, M., Bertoldo, A., et al. (2017). High prevalence of erectile dysfunction in diabetes: A systematic review and meta-analysis of 145 studies. *Diabetic Medicine, 34*(9), 1185–1192.

Kramer, L. (1989). *Reports from the Holocaust: The making of an AIDS activist.* St. Martin's Press.

Kuhn, D. (2002). Intimacy, sexuality and residents with dementia. *Alzheimer's Care Quarterly, 3*(2), 165–176.

Lee, D., & Tetley, J. (2021). Sex and ageing in heterosexual men. In P. Hafford-Letchfield, P. Simpson, & P. Reynolds (Eds.), *Sex and diversity in later life: Critical perspectives* (pp. 79–101). Policy Press.

Lewis, R., Mitchell, K. R., Mercer, C. H., Datta, J., Jones, K. G., & Wellings, K. (2020). Navigating new sexual partnerships in midlife: A socioecological perspective on factors shaping STI risk perceptions and practices. *Sexually Transmitted Infections, 96*, 238–245.

Lyons, A., Heywood, W., Fileborn, B., Minichiello, V., Barrett, C., Brown, G., et al. (2017). Sexually active older Australian's knowledge of sexually transmitted infections and safer sexual practices. *Australian and New Zealand Journal of Public Health, 41*(3), 259–261.

Macia, E., Duboz, P., & Chevé, D. (2015). The paradox of impossible beauty: Body changes and beauty practices in aging women. *Journal of Women & Aging, 27*(2), 174–187.

Magnan, M. A., Reynolds, K. E., & Galvin, E. A. (2006). Barriers to addressing patient sexuality in nursing practice. (Research). *Dermatology Nursing, 18*(5), 448–454.

Mahieu, L., De Casterlé, B., Acke, J., Vandermarliere, H., Van Elssen, K., Fieuws, S., et al. (2016). Nurses' knowledge and attitudes toward aged sexuality in Flemish nursing homes. *Nursing Ethics, 23*(6), 605–623.

Marmot, M., Allen, J., Boyce, T., Goldblatt, P., & Morrison, J. (2020). Health equity in England: The Marmot Review 10 years on. *Institute of Health Equity.* https://www.health.org.uk/publications/reports/the-marmot-review-10-years-on.

Moore, A., & Reynolds, P. (2016). Against the ugliness of age: Towards an erotics of the ageing sexual body. *Inter Alia: A Journal of Queer Studies, 11*, 88–105.

Morley, J. E., & Tolson, D. T. (2012). Sexuality and ageing. In A. J. Sinclair, J. E. Morley, & B. Vellas (Eds.), *Principles and practice of geriatric medicine* (5th ed., pp. 93–102). John, Wiley & Sons Ltd.

National Health Service. (2019). The NHS long term plan. https://www.longtermplan.nhs.uk/publication/nhs-long-term-plan

Naumova, I., & Castelo-Branco, C. (2018). Current treatment options for postmenopausal vaginal atrophy. *International Journal of Women's Health, 10*, 387–395.

Nolan, M. R., Brown, J., Davies, S., Nolan, J., & Keady, J. (2006). *The Senses Framework: Improving care for older people through a relationship-centred approach.* University of Sheffield. Getting Research into Practice (GRiP) Report No 2. Project Report. http://shura.shu.ac.uk/280.

Nursing and Midwifery Council. (2018). The Code: Professional standards of practice and behaviour for nurses, midwives, and nurse associates. https://www.nmc.org.uk/globalassets/sitedocuments/nmc-publications/nmc-code.pdf

O'Brien, K., Roe, B., Low, C., Deyn, L., & Rogers, S. (2012). An exploration of the perceived changes in intimacy of patients' relationships following head and neck cancer. *Journal of Clinical Nursing, 21*(17–18), 2499–2508.

Pryzbylo, E. (2021). Aging asexually: Exploring desexualization and aging intimacies. In P. Hafford-Letchfield, P. Simpson, & P. Reynolds (Eds.), *Sex and diversity in later life: Critical perspectives* (pp. 181–198). Policy Press.

Public Health England. (2020). New STI diagnoses and rates by gender, sexual risk, age group and ethnic group, 2014 to 2018. https://www.gov.uk/government/statistics/sexually-transmitted-infections-stis-annual-data-tables

Roper, N., Logan, W., & Tierney, A. (1980). *The elements of nursing.* Churchill Livingston.

Royal College of Nursing. (2018). Older people in care homes: Sex, sexuality and intimate relationships. An RCN discussion and guidance document for the nursing workforce. https://www.rcn.org.uk/professional-development/publications/pub-007126

Royal Society of Chemistry. (n.d.). LGBT+ toolkit. https://www.rsc.org/new-perspectives/talent/inclusion-and-diversity/resources/lgbt-toolkit

Saunamäki, N., & Engström, M. (2014). Registered nurses' reflections on discussing sexuality with patients: Responsibilities, doubts and fears. *Journal of Clinical Nursing, 23*(3–4), 531–540.

Schaller, S., Traeen, B., & Lundin Kvalem, I. (2020). Barriers and facilitating factors in help-seeking: A qualitative study on how older adults experience talking about sexual issues with healthcare personnel. *International Journal of Sexual Health, 32*, 65–80.

Schouten, M., van Velde, A. J., Snijdewind, I. J., Verbon, A., Rijnders, B. J., & van der Ende, M. E. (2013). Late diagnosis of HIV positive patients in Rotterdam, the Netherlands: Risk factors and missed opportunities. *Nederlands Tijdschrift voor Geneeskunde, 157*(15), A5731.

Simpson, P. (2015a). Ageing sexuality. In C. Richards, & M. J. Barker (Eds.), *The Palgrave handbook of the psychology of sexuality and gender* (pp. 375–390). Palgrave Macmillan.

Simpson, P. (2015). *Gay male ageing and ageism: Over the rainbow?.* Palgrave Macmillan.

Simpson, P. (2016). Ageisms and lesbian, gay, bisexual, trans and queer cultures. In A. E. Goldberg (Ed.), *The SAGE encyclopedia of LGBTQ studies.* SAGE Publications. doi:10.4135/9781483371283.n24.

Simpson, P. (2021). At YOUR Age???!!! The constraints of ageist erotophobia on older people's sexual and intimate relationships. In P. Simpson, P. Hafford-Letchfield, & P. Reynolds (Eds.), *Desexualisation: The limits of sex and intimacy in later life* (pp. 35–51). Policy Press.

Simpson, P., Brown Wilson, C., Brown, L. J. E., Dickinson, T., & Horne, M. (2016). The challenges of and opportunities involved in researching intimacy and sexuality in care homes accommodating older people: A feasibility study. *Journal of Advanced Nursing, 73*(1), 127–137.

Simpson, P., Brown Wilson, C., Horne, M., Brown, L. J. E., & Dickinson, T. (2018). 'We've had our sex life way back': Older care home residents, sexuality and intimacy. *Ageing and Society, 38*(7), 1478–1501. doi:10.1017/S0144686X17000101.

Simpson, P., Horne, M., Brown, L. J. E., Wilson, C. B., Dickinson, T., & Torkington, K. (2017). Old(er) care home residents and sexual/intimate citizenship. *Ageing & Society, 37*(2), 243–265.

Sinković, M., & Towler, L. (2019). Sexual aging: A systematic review of qualitative research on the sexuality and sexual health of older adults. *Qualitative Health Research, 29*(9), 1239–1254.

Slevin, K., & Mowery, C. (2012). Exploring embodied aging and ageism among old lesbians and gay men. In L. Carpenter, & & J. DeLamater (Eds.), *Sex for life course. From virginity to Viagra: How sexuality changes throughout our lives* (pp. 260–277). University Press.

Smith, J. M. (2012). Toward a better understanding of loneliness in community-dwelling older adults. *Journal of Psychology, 146*(3), 293–311. doi:10.1080/00223980.2011.602132.

Smith, M. L., Bergeron, C. D., Goltz, H. H., Coffey, T., & Boolani, A. (2020). Sexually transmitted infection knowledge among older adults: Psychometrics and test–retest reliability. *International Journal of Environmental Research and Public Health, 17*(7), 2462.

Social Care Institute for Excellence. (2015). Care act guidance on strength-based approaches. https://www.scie.org.uk/strengths-based-approaches/guidance

Spandler, H., & Carr, S. (2022). Lesbian and bisexual women's experiences of aversion therapy in England. *History of the Human Sciences.* 10.1177%2F09526951211059422.

Steptoe, A., Jackson, S., & Wardle, J. (2016). Sexual activity and concerns in people with coronary heart disease from a population-based study. *Heart, 102*(14), 1095–1099.

Tao, Y., Chen, M. Y., Tucker, J. D., Ong, J. J., Tang, W., Wong, N. S., & Zhang, L. (2020). A nationwide spatiotemporal analysis of syphilis over 21 years and implications for prevention and control in China. *Clinical Infectious Diseases, 70*(1), 136–139.

Tavoschi, L., Dias, J. G., Pharris, A., Schmid, D., Sasse, A., Van Beckhoven, D., & Maly, M. (2017). New HIV diagnoses among adults aged 50 years or older in 31 European countries, 2004–15: An analysis of surveillance data. *The Lancet HIV, 4*(11), e514–e521.

Taylor, B., & Davis, S. (2006). Using the Extended PLISSIT model to address sexual healthcare needs. *Nursing Standard, 21*(11), 35–40.

Taylor, J. (2018). Out of the darkness and into the shadows: The evolution of contemporary bisexuality. *Canadian Journal of Human Sexuality, 27*(2), 103–109.

The Care Quality Commission (CQC). (2020). Relationships and Sexuality in Adult Social Care Services. https://www.cqc.org.uk/sites/default/files/20190221-Relationships-and-sexuality-in-social-care-PUBLICATION.pdf

Træen, B., Hald, G., Graham, C., Enzlin, P., Janssen, E., Kvalem, I., et al. (2017). Sexuality in older adults (65)—An overview of the literature, Part 1: Sexual function and its difficulties. *International Journal of Sexual Health, 29*(1), 1–10.

Treais, J. (2016). *The lives of older lesbians: Sexuality, identity and the lifecourse.* Palgrave Macmillan.

Ussher, J. M., Perz, J., Kellett, A., Chambers, S., Latini, D., Davis, I. D., et al. (2016). Health-related quality of life, psychological distress, and sexual changes following prostate cancer: A comparison of gay and bisexual men with heterosexual men. *Journal of Sexual Medicine, 13*(3), 425–434.

Verschuren, J., Enzlin, P., Dijkstra, P., Geertzen, J., & Dekker, R. (2010). Chronic disease and sexuality: A generic conceptual framework. *Journal of Sex Research: Annual Review of Sex Research, 47*(2–3), 153–170.

Wandera, S. O., Kwagala, B., & Maniragaba, F. (2020). Prevalence and determinants of recent HIV testing among older persons in rural Uganda: A cross-sectional study. *BMC Public Health, 20*(1), 144.

Wilson, K. D. A., Dray-Spira, R., Aubrière, C., Hamelin, C., Spire, B., & Lert, F. ANRS-Vespa2 Study Group. (2014). Frequency and correlates of late presentation for HIV infection in France: Older adults are a risk group–results from the ANRS-VESPA2 Study, France. *AIDS Care, 26*(1), S83–S93.

Wiskerke, E., & Manthorpe, J. (2019). Intimacy between care home residents with dementia: Findings from a review of the literature. *Dementia, 18*(1), 94–107.

Wiskerke, E., & Manthorpe, J. (2018). New relationships & intimacy in long-term care: The views of relatives of residents with dementia and care home staff. *Dementia, 17*(4), 405–422. doi:10.1177/1471301216647814.

World Association for Sexual Health. (2014). Declaration of sexual rights. http://www.worldsexology.org/wp-content/uploads/2013/08/declaration_of_sexual_rights_sep03_2014.pdf

World Health Organization. (2004). *ICD-10: International statistical classification of diseases and related health problems, tenth revision* (2nd ed.). World Health Organization.

World Health Organization. (2006). Defining sexual health: Report of a technical consultation on sexual health, 28–31 January 2002. https://www.who.int/reproductivehealth/publications/sexual_health/defining_sexual_health.pdf

Youssef, E., Wright, J., Delpech, V., Davies, K., Brown, A., Cooper, V., et al. (2018). Factors associated with testing for HIV in people aged ≥ 50 years: A qualitative study. *BMC Public Health, 18*(1), 1156.

27

Pain and Older People

Pat Schofield, Margaret Dunham

CHAPTER OUTLINE

OVERVIEW OF CHAPTER

In this chapter we aim to discuss the experience of pain, particularly from the perspective of the older adult. We explore the physiology of pain and the types of pain you are likely to see in clinical practice. Our focus is on the syndromes particularly seen among the older population, including types of pain and comorbidities or consequences such as falls and frailty. This is followed by a section that discusses the latest recommendations on pain assessment and the tools validated for use in this population. How to manage pain in the older population is discussed based on the newly published British Pain Society/British Geriatric Society Guidelines. Finally, we discuss the recent COVID-19 pandemic, which impacted the experience and management of pain. Throughout the chapter we encourage thinking around the nursing contribution to supporting older people who experience pain.

NATURE OF PAIN

Everyone experiences pain intermittently. Although pain is a common experience for people receiving care in hospital, its ubiquitous nature is a significant challenge for the wider health care team and for older people in particular. McCaffrey's (1968, p. 95) seminal definition of pain as 'whatever the experiencing person says it is, existing whenever the experiencing person say it does' appreciates the wide variety of pain.

Pain was recently redefined by the International Association for the Study of Pain (IASP) as 'an unpleasant sensory and emotional experience associated with, or resembling that associated with, actual or potential tissue damage' (Raja et al., 2020, p. 1976).

This new definition was driven largely by the need to accommodate the heterogeneity of expression and experience for each individual; the definition emphasises the psychological and emotional parameters in addition to physical parameters. Due to its personal and subjective nature, pain is also described as 'one of the most challenging problems in medicine' (Melzack & Wall, 1988).

Pain Physiology

The complexity of each person's pain experience is challenging for the nursing team in particular because it prevents a one-size-fits-all approach to assessment and management. The physiological basis for experiencing pain in an aged nervous system suggests older people have a lower sensitivity to pain and thus a higher pain threshold (Lautenbacher et al., 2017). However, pain is not just a physiological response to external stimuli; it is a uniquely personal, highly complex and evolving experience. Pain is multifaceted, with sensory, cognitive and motivational determinants (Melzack & Casey 1968). The complex and subjective nature of pain experience makes consensus about measuring pain and its effects a considerable challenge for researchers and clinicians, as there is a need for an awareness of the whole range of measures and flexibility in the application of each tool.

Various theories have been developed to account for the way the experience of pain is potentially modifiable by factors such as environment, context, thoughts and feelings. Gate control theory, proposed by Ronald Melzack and Patrick Wall, was a novel approach to understanding the complex nature of pain and its expression (Melzack & Wall 1965, 1988), considering particular nerve fibres, transmission of pain and the factors that affect this process.

The gate in gate control theory represents the control over the transmission of pain messages, via the substantia gelatinosa in the dorsal horn of the spinal cord to higher centres in the brain (Mendell, 2014). This gate can be opened by painful stimuli, leading to a chemical response at the synapse, with messages ascending via the spinothalamic tract to the brain, where they are perceived as pain. Larger nerve fibres and inhibitory interneurons can modify the stimuli received in the brain. Thus, the balance between the effects of nociceptor stimulation and inhibition of input from large fibres is thought to inform the degree of painful experience.

It has also been noted the gate is influenced by external and internal factors, including emotions such as fear and anxiety (Zhuo, 2016). People who are experiencing anxiety or fear may have more pain because the gate is opened or partially opened, allowing pain impulses to pass through and ascend to the brain (Geva et al., 2014). Conversely, reducing distressing input may relieve or modify the painful experience to a more acceptable level (Bushnell et al., 2013).

In an extension to gate control theory, pain has been conceptualised in the form of a biopsychosocial model where the physical, psychological, social, cognitive, affective and behavioural aspects are all acknowledged (Darnall et al., 2017; Gagliese et al., 2018). This biopsychosocial model of pain offers an approach to appreciating the complex way pain affects people's lives.

The neuromatrix model is a theoretical model that explains the nature of pain, including chronic pain, that may account for some of the chronic pain people experience in the apparent absence of injury or disease (Melzack, 1999). It builds on Melzack and Wall's (1965) gate control theory. The central tenet to these theories is the role the brain plays in the interpretation and modulation of painful stimuli across the sensory, cognitive and affective elements. This all reinforces the subjective nature of pain.

TYPES OF PAIN

Pain is often described as acute or chronic; requirements for the treatment of each are quite distinct (Schug & Goddard, 2014). However, much of our understanding of the nature and expression of pain is informed by the experience of acute pain. Furthermore, pain may be a combination of acute and chronic pain, which poses an additional, significant challenge for observation and planning appropriate interventions.

Acute Pain

Acute pain is usually a normal response to injury, disease or surgical intervention (Treede, 2016). It can be defined as a response to an acute noxious stimulus. The experience of acute pain acts as a warning—a deterrent to avoid the painful experience, or it signals the need to seek help and is usually transient, meaning it resolves as healing takes place. In acute pain, particular primary afferent nociceptors (i.e., small Aδ nerve fibres) produce pain when stimulated by thermal, mechanical or noxious chemical input (Smith, 2018). Sometimes known as fast fibres, stimulation of Aδ nerve fibres can provoke a rapid response to withdraw from the source of the pain. The receptor sites for these afferent nociceptors are situated in the skin and viscera. An early experience of acute pain can become an informative and protective experience for an individual.

Chronic Pain

Chronic pain can be enduring, often with no identifiable cause. Even when the cause is known, it is not always easily managed and appears to serve no useful or protective function. The IASP defines chronic pain as 'pain that persists or recurs longer than 3 months' (Schug et al., 2019). Chronic pain is frequently associated with distress; it limits activities of daily living, can be a considerable cause of suffering and is acknowledged as a disease in its own right (Treede et al., 2019). The causes of chronic pain are multiple and complex. For example, arthritis, rheumatoid arthritis, poststroke pain, and joint pain are just a few of the over 200 recognised pain syndromes. Repeated exposure to acute pain that is poorly managed, including some surgical procedures, and the associated inflammatory response can initiate an extended or exaggerated chemical response in the nociceptors, affecting the threshold at which they mediate pain. This is sometimes termed peripheral sensitisation (Kuner & Flor, 2017).

Acute and Chronic (Mixed) Pain and Cancer Pain

The transition of acute to chronic pain may be gradual, and the causes are not fully understood. The risk of developing chronic pain following surgery is now widely recognised. A recent pan European study of over 3,000 people following surgery noted a significant risk of developing chronic pain after surgical procedures (Fletcher et al., 2015). The development of chronic pain following surgery occurs in approximately 10% of people and is associated with poorly controlled acute postoperative pain and overprescription of opioids (Glare et al., 2019).

There is growing appreciation that as early cancer diagnosis improves, older people are living longer following cancer treatment. Pain after cancer diagnosis and treatment may be a significant problem for older people and those who experience complex health problems in particular (Paice, 2011). Similar to younger adults, older people may experience pain due to cancer or its treatment, including surgery, radiotherapy and chemotherapy. However, older people may be more vulnerable to the development of chronic pain following cancer treatment (Dunham et al., 2013; Gagliese et al., 2009).

IS PAIN DIFFERENT FOR OLDER ADULTS?

For decades we have believed pain is a normal part of the ageing process, something older adults 'get used to' or 'learn to live with' (Gagliese et al., 2009). Older adults are deemed to be stoical, not wishing to complain. There is a classic quote in the literature where the patient goes to the doctor with a pain in their leg to be told it is part of getting older. 'But my other leg is the same age', says the patient in response. This illustrates an attitude that permeates among health professional and patients (Dunham et al., 2020) that patients of a certain age should expect to live with pain. Nevertheless, over the past two decades we have seen a proliferation of publications in

the field of pain and ageing around tenfold and on average 10 articles per week (Gibson & Lussier, 2012). So health care professionals and scientists are recognising pain and ageing are an important speciality in their own right, a giant step from the seminal article of Melding (1991), who asked the question, 'Is there such a thing as geriatric pain?'

Older adults are not simply a chronologically older version of their younger counterparts. We cannot apply the same principles of assessing and managing pain in younger adults to older populations; it does not work that way. The sooner we acknowledge this and focus on applying clinically relevant research to older adults and find the best strategies to deal with pain for this group, the sooner we move away from the terrifying epidemiological figures that demonstrate 40% of older adults living in the community have poorly controlled chronic pain—which increases significantly to 80% in nursing home populations (Schofield, 2013). Recent epidemiological studies such as the English Longitudinal Study of Ageing (Yiengprugsawan & Steptoe, 2018), the Irish Longitudinal Study of Ageing (O'Sullivan et al., 2017) and National Health—USA (Patel et al., 2013) demonstrate although increased longevity is a celebration of medical science, it is at the cost of increased incidence of poorly controlled chronic pain.

Sensory Components of Pain

Pain is recognised as having a sensory component (i.e., intensity) and an affective component (i.e., unpleasantness) (Talbot et al., 2019). The sensory component of pain applies to the type and intensity of the sensation. The type is described in words such as *dull, aching, throbbing*, and the intensity is often described in magnitude terms using pain scales such as a visual analogue or numerical rating scale (Huskisson, 1974). We don't fully understand the experience of pain in older adults. But it has been suggested ageing is associated with increased pain, increased pain thresholds and poor functioning of endogenous inhibition mechanisms (Lautenbacher, 2012: Lautenbacher et al., 2017). This suggests for older adults, pain systems are activated later, and consequently they show signs of pain insensitivity. In contrast the lack of pain inhibition mechanisms would result in pain escalation over time. Thus, older adults often display more prevalent pain syndromes (Lautenbacher, 2012). Although the findings of these studies appear to be robust, functional changes in the central nervous system that possibly cause or maintain increased thresholds and inhibitory deficits are still unknown (Farrell, 2012).

A recent study by González-Roldán et al. (2020) looked at pressure pain thresholds in 75 adults on the Balearic islands in Spain. The sample included 38 healthy older adults. The older adults reported a higher pressure pain index and subjective pain rating index than their younger counterparts. The sample was small, but the authors suggested their study contributes to the understanding of the evolution of cortical networks in ageing and the relevance to pain perception. They concurred with the work of Lautenbacher (2012) in that the pain systems are activated later, but over time the dysfunction of the modulatory system and evaluation processes lead to increased pain perception. The authors suggested the results of their study could explain the increased vulnerability to chronic pain in older adults and that older adults with health conditions could be more susceptible to chronic pain disorders.

Affective Components of Pain

Chronic pain is much more than a sensory experience. It includes emotional responses (i.e., affective elements), attitudes and beliefs (i.e., cognitive elements), and responses to pain by patients, family members and carers (i.e., behavioural components). When pain is present, older adults may limit their activities. This is partly due to the restrictions that may occur as a result of the pain and disability but also as a result of fear of further injury or falling (Hübscher et al., 2010; Martin et al., 2005; Tse & Vong, 2012). Ageing-associated brain changes impact the experience of pain. Therefore, dysfunctional brain changes associated with ageing can cause impaired descending inhibition as described by gate control theory. This impairment can affect the modulation of sensory input such as fear, depression, anxiety and dysfunctional coping, which influence the experience of pain and disability (Karp et al., 2008).

Depression and anxiety are fairly common in older adults, with estimates of around 65% of the older population being anxious (Lenze et al., 2000). Affective and anxiety disorders share the same neurotransmitters and brain areas as persistent pain. These conditions coexist and subsequently exacerbate each other. Detrimental effects of persistent pain in older adults include mood disturbance, functional impairment, poorer sleep and reduced quality of life (Gibson & Weiner, 2005).

PAIN SYNDROMES

A syndrome is a collection of signs and symptoms correlated with one another and often associated with a particular disease. An example is pain.

Cardiac Syndromes

Advancing age is a risk factor for the development of coronary artery disease. Acute cardiac syndromes are the leading cause of death and include unstable angina and acute myocardial infarction. When an older adult presents in the emergency department without chest pain, it is a common cause of misdiagnosis and undertreatment. Adults under 65 are more likely to complain of chest pain and subsequently survive an incident. A recent systematic review of acute coronary syndromes in older adults (Gillis et al., 2014) identified 149 studies between 2000 and 2012 and found older adults with acute cardiac syndromes are less likely to report chest pain on arrival to an emergency department. They also found older adults have higher in-hospital mortality rate than adults younger than 65. However, older adults who do not report chest pain on arrival are twice as likely to die compared with older adults with chest pain. Nevertheless, older adults with silent myocardial infarctions are perceived to be fairly prevalent. A study by Goch et al. (2009) examined the differences in clinical presentation and treatment of myocardial infarction between adults over 75 and their younger counterparts admitted to a cardiac ward in Poland. They found dyspnoea, fatigue and other heart failure symptoms were more commonly reported than chest pain and attributed the differences to comorbidities such as ischemic heart disease, hypertension, diabetes mellitus, chronic obstructive pulmonary disease, chronic renal failure and digestive system disorders along with joint and bone disorders, which they suggested confounded the clinical picture and caused it to be uncharacteristic. They also found in the early hours of the infarction, older adults were less likely to complain of chest pain. They highlighted in previous studies, over 75% of adults over 85 did not present with chest pain. The authors suggested this is attributed to the altered pain perception associated with ageing, a phenomenon that could be the result of permanently ischemic sensory nerves, ischemic dysfunction of the cerebral cortex and dysfunction of the autonomic nervous system.

Musculoskeletal Pain

One of the most common pain problems in older adults is musculoskeletal pain. A recent systematic review for the UK National Guidelines (Schofield et al., 2022) demonstrated common pain syndromes in this population include knee, hip and back pain. Osteoporosis and osteoarthritis are also common pain syndromes in this group. An interesting survey that spanned Europe demonstrated musculoskeletal pain as prevalent in almost 36% of 61,157 participants over 50 who resided in Austria, Belgium, Czech Republic, Denmark, Estonia, France, Germany, Italy, Luxembourg, the Netherlands, Slovenia, Spain, Sweden and Switzerland. Researchers used the Survey of Health, Ageing and Retirement in Europe and found most of the participants with chronic musculoskeletal pain were women (Cimas et al., 2018).

Musculoskeletal pain often comes with side effects, as demonstrated by Eggermont and colleagues (2009) in their Boston Mobilize study, which included the occurrence of life-threatening falls. They demonstrated chronic pain in the older population is associated with interference in activities of daily living and subsequently an increased risk of falls. In the United States, where this study took place, falls account for one of the top 10 causes of mortality. Figures are similar in the United Kingdom, with over 5,000 fall-related deaths in adults over 75 in 2010 and a 70% increase in 2017 (Age UK, 2019). Although we are aware musculoskeletal pain exists in older adults, there is also evidence the incidence of musculoskeletal pain decreases in very old adults (Brattberg et al., 1996), when this syndrome is replaced by other syndromes such as abdominal pain.

Abdominal Pain

Acute abdominal pain is a common complaint among older adults who present in the emergency department. Presentation of abdominal pain in the older population is often different to that of their younger counterparts. Older adults tend to present later in their disease process for a number of reasons: they are afraid of losing independence, they may not have transport, they lack support to care for their spouse or pet, or they fear death (Rothrock et al., 1992). Abdominal pain may be due to constipation or urinary tract infections missed in the community that become significant for the older person. It is important to look for the hidden signs.

Studies suggest among older adults who present to a hospital with abdominal pain, 50% are admitted. Thirty to 40% of cases result in surgery for underlying conditions. Fenyö (1982) highlighted if a diagnosis is delayed, there is a 19% increased chance of mortality compared to 8% when a diagnosis is made promptly, supporting the need for early diagnosis in this population. But the diagnosis and progression of disease may be different in an older adult compared to their younger counterparts and perhaps confounded by cognitive decline that prevents effective communication. An older adult is more likely to present with symptoms other than pain such as fever, fatigue, anorexia or altered mental status. For example, in one study of older adults who were acutely ill, 40% had empyema of the gallbladder, gangrenous cholecystitis or free perforation, and 15% had concomitant subphrenic or hepatic abscess (Chang & Wang, 2007). However, of these patients, more than one third were afebrile, and one quarter did not have abdominal tenderness. Furthermore, they reported 10% of older adults admitted to an emergency department with non-specific abdominal pain were diagnosed with underlying malignancy within 1 year (Chang & Wang, 2007).

Of great concern is the issue of peptic ulceration. With the high use of non-steroidal anti-inflammatory (NSAID) drugs prescribed for this population, the real worry is it has been demonstrated 35% of older adults with peptic ulceration do not present with abdominal pain. They are more likely to present with melaena. The Oxford Pain website (2004) clearly highlights how the risk of an NSAID-related adverse event is age-related. For individuals over 75, an annual risk of a gastrointestinal bleed with an NSAID is 1 in 110, and the annual risk of death from a gastrointestinal bleed is 1 in 650. Nurses must try to avoid NSAID prescribing in older adults and should consider alternative options such as transcutaneous electrical nerve stimulation, relaxation, exercise and self-management. Celecoxib can be used but with caution, and any NSAID use should be for only a short duration and carefully monitored (Schofield et al., 2022).

Frailty, Falls and Pain

It is interesting frailty and pain seem to coexist and are often present with increasing age (see Chapter 6 for a discussion of new perspectives on frailty in old age). Both pain and frailty increase the potential for falls, which can cause functional limitations, increased potential for dependence and ultimately death. A recent study from Spain of 1,505 older individuals highlighted those with frequent chronic pain were more likely to become frail. The risk of frailty increased as the number of pain sites increased. Furthermore, investigators found a higher pain intensity along with number of locations were linked to higher risk of exhaustion. Functional impairment, decreased quality of life, an increase in the potential for cognitive impairment and other comorbidities such as cardiovascular disease, lung disease, diabetes, musculoskeletal disease and depression are all associated with pain and frailty (Rodríguez-Sánchez et al., 2019).

Falling is common in community-dwelling older adults; about 5% of falls result in fractures. A recent systematic review of 71 papers by Stubbs et al. (2014) found the annual prevalence of recurrent falls in individuals reporting pain (12.9%) was higher than the pain-free control group (7.2%, $P < 0.001$) in a population of 9,581 older adults. Another study by Wade et al. (2017) explored data in the English Longitudinal Study of Ageing (waves 2 and 6) with an 8-year follow-up. A total of 5,316 participants provided data for the analysis. The authors concluded pain was associated with an increased risk and intensity of frailty in older men and women.

Socioeconomic factors contribute to the occurrence of frailty, although Wade et al.'s (2017) study was unable to demonstrate the relationship between pain and frailty. This is an area of research that receives much interest.

The work is clearly points toward some kind of relationship between pain, frailty and falls. With an increasing demographic of older adults and awareness poorly controlled chronic pain exists in 40% of the older population living in the community and 80% of those living in care homes (Schofield et al., 2020), more work to understand the pain, frailty, and falls relationship needs to be done. It is clear this is an issue to be addressed. Falls are life-limiting and life-threatening to older adults and costly to the health and social care system, so in order to prevent falls we should manage pain more effectively and maybe see a reduction in frailty as a consequence. As recommended by Rodríguez-Sánchez et al. (2019, p. 79), 'Future research should establish if effective pain management, especially within the context of chronic diseases, could reduce frailty risk'.

EXPERIENCE OF PAIN

We know pain is generally an unpleasant experience and requires attention or management. The experience of pain can interfere with normal daily function, and it may also affect thinking (Oosterman et al., 2013). Oosterman and colleagues assessed 22 younger and 24 older adults living with chronic pain and observed any possible association between pain and cognition may be moderated by age. They proposed pain has a reduced effect on cognitive performance as people age.

In a 2014 study of 79 older adults with osteoarthritis, no significant relationship between pain and executive (i.e., cognitive) function was noted (Morone et al., 2014). However, there is a possibility the ageing brain results in a corresponding decline in pain reporting (Cruz-Almeida et al., 2019).

What is apparent is people's experiences are unique. Older people report their pain experience from a cognitive, sensory, motivational or affective viewpoint, frequently in terms that relate the constraint of living with chronic pain (Gagliese et al., 2018; Schofield, 2018). The perception of pain may be stated using sensory terminology such as burning, stabbing and aching (Schofield, 2018), reflecting the unpleasant nature of pain. Motivational and emotional (i.e., affective) elements of the pain experience may relate to the limiting influence on activities of daily living (Dueñas et al., 2020). The cognitive aspect of pain includes the meaning people ascribe to their pain and the causal influences and other determinants or factors that inform the experience of pain.

The report of the individual experiencing pain may be considerably different from the report of the carer or health professional. In a study of older people and their family caregivers, the caregivers interviewed were more likely to think pain was inevitable in contrast with the older people, who were slightly more optimistic about their pain and its successful management (McPherson et al., 2014). Some of the participants did not want to 'bother' people with their pain, or they wanted to protect their family members from sharing in their pain and distress.

There is a tendency for older people's pain to be underrecognised and undertreated and sometimes dismissed. For older people living with cancer or in receipt of specialist palliative care, pain is a significant concern and may be of particular concern for those who have complex biopsychosocial needs (Dunham et al., 2013). The experiences of older people living with chronic pain post-cancer treatment were studied by Dunham et al. (2017). They noted older people's reluctance to report their pain; two of the themes identified were dislike of analgesia and denial of pain. For the older people studied, blaming their pain on old age was preferable to the possibility the pain was a sign of the cancer returning. The management of pain in end-of-life care is discussed in Chapter 34.

These interrelated aspects of the pain experience all inform behaviour and the report or expression of pain. Older people's descriptions of pain acknowledge it is more than a sensory experience and may include influencing variables such as culture, mood and prior pain experiences to inform the present.

ASSESSMENT OF PAIN

Melzack once said 'that to describe pain solely in terms of intensity is like specifying the visual world only in terms of light flux without regard to pattern, colour, texture, and the many other dimensions of visual experience' (Melzack & Wall, 1988, p. 37).

That suggests pain assessment is a complex process that should take a holistic perspective; it is not just about intensity. The first thing to consider is whether the pain is acute or chronic. The approach to assessment varies according to the type of pain. If the patient is in the emergency department with, for example, a fractured femur, the priority is to determine the intensity of pain and subsequently manage it to an acceptable level. In chronic pain, however, there is more time to carry out a comprehensive assessment before a management plan is developed.

Dame Cicely Saunders (1964) first espoused the concept of 'total pain'. It encompasses physical, psychological, spiritual and social aspects. Although it was originally developed for cancer pain, it is appropriate to apply to any type of pain. Below we consider each aspect.

Physical Aspect

Pain is an unpleasant sensory experience. Trauma or damage can cause a set of physiological responses, transmitting into the nervous system and up to the brain, where they are perceived as pain. We have discussed the particular issue that relates to the physiological experiences of the older adult. We also know the complexities surrounding the acute or chronic pain experience and how acute pain can have a physiological explanation, whereas chronic pain does not. We also know other important factors influence this experience, including age, gender, culture and social class, that need to be understood when assessing pain.

Age is a complex issue. Do younger or older adults feel more pain? Stoicism and expectations that pain is part of getting older are beliefs common among health professionals and older adults. In terms of gender, evidence in the literature demonstrates women are more likely to complain, a concept influenced by social norms during childhood and development (Myers et al., 2003). A recent study from Brazil highlighted that a higher degree of femininity or female social roles are associated with lower thresholds and less tolerance to pain along with an increased tendency to report pain. This is irrespective of pain type, ethnicity or sexual orientation (Nascimento et al., 2020). It has been many years since Zborowski (1952) highlighted the cultural responses to pain, but cultural differences and influences have been the focus of many researchers since that time, demonstrating vast cultural differences in how pain is perceived (Chan et al., 2011; Kolmar & Kamal, 2018; Leong et al., 2016), in particular end-of-life pain.

Psychological and Spiritual Aspect

Beliefs about pain and the meaning of the experience have the potential to influence how well an individual copes with pain. Modifying thoughts and beliefs is the key principle that underpins cognitive-behavioural approaches to pain management. Negative beliefs can impact willingness to seek help along with psychological well-being and functional ability. When an older adult stoically accepts pain as part of the normal ageing process, they also report loss of independence and control along with loneliness, disability and symptoms of depression (Ferreira et al., 2016; Makris et al., 2017; Miro et al., 2014; Nicholas et al., 2017; Tse et al., 2012).

Subsequently, these beliefs lead to a feeling of hopelessness that in turn impacts coping mechanisms. Fear-avoidance beliefs have been found to affect older adults' willingness to engage in pain treatment (Camacho-Soto et al., 2012; Holden et al., 2012), an important consideration for planning management strategies for older adults.

Social Aspect

Health inequalities are widely reported in the literature. It is well documented that people from Black and minority ethnic group communities often experience poorer health and more long-term health conditions than their White British counterparts (NHS England, 2016). Similarly, pain is frequently less well identified and managed in in people who are economically socially marginalised, including ethnic minorities and older people (Craig et al., 2020). These social inequalities persist into old age. Similarly, social isolation is well documented as an important factor reported by older adults with pain as a result of restricted social interaction, reduced activity and ability to engage in normal hobbies (Makris et al., 2014).

MEASUREMENT OF PAIN

Assessment refers to gaining a complete understanding of the total pain experience, not just intensity. A range of instruments and scales are used in health care research to measure pain or the effects of pain (Table 27.1).

These scales are often used to measure chronic pain experience in pain clinics. The research regarding reliability and validity is variable, and questionnaires can be time consuming to complete and analyse. Furthermore, the use of lengthy questionnaires can be burdensome for older adults to complete.

PAIN INTENSITY MEASURES

A number of pain scales have been well researched in practice and laboratory settings (Schofield, 2018).

Visual Analogue Scale

The visual analogue scale (Scott & Huskisson, 1979) consists of 10 cm line with 'no pain' at one end and 'worst pain imaginable' at the other. The patient is required to insert a

TABLE 27.1	Scales Used to Measure Pain or the Effects of Pain	
Quality-of-life tools	EORTC and EQ-5D comprise function and symptom scales, including pain (Devlin et al., 2018; Fredheim et al., 2007; Vartiainen et al., 2017)
Coping tools	Coping strategies questionnaire (Monticone et al., 2014)
Confidence/self-efficacy tools	(Cheng et al., 2020; Gaumer Erickson & Noonan, 2021)
Anxiety and depression scales	(Beck et al., 1996; Harris & Joyce, 2008; Turk et al., 2015)

line vertically through the horizontal line. This is the most reliable and valid scale for measuring pain intensity.

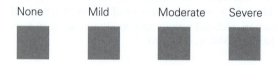

The distance is then measured and a pain score obtained. The scale should be applied horizontally, not vertically.

Though potentially helpful in measuring acute pain, as a two-dimensional graphic, the visual analogue scale does not allow for the holistic interpretation of the impact of chronic pain (Wewers & Lowe, 1990). Another issue is the user needs to have the visual acuity, manual dexterity and cognitive ability to support completion of the scale (Herr & Garand, 2001).

Verbal Descriptors

The verbal descriptors scale (Gracely & Dubner, 1987) consists of a series of boxes that indicate a level of pain.

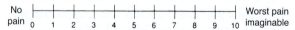

Descriptors of pain intensity are useful, but the words may have a different meaning to each person. Unlike numeric values, the difference between mild and moderate is not the same as that between moderate and severe, so attribution and appreciation of pain magnitude is subjective (Jensen et al., 2017). It's important to have only the four options as too many can be confusing for the patient. You can simply ask, 'Is your pain, none, mild, moderate or severe?'

Numerical Rating Scale

This numerical rating scale (Jensen et al., 2003) is essentially the visual analogue scale with numbers along the scale.

The numerical rating scale is quite easy to use, although it has been suggested patients tend to mark nearest a number, thus not giving a true reading (Ware et al., 2006). Also, it may not be suitable for people with cognitive impairment. As with other linear scales, it does not identify the many aspects of the lived experience of pain, which would be identified using a thorough nursing assessment.

These are the most commonly used scales with adults. The brief pain inventory was developed for use with cancer pain and has subsequently been validated in multiple languages and contexts and for older people (Cleeland & Ryan 1994; Ersek et al., 2006; Tan et al., 2004). Other scales, including the Faces scale, tend to be used with children and are not appropriate for older adults (Kim & Buschmann, 2006).

The best scales for working with older adults are the verbal descriptors and the numerical rating scale (Schofield, 2018). They can be used in older adults with no, mild or moderate cognitive impairment and are interchangeable, so if the patient does not understand the concept of the verbal rating scale, you can switch to the numerical rating scale.

Box 27.1 describes some key considerations when using pain scales with older adults.

BOX 27.1   Key Considerations When Using Pain Scales With Older Adults

1. Direct enquiry about the presence of pain
   - Including the use of alternative words to describe pain
2. Observation for signs of pain
   - Especially in older people with cognitive or communication impairment
3. Description of pain to include:
   a) Sensory dimension
      - Nature of the pain (e.g., sharp, dull, burning, etc.)
      - Pain location and radiation (e.g., by patients pointing to the pain on themselves or by using a pain map)
      - Intensity, using a standardised pain assessment scale
   b) Affective dimension
      - Emotional response to pain (e.g., fear, anxiety, depression)
      - Impact: Disabling effects of pain at the level of functional activities (e.g., activities of daily living)
      - Participation (e.g., work, social activities, relationships)
4. Measurement of pain
   - Using standardised scales in a format that is accessible to the individual
5. Identifying the cause of pain
   - Examination for tender areas and investigation (e.g., using X-rays, blood tests) to establish the cause of pain (Hadjistavropoulos et al., 2007)
6. Whichever scale is selected:
   Listen carefully. What words are used?
   - The patient may deny pain but admit to discomfort, aching, soreness using local language
   - Do you hurt anywhere?
   - Are you uncomfortable?
   - How does it affect you?
   - Believe the patient.
7. Record the pain regularly.
   - Depending on the type/cause of pain, act on the pain score and monitor the effects of interventions.

Communication of Pain

Fordyce (1976) highlighted the concept of pain behaviours. These behaviours can be verbal (e.g., verbal descriptions of the intensity, location and quality of pain; vocalisations of distress; moaning or complaining) or non-verbal (e.g., withdrawing from activities, taking pain medication, pain-related body postures or facial expressions). Recognition of these behaviours resulted in the introduction of the operant model of pain management, which later led to the cognitive-behavioural model (Tang, 2018). Pain behaviours have informed the development of many of the pain assessment tools used with older adults with cognitive impairments. Behavioural indicators can be classed as intuitive signs.

- Facial expression (e.g., grimace)
- Verbal expression (e.g., groaning, moaning)
- Protected position (e.g., rigid, limited movement)
- Restlessness or agitation
- Physiological signs (e.g., clammy, sweating, pale, elevated blood pressure, tachycardia)

Any patient who displays changes in behaviour, including the above indicators, could indicate they are experiencing pain. These are simple signs to note. Physiological signs occur only in acute pain and cannot be relied on to assess chronic pain. Ahn and Horgas (2013) explored nursing home residents in Florida (n = 56,577) and concluded those with severe pain were less likely to wander but more likely to display aggressive and agitated behaviours.

Evidence for Pain-Assessment Scales

A recent systematic review identified the most appropriate pain assessment scales for use with older people (Schofield, 2018). In terms of behavioural pain assessment scales, 12 scales were identified:

- Abbey
- PAINAD
- Pain assessment scale for seniors with severe dementia
- Disability distress scale
- Pade
- Universal pain assessment tool
- Doloplus
- NoPain
- Checklist of nonverbal pain indicators
- Assessment of discomfort in dementia
- Mobilization-observation-behavior-intensity-dementia pain scale
- COOP

In 2007 the United Kingdom's national guidelines for chronic pain management in older people recommended the use of the Abbey pain or Doloplus scale. Both scales

BOX 27.2	Commonly Used Behavioural Pain Scales
Abbey pain scale	https://www.aci.health.nsw.gov.au/__data/assets/pdf_file/0018/212922/Abbey_Pain_Scale_Final.pdf
PAINAD	http://dementiapathways.ie/_filecache/04a/ddd/98-painad.pdf
Doloplus	http://www.doloplus.fr/en/the-doloplus-scale

had fairly good evidence supporting their use and were simple and quick to complete (Collett et al., 2007). However, there has been no further research to support the development or adaptation of the Abbey pain scale. The recommendation from the 2018 United Kingdom guidelines for pain assessment in older people is the Doloplus or PainAd scale, as they now have more evidence (Jordan et al., 2011; Pickering et al., 2010; Schofield, 2018). However, the Abbey scale is still popular in care settings, perhaps because familiarity and ease of use (Corbett et al., 2016).

See Box 27.2 for details on these scales, which have similar properties. Interestingly, recent survey studies across Europe demonstrated these scales are not widely used in practice (Giménez-Llort et al., 2020; Zwakhalen et al., 2018) indicating more work needs to be done in terms of implementation. One approach to improving pain assessment in practice is the development of the Pain Assessment app, which incorporates a pain algorithm or pathway and the Abbey pain scale. It was evaluated with paramedics and proved positive at helping quickly and efficiently diagnose pain in older adults with dementia (Docking et al., 2018).

It's important to assess pain, regardless of age or cognitive ability. A number of validated pain scales can be used to measure intensity, including some well-validated behavioural pain scales. When carrying out pain assessment, it is important to be respectful to the cultural needs of older adults, be patient, change your language to match the person you are with and trust your intuition. If you think pain is present, it probably is. Communicate with formal and informal carers. They can be a good source of information. Act on the pain score, manage the pain and reassess the impact of your intervention. Remember these scales provide information on only one aspect of pain. Other important factors to consider include the quality, location, distribution and impact of the pain on quality of life, mood, function and coping.

BARRIERS TO ASSESSMENT AND MANAGEMENT

We know pain is poorly assessed and managed in the older population. This is not something specific to the United Kingdom. Studies across Europe also report this as an issue. For example, Zwakhalen et al. (2018) undertook a survey that included nurses, health care and social care workers in seven countries (n = 415 responses, UK n = 28, Netherlands n = 139, Germany n = 147, Denmark n = 9, Belgium n = 35, Switzerland n = 18, Austria n = 39) and reported the following results:

- Only 25% of respondents used guidelines.
- Different scales were used across countries.
- There was dissatisfaction about the current knowledge of pain assessment in cognitively impaired older adults.
- There seemed to be an international struggle to interpret findings of the observational pain scales available.

Almost half the staff were in hospital settings (48.5%). Similar results were found in a survey of Spanish older people (Giménez-Llort et al., 2020). Another study looked at residents and staff in care homes (Schofield, 2006) and highlighted the following themes:

- Reluctance to report pain
- Acceptance that being in pain is normal
- Low expectation from medical interventions
- Fear of chemical/pharmacological interventions
- Age-related perceptions of pain
- Lack of awareness of potential strategies

However, for older people from Black and ethnic minority backgrounds, a small but growing body of evidence supports the need to address disparities of care provision; these disparities extend to appreciation of the prevalence, management and consideration of pain-related conditions (Burton & Shaw, 2015; Campbell & Edwards, 2012).

A number of guidelines have been implemented around the world (e.g., United States, Australia, United Kingdom), but clearly the results of previous studies suggest they are not being implemented. A study by Tai-Seale et al. (2011) looked at the reasons behind poor implementation of national guidelines and suggested from a review of the literature there are three main reasons:

- Reluctance of the older person to discuss their pain; pain is to be expected or the person does not want to be labelled a complainer (Pautex & Gold, 2006).
- Gender and racial disparities: Women were given less opioids than men (McDonald, 1994); Black and minority ethnic patients were prescribed less analgesia; physicians' perceptions of minority patients regarding drug-seeking behaviour (Martin, 2000)

- Hot-cold empathy gap: The physician does not understand the behaviour of the patient, thus underestimates the behaviour and therefore undertreats it (Loewenstein, 2005)

Tai-Seale et al. (2011) recorded 385 primary care physician interactions with patients and noted the following about discussions regarding pain with older adults:

- 2–3 minutes duration
- 48% of visits to GP involved pain discussion
- Gender and race influenced discussion
- Physician effect
- Severity of pain
- Time constraints

With time constraints pain assessment is difficult and challenging. These barriers recur throughout the literature, suggesting governments need to urgently address the lack of education of all health professionals to equip them with the tools and skills to assess pain efficiently and manage it effectively.

Painchek® is one recent commercially produced approach which uses artificial intelligence to assess the micro-facial features of pain for older adults who do not reliably report their pain. This is gaining popularity, but more research needs to be done to assess its effectiveness, usefulness and acceptability. See: https://www.painchek.com/uk/.

MANAGEMENT AND INTERVENTION

What should pain management for older people consist of? The first and most important consideration is what is meant by 'old'. The definition of older people varies depending on context; age may be chronological or physiologically determined (Gagliese & Melzack, 1997). The use of the term *elderly* is both pejorative and problematic; clearly the risk of some health disorders increases with age. The general principles of pain management are similar across adult populations, with the physiological health of the individual being the most important influencing factor. A major risk for older people is people with cognitive impairment or communication problems are at greater risk of under treatment. An overcautious approach to treatment initiatives based solely on chronological age may deny people optimum treatment (Pickering et al., 2006).

Ageing is a major risk factor for many chronic systemic diseases. As people age the potential for living with multiple comorbidities increases (Tracy & Morrison, 2013). However, cellular decline, or senescence, is affected by many factors, including diet, exercise and environment, not just chronological age.

Pharmacological Management

The neurological changes of ageing, including some reduced sensitivity at the pain-receptor level, may be a factor in considering which approach to pain management is indicated (Cole et al., 2010). Another important factor, alongside other physiological changes, is renal and hepatic health, which should inform medication dose and monitoring (see Chapter 31 for a more detailed discussion). Some groups of analgesic drugs are contraindicated regardless of age for individuals living with renal failure, cardiovascular disease and other chronic disease (Mercadante, 2015). Cognitive decline may limit engagement with treatment benefits or adverse effects. Prescribing for older people can be a challenging proposition. There is limited data to support the effective use of analgesic drugs in older populations because of the lack of uniformity in ageing populations, and individuals over 60 have largely been excluded from clinical drug trials (Crome et al., 2011).

There are different approaches to pain prescribing, depending on the type of pain. Analgesics for people with acute pain are generally not effective for people with chronic pain. Classifications of analgesics fall into three broad categories: opioids, non-opioids and adjuvant drugs. Paracetamol in particular is an effective non-opioid analgesic and is generally considered a safer alternative to non-steroidal anti-inflammatory drugs such as ibuprofen. However, both are regarded unsuitable for long-term use in chronic pain (Altman, 2010; Roberts et al., 2016).

Opioids can be described as strong or weak because of their effect at the nociceptor (i.e., opioid) receptor sites and their metabolised state after passing through the gut and liver (Mercadante, 2015). A growing number of synthetic opioids and other drugs mimic some of the effects of opioids, often called partial agonists (Karila et al., 2019). However, the use of opioids in older people is controversial and sometimes excessively cautious (Spitz et al., 2011).

Prescribing of analgesia for acute pain has largely followed the three-step World Health Organisation analgesia ladder, with opioids as the top tier of treatment. However, given current concern for opioid misuse, the strategy of using a multimodal approach is now widely accepted (American Geriatrics Society, 2009; Ng & Cashman, 2018). The multimodal approach proposes a combination of analgesics for acute pain, minimising the need for opioids.

The use of specific opioids for older people may be beneficial for acute pain only if used in the short term (Chaparro et al., 2013). In low doses, morphine has been demonstrated to be a useful opioid for biomechanical pain (Lee et al., 2015). Codeine, a weak opioid, may be useful when combined with paracetamol for non-cancer pain such as osteoarthritis (Conaghan et al., 2011). However, adverse cardiac events have been noted in older people taking codeine. Buprenorphine, a synthetic opioid administered via transdermal patch, may have some usefulness for chronic pain in older people (Plosker, 2011). Recommendations for analgesia urge greater caution in the use of opioids for the management of chronic pain (Faculty of Pain Medicine, 2009).

Adjuvant medication such as antidepressants and anticonvulsants is more frequently recommended for chronic pain (National Institute for Health and Care Excellence, 2020). However, both groups of drugs have an array of side effects that may be more pronounced in older people. The tricyclic antidepressants may cause dry mouth, blurred vision, constipation, confusion, sedation and delirium, among others. The anticonvulsants have a similarly long list of potential side effects, including sedation and drowsiness, with gabapentin and pregabalin having the fewest adverse events (National Institute for Health and Care Excellence, 2016). However, caution for individuals with renal impairment is advised because of their limited hepatic metabolism (Fleet, 2018).

Non-Pharmacological Management

Pharmacological solutions may be only partially effective, so other options should be available to complement existing regimes. Non-pharmacological strategies may be useful where drug interventions are ineffective or identified as clinically inappropriate. Non-pharmacological management methods include physical, psychological and psychosocial approaches to manage pain (Abdulla et al., 2013). Health professionals may be able to offer advice and support for engagement with a variety of non-pharmacological strategies or complementary therapies, including exercise, relaxation techniques, imagery, manual therapies and stimulation such as art or music therapy.

Keeping active and engaging with exercise on a regular basis can be a considerable factor in the prevention of pain (Geneen et al., 2015). However, there are still relatively few studies of exercise as an intervention for older people with pain (Geneen et al., 2015; Hasegawa et al., 2013; Irandoust & Taheri, 2015; Nicholas et al., 2013; Tse et al., 2013; Tse et al., 2014). If exercise is an option, the primary consideration must be the capacity, utility and preference of the individual. Exercise can be a social activity; engagement with others as well as the exercise regime may be an important factor in an older person's engagement with any recommended activity.

Psychological strategies are founded in the understanding of adverse psychological influences on pain experience. In a recent systematic review, behavioural therapies were found to have a small effect on older people (de C Williams et al., 2020). Cognitive behavioural therapy for older people has a small but growing evidence base (Andersson et al., 2012; Broderick et al., 2016; Nicholas et al., 2017). Similarly, evidence for pain management programmes is scant, but they may be beneficial (Darchuk et al., 2010; Eccleston et al., 2016; Ehrenbrusthoff et al., 2012).

THE POST-PANDEMIC WORLD

There is no doubt the impact of COVID-19 has been highly significant around the world, with no country escaping a level of infection. As a result of self-isolation and lockdown, patients have been unable to seek help for their chronic pain problems, and many surgical procedures have been postponed. Furthermore, redeployment of many pain clinic staff into intensive care and COVID-19 wards impacted pain services. We don't know at this stage what the impact of long COVID-19 will be, with many reports of diverse problems from the disease. Originally it was believed respiratory symptoms were a result, but we are now learning of other sequalae and even the suggestion of an increase in chronic pain (Matielo-Alonson et al., 2021). The pandemic focused the minds of health professionals to adopt new ways of delivering services, which is exciting. We are seeing online services, ehealth and mhealth being introduced and patients more engaged with these approaches.

NURSING REFLECTIONS

The past 30 years has seen major changes in the management of pain across the United Kingdom and the rest of the world. We have seen an increasing recognition of the need for a multidisciplinary approach to pain management and with that the unique contribution of the nurse as the patient advocate. Pain assessment is now widely recognised as being fundamental to the whole pain management process and is largely implemented in clinical areas by nursing staff on the frontline of care. Increasingly, we have seen nurses take on the role of care delivery, prescribing drugs for their patients and taking on other roles such as delivering acupuncture and self-management training. This is an exciting time for nurses in the field and an opportunity for advanced roles as long as they don't lose sight of the important contribution of nursing as the patient advocate.

CONCLUSION

Effective management of pain is a basic human right and limited only by our own knowledge. It is the responsibility of the nurse to advocate for the individual needs of the patient regardless of age, gender or sociocultural background.

KEY LEARNING POINTS

- Diagnosis and management of pain should always be informed by an individualised holistic assessment.
- Listening to the person's needs and taking account of their personal and family circumstances and general well-being is of utmost importance.
- The nurse, as part of a multidisciplinary health and social care team, has an important part to play in building a trusting relationship with older adults to enable an understanding of the experience of pain and appreciate the unique way pain affects a person's life.
- The nursing role as advocate for the person living with pain is fundamental to good pain management practice.
- The nurse can direct, support and sustain good care that enhances quality of life and supports independence by addressing the needs of older adults in pain.

REFERENCES

Abdulla, A., Adams, N., Bone M, Elliott, A. M., Gaffin, J., Jones, D., et al. (2013). Guidance on the management of pain in older people. *Age and Ageing, 42*(Suppl 1), 1–57.

Age UK. (2019). Falls in later life: a huge concern of older people. https://www.ageuk.org.uk/latest-press/articles/2019/may/falls-in-later-life-a-huge-concern-for-older-people/

Ahn, H., & Horgas, A. (2013). The relationship between pain and disruptive behaviors in nursing home resident with dementia. *BMC Geriatrics, 13*(1), 14.

Altman, R. D. (2010). Pharmacological therapies for osteoarthritis of the hand. *Drugs & Aging, 27*(9), 729–745.

American Geriatrics Society Panel on Persistent Pain in Older Persons. (2009). Pharmacological management of persistent pain in older persons. *Journal of the American Geriatrics Society, 57*, 1331–1346.

Andersson, G., Johansson, C., Nordlander, A., & Asmundson, G. J. (2012). Chronic pain in older adults: A controlled pilot trial of a brief cognitive-behavioural group treatment. *Behavioural and Cognitive Psychotherapy, 40*(2), 239–244.

Beck, A. T., Steer, R. A., & Brown, G. K. (1996). Beck depression inventory (BDI-II)10: Pearson, Article s15327752j-pa6703_13. https://www.ismanet.org/doctoryourspirit/pdfs/Beck-Depression-Inventory-BDI.pdf.

Brattberg, G., Parker, M. G., & Thorslund, M. (1996). The prevalence of pain among the oldest old in Sweden. *Pain, 67*(1), 29–34.

Broderick J. E., Keefe F. J., Schneider S., Junghaenel D. U., Bruckenthal P., Schwartz J. E., et al. (2016). Cognitive behavioral therapy for chronic pain is effective, but for whom? *Pain,* 157(9):2115–2123. doi: 10.1097/j.pain.0000000000000626. PMID: 27227692.

Burton, A. E., & Shaw, R. L. (2015). Pain management programmes for non-English-speaking black and minority ethnic groups with long-term or chronic pain. *Musculoskeletal Care, 13*(4), 187–203.

Bushnell, M. C., Čeko, M., & Low, L. A. (2013). Cognitive and emotional control of pain and its disruption in chronic pain. *Nature Reviews Neuroscience, 14*(7), 502–511.

Camacho-Soto, A., Sowa, G. A., Perera, S., & Weiner, D. K. (2012). Fear avoidance beliefs predict disability in older adults with chronic low back pain. *Physical Medicine and Rehabilitation, 4*(7), 493–497.

Campbell, C. M., & Edwards, R. R. (2012). Ethnic differences in pain and pain management. *Pain Management, 2*(3), 219–230. https://doi.org/10.2217/pmt.12.7.

Chang, C. C., & Wang, S. S. (2007). Acute abdominal pain in the elderly. *International Journal of Gerontology, 1*(2), 77–82.

Chaparro, L. E., Furlan, A. D., Deshpande, A., Mailis-Gagnon, A., Atlas, S., & Turk, D. C. (2013). Opioids compared to placebo or other treatments for chronic low-back pain. *Cochrane Database of Systematic Reviews, 8*, 1465–1858. https://doi.org/10.1002/14651858.CD004959.pub4.

Cimas, M., Ayala, A., Sanz, B., Agulló-Tomás, M. S., Escobar, A., & Forjaz, M. J. (2018). Chronic musculoskeletal pain in European older adults: Cross-national and gender differences. *European Journal of Pain, 22*(2), 333–345.

Chan, W. L., Hui, E., Chan, C., Cheung, D., Wong, S., Wong, R., Li, S., et al. (2011). Evaluation of chronic disease self-management programme (CDSMP) for older adults in Hong Kong. *The Journal of Nutrition, Health & Aging, 15*(3), 209–214.

Cheng, S. T., Chen, P. P., Chow, Y. F., Chung, J. W., Law, A. C., Lee, J. S., et al. (2020). Developing a short multidimensional measure of pain self-efficacy: The chronic pain self-efficacy scale-short form. *The Gerontologist, 60*(3), e127–e136.

Cleeland, C. S., & Ryan, K. M. (1994). Pain assessment: Global use of the Brief Pain Inventory. *Annals, Academy of Medicine, Singapore, 23*(2), 129–138.

Cole, L. J., Farrell, M. J., Gibson, S. J., & Egan, G. F. (2010). Age-related differences in pain sensitivity and regional brain activity evoked by noxious pressure. *Neurobiology of Aging, 31*(3), 494–503.

Collett, B., O'Mahoney, S., Schofield, P., Closs, S. J., & Potter, J. (2007). The assessment of pain in older people. *Clinical Medicine, 7*(5), 496.

Crome, P., Lally, F., Cherubini, A., Oristrell, J., Beswick, A. D., Clarfield, A. M., et al. (2011). Exclusion of older people from clinical trials. *Drugs & Aging, 28*(8), 667–677.

Conaghan, P. G., O'Brien, C. M., Wilson, M., & Schofield, J. P. (2011). Transdermal buprenorphine plus oral paracetamol vs an oral codeine-paracetamol combination for osteoarthritis of hip and/or knee: a randomised trial. *Osteoarthritis and Cartilage, 19*(8), 930–938.

Corbett, A., Nunez, K. M., Smeaton, E., Testad, I., Thomas, A. J., Closs, S. J., et al. (2016). The landscape of pain management in people with dementia living in care homes: A mixed methods study. *International Journal of Geriatric Psychiatry, 31*(12), 1354–1370.

Craig, K. D., Holmes, C., Hudspith, M., Moor, G., Moosa-Mitha, M., Varcoe, C., et al. (2020). Pain in persons who are marginalized by social conditions. *Pain, 161*(2), 261–265.

Cruz-Almeida, Y., Fillingim, R. B., Riley, J. L., III, Woods, A. J., Porges, E., Cohen, R., et al. (2019). Chronic pain is associated with a brain aging biomarker in community-dwelling older adults. *Pain, 160*(5), 1119–1130.

Darchuk, K. M., Townsend, C. O., Rome, J. D., Bruce, B. K., & Hooten, W. M. (2010). Longitudinal treatment outcomes for geriatric patients with chronic non-cancer pain at an interdisciplinary pain rehabilitation program. *Pain Medicine, 11*(9), 1352–1364.

Darnall, B. D., Carr, D. B., & Schatman, M. E. (2017). Pain psychology and the biopsychosocial model of pain treatment: ethical imperatives and social responsibility. *Pain Medicine, 18*(8), 1413–1415.

de C Williams, A. C., Fisher, E., Hearn, L., & Eccleston, C. (2020). Psychological therapies for the management of chronic pain (excluding headache) in adults. *Cochrane Database of Systematic Reviews, 8*(8):CD007407.

Devlin, N. J., Shah, K. K., Feng, Y., Mulhern, B., & van Hout, B. (2018). Valuing health-related quality of life: An EQ-5 D-5 L value set for England. *Health Economics, 27*(1), 7–22.

Docking, R. E., Lane, M., & Schofield, P. A. (2018). Usability testing of the iPhone app to improve pain assessment for older adults with cognitive impairment (Prehospital Setting): A qualitative study. *Pain Medicine, 19*(6), 1121–1131.

Dueñas, M., Salazar, A., de Sola, H., & Failde, I. (2020). Limitations in activities of daily living in people with chronic pain: Identification of groups using clusters analysis. *Pain Practice, 20*(2), 179–187.

Dunham, M., Allmark, P., & Collins, K. (2017). Older people's experiences of cancer pain: A qualitative study nursing older people. *Nursing Older People, 29*(6), 28–32.

Dunham, M., Ingleton, C., Ryan, T., & Gott, M. (2013). A narrative literature review of older people's cancer pain experience. *Journal of Clinical Nursing, 22*(15–16), 2100–2113.

Dunham.M., Schofield, P. A., & Knaggs, R. (2020). Evidence-based clinical practice guidelines on the management of pain in older people—a summary report. *British Journal of Pain, 16*(1), 6–13.

Ehrenbrusthoff, K., Ryan, C. G., Schofield, P. A., & Martin, D. J. (2012). Physical therapy management of older adults with chronic low back pain: a systematic review. *Journal of Pain Management, 5*(4), 317–329.

Eccleston, C., Tabor, A., Edwards, R. T., & Keogh, E. (2016). Psychological approaches to coping with pain in later life. *Clinics in Geriatric Medicine, 32*, 763–771.

Eggermont, L. H., Bean, J. F., Guralnik, J. M., & Leveille, S. G. (2009). Comparing pain severity versus pain location in the MOBILIZE Boston study: chronic pain and lower extremity function. *Journals of Gerontology Series A: Biomedical Sciences and Medical Sciences, 64*(7), 763–770.

Ersek, M., Turner, J. A., & Kemp, C. A. (2006). Use of the chronic pain coping inventory to assess older adults' pain coping strategies. *The Journal of Pain, 7*(11), 833–842.

Faculty of Pain Medicine. (2009). Opioids aware: A resource for patients and healthcare professionals to support prescribing of opioid medicines for pain. *Royal College of Anaesthetists.* https://www.rcoa.ac.uk/faculty-of-pain-medicine/opioids-aware.

Farrell, M. J. (2012). Age-related changes in the structure and function of brain regions involved in pain processing. *Pain Medicine, 13*(Suppl. 2), S37–S43.

Fenyö, G. (1982). Acute abdominal disease in the elderly: Experience from two series in Stockholm. *The American Journal of Surgery, 143*(6), 751–754.

Ferreira, K., Bastos, T., & de Andrade, D. (2016). Prevalence of chronic pain in a metropolitan area of a developing country: a population-based study. *Arquivos de Neuro-Psiquiatria, 74*(12), 990–998.

Fleet, J. L., Dixon, S. N., Kuwornu, P. J., Dev, V. K., Montero-Odasso, M., Burneo, J., & Garg, A. X. (2018). Gabapentin dose and the 30-day risk of altered mental status in older adults: A retrospective population-based study. *PloS One, 13*(3), e0193134.

Fletcher, D., Stamer, U. M., Pogatzki-Zahn, E., Zaslansky, R., Tanase, N. V., Perruchoud, C., et al. (2015). Chronic post-surgical pain in Europe: An observational study. *European Journal of Anaesthesiology, 32*(10), 725–734.

Fordyce, W. E. (1976). *Behavioral methods for chronic pain and illness.* CV Mosby.

Fredheim, O. M. S., Borchgrevink, P. C., Saltnes, T., & Kaasa, S. (2007). Validation and comparison of the health-related quality-of-life instruments EORTC QLQ-C30 and SF-36 in assessment of patients with chronic nonmalignant pain. *Journal of Pain and Symptom Management, 34*(6), 657–665. https://doi.org/10.1016/j.jpainsymman.2007.01.011.

Gagliese, L., Gauthier, L. R., Narain, N., & Freedman, T. (2018). Pain, aging and dementia: Towards a biopsychosocial model. *Progress in Neuro-Psychopharmacology and Biological Psychiatry, 87,* 207–215.

Gagliese, L., Jovellanos, M., Zimmermann, C., Shobbrook, C., Warr, D., & Rodin, G. (2009). Age-related patterns in adaptation to cancer pain: A mixed-method study. *Pain Medicine, 10*(6), 1050–1061.

Gagliese, L., & Melzack, R. (1997). Chronic pain in elderly people. *Pain, 70,* 3–14.

Gaumer Erickson, A. S., & Noonan, P. M. (2021). Self-efficacy assessment suite: Technical report. *College & Career Competency Framework.* http://www.researchcollaboration.org/uploads/Self-EfficacyQuestionnaireInfo.pdf.

Geneen, L. J., Martin, D. J., Adams, N., Clarke, C., Dunbar, M., Jones, D., et al. (2015). Effects of education to facilitate knowledge about chronic pain for adults: A systematic review with meta-analysis. *Systematic Reviews, 4*(1), 132.

Geva, N., Pruessner, J., & Defrin, R. (2014). Acute psychosocial stress reduces pain modulation capabilities in healthy men. *Pain, 155*(11), 2418–2425.

Gibson, S. J., & Lussier, D. (2012). Prevalence and relevance of pain in older persons. *Pain Medicine, 13*(Suppl. 2), S23–S26.

Gibson, S. J., & Weiner, D. K. (2005). *Pain in older persons*: ASP Press.

Gillis, N. K., Arslanian-Engoren, C., & Struble, L. M. (2014). Acute coronary syndromes in older adults: A review of literature. *Journal of Emergency Nursing, 40*(3), 270–275.

Giménez-Llort, L., Bernal, M. L., Docking, R., Muntsant-Soria, A., Torres-Lista, V., Bulbena, A., et al. (2020). Pain in older adults with dementia: A survey in Spain. *Frontiers in Neurology, 11.* doi:10.3389/fneur.2020.592366.

Glare, P., Aubrey, K. R., & Myles, P. S. (2019). Transition from acute to chronic pain after surgery. *The Lancet, 393*(10180), 1537–1546.

Goch, A., Misiewicz, P., Rysz, J., & Banach, M. (2009). The clinical manifestation of myocardial infarction in elderly patients. *Clinical Cardiology: An International Indexed and Peer-Reviewed Journal for Advances in the Treatment of Cardiovascular Disease, 32*(6), E45–E50.

González-Roldán, A. M., Terrasa, J. L., Sitges, C., van der Meulen, M., Anton, F., & Montoya, P. (2020). Age-related changes in pain perception are associated with altered functional connectivity during resting state. *Frontiers in Aging Neuroscience, 12,* 116.

Gracely, R. H., & Dubner, R. (1987). Reliability and validity of verbal descriptor scales of painfulness. *Pain, 29*(2), 175–185.

Hadjistavropoulos, T., Herr, K., Turk, D. C., Fine, P. G., Dworkin, R. H., Helme, R., et al. (2007). An interdisciplinary expert consensus statement on assessment of pain in older persons. *The Clinical Journal of Pain, 23,* S1–S43.

Harris, C. A., & Joyce, L. D. (2008). Psychometric properties of the Beck Depression Inventory-(BDI-II) in individuals with chronic pain. *Pain, 137*(3), 609–622.

Hasegawa, M., Yamazaki, S., Kimura, M., Nakano, K., & Yasumura, S. (2013). Community-based exercise program reduces chronic knee pain in elderly Japanese women at high risk of requiring long-term care: A non-randomized controlled trial. *Geriatrics & Gerontology International, 13*(1), 167–174.

Herr, K. A., & Garand, L. (2001). Assessment and measurement of pain in older adults. *Clinics in Geriatric Medicine, 17*(3), 457–478. https://doi.org/10.1016/s0749-0690(05)70080-x.

Hübscher, M., Vogt, L., Schmidt, K., Fink, M., & Banzer, W. (2010). Perceived pain, fear of falling and physical function in women with osteoporosis. *Gait & Posture, 32*(3), 383–385.

Huskisson, E. C. (1974). Measurement of pain. *The Lancet, 304*(7889), 1127–1131. https://doi.org/10.1016/S0140-6736(74)90884-8.

Holden, M. A, Nicholls, E. E., Young, J., Hay, E. M., & Foster, N. E. (2012). Role of exercise for knee pain: What do older adults in the community think?. *Arthritis Care Research, 64*(10), 1554–1564.

Irandoust, K., & Taheri, M. (2015). The effects of aquatic exercise on body composition and nonspecific low back pain in elderly males. *Journal of Physical Therapy Science, 27*(2), 433–435.

Jensen, M. P., Keefe, F. J., Lefebvre, J. C., Romano, J. M., & Turner, J. A. (2003). One-and two-item measures of pain beliefs and coping strategies. *Pain, 104*(3), 453–469.

Jensen, M. P., Tomé-Pires, C., de la Vega, R., Galán, S., Solé, E., & Miró, J. (2017). What determines whether a pain is rated as mild, moderate, or severe? The importance of pain beliefs and pain interference. *The Clinical Journal of Pain, 33*(5), 414–421. https://doi.org/10.1097/AJP.0000000000000429.

Jordan, A., Hughes, J., Pakresi, M., Hepburn, S., & O'Brien, J. T (2011). The utility of PAINAD in assessing pain in a UK population with severe dementia. *International Journal of Geriatric Psychiatry, 26*(2), 118–126.

Karila, L., Marillier, M., Chaumette, B., Billieux, J., Franchitto, N., & Benyamina, A. (2019). New synthetic opioids: Part of a new addiction landscape. *Neuroscience & Biobehavioral Reviews, 106*, 133–140.

Karp, J. F., Shega, J. W., Morone, N. E., & Weiner, D. K. (2008). Advances in understanding the mechanisms and management of persistent pain in older adults. *British Journal of Anaesthesia, 101*(1), 111–120.

Kim, E. J., & Buschmann, M. T. (2006). Reliability and validity of the Faces Pain Scale with older adults. *International Journal of Nursing Studies, 43*(4), 447–456.

Kolmar, A., & Kamal, A. H. (2018). Developing a path to improve cultural competency in Islam among palliative care professionals. *Journal of Pain and Symptom Management, 55*(3), e1–e3.

Kuner, R., & Flor, H. (2017). Structural plasticity and reorganisation in chronic pain. *Nature Reviews Neuroscience, 18*(1), 20.

Lautenbacher, S. (2012). Experimental approaches in the study of pain in the elderly. *Pain Medicine, 3*(Suppl. 2), S44–S50.

Lautenbacher, S., Peters, J. H., Heesen, M., Scheel, J., & Kunz, M. (2017). Age changes in pain perception: A systematic-review and meta-analysis of age effects on pain and tolerance thresholds. *Neuroscience & Biobehavioral Reviews, 75*, 104–113.

Lee, J., Lakha, S. F., & Mailis, A. (2015). Efficacy of low-dose oral liquid morphine for elderly patients with chronic non-cancer pain: Retrospective chart review. *Drugs-Real World Outcomes, 2*(4), 369–376.

Lenze, E. J., Mulsant, B. H., Shear, M. K., Schulberg, H. C., Dew, M. A., Begley, A. E., et al. (2000). Comorbid anxiety disorders in depressed elderly patients. *American Journal of Psychiatry, 157*(5), 722–728.

Leong, M., Olnick, S., Akmal, T., Copenhaver, A., & Razzak, R. (2016). How Islam influences end-of-life care: education for palliative care clinicians. *Journal of Pain and Symptom Management, 52*(6), 771–774.

Loewenstein, G. (2005). Hot-cold empathy gaps and medical decision making. *Health Psychology, 24*(4S), S49–S56.

Makris, U. E., Abrams, R. C., Gurland, B., & Reid, M. C. (2014). Management of persistent pain in the older patient: A clinical review. *Journal of the American Medical Association, 312*(8), 825–836.

Makris, U. E., Higashi, R. T., Marks, E. G., Fraenkel, L., Gill, T. M., Friedly, J. L., et al. (2017). Physical, emotional, and social impacts of restricting back pain in older adults: A qualitative study. *Pain Medicine, 18*(7), 1225–1235.

Martin, M. L (2000). Ethnicity and analgesic practice: an editorial. *Annals of Emergency Medicine, 35*(1), 77–79.

Martin, R. R., Hadjistavropoulos, T., & McCreary, D. R. (2005). Fear of pain and fear of falling among younger and older adults with musculoskeletal pain conditions. *Pain Research and Management, 10*(4), 211–218.

Matielo-Alonson, H., da Silva Oliveiro, V. R., de Oliveiro, V. T., & Dale, C. S (2021). Pain in COVID era. *Frontiers in Physiology*. https://doi.org/10.3389/fphys.2021.624154.

McCaffery M. (1968). Nursing practice theories related to cognition, bodily pain, and man-environment interactions. Los Angeles: UCLA Students Store.

McDonald, D. D. (1994). Gender and ethnic stereotyping and narcotic analgesic administration. *Research in Nursing & Health, 17*(1), 45–49.

McPherson, C. J., Hadjistavropoulos, T., Devereaux, A., & Lobchuk, M. M. (2014). A qualitative investigation of the roles and perspectives of older patients with advanced cancer and their family caregivers in managing pain in the home. *BMC Palliative Care, 13*(1), 39.

Melding, P. S. (1991). Is there such a thing as geriatric pain?. *Pain, 46*(2), 119–121.

Melzack, R. (1999). *Pain: An overview.* Wiley. https://doi.org/10.1034/j.1399-6576.1999.430903.x.

Melzack, R., & Casey, K. L. (1968). Sensory, motivational, and central control determinants of pain. A new conceptual model. *The Skin Senses, 1*, 423–443.

Melzack, R., & Wall, P. (1965). Pain mechanisms: A new theory. *Science, 150*(3699), 971–979. doi:10.1126/science.150.3699.971.

Melzack, R., & Wall, P. D. (1988). *The challenge of pain.* Penguin.

Mendell, L. M. (2014). Constructing and deconstructing the gate theory of pain. *Pain, 155*(2), 210–216.

Mercadante, S. (2015). Opioid metabolism and clinical aspects. *European Journal of Pharmacology, 769*, 71–78.

Miro, J., Gertz, K., Carter, G., & Jenson, M. (2014). Pain location and functioning in persons With spinal cord injury. *PM&R, 6*(8), 690–697.

Monticone, M., Ferrante, S., Giorgi, I., Galandra, C., Rocca, B., & Foti, C. (2014). The 27-item coping strategies questionnaire—revised: Confirmatory factor analysis, reliability and validity in Italian-speaking subjects with chronic pain. *Pain Research and Management, 19*(3), 153–158.

Morone, N. E., Abebe, K. Z., Morrow, L. A., & Weiner, D. K. (2014). Pain and decreased cognitive function negatively impact physical functioning in older adults with knee osteoarthritis. *Pain Medicine, 15*(9), 1481–1487. https://doi.org/10.1111/pme.12483.

Myers, C. D, Riley, J. L., III, & Robinson, M. E (2003). Psychosocial contributions to sex-correlated differences in pain. *Clinical Journal of Pain, 19*(4), 225–232.

Nascimento, M. G., Kosminsky, M., & Chi, M. (2020). Gender role in pain perception and expression: An integrative review. *Brasilian Journal of Pain, 3*(1), 58–62.

National Institute for Health and Clinical Excellence. (2016). Low back pain and sciatica in over 16s: Assessment and management. *NICE Guideline* [NG59]. https://www.nice.org.

uk/guidance/ng59/resources/low-back-pain-and-sciatica-in-over-16s-assessment-and-management-pdf-1837521693637.

National Institute for Health and Care Excellence. (2020). Chronic pain: assessment and management. *Evidence Review for Pharmacological Management*. https://www.nice.org.uk/guidance/ng193/documents/evidence-review-10.

NHS England. (2016). Accessible information and communication. https://www.england.nhs.uk/wp-content/uploads/2016/11/nhse-access-info-comms-policy.pdf.

Ng, L., & Cashman, J. (2018). The management of acute pain. *Medicine, 46*(12), 780–785.

Nicholas, M. K., Asghari, A., Blyth, F. M., Wood, B. M., Murray, R., McCabe, R., et al. (2013). Self-management intervention for chronic pain in older adults: A randomised controlled trial. *Pain, 154*(6), 824–835.

Nicholas, M., Asghari, A., Blyth, F., Wood, B., Murray, R., McCabe, R., et al. (2017). Long-term outcomes from training in self-management of chronic pain in an elderly population: A randomized controlled trial. *Pain, 158*(1), 86–95.

Oosterman, J. M., Gibson, S. J., Pulles, W. L., & Veldhuijzen, D. S. (2013). On the moderating role of age in the relationship between pain and cognition. *European Journal of Pain, 17*(5), 735–741.

O'Sullivan, K., Kennedy, N., Purtill, H., & Hannigan, A. (2017). Understanding pain among older persons: Part 1—the development of novel pain profiles and their association with disability and quality of life. *Age and Ageing, 46*(1), 46–51.

Oxford Pain. (2004). http://www.bandolier.org.uk/booth/pain-pag/index2.html

Paice, J. A. (2011). Chronic treatment-related pain in cancer survivors. *Pain, 152*(3), S84–S89.

Patel, K. V., Guralnik, J. M., Dansie, E. J., & Turk, D. C. (2013). Prevalence and impact of pain among older adults in the United States: Findings from the 2011 National Health and Aging Trends Study. *Pain, 154*(12), 2649–2657.

Pautex, S., & Gold, G. (2006). Assessing pain intensity in older adults. *Geriatrics Aging, 9*(6), 399–402.

Pickering, G., Gibson, S. J., Serbouti, S., Odetti, P., Gonçalves, J. F., Gambassi, G., et al. (2010). Reliability study in five languages of the translation of the pain behavioural scale Doloplus. *European Journal of Pain, 14*(545), e1–10.

Pickering, G., Jourdan, D., & Dubray, C. (2006). Acute versus chronic pain treatment in Alzheimer's disease. *European Journal of Pain, 10*, 379–384.

Plosker, G. L. (2011). Buprenorphine 5, 10 and 20 μg/h transdermal patch. *Drugs, 71*(18), 2491–2509.

Raja, S. N., Carr, D. B., Cohen M., Finnerup, N. B., Flor, H., Stephen Gibson, S., et al. (2020). The revised International Association for the Study of Pain definition of pain: concepts, challenges, and compromises. *Pain, 161*(9), 1976–82. https://doi.org/10.1097/j.pain.0000000000001939.

Roberts, E., Nunes, V. D., Buckner, S., Latchem, S., Constanti, M., Miller, P., et al. (2016). Paracetamol: not as safe as we thought? A systematic literature review of observational studies. *Annals of the Rheumatic Diseases, 75*(3), 552–559.

Rodríguez-Sánchez, I., García-Esquinas, E., Mesas, A. E., Martín-Moreno, J. M., Rodríguez-Mañas, L., & Rodríguez-Artalejo, F. (2019). Frequency, intensity and localization of pain as risk factors for frailty in older adults. *Age and Ageing, 48*(1), 74–80.

Rothrock, S. G., Greenfield, R. H., & Falk, J. L. (1992). Acute abdominal emergencies in the elderly: Clues to identifying serious illness. Part I-Clinical assessment and diagnostic studies. *Emergency Medicine Reports, 13*, 177–184.

Saunders, C. (1964). The symptomatic treatment of incurable malignant disease. *Prescribers' Journal, 4*(4), 68–73.

Schofield, P., Dunham, M., Martin, D., Bellamy, G., Francis, S.-A., Sookhoo, D., et al. (2022). Evidence-based clinical practice guidelines on the management of pain in older people—A summary report. *British Journal of Pain, 16*(1), 6–13.

Schofield, P. (2006). Pain management of older people in care homes: A pilot study. *British Journal of Nursing, 15*(9), 509–514.

Schofield, P. (2013). Managing chronic pain in older people. *Nursing Times, 109*(30), 26–27.

Schofield, P. (2018). The assessment of pain in older people: UK national guidelines. *Age and Ageing, 47*(Suppl. 1), i1–i22.

Schug, S. A., & Goddard, C. (2014). Recent advances in the pharmacological management of acute and chronic pain. *Annals of Palliative Medicine, 3*(4), 263–275.

Schug, S. A., Lavand'homme, P., Barke, A., Korwisi, B., Rief, W., & Treede, R. D. (2019). IASP Taskforce for the Classification of Chronic Pain. The IASP classification of chronic pain for ICD-11: Chronic postsurgical or posttraumatic pain. *Pain, 160*(1), 45–52.

Scott, J., & Huskisson, E. C. (1979). Vertical or horizontal visual analogue scales. *Annals of the Rheumatic Diseases, 38*(6), 560.

Smith, E. S. (2018). Advances in understanding nociception and neuropathic pain. *Journal of Neurology, 265*(2), 231–238.

Spitz, A., Moore, A. A., Papaleontiou, M., Granieri, E., Turner, B. J., & Reid, M. C. (2011). Primary care providers' perspective on prescribing opioids to older adults with chronic non-cancer pain: A qualitative study. *BMC Geriatrics, 11*(1), 35.

Stubbs, B., Schofield, P., Binnekade, T., Patchay, S., Sepehry, A., & Eggermont, L. (2014). Pain is associated with recurrent falls in community-dwelling older adults: Evidence from a systematic review and meta-analysis. *Pain Medicine, 15*(115), 28.

Tai-Seale, M., Bolin, J., Bao, X., & Street, R. (2011). Management of chronic Pain among older patients: Inside primary care in the U.S. *European Journal of Pain, 15*(10), 1087.e1–1087.e8.

Talbot, K., Madden, V. J., Jones, S. L., & Moseley, G. L. (2019). The sensory and affective components of pain: Are they differentially modifiable dimensions or inseparable aspects of a unitary experience? A systematic review. *British Journal of Anaesthesia, 123*(2), e263–e272.

Tan, G., Jensen, M. P., Thornby, J. I., & Shanti, B. F. (2004). Validation of the Brief Pain Inventory for chronic nonmalignant pain. *The Journal of Pain, 5*(2), 133–137.

Tang, N. K. (2018). Cognitive behavioural therapy in pain and psychological disorders: Towards a hybrid future. *Progress in Neuro-Psychopharmacology and Biological Psychiatry, 87*, 281–289.

Tracy, B., & Morrison, R. S. (2013). Pain management in older adults. *Clinical Therapeutics, 35*(11), 1659–1668.

Treede, R. D. (2016). Gain control mechanisms in the nociceptive system. *Pain, 157*(6), 1199–1204.

Treede, R. D., Rief, W., Barke, A., Aziz, Q., Bennett, M. I., Benoliel, R., et al. (2019). Chronic pain as a symptom or a disease: The IASP Classification of Chronic Pain for the International Classification of Diseases (ICD-11). *Pain, 160*(1), 19–27.

Tse, M. M., & Vong, S. (2012). Pain beliefs and pain-related profiles of older persons living in nursing homes. *Journal of Pain Management, 2,* 141–151.

Tse, M. M. Y., Vong, S. K. S, & Ho, S. S. (2012). The effectiveness of an integrated pain management program for older persons and staff in nursing homes. *Archives of Gerontology and Geriatrics, 54*(2), e203–e212.

Tse, M. M., Vong, S. K., & Tang, S. K. (2013). Motivational interviewing and exercise programme for community-dwelling older persons with chronic pain: a randomised controlled study. *Journal of Clinical Nursing, 22*(13–14), 1843–1856.

Tse, M. M. Y., Tang, S. K., Wan, V. T. C., & Vong, S. K. S. (2014). The effectiveness of physical exercise training in pain, mobility, and psychological well-being of older persons living in nursing homes. *Pain Management Nursing, 15*(4), 778–788.

Turk, D. C., Dworkin, R. H., Trudeau, J. J., Benson, C., Biondi, D. M., Katz, N. P., et al. (2015). Validation of the hospital anxiety and depression scale in patients with acute low back pain. *The Journal of Pain, 16*(10), 1012–1021.

Vartiainen, P., Mäntyselkä, P., Heiskanen, T., Hagelberg, N., Mustola, S., Forssell, H., et al. (2017). Validation of EQ-5D and 15D in the assessment of health-related quality of life in chronic pain. *Pain, 158*(8), 1577–1585.

Wade, K. F., Marshall, A., Vanhoutte, B., Wu, F. C., O'Neill, T. W., & Lee, D. M (2017). Does pain predict frailty in older men and women? Findings from the English Longitudinal Study of Ageing (ELSA). *The Journals of Gerontology: Series A, 72*(3), 403–409.

Ware, L. J., Epps, C. D., Herr, K., & Packard, A. (2006). Evaluation of the revised faces pain scale, verbal descriptor scale, numeric rating scale, and Iowa pain thermometer in older minority adults. *Pain Management Nursing, 7*(3), 117–125.

Wewers, M. E., & Lowe, N. K. (1990). A critical review of visual analogue scales in the measurement of clinical phenomena. *Research in Nursing & Health, 13*(4), 227–236.

Yiengprugsawan, V., & Steptoe, A. (2018). Impacts of persistent general and site-specific pain on activities of daily living and physical performance: A prospective analysis of the English Longitudinal Study of Ageing. *Geriatrics & Gerontology International, 18*(7), 1051–1057.

Zborowski, M. (1952). Cultural components in response to pain. *Journal of Social Issues, 8*(4), 16–30.

Zhuo, M. (2016). Neural mechanisms underlying anxiety–chronic pain interactions. *Trends in Neurosciences, 39*(3), 136–145.

Zwakhalen, S., Docking, R. E., Gnass, I., Sirsch, E., Stewart, C., Allcock, N., et al. (2018). Pain in older adults with dementia. *Der Schmerz, 32*(5), 364–373.

28

Delirium: Diagnosis, Management and Care for Older People

Emma Vardy, Rachel Kirby, Lindsay Dingwall

CHAPTER OUTLINE

Delirium is a common and underrecognised condition that is associated with poor outcomes and high mortality rates. Delirium in older adults requires skilled management and care. It is often said good delirium care is simply good care; this is pertinent to the nursing of older adults. Since the turn of the century, much progress has been made in defining and diagnosing delirium and in the development of definitions and assessment tools. In addition, models of care have been described. Central to enhancing delirium diagnosis and care is education and embedding good practice. In this chapter we provide a comprehensive overview of delirium, from definition and pathophysiology to diagnosis and management. A variety of care settings are considered, including those in hospital and in the community. In developing a solid understanding of the principles of delirium assessment and nursing care, nurses will improve individual practice and contribute to the education and improved practice of others.

DELIRIUM DEFINED

Delirium describes a condition of altered mental status as a result of illness, stress or drug intoxication (Meagher et al., 2008). Delirium has no single identifying feature; characterisation requires clinical symptoms and signs as well as context. Two key features distinguish delirium from other differential diagnoses: acute onset and the fluctuation of symptoms.

Two key classifications describe delirium: ICD 11 and DSM-V. DSM-V (American Psychiatric Association, 2013) define delirium as follows:

- A disturbance in attention (i.e., reduced ability to direct, focus, sustain and shift attention) and awareness (i.e., reduced orientation to the environment).
- A disturbance that develops over a short period of time, usually hours to a few days, and represents a change from baseline attention and awareness; tends to fluctuate in severity during the course of a day.
- An additional disturbance in cognition (e.g., memory deficit, disorientation, language, visuospatial ability or perception).
- A disturbance not better explained by a pre-existing, established or evolving neurocognitive disorder and do not occur in the context of a severely reduced level of arousal such as coma.
- Evidence from the history, physical examination or laboratory findings that the disturbance is a direct physiological consequence of a medical condition, substance intoxication or withdrawal, or exposure to a toxin or due to multiple aetiologies.

An aspect of practical significance in applying the DSM-V criteria is the detection of underlying causes. In older people it is common to identify multiple causes, some of which may interact, such as dehydration causing constipation and leading to urinary retention and pain. Similarly, over the course of delirium, other precipitating factors may emerge.

Delirium is described in clinical practice using terminology such as acute confusion, toxic encephalopathy, acute brain dysfunction and altered mental status. However, a recent review made the case for use of the term *delirium* as a clinical state characterised by features described in diagnostic systems such as the DSM-V and acute encephalopathy as the rapid development of a pathobiological process in the brain, one feature of which may be delirium (Slooter et al., 2020). The reason for using clear terminology is it facilitates clinical communication between nursing and other health care professionals. *Delirium* is increasingly recognised by the general public and simplifies data collection and clinical coding in health care organisations. Alternative definitions should be avoided where possible.

DELIRIUM SUBTYPES

Delirium is categorised into motor subtypes based on clinical signs and symptoms. The features of hyperactive, hypoactive and mixed delirium are detailed in Table 28.1 (Meagher, 2009). The hypoactive subtype is more frequently associated with poorer outcomes in terms of mortality. The cause of this association is not fully understood but may be in part due to poorer recognition and delayed assessment.

TABLE 28.1	**Features of Delirium and Motor Subtypes**		
Symptom	**Hyperactive Delirium**	**Hypoactive Delirium**	**Mixed Delirium**
Physical activity	Increased and may include pacing, fidgeting and overactivity; unable to remain still	Decreased; may sit still more; reduction in movements; reduced speed of movements	Increased and decreased
Awareness of surroundings	Hyperalert	Reduced awareness; less emotion in response to surroundings; passive attitude	Both increased and decreased alertness
Level of arousal	Mental restlessness; agitation	Reduced alertness and/or withdrawal	Increased and decreased
Speech	Disorganised thinking may be evident	Reduced amount of speech and speed; reduced verbal output; pauses	Increased and decreased
Mobility	Increased	Reduced and reduced speed	Increased and decreased

Source: Adapted from Meagher (2009).

DISTINGUISHING DELIRIUM FROM DEMENTIA

An important distinction in clinical practice is the difference between delirium and dementia. Understanding the distinction is important to ensure an older person is not mislabelled as having a diagnosis of dementia. Mistaking a person as having dementia may cause distress to the person and their family and may influence clinical decision making. It is important to understand the similarities and distinguishing features of dementia and delirium as detailed in Table 28.2.

Distinguishing delirium from dementia in practice can be difficult. In particular Lewy body dementia has certain features in common with delirium, such as fluctuation of symptoms of confusion and periods of reduced arousal. Not infrequently, delirium occurs in the context of dementia, either diagnosed or undiagnosed. In general, making a diagnosis of dementia in an older person with delirium is not recommended, although there is evidence informant-based tools can be used to make a diagnosis of delirium in the context of dementia (Jackson et al., 2016).

DELIRIUM AND DIFFERENTIAL DIAGNOSIS

Distinguishing delirium from the progression of dementia is important. However, there are other differential diagnoses. Depression may be mistaken for hypoactive delirium and vice versa. Attention may be impaired in delirium, but orientation is normal (Fong et al., 2009b). The distinguishing features are the presentation of depression tends to be insidious, fluctuations of features are absent, level of consciousness is unaffected and there may be a history of previous episodes of depression (Martins & Fernandes, 2012). Hallucinations are rare in depression (Fong et al., 2009b).

Psychotic disorders, for example due to schizophrenia, bipolar or depressive disorder, share a number of features with delirium, particularly acute onset and hallucinations. Distinguishing the two may be difficult. Previous episodes and psychiatric history can provide clues. However, it should be recognised primary psychosis, as opposed to psychosis due to a secondary cause such as dementia, though rare, may occur in older people (Martins & Fernandes, 2012). Disturbance of thought and delusions may be present in both, but individuals with delirium tend to be less well formed and less complex and may be influenced by environment. Hallucinations tend to be visual in delirium vs. auditory in psychosis (Martins & Fernandes, 2012). Orientation is usually normal in psychotic disorders (Fong et al., 2009b).

It is worth mentioning delirium can mimic stroke in presentation. This is due to acute onset of symptoms and occurs where effects on mobility predominate. Where stroke is suspected, distinction should be made by a specialist in stroke medicine given the urgency of treatment in the context of stroke.

PATHOPHYSIOLOGY

The pathophysiology of delirium is not fully understood. As there are a number of different precipitating causes for delirium, so too it is likely there are a number of causative mechanisms. To date those described include brain energy metabolism, inflammation, disturbance of neurotransmitters, vascular dysfunction and interactions between systemic

TABLE 28.2	Distinguishing Clinical Characteristics of Delirium and Dementia	
Feature	**Delirium**	**Dementia**
Onset	Rapid (hours, days)	Slow (months, years)
Symptoms	Fluctuates over course of day and night	Relatively stable with the exception of dementia with Lewy bodies
Duration	Hours, days, weeks, months	Months to years
Orientation	Disorientation and disturbed thinking are intermittent	Persistent disorientation
Attention	Impaired	Normal other than late stages
Memory	Impaired	Impaired
Hallucinations	Mainly visual when present	Usually absent other than in severe dementia and/or dementia with Lewy bodies
Level of consciousness	Fluctuates, with inability to concentrate	Alert, stable
Impact on sleep–wake cycle	Sleep–wake cycle may be reversed	Sleep may be fragmented

features and the brain. Some of these are hypotheses, and some have a greater evidence base.

BRAIN ENERGY METABOLISM

The cerebral metabolic insufficiency hypothesis speculates delirium is caused by a failure to meet the energy requirements of the brain (Engel & Romano, 1959). This hypothesis would explain why hypoxia, hypoglycaemia and reductions in cerebral blood flow, for example in stroke, cause delirium. Although there is some data that supports it, no research has confirmed a direct causative link (Wilson et al., 2020).

INFLAMMATION

Peripheral inflammation is a known trigger for delirium, but most of the evidence has been provided in studies on animals rather than humans (Wilson et al., 2020).What is unclear is why some people appear to have greater vulnerability to peripheral inflammation than others.

Disruption of the blood brain barrier is presumed to be key to inflammation-induced delirium, although there is no evidence to support this (Wilson et al., 2020). The effect of inflammation on coagulation may offer a further mechanism for the development of delirium, but again there is no evidence that confirms this idea.

NEUROTRANSMITTERS, NEURAL NETWORKS AND BRAIN CONNECTIVITY

Some neurotransmitters have been implicated in the pathology of delirium: acetylcholine, dopamine, noradrenaline and gamma-aminobutyric acid (GABA) (Wilson et al., 2020). Anticholinergic drugs have been observed to precipitate a delirium. Medications have varying degrees of anticholinergic effects, and a number of scales measure anticholinergic burden. There is evidence as burden of anticholinergic medication increases, so too does risk of delirium (Wilson et al., 2020). Observations have led to trials of treatment of delirium with acetylcholinesterase inhibitor drugs, but studies to date have not been successful. Dopamine depletion has been hypothesised to be linked to delirium. People with Parkinson's disease, with loss of dopamine-producing neurones, are at particular risk (Vardy et al., 2015). Antipsychotic medications that are dopamine agonists are frequently used to treat delirium, but meta-analyses have not confirmed effectiveness in either prevention or treatment (Neufeld et al., 2016). An extension of the neurotransmitter hypothesis for delirium is the concept of brain network disintegration as the final common pathological pathway for delirium, through collation of evidence from brain imaging and electroencephalogram data (Van Montfort et al., 2019).

INTERACTION BETWEEN BRAIN AND SYSTEMIC TRIGGERS

The vulnerable brain hypothesis attempts to describe why older people, those with frailty and those with cognitive impairment may develop delirium in relation to a relatively innocuous insult such as constipation or urinary retention, yet younger and more physiologically resilient individuals develop delirium only in the context of severe illness such as sepsis. Previously this was seen as a rather clear delimitation; that is, the brain is vulnerable, or it is not. Study of the relationship between cognitive impairment and delirium has shown it to be much more linear; with progression of cognitive impairment, the risk of delirium increases (Davis et al., 2015). Brain vulnerability is likely a result of a combination of these processes (Wilson et al., 2020). Some are known to be influenced by age, including brain network connectivity with degeneration of cholinergic and noradrenergic neurones, changes in brain vasculature and increased vulnerability to circulating inflammatory factors (Wilson et al., 2020).

RISK FACTORS

A number of risk factors predispose the development of delirium. A comprehensive review by Wilson et al. (2020) helpfully categorised risk factors as pre-morbid, factors related to presenting illness and factors related to hospital admission, summarised in Table 28.3.

PRECIPITATING FACTORS

Precipitating factors are clinical or physiological events that, particularly in the context of predisposing risk factors, are commonly identified to occur at the time of development of delirium. In Table 28.3, many of the factors related to present illness and hospital admission are also precipitating factors. A simple mnemonic that aids assessment and identification of one or more precipitating factors is PINCH ME, described on page 6.

PREVALENCE OF DELIRIUM IN OLDER PEOPLE

The prevalence of delirium in older people is dependent on setting. A systematic review by Siddiqi et al. (2006) concluded a prevalence of 10%–31% in medical inpatients on admission and of 3%–29% in hospitals. Prevalence very much depends on the type of inpatient setting. Ryan et al. (2013) carried out a point prevalence study at a tertiary

TABLE 28.3 **Risk Factors for Delirium**

Pre-Morbid	Related to Present Illness	Related to Hospital Admission
Age	Hip fracture	Pain
Dementia	Severe illness	Infection
Multimorbidity	Sepsis	Immobility
Polypharmacy	Infection, including COVID-19	Opioids
Frailty	Dehydration	Steroids
Sensory impairment (e.g., visual, hearing)	Electrolyte imbalance	Sleep deprivation
	Acute kidney injury	Physical restraints
Depression	Liver dysfunction	Psychoactive drugs
Alcohol use	Alcohol or drug withdrawal	Benzodiazepine initiation or withdrawal
Poor nutrition	Hypoxia	
History of delirium	Prolonged ventilation	Anticholinergic agents
		Nicotine withdrawal
		Ward moves

referral, level 1 trauma centre with 407 acute adult inpatient beds and found prevalence on wards to vary between 7% (general surgery, $n = 83$) and 53% (geriatric medicine, $n = 15$). Point prevalence estimates in palliative settings vary from 4%–12% in the community, 9%–57% in hospital services, and 6%–74% in inpatient palliative care units, with prevalence of delirium prior to death across all settings of 42%–88% (Watt et al., 2019).

There is limited literature on the prevalence of delirium in the care home setting. Reported prevalence in nursing homes in the Netherlands was 8.9% in nursing homes and 8.2% in residential homes (Boorsma et al., 2012). An Italian study found a higher prevalence of 36.8% in nursing homes (Morichi et al., 2018).

FRAILTY AND DELIRIUM

Frailty is a condition of functional decline and is a continuum from healthy ageing to a state of disability and death (Rahman, 2018). It is associated with a vulnerability to endogenous and exogenous stressors with links to poorer health outcomes and ultimately death (Rahman, 2018). The hypothesis that frailty underlies and predisposes people to delirium was tested through systematic review and meta-analyses. An examination of limited literature confirmed frailty predisposes to delirium (Persico et al., 2018). Risk of developing delirium was 2.2 times higher in individuals classed as frail. In clinical practice, frailty should be considered a risk factor for delirium, and similarly delirium should prompt assessment for frailty.

COVID-19 AND DELIRIUM

Delirium is a presenting feature of COVID-19, manifest either as new confusion or new drowsiness, particularly in older people. A systematic review and meta-analysis of coronavirus cases showed 30% prevalence of confusion among 3,359 patients (Rogers et al., 2020). A United Kingdom study of 20,133 patients with COVID-19 showed confusion to be the fifth most common symptom, affecting 20% of patients (Docherty et al., 2020). With age, as typical symptoms of COVID-19 become less prevalent, atypical symptoms such as confusion and malaise predominate (Hall et al., 2020). One study of 322 hospitalised patients and 535 community-based older adults with COVID-19 found 25.2% of the hospital cohort and 35.6% of the community sample had delirium, with higher rates in individuals with frailty (Zazzara et al., 2020). The pathophysiology of delirium is not fully understood in the context of COVID-19, but delirium appears to confer a particularly bleak prognosis when present (Marengoni et al., 2020).

OUTCOMES

Outcomes for older people with delirium are universally poor. These include morbidity such as increased falls and skin pressure damage, prolonged length of acute hospital inpatient stay, increased risk of developing dementia, increased rates of cognitive decline in individuals with a pre-existing diagnosis of dementia, increased rate of institutional care and increased risk of death. The risk of complications and death continue after an older person has been discharged from hospital and/or recovered from delirium. One study showed the incidence of death to be 38% for older people diagnosed with delirium versus 27.5% in individuals without delirium after 22.7 months (Witlox et al., 2010).

The relationship between delirium and dementia is complex. Delirium is a common reason for admission to hospital for older adults living with dementia, complicating

24%–89% of inpatient stays (Sampson et al., 2009). Strong evidence showed delirium increased the risk of developing dementia by as much as six-fold at a 6-year follow-up (MacLullich et al., 2009). Delirium has also been shown to accelerate decline in cognition in older adults with a diagnosis of Alzheimer's dementia (Fong et al., 2009a).

DIAGNOSIS OF DELIRIUM

A diagnosis of delirium is made based on history and examination. Examination includes both physical and cognitive examination. This approach enables a diagnosis and at the same time assessment for one or more underlying causes. Though not all of these aspects may be completed by nursing staff, dependent on role and experience, an understanding of all aspects is helpful.

History

It is important to establish whether a person is more confused or drowsy than normal. Due to the nature of delirium, history from a carer, relative or someone who knows the person well is almost always required. Key questions to ask include whether any change is acute, whether symptoms fluctuate, whether there is evidence of hallucinations and other questions to help distinguish delirium from differentials. Hallucinations should be asked about gently and sensitively—for example, 'Have you seen anything strange or unexpected recently that perhaps others haven't seen?'

It is crucial not to overlook symptoms of hypoactive delirium, such as reduced activity and sleepiness, as hypoactive delirium is frequently underdiagnosed and consequentially associated with worse outcomes (O'Keeffe, 1999). It is also important to assess for other signs of delirium such as reduced mobility or reduced intake of food or fluid. Questions on admission to a new environment about what is normal for an individual and any worsening of existing cognitive symptoms are essential. Ask questions to try and identify the underlying physical cause of delirium. The PINCH ME mnemonic is helpful to remember causes:

Pain
Infection/ intoxication/ intracerebral
Nutrition
Constipation
Hydration/hypoxia
Sensory impairment (e.g., poor eyesight, deafness)
Medications
Environmental (e.g., unfamiliar environment, disruption of sleep–wake cycle)

Pain results from a number of causes. One important type of pain that should not be overlooked is chest pain due to myocardial infarction. Infection may be urinary, respiratory (including COVID-19), soft tissue, hepatobiliary

or neurological. Assessment for intoxication should include questions around alcohol intake. Intracerebral causes include ischaemic or haemorrhagic. Management of alcohol withdrawal is not considered further in this chapter. Medication history should include changes to prescription medications, over-the-counter medications and any abrupt medication withdrawal. Medications classically associated with delirium include anticholinergic medications, steroids and opiates. Anticholinergic medications are known to have a cumulative effect in delirium development; older people on multiple anticholinergic medications are at greater risk (Egberts et al., 2020). Withdrawal of benzodiazepines may induce delirium; establish whether any medications have been stopped recently. If an individual is a smoker and is unable to smoke in a health care environment, nicotine withdrawal should be considered.

EXAMINATION

Physical examination should focus on identifying the underlying cause of delirium, including assessment of hydration status, source of any pain, assessment for infection and urinary retention. Constipation may require confirmation using rectal examination. Neurological examination should be based on history.

Various tools are available to assess cognition in delirium. Some are screening tools and require further tests to confirm diagnosis. In general, given the associated poor outcomes if delirium is suspected, it should be treated as such until proven otherwise.

SCREENING TOOLS FOR DELIRIUM

Screening tools for delirium can be used as the first step to making a diagnosis to monitor individuals at high risk of developing delirium. Some tools can also be used to monitor delirium. A wide array of screening tools is available (see Table 28.4); a review compared five of the most widely used to determine the benefits of each in a hospital setting (Hendry et al., 2016). Tests included were the abbreviated mental test (AMT10 or AMT4), 4-As test (4AT), brief confusion assessment method (bCAM), months of the year backward (MOTYB), and single question in delirium (SQiD). All involve questions directed toward the older person and/or an informant. The informant may be the next of kin, a carer or another individual who is familiar with the older adult at their cognitive and functional baseline. This review focused on screening tools in a hospital setting. Application is less established in the community setting, as there is less research in this area. In the hospital setting, the most favoured tests were the AMT4, AMT10, MOTYB and 4AT, all of which had sensitivity above 86% (Hendry et al.,

TABLE 28.4 Summary of Screening Tools for Delirium

Screening Tool	Questions to Patient	Questions to Informer	Sensitivity	Specificity
AMT4	Age Date of birth Year Place	Nil	92.7%	53.7%
AMT10	Age Time (to nearest hour) Year Home address Recognise two people's jobs Date of birth Year World War 1 started Current prime minister Count backward from 20 to 1 Recall a given address	Nil	86.6%	63.5%
bCAM	Evidence of inattention (e.g., MOTYB); evidence of disorganised thinking	Altered mental status changes or a fluctuating course; altered level of consciousness	70.3%	91.4%
MOTYB	Listing months of the year backward	Nil	91.3%	49.7%
4AT	AMT4 questions MOTYB	Altered mental status changes or a fluctuating course; altered level of consciousness	86.7%	69.5%
SQiD		Is this patient more confused than before?	91.4%	61.3%

Source: From Hendry et al. (2016).

2016). The bCAM was discounted as a reliable screening tool in the clinical setting due to low sensitivity. Of note, the bCAM takes 1–2 minutes to perform, compared with the CAM, which takes 10–15 minutes and requires specialised training (Inouye et al., 1990). The SQiD was considered a good screening tool but relies on information from an informant, which is not always easy to obtain. Although the authors demonstrated that no test was 100% sensitive and 100% specific—in other words, there's not a perfect test—they concluded the 4AT to be the preferred screening test. The 2019 Scottish Intercollegiate Guidelines Network (SIGN, 2019) also endorsed the use of 4AT as the screening method of choice in the emergency department or in acute hospital admissions. The primary benefit of the 4AT is speed of completion and lack of specific training to use and interpret (Rapid Clinical Test for Delirium, 2020). The test takes into account individuals who are unable to communicate, and as a consequence no person is deemed untestable. For older people who are well known to the assessor, for example as applied by a carer or nurse in a nursing or residential home, the SQiD may be used as a rapid assessment, since the assessor may also act as the informant. The SQiD may miss people with hypoactive delirium, so the modified SQiD asks the informant, 'Has the patient been more confused or drowsy in the last 3 days?' In one study the modified SQiD was found to have 86% sensitivity and 88% specificity, showing a significant improvement in specificity compared to the original (Burn et al., 2019). The modified SQiD and 4AT are recommended in assessing for new confusion as part of the United Kingdom–based hospital National Early Warning System 2 (NEWS2), endorsed by the Royal College of Physicians and designed to recognise a deteriorating patient early and trigger urgent medical review (Royal College of Physicians (RCP), 2020).

A nursing specific screening tool called the nursing delirium screening scale (NuDESC) is designed for the nursing team to perform at the point of care. It assesses for symptoms in keeping with delirium: disorientation, inappropriate behaviour, inappropriate communication, hallucination and psychomotor retardation. The NuDESC has been shown to be highly sensitive (90%) with specificity at 72% (Hargrave et al., 2017).

The CAM-ICU tool is designed for use for patients who are sedated and/or intubated in an intensive care unit (ICU) setting (El-Menyar et al., 2017).

DIAGNOSIS AND INVESTIGATIONS

No single blood test, imaging tool or other investigation diagnoses delirium, so any investigations performed are designed to diagnose the underlying causes of delirium.

As a standard, the following routine tests as proposed by the SIGN guidelines (SIGN, 2019) should be strongly considered for older people with a clinical diagnosis of delirium to investigate the cause:

- Bedside tests
  - Observations such as blood pressure, temperature, pulse, oxygen saturations, level of consciousness
  - ECG to assess for possibility of myocardial infarction
  - Blood glucose
  - Bladder scan for urinary retention
  - Pain assessment tools such as the Abbey pain scale in people with pre-existing dementia
- Blood tests
  - Full blood count
  - Urea and electrolytes
  - Liver function tests
  - Bone profile, including calcium
  - Magnesium
  - C reactive protein
  - Blood culture (if infection is evident)
  - Arterial blood gas if hypoxic
- Microbiology tests
  - Urine microscopy, culture and sensitivity if there are symptoms suggestive of infection such as dysuria or urinary frequency
  - Sputum culture, wound swab (dependent on other clinical findings)
- Radiology tests
  - Chest X-ray

Other investigations that should not be performed as standard but may be considered include the following (SIGN, 2019):

- CT brain scan where there is clinical suspicion of an intracranial cause such as a history or evidence of trauma, focal neurology on examination or reduced level of consciousness not adequately explained by other causes; this should be arranged urgently if the patient is anticoagulated; brain imaging may also be considered if an alternative cause is not identified
- Lumbar puncture to sample cerebrospinal fluid when meningitis or encephalitis is considered
- Electroencephalogram when epileptic activity or non-convulsive status epilepticus is suspected

NURSING CARE OF AN OLDER PERSON WITH DELIRIUM

Despite the prevalence of delirium in acutely ill older people, delirium is at risk of being overlooked or wrongly attributed to symptoms of dementia (Blevins & DeGennaro, 2018). Prompt recognition of delirium by nurses may reduce the long-term consequences of delirium and minimise distress to older people and their families. Although successful detection and management of delirium is vital, skilled nursing care can prevent or reduce the risk of delirium onset. In this section we focus on the elements of care that contribute to risk reduction, detection, and management of delirium.

PHYSIOLOGICAL CARE

One of the most important nursing interventions in delirium management is robust nursing assessment throughout the patient journey, regardless of the care setting. The nursing contribution to assessing frailty in all care settings improves the effectiveness of primary prevention strategies for delirium through identifying individuals at highest risk and through early detection of the signs of delirium (British Geriatrics Society, 2019).

All countries have unique legislation and guidance to treat people who lack capacity to consent. Older people with delirium may have fluctuating capacity to understand, retain or weigh up information, and communicate their wishes, so ongoing assessment must be part of care (National Institute of Health & Care Excellence (NICE), 2019). When a person does lack capacity to consent to a health care procedure, the practitioner primarily responsible for their care has a duty to act in their best interest.

Nurses have an important role in routine measurement of vital signs and other assessments of physical health. This is seen in the assessment for acute confusion contained in the United Kingdom–based NEWS2.

While delirium usually improves if the underlying causes are identified and treated, nurses must be watchful for emergent triggers and pay careful attention to pain management, sleep hygiene, sensory impairment, food and fluid intake, elimination needs and activity.

HYDRATION

Failure to manage fluid balance can result in more severe delirium, pressure ulcer development and low blood pressure with an increased fall risk. The effects of acute illness such as pyrexia, vomiting and reduced self-care skills can trigger dehydration and electrolyte disturbances. Normal ageing reduces the effectiveness of the body's protective mechanisms to prevent dehydration, and older people are less able to conserve fluids and concentrate urine effectively. Older people's reduced thirst signals and fear of incontinence may reduce motivation to request fluids. Nurses must be alert to the signs of dehydration, including fragile skin, dry mouth and lips, sunken eyes and dark, concentrated urine. Where possible nurses should support an older person to re-establish and maintain normal oral diet and fluids. For a tailored daily intake, people aged 60 and over should have fluid goals based on 30 mL/kg per day (British Association for Parenteral & Enteral Nutrition, 2016). Good practice in fluid management requires a person-centred approach with 24-hour intake and output measurement, offering a full glass of fluid at routine events such as medication rounds and visiting times, keeping preferred fluids available and giving assistance as required. To encourage sleep, caffeinated drinks, including some fizzy juices, should be avoided especially later in the day.

If adequate oral intake cannot be achieved, subcutaneous fluids, or hypodermoclysis, may be suitable for mild to moderate dehydration, providing there are no contraindications (e.g., heart failure or chronic kidney disease). Relatively small volumes of isotonic or hypotonic solutions (e.g., 0.9% sodium chloride) totalling up to 2 L over 24 hours may be prescribed and infused. Before treatment is considered, blood tests should be taken to establish urea and electrolytes and to evaluate need for treatment and correct fluid management. Maintenance of good oral hygiene and strict monitoring of all fluid intake and output is essential.

NUTRITION

People who are unwell with delirium may have reduced intake of oral nutrition. Encouragement, adhering to usual routines and tastes, and assistance as necessary may suffice. If the older person has dentures, they should be appropriately fitted to support nutrition. Family has an important role to play in optimising nutrition. Should these measures not be effective, the dietetic team may be able to assist through the prescription of high-calorie drinks to ensure adequate calorific intake is maintained, even when nutritional intake is poor.

If the older person is unable to reach adequate daily fluid or calorific intake orally, a decision must be made about alternative feeding options. In some situations, the use of a nasogastric tube (NGT) can be considered as a short-term alternative feeding method. This must be a carefully considered decision, as NGT feeding carries risks such as discomfort and distress at the time of insertion, aspiration pneumonia and, for individuals with delirium, increased risk of tube coming/being pulled out. NGT feeding is uncommon in the context of delirium.

BLADDER AND BOWEL MANAGEMENT

The normal ageing process and the presence of frailty and polypharmacy increase the risk of urinary incontinence for many older people. The presence of delirium or its causes may tip an older person into incontinence. Despite the risks of incontinence to skin integrity, indwelling urinary catheters (IUCs) should be avoided, or if required, they should be removed as soon as clinically indicated. Unrecognised urinary retention may be a factor in delirium; although bladder decompression through IUC addresses retention, IUCs limit mobility and are portals for infection such as urinary tract infections and bacteraemia. The introduction of an unfamiliar or uncomfortable object to an older person with reduced cognition can increase stress and the risk of self-removal of the catheter, causing potential damage to the urethra (Rosen et al., 2015). Instead, regular toileting can reduce episodes of incontinence by pre-empting when an older person needs to empty their bladder. Maintaining a fluid balance chart to include fluid intake, times of voiding and the amount of urine passed can inform individually scheduled toileting when an older person lacks the cognition to ask for the toilet or to respond to prompts from staff to use it.

Research suggests 17%–40% of adults over 65 may have chronic constipation, which is a frequently overlooked factor in delirium management (Rosen et al., 2015). Constipation is caused by many factors, including reduced nutritional intake, reduced mobility, dehydration and medication side effects, for example from opiates. Medication should be reviewed to identify any that contribute to constipation and alternatives considered. All older people who receive opiates should be prescribed a stool softener unless contraindicated, and the frequency and consistency of their bowel movements should be documented. Laxatives must be prescribed with caution and titrated frequently. Overtreatment can cause iatrogenic diarrhoea, precipitating dehydration and exacerbating delirium. The National Institute for Health and Care Excellence recommends non-pharmacological strategies such as encouraging mobilisation and providing an optimum food and fluid intake (NICE, 2019).

PAIN MANAGEMENT

Interactions between pain and delirium are complex, and the presence of delirium interferes with self-reported pain. Under- or overtreatment of pain can precipitate a delirium. Obtaining a comprehensive physical and mental health history is important in the management of pain. For example, does the person have a condition associated with pain, such as arthritis or malignancy, or are there new signs of injury or disease (Fischer et al., 2019)? Any pain-associated conditions, such as depression and insomnia, should be addressed at the same time (Sampson et al., 2020). Nurses should also anticipate when pain is likely, for example post-surgery or trauma, and act to manage it (NICE, 2019). Individuals who report pain at rest are three times more likely to have a comorbidity of delirium than those who experience pain on activity, but hyperactive delirium may exacerbate movement-related pain.

Delirium presentation can make pain assessment difficult, especially if the older person was admitted with delirium without the opportunity to participate in their own assessment. Non-verbal behavioural signs of pain therefore become the most important aspect of pain communication and nursing assessment. The American Geriatrics Society (2002) lists behaviours similar to those found in people living with dementia who have pain (American Geriatrics Society, 2002):

- Facial expressions: Grimacing, rapid blinking
- Verbalisations/vocalisations: Signing, moaning, wincing, crying
- Body movements: Rubbing, stiffness, limited movement, guarding an area
- Changes in interpersonal interactions: Withdrawn behaviour, aggression
- Changes in activity patterns or routines: Increased wandering or walking with purpose, trying to leave the environment, increased restlessness
- Mental status change: Increased confusion

There are no standardised tools to measure pain in the context of delirium as the validity of commonly used pain scales such as the numerical rating scale, visual analogue scale and faces pain scale have not been demonstrated through research (Fischer et al., 2019). The SIGN guidelines recommend the use of observational tools more commonly used for people living with dementia (SIGN, 2019). Assessment may not be accurate because observation tools may be biased toward hyperactive delirium, and the symptoms of delirium may overlap with symptoms of pain. The older person may receive unnecessary pain relief with the side effects associated with analgesics. Few studies provide clear evidence of the effect of prescribing opiates in older people (Sampson et al., 2020). Further information on the management of pain in older people is provided in a comprehensive review (Abdulla et al., 2013).

Special care is required when prescribing analgesia in older people as they are more sensitive to some of the side effects. Although opiates are known to precipitate delirium in some older adults, withholding opiate medications for fear of delirium is clinically inappropriate. That said, all prescribed analgesia should be titrated to the lowest effective dose (Clegg & Young, 2011). This requires continuous assessment of pain effectiveness. Non-pharmaceutical multidisciplinary therapies can contribute to pain management either alone or in combination with prescribed modifications, including massage and relaxation, physiotherapy, acupuncture or the application of hot and cold packs. Whichever interventions are used, evaluation of their effectiveness is important.

SENSORY IMPAIRMENT

Impairments such as poor vision or hearing are common in older adults (Cimarolli & Jopp, 2014). Sensory loss and limited mobility restrict or distort how a person perceives and interprets their surroundings. Treating modifiable sensory impairments such as earwax or eye infections assist in optimising hearing and eyesight. Fundamental measures include supporting the person to maintain and use their glasses or hearing aids as required (SIGN, 2019). Additional strategies include having good light sources and using aides to communication such as clear signage, magnifiers and communication boards. In patients with prescriptions for hearing aids and glasses, they should be provided daily to the patient. It is important to ensure hearing aids are in working order—for example, have the battery replaced if required and are correctly fitted in the ear.

SLEEP HYGIENE

Poor sleep patterns and sleep hygiene are recognised contributing factors to the onset of delirium. Environmental factors such as high noise levels and inappropriate lighting are likely to cause fragmented sleep patterns (Social Care Institute for Excellence, 2015). Staff should consider and attempt to reduce nighttime noise and, where possible, aim to promote sleep by administering medications and delivering care outside sleeping hours (NICE, 2019). Earplugs and eyeshades are measures to reduce noise and visual stimuli, although they can increase sensory impairment. Interventions should be decided on an individual basis and monitored closely. It is also helpful to minimise caffeinated drinks during the evening. Despite benzodiazepines being prescribed and given as sleeping tablets, new prescriptions should be avoided in older people with or at risk of delirium. Although they aid sleep, the sleep is often poor quality and the benefit is counteracted by the pro-deliriogenic effect of benzodiazepines.

MOBILITY

Mobilisation should be encouraged for people with or at risk of delirium. There should be emphasis on early mobilisation, such as after a hip fracture or a fall, or maintenance of mobility for individuals without a contraindication to mobilising. Encouragement of mobility can be achieved by small regular interventions such as encouragement to mobilise to the bathroom as opposed to using a commode at the bedside. Delirium is considered to be a neurocognitive disorder, but Gual et al. (2020) hypothesised it to be a motor disorder, as the inattention frequently present in delirium has a deleterious effect on safe mobilisation. They concluded physical exercise can prevent delirium and treat frailty. It is important to consider what factors affect mobility, such as the presence of lines and catheters, pain and walking aids. For older people with reduced mobility, physiotherapy assessment helps establish loss of muscle mass, gait abnormalities and specific mobility problems. If an older person has had a deterioration in their mobility, a new walking aid may be needed to re-establish independent mobilising.

PSYCHOLOGICAL CARE

The psychological effects of delirium can be significant and frightening to an older person, family and carers. An older adult may be unable to process or may misinterpret their surroundings, have auditory or visual hallucinations or develop paranoid thoughts. These symptoms may not be so apparent in people with hypoactive delirium, but they may still be distressed with psychotic symptoms. An older person may lack the attention to follow conversations and process information or could perceive people are trying to harm them or poison them and refuse food, fluids and medication. It was once thought that people did not remember their delirium experiences, but one study reported recall of experiences correlated with severe delirium and heightened perceptual disturbances (Grover et al., 2014).

How nurses react to and communicate with people with delirium is important and must adhere to best practice principles. Providing a supportive care environment is essential and includes greater involvement and communication with the older person and their family.

Despite the increased risk of falls and associated harms in the presence of delirium, restraint should be avoided. Restraint is defined as 'the intentional restriction of a person's voluntary movement or behaviour' (Royal College of Nursing, 2008). The means when used, whether chemical, physical or psychological, restraint may worsen delirium. Acute illness is already associated with functional and cognitive decline (Brummel et al., 2015), but immobility that results from restraints such as bed rails, bed tilts or sedatives may prevent a person with delirium from eating, drinking and eliminating without assistance. Instead of restraint, nurses should use strategies for optimum communication, safety and activity.

Staff must avoid arguing with or confronting an older person with delirium. Reassuring communication involves not disputing psychological symptoms (e.g., hallucinations or misperceptions) but verifying the older person's fear and providing consistent and calm explanation of delirium and its symptoms. It is helpful to aid understanding through the use of simple sentences and explanations in plain language, making good eye contact and therapeutic touch. One piece of information should be provided at a time, and the older person's responses and understanding checked regularly. The presence of delirium means all individuals who care for the older person consistently remind them of where they are, explain who the staff are, explain why they feel confused and provide reassurance of safety.

Introduction of cognitively stimulating activities is helpful in preventing delirium and aiding recovery. Providing one-on-one care may be needed after appropriate assessment. Meaningful activity throughout the day provides distraction from distressing symptoms and improves the effectiveness of sleep hygiene activities. An important part of care is facilitating regular visits from family and friends and encouraging them to bring in photographs and personal items such as a bedside clock and clothing. Staff should use family knowledge to develop person-centred daily activities, including physical activity. In the absence of relatives, one-on-one carers trained in delirium are helpful; among other things, trained support people can provide social interaction, assist with dietary and fluid intake, encourage activity and report progress to staff.

If an older person's psychiatric symptoms are distressing or threaten their safety and the safety of others, pharmacological treatment may be needed.

IMPORTANCE OF THE ENVIRONMENT AND FAMILY IN THERAPEUTIC CARE

The impact of a stable and comfortable clinical environment cannot be underestimated. Staffing should be organised to enhance consistency and minimise the number of people who interact with an older adult with delirium. Clinical interventions should be avoided at night if possible, and changes in environment should be avoided, especially at night. It is not uncommon for patients, particularly older patients, to be moved multiple times during a hospital stay (Royal College of Physicians [RCP], 2012). Ward transfers contravene best practice (NICE, 2019). Nurses should coordinate nursing activities (e.g., medication administration, vital signs) to minimise sleep interruption. Nursing people with delirium in single rooms is preferable to avoid overstimulation and decrease environmental noise (Blandfort et al., 2020), but the patient should be within sight of nurses.

The clinical area should have clear signage, dementia-friendly clocks, large-print calendars and patient care boards that list the date and the name of the health care personnel who work with the older person. To improve orientation and promote sleep, natural sunlight is important during the day, with reduced lighting in an older person's room and on the unit at night. Ensuring safety is important; night-lights in the room and leaving the bathroom door open are useful to reduce hallucinations and falls.

People with hyperactive delirium who are restless or distressed may try to leave the clinical environment. Nurses should consider the use of a motion sensor alarm on the bed, chair or floor. The sensor should be silent in the room, and nurses must take care when responding not to alarm the older person, which could increase distress and combative behaviour. For older adults who are keen to walk, one-to-one carers to accompany them reduces distress and promotes activity. Introducing familiar objects, including personal nightclothes and toiletries, can contribute to orientation strategies and help the older person recognise their 'own' area. Any clinical equipment not in use should be removed, such as monitors and pumps.

The attitudes of health care staff contribute to the clinical environment (RCP, 2012). A collaborative approach to care with older adults and their relatives reduces staff stress and positively influences the patient journey. Acting on family members' reporting of early warning signs of an episode of delirium can reduce the severity of the episode. Inviting families to share biographic knowledge creates therapeutic relationships and increases perceptions of safety (Dewar et al., 2013). Asking families to complete a 'getting to know me' document (Robertson & Fitzpatrick, 2021) helps health care staff deliver person-centred care. Older people and families value a reciprocal relationship, and staff sharing information about delirium presentation, causes, treatment and non-pharmaceutical interventions is appreciated (NICE, 2019).

Flexible visiting times and overnight stays facilitate families who wish to support an older adult with fundamental care and meaningful activity, including cognitive stimulation and mobilising during daytime hours. Informal caregivers may not have had formal training as a health or social care provider, so staff must continue to educate, support and supervise their involvement. Family can become fatigued and stressed; staff must check frequently on their well-being and offer breaks. Caregiver stress is reduced by receiving timely and relevant information about an older person's progress and knowing they are making a difference for the older person and the staff (Dewar et al., 2013).

Older people who recover from delirium sometimes report post delirium stress if they recall any aspects of their hallucinations and confusion (SIGN, 2019). Although some express feelings of fear the condition will recur or embarrassment at acting out of character, others are curious about their experiences. They should have the opportunity to talk about it. Early in the delirium journey, staff can suggest the family keep a journal about the older person's delirium experiences to help them make sense of what happened after recovery.

MEDICAL TREATMENT OF UNDERLYING CAUSES

Delirium is a medical emergency that is associated with poor outcomes, including increased risk of death. The possible underlying aetiology list is broad. It is not possible to discuss all aspects of delirium treatment, familiarity with some of the more common causes and treatments is helpful. Some, such as dehydration, pain and constipation, have already been discussed. In the initial approach to an individual with delirium, life-threatening conditions should be diagnosed and treated. SIGN includes in its life-threatening emergencies section hypoxia, hypoglycaemia, hypotension and acute intoxication or withdrawal (SIGN, 2019).

INFECTION

Sepsis in older people can be diagnostically challenging as older patients have a reduced febrile response and the primary presenting symptoms may be atypical, including delirium, reduced consciousness, fatigue and urinary incontinence (Juneja, 2012). Older people may be prescribed medications that affect their responses, such as beta-blockers, and mask sepsis associated tachycardia.

Infection should be treated with appropriate antibiotics. A common incorrect presumption is urinary tract infection is diagnosed on the basis of a positive urinary dipstick. This should be avoided and careful assessment for signs and symptoms made, together with any laboratory results if available, before diagnosis is made and treatment provided.

CARDIAC

Myocardial infarction is a less common yet important cause of delirium. One study showed 5% of individuals over 70 who experienced ST-elevation myocardial infarction (STEMI) presented with delirium as their primary complaint. Individuals who presented with delirium had longer prehospital waits, longer waits for assessment in hospital, reduced chance of reperfusion therapy and higher mortality at 1 month. For this reason, an electrocardiogram is an important investigation in the assessment of delirium (Grosmaitre et al., 2013).

MULTIPLE CAUSES

It is important to treat each individual aetiology that provokes delirium in accordance with best practices. Often, multiple causes for delirium are identified and must be treated simultaneously. Even after the initial assessment and identification of causes, an older adult with delirium must be reassessed daily to see whether it remains present and to identify any new contributing causes.

NON-PHARMACOLOGICAL INTERVENTIONS TO PREVENT DELIRIUM AND TREAT DISTRESS IN DELIRIUM

There is a significant overlap between interventions considered to be preventative measures for delirium and those considered supportive. Most research into non-pharmacological interventions focuses on the outcome in terms of prevention of delirium as opposed to treatment of the delirium once it has occurred. A Cochrane study assessed the use of non-pharmacological intervention: a multicomponent delirium prevention intervention compared against standardised care within an acute hospital setting (Siddiqi et al., 2016). The parameters considered were prevention of delirium, duration and severity of delirium, length of admission, return to independent living and inpatient mortality. The study showed the multicomponent delirium prevention intervention had a moderate effect on reducing the incidence of delirium compared to standard care (30%), but the evidence was less clear for reduction of severity, length of hospital admission, admission to long term care and mortality following the onset of delirium. The Cochrane study showed some evidence the interventions may reduce pressure ulcers and improve cognition in the long term. This reinforces the importance that the primary aim of treatment should be delirium prevention.

Despite absence of evidence these interventions improve outcomes once delirium develops, it remains the case that the correct management of delirium includes good supportive care for the symptoms of delirium while preventing development of conditions that exacerbate the existing delirium, such as sleep deprivation and constipation. Holistic nursing care that meets deficits in independent management of activities of daily living is the basis of delirium management for nursing staff.

The latest National Institute for Health and Care Excellence guidelines advise a multicomponent intervention should be patient-specific, determined within 24 hours of admission for all patients at risk of delirium and applied by a multidisciplinary team who are competent in management of delirium (NICE, 2019).

MEDICAL THERAPIES TO TREAT DISTRESS IN DELIRIUM

Delirium affects multiple neurochemical pathways, including the dopaminergic and cholinergic pathways, and it is hypothesised that targeting these pathways through pharmacological therapy alleviates the symptoms of delirium (Wilson et al., 2020). Given that delirium affects multiple neurological pathways, and treatments focus only on a specific target, this is thought to be an oversimplification.

A Cochrane analysis assessed the role of antipsychotics in treating delirium (Siddiqi et al., 2016) and identified three low-quality studies that assessed either haloperidol (a first-generation antipsychotic) or olanzapine (a second-generation antipsychotic) as a treatment. Due to the low quality of the research, it was not possible to establish whether there was any benefit in treatment of delirium, including duration and severity. These outcomes were further echoed in a larger systematic review of antipsychotics that included 10 randomised control studies and eight observational studies and compared haloperidol against placebo and against second-generation antipsychotics (olanzapine, risperidone and quetiapine) to determine the effect on delirium. The authors concluded that neither haloperidol or second-generation antipsychotics when compared to the placebo affected length of hospital admission, duration of delirium, mortality and sedation, and they could not establish whether they affected severity of delirium or cognitive function (Nikooie et al., 2019).

It is also important the side effects and risks associated with these medications for the treatment of delirium are considered. The British National Formulary (2020b) notes that with all antipsychotics, caution should be used for individuals with cardiovascular disease and those with predisposition to seizures or closer angle glaucoma and prostatic hypertrophy (i.e., increased risk of urinary retention). They also advise caution for people who are prone to falling, as gait dyspraxia may be exacerbated. These conditions are more prevalent in older adults compared to the younger population and can have significant consequences. In individuals with cardiovascular conditions, antipsychotics may cause QT prolongation on the electrocardiogram, which increases the risk of life-threatening arrythmias. Antipsychotics can also interact with other medications that prolong the QT interval.

Nikooie et al. (2019) considered the potential complications of antipsychotics and concluded most trials that assessed for complications were focused on individuals who are critically ill. The analysis found no evidence of neurological complications with short-term use of antipsychotics but did find evidence of QT prolongation associated with second-generation antipsychotics compared with haloperidol and placebo. One palliative care study showed a higher rate of mortality was associated with use of haloperidol or risperidone vs. a placebo.

The lack of established efficacy and potential side effects, particularly in older people, means antipsychotics should not be prescribed for delirium other than in cases of severe agitation where the person is at risk of harm to themselves or others. Current guidelines recommend the use of antipsychotics to treat distress only when verbal and non-verbal techniques fail (NICE, 2019). The National Institute for Health and Care Excellence guidelines also state antipsychotics should not be given to individuals with Parkinson's disease or Lewy body dementia, as the severe extrapyramidal side effects outweigh any potential treatment benefit (NICE, 2019).

Antipsychotics are the most studied drug class for preventing delirium. Other studied drugs include cholinesterase inhibitors, dexmedetomidine (a sedative) and benzodiazepines. The SIGN guidelines (SIGN, 2019) discuss the role of anticholinesterases for delirium treatment and were unable to detect a difference between their use vs. a placebo. Anticholinesterases are not currently recommended in the treatment of delirium. Dexmedetomidine is a sedative that does not affect respiratory function and has been studied for the treatment of delirium in ICU patients, for whom research is limited. In one small study of patients intubated for severe delirium/agitation, dexmedetomidine was shown to increase ventilator-free days compared to standard care (Reade et al., 2016). Another study showed it achieved satisfactory sedative levels in ICU patients with delirium resistant to haloperidol (Carrasco et al., 2016). Dexmedetomidine carries significant risk of side effects, including arrythmias and hypo- and hypertension respiratory depression, so it must be used with caution in older adults or those with cardiovascular or cerebrovascular disease (British National Formulary [BNF], 2020a). Although it is licensed, its use is reserved for limited cases in ICUs under direct supervision of health care professionals with adequate anaesthetic experience.

There is limited research into benzodiazepines as treatment for delirium, and they are known to be a risk factor for the development of delirium. One Cochrane review to assess their role in non-alcohol related delirium concluded the limited studies fail to show any benefit in the treatment of delirium (Lonergan et al., 2009).

There is lack of proven efficacy for any medication to treat agitation and distress due to delirium. Given concerns over safety, medication should be prescribed only in exceptional circumstances for severe delirium. For this reason the recommendations for first- and second-line medications as well as dosages vary between guidelines, and we do not provide specific guidance in this chapter. The presence of comorbidities and associated drug therapies must be considered before starting medication. For example, antipsychotic medications are contraindicated in Parkinson's disease and Lewy body dementia (NICE, 2017). Benzodiazepines may be considered but may cause side effects in people with Parkinson's disease or Lewy body disease. Medication used should be prescribed in the lowest possible dose for the shortest time possible and should involve specialist guidance.

If commenced, medication prescribed for delirium should be reviewed daily and stopped as soon as clinically indicated. In some situations, antipsychotic therapy for delirium is required beyond discharge or transfer from hospital; in these cases a clear plan for early medication review and follow-up in the community should be agreed with the primary care or mental health team.

MANAGEMENT OF DELIRIUM IN DIFFERENT CARE SETTINGS

We have discussed the role of excellent nursing care in both prevention and management of delirium. Physiological and psychological interventions form the mainstay of treatment, including addressing modifiable risk factors and managing the distress caused by delirium. Most aspects of nursing care can be provided in any care setting for patients with delirium. The decision of where to treat an older person with delirium should be made by an experienced clinician, taking into account local resources and a risk–benefit balance. In some cases an older person needs to be taken to hospital for management of either the symptoms of delirium or the underlying aetiology. However, in other cases it is possible to safely manage the older person with delirium in their own home or care home setting, with increased support. The decision of where the older person is treated may change as the clinical course evolves.

MANAGEMENT OF DELIRIUM IN AN INTENSIVE CARE SETTING

Although we typically imagine ICUs more commonly manage younger patients, in fact people over 65 account for 45%–52% of admissions and 60% of ICU days (Marik, 2006). Given the risk of delirium being significantly higher in ICUs compared with other settings due to the amount of interventions, use of pro-delirogenic medications and disruption to the sleep–wake cycle, it is important to consider the care and management of an older patient with delirium in an ICU.

Supportive care remains the mainstay of delirium treatment and prevention in the ICU. Nursing is on a reduced nurse-to-patient ratio in an ICU, which allows for familiarity to develop. This helps with the reorientation as the older person spends more direct time being nursed, given their higher care needs, compared to in the community or in a standard hospital bed. Early reduction in the use of sedatives and promotion of spontaneous breathing trials in an ICU programme called awakening and breathing coordination of daily sedation and ventilator removal trials, choice of sedative or analgesic exposure, delirium monitoring and management, and early mobility and exercise (ABCDE) showed promising effects in reducing length of sedation, hospital and intensive care stay and improved rates of mortality (Balas et al., 2014).

The use of medications to treat delirium syndrome is more freely used in the ICU setting. The Scottish Intensive Care Society advised the use of medications if no organic cause is found and preventative measures have been ineffective; as a first line the society advises haloperidol (Northwick et al., 2006). This differs from care in the community or other wards where medications are seldom used and only for symptomatic relief. The accepted use of medications to treat delirium in the ICU is likely due to a combination of close monitoring of potential side effects, including the use of cardiac monitoring as standard care, increased risk of agitation for preventing or removing life-saving treatment, and the significance of the delirium due to the number of driving factors in the ICU. The use of mechanical, pharmacological or physical restraints is a controversial area of practice but is probably more freely used than in other settings given the risk for harm. The British Association of Critical Care Nurses produced guidelines on the use of restraints and advised the United Kingdom is less accepting of restraints because they result in failure to perform the 'professional obligation to ensure that patient freedom, dignity and autonomy are maintained' (Bray et al., 2004, p. 200). The association also advised restraints should never be used in place of human and environmental resources and should be used only when other methods of treatment fail. The decision must be made following a detailed patient-specific assessment and be regularly reviewed (Bray et al., 2004). An older person's family should be engaged in discussion and decision making around the use of restraints, including the rationale behind the chosen method of any sedation.

MANAGEMENT OF DELIRIUM IN END-OF-LIFE CARE

Delirium is a common symptom experienced as a person nears death; some studies report incidence of delirium in up to 88% of people with terminal illness (Harris, 2007). As with management of all cases of delirium, assessing and treating the underlying aetiology should be a primary aim. For end-of-life care, the use of certain medications, such as

analgesia, may be the precipitating factor. It is often the case that the terminal stage of illness is the underlying aetiology. Treatment for the older person and their family is the provision of high-quality palliative care. The presence of family at the end of life is particularly helpful for reorientation and the distress associated with delirium.

As an older person approaches the terminal stage of disease, management of delirium may differ from that used with terminally ill patients. When an individual enters their final days of life, they may experience terminal anguish, or delirium with overwhelming anxiety. In this situation symptom-control medications are used, even though it may result in oversedation (Barraclough, 1997). In the final stages, it is common for a person to be kept on a continuous infusion of medications, typically benzodiazepine or haloperidol, to ease anxiety, and the side effects are accepted in order to minimise distress in terminal disease.

There is some debate around the best medication to use. One study compared the use of placebo with haloperidol or risperidone showed worsening of behavioural, communication and perceptual problems in the haloperidol or risperidone group as compared to a placebo (Agar et al., 2017). Whichever medications are prescribed, the older person should be carefully monitored for signs of distress. Proactive increases in medication are used until adequate symptom relief is achieved. The doctrine of double effect provides an ethical clause in palliative care; it advises that if a health care worker is aiming for moral good, such as with symptom control, any morally bad side effect, such as hastening death, can be tolerated (Palliative Care: Education & Training, 2020). In practice this means the side effects of medications and treatments that hasten death are accepted as they alleviate suffering—for example, the use of benzodiazepines to reduce terminal anguish.

DISCHARGE PLANNING AND FOLLOW-UP

Persistent delirium at discharge occurs in approximately 30% of older people (Verloo et al., 2016) and causes concerns about the safety of discharge. Early supported discharge may resolve delirium symptoms when an older person returns home to a familiar environment and routines. It should be explained to family members what to do if delirium does not resolve or recurs, and they should be supported to continue with the non-pharmaceutical interventions used during admission. The management of delirium should involve discharge planning that includes post-discharge follow-up in the community (MacLullich et al., 2013). The potential association with future dementia risk necessitates periodic cognitive function assessment, and the SIGN guidelines recommend seeking primary care review if cognitive symptoms persist in the following months (SIGN, 2019). Developing delirium increases the risk of future episodes of delirium. Multidisciplinary information sharing between care settings is vital.

CONCLUSION

Delirium is a common condition in older people but is often under-recognised and under-diagnosed. The presenting complaint may not always be acute confusion and hence the diagnosis should always be sought in those with frailty and common presentations in that group such as reduced mobility and falls. Similarly attributed causes for

delirium with little clinical evidence such as urinary tract infection should be questioned and confirmed. Given high prevalence, the distress caused and delirium as a common reason for deterioration in the health of the older person there has been an increase in the number of guidelines and the amount of research taking place. The overview here is comprehensive but we would encourage the interested reader to explore current literature at the time of reading for any new developments in the field. As mentioned at the start of this chapter good delirium care is good care, and there is a great deal of satisfaction to be gained in provision of high standard nursing care.

KEY LEARNING POINTS

- Delirium is a commonly occurring but poorly understood and underrecognised condition that has consistently poor outcomes in older adults.
- Delirium is multifactorial in nature. The components that contribute to delirium are frequently interrelated.
- Many delirium triggers are modifiable. Prevention strategies may overlap with treatment.
- Nursing interventions to reduce the risk of developing delirium and to treat delirium must be acted on throughout the care journey of an older person.

- Person-centred care is the recommended aim for best practice in caring for older people. In the care of delirium, this approach extends to include the family through relationship-centred care.
- Using clinical and biographic knowledge alongside assessment tools, nurses can play a central role in the detection, treatment and prevention of delirium and to improve physical, psychological and social outcomes for older adults.

REFERENCES

4AT—*Rapid Clinical Test for Delirium.* https://www.the4at.com.
Abdulla, A., Adams, N., Bone, M., Elliott, A. M., Gaffin, J., Jones, D., Knaggs, R., Martin, D., Sampson, L., & Schofield, P., British Geriatric Society. (2013). Guidance on the management of pain in older people. *Age & Ageing, 42*(Suppl 1) i1–57.
Agar, M., Lawlor, P., Quinn, S., Draper, B., Caplan, G., Rowett, D., Sanderson, C., Hardy, J., Le, B., Eckermann, S., McCaffrey, N., Devilee, L., Fazekas, B., Hill, M., & Currow, D. (2017). Efficacy of oral risperidone, haloperidol, or placebo for symptoms of delirium among patients in palliative care: A randomised clinical trial. *JAMA Internal Medicine, 177*(1), 34–42.
American Geriatrics Society. (2002). Clinical practice guidelines: The management of persistent pain in older persons. *Journal of the American Geriatrics Society, 50,* S205–S224.
American Psychiatric Association. (2013). *American psychiatric diagnostic and statistical manual of mental disorders* (5th ed.). American Psychiatric Association.
Balas, M. C., Vasilevskis, E. E., Olsen, K. M., Schmid, K. K., Shostrom, V., Cohen, M. Z., Peitz, G., Gannon, D. E., Sisson, J., Sullivan, J., Stothert, J. C., Lazure, J., Nuss, S. L., Jawa, R. S., Freihaut, F., Ely, E. W., & Burke, W. J. (2014). Effectiveness and safety of the awakening and breathing coordination, delirium monitoring/management, and early exercise/mobility bundle. *Critical Care Medicine, 42*(5), 1024–1036.

Barraclough, J. (1997). ABC of palliative care: Depression, anxiety, and confusion. *BMJ, 315,* 1365.
Blandfort, S., Gregersen, M., Rahbek, K., Jull, S., & Damsgaard, E. M. (2020). Single-bed rooms in a geriatric ward prevent delirium in older patients. *Aging—Clinical & Experimental Research, 32,* 141–147.
Blevins, C., & DeGennaro, R. (2018). Educational intervention to improve delirium recognition by nurses. *American Journal of Critical Care, 27*(4), 270–278.
Boorsma, M., Joling, K. J., Frijters, D. H. M., Ribbe, M. E., Nijpels, G., & van Hout, H. P. J. (2012). The prevalence, incidence and risk factors for delirium in Dutch nursing homes and residential care homes. *International Journal of Geriatric Psychiatry, 27*(7), 709–715.
Bray, K., Hill, K., Robson, W., Leaver, G., Walker, N., O'Leary, M., Delaney, T., Walsh, D., Gager, M., & Waterhouse, C. (2004). British Association of Critical Care Nurses position statement on the use of restraint in adult critical care units. *Nursing in Critical Care, 9*(5), 199–212.
British Association for Parenteral and Enteral Nutrition. (2016). *Nutrition support: Assessment and planning.* https://bapen. org.uk/screening-and-must/81-nutrition-suort
British Geriatrics Society. (2019). *CGA in primary care settings: Patients presenting with confusion and delirium.* https://www.bgs.org.uk/resources/14-cga-in-primary-care-settings-patients-presenting-with-confusion-and-delirium

British National Formulary (BNF) (2020a). DEXMEDETOMI-DINE | Drug | BNF Content Published By NICE. [online] https://bnf.nice.org.uk/drug/dexmedetomidine.html

British National Formulary (BNF). (2020b). HALOPERIDOL | Drug | BNF Content Published By NICE. [online] https://bnf.nice.org.uk/drug/haloperidol.html#cautions.

Brummel, N. E., Balas, M. C., Morandi, A., Ferrante, L. E., Gill, T. M., & Ely, E. W. (2015). Understanding and reducing disability in older adults following critical illness. *Critical Care Medicine, 43*(6), 1265–1275.

Burn, E., Hartley, C., Cabada, J., Skelly, R., & Gordon, A. (2019). Is the modified single question in delirium as good as the confusion assessment method as diagnosing delirium. *Age & Ageing, 48*(Suppl. 2) ii31–ii31.

Carrasco, G., Baeza, N., Cabré, L., Portillo, E., Gimeno, G., Manzanedo, D., & Calizaya, M. (2016). Dexmedetomidine for the treatment of hyperactive delirium refractory to haloperidol in nonintubated ICU patients. *Critical Care Medicine, 44*(7), 1295–1306.

Cimarolli, V., & Jopp, D. S. (2014). Sensory impairments and their associations with functional disability in a sample of the oldest-old. *Quality of Life Research, 23*(7), 1977–1984.

Clegg, A., & Young, J. B. (2011). Which medications to avoid in people at risk of delirium: A systematic review. *Age & Ageing, 40*(1), 23–29.

Davis, D., Skelly, D., Murray, C., Hennessy, E., Bowen, J., Norton, S., Brayne, C., Rahkonen, T., Sulkava, R., Sanderson, D., Rawlins, J., Bannerman, D., MacLullich, A., & Cunningham, C. (2015). Worsening cognitive impairment and neurodegenerative pathology progressively increase risk for delirium. *The American Journal of Geriatric Psychiatry, 23*(4), 403–415.

Dewar, B., Bond, P., Miller, M., & Goudie, K. (2013). Staff, patients and families experiences of giving and receiving care during an episode of delirium in an acute hospital care setting. *Healthcare Improvement Scotland*. www.healthcare-improvmentscotland.org

Docherty, A., Harrison, E., Green, C., Hardwick, H., Pius, R., Norman, L., Holden, K., Read, J., Dondelinger, F., Carson, G., Merson, L., Lee, J., Plotkin, D., Sigfrid, L., Halpin, S., Jackson, C., Gamble, C., Horby, P., Nguyen-Van-Tam, J., Ho, A., & Semple, M. (2020). Features of 20 133 UK patients in hospital with Covid-19 using the ISARIC WHO Clinical Characterisation Protocol: Prospective observational cohort study. *BMJ, 369*, m1985.

Egberts, A., Moreno-Gonzalez, R., Alan, H., Ziere, G., & Mattace-Raso, F. U. S. (2020). Anticholinergic drug burden and delirium: A systematic review. *Journal of the American Medical Directors Association, 22*(1), 65–73.

El-Menyar, A., Arumugam, S., Al-Hassani, A., Strandvik, G., Asim, M., Mekkodithal, A., Mudali, I., & Al-Thani, H. (2017). Delirium in the intensive care unit. *Journal of Emergencies, Trauma, & Shock, 10*(1), 37.

Engel, G. L., & Romano, J. (1959). Delirium, a syndrome of cerebral insufficiency. *Journal of Chronic Diseases, 9*, 260–277.

Fischer, T., Hosie, A., Luckett, T., Agar, M., & Phillips, M. (2019). Strategies for pain assessment in adult patients with delirium: A scoping review. *Journal of Pain & Symptom Management, 58*(3), 487–502.

Fong, T., Jones, R., Shi, P., Marcantonio, E., Yap, L., Rudolph, J., Yang, F., Kiely, D., & Inouye, S. (2009a). Delirium accelerates cognitive decline in Alzheimer disease. *Neurology, 72*(18), 1570–1575.

Fong, T., Tulebaev, S., & Inouye, S. (2009b). Delirium in elderly adults: Diagnosis, prevention and treatment. *Nature Reviews Neurology, 5*(4), 210–220.

Grosmaitre, P., Le Vavasseur, O., Yachouh, E., Courtial, Y., Jacob, X., Meyran, S., & Lantelme, P. (2013). Significance of atypical symptoms for the diagnosis and management of myocardial infarction in elderly patients admitted to emergency departments. *Archives of Cardiovascular Diseases, 106*(11), 586–592.

Grover, S., Ghosh, A., & Ghormode, D. (2014). Experience in delirium: Is it distressing? *The Journal of Neuropsychiatry & Clinical Neurosciences, 27*(2), 139–146.

Gual, N., Garcia-Salmones, M., Britez, L., Crespo, N., Udina, C., Pérez, L. M., & Inziteri, M. (2020). The role of physical exercise and rehabilitation in delirium. *European Geriatric Medicine, 11*, 83–93.

Hall, M., Pritchar, M., Dankwa, E., Kenneth Baillie, J., Carson, G., Citarella, B., Docherty, A., Donnelly, C., Dunning, J., Fraser, C., Hardwick, H., Harrison, E., Holden, K., Kartsonaki, C., Kennon, K., Lee, J., Mclean, K., Openshaw, P., Plotkin, D., Rojek, A., Merson, L. (2020). *COVID-19 evidence and reports – ISARIC.* [online] ISARIC. https://isaric.org/research/covid-19-clinical-research-resources/evidence-reports

Hargrave, A., Bastiaens, J., Bourgeois, J., Neuhaus, J., Josephson, S., Chinn, J., Lee, M., Leung, J., & Douglas, V. (2017). Validation of a nurse-based delirium-screening tool for hospitalized patients. *Psychosomatics, 58*(6), 594–603.

Harris, D. (2007). Delirium in advanced disease. *Postgraduate Medical Journal, 83*(982), 525–528.

Hendry, K., Quinn, T., Evans, J., Scortichini, V., Miller, H., Burns, J., Cunnington, A., & Stott, D. (2016). Evaluation of delirium screening tools in geriatric medical inpatients: A diagnostic test accuracy study. *Age & Ageing, 45*(6), 832–837.

Inouye, S., van Dyck, C., Alessi, C., Balkin, S., Siegal, A., & Horwitz, R. (1990). Clarifying confusion: The confusion assessment method. A new method for detection of delirium. *Annals of Internal Medicine, 113*(12), 941–948.

Jackson, T., MacLullich, A., Gladman, J., Lord, J., & Sheehan, B. (2016). Diagnostic test accuracy of informant-based tools to diagnose dementia in older hospital patients with delirium: A prospective cohort study. *Age & Ageing, 45*(4), 505–511.

Juneja, D. (2012). Severe sepsis and septic shock in the elderly: An overview. *World Journal of Critical Care Medicine, 1*(1), 23.

Lonergan, E., Luxenburg, J., & Areosa Sastre, A (2009). Benzodiazepines for delirium. *Cochrane Database of Systematic Reviews*(4), Article CD006379 2009.

MacLullich, A., Beaglehole, A., Hall, R., & Meagher, D. (2009). Delirium and long-term cognitive impairment. *International Review of Psychiatry, 21*(1), 30–42.

MacLullich, A. M. J., Anand, A., & Davis, D. H. J. (2013). New horizons in the pathogenesis, assessment and management of delirium. *Age & Ageing, 42*(6), 667–674.

Marengoni, A., Zucchelli, A., Grande, G., Fratiglioni, L., & Rizzuto, D. (2020). The impact of delirium on outcomes for older adults hospitalised with COVID-19. *Age & Ageing, 49*(6), 923–926.

Marik, P. (2006). Management of the critically ill geriatric patient. *Critical Care Medicine, 34*(Suppl), S176–S182.

Martins, S., & Fernandes, L. (2012). Delirium in elderly people: A review. *Frontiers in Neurology, 2012*(3), 101.

Meagher, D. (2009). Motor subtypes of delirium: Past, present and future. *International Review of Psychiatry, 21*(1), 59–73.

Meagher, D., MacLullich, A., & Laurila, J. (2008). Defining delirium for the International Classification of Diseases, 11th Revision. *Journal of Psychosomatic Research, 65*(3), 207–214.

Morichi, V., Fedecostante, M., Morandi, A., Di Santo, S. G., Mazzone, A., Mossello, E., Bo, M., Bianchetti, A., Rozzini, R., Zanetti, E., Musicco, M., Ferrari, A., Ferrara, N., Trabucchi, M., Cheruini, A., & Bellelli, G. (2018). A point prevalence study of delirium in Italian nursing homes. *Dementia Geriatric Cognitive Disorders, 46*(1-2), 27–41.

National Institute for Clinical Excellence. (2017). *Parkinson's disease in adults. NICE guideline 71.* https://www.nice.org.uk/guidance/ng71

National Institute of Health and Care Excellence (NICE). (2019). *Delirium: Prevention, diagnosis and management CG103.* https://www.nice.org.uk/guidance/cg103ng70

Neufeld, K., Yue, J., Robinson, T., Inouye, S., & Needham, D. (2016). Antipsychotic medication for prevention and treatment of delirium in hospitalized adults: A systematic review and meta-analysis. *Journal of the American Geriatrics Society, 64*(4), 705–714.

Nikooie, R., Neufeld, K., Oh, E., Wilson, L., Zhang, A., Robinson, K., & Needham, D. (2019). Antipsychotics for treating delirium in hospitalized adults. *Annals of Internal Medicine, 171*(7), 485.

Northwick, M., Bourne, R., Craig, M., Egan, A., & Oxley, J. (2006). *Detection, prevention and treatment of delirium in critically ill patients.* [online] https://www.scottishintensivecare.org.uk/uploads/2014-07-24-19-57-26-UKCPADelirium-Resourcepdf-92654.pdf

O'Keeffe, S. (1999). Clinical significance of delirium subtypes in older people. *Age & Ageing, 28*(2), 115–119.

Palliative Care: Education and Training. (2020). *Ethical framework of palliative sedation: The principle of double effect.* https://palliative.stanford.edu/palliative-sedation/ethical-framework-of-palliative-sedation-the-principle-of-double-effect

Persico, I., Cesari, M., Morandi, A., Haas, J., Mazzola, P., Zambon, A., Annoni, G., & Bellelli, G. (2018). Frailty and delirium in older adults: A systematic review and meta-analysis of the literature. *Journal of the American Geriatrics Society, 66*(10), 2022–2030.

Rahman, S. (2018). *Living well with frailty: From assets and deficits to resilience.* Routledge.

Reade, M. C., Eastwood, G. M., Bellomo, R., Bailey, M., Bersten, A., Cheung, B., Davies, A., Delaney, A., Ghosh, A., van Haren, F., Harley, N., Knight, D., McGuiness, S., Mulder, J.,

O'Donoghue, S., Simpson, N., & Young, P. DahLIA Investigators; Australian and New Zealand Intensive Care Society Clinical Trials Group. (2016). Effect of dexmedetomidine added to standard care on ventilator-free time in patients with agitated delirium: A randomized clinical trial. *JAMA: Journal of the American Medical Association, 315*(14), 1460–1468.

Robertson, E. M., & Fitzpatrick, J. M. (2021). 'Five things about me'—enhancing person-centred care for older people. *Nursing Older People, 34*(1), 21–27.

Rogers, J., Chesney, E., Oliver, D., Pollak, T., McGuire, P., Fusar-Poli, P., Zandi, M., Lewis, G., & David, A. (2020). Psychiatric and neuropsychiatric presentations associated with severe coronavirus infections: A systematic review and meta-analysis with comparison to the COVID-19 pandemic. *The Lancet Psychiatry, 7*(7), 611–627.

Rosen, T., Connors, S., Sunday, C., Halpern, A., Stern, M. E., DeWald, J., Lachs, M. S., & Flomenbaum, N. (2015). Assessment and management of delirium in older adults in the emergency department: Literature review to inform development of a novel clinical protocol. *Advanced Emergency Nursing Journal, 37*(3), 183–196.

Royal College of Nursing. (2008). *"Let's talk about restraint" Right, risk and responsibility.* Royal College of Nursing.

Royal College of Physicians (RCP). (2012). *Hospitals on the edge? The time for action,* https://www.rcplondon.ac.uk/guidelines-policy/hospitals-edge-time-action

Royal College of Physicians (RCP). (2020). *National Early Warning Score (NEWS) 2 Standardising the assessment of acute-illness severity in the NHS. Additional implementation guidance.* https://www.rcplondon.ac.uk/projects/outputs/news2-additional-implementation-guidance

Ryan, D., O'Regan, N., Caoimh, R., Clare, J., O'Connor, M., Leonard, M., McFarland, J., Tighe, S., O'Sullivan, K., Trzepacz, P., Meagher, D., & Timmons, S. (2013). Delirium in an adult acute hospital population: Predictors, prevalence and detection. *BMJ Open, 3*(1), e001772.

Sampson, E., Blanchard, M., Jones, L., Tookman, A., & King, M. (2009). Dementia in the acute hospital: Prospective cohort study of prevalence and mortality. *British Journal of Psychiatry, 195*(1), 61–66.

Sampson, E. L., West, E., & Fischer, T. (2020). Pain and delirium: Mechanisms, assessment, and management. *European Geriatric Medicine, 11*, 45–52.

Scottish Intercollegiate Guidelines Network (SIGN). (2019). 157: Guidelines on risk reduction and management of delirium. *Medicina, 55*(8), 491.

Siddiqi, N., Harrison, JK., Clegg, A., Teale, EA., Young, J., Taylor, J., & Simpkins, S. A. (2016). Interventions for preventing delirium in hospitalised non-ICU patients. *Cochrane Database of Systematic Reviews, 2016*(3), CD005563.

Siddiqi, N., House, A., & Holmes, J. (2006). Occurrence and outcome of delirium in medical in-patients: A systematic literature review. *Age & Ageing, 35*(4), 350–364.

Slooter, A., Otte, W., Devlin, J., Arora, R., Bleck, T., Claassen, J., Duprey, M., Ely, E., Kaplan, P., Latronico, N., Morandi, A., Neufeld, K., Sharshar, T., MacLullich, A., & Stevens, R. (2020). Updated nomenclature of delirium and acute encephalopathy: Statement of ten Societies. *Intensive Care Medicine, 46*(5), 1020–1022.

Social Care Institute for Excellence. (2015). *Dementia-friendly environments: Noise levels*. https://www.scie.org.uk/dementia/suorting-people-with-dementia/dementia-friendly-environments/noise.asp

Van Montfort, S., van Dellen, E., Stam, C., Ahmad, A., Mentink, L., Kraan, C., Zalesky, A., & Slooter, A. (2019). Brain network disintegration as a final common pathway for delirium: A systematic review and qualitative meta-analysis. *NeuroImage: Clinical, 23*, 101809.

Vardy, E. R., Teodorczuk, A., & Yarnall, A. J. (2015). Review of delirium in patients with Parkinson's disease. *Journal of Neurology, 262*(11), 2401–2410.

Verloo, H., Goulet, C, Morin, D., & von Gunten, A. (2016). Association between frailty and delirium in older adult patients discharged from hospital. *Clinical Interventions in Aging, 18*(11), 55–63.

Watt, C. L., Momoli, F., Ansari, M. T., Sikora, L., Bush, S. H., Hossie, A., Kabir, M., Rosenberg, E., Kanji, S., & Lawlor, P. G. (2019). The incidence and prevalence of delirium across palliative care settings: A systematic review. *Palliative Medicine, 33*(8), 865–877.

Wilson, J., Mart, M., Cunningham, C., Shehabi, Y., Girard, T., MacLullich, A., Slooter, A., & Ely, E. (2020). Delirium. *Nature Reviews Disease Primers, 6*, 90.

Witlox, J., Eurelings, L., de Jonghe, J., Kalisvaart, K., Eikelenboom, P., & van Gool, W. (2010). Delirium in elderly patients and the risk of postdischarge mortality, institutionalization, and dementia. *JAMA: Journal of the American Medical Association, 304*(4), 443.

Zazzara, M., Penfold, R., Roberts, A., Lee, K., Dooley, H., Sudre, C., Welch, C., Bowyer, R., Visconti, A., Mangino, M., Freidin, M., El-Sayed Moustafa, J., Small, K., Murray, B., Modat, M., Graham, M., Wolf, J., Ourselin, S., Martin, F., Steves, C., & Lochlainn, M. (2020). Probable delirium is a presenting symptom of COVID-19 in frail, older adults: A cohort study of 322 hospitalised and 535 community-based older adults. *Age & Ageing, 50*(1), 40–48.

29

Care of the Person Living With Dementia

Katie A. Davis, Rachel S. Price

CHAPTER OUTLINE

A note on terminology: Throughout this chapter, you will see the use of the term *person living with dementia*. Over the past 20 years, terminology has changed to recognise the person should be identified first. *Demented, sufferer* and even *dementia patients* are outdated and should no longer be used by health care professionals, the general public or the media.

Dementia is not a disease but a syndrome that can affect memory, orientation, thinking, comprehension, language, learning capacity and judgement. Dementia is caused by diseases of the brain and can interfere significantly with an individual's ability to engage and sustain everyday activities of daily living. Each person living with dementia experiences associated symptoms in an unique way, depending on the nature of the dementia syndrome and which part of their brain is affected. The experience of living with dementia can be challenging for individuals with the condition and for those providing care, but there is evidence personalised dementia care can reduce these challenges and enhance quality of life.

The medical model of dementia presents a view that the condition is a clinical syndrome where the person living with dementia is defined by their illness or disease; they are dependent and need to be cured. As a result, the person is more likely to lose their identity, with the focus more intent on the process, causes and symptoms of disease rather than the person living with dementia. The medical model view holds relevance in presenting the biological processes that arise as a result of the onset of a dementia. However, the work of the late Tom Kitwood and the Bradford Dementia Group in the late 1990s presented a new culture of dementia care where there was a shift from understanding dementia as a singular medical construct. This shift was aligned with the principles of person centredness, which were developed by Carl Rogers and promoted a move away from traditional medical models of care. Kitwood's concept of personhood has been established for over 20 years, and the psychosocial perspective of dementia has matured to include the concepts of citizenship and human rights.

The adoption of a personalised approach in dementia care ensures power is redistributed from the hands of the health care professionals and medicine to a partnership approach to care. The person with dementia's skills, life history, feelings, emotions and perceptions are promoted with an emphasis on high-quality communication. The person living with dementia should be at the centre of decision making with regard to their care and their views and wishes respected at all stages of the care process.

This chapter begins by introducing the reader to what dementia is and challenges commonly held assumptions. Common types of dementia are presented, with an exploration of how dementia is recognised, assessed and diagnosed. The chapter introduces current perspectives of dementia, including personhood, citizenship and human rights. Supporting people living with dementia and their care partners is discussed from a four-country perspective.

UNDERSTANDING DEMENTIA

Dementia is an umbrella term used to describe a wide-ranging series of symptoms that arise through chemical change, structural change or sometimes both within the brain (World Health Organization, 2021). The onset of these cognitive changes varies significantly from person to person. Cognitive changes are dependent on the aetiology, and the impact of these changes varies depending on a whole host of variables such as premorbid education, social activity, physical health status, gender, ethnicity, genetics and support networks.

Assumptions are often made that dementia is a disease of memory and that the person with dementia will be 'forgetful'. Memory impairment is a common symptom of dementia, but it is important to understand cognition features many complex operations, including language, perception and motor control, in addition to the primary operation of activating, storing and retrieving memories. Therefore, some people living with dementia retain an operational and functional working memory but face other significant challenges with language and perception.

A common experience for people living with dementia is they are aware something has changed, usually related to some element of everyday living. People may become aware certain everyday tasks or activities, such as paying bills, remembering dates or appointments or even knowing how to sequence the activity of getting dressed, are more challenging. Assumptions are often made that these difficulties have arisen because of tiredness, stress or just 'old age', yet they can be the first indicators of changes in the brain that potentially indicate signs of an emerging dementia.

Dementia is not a normal part of ageing, although it is more prevalent in individuals over 65. The ageing brain can routinely experience changes in cognitive function. An older person may forget the name of a person they rarely see, their interests may change or they may experience a fleeting lapse in memory but are able to recall the missing knowledge and information quite easily. In contrast, an ageing brain that is developing a more significant cognitive impairment that may be the result of a developing dementia syndrome, would in the same circumstances forget the

names of people they are close to, forget things more readily or find it challenging to recall new information in addition to losing interest and motivation to engage in social activity and hobbies.

It is essential any changes in cognitive function, especially in an older person, are investigated. It is recognised there are a group of conditions that potentially mimic the onset and progression of dementia and if treated reverse the person's cognitive change (see Table 29.1). If treatable causes for cognitive impairment are attributed to the onset of a dementia syndrome without further clinical investigation, there is a danger they can lead to prolonged and distressing cognitive dysfunction that results in significant morbidity and mortality as the underlying condition is not identified and not treated effectively.

It is estimated around 55 million people worldwide live with dementia. Estimations predict this figure will rise to around 139 million by 2050 (World Health Organization, 2021). In the United Kingdom, approximations indicate there are 850,000 people with a dementia diagnosis (Wittenberg et al., 2019), but this is a conservative estimate as many people are living with cognitive problems and neurological impairment who have yet to be diagnosed.

Current government and charitable spending on dementia research is 12 times lower than investment into cancer research, for example. Spending on dementia care and research is far below expectation, particularly due to the economic burden in terms of health and social care costs. These figures exclude the 1.5 billion hours of unpaid care provided to people with dementia living in the community, which amounts to around £24.2 billion per year (Wittenberg et al., 2019).

Dementia is currently not preventable in most cases or curable at all. However, medications are available that have the potential to slow down the progression of the disease in certain cases and medications to relieve the behavioural and psychological symptoms that may arise as the person's dementia progresses. There are also a range of alternative therapies such as aromatherapy, massage, bright light therapy and nerve stimulation that may have some benefit in supporting people living with dementia, but more research is needed to determine the efficacy of these interventions and to fully understand their effects in minimising the symptoms of the disease.

As a progressive disease, the early symptoms of dementia may present only mildly and are less impactful on everyday life and activity. However, as the disease progresses, the symptoms become more noticeable and progressively interfere with everyday life. At the most severe stage of the disease, the person with dementia is almost fully reliant on the care of others to meet even the most basic needs such as maintaining personal care, toileting, eating and drinking, communicating and mobilising.

TABLE 29.1	Common Reversible Causes for the Onset of Cognitive Impairment
Linked to many of the factors below	Delirium is an acute worsening in cognitive function that occurs over a very short period. Delirium is a sign the individual has an underlying physical health problem that needs treatment. This condition is often misdiagnosed as dementia as it presents with symptoms such as acute confusion, restlessness, agitation, poor concentration, lethargy, drowsiness and at times delusions and hallucinations.
Neurological	Abrasions or lesions in the intercranial space Hydrocephalus (normal pressure type)
Endocrine	Underactive (hypo) or overactive (hyper) thyroid Too little production of hormone parathyroid (hypoparathyroidism)
Nutritional	Vitamin deficiency, particularly vitamin B12 and folate
Vascular/collagen protein	Systemic lupus erythematosus Cerebral vasculitis
Infectious disease	Chest/urine and other bacterial systemic infection Autoimmune deficiency syndrome (AIDS) Neurosyphilis
Drug/metabolic	Tranquillizers Hypnotics Antipsychotics Antihypertensives Anticholinergics Alcohol toxicity Drug/substance use
Psychiatric disorder	Late-onset schizophrenia Depression Grief disorder
Miscellaneous	Sleep deprivation Sleep apnoea Chronic obstructive airway disease

The progression of dementia should be viewed as a continuum with three key stages (Table 29.2). The initial stage relates to the pre-clinical phase, where there are no physical symptoms, but the changes in the brain have started to occur. The person is often unaware of any changes to their cognitive function and to the damage occurring in their brain. The early stage occurs when there is a noticeable change in cognitive function where some everyday activities become more challenging to complete, but overall, the person can maintain activities of daily living independently. The middle stage of the progression of dementia is where the symptoms begin to interfere with many activities of daily living and there is a need for increased levels of support and care. The late stage of the dementia progression is where the symptoms of the syndrome are so marked that they interfere with almost every element of daily living, and the person requires a high level of care and support to meet the most basic needs.

COMMON TYPES OF DEMENTIA

The International Statistical Classification of Diseases and Related Health Problems 10th Revision (ICD-10; World Health Organisation, 2016) reports dementia as a syndrome that arises as a result of disease in the brain, usually of a chronic or progressive nature. Dementia can be caused by a multitude of medical conditions or diseases and their impact on the brain. For example, in adults over the age of 65, neurogenerative diseases such as Alzheimer's disease and dementia with Lewy bodies are the most common causes; in younger adults, brain tumours and traumatic brain injury are a common cause (Gale et al., 2018). Dementia can present with a multitude of clinical features (Table 29.3), which may present

TABLE 29.2   Three Stages of Dementia

Stage	Early	Middle	Late
Signs and Symptoms	• Forgetfulness • Losing track of the time • Becoming lost in familiar places	• Becoming forgetful of recent events and people's names • Becoming lost at home • Having increasing difficulty with communication • Needing help with personal care • Experiencing behaviour changes, including wandering and repeated questioning	• Becoming unaware of time and place • Having difficulty recognising relatives and friends • Having an increasing need for assisted self-care • Having difficulty walking • Experiencing behaviour changes that may escalate and include aggression

Source: Adapted from World Health Organization (2016).

TABLE 29.3   Common Clinical Features of Dementia

Clinical Feature	Clinical Characteristics
Impaired memory	Changes in storing information for short periods, adding up money and taking longer to figure things out (working memory) Recalling past events, forgetting what lunch was, forgetting where the car is parked (episodic memory) Forgetting familiar objects or people, struggling to find the right words in conversation (semantic memory) Struggling to do things that you have done for years, actions or sequences become more difficult to undertake—for example getting dressed or knowing how to make a hot drink (procedural memory) Forgetting appointments or significant dates, forgetting to pay bills on time or attend social events (prospective memory)
Impaired judgement	Difficulty in making decisions, solving problems and understanding potential outcomes; comprehending a situation to make a choice or to take or not act
Movement disorder	Loss of posture and the ability to maintain posture; changes in mobility; stiffness and rigidity; tremor; slowed down movement; lack of spontaneous movement; falls and fear of falling
Language and communication difficulties	Word-finding problems; naming objects and people; reduced verbal expression; lack of fluency; incomprehensive speech; reduced participation in interaction and communication; impairment to the arrangement of words; problems creating and constructing phrases
Hallucinations and delusions	Changes in perception in the senses (e.g., visual, auditory, tactile, olfactory) that result in sensory experiences caused by stimuli produced by the individual in isolation and not occurring from external events; delusions are ideas and beliefs based on the individual's own experience but that may have no basis in fact or reality
Incontinence	Urinary incontinence is more prevalent in some early manifestations of dementia, but as the disease progresses in all conditions, the incidence increases; bowel and bladder incontinence are more likely; contributing factors may be related to mobility issues, loss of sensation or loss of urgency, infection, constipation, disorientation, premorbid bladder and bowel conditions
Eating difficulty	Loss of appetite; increases in appetite; changes in food preference—for example, prefers savoury to sweet foods or vice versa; constipation and digestive problems; dehydration; oral problems such as thrush, ill-fitting dentures, ulcers
Sleep–wake disturbances	Insomnia; problems maintaining sleep; nocturnal disturbance and increased nocturnal activity; interrupted REM sleep; altered circadian rhythm; daytime sleepiness

TABLE 29.3	Common Clinical Features of Dementia—cont'd
Clinical Feature	**Clinical Characteristics**
Agitation and/ or aggressive behaviour	Verbal or physical aggression is a form of communication; a sign a need is being unmet
Changes to personality	Changes to emotional response, conscientiousness, self-awareness; becoming more easily upset, worried or angry; difficulty expressing or understanding emotions; apathy, impulsive behaviour; withdrawn; more compulsive; irritability; disinhibition; compulsive behaviour
Depression*	Prominent signs are irritability, delusions and hallucinations; anxiety; slowed down thinking and movement (psychomotor retardation); low energy; poor appetite; loss of enjoyment or feelings of pleasure; cognitive decline; increased behavioural symptoms Less prominent but still present are sadness and low mood; feelings of guilt and hopelessness

*Depression in dementia is very common and often under-recognised and undertreated.
Source: Adapted from Antunes et al. (2017).

with differing degrees of severity or may not be present at all depending on what parts of the brain are affected. We explore some of the common types of dementia below.

Alzheimer's Disease

Alzheimer's disease is the most common cause of dementia. The pathology of the disease relates to the accumulation of plaques—fragments of a protein called beta-amyloid—and tangles that occur outside the neurons present in the brain. These plaques and tangles are made up of malformed strands of a protein called Tau that is present inside the neuron cells.

A build-up of the beta-amyloid and Tau proteins in the brain contribute to the death of brain cells and damage to the tissue and structure of the brain. Imaging of the brain of a person with Alzheimer's highlights brain shrinkage and atrophy as a result of the loss of the neuronal brain cells.

The early manifestation of Alzheimer's disease presents with problems with memory and new learning particularly because the disease is thought to start in the hippocampus, which is the part of the brain that plays an integral role in supporting day-to-day memory. In the early stages, long-term memory can remain unaffected, so the individual may experience problems recalling what they ate for breakfast but can recall clearly an event from their childhood. As the disease progresses and more damage occurs within the brain from the death of neuronal brain cells, Alzheimer's dementia becomes more challenging, especially in recalling information from memory. The person may forget about recent conversations, forget birthdays and anniversaries, and find it difficult to remember names or even where things are around the house.

Alzheimer's disease progression develops with more and more noticeable memory problems in addition to impairments in language and communication, visuospatial skill, concentration, sequencing tasks effectively and remaining orientated to time. The person with Alzheimer's type dementia may also experience changes in their mood and become depressed, anxious or irritable. In the later stages, when the disease is more severe, the person requires much more support with maintaining fundamental activities of daily living and becomes less aware of what is happening around them. They may experience significant changes in behaviour, such as aggression, agitation, restlessness, hallucinations and delusional ideation and disturbances to sleep–wake cycle in addition to physical changes such as frailty, weight loss, nutritional challenges, mobility decline and swallowing difficulties.

It is valuable to recognise that although there are common symptoms and stages present in Alzheimer's disease, no experience is the same. Each person's lived experience of Alzheimer's disease is very different. The progression of Alzheimer's disease is a downward trajectory over the course of many years with a time line of cognitive decline that spans around 10 to 15 years from the early identification of cognitive deficit to the very severe and end-of-life stage of the disease (Raket & Lundbeck, 2019).

Age is the most significant risk factor for developing Alzheimer's disease; people over the age of 65 are mainly affected. However, younger people can also develop Alzheimer's disease, known as young onset dementia, Alzheimer's type.

Other risk factors for Alzheimer's disease include gender. Twice as many women than men are diagnosed with the disease. This is linked to life expectancy, with women living longer than men and a potential link to the hormone oestrogen, which dramatically reduces in women after menopause.

Genetics also may play a role in developing Alzheimer's disease, but to date little evidence supports that Alzheimer's disease is inherited. Familial Alzheimer's disease is documented to have occurred in some family groups, but this is rare and still not fully understood.

Lifestyle factors such as diabetes, high cholesterol, obesity, smoking, high blood pressure, previous incidence of stroke and heart disease are factors linked to an increased prevalence of Alzheimer's disease and other dementias. Engaging in an active, healthy lifestyle has the potential to minimise the risk of developing Alzheimer's disease, but even some individuals who have sustained healthy living develop this form of dementia.

Vascular Dementia

Vascular dementia accounts for one-third of all dementias and is widely recognised as the second most common subtype of dementia after Alzheimer's disease. As an umbrella term, vascular dementia is used to identify a diagnostic subset of conditions that ultimately cause cell death in the brain, which leads to cognitive and functional change. There are several reasons why vascular dementia develops from an aetiological perspective, but three main contributing factors relate to the onset of vascular dementia.

Stroke-Related Vascular Dementia

A stroke is an interruption of blood flow to the brain that arises through blockage from a clot or other matter such as fatty deposits (i.e., ischemic stroke) or through a blood vessel fracture, causing the oxygenated blood to leak (i.e., haemorrhagic stroke). Both events reduce the supply of oxygenated blood to essential parts of the brain, and cell death occurs.

Small Vessel Disease

Small arteries, venules, arterioles and capillaries are essential in maintaining adequate blood supply to the subsurface of the brain. Damage to this vascular pathway can arise through disease and inflammation, causing reduced blood supply to the brain. The brain becomes impaired, elimination of waste becomes less effective and affected parts of the brain do not receive adequate oxygenation to prevent cell death.

The walls of the small vessels in the brain thicken, becoming stiffened and contorted, which consequently means the blood supply is unable to pass freely through the vessels to keep the brain perfused with oxygen.

Transient Ischemic Attack (Mini Stroke)

A transient ischemic attack (TIA), or mini stroke, occurs when the blood vessels in the brain become blocked but then spontaneously clear, allowing blood flow to resume without any intervention. Although a TIA and associated symptoms tend to resolve within 24 hours, its occurrence is a medical emergency. A clinical evaluation is needed to confirm changes in the ischemic mechanisms in the brain and to initiate tailored therapy to reduce the risk of further vascular events (Cereda & Olivot, 2018).

Mixed Type Dementia

Mixed dementia is the coexistence of two forms of dementia simultaneously. It usually refers to an individual who experiences vascular dementia in addition to Alzheimer's disease. However, it is valuable to recognise that coexisting pathologies can be present in other forms of dementia. Parkinson's disease, dementia with Lewy bodies and Alzheimer's disease all account for mixed types of dementia. Although diagnostic criteria differ, the term *mixed dementia* predominantly refers to the development of vascular and Alzheimer's disease.

For an individual with a mixed type of dementia, amyloid plaques and neurofibrillary tangles associated with Alzheimer's disease are often present in addition to cerebral damage due to small vessel disease, stroke or TIA that contributes to the onset of vascular dementia.

The coexistence of vascular dementia and Alzheimer's disease is complex; patients with Alzheimer's disease are often found to have cardiovascular lesions in the brain associated with vascular events and cell death as a result of stroke, infarct and small vessel disease. In contrast, individuals with vascular dementia are often found to have the amyloid plaques and neurofibrillary tangles associated with Alzheimer's disease. Recognising the difference between the conditions presents a significant challenge. However, with advances in neuro imaging, the development of diagnostic criteria and better understanding of the symptoms that manifest in mixed type dementia, it is possible to identify the dominant contributor to the mixed dementia presentation and treat and support accordingly.

Lewy Body Dementia

Lewy body dementia can be subcategorised into Parkinson's disease dementia or dementia with Lewy bodies. Although these forms of dementia are less familiar than Alzheimer's disease and vascular dementia, they often occur more often in the older population than expected.

Lewy body dementia is caused by abnormal protein deposits in the brain known as alpha-synuclein. These deposits were named Lewy bodies after Dr Friedrich Lewy, a German neurologist. Dr Lewy was the first to identify these microscopic protein deposits, which he linked to the death of brain cells, particularly in the cerebral and limbic cortex, hippocampus, midbrain, brainstem and olfactory (i.e., sense of smell) channel.

Alpha-synuclein has an important function in the brain, particularly within the nerve cells, which is where the brain synapses (i.e., nerve cells) transfer electrical information from one cell to another. When these nerve cells become impaired because the alpha-synuclein protein forms into clumps within the cell, the synapses are not as effective, which can lead to cell death. The build-up of the alpha-synuclein protein impairs cognitive function and ultimately leads to widespread brain damage.

Parkinson's disease dementia and dementia with Lewy bodies, both of which come under the umbrella of Lewy body dementia, typically present with cognitive impairment and problems with movement and coordination. To differentiate between the two conditions, diagnosticians look for what symptoms occur and in what time frame. In both conditions, as time and the disease progress, symptoms become more similar.

Initially, dementia with Lewy bodies presents similar to Alzheimer's disease with memory problems, language and communication difficulties, and visuospatial impairment becomes more challenging. However, symptoms such as impaired rapid eye movement (REM) sleep, visual hallucinations, slowed and unsteady movement, sensitivity to antipsychotic medications (which are often prescribed to treat hallucinations), altered consciousness, alertness and attentiveness become more prominent as dementia with Lewy bodies progresses.

Parkinson's disease dementia presents initially as a disorder of movement, with the main symptoms being muscle stiffness and rigidity, slowed movement, tremor and an unsteady gait. Falls are a significant risk, particularly for an older person with Parkinson's disease. Initially the symptoms of Parkinson's dementia are associated with motor function becoming impaired. The difference between Parkinson's dementia and dementia with Lewy bodies is that cognitive impairment is more evident in the early onset of dementia with Lewy bodies. Not everyone who develops Parkinson's disease develops dementia. Current diagnostic criteria advocates that if cognitive symptoms and impairment emerge within a year of the motor symptoms of Parkinson's disease occurring, a diagnosis of Parkinson's dementia can be made.

Frontotemporal Dementia

Frontotemporal dementia refers to a category of dementia that primarily impacts the frontal and temporal lobes of the brain. The frontal lobes have many vital functions but are commonly associated with judgement, impulse control, language and problem solving. Changes in personality are notable, and motor function can become impaired if the frontal and temporal lobes are damaged. Damage to

the frontal area of the brain can set off a swell of further changes to the rest of the brain, and damage to other parts of the brain can interfere with frontal lobe function, as this area acts as a pivotal point in managing the 'traffic' of the nervous system.

The temporal lobes play an important role in processing information and encoding memory in addition to processing emotions, language, and visual and auditory perception. The temporal lobes are situated to the right and the left of the brain. Damage to the left temporal lobe results in decreased verbal and visual comprehension and increased challenge in understanding the speech and communication of others. Damage to the right temporal lobe may impact an individual's ability to recognise visual stimuli such as familiar faces or pictures, and there may be challenges to finding words to inform communication. The temporal lobes play a significant part in sexuality and sexual behaviour, and more significant damage to both lobes can result in hypersexualised behaviour. This can be very distressing for an individual and their care partners and may result in the use of psychoactive medications and early entry to a care facility.

Like other dementias, there are multiple variants of frontotemporal dementia, and these different manifestations arise depending on where within the frontal and temporal lobes the nerve cell damage occurs. Behaviour variant frontotemporal dementia occurs when nerve cell damage arises predominantly in the frontal lobe of the brain, leading to problems with insight and judgement, the ability to empathise with others and understanding of social norms and values. Primary progressive aphasia is another significant form of frontotemporal dementia. The term *aphasia* refers to a language disorder that involves the impairment of comprehension, writing and speaking. *Primary progressive* relates to the way the symptoms present. Specifically, the initial symptoms present as language disfunction rather than symptoms most typically associated with dementia such as memory loss. Frontotemporal dementia can also manifest with disturbances of motor function, as neurone damage and degeneration of the brain results in changes to motor and muscle function. The individual may become stiff and uncoordinated in their limbs, and there may be changes in posture, mobility and changes in eye movement.

Frontotemporal dementia is less common in older adults, and onset is often within the 45–65 years of age range, but like many of the dementias, the onset can occur at any age. Individuals with younger onset dementias may require access to older people's mental health services because of their knowledge and skills in supporting people with dementia and cognitive impairment.

RECOGNISING, ASSESSING AND DIAGNOSING DEMENTIA

Diagnosing dementia can be difficult, particularly during the early stages, as the symptoms can be the result of other conditions such as depression, delirium or a thyroid deficiency (Alzheimer's Society, 2014). Despite this challenge, an early diagnosis of dementia is advocated by organisations such as the Alzheimer's Society and the Social Care Institute for Excellence as it allows people living with dementia time to plan ahead and to obtain answers to questions about their condition (Alzheimer's Society, 2014; Social Care Institute for Excellence, 2015).

Dementia is a progressive condition, but it varies from person to person in the time it takes for an individual to progress through the three stages (Pulsford & Thompson, 2012) described in Table 29.2. In the early stages of dementia, the person may develop coping mechanisms to help manage the early symptoms of their condition. For example, they may try and cover up evidence of their forgetfulness by 'explaining away' the situation (Hobson, 2019). Depression, which is characterised by persistent low mood, is common in the early stages as the person begins to realise and accept something is wrong (Orgeta et al., 2015). In the middle stage of dementia, the individual's condition has progressed and becomes more noticeable. Some assistance may be required for activities of daily living, and communication difficulties may lead to frustration for people living with dementia and their care partners (Hobson, 2019). The late stages of dementia bring further dependence on others to ensure the person with dementia's needs are met. It is important to note that an early diagnosis of dementia does not mean a person is in the early stages of the condition. They may not be diagnosed until they are in the middle or later stages when symptoms are more prevalent.

Although fluent verbal communication can be very challenging in the late stage of dementia, people in the late stages can still have episodes of awareness and clarity. It is important to recognise their strengths and maintain independence as far as possible (Hobson, 2019). The impact of dementia varies depending on the disease and on an individual's life circumstances. People living with dementia who are of working age may need to navigate additional responsibilities such as child-rearing and financial obligations in addition to challenges such as the lack of services tailored to younger people living with dementia (Pulsford & Thompson, 2012).

Assessing for Dementia

No one single test can confirm a diagnosis of dementia. Health care professionals use a combination of tests to assess an individual for dementia. A complete and extensive history of the individual and presenting symptoms along with a physical examination can help rule out other causes of cognitive decline as described in Table 29.1. Following this, paper-based tests of cognitive function are often used to support or rule out a dementia diagnosis. A number of tests are used throughout the NHS and in private practice in the United Kingdom. Four of the most popular are as follows:

- The mini-mental state exam (MMSE) is widely used as a test of cognitive function. It tests memory, language, visual-spatial skills, attention and orientation. The MMSE is relatively quick and easy to use but is copyrighted, so the correct permissions should be granted before use (https://patient.info/doctor/mini-mental-state-examination-mmse).
- The Montreal cognitive assessment test (MOCA) takes around 10 minutes to complete and assesses language, short-term memory, orientation and executive function. It has been shown to be better at identifying early stage dementia than the MMSE (https://www.mocatest.org/the-moca-test).
- The six item cognitive impairment test (6CIT) takes less than 5 minutes to administer and is commonly used by GPs and in primary care settings. It is comparable to the MMSE but is free to use by health care professionals (https://patient.info/doctor/six-item-cognitive-impairment-test-6cit).
- Addenbrooke's cognitive examination III (ACE-III) takes around 15–20 minutes to administer (with training) but has shown high sensitivity to identifying early onset dementia as part of a full clinical assessment. The ACE-III is commonly used in memory clinics (https://www.quest.scot.nhs.uk/hc/en-gb/articles/115004522689-Addenbrooke-s-Cognitive-Examination-ACE-III).

Many of the paper-based tests include the clock drawing test (see Fig. 29.1). This test involves asking the person to draw a clock face and put the hands to a time (e.g., ten to two). It is a particularly useful test (Eknoyan, et al., 2012). If drawn accurately, it 'virtually excludes dementia because a wide range of cognitive skills are used' (Barrett & Burns, 2014, p. 14).

If a diagnosis is still uncertain, the individual may be referred for a brain scan. Although not conclusive, a brain scan such as an MRI, CAT or PET can identify changes to the structural integrity of the brain, which in turn could support a dementia diagnosis. It is important to note brain imaging is not recommended if the diagnosis is already clear and dementia is in the later stages of severity.

DECISION MAKING, CAPACITY AND CONSENT

Assumptions that people living with dementia are not capable of making decisions and shouldn't remain autonomous

Healthy Brain

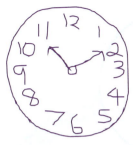

Brain affected by dementia

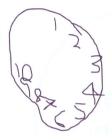

Fig. 29.1 The clock drawing test.

in deciding for themselves what their needs and wishes are result in paternalistic care. This approach may have good intentions in trying to do what seems to be in the individual's best interests, but it excludes the voice of the person living with dementia.

As dementia is a progressive condition, there are times when the individual may find it increasingly difficult to engage in the decision-making process and feel challenged by understanding, communicating, retaining and weighing up information. Decision making can become increasingly challenging as the syndrome progresses, and questions may be raised about the individual's abilities to manage everyday activities such as driving, finances and maintaining independence.

People living with dementia should be supported under a presumption they have capacity and as such have the right to make their own decisions unless there is evidence of mental impairment with the potential to impact decision-making ability. Dementia is a condition that impacts decision making, but it is important to understand the individual's lived experience of the disease and to be clear about what decision, if any, they need support with at a specific time. Consideration needs to be given to how information is delivered and how the individual can communicate their wishes and requirements as effectively as possible.

As with any autonomous individual with capacity, a person with dementia has the right to make unwise decisions.

Even if a decision places an individual at risk or is challenged by family and care providers, it does not mean the person lacks capacity. People living with dementia who have mental capacity are as capable as anyone to make unwise decisions. This should not suggest the individual doesn't have the ability to weigh up the risks and benefits of a specific decision.

The Mental Capacity Act (2005) (see Fig. 29.2) is a statutory framework that supports individuals who have a form of mental impairment that limits their ability to make some or all decisions autonomously about their own lives. In addition, it provides a clear framework for helping individuals who lack capacity to remain empowered to participate and be considered fully in the decision-making process, removing prescriptive and paternalistic approaches to care in favour of a person-centred, collaborative approach to establishing what is in the individual's best interest. The act is applicable in England and Wales. Similar acts apply in Northern Ireland (Mental Capacity Act [NI], 2016) and Scotland (Adults with Incapacity [Scotland] Act, 2000).

Planning, organising and delivering care in the best interests of people living with dementia should be considered when an individual has been identified to lack capacity related to a specific decision. Family, carers, health professionals and social care providers in addition to people who know the person with dementia well should be included in discussions about the best interests for the person with dementia if found to lack the capacity to make a specific decision. The best interest process elicits insight into the views and wishes of the individual before they lost the capacity to make the decision autonomously.

The person living with dementia should be involved as much as possible in the process of decision making and should be included in meetings and discussions about their care. Cultural and religious beliefs should be considered in addition to any advanced directives or guidance written by the person with dementia that highlighted their wishes before the disease progressed. The Mental Capacity Act (2005) provides guidance for how people living with dementia can make advanced decisions about their care and treatment prior to the disease progressing to a stage where they are unable to make decisions autonomously. These advanced decision-making plans can include wishes to decline particular treatments or interventions in the future, identifying and registering a lasting power of attorney to oversee finances or health care and specific statements about prospective care and how their needs should be met.

Although an advanced statement of wishes is not a legally binding document, it is a template for individuals who provide future care to respect and proactively attempt to comply with in order to deliver the most effective

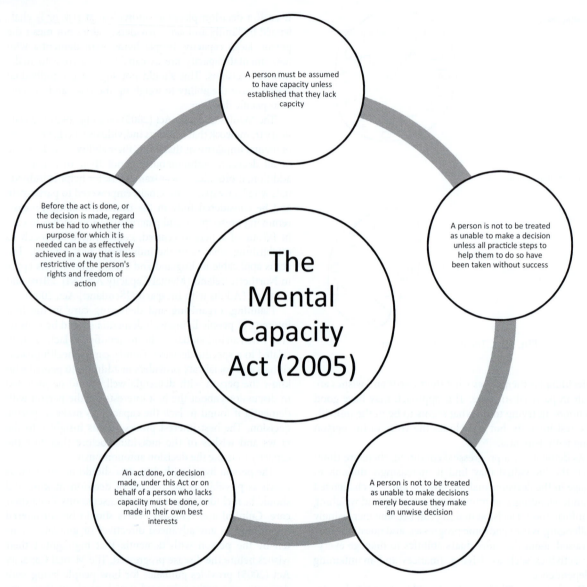

Fig. 29.2 Principles of the Mental Capacity Act (2005).

person-centred care possible. The identification and registration through the Court of Protection of a power of attorney for health and finances is a legal framework under which the best interests and wishes of the person with dementia can be delivered by proxy.

It is essential in circumstances where the person with dementia lacks capacity to decide on a specific issue that any best-interest decision must restrict their rights and freedoms as little as possible. A balance needs to be struck between trying as much as possible to maintain the individual's autonomy and limiting any potential risks or harms that may arise if decisions are not taken on behalf of the person.

PERSPECTIVES OF DEMENTIA

Until the 1990s, dementia was predominately viewed from a biomedical perspective concerned with the limited neurological aspects of the syndrome (Bartlett & O'Connor, 2010; Kitwood, 1997). Dementia was considered to be a neurodegenerative disorder with irreversible decline, eventually leading to death (Bartlett & O'Connor, 2010; Goldsmith, 1996). It was suggested that by adopting this medicalised view of dementia, health care professionals and carers could distance themselves from the person living with dementia and reduce the burden of emotional attachment (Goldsmith, 1996; Kitwood & Bredin, 1992). Although limited in its view, the biomedical perspective of dementia contributed to scientific research that supported developments in diagnosis and treatment (Bartlett & O'Connor, 2010).

Kitwood and Personhood

In the early 1980s, reports were published that began to challenge this biomedical focus on the condition and highlighted the humanity of people living with dementia (Keady & Nolan, 2013). There was a notable move from a focus on dementia as a condition to a focus on the person living with dementia. This was further enhanced by the work of Tom Kitwood and his concept of personhood. Kitwood acknowledged the benefits of the medical perspective of dementia and its contributions (Goldsmith, 1996) but suggested the use of personhood to adopt a more holistic view of dementia in which the *person* living with dementia is recognised before the person with dementia. Kitwood (1997) defined personhood (p. 8) as 'a standing or status that is bestowed upon one human being, by others, in the context of relationship and social being. It implies recognition, respect and trust.'

Kitwood (1997) suggested personhood is measurable and identified five defining attributes presented using the following equation:

$$D = P + B + H + NI + SP$$

- *D* stands for dementia presentation with acknowledgment of the disease process and how it leads to cognitive impairment but emphasises the uniqueness of each individual and how dementia impacts each person differently.
- *P* acknowledges the individual personality of each person.
- *B* stands for biography and recognises how an individual's personal history affects the language they use, their interactions with others and their behaviour.
- *H* considers the individual's health status, which acknowledges the individual may be living with other conditions besides dementia.
- *NI* stands for neurological impairment, which identifies the type of dementia a person is living with.
- *SP* stands for social psychology, which acknowledges how the person living with dementia is affected and

influenced by their environment and the actions of the people close to them.

Kitwood (1997) also proposed everyone has six fundamental psychological and social human needs, and these needs should be met in order to enhance the person living with dementia's personhood:

- Love: Loving and being loved is a fundamental human need.
- Attachment: This considers our connections in life to someone or something.
- Comfort: Comfort means different things for different individuals but commonly reflects physical needs such as warmth, cleanliness, being free from pain and having nutritional needs met. Comfort can also mean an emotional connection or bond with another person.
- Identity: Identity defines who each person is as a unique individual, from their food and drink preferences to haircuts and choice of clothes.
- Occupation: This reflects the need to be engaged in activities and have purpose in our day to day lives.
- Inclusion: This means not being left out of anything that has meaning to us; it's a need to be a part of something.

There can be a detrimental effect on the person living with dementia's personhood if these needs are not met or considered. Kitwood (1997) coined the term malignant social psychology to describe behaviours of the caregiver that can lead to erosion and loss of the person living with dementia's personhood, including disempowerment, infantilisation and ignoring. This poor practice, or the malignancy, can be instigated by a single person, and if they are in a position of power or influence, others may copy this behaviour, which introduces the social element of malignant social psychology (Hobson, 2019). To facilitate the maintenance of personhood, Kitwood (1997) recommended the concept of person-centred care.

The concept of personhood contributed to dementia research and practice in three specific ways (Bartlett & O'Connor, 2010). First, it moved the perception of dementia as a disease to a holistic understanding of the condition (Bartlett & O'Connor, 2010). Second, personhood highlights the importance of an individual's personal biography that contributes to their unique experience of living with dementia and their care (Bartlett & O'Connor, 2010). The third contribution is consideration of language and discourse used when discussing dementia and people living with it. Terms such as *demented patient* and *suffers with dementia* are no longer used as they do not put the person at the centre of the discussion and imply it is not possible to live well with dementia (Bartlett & O'Connor, 2010). Campaigns by organisations such as the Dementia Engagement and Empowerment Project (DEEP) and the Alzheimer's

Society aim to educate and provide guidance to ensure the language used with people living with dementia is person-centred (Alzheimer's Society, 2018; DEEP, 2014). Personhood is arguably one of the most significant concepts for dementia care, practice and research (Brooker, 2004). However, Bartlett and O'Connor argued personhood focuses too narrowly on the immediate environment of a person living with dementia and does not consider dementia from a broader societal view (Bartlett & O'Connor, 2010).

Citizenship

Citizenship is defined as 'a status bestowed on those who are full members of a community. All who possess the status are equal with respect to the rights and duties which the status bestow' (Marshall, 1992, p. 18).

Bartlett and O'Connor (2010) suggested people living with dementia are acknowledged and viewed as active members of society, taking the concept of personhood and expanding it toward a model of social citizenship. Citizenship studies previously focused on working-age adults and individuals with a physical disability, but there is an increasing focus on older adults and those with a cognivitve impairment (Bartlett, 2016). Bartlett (2016) acknowledged the idea of social citizenship is still developing for people living with dementia but has gained traction over the past 10 years. In recognising dementia activism and the evolution of dementia-friendly communities, further thought and understanding can be appropriated to the idea of social citizenship for people living with dementia.

In the United Kingdom and worldwide, groups of people living with dementia are actively campaigning and advising on policy, raising awareness and educating the public (Bartlett, 2014; Weaks et al., 2012). The Scottish Dementia Working Group (see Box 29.1) was co-founded in 2002 by Professor Heather Wilkinson and James McKillop, a person living with dementia (Weaks et al., 2012). The group actively campaigns as a collective with the lived experience of dementia and aims to influence decisions made about people living with dementia at local, national and international levels. Early Dementia Users Cooperative Aiming to Educate (EDUCATE), a group of people living with dementia based in Stockport, England, use the power of their collective voice to educate health and social care professionals, students and the general public on dementia (Perry & Chaplin, 2014). These two groups are just a snapshot of the hundreds of active groups of people living with dementia campaigning to have their voices heard in the United Kingdom.

Outside the United Kingdom, the European Working Group of People Living with Dementia (EWGPWD) is one of many groups in Europe actively campaigning for the rights of people living with dementia. The EWGPWD works closely with Alzheimer Europe, an umbrella organisation of

> ### BOX 29.1   Scottish Dementia Working Group
>
> The Scottish Dementia Working Group (SDWG) is a campaigning group for people living with dementia, managed by people living with dementia (Alzheimer Scotland, 2021). The idea for the group began when Professor Heather Wilkinson met James McKillop, a person living with dementia, in the early 2000s. From this early meeting, a small steering group was formed to explore the creation of the group, and numbers of people passionate about having their voices heard grew rapidly (Weaks et al., 2012). The SDWG works under the umbrella of Alzheimer Scotland and is the 'independent voice of people with dementia within Alzeimer Scotland' (Alzheimer Scotland, 2021). Membership is open to anyone with a diagnosis of dementia in Scotland. The SDWG is active at local and national levels in Scotland and has had significant success in contributing to the Scottish government's policies on dementia. As well as campaigning, members are involved in raising awareness and training health care professionals and are actively involved in research (Alzheimer Scotland, 2021; Weaks et al., 2012). The SDWG has produced numerous publications, including booklets and DVDs on living with dementia. The SDWG also works closely with the National Dementia Carers Action Network (Scotland) (Alzheimer Scotland, 2021).

European Alzheimer's associations, producing projects and organising activities relevant to people living with dementia (Alzheimer Europe, 2019). The EWGPWD aims to ensure its voice is heard and acknowledged across education, research and policy and has presented at the European parliament, participated in public involvement work and co-authored articles in peer-reviewed journals (Alzheimer Europe, 2019).

Alongside activist groups, there are also peer-support groups for people living with dementia throughout the United Kingdom and Europe. People living with dementia have provided a positive reaction to involvement in peer-support groups, where they can interact with people who also have lived experience of dementia and develop new friendships and relationships (Clarke et al., 2013). This contributes to the maintenance of personhood in people living with dementia and drives the model of social citizenship. There has been a significant rise in dementia activism in recent years from both individuals and groups of people living with dementia. The voices of people living with dementia are becoming more prominent and rightly acknowledged and are a consideration health care professionals should acknowledge in the delivery of care.

Human Rights and Dementia as a Disability

Cahill (2018) argued that despite the substantial contribution and reframing of dementia personhood achieved, there was no call for legislative or political change to protect and enshrine the rights of people living with dementia. Traditionally, the rights, needs and wants of people living with dementia have been a low priority on a national and global scale (Cahill, 2018). People living with dementia retain the same rights as anyone else in society, but the nature of their illness means they often have great difficulty in protecting their own rights (Scottish Government, 2013). 'The voices of older people living with dementia and those who look after them need to be heard in a meaningful way,' said Rosa Kornfield-Matte (Scottish Government, 2013, p. 1).

In 2015 Rosa Kornfield-Matte, the United Nations Independent Expert on the Enjoyment of All Human Rights by Older People, called on all member states to adopt a human rights-based approach to dementia (Cahill, 2018). Despite this call to action, a human rights-based approach to dementia has not been embedded in the majority of countries' policies (Cahill, 2018). People living with dementia have not always been at the forefront of human rights debates in the way other stigmatised groups are, (Mental Health Foundation, 2015) and dementia is not typically recognised as a disability.

Like citizenship studies, dementia does not often feature in research and reports exploring disabilities (Cahill, 2018). People living with dementia do not tend to identify as being disabled, and the focus is often on dementia as a health condition as opposed to considering dementia as a disability (Shakespeare et al., 2019). However, by framing dementia as a disability, people living with dementia can secure the same human rights protections as other stigmatised and marginalised groups (Cahill, 2018; Mental Health Foundation, 2015). The World Health Organization (2015) advocates for people living with dementia to demand their human rights are recognised rather than wait for legislation, policies and services to catch up. Having their human rights acknowledged should ensure people living with dementia have the right to health care from properly trained health care professionals (World Health Organization, 2015). Health care professionals should ensure people living with dementia can access timely and accessible support and that the person is centred within care and treatment decisions. Beyond the advocacy of health care professionals, people living with dementia are active in calling for their voices to be heard and their rights acknowledged through dementia activism.

Dementia Activism

Groups such as the Scottish Dementia Working Group (see Box 29.1) have helped establish the creation of a United Kingdom–wide network of groups committed to advocating for the rights of people living with dementia (Thomas & Milligan, 2018). DEEP, the UK network of dementia voices, originally began with 17 member groups and now of consists of over 80 groups of people living with dementia. DEEP is an active promotor and advocate of human rights for people living with dementia (Hare, 2016) and supports individuals hoping to start a group. DEEP is an independent organisation that does not fall under the influence of any particular services or organisations, and with peer support, they support groups who are aiming to develop their influence and activism in dementia policy and services at local and national levels (Innovations in Dementia and ECRED, 2016).

On an international stage, Dementia Alliance International (DAI) is a worldwide, non-profit organisation with a commitment to eradicating stigma and discrimination and furthering the human rights agenda for people living with dementia (DIA, 2016; Thomas & Milligan, 2018). DAI began with the aim to establish one collective voice of advocacy to argue for rights of individuals living with dementia and is free to anyone with a diagnosis of dementia (DIA, 2016). DAI published a report that advocated for the human rights of people living with dementia on a global scale and offers advice to individuals and organisations on how they can support and advocate for their human rights (DIA, 2016). DAI adopted the disability movement's 'nothing about us without us' motto to lobby for people living with dementia to be heard and included on the world stage (DIA, 2016). Health care professionals may signpost people living with dementia to these organisations for further support and information on living well with dementia and ensuring their human rights and needs are met.

SUPPORTING PEOPLE LIVING WITH DEMENTIA

In the United Kingdom, the four countries have each adopted dementia strategies that recognise the need to improve the care of people living with dementia. In 2012 the Prime Minister's Challenge on Dementia (Department of Health, 2012) was launched with the aim to make England a leading country for dementia care, support and research. This initial challenge set out three key areas for investment:

- Driving improvements in health and care
- Creating dementia-friendly communities that understand how to help
- Better research

In Scotland the National Dementia Strategy (2017–2020) aimed to transform the services available to people living with dementia and improve the outcomes of people affected by the condition (Scottish Government, 2017). The Welsh and Northern Irish governments have similar strategies and action plans in place (Department of Health, Social Services and Public Safety (NI), 2011; Welsh Government, 2018).

Although aimed at each country's specific populations, these policies have similar goals to actively improve dementia care but also include the voices of individuals with lived experience of dementia in their guidance. As we have highlighted throughout this chapter, the person living with dementia should be at the centre of all decision making, with their views and wishes respected at all times. Nurses encounter and work with people living with dementia across all types of care settings, including primary care, acute hospitals, mental health settings and in the community. Caring for a person living with dementia should be personalised, timely and appropriate. As highlighted earlier in the chapter and reinforced by the Mental Capacity Act (2005), the person living with dementia should be assumed to have capacity unless there is evidence to support otherwise. A diagnosis of dementia does not mean the person cannot make decisions about their care, and it is important to remember capacity is fluid. A person in the advanced stages of dementia may no longer be able to make decisions about their care but could still make decisions about what they eat for breakfast. The nurse should take this approach at all stages of the nursing process.

Dementia-Friendly Environments

Dementia-friendly environments are places and spaces that promote the acceptance and inclusion of people living with dementia (Handley et al., 2017). A dementia-friendly environment includes considerations for practical aspects of the space. Physical aspects such as signage and furnishings should consider that some people living with dementia have difficulty with language and linguistics, so signs that depict pictures instead of words improve accessibility. Perception is also a cognitive function that can be affected by dementia, and therefore careful consideration of furnishings should be implemented. A black rug may look like a hole, a shiny floor may look wet, or a stripey carpet may look like steps.

A dementia-friendly environment also includes the perceptions and understanding of the people who interact in it. Initiatives in the United Kingdom such as Dementia Friends (Alzheimer's Society, Alzheimer Scotland) and continued activism by DEEP aim to ensure the general public has an understanding of what it is like to live with dementia and thus increase understanding and acceptance.

Current policy in the United Kingdom is driving the push for dementia-friendly environments not just in public spaces but also in care environments. Best-practice care for people living with dementia is dependent on staff knowledge and skills as well as the care environment.

In the Community

Dementia care often begins in the community, with diagnosis as the first step. A diagnosis of dementia can be made by a person's GP, but often individuals are initially referred to a memory service or clinic for further investigation. Memory clinics were first set up in the United Kingdom in the 1980s and were initially focused on recruiting people with Alzheimer's disease into clinical drug trials (Burns et al., 2014). Present-day memory clinics have a wider focus and aim to diagnose and support people living with dementia across the spectrum. As described earlier in the chapter, various tests can be carried out to suggest a diagnosis of dementia or rule out other conditions that present with similar symptoms.

An early diagnosis ensures individuals can access post-diagnostic support and advanced care planning. Post-diagnostic support is often provided by nurses or other allied health professionals on community mental health teams. Individuals with Alzheimer's disease may be started on a medication regime and monitored regularly. It is also an opportunity for individuals diagnosed with dementia and their care partners to be signposted to additional services hosted by the NHS or third-sector organisations. An example of the services available to people living with dementia in the community is the Open Doors Network in Salford, Greater Manchester. As described in Box 29.2, the service aims to provide peer support and other services to people living with dementia to support them to live well.

The Scottish Government guarantees a year of post-diagnostic support to every person diagnosed with dementia. This post-diagnostic support is based on five key pillars (Simmons, 2011):

- Understanding the illness and managing symptoms
- Planning for future decision-making
- Supporting community connections
- Peer support
- Planning for future care

This support is provided by a variety of professionals, depending on the geographical location, but is consistent in aiming to address and provide a high level of support to people living with dementia.

Appropriate support in the community can help reduce hospital admissions and enable people living with dementia to live well, but a key part of this support is to plan for the future. As we know, dementia is a degenerative condition, and it is important for people living with dementia to plan for their care in the future, including legal considerations such as appointing a power of attorney should they not have capacity to make decisions about their care or finances but also what their care should look like in the future. It is entirely possible for people to live in their own homes in the advanced stages of dementia with the

BOX 29.2 Open Doors Network

Open Doors aims to support the delivery, development and innovation of dementia services in Salford and is funded and supported by Greater Manchester Mental Health NHS Foundation Trust (GMMH), as described in its supporting literature: 'The Open Doors Service is based upon the promotion of living well with dementia and aims to literally 'open doors' for people living with dementia, whose goals are to support the delivery, development and innovation of dementia services within Salford' (Greater Manchester Mental Health NHS Foundation Trust, 2018).

Open Doors, as part of GMMH, was the first NHS trust in the United Kingdom to employ a person living with dementia in their services to truly ensure a voice for people living with dementia. Mike Howorth was a person living with Alzheimer's disease who was employed by GMMH NHS Foundation Trust in 2010. In his role, Mike developed networks across the city of Salford and took on duties such as role modelling, leading the dementia café and taking part in research and educational opportunities (Howorth et al., 2012). Among the services developed by Open Doors are a dementia café, two support groups, a book club and a dining club. The project also takes an active part in research both within GMMH and with local universities (Greater Manchester Mental Health NHS Foundation Trust, 2018).

charter encourages hospitals to self-assess their services and supports the trusts to make the necessary adjustments toward becoming dementia-friendly. Embedded within the charter are seven key themes trusts are encouraged to assess themselves against:

- Staffing: Care is provided by staff who are appropriately trained in dementia care and should be a fundamental part of the hospital's training strategy.
- Partnership: People living dementia and their care partners should have choice and control in their care decisions.
- Assessments: A full and accurate assessment of the person living with dementia's needs should be carried out and care delivered accordingly.
- Care: Care is person-centred and meets the individual needs of the person living with dementia.
- Environment: The hospital environment is safe, comfortable and supportive and promotes independence.
- Governance: Care is continuously assessed for quality, and systems are in place to support and improve it.
- Volunteering: Trained volunteers are available to assist people living with dementia but not as a substitute for paid staff.

People living with dementia who are in the later stages of the disease may have difficulty communicating. Their needs may not be met, and resulting frustration can result in challenging behaviours. Health care professionals with appropriate training and education in dementia will recognise these behaviours are a form of communication and strive to treat the underlying cause. This could be meeting toileting needs, promoting independence, supporting mobility or recognising pain (Handley et al., 2017). Personalised care involves identifying, understanding and meeting an individual's needs and treating them from a holistic perspective and not writing off challenging behaviours as 'because they have dementia' (Fig. 29.1 and Fig. 29.2).

Specialist dementia nurses are now commonly found in hospital environments, and with their high degree of knowledge and skills in dementia care can support staff to use their resources appropriately and meet challenges. Specialist dementia nurses can support staff in identifying and ensuring the needs of the person living with dementia are met and reducing incidents of pain and distress. They can also be a source of information and support for people living with dementia and their care partners during a hospital stay (Rahman & Harrison Dening, 2016).

right support, or the person may stipulate they would like to move into a care or nursing home if they can no longer have their needs met at home. Addressing these plans as soon as possible after diagnosis emphasises the right to the person living with dementia to be heard and for their care to be personalised. Writing down what is important to them, whether it is listening to a particular type of music, eating a certain food or having contact with a loved one, can enable care professionals and care partners to ensure a high level of personalised care as the condition progresses.

In Hospital

It is estimated that one in four people in acute hospitals are living with a form of dementia (Alzheimer's Society, 2009). People living with dementia are often admitted to hospital for reasons other than their dementia (Handley et al., 2017), and it is crucial all staff have an understanding of the needs of people living with dementia.

The National Dementia Action Alliance launched the Dementia-Friendly Hospital Charter in 2015 as a response to the Prime Minister's Challenge on Dementia, asking acute hospital trusts to commit to creating dementia-friendly hospitals (National Dementia Action Alliance, 2015). The

SUPPORTING THE CARE PARTNERS OF PEOPLE LIVING WITH DEMENTIA

Until recently, research in dementia care tended to focus on the experiences of the care partners of people living with dementia. Although this imbalance is being addressed with activism by people living with dementia, it is still important to consider the immense pressure and difficulties that can be put on the care partners of people living with dementia. People who live with a partner who is living with dementia have reported three noticeable impacts on their lives (Egilstrod et al., 2019):

- Changes in everyday life, including changes in their partner's personality and behaviour.
- Transformation to a new marital relationship in everyday life, including changes in marital roles, increased responsibility and management of household chores, and feelings of guilt in trying to meet their own needs
- Planning the future, including denial about the future, re-planning and fear.

These findings show how partners struggle with both emotional and practical challenges in their lives due to their partner living with dementia. Many services provide support for care partners as well as individuals living with dementia. A specialist service for families available throughout the United Kingdom is admiral nurses (see Box 29.3).

Care partners may also fall ill and require hospital treatment, and assessing both the care partner's and the person living with dementia's needs can ensure positive outcomes, such as the experience described below.

Following a fall breaking my wrist and injuring my leg, I was told I needed to be admitted to hospital to have a plate inserted in my wrist. I explained that I could not leave my husband as he had dementia and the staff nurse found a room with two beds so he could stay with me. A dementia nurse stayed with him while I had my operation. We were treated with kindness and compassion, something I will never forget (Davis, 2019).

CONCLUSION AND LEARNING POINTS

This chapter gives an overview of dementia and presents the argument for nursing a person living with dementia from a holistic and personalised perspective.

BOX 29.3　Role of Admiral Nurses

Dementia UK is a national charity that provides support to families affected by dementia through providing specialist dementia nurses known as admiral nurses. Admiral nurses provide specialist support to people with dementia and their families who are facing high levels of complexity from peri-diagnosis through to post-bereavement, using a biopsychosocial approach to care (Harrison Dening et al., 2017; Harrison Dening & Aldridge, 2019). The aim of admiral nursing services is to operate within the multidisciplinary team to provide high-quality, integrated, post-diagnostic support and in doing so improve the experience of dementia for people affected by the disease and family carers throughout their disease trajectory.

The admiral nurse model is twofold. It is the direct face-to-face clinical work with families, and it provides professional, supportive education and consultancy to other professionals across all aspects of service provision within the field of dementia. Admiral nurses offer informal and formal training, education and supervision to promote best practices in dementia care and are also actively involved in the strategic design and development of services.

Admiral nurses work across all health and social care settings, including primary care networks, acute services, hospices, domiciliary care, care homes and third-sector organisations. Admiral nurses also provide clinics across the country as well as specialist services such as young onset and learning disability roles. Within every setting admiral nurses work, they work closely with existing services with a key aim is to support greater integration and joint working of services for people with dementia and their carers. Admiral nurses ensure appropriate interagency working is undertaken and work closely with tier 1 and 2 agencies such as local authority services, health services, police and independent, private and voluntary agencies within both primary and secondary services.

KEY LEARNING POINTS

- Dementia is an umbrella term that is used to describe different syndromes that arise through disease in the brain.
- Each person living with dementia experiences symptoms of the disease in a unique and individual way. Care should be delivered in an individualised and person-centred way.

- Dementia is not curable; it is a progressive and life limiting condition. More research and funding are needed to improve treatment and support.
- Although associated with older age groups, dementia can also occur in younger people.
- Diagnosing dementia can be challenging, no single test can be applied to inform diagnosis. Consideration must

be given made to the individual's history and physical health in addition to the application of cognitive testing tools to support diagnosis.

- People living with dementia face challenges not only with the symptoms of the condition but face social exclusion, stigmatisation, and isolation. The development of dementia friendly communities and moving away from the medical model view of dementia serves to improve opportunities and maintain the individual's personhood (Kitwood, 1997).

- Carers of people living with dementia face ongoing emotional and practical challenges. Carers should have access to support to be enabled to continue supporting the person living with dementia.

ACKNOWLEDGEMENTS

We thank Dr Emily Oliver for her account of the work of admiral nurses. We also thank all people involved in dementia activism who continue to push and inform our work and ensure the voice of people living with dementia is heard.

RECOMMENDED READING

Bartlett, R., & O'Connor, D. (2010). *Broadening the dementia debate: Towards social citizenship*. Policy Press.
Builds on Kitwood's concept of personhood and advocating for a citizenship approach for dementia care and research that ensures the voices of people living with dementia are recognised. Essential reading for anyone involved in dementia care.

Bryden, C. (2015). *Nothing about us, without us!: 20 years of dementia advocacy*. Jessica Kingsley Publishers.

Cahill, S. (2018). *Dementia and human rights*. Policy Press.
Advocates for a human rights approach for dementia care and practice. This book advocates for dementia to be viewed as a disability, thus ensuring people living with the condition are protected under disability laws. A must read for students, practitioners and policy makers.

Department of Health. (2012). *Prime Minister's challenge on dementia: Delivering major improvements in dementia care and research by 2015*. Department of Health.

Department of Health, Social Services and Public Safety (NI). (2011). *Improving dementia services in Northern Ireland—A regional strategy*. Department of Health.

Kitwood, T. (1997). *Dementia reconsidered: The person comes first*. Open University Press.
This seminal work changed the face of dementia care and puts the person at the heart of practice and research.

Mitchell, W. (2019). *Somebody I used to know*. Bloomsbury Publishing.

Scottish Government. (2017). *Scotland's national dementia strategy 2017-2020*. Scottish Government.

Swaffer, K. (2016). *What the hell happened to my brain?: Living beyond dementia*. Jessica Kingsley Publishers.
This refers to the books listed in the recommended reading section that are written specifically by people living with dementia and authors Bryden, Mitchell and Swaffer.

Welsh Government. (2018). *Dementia action plan for Wales 2018-2022*. Welsh Government.
Current policy on dementia care that informs research and practice and drives the need for personalised dementia care.

REFERENCES

Adults with Incapacity (Scotland) Act. (2000). legislation.gov.uk.

Antunes, AP., Dias, MC., & Verdelho, A. (2017). Neuropsychiatric symptoms in reversible dementias (Chapter 6). From: Verdelho, A. & Goncalves-Pereira, M. (2017). *Neuropsychiatric Symptoms of Cognitive Impairment and Dementia*. Switzerland: Springer International Publishing.

Alzheimer Europe. (2019). European Working Group of People with Dementia—EWGPWD. Alzheimer Europe. https://www.alzheimer-europe.org/Alzheimer-Europe/Who-we-are/European-Working-Group-of-People-with-Dementia.

Alzheimer Scotland. (2021). Scottish dementia working group. Alzheimer Scotland. https://www.alzscot.org/our-work/campaigning-for-change/have-your-say/scottish-dementia-working-group.

Alzheimer's Society. (2009). *Counting the costs. Caring for people with dementia on hospital wards*. Alzheimer's Society.

Alzheimer's Society. (2014). *Dementia UK: Update* (2nd Ed.). Alzheimer's Society.

Alzheimer's Society. (2018). *Positive language: An Alzheimer's society guide to talking about dementia*. Alzheimer's Society.

Barrett, A., & Burns, A. (2014). *Dementia revealed what primary care needs to know*. Department of Health.

Bartlett, R. (2014). The emergent modes of dementia activism. *Ageing and Society, 34*(04), 623–644.

Bartlett, R. (2016). Scanning the conceptual horizons of citizenship. *Dementia, 15*(3), 453–461.

Bartlett, R., & O'Connor, D. (2010). *Broadening the dementia debate: Toward social citizenship*. Policy Press.

Brooker, D. (2004). What is person-centred care in dementia? *Reviews in Clinical Gerontology, 13*(3), 215–222.

Burns, A., Wilkinson, A., & Peachey, S. (2014). *Best practice in memory services: Learning from across England*. NHS England.

Cahill, S. (2018). *Dementia and human rights*. Policy Press Bristol.

Cereda, C. W., & Olivot, J. M. (2018). Emergency department (ED) triage for transient ischemic attack (TIA). *Current Atherosclerosis Reports, 20*(11), 56.

Clarke, C., Keyes, S., Wilkinson, H., Alexjuk, J., Wilcockson, J., Robinson, L., Reynolds, J., McClelland, S., Hodgson, P.,

Corner, L., & Cattan, M. (2013). *Healthbridge: The national evaluation of peer support networks and dementia advisers in implementation of the National Dementia Strategy for England*. Department of Health.

Davis, K. A. (2019). *Co-researching with people living with dementia: A co-operative inquiry*. PhD. The University of Manchester.

DEEP. (2014). *Dementia words matter: Guidelines on language about dementia*. DEEP.

Dening, K. H., Aldridge, Z., Pepper, A., & Hodgkison, C. (2017). Admiral nursing: Case management for families affected by dementia. *Nursing Standard, 31*(24), 42.

Department of Health. (2012). *Prime Minister's challenge on dementia: Delivering major improvements in dementia care and research by 2015*. Department of Health.

Department of Health, Social Services and Public Safety (NI). (2011). *Improving dementia services in Northern Ireland—A regional strategy*. Department of Health, Belfast.

DIA. (2016). *The human rights of people living with dementia: From rhetoric to reality*. Dementia International Alliance.

Egilstrod, B., Ravn, M. B., & Schultz Petersen, K. (2019). Living with a partner with dementia: A systematic review and thematic synthesis of spouses' lived experiences of changes in their everyday lives. *Aging & Mental Health, 23*(5), 541–550.

Eknoyan, D., Hurley, R. A., & Taber, K. H. (2012). The clock drawing test task: common errors and functional neuroanatomy. The Journal of Neuropsychiatry and Clinical Neurosciences, July, https://doi.org/10.1176/appi.neuropsych.12070180.

Gale, S. A., Acar, D., & Daffner, K. R. (2018). Dementia. *The American Journal of Medicine, 131*(10), 1161–1169.

Goldsmith, M. (1996). *Hearing the voice of people with dementia: Opportunities and obstacles*. Jessica Kingley Publishers.

Greater Manchester Mental Health NHS Foundation Trust (2018). Reach beyond and open doors project. https://www.gmmh.nhs.uk/reach-beyond-and-open-doors-project/.

Handley, M., Bunn, F., & Goodman, C. (2017). Dementia-friendly interventions to improve the care of people living with dementia admitted to hospitals: A realist review. *BMJ Open, 7*, e015257.

Hare, P. (2016). Dementia without walls: Reflections on the Joseph Rowntree Foundation programme. *Working with Older People, 20*(3), 134–143.

Harrison Dening, K., & Aldridge, Z. (2019). Admiral nurse case management: A model of caregiver support for families affected by dementia. *OBM Geriatrics, 3*(2), 1902053.

Hobson, P. (2019). *Enabling people with dementia: Understanding and implementing person-centred care* (3rd Edn.). Springer.

Howorth, M., Keady, J., Riley, C., & Drummond, G. (2012). The open doors network: Dementia and self-growth. *British Journal of Mental Health Nursing, 1*(2), 108–111.

Innovations in Dementia and ECRED. (2016). *Making an impact together: Sharing the learning on dementia activism from and across the DEEP network*. Innovations in Dementia and ECRED (The University of Edinburgh), Edinburgh.

Keady, J., & Nolan, M. (2013). Person- and relationship-centred dementia care: Past, present and future. In T. Dening, & A. Thomas (Eds.), *Oxford textbook of old age psychiatry* (2nd Edn.). Oxford University Press.

Kitwood, T. (1997). *Dementia reconsidered: The person comes first*. Open University Press.

Kitwood, T., & Bredin, K. (1992). Toward a theory of dementia care: Personhood and well-being. *Ageing and Society, 12*(3), 269–287.

Marshall, T. H. (1992). Citizenship and social class. In T. H. Marshall, & T. Bottomore (Eds.), *Citizenship and social class*. Pluto Press.

Mental Capacity Act. (2005). legislation.gov.uk.

Mental Capacity Act (Northern Ireland). (2016). legislation.gov.uk.

Mental Health Foundation. (2015). Dementia, rights, and the social model of disability: A new direction for policy and practice? Mental Health foundation.

National Dementia Action Alliance. (2015). *Dementia-friendly hospital charter*. NDAA.

Orgeta, V., Qazi, A., Spector, A., & Orrell, M. (2015). Psychological treatments for depression and anxiety in dementia and mild cognitive impairment: Systematic review and meta-analysis. *British Journal of Psychiatry, 207*(4), 293–298.

Perry, M., & Chaplin, R. (2014). Learning from people with dementia: EDUCATE's story. *Journal of Dementia Care, 22*(6), 24–26.

Pulsford, D., & Thompson, R. (2012). *Dementia: Support for family and friends*. Jessica Kingsley Publishers.

Rahman, S., & Harrison Dening, K. (2016). The need for specialist nurses in dementia care. *Nursing Times, 112*(16), 14–17.

Raket, L. L., & Lundbeck, H. (2019). Statistical disease progression modelling in Alzheimer disease. *Frontiers in Big Data: Medicine and Public Health*. https://doi.org/10.3389/fdata.2020.00024.

Scottish Government. (2013). *Scotland's national dementia strategy 2013-2016*. Scottish Government.

Scottish Government. (2017). *Scotland's national dementia strategy 2017-2020*. Scottish Government.

Shakespeare, T., Zeilig, H., & Mittler, P. (2019). Rights in mind: Thinking differently about dementia and disability. *Dementia, 18*(3), 1075–1088.

Simmons, H. (2011). *Getting post-diagnostic support right for people with dementia*. Alzheimer Scotland.

Social Care Institute for Excellence (2015). Why early diagnosis of dementia is important. https://www.scie.org.uk/dementia/symptoms/diagnosis/early-diagnosis.asp.

Thomas, C., & Milligan, C. (2018). Dementia, disability rights and disablism: Understanding the social position of people living with dementia. *Disability and Society, 33*(1), 115–131.

Weaks, D., Wilkinson, H., Houston, A., & McKillop, J. (2012). *Perspectives on ageing with dementia*. Joseph Rowntree Foundation.

Welsh Government. (2018). *Dementia action plan for Wales 2018-2022*. Welsh Government.

Wittenberg, R., Knapp, M., Hu, B., Comas-Herrera, A., King, D., Rehill, A., Shi, C., Banerjee, S., Patel, A., Jagger, C., & Kingston, A. (2019). The costs of dementia in England. *International Journal of Geriatric Psychiatry, 34*(7), 1095–1103.

World Health Organization. (2015). *Ensuring a human rights-based approach for people living with dementia*. World Health Organisation Geneva.

World Health Organization. (n.d.). Dementia. World Health Organisation. https://www.who.int/news-room/fact-sheets/detail/dementia.

World Health Organisation. (2016). *The international statistical classification of diseases and related health problems, 10th Revision (ICD-10)*. The World Health Organisation.

World Health Organization. (2021). *Dementia: FactSheet*. World Health Organisation.

30

Depression in Older People

Colin Hughes

CHAPTER OUTLINE

Throughout this chapter the role of the nurse is explored in relation to the care of older people, including the assessment, formulation, treatment and implementation of patient-centred care. The role of the nurse in health promotion, prevention through early intervention and detection is discussed, but it is noted that working effectively with the patient and their carers often involves a multidisciplinary team. The nurse has an important role within the multidisciplinary team, particularly in coordinating the biopsychosocial, recovery-orientated, multidimensional approach to assessment and care required by older adults and their carers. The nurse's role in the treatment of depression in older people is looked at, including the generic nursing approach as well as more specific evidence-based approaches such as cognitive behavioural psychotherapy and interpersonal therapy.

Depression is a leading cause of disability worldwide and a major contributor to the global burden of disease (WHO, 2021). It is a common illness throughout the world and in 2019 there were an estimated 280 million people living with this common mental health condition (WHO, 2022). In addition, depression can be long-lasting, with mild to severe presentations. At its worst, depression leads to suicide, with close to 700,000 people dying from suicide every year (WHO, 2021). Globally the population is ageing rapidly; between 2015 and 2050, the proportion of the world's population over 60 will double from 12% to as much as 22% (WHO, 2021).

Depression in older adults causes significant suffering and has a negative impact on a person's daily functioning. Approximately 6.6% of all disability in people over 60 is due to mental and neurological disorders, the most common being dementia and depression, which affect 5% and 7% of the world's older population, respectively (WHO, 2021). Depression is also acknowledged to be both underdiagnosed and undertreated in primary care settings, often due to comorbid presentations (WHO, 2021). Unfortunately, when it occurs, prognosis can be poor, with associated increased mortality rates. As well as having a negative impact on a person's functioning and the number of years living with disability, depression adds to the disability created by a physical disorder and frailty in general. Older people with depression and depressive symptoms, when compared to those suffering from chronic medical conditions such as diabetes, hypertension or lung disease, have poorer functioning, and the experience of depression increases the person's perception of poor health (WHO, 2021). Depression necessitates an increased use and reliance on care services and reduces an older patient's quality of life. The negative impact on carers must also be considered.

There are effective treatments for mild to severe presentations of depression, from low-intensity interventions offered by psychological well-being practitioners, such as behavioural activation, to high-intensity cognitive behavioural psychotherapy (CBP/CBT), interpersonal psychotherapy and antidepressant medication. Psychosocial treatments are also effective for mild depression, and although medication can be an effective treatment approach for moderate to severe depression, it should not be the first line of treatment for mild depression (WHO, 2021). This chapter is concerned solely with depression in older people and the role of nurses in effective assessment and treatment.

CLASSIFICATION OF DEPRESSION

There are two main classification systems for depression and all mental health disorders: the *Diagnostic and Statistical Manual-5* (DSM-5) (APA, 2013) and the *International Classification of Diseases* (ICD-10/11) (WHO, 1992). In the United Kingdom and Europe, the adopted system of classification is the ICD (currently ICD-11) (WHO, 2018).

Unlike the older ICD-10 classification system from the WHO (1992), in the ICD-11, mood disorders are not independently diagnosable, but their pattern over time is used as a basis for determining which mood disorder best fits the clinical presentation of the patient (Reed et al., 2019). Mood disorders in the ICD system are subdivided into specific depressive disorders: single episode, recurrent, dysthymic, mixed depression and anxiety. Please see Table 30.1 for a table of categories and symptoms. The ICD-11 includes three distinct bipolar disorders: bipolar type I disorder, bipolar type II disorder and cyclothymia (see Table 30.2 and the WHO [2022] online classification database). Precedence was given within the revised ICD-11 to clinical utility to facilitate diagnosis. Care was taken to ensure its validity and harmonise it with the DSM-5 (APA, 2013; Chakrabarti, 2018). The mood disorders section is designed to be easier to use while being more precise (Chakrabarti, 2018).

Within the ICD-11, the diagnostic guideline for a diagnosis of depression requires a minimum of five out of 10 symptoms. This brings the WHO system of classification more in line with that of the DSM-5 (APA, 2013). One of these symptoms must be depressed mood or a markedly diminished interest or pleasure in activities. The ICD-11 classifies a single depressive episode by the presence or history of one depressive episode when there has been no previous history of depression.

The key symptomology of depression for all ages is described in the DSM-5 (APA, 2013) and shows how a depressive episode is classified. The DSM is now in its fifth iteration (APA, 2013).

PREVALENCE

Some key facts in relation to depression in older people are as follows (WHO, 2017):

- The global population is ageing rapidly. Between 2015 and 2050, the proportion of the world's population over 60 will nearly double.
- Approximately 15% of individuals 60 and over experience a mental health problem.

In real terms, this means an increase from an estimated 900 million to 2 billion people over the age of 60 (WHO, 2017). Given the ageing nature of the population, it is understandable that the mental health of older people is becoming a public health concern. According to Horackova et al. (2019), depression is a leading cause of disability associated with cognitive and physical decline, poor quality of life and increased mortality.

The prevalence of depression across Europe is variable, but some studies suggest a higher burden of later life depression (LLD) in Southern and Central Eastern Europe. The reasons for this variation are currently unclear (Horackova et al., 2019). A study of approximately 30,000 individuals suggested that 30% of Europeans over 65 may have LLD, associated strongly with somatic comorbidities and reduced physical and cognitive functioning (Horackova et al., 2019). Although depression in general and LLD in particular are underdiagnosed and undertreated, individuals with somatic symptoms are more likely to gain access to mental health services. This indicates individuals with comorbidity are more likely to be in contact with health services and therefore more likely to be referred, diagnosed and treated for depression. People with LLD without comorbid somatic symptoms are less likely to access health services and therefore much less likely to be diagnosed and less likely to gain access to appropriate treatment (Horackova et al., 2019).

BARRIERS TO EFFECTIVE ASSESSMENT AND CARE

Research has consistently found depression is underdiagnosed and undertreated across all populations (Williams et al., 2017). This is seen in older populations, as individuals are often reluctant to discuss emotional problems and sometimes blame themselves for 'not being happier' (Bor, 2015). Despite the readily available and evidence-based approaches to care for depression, many older people remain untreated. Patients, health care providers and the service system are all barriers to accessing effective treatment (Ell, 2006). Although Luck-Sikorski et al. (2017) found older adults preferred a psychotherapeutic approach to treatment rather than antidepressants, interestingly, with increasing age, less people access psychological therapy (Stark et al., 2018). Also, we know older adults tend to seek less professional help than younger adults (MacKenzie et al., 2009). There are various reasons behind these barriers to seeking assistance with depression—for example,

TABLE 30.1 ICD-11 Classification

Single Episode Depressive Episode (see Case Study 30.1)	Recurrent Depressive Disorder (see Case Study 30.2)	Dysthymic Disorder (see Case Study 30.3)	Mixed Depressive and Anxiety Disorder (see Case Study 30.4)
Single episode depressive disorder is characterised by the presence or history of one depressive episode when there is no history of prior depressive episodes. A depressive episode is characterised by a period of almost daily depressed mood or diminished interest in activities lasting at least 2 weeks, accompanied by other symptoms such as difficulty concentrating, feelings of worthlessness or excessive or inappropriate guilt, hopelessness, recurrent thoughts of death or suicide, changes in appetite or sleep, psychomotor agitation or retardation, and reduced energy or fatigue. There have never been any prior manic, hypomanic or mixed episodes that would indicate the presence of a bipolar disorder.	Recurrent depressive disorder is characterised by a history or at least two depressive episodes separated by at least several months without significant mood disturbance. A depressive episode is characterised by a period of almost daily depressed mood or diminished interest in activities lasting at least 2 weeks, accompanied by other symptoms such as difficulty concentrating, feelings of worthlessness or excessive or inappropriate guilt, hopelessness, recurrent thoughts of death or suicide, changes in appetite or sleep, psychomotor agitation or retardation, and reduced energy or fatigue. There have never been any prior manic, hypomanic, or mixed episodes that would indicate the presence of a bipolar disorder.	Dysthymic disorder is characterised by a persistent depressive mood (i.e., lasting 2 years or more) for most of the day, for more days than not. In children and adolescents, depressed mood can manifest as pervasive irritability. The depressed mood is accompanied by additional symptoms such as markedly diminished interest or pleasure in activities, reduced concentration and attention or indecisiveness, low self-worth or excessive or inappropriate guilt, hopelessness about the future, disturbed sleep or increased sleep, diminished or increased appetite, or low energy or fatigue. During the first 2 years of the disorder, there has never been a 2-week period during which the number and duration of symptoms were sufficient to meet the diagnostic requirements for a depressive episode. There is no history of manic, mixed or hypomanic episodes.	Mixed depressive and anxiety disorder is characterised by symptoms of both anxiety and depression more days than not for a period of 2 weeks or more. Depressive symptoms include depressed mood or markedly diminished interest or pleasure in activities. There are multiple anxiety symptoms, which may include feeling nervous, anxious or on edge; not being able to control worrying thoughts; fear that something awful will happen; having trouble relaxing; muscle tension; or sympathetic autonomic symptoms. Neither set of symptoms considered separately is sufficiently severe, numerous or persistent to justify a diagnosis of another depressive disorder or an anxiety or fear-related disorder. The symptoms result in significant distress or significant impairment in personal, family, social, educational, occupational or other important areas of functioning. There is no history of manic or mixed episodes that would indicate the presence of a bipolar disorder.

Source: World Health Organisation (WHO) (2019).

older people report thinking depression in old age is a normal fact of life. There can be fear of being stigmatised for seeking help. Others report difficulty with getting to appointments and a lack of knowledge and understanding when it comes to accessing help (Stark et al., 2018). In addition, cost and insurance are issues in countries without access to state-funded health care (Stark et al., 2018).

When older adults access treatment, they tend to do so via a primary care provider. Within this environment, the primary treatment approach is antidepressant medication (Seitz et al., 2010). According to Frost et al. (2019), 87.1% of older adults being treated receive antidepressant medication. Frost et al. (2019) point out that antidepressants have certain limitations in older adults, for example, increased age is associated with antidepressants being less effective and having more potential side effects. In addition, the impact of the pharmacokinetics and pharmacodynamics of antidepressants have not been comprehensively studied

TABLE 30.2 ICD-11 Classification		
Bipolar I (see Case Study 30.5)	**Bipolar II (see Case Study 30.6)**	**Cyclothymic (see Case Study 30.7)**
Bipolar type I disorder is an episodic mood disorder defined by the occurrence of one or more manic or mixed episodes. A manic episode is an extreme mood state lasting at least 1 week unless shortened by a treatment intervention characterised by euphoria, irritability or expansiveness and by increased activity or a subjective experience of increased energy accompanied by other characteristic symptoms such as rapid or pressured speech, flight of ideas, increased self-esteem or grandiosity, decreased need for sleep, distractibility, impulsive or reckless behaviour, and rapid changes among different mood states (i.e., mood lability). A mixed episode is characterised by the presence of several prominent manic and several prominent depressive symptoms consistent with those observed in manic episodes and depressive episodes, which either occur simultaneously or alternate very rapidly (from day to day or within the same day). Symptoms must include an altered mood state consistent with a manic and/or depressive episode (i.e., depressed, dysphoric, euphoric or expansive mood) and be present most of the day, nearly every day, during a period of at least 2 weeks, unless shortened by a treatment intervention. Although the diagnosis can be made based on evidence of a single manic or mixed episode, typically manic or mixed episodes alternate with depressive episodes over the course of the disorder.	Bipolar type II disorder is an episodic mood disorder defined by the occurrence of one or more hypomanic episodes and at least one depressive episode. A hypomanic episode is a persistent mood state lasting for at least several days characterised by persistent elevation of mood or increased irritability as well as increased activity or a subjective experience of increased energy accompanied by other characteristic symptoms such as increased talkativeness, rapid or racing thoughts, increased self-esteem, decreased need for sleep, distractibility and impulsive or reckless behaviour. The symptoms represent a change from the individual's typical mood, energy level and behaviour but are not severe enough to cause marked impairment in functioning. A depressive episode is characterised by a period of depressed mood or diminished interest in activities occurring most of the day, nearly every day, during a period lasting at least 2 weeks accompanied by other symptoms such as changes in appetite or sleep, psychomotor agitation or retardation, fatigue, feelings of worthless or excessive or inappropriate guilt, feelings of hopelessness, difficulty concentrating and suicidality. There is no history of manic or mixed episodes.	Cyclothymic disorder is characterised by a persistent instability of mood over a period of at least 2 years, involving numerous periods of hypomanic (e.g., euphoria, irritability or expansiveness, psychomotor activation) and depressive (e.g., feeling down, diminished interest in activities, fatigue) symptoms that are present during more of the time than not. The hypomanic symptomatology may or may not be sufficiently severe or prolonged to meet the full definitional requirements of a hypomanic episode (see bipolar type II disorder), but there is no history of manic or mixed episodes (see bipolar type I disorder). The depressive symptomatology has never been sufficiently severe or prolonged to meet the diagnostic requirements for a depressive episode (see bipolar type II disorder). The symptoms result in significant distress or significant impairment in personal, family, social, educational, occupational or other important areas of functioning.

Source: World Health Organisation (WHO) (2019).

in very old age groups, individuals with medical comorbidities or those with poor nutritional intake (Avasthi & Grover, 2018).

As stated, older people express a preference for talking therapies. In the United Kingdom, the Improving Access to Psychological Therapies (IAPT) initiative was launched in 2008 (Clark et al., 2009). Layard and Clark (2015) reported that less than 5% of adults had access to an empirically supported psychological therapy. Since the launch of IAPT, approximately 537,000 patients have been treated per year, and from the data collected on these patients, around 50% have recovered, and two-thirds show a benefit from the evidence-based interventions (Clark, 2018). Despite this, in the United Kingdom older people's access to this service is poor, with recorded referrals as low as 3.5%, which decreases with greater

CASE STUDY 30.1

Michael Hughes is a 71-year-old who lives with his wife in their own house. He has cardiac problems that resulted in the placement of two stents and minor cardiac damage. He also has reduced blood oxygen levels due to a diagnosis of asbestosis and vasculitis. He had a successful double knee replacement 2 years ago. He has three children: two girls, aged 35 and 30, and one boy, aged 26. He has a very good relationship with his elder daughter and his son but is estranged from his youngest daughter. They were previously very close but fell out about a year ago over her relationships. He experiences pain from his knees when climbing stairs or walking long distances, but due to his low oxygen level, he is quite breathless and as a result can stand only for short periods and walk only short distances. He was prescribed portable oxygen by his doctor 3 months ago but finds it difficult to manage, so he tends not to use it. He feels tired all the time and is irritable. He reports feeling guilty about the breakdown in the relationship with his daughter. He notes reduced energy and worries at night, which disrupts his sleep. This is made worse because he finds himself napping throughout the day. One of his great loves in life was being a member of the local golf club, and he had planned to play as often as possible during retirement. However, due to his failing health, he has had to give up his membership, a decision he made 1 month ago. Following this he noted problems with his memory, which he is worried might be an indication of dementia. He also reports an inability to concentrate when speaking to others, watching television or reading the paper. Over the past 2 weeks, he has spent his time staring out of the window, thinking about what he has lost and that nothing can repair this relationship or his health. This has led to fleeting thoughts that his life is not worth living. He reports no suicidal intent, stating, 'That would kill my wife, and I couldn't do that to her'. He has no feelings of being worthless or low self-esteem. He reports reduced energy and fatigue. Mr Hughes reluctantly saw his GP, initially about complaints of low energy, fatigue and disrupted sleep. The GP recognised depression and prescribed an antidepressant, referring Mr Hughes to his local community mental health team for assessment and treatment.

Plan: Following biopsychosocial assessment, discuss with multidisciplinary team (MDT), create problem statement and formulation (a shared understanding of the problem(s)). Create behaviourally defined value orientated SMART goals. Work to develop trust and a therapeutic relationship. Consider the use of behavioural activation/facilitated self-help as described. Consider in consultation with the MDT the impact of cardiac problems, knee replacement and other physical health problems. May have to seek advice as required on goals for physical wellbeing (consult with MDT/Physiotherapy/Doctor for assessment of this and review of prescribed oxygen). Take small steps to promote increased activity and connection with others, building up slowly (review regularly with the MDT). Use basic problem solving, and if advised by the MDT note as part of the schedule when medications including oxygen should be taken. Use psychoeducation to help the patient understand why he feels the way he does and how the activity schedule can help.

CASE STUDY 30.2

Patricia Smith is a 65-year-old lady who lives alone in her own home. Her husband died 5 years ago as a result of a heart attack. She has three daughters, two of whom live nearby. The other has moved out of the country. She was to have a knee replacement 2 years ago, but unfortunately this surgery has not taken place. Due to the altered biomechanics of her walk and the pain from her knee, she now has severe lower back pain (referred pain from her hip) and has been informed she also needs hip surgery. She has lived with persistent and chronic severe pain for the past 3 years, which has had a negative impact on her mobility and ability to rest. Since her husband died, she has consistently attended her GP with various minor ailments and increased her reliance on her two daughters who live nearby. She has reported her mood has been depressed since she lost the 'love of her life and constant companion'. Three months ago she stopped going to the local shops, which she did every day with her friend. At the same time, she stopped going to the local bingo club with her friend three times a week. She reported these were things she used to like to do and looked forward to, but more recently she has felt 'what is the point'. She had a period of depression following the death of her husband, which she was successfully treated for. She had a recurrence of her low mood 3 years ago, but since successful treatment of this second episode via her GP, she has reported no problems over the past 18 months. She now reports a low mood every day accompanied by feeling worthless, stating this must be because 'no one is helping me with my knee, my hip or my pain'. She has no hope anything will change and has expressed thoughts she would be better off dead

Continued

CASE STUDY 30.2—cont'd

(although she does not report any plan). Ms Smith also reports a much-reduced appetite, noting her clothes are 'hanging off me' and feeling 'tired all the time'. The GP started her on an antidepressant and referred her to a local community health team and psychiatrist for review and treatment.

Plan: Following biopsychosocial assessment, discuss with multidisciplinary team (MDT), create problem statement and formulation (a shared understanding of the problem(s)). Create behaviourally defined value orientated SMART goals. Work to develop trust and the therapeutic relationship. Consider the use of behavioural activation,

be aware of the patient's pain management. Ensure this is discussed with the MDT, reviewed and included in the care plan. Take small steps to promote increased activity and connection with others. In addition to medication review for pain, use basic problem solving to assist with pain management. This may include managing expectations with reference to what activity is reasonable and practical steps such as frequent resting when walking. Remember to start with small steps and build up slowly (review regularly with MDT). Use psychoeducation to help Ms Smith understand why she feels the way she does and how the activity schedule can help.

CASE STUDY 30.3

Anne Rogan, 69, lives with her husband, who retired at age 65 after a successful career as an accountant. They have one child, a 38-year-old son. Her son is married with two children, but they live far away, and they see each other only a few times per year. They are in contact by telephone on a regular basis. Ms Rogan reported having a very happy married life. She had a part-time job as a medical secretary and looked after the home. She reported finding her husband's retirement difficult. She had initially looked forward to spending more time together but found he slowly began to take over the roles in the house she had considered her domain. They began to have difficulties, and 2 years ago Ms Rogan began to experience problems with her mood. She began to do less and less around the house and slowly stopped going out. She reported feeling low persistently for the past 2 years and cannot remember a day over those 2 years when she felt joy or happiness. She reports feeling only low in mood and poor concentration, which she reports is only getting worse. In addition, she experiences feelings of guilt, worthlessness, low self-esteem, low energy and fatigue 'all the time'. She is not getting on with her husband and worries the relationship may break down. As a result she

feels very disempowered and hopeless. She has been to see the GP, who started her on a course of antidepressants and referred her to the mental health older person team for assessment and treatment with a psychiatrist.

Plan: Following biopsychosocial assessment, discuss with multidisciplinary team (MDT). Query with the MDT team possible referral on to high intensity CBT/CBP. If not considered necessary (keep under review) create problem statements and formulation (a shared understanding of the problem(s)). Create behaviourally defined value orientated SMART goals. Work to develop trust and therapeutic relationship. Consider the use of behavioural activation and basic problem solving. Use psychoeducation to help Ms Rogan understand why she feels the way she does and how the activity schedule can help. Take small steps to promote increased activity and connection with others. If there is no improvement, review formulation with patient and MDT and consider onward referral for high intensity CBT/CBP treatment. If this is not suitable due to deteriorating mood discuss other options with MDT, i.e., medication review or consideration of electroconvulsive therapy (this will be a decision made by the Psychiatrist and MDT, in conjunction with the patient).

CASE STUDY 30.4

Francis Cunningham is 81 and reported being an active man his entire life. He lives with his partner in a shared flat in the centre of town. They co-own the flat and have no children but own one cat and two dogs. Mr Cunningham reported he loves their pets but especially used to love taking the two dogs for long walks twice a day. Unfortunately, after feeling breathless 2 year ago while out with the dogs, he

'had to sit down or collapse'. A passerby offered help, which resulted in his admittance to hospital, where he was diagnosed with angina. The angina has been treated and is well managed, but since that time Mr Cunningham has worried he will have a heart attack, and no one will be around to help him and as a result he will die alone. He reports constantly seeking reassurance from his partner and his GP but feels

CASE STUDY 30.4—cont'd

they do not take his 'problem' seriously enough. He is so worried about having a heart attack that he rarely goes for walks with the dogs anymore and rarely leaves the house alone. He reports thinking something bad will happen. He is always on the alert, cannot control his worrisome thoughts and is nervous and on edge all the time. In addition, because he can no longer do the things he used to like doing the way he used to, his mood is depressed and has been for more than 3 weeks. He is more irritable, argues more with his partner and has a significantly reduced activity level. His GP prescribed an antidepressant and referred him to the local community mental health team for assessment, psychological support and treatment (i.e., low intensity treatments such as basic problem solving, exposure treatment and behavioural activation).

Plan: Following biopsychosocial assessment, discuss with multidisciplinary team (MDT). Query with the MDT team possible referral to high intensity CBT/CBP. If not considered necessary (keep under review) create problem statements and formulation (a shared understanding of the problem(s)). Work to develop trust and therapeutic relationship. Create behaviourally defined value orientated SMART goals. Consider the use of behavioural activation and basic problem solving. Use psychoeducation to help Mr Cunningham understand why he feels the way he does and how the activity schedule can help. Consider the use of further low intensity interventions. Review progress and discuss with patient and MDT.

CASE STUDY 30.5

Michaela Boyle, 75, lives with her partner and has become increasingly euphoric over the past week. This manifests as a state of irritability with her partner and others, increased energy cleaning the house and working in the garden without rest and difficulty keeping to one topic during conversations. However, her partner says this mood has been a problem 'on and off' over the past 10 years, reporting periods of very high energy and activity and euphoria with irritability and being difficult to have conversations with as she bounds from topic to topic. Ms Boyle reports that when this happens, she feels full of energy and creativity almost 'able to do anything'. Her GP referred her to her psychiatrist for assessment and treatment. Her psychiatrist from the home treatment team assessed her, and Michaela agreed to be admitted to the local acute mental health inpatient unit for assessment and treatment. She has also been started on an antipsychotic and antidepressant.

Plan: Following biopsychosocial assessment, discuss with multidisciplinary team (MDT), create problem statement and formulation (a shared understanding of the problem[s]). Create behaviourally defined value orientated SMART goals. Work to develop trust and therapeutic relationship. Include the patient as much as possible in decisions with regards to her treatment. Remember to review for capacity to make each decision. Consider use of behavioural activity schedule to collaboratively schedule activities on the ward suitable for and acceptable to the patient. Use psychoeducation with reference to medication and monitor the effect of this, monitor physical health. If possible and with permission discuss patients' premorbid personality to assist in ongoing assessment. As condition improves reformulate, create new goals, consider high intensity intervention such as CBT/CBP for psychosis (discuss this with MDT). If not suitable consider increased social engagement and structured management.

CASE STUDY 30.6

Sean Wilson, 65, lives with his wife and has become increasingly depressed over the past month. He worries about their physical and financial security so much he demands his wife stays with him constantly. The worries about safety also concern the home; he feels the roof will collapse or there will be a fire that will consume the house and everyone in it. He finds these thoughts race quickly through his mind without pause. As a result, he constantly unplugs appliances around the house. He does

report being able to continue to work as a supervisor in the civil service but finds it increasingly stressful as he worries about his wife and home. He also reports finding his work mates 'not up to the task' and has come into conflict with them as a result of dismissive comments he has made towards them. He reports feeling energised with an elevated sense of self-worth. His concentration in work is impacted, and he reports feeling increased energy all the time. He reports increased irritability with his

Continued

CASE STUDY 30.6—cont'd

family and has become more impulsive. In addition, his increased energy is accompanied by a decreased need for rest and sleep. His GP referred him to his psychiatrist for assessment and treatment. His psychiatrist from the home treatment team has started him on an antipsychotic and antidepressant. The home treatment team engage with him on a daily basis with behavioural activation, and hospital admission is being kept under review.

Plan: Following biopsychosocial assessment, discuss with multidisciplinary team (MDT), create problem statement and formulation (a shared understanding of the problem(s)). Create behaviourally defined value orientated SMART goals. Include the patient as much as possible in treatment decisions. Remember to review for capacity to make each decision.

Home treatment: engage with frequent visits, to continually assess. Develop trust and therapeutic relation-

ship. In collaboration with the patient and his family and the MDT consider referral to high intensity CBT/CBP. If not suitable or desired, continue to develop the relationship. Provide psychoeducation on condition and medication, to develop understanding and monitor physical health and review regularly with MDT. Consider use of behavioural activation to establish a routine. Consider engagement in group activities to promote social engagement and physical activity. Activity chart can be used to organise this. Continue to monitor and review. Do not directly challenge thoughts but acknowledge Sean's perspective. When appropriate use strategies to encourage 'balanced' thinking. As condition improves reformulate and create new goals. Consider high intensity intervention such as CBT/CBP for psychosis (discuss this with MDT). If not suitable consider increased social engagement and structured management.

CASE STUDY 30.7

Clare French, 70, with her partner and has become increasingly euphoric over the past month, but her partner says this mood has been a problem 'on and off' over the past 3 years, reporting periods of very high energy and activity followed by a depressive phase when she is constantly tired and withdrawn. Ms French reports this 'up and down' feeling, while good when it is 'up', is difficult to manage. She reports if she had a choice, she would like to be 'up' all the time as she feels full of energy and creativity almost 'able to do anything'. Her GP referred her to her psychiatrist for assessment and treatment. Her psychiatrist from the home treatment team assessed her, and she agreed to be admitted to the local acute mental health inpatient unit for assessment and treatment. In addition, she has been started on an antipsychotic and antidepressant.

Plan: Following biopsychosocial assessment, discuss with multidisciplinary team (MDT), create problem statement and formulation (a shared understanding of the problem(s)). Create behaviourally defined value orientated SMART goals. Work to develop trust and therapeutic relationship. Include the patient as much as possible in decisions with regards to her treatment. Remember to review for capacity to make each decision. Consider use of behavioural activity schedule to schedule activities collaboratively on the ward, suitable for and acceptable to the patient. Use psychoeducation with reference to medication and monitor this closely for effect. Monitor physical health. As condition improves reformulate and create new goals. Consider high intensity intervention such as CBT/CBP for psychosis (discuss this with MDT). If not suitable consider increased social engagement and structured management.

age (Frost et al., 2019). Individuals 85 or older are five times less likely to be referred despite their preference for psychological therapies than their 55- to 59-year-old counterparts, and one-third more likely to be prescribed antidepressants despite the lack of research on treatment benefit (Frost et al., 2019).

Older people are no less prone to experiencing poor mental well-being than others in the general population, although poor mental well-being can present differently in an older person. The Department of Health England estimated 40% of older people who attend GP outpatient

clinics have a mental health problem and 50% of those in general hospitals and 60% of those in care homes (Social Care Institute for Excellence, 2006). In a typical day in a 500-bed hospital, individuals over 65 occupy 330 of the beds, of which 220 patients have a mental health problem: 100 with depression, 100 with dementia and 66 with delirium (Burns, 2015). It is particularly concerning to note that in 2016, 1.6 million people in the United Kingdom, or 2.4% of the population, were 85 years of age or over. This number is forecast to double in just 25 years, and the number of people 75 or over is expected to double in the next 30 years (Royal College of Psychiatrists, 2018). Knowing the preference for evidence-based treatment approaches, why does the older population appear to have difficulty getting access to treatment? We can see the impact of discrimination and ageism, both direct and indirect. Indirect age discrimination is apparent where services have neutral arrangements that apply to all—for example, a health service that trains and employs practitioners with generalist skills in the belief these skills are equally relevant to all. We know older people have complex and complicated mental health needs that require specialist skills. A generic service puts older people at a disadvantage (The Royal College of Psychiatrists, 2018). An example of direct discrimination is where an older person is denied a referral to a CBP service or counselling service simply because they are over 65, on the basis they are too old.

Ageism in society as a whole is a problem, and we see this impact the commissioning and running of mental health services. According to Age Concern and Help the Aged (2009), 60% of individuals over 65 believe age discrimination exists in their daily lives, with 53% believing once a person reaches old age, people tend to treat them as though they are children. A 2018 survey on attitudes toward older people (Royal Society for Public Health [RSPH], 2018) found ageism was widespread, with 47% of respondents reporting older people find it difficult to learn new skills and 64% reporting forgetfulness is a part of growing older. In addition, according to the RSPH (2018), two out of five young people in the 18 to 24 age group believe you cannot escape dementia as you get older, and 25% of 18- to 34-year-olds think it is completely normal to become depressed and unhappy when a person is old. With this information, is it surprising older people find it difficult to access the help, support and treatment they require from their health services?

We also see unconscious bias with older people in health care settings when they are stereotyped as ill, dependant and incompetent. The fact that older people, when assessed are often ill and therefore dependent, reinforces this stereotype (Swift et al., 2017). According to the organisation 'Independent Age' people from every age group believe that older people are unlikely to recover from a mental health condition. It is therefore unsurprising that attitudes such as these may influence the decisions of doctors and other health care professionals in relation to older people. Linden and Kurtz (2009), cited in Swift et al. (2017), provided 121 doctors with two identical case studies of patients with depression. The doctors were asked in the study to assess, diagnose and prescribe treatment. Other than the indicated age, these cases were identical (Linden & Kurtz, 2009).

In one case study, the age of the patient was 39; in the other, the age was 81. In the case of the younger age profile, the doctors were more likely to diagnose depression. The older person was much more likely to be diagnosed with dementia or a physical illness (Linden & Kurtz, 2009). The younger person was prescribed relevant psychotherapy, pharmacotherapy and inpatient care, while the older person was prescribed supportive counselling. This is as an example of direct age discrimination: doctors treating the age of the person, not the underlying problems.

According to Ell (2006), barriers to care for depressed older people include detection, individual choice, health care and systemic barriers. Frost et al. (2019) largely consider the same areas but from a health care professional's perspective, identifying the following as important barriers: avoiding medicalisation of what is perceived to be a social problem, negative assumptions regarding older people's mental health, a focus on physical rather than psychological well-being, the variation of service provision across areas and a variation in health care professionals' skill sets.

It is fair to say primary care services do not currently attend well enough to older people's psychological well-being, at least to the same extent as to their physical well-being. This is complicated by a lack of referral options (Frost et al., 2019). Further training for health care practitioners as well as an increase in service provision and consistency of what is offered across jurisdictions are required. Most GPs report that depression is an important area of their practice and suggest it can be well managed in primary care, but it requires greater priority to address the complex and often complicated needs of older adults. This requires additional training and investment in specialist psychological therapies suitable for older people, such as the model successfully implemented by the Department of Health England in 2007 through IAPT in adult services. A similar targeted programme aimed at older populations is required.

Depression in older people may go unrecognised and undertreated even though it is more common in older populations than dementia (Allan et al., 2014). Reasons for this include the following (Donaghy, 2019; Vieira et al., 2014):

- Low mood seen as part of the normal aging process
- Screening tests not routinely used
- Lack of recognition by services users, carers and professionals
- Overlapping symptoms such as physical ill health
- Misdiagnosis as dementia

All health care professionals need to be aware of these issues to ensure depression is both detected and treated.

HEALTH PROMOTION

Given what we know about LLD and patients' access to screening, assessment and treatment, it is important that all professionals and the general public begin to address this problem. To do this, we can

- Promote help-seeking behaviour in older adults.
- Ensure professionals adopt a non-stigmatising approach to assessment and care (embed in training/educational programmes and reinforce through yearly CPD).
- Be clear that mental health treatment is more than simply a biomedical problem.
- Ensure general practitioners and practice nurses increase their understanding of LLD, and that evidence-based treatment and screening are routinely available.
- Reinforce the importance of prevention. This requires an educational programme beyond the health service and should be embedded in public health initiatives.

According to the National Service Framework for Older People standard eight (Department of Health, 2001), the promotion of health and active life in older age and modification of risk factors for disease even later in life can have a positive impact on physical and psychological well-being. We see this approach carried through to the Northern Ireland service framework (DOHNI, 2013). These benefits include increased or maintained levels of functioning, a longer life, disease prevention and an improved sense of well-being (Department of Health [DOH], 2001). In addition, this framework emphasises cultural sensitivity when considering methods of health promotion. For example it would be inappropriate to advise a strict Muslim woman to engage in a form of exercise that requires the adoption of scant clothing or to be in the same room as men. It is important that when engaging with or suggesting health promotion exercises, consultation takes place with local Black and minority ethnic communities and that agencies work collaboratively to identify and develop appropriate and accessible forms of exercise and physical activity' (DOH, 2001, p. 108). It is recommended that the issue of inclusivity is considered as well as the impact gender, culture, religion, etc. have on a server user's psychological well-being. We must aim to ensure a safe and supportive environment (Ostlin et al., 2007).

Older people should have access to mainstream health promotion and disease prevention programmes, and this access must be determined by need and not age. These programmes must be tailored to cultural diversity and should include a multi-agency and multisector approach (DOH, 2001). Nurses have an important role in advocating for older people in terms of both informing them about the interventions/opportunities available and ensuring these opportunities are in line with the National Service Framework (DOH, 2001; DOHNI, 2013). The multi-agency approach requires a coordinator to ensure interventions are optimised, a role for which the nurse is uniquely qualified. For example, coordinating between the GP and specialist medicine to ensure physical health is optimised along with the consideration of disability or mobility issues. This may require input from physiotherapy or occupational therapy, who may suggest the use of various medical aids or specialist adaptions in the person's home. Coordination ensures barriers to functioning and psychological well-being are mitigated against. For individuals who have significant physical disability and who have a carer, consider how to best support them. Often family carers experience significant social strain, including physical, psychological and financial strain, associated with their caring role (Al-Janbi et al., 2019). This strain, often called spill-over, can not only negatively impact the carer and family but also the older person themselves. The use of health promotion strategies for the carer are important; ensuring carers are listened to and supported helps optimise outcomes for the person. In terms of depression, avoidance and withdrawal from specific activities, in particular those that were once enjoyed, are a significant feature of the condition (Hughes et al., 2014). Withdrawal reinforces low mood through the removal of diverse sources of social support and possible positive reinforcement (see section on behavioural activation). Nurses can assist by identifying sources of social support and incorporating them into the treatment plan. Examples are the use of leisure facilities, lunch clubs, day centres and befriending services. Social support can help not only in treating an older person's depression but also in maintaining their mood, thus contributing to relapse prevention.

A carer can encounter financial strain, but poverty may also be an issue for an older person. There are 2 million older people living in poverty. Nearly one million (920,000) older people would not be able to cover the cost of an additional and unexpected £200 bill (Age UK, 2021). According to the Age UK (2019) report *Struggling On*, individuals with health care needs are particularly likely to struggle with financial hardship as a result of having to spend more on heating, laundry, transport and care. In short this emphasises the need for a holistic assessment process that covers every aspect of an individual's life, and a multidisciplinary collaborative approach to care.

ASSESSMENT

Comprehensive geriatric assessment (Ellis, 2011) is fundamental to the process of assessment, formulation, planning, implementing and review of care. The needs of an older person are often complex, and assessment should be a multidisciplinary process, involving collaboration with the service user, carers and family. A biopsychosocial approach (Engel, 1977; Wade & Halligan, 2017) to assessing an individual considers the biological background (i.e., current physical signs and symptoms as well as genetic history), psychological contributors (i.e., mental health aspects) and social aspects, all which contribute to the health and recovery of the service user.

A biopsychosocial approach (Engel, 1977; Wade & Halligan, 2017) should be taken by clinical staff responsible for assessment, regardless of profession (i.e., nurse, doctor, therapist etc.) or field (e.g., general medicine, mental health). A registered general nurse (RGN), for example, working in primary or secondary care should be competent in identifying indicators of delirium and dementia and have a basic understanding of depression and anxiety, how to identify them and the impact they have on physical well-being. This knowledge should be comprehensive enough to enable the nurse to identify when more specialist input is required. Nurses who work in the mental health field must take into consideration the physical and biological signs and symptoms of the service user, again drawing on the skills of the multidisciplinary team. It is important that nurses (RGNs and RMNs) recognise any deficits in their knowledge and skills in relation to adopting a biopsychosocial approach and seek additional training to increase their competency.

Following assessment, the team generally decides if onward referral to a more specialist team is required. Examples include an older people's medicine multidisciplinary team referring an older person to an old age psychiatry service and a mental health team making an onward referral of a service user who is exhibiting symptoms of major depression to a nurse trained in CBP.

As with all health care professionals, nurses must use all the tools at their disposal when it comes to the immediate and ongoing assessment of a patient. It is important to remember that although there is a distinct period of assessment—usually the first to third sessions are used to arrive at a comprehensive assessment—each subsequent treatment session should also be considered a form of assessment. This is to ensure new information can be incorporated into the original assessment, and if required the course of therapy or treatment can be modified. As with all other treatments and interactions with others (e.g., patients, family and carers), the nurse must attend to and be competent in the three core levels of the person-centred approach. They must be completely genuine, non-judgemental and valuing and attempt to understand the patient's experience. These are Rogers' (1956) core conditions:

- Empathy
- Unconditional positive regard
- Congruence

The aim of a mental health nursing assessment is to arrive at an overall formulation or nursing diagnosis that should be agreed jointly between the patient and nurse. Once it has been established, the goals for treatment can be determined, and the treatment approaches to address those goals can be agreed in the form of a treatment plan. It is important for goals to be specific, measurable, achievable, realistic and time-limited (SMART) and also value directed. Value directed simply means a goal needs to be tied to an area in life important to the patient. This aids with motivation.

An example is 'I will get up each morning at 9:00 a.m. and make and eat breakfast with my partner because they are important to me'. The valued areas could be family, friends, hobbies, spirituality, community engagement and employment; these will be personal to the patient.

In modern nursing it is also important to evidence any formulation/diagnosis with both diagnostic criteria and psychometric tests. This includes ICD-10/11 (WHO, 1992) and the DSM-5 (APA, 2013) for the diagnostic criteria and the geriatric depression scale (Stiles & McGarrahan, 1998), the patient health questionnaire (PHQ-9) (Kroenke et al., 2001) and the Becks depression inventory or the Becks depression inventory II (Becks et al., 1996), for psychometric tests. Here we focus on the geriatric depression scale and PHQ-9. The use of the patient history (e.g., personal, family, mental health) and if required collateral history from carers, in conjunction with the appropriate application of relevant psychometrics and diagnostic criteria, guides the formulation and treatment for the patient.

Nurses encounter patients in a variety of settings, both in hospitals (e.g., medical and mental health wards) and the community (e.g., at home, in residential or care homes). Assessment and treatment usually but not always involve more than one discipline; however, this depends on each patient assessment. Care is agreed and delivered collaboratively. With this in mind, it is important to stress the importance of working in an interdisciplinary way.

The first interview with the patient is very important and should be used to gain specific information on the patient's main problem or difficulty. This is a skill in which all mental health nurses should be competent. It should be done by exploring a recent example of the problem and focusing on the antecedents or triggers, followed by the patient's emotional and physical responses and the behaviours they engaged in to manage the problem. This can best be accomplished by examining a recent example of the difficulty when a shift in mood was first noticed. The example should then be explored by reviewing the situation or environment and the thoughts or images the person experienced and the resulting physical and emotional responses. Having identified the behaviours used to try and address the problem, the consequences or outcome of these coping strategies should be discussed. Did they work? If so, would they work in the medium to long term? The overall aim is to examine the problem in terms of frequency (i.e., how often do they experience the problem), intensity (i.e., how much distress do they experience), duration (i.e., how long does the problem/experience last each time it occurs) and onset, both in terms of when they remember experiencing the problem for the first time and what happens just before the problem occurs. In addition, involvement of others and the environment is important. Who was involved at the time of the problem? Who, if anyone, makes it better or worse? What happens? What helps, and what does not? Where does it occur? Where does it not occur? When is it most likely to occur? On completion of this process, if the problem appears complex (refer to the ICD and DSM classifications for help), it must be discussed with the multidisciplinary team. Very complex problems may need to be addressed by senior mental health nurses or even specialist mental health services such as CBP teams.

Example: When I think about getting up and leaving the house (antecedent/situation), I think, 'What is the point? No one wants me around. I am useless, stupid, boring and a bother to others (negative thoughts). I feel low in my mood and angry with myself (resultant emotions). I have no energy and am sore all the time (physical responses). I lie in bed and ruminate, don't get up, don't wash and don't engage with anyone (resultant coping behaviour). As a result I feel in the short term a little better, but then I feel worse because I don't get up or washed or engage with anyone, and I begin to feel even worse (consequence/outcome medium to long term).

It is important to note that quite often the nurse or other health care professional views the assessment process as a data-gathering or fact-finding process. Although this is important, the assessment process is also about establishing and developing a therapeutic relationship. The therapeutic relationship is important to aid in building trust, which allows for a better flow of information and is helpful when it comes to treatment implementation. Often the treatment involves engaging in an activity that has been avoided, and as such the nurse needs to encourage and support the patient to re-engage. In addition, the assessment process affords the opportunity to identify what the patient wishes to achieve across a variety of dimensions in their life, such as relationships, work, hobbies, social interaction, spirituality, family, physical well-being and intimate relationships. Hughes et al. (2014) recommend a four-step approach to assessment:

Step 1: Focuses on the patient's current problems. The aim here is to obtain a detailed problem list.

Step 2: Asks the patient to prioritise their problems and identify the problem they wish to focus on initially. Looks at the problem by identifying the internal and external triggers and the impact they have on the person's thinking. Identifies what type of thoughts the person is having. A depressed person usually reports a negative thought pattern that is usually past focused and results in ruminative thinking. This in turn is responsible for the depressed state (emotional reaction) as well as the associated physical symptoms. It is also important to identify any behaviour the person employs to help manage these thoughts and feelings. These behaviours need to be broken down into behaviours that are useful and should be retained and behaviours that are less helpful and need to be dropped.

Step 3: Focuses on helpful and less helpful behaviours. All the behaviours the patient employs are behaviours they are using to help themselves, so when unhelpful behaviours are identified, they need to be discussed with the patient. It is important to help the patient arrive at their own conclusion as to why an unhelpful behaviour remains there. The self-discovery or reflective process helps the patient when it comes to dropping these less helpful behaviours and adopting new behaviours when moving on to treatment.

Step 4: Considers the onset of the problems by asking the person to identify when they first noticed having difficulty with their mood. This involves a history and detailed exploration of the person's life course. A comprehensive mental state examination should be undertaken to observe appearance, speech, thought content, mood, perceptual abnormality and insight. As part of step four it is important to develop a risk management plan. The risk management plan must be a living document that is reviewed briefly at each appointment and if necessary updated.

Geriatric Depression Scale

Various psychometrics can be used as part of the assessment of an older person. One is the geriatric depression scale, created by Yesavage et al. (1982), which has been extensively tested with older populations. In includes an original 30-item psychometric as well as a shorter, 15-item geriatric depression scale developed in 1986 (Sheikh & Yesavage, 1986). Nurses in different settings are helped in detecting depression by the routine use of the geriatric depression scale, developed specifically for detecting probable depression in older people.

The questions on the geriatric depression scale concentrate on the thoughts and feelings of depression as they have been experienced over the past week (Stiles & McGarrahan, 1998). It avoids asking about physical symptoms, as they could be due to physical illness rather than depression. The original validation study was with psychiatric outpatients and inpatients (Yesavage et al., 1982). However, the geriatric depression scale adequately detects depression in medical patients (Jackson & Baldwin, 1993) and the 15-item GDS is recommended for use in primary care (Mitchell et al., 2010).

The short form of the geriatric depression scale (Sheikh & Yesavage, 1986) (see Box 30.1) is especially useful for patients experiencing fatigue, physical illness and poor concentration or those with mild to moderate cognitive impairment or a shorter attention span (Greenberg, 2007). Scores of six or more indicate probable depression (Sheikh & Yesavage, 1986). The 15-item psychometric is well established as a screening instrument for older people who live at home (Arthur et al., 1999), primary care attenders (D'Ath et al., 1994), psychiatric outpatients (Almeida & Almeida, 1999) and medical patients (Pomeroy et al., 2001). It also remains effective for individuals over 85 (De Craen et al., 2002). The total score on the 15-item version appears to correlate with severity of depression (Almeida & Almeida, 1999). The geriatric depression scale has been found to have 92% sensitivity and an 89% specificity when evaluated against diagnostic criteria and displays good psychometric properties (Greenberg, 2012). Updated versions, including in the various languages can be found at https://www.stanford.edu/~yesavage/GDS.html. A free app for the 15-item geriatric depression scale is available on the Stanford website.

Patient Health Questionnaire

The geriatric depression scale is not the only psychometric available for use in the assessment of depression. Whichever tool or psychometric is used, it is important to obtain the necessary permissions from the copyright holder. In the Improving Access to Psychological Therapy programme run by the Department of Health England, there are a variety of permission-free tools available. One is the PHQ-9 (Kroenke et al., 2001). Like the geriatric depression scale, different language versions are available. The PHQ-9 (Kroenke et al., 2001), according to Levis et al.'s (2019) meta-analysis for pooled data, indicated the sensitivity for a cut-off score of 10 was 0.88 (95% CI 0.70–0.84) Overall, Levis et al. (2019) indicated the PHQ-9 compared well with semi-structured interviews. In addition, Phelan et al.'s (2010) study on the accuracy of the PHQ-9 for older populations found it compares well with both the PHQ-2 and the 15-item geriatric depression scale in identifying depression among primary care older adults. Hence the PHQ-9 is an accurate tool for this population. Although the use of appropriate psychometrics is recommended, clinical judgement remains essential in the assessment of mood in an older person.

Assessment of Risk and Risk Management

Consideration of risk is an important area for nurses and is generally seen as a core competency. Specific training should be provided. The nurse must be aware of and implement national guidelines and local policies regarding risk, including on vulnerable adults, adult safeguarding (see Chapter 14), safeguarding children and relevant risk assessment and management tools.

It is important to remember that asking about suicide, suicide intent or active plans does not increase the likelihood of a patient completing suicide. Being asked the question allows the patient to give an open and honest answer, which in turn can aid in treatment decisions. The person may need urgent treatment in hospital, or an intensive supportive package may need to be arranged immediately to maintain the person safely in the community. The following questions can be very useful in risk assessment: Do you ever think life is not worth living? Do you have thoughts of suicide? Do you have any active plans for suicide? If so, can you describe them? Areas of note that can increase risk are

---

BOX 30.1 The Geriatric Depression Scale (short form)

Choose the best answer for how you have felt over the past week

1. Are you basically satisfied with your life?   yes/no
2. Have you dropped many of your activities and interests?   yes/no
3. Do you feel that your life is empty?   yes/no
4. Do you often get bored?   yes/no
5. Are you in good spirits most of the time?   yes/no
6. Are you afraid that something bad is going to happen to you?   yes/no
7. Do you feel happy most of the time?   yes/no
8. Do you often feel helpless?   yes/no
9. Do you prefer to stay at home, rather than going out and doing new things?   yes/no
10. Do you feel you have more problems with memory than most?   yes/no
11. Do you think it is wonderful to be alive?   yes/no
12. Do you feel pretty worthless the way you are now?   yes/no
13. Do you feel full of energy?   yes/no
14. Do you feel that your situation is hopeless?   yes/no
15. Do you think that most people are better off than you are?   yes/no

The following answers score one point:
No to 1, 5, 7, 11, 13
Yes to 2, 3, 4, 6, 8, 9, 10, 12, 14, 15
A score of six or more indicates probable depression (this cut-off can be changed depending on aims of use)

Reproduced with permission from Sheikh & Yesavage 1986.

loss of a person's environment, someone important or control (i.e., divorce, death), all which can impact n self-esteem and quality of life. Physical health issues such as chronic pain (something that can be poorly managed in older populations), a new diagnosis of physical ailments, dementia and cognitive decline can all lead to a sense of hopeless.

Suicide is a public health concern around the world. Suicide rates increase in later life and are as high as 48.7/100,000 among older White males in the United States (Conejero et al., 2018). We have spoken here about active risk and active plans. A passive form of suicide is also seen in older populations. However, according to Van Orde et al. (2014), passive suicidal ideation is rarer in people over 60 and is usually a problem only when paired with other significant risk factors and increased psychological distress. Self-neglect of food and fluids should act as a trigger for further investigation, as inadequate food and fluid intake can put an older person at considerable risk.

Critical thinking is also required in the collection of information from the patient and carer and from pre-existing records. However, the use of pre-existing records should be treated with care to avoid bias in the data collection process. The information gathered during assessment is used to create a working hypothesis or diagnosis—an understanding of the patient's problem. It is only with this shared understanding nurses can move forward to create the treatment plan. Maslow's (1954) hierarchy of needs is a useful guide in this process. Basic physiological needs must be met before higher needs such as self-esteem and self-actualisation (Tony-Butler & Thayer, 2020).

Guidance from the National Institute of Health and Care Excellence NICE (2022) reiterates that in terms of diagnosis, a comprehensive assessment must not simply rely on a symptom count using ICD or DSM criteria. When assessing a patient for depression, level of functioning and disability associated with depression must be considered. The development, course and severity of a patient's depression and their symptoms and functional impairment need to be considered in addition to the following (NICE, 2009a; 2018a):

- History of depression
- Coexisting mental health disorders
- Coexisting physical health disorders
- History of elevated mood; is the depression part of bipolar disorder?
- Past experience and response to previous treatments
- Quality of interpersonal relationships
- Living conditions
- Employment/financial situation
- Social isolation

Planning follows assessment and diagnosis, which includes the creation of value-directed goals. Once these have been agreed collaboratively with the patient, the interventions or treatment can also be agreed collaboratively. Interventions should focus on addressing the patient's goals and through this the underlying problem. Once implemented, progress can then be evaluated using objective measures such as psychometrics and subjective measures. If no progress is observed or reported, the formulation, goals and interventions will need to be reviewed to see what needs to be adjusted to achieve the desired outcome. This process is an iterative one designed to maximise positive outcomes for the patient.

Nursing Assessment and Management of Depression in Older People

Depression can occur due to major life changes such as the following:

- Bereavement, grief or painful events
- Loneliness
- Loss of role or reduced sense of purpose
- Physical ill health or medical conditions such as
  - Stroke
  - Heart disease
  - Cancer
  - Parkinson's disease
  - Diabetes
  - Thyroid disorders
  - B12 deficiency
  - Lupus
  - Multiple sclerosis
  - Dementia
  - Chronic pain
  - Chronic fatigue
- Past mental ill health
- Fears (e.g., fear of death, financial worries abuse or neglect).

Any medical problem, particularly if it is painful, impacts functioning and if disabling or life threatening and can lead to depression or make the symptoms of depression worse

If a person has communication difficulties due to language issues, sensory and/or cognitive impairment, the nurse needs to consider a tripartite assessment that includes a family member or carer (NICE, 2022).

In addition, various medications can be prescribed for physical problems associated with depression. It is therefore useful for the nurse to obtain a comprehensive list of all medications taken by the patient and to identify those with a potential side effect of depression. This information can be taken into account by the multidisciplinary team when discussing the treatment plan. It is important to note that depression can be a complex condition, and many factors contribute to its development. However, caution needs to be taken before altering medications such as beta blockers and proton pump inhibitors, both of which are associated with depression. Medications should be altered only if there is a suitable alternative and only after consultation with the multidisciplinary team.

There is significant undertreatment of depression in older people (Barry et al., 2012). The NICE (2009b) recommends particular attention is paid to individuals with a physical health need, an area all nurses are in a position to address. Due to this underidentification and therefore undertreatment, we see increased mortality and morbidity, institutionalisation, reduced health, physical dependence and longer hospital stays (Gotlib & Hammen, 2009). Individuals who are experiencing depression report experiencing increased pain, which can impact recovery from illness. Engaging in treatments such as physical therapy can be more challenging, resulting in poorer outcomes (Gureje et al., 2007).

One important area for nurses to be aware of is delirium (see Chapter 28). It is often confused with depression or mild cognitive impairment and dementia, as there is an overlap of symptoms between these conditions. Sometimes patients do not fully disclose information for fear of being labelled 'mentally ill' and of how they may subsequently be treated (Thomas, 2013). It is imperative nurses are informed and knowledgeable about what Thomas (2013) labelled the three Ds—depression, dementia and delirium—in order to be able to accurately distinguish between the three (see Box 30.2).

The nursing role is not only that of physical care provider but also one that involves giving advice and providing education and counselling in order to manage the psychosocial aspects of care within a holistic framework. The Nursing and Midwifery Council (NMC, 2018) is clear when it demands that all nurses must recognise and interpret signs of normal and deteriorating physical and mental health and respond appropriately and promptly. Despite this directive, depression, especially in people over 60, continues to go unidentified and undertreated. One possible reason is nurses who are not trained in mental health care may feel unskilled and uncertain and subsequently lack confidence in asking questions focused on psychological well-being.

Nurses need to be aware of the issues raised by the lack of recognition of depression, its underreporting and the impact of physical well-being on depression identification and treatment. When assessing a patient, it is important to listen actively and ask not only about mood but also about levels of functioning and ability to experience pleasure. Lack of sleep can also be an indicator of depression, as can mood and other issues such as appetite and energy level (see Chapter 25). Another consideration where there is a

---

BOX 30.2 Three Ds

Depression: A functional disorder that causes impairment without any physical cause. Three core symptoms occur most days most of the time for 3 weeks:
- Depressed mood
- Loss of pleasure and enjoyment (i.e., anhedonia)
- Reduced energy leading to fatigue and reduced activity
- Sleep disturbance (too much or too little)
- Guilt
- Thoughts of life not worth living
- Suicide
- Self-harm
- Irritability
- Psychomotor retardation
- Reduced self-care
- Changes in appetite (over- or undereating)

Delirium: Affects 6%–56% of people admitted to medical units and is a common cause of mortality and morbidity in older people (Rai et al., 2014). The term *acute confusional state* is often used when describing delirium because of a systemic illness. It is essential to identify and treat the underlying cause of the delirium, such as infection. It is often characterised by
- Rapid onset
- Short duration (about 1 week)
- Impaired ability to think and concentrate; levels of confusion and consciousness can be changeable

Dementia: An organic disorder where the brain's physical structure is the cause of the illness. Age is a known risk factor. Symptoms include
- Short-term memory loss
- Problems with reasoning and communication
- Progressive loss of functional abilities, including a reduction in a person's ability to carry out daily activities such as shopping, washing, dressing and cooking (NICE, 2018b).

---

lack of recognition is loss—for example, the loss a person experiences due to the death of a loved one or friend and the resulting grief reaction. It is important to note that bereavement-related grief and major depression share some features (Pies, 2014). The ICD-11 and DSM-5 give diagnostic criteria for prolonged grief disorder and include it in the section for major depressive disorder. These diagnostic systems note that any significant loss may include symptoms of a depressive episode, and although it may be an understandable response, the presence of a major depressive episode should be carefully considered (Kavan & Barone, 2014).

Nurses also need to be aware of cognitive impairment (see Chapter 29) and the link between depression and dementia (Byers & Yaffe, 2011). Earlier life depression or depressive symptoms are associated with a twofold or greater increased risk of developing dementia in later life. Interestingly, studies of the link in later life are unclear (Byers & Yaffe, 2011).

Nursing assessment should include asking the person about whether they have had any thoughts about life not being worth living or about suicide, self-harm or self-neglect. This can be a sensitive area and one nurses find difficult to broach. For individuals who have a diagnosis of depression or exhibit depressive symptoms, these questions should feature in every interaction in order to maximise the patient's safety.

According to Conejero et al. (2018), risk factors for increased vulnerability in regard to suicide and self-harm include

- Mental and neurocognitive disorders
- Social isolation
- Feeling disconnected
- Loss of relatives
- Chronic physical illness
- Physical and psychological pain
- Neurocognitive impairment and altered decision making
- History of previous self-harm and suicide attempts.

If a patient presents as being at risk, it should be brought to the attention of the multidisciplinary team and a risk management plan agreed on. This plan should be strengths based and include the patient in its creation. It should be a living document that can be updated as the clinical presentation of the patient changes.

MORE EFFECTIVE IDENTIFICATION AND MANAGEMENT OF DEPRESSION

In terms of the effective identification and management of depression in older people, although all professions are important, nursing has a particular role to play. Nurses, including RGNs and registered mental health nurses, are found in every area of the health service and make up a significant proportion of the workforce. They are ideally placed to identify depression and low mood in older people and to ensure timely assessment and treatment. They also have a role in educating the wider public that old age does not go hand in hand with depression and that depression it is not a normal part of ageing. The loss of loved ones, friends, social outlets and so on can create vulnerability that may then result in depression. Awareness in the general public and for professionals who do not specialise in mental health is therefore essential.

The greatest risk to the population is the stigma associated with depression together with ignorance of its signs and symptoms and a lack of understanding that it is an illness like any other with safe and effective treatments. The level of knowledge a professional requires depends on their field of nursing and role, but a basic understanding of the signs and symptoms and knowing who to pass this information to is essential. Similarly, the general public should have a basic understanding of depression to aid in reducing the stigma of mental ill health and improving the efficiency by which older people and adults in general access assessment and treatment. Professionals of all fields should have access to and competency in the use of psychometrics such as those promoted by the IAPT initiative (PHQ-9) (Kroenke et al., 2001), generalised anxiety disorder 7 (Spitzer et al., 2006) and the geriatric depression scale.

Although there have been impressive strides forward in terms of understanding and treating depression, it remains a relentless illness that continues to place a significant burden on the individual, their family and society as a whole (Kraus et al., 2019). Kraus et al. (2019) demonstrated that early recognition and treatment are of extreme importance, as duration of untreated depression correlates with worse outcomes.

According to Short (2017), up to 90% of patients with depression are treated in primary care. These patients usually present as complex cases that necessitate input from a number of specialisms, which can result in fragmented treatment. A joined-up approach is necessary, especially for older people. We can see this with the development of care pathways, or a collaborative care approach (Short, 2017), that can be coordinated by one professional, usually the care manager. An important element of the collaborative care approach is the timely use of behavioural activation (see "Behavioural Activation"). Using a care pathway or collaborative care approach includes routine screening for depression using appropriate psychometrics and comprehensive assessment inclusive of a mental state exam and if warranted a cognitive assessment. Following this, treatment is considered jointly by the patient and their carers, if possible. The importance of the care coordinator role, one the nurse is ideally placed to fulfil, was highlighted initially in the National Service Framework for Older People (Department of Health, 2001).

Generally, a diagnosis of depression in an older person can be made using the DSM or ICD classification criteria. That said, the criteria of 'markedly diminished interest or pleasure' can overlap with the apathy often seen in dementia. Weight loss or a change in a patient's appetite can be indicative of a physical illness or neurocognitive disorder (Blackburn et al., 2017). Sleep disturbance can as also result from drug use, chronic pain or physical illness. As a result, screening for depression can be useful, with, for example, the geriatric depression scale. It should be noted, however, that the reliability of the geriatric depression scale diminishes when the patient is experiencing cognitive impairment. If this is the case, the Cornell scale for depression in dementia is preferred (Blackburn et al., 2017). The Cornell scale is a tripartite psychometric that not only involves the patient and interviewer but also a family member or carer. Screening is most efficient when targeted at high-risk populations. The purpose of screening is to lead to a full assessment and if appropriate suitable treatment agreed collaboratively. Screening is effective only when it is part of a care pathway/collaborative care approach and leads to appropriate care and treatment.

The NICE (2009a, 2018a) recommends all professionals are alert to possible depression, particularly if the person has a history of depression or chronic physical ill health, as is often the case in older people. The NICE guidance (2009a, 2018a) recommends asking people who may have depression two questions:

- During the last month, have you often been bothered by feeling down, depressed or hopeless?
- During the last month, have you often been bothered by having little interest or pleasure in doing things?

In addition, if the clinician is not competent to conduct a mental health assessment, the person should be referred to a professional who is competent (NICE, 2018a). If the clinician is competent, the service user's mental state should be reviewed along with associated functional, interpersonal and social difficulties (NICE, 2009a).

GENERAL APPROACHES TO SUPPORT AND TREATMENT BY NURSES

When considering the treatment of an older person with depression, the available evidence should be used. The NICE (2022) guidance provides the best guide. See Case Studies 30.1 to 30.7.

All interventions must be provided by practitioners who are competent to deliver psychological and psychosocial interventions based on the appropriate treatment manuals and evidence base (NICE, 2018). This is of particular importance for nurses as their initial training may not provide the required level of training to deliver these interventions. Additional training may be necessary to be deemed competent. The current Nursing and Midwifery Council guidance on training programmes has in part recognised this and directed there be an increase in the provision of psychological and psychosocial interventions in training programmes (Nursing and Midwifery Council, 2019).

Regardless, practitioners who deliver relevant interventions should

- Receive regular competent supervision
- Routinely use outcome measures (e.g., relevant appropriate psychometric) to review treatment progress and outcomes
- Monitor and evaluate both patient adherence to treatment and practitioner adherence/competence using recordings

Nurses should adopt a stepped approach to treatment and use both low-intensity approaches such as facilitated self-help, used by a majority of nurses, and high-intensity interventions (i.e., more specialised approaches) such as intensive CBP.

For patients with sub-threshold depressive symptoms or mild to moderate depression, one or more of the following should be considered:

- Individual guided or facilitated self-help using principles of CBP, usually based around a manual
  - Book (i.e., bibliotherapy)
  - Computerised CBP
- A structured group activity

NICE (2009a) does not routinely recommend the use of antidepressant medication for individuals with mild depression or persistent sub-threshold depression, but they should be considered for those with a history of moderate or severe depression, or if there have been persistent sub-threshold symptoms. Rather, medication should be considered only for individuals with a past history of depression, severe depression or sub-threshold depressive symptoms that have been present for at least 2 years or persist after other interventions (NICE, 2009a).

For individuals with moderate or severe depression, a combination of medication and a high-intensity psychological intervention is recommended (NICE, 2018). For high-intensity psychological intervention, the NICE guidance indicates CBP or interpersonal therapy. Both treatments require additional training and supervision; people with this training are considered psychotherapists. It is important the nurse is competent in the delivery of the low-intensity intervention and is under regular supervision to ensure that if the patient requires a more intense high-intensity intervention, it is identified in a timely manner and an appropriate referral is made.

It is not unusual to experience anxiety when depressed. In this case, it is important to treat the depression first. Basic steps must be considered. If the patient is experiencing the sleep disturbance that is likely with depression, sleep hygiene should be offered as follows:

- Conduct an investigation into the current sleep cycle. Use a sleep diary to help.
- Educate the patient about what is meant by good sleep.
- Offer individual self-help.
- Advise the patient to

- Avoid sleeping throughout the day.
- Exercise throughout the day except in the hour or so before going to bed.
- Limit or stop the use of caffeine and nicotine products as well as any alcohol or other stimulants prior to going to bed.
- Ensure the environment is suitable to sleep. The room should be dark and the right temperature, the mattress should be comfortable, ambient noise should be reduced and electrical items removed from the room.
- Engage in an appropriate bedtime routine with regular sleep and wake times, and engage in relaxing activities before going to bed.
- Only use the bedroom for sleep and intimate activities.

For individuals with mild depression, those deemed as not requiring formal intervention or those who simply do not wish to have an intervention, self-help with support should be offered. The principles of CBP should be followed when providing self-help (NICE, 2018a).

Self-help should include the following (NICE, 2018a):
- Age-appropriate written, audio or digital material
- Support from a practitioner trained in the facilitation of self-help interventions to assist and support completion of tasks and review of progress
- Up to 10 sessions (which can be face to face, online or by telephone)
- An initial session of up to 30 minutes and further sessions of up to 15 minutes
- Follow-up of between 9 to 12 weeks
- Consideration of an age-appropriate physical exercise programme as an initial treatment for individuals with less severe depression

Physical activity programmes should (NICE, 2018a):
- Be group-based and delivered by a competent practitioner
- Consist of 45 minutes of aerobic exercise of moderate intensity biweekly for 4 to 6 weeks, then weekly for a further 6 weeks
- Have eight people per group

With reference to all interventions, the use of support groups and organisations can also be considered both a stand-alone approach to improve psychological well-being and a part of wider treatment approaches. Community referrals, or social prescribing, where the patient can be referred to local non-clinical services, has been shown to improve quality of life as well as reduce the requirement for health service involvement (Aggar et al., 2021).

The next step up from providing self-help for individuals with mild to moderate depression or persistent sub-threshold depression is to provide low-intensity interventions. These should comprise individual guided self-help, which in turn includes behavioural activation and problem-solving techniques.

Behavioural Activation

In relation to behavioural activation, behavioural theorists focus on exposing patients to diverse sources of positive reinforcement and minimising corresponding exposure to unhelpful sources of negatively reinforcing avoidance behaviour (Polenick & Flora, 2013). Behavioural activation treatment is designed to facilitate structured increases in enjoyable activities that increase the opportunity to be exposed to positive reinforcers.

Lewinsohn and Graf (1973) found a significant association between self-reported mood and pleasant activities, with depressed patients engaging in fewer activities and identifying fewer activities as pleasant than non-depressed individuals. Following from this work, Jacobson et al. (1996) and Dimidjian et al. (2011) found the behavioural component alone was as effective as the entire CBP package in terms of treatment and relapse prevention. For older people, later life is associated with difficult losses in many domains that would have once offered a source of positive reinforcement. Such losses include death of loved ones or friends, the loss of a job or social role, impaired physical functioning and reduced physical or cognitive health (Polenick & Flora, 2013).

For details of behavioural activation and other resources on low-intensity interventions see the University of Cedar's low-intensity CBP workbooks (cedar.Exeter.ac.uk/iapt/lihandbook/resources).

According to Richards and Whyte (2011), there are six steps involved in the implementation of behavioural activation. See Box 30.3 for the six-step guide and a behavioural activation worksheet.

Interpersonal Therapy

In addition to the above recommended treatments, interpersonal therapy should also be offered to individuals with less severe depression who would like help for interpersonal difficulties, grief, disputes or role transitions or those for whom the previous interventions were unsuccessful (NICE, 2018a). Interpersonal therapy makes a link between the service user's mood (or depression) and any disturbing life events that can be identified as a trigger or follow on from the experience of the mood disturbance (Markowitz & Weissman, 2004).

Depression often follows the death of a loved one or some other life upheaval. These are disturbing changes in a person's interpersonal environment. According to interpersonal theorists, if the patient can resolve their life problem, their mood disorder should also resolve (Markowitz & Weissman, 2004). Much like CBP, interpersonal therapy is a time-limited treatment (12 to 16 weeks in length). It has three distinct phases: beginning (one to three sessions), middle and end phases (three sessions). The beginning

BOX 30.3	**Six-Step Guide to Behavioural Activation**

Step 1	Educate the patient as to what behavioural activation is, and ask them to keep a baseline weekly or daily diary of their activity.
Step 2	Ask the patient to create three lists: necessary activities, pleasurable activities and routine activities. They may need help with this.
Step 3	Ask the patient to rank the items in each list from the easiest to do to the most difficult.
Step 4	On a blank activity schedule, using the ranked lists from Step 3, create a timetable of activities for the coming week. Start with the easiest items for each week, but be sure the entire schedule is completed. Ask the patient to predict the impact this activity will have on their mood by assigning a rating to each item—for example, 1–10, with 10 the worst and 1 the best.
Step 5	The patient follows the activity schedule for the coming week, only this time they note how they actually feel when they engage with the activity. They need to re-rate using the scale from Step 4.
Step 6	Review how the week went to see if the predicted rating is different from the actual rating. Note any differences. Based on this information and the lists from Step 3, create another schedule and repeat Steps 4 and 5. To begin with, progress can be very slow. It is important the practitioner provides positive reinforcement; this homework can never go wrong. The patient and practitioner can just learn new information.

Hierarchy of Activities

Routine Activity	Rank (from easiest to most difficult)	Pleasurable activity	Rank (from easiest to most difficult)	Necessary activity	Rank (from easiest to most difficult)

Behavioural Activation

Once you have listed the activities you deem to be necessary, routine and pleasurable, rank each category from easiest to most difficult. Using this ranking, populate your behavioural activation diary with a selection of activities from the three categories. Note the impact you think this has on your mood using a mood rating from 1 to 10, with 10 being the most depressed you can be. Then adhere precisely to this diary over the coming week and note the intensity of your mood. Remember to follow this for at least 2 weeks before restructuring the diary.

Weekly Behavioural Activity Diary Rate Mood from 1 to 10, with 10 the worst

Time	Monday	Tuesday	Wednesday	Thursday	Friday	Saturday	Sunday
8:00–9:00 a.m.							
9:00–10:00 a.m.							

Continued

BOX 30.3   Six-Step Guide to Behavioural Activation—*cont'd*

Weekly Behavioural Activity Diary Rate Mood from 1 to 10, with 10 the worst

Time	Monday	Tuesday	Wednesday	Thursday	Friday	Saturday	Sunday
10:00–11:00 a.m.							
11:00 a.m.–12:00 p.m.							
12:00–1:00 p.m.							
1:00–2:00 p.m.							
2:00–3:00 p.m.							
3:00–4:00 p.m.							
4:00–5:00 p.m.							
5:00–6:00 p.m.							
6:00–7:00 p.m.							
7:00–8:00 p.m.							
8:00–9:00 p.m.							
9:00–10:00 p.m.							
10:00–11:00 p.m.							
11:00 p.m.–12:00 a.m.							

Source: Richards & Whyte (2011).

phase is focused on the interpersonal therapist identifying the target (i.e., depression or major depressive disorder) and the interpersonal context (i.e., the disturbing change in the patient's interpersonal environment). This requires the use of appropriate psychometrics and a diagnostic criterion such as the DSM or ICD. The therapist must also create an interpersonal inventory, or a review of the patient's patterns in relationships and ability to connect. There is a requirement to evaluate the number and quality of current relationships, which becomes the focus of treatment—for example, bereavement or complex grief, a dispute with a significant other or role transition. In the absence of any of these, the focus becomes interpersonal deficits in the absence of a current life event (Markowitz & Weissman, 2004).

As with behavioural activation or low-intensity interventions, interpersonal therapy requires the individual practitioner be competent in the delivery of the approach. Additional training for nurses and other health care practitioners is needed, along with ongoing supervision to ensure competence.

The approach used with the patient is determined by the outcome of the collaborative assessment. Higher order interventions such as interpersonal therapy and CBP, which require specialist training, are considered only if lower intensity interventions are not successful or deemed not adequate. When using any psychological therapy approach, the practitioner should have the appropriate training and competency and ongoing supervision to ensure they have the support they need.

Medication

When considering the use of antidepressants for older people, it is important to evaluate the person's response to previous treatment, other medical problems, other medications, risk of overdose and type of depression (Wiese, 2011). When an antidepressant is prescribed, consideration must be given to the side effect profile and the risk of drug interactions, with the aim of reducing the negative impact of both. The names and types of antidepressants commonly used in older people are as follows:

- Selective serotonin reuptake inhibitors (SSRIs)
  - Citalopram
  - Escitalopram
  - Sertraline
- Tricyclic
  - Desipramine: Anticholinergic (may cause cardiovascular side effects)

- Nortriptyline: Anticholinergic (may cause cardio-vascular side effects)
- Others
  - Buproprion (can cause seizures)
  - Mirtazapine
  - Moclobemide (do not combine with MAOB inhibitors or tricyclics)
  - Venlafaxine (may increase blood pressure)

The newer antidepressants, such as buproprion, mirtazapine, moclobemide and the selective norepinephrine reuptake inhibitor venlafaxine, are considered relatively safe for older people. It is recommended, however, to start with a lower dose before titrating upward to reach a therapeutic effect. It is important to monitor for side effects and drug interactions. Citalopram, escitalopram and sertraline (SSRIs) are the best tolerated medications in older people (Wiese, 2011); fluoxetine, paroxetine and fluvoxamine have greater risks in terms of drug interactions, so special consideration is needed if the person is taking multiple medications (Wiese, 2011). Other antidepressants classes, such as monoamine oxidase inhibitors, are not considered to be first- or second-line options for older people due to their side effects. Tricyclics are best considered as second-line treatments, with close monitoring due to their side effect profile.

Above all it must be remembered the use of an antidepressant should be carefully considered, and if it is required, the patient should be monitored closely. According to the NICE (2018a) guidance, when prescribing an antidepressant medication, the practitioner must first

- Explain the reasons for offering the medication.
- Discuss the harms and benefits.
- Discuss any concerns the person may have about taking or stopping the medication.
- Make sure the person has all the relevant information.

The patient should know how long to expect before the medication is likely to have an effect, which is typically within 3 weeks. They should also know to seek a medication review if there is no improvement within 3 to 4 weeks and that it is important to follow the prescribing advice. The patient must be aware of the following (NICE, 2018):

- Treatment may need to continue after remission of their depression.
- The medication is not addictive.
- There is the possibility of interactions with other medications.
- Stopping the medication can impact their mood. A management plan should be incorporated into their recovery plan.

In terms of side effects, the patient should be aware they may feel unsteady, agitated/restless, irritable, anxious or confused. They may also experience altered sensations, sleep may be impacted and they may have an upset stomach (NICE, 2018a; Wiese, 2011).

They should be informed side effects are usually mild and go away after a week, but they can also unfortunately be quite severe, especially if the antidepressant is suddenly stopped. When stopping an antidepressant, the half-life of the medication should be considered (i.e., how long the active drug remains in a person's system), and a slow reduction over time should be considered and managed. If a patient is on a reducing-to-stop dose, they should be monitored closely to allow for adjustments to the dose reduction according to the symptoms. When reducing doses, nurses should be aware of the following:

- Fluoxetine has a prolonged duration of action and can usually be stopped with a dose reduction regime.
- Venlafaxine and paroxetine are known to have discontinuation symptoms, so patients who were taking these medications need to be closely monitored.

If a patient experiences discontinuation symptoms, they should be reminded it is not uncommon, relapse doesn't usually happen and even if they restart their medication or need to increase the dose, symptoms can take up to 3 weeks to disappear (NICE, 2018a).

Mild discontinuation symptoms should be monitored and reassurance given to the patient that what they are experiencing is common and to be expected. If the symptoms are severe, consider restarting the original medication. Alternatively, another antidepressant from the same class but with a longer half-life can be considered. The dose can then be reduced gradually while monitoring symptoms.

For individuals with a psychotic type of depression and who are prescribed an antipsychotic, the following should be undertaken:

- A fasting blood glucose or HbA1c and fasting lipids along with weight measurement before starting, then annual fasting blood glucose or HbA1c and fasting lipids
- Weekly monitoring of weight for the first 6 weeks, and then at 12 weeks, 1 year, and then annually
- EEG monitoring—baseline and at final dose for individuals with cardiovascular disease and for those on other medications known to prolong the cardiac QT interval
- At each review, check for side effects inclusive of extrapyramidal- and prolactin-related effects such with high prolactin level; excess body and facial hair; loss of interest in sex
- Other extrapyramidal side effects can be parkinsonian symptoms and acute dystonia; patient should be reminded to discuss these important side effects with their health care professional

- If rapid or excessive weight gain or abnormal lipid or blood glucose levels are found, investigate and treat as necessary (NICE, 2018a)
- Consider if the medication is needed in view of physical and psychological health risks
- If a decision is made to stop medication, it should be managed by specialist mental health services and done gradually

The patient should be cautioned against taking alternative medications. One such example is St John's wort, which may be useful but can have serious interactions with medications such as anticonvulgants and anticoagulants. In addition, there will be uncertainty about the dose of active ingredient contained in each preparation.

The first-line treatment for less severe depression and the lower half of moderate depression is lower-intensity psychological interventions and not medication. Overall, patients should be offered a psychological intervention before an antidepressant is considered. For more severe depression, a combined antidepressant and psychological intervention is appropriate (NICE, 2018a).

Electroconvulsive Therapy

Modern electroconvulsive therapy is one of the most controversial treatments used, despite its history of efficacy and safety (Amarjothi et al., 2007). Although there is uncertainty in terms of its mode of action, it is thought electroconvulsive therapy affects several 5HT receptors in the central nervous system. 5-hydroxtryptamine is one of the most important neurotransmitters involved in depression, so this impact may be responsible for the efficacy of electroconvulsive therapy. According to Nobler et al. (2001), electroconvulsive therapy decreases glucose metabolism, particularly in the frontal and parietal cortex. It also reduces neuronal activity in some cortical regions; this has the antidepressant effect (Nobler et al., 2001). Although it is a proposed theory, Amarjothi et al. (2007) highlighted a weakness, explaining that benzodiazepines and anticonvulsant medications bring about similar neuronal changes but do not improve depressive symptoms.

In older populations electroconvulsive therapy is usually used only for major depressive disorder and has a recovery rate of approximately 80% (Mulsant et al., 1991). It is known to be well tolerated by patients and particularly effective with severe depression associated with a high degree of risk (i.e., suicide), psychomotor retardation, delusions and life-threatening food and fluid refusal. The patient requires a full physical review including a review by a senior anaesthetist. Cognitive function and mental state must be reviewed after each treatment. It should be conducted in a purpose-built suite with access to immediate medical support should resuscitation be required.

A course of electroconvulsive therapy consists of between 6 and 12 sessions biweekly until improvement. At each session the patient is given an anaesthetic, and when unconscious a muscle relaxant is given to help modify the fit and reduce the risk of possible physical injury. The patient's vital signs, heart rate and brain activity (electroencephalogram) are monitored throughout each session. If there is no improvement between the sixth and eighth sessions, the treatment may be stopped. Adverse cognitive side effects have been noted, although they have been mitigated against with modern electroconvulsive therapy. However, there is a short-term memory loss of the events leading up to the treatment. Some report longer-term memory loss of as much as several years. Others report difficulty remembering the few days after the treatment, and still others report permanent memory impairment, although this is probably not due only to the electroconvulsive therapy treatment (Amarjothi, 2007). ECT is effective and safe and can be life saving. Psychotic, severe or treatment resistant depression are the most common types of condition for this treatment, and it is well tolerated by the older population. There is no good evidence to suggest it has a prophylactic benefit.

The nurse has a role in education and advocacy for the patient and in physically preparing them for treatment. They may be involved in the preparation of the electroconvulsive therapy suite and its equipment and in the patient's treatment and recovery.

CONCLUSION

The nurse has an important part to play in the identification, assessment and treatment of older adults with depression. This role is one every nurse, regardless of specialism, must be aware of and one that must be embraced. For nurses with an interest or specialism in mental health, there are opportunities to expand knowledge and competency in the treatment of depression, from exercise and education to facilitated self-help and providing low- and high-intensity psychological therapies. Ultimately nurses see older people in a variety of settings and for a variety of reasons and are in a unique and privileged position to ensure depression in older adults is identified and treated. Nurses have always made a difference to the lives of their patients and can make a significant difference for those who suffer from depression.

KEY LEARNING POINTS

- Conduct a comprehensive biopsychosocial assessment inclusive of risk.
- Rule out any physical reasons for low mood or confusion, such as delirium and dementia.
- Once assessed, use the diagnostic criteria of the ICD and/or the DSM to confirm the diagnosis.
- Use appropriate psychometric tools to aid in diagnosis and monitor treatment progression.
- Establish a clear collaborative understanding of the problem (i.e., problem statements and formulation).

- Establish clearly defined behavioural goals. Ensure they are created with the patient and not for the patient.
- Make sure the goals are value directed. (Why would the patient identify a certain goal as important? Perhaps because of family, friends, hobbies, spirituality, etc.)
- Use the appropriate step in the stepped approach to care.
- It is essential the health care professional receives good quality clinical supervision from a competent practitioner.

REFERENCES

Age Concern, Help the Aged. (2009). *One Voice: Shaping our Ageing Society*. Age Concern.

Age UK. (2021). Number of pensioners living in poverty tops two million, with Black and Asian older people most at risk: accessible: https://www.ageuk.org.uk/latest-press/articles/2021/number-of-pensioners-living-in-poverty-tops-two-million/

Aggar, C., Thomas, T., Gordon, C., Bloomfield, J., & Baker, J. (2021). Social Prescribing for individuals living with mental illness in an Australian Community setting: A pilot study. *Community Mental Health Journal, 57*, 189–195.

Al-Janabi, H., McLoughlin, C., Oyebode, Jan R., Efstathiou, N., & Calvert, M. (2019). Six mechanisms behind carer wellbeing effects: A qualitative study of healthcare delivery. *Social Science and Medicine, 235*, Article 112382.

Allan, C. E., Valkanova, V., & Ebmeier, K. P. (2014). Depression in older people is underdiagnosed. *Practitioner, 258*(1771), 19–22.

Almeida, O. P., & Almeida, S. A. (1999). Short versions of the geriatric depression scale: a study of their validity for the diagnosis of a major depressive episode according to ICD-10 and DSM-IV. *International JJournal of Geriatric Psychiatry, 14*, 858–865.

Amarjothi, S., Krishna, M., & Barnes, R. (2007). ECT in the Elderly. *Geriatric Medicine*. Retrieved from https://www.gmjournal.co.uk/media/21426/apr07p23.pdf.

American Psychiatric Association (APA). (2013). *Diagnostic and Statistical Manual of Mental Disorders* (5th ed). Arlinghton, VA: APA.

Andreas, A., Schulz, H., Volkert, J., Dehoust, M., Sehner, S., Suling, A., Ausin, B., Canuto, A., Crawford, M., Da Ronch, C., Grassi, L., Hershkovitz, Y., Munoz, M., Quirk, A., Rotenstein, O., Belen, A., Santos-Olmo, A. B., Shalev, A., Strehle, J., & Harter, M. (2017). Prevalence of mental disorders in elderly people: the European MentDis_ICF65+ study. *The British Journal of Psychiatry, 210*, 125–131.

Arthur, A., Savva, G.M., Barnes, L.E., Borjian-Boroojeny, A., Dening, T., Jagger, C., Matthews, F.E., Robinson, L., Brayne, C., & the Cognitive Function and Aging Studies Collaboration (2019). Changing prevalence and treatment of depression among older people over two decades. *British Journal of Psychiatry, 216*, 49–54.

Arthur, A., Jagger, C., Lindesay, J., Graham, C., & Clarke, L. (1999). Using an annual over-75 health check to screen for depression: validation of the short Geriatric Depression Scale (GDS15) within general practice. *International Journal of Geriatric Psychiatry, 14*, 431–439.

Avasthi, A., & Grover, S. (2018). Clinical practice guidelines for management of depression in elderly. *Indian Journal of Psychiatry, 60*(3), S341–S362.

Baral, P. (2020). Depression in the older person. *Geriatric Medicine Journal*. https://www.gmjournal.co.uk/depression-in-the-older-population.

Barry, L. C., Abou, J. J., & Gill, M. B. (2012). Under-treatment of depression in Older Persons. *Journal of Affective Disorders, 136*(3), 789–796.

Beck, A. T., Steer, R. A., & Brown, G. K. (1996). *Manual for Beck depression inventory-II*. Psychology Corporation.

Blackburn, P., Wilkins-Ho, M., & Iiese, B. (2017). Depression in older adults: Diagnosis and Management. *British Columbia Medical Journal, 59*(3), 171–177.

Bor, J. S. (2015). Among the elderly, many mental illnesses go undiagnosed (pp. 5). Health Affairs.

Burns, A. (2015). Better access to mental health services for older people. Retrieved from: https://www.england.nhs.uk/blog/mh-better-access/

Butler-Tony, T. J., & Thayer, J. M. (2020). *Nursing process*. StatePearls Publishing.

Byers, A. L., & Yaffe, K. (2011). Depression and risk of developing dementia. *Nature Reviews Neurology, 7*, 323–331.

Chakrabarti, S. (2018). Mood Disorders in the International Classification of Diseases-11: Similarities and differences with the Diagnostic and Statistical Manual of Mental Disorders 5 and the International Classification of Disease-10. *Indian Journal of Social Psychiatry, 34*(S1), 17–22.

Clarke, D. M. (2018). Realising the Mass Public Benefit of Evidence-Based Psychological Therapies: The IAPT Program. *Annual Review of Clinical Psychology, 7*(14), 159–183.

Clark, D. M., Layard, R., Smithies, R., Richards, R. A., Suckling, R., & Wright, B. (2009). Improving access to psychological therapy: An evaluation of two UK demonstration sites. *Behaviour Research Therapy, 4*(11), 910–920.

Conejero, I., Olie, E., & Calati, R. (2018). Suicide in older adults: Current perspectives. *Clinical Interventions in Aging, 13*, 691–699.

Cox, D., & D'Oyley, H (2011). Cognitive-Behavioural therapy with older adults. *BC Medical Journal, 53*(7).

D'Ath, P., Katona, P., & Mullan, E. (1994). Screening, detecting and management of depression in elderly primary care attenders I: The acceptability and performance of the 15 item Geriatric Depression Scale (GDS-15) and the development of shorter versions. *Family Practice, 11*, 260–266.

De Craen, A. J. M., Heeren, T. J., & Gussekloo, H. J. (2002). Accuracy of the 15-item geriatric depression scale (GDS-15) in a community sample of the oldest old. *International Journal of Geriatric Psychiatry, 18*(1), 63–66.

Dimidjian, S., Barrera, M., Martell, C., Munoz, R. F., & Lewinsohn, P. M. (2011). The origins and current status of behavioural activation treatments for depression. *Annual Review Clinic Psychology, 7*, 1–38.

DoH. (2001). National service framework for older people. Department of Health.

DoH. (2019). The Community Mental Health Framework for Adults and Older adults. National Collaborating Centre for Mental Health. Retrieved from https://www.england.nhs.uk/wp-content/uploads/2019/09/community-mental-health-framework-for-adults-and-older-adults.pdf

DoHNI. (2013). *Service framework for older people*. Department of Health, Social Services and Public Safety.

Donaghy, G. (2019). *Mental diagnosis of people aged 65 and over. Evidence summary*. Voluntary Health Scotland.

El Khoury, J. R., Baroud, E. A., & Khoury, B. A. (2020). The revision of the categories of mood, anxiety and stress-related disorders in the ICD-11: A perspective from the Arab region. *Middle East Current Psychiatry, 27*, 7.

Ellis, G. (2011). Comprehensive geriatric assessment for older adults admitted to hospital: Meta-analysis of randomised controlled trails. *British Medical Journal, 343*. https://doi.org/10.1136/bmj.d6553.

Ell, D. (2006). Depression care for the elderly: Reducing barriers to evidenced based practice. *Home Health Care Services Quarterly, 25*(1-2), 115–148.

Engel, G. L. (1977). The need for a new medical model: A challenge for biomedicine. *Science, 196*, 129–136.

Ettman, C. K., Adballa, S. M., Cohen, G. H., Sampson, L., Vivier, P. M., & Galea, S. (2020). Prevalence of depression symptoms in US adults before and during the COVID-19 pandemic. *JAMA Network Open, 3*(9), Article e2019686. https://doi.org/10.1001/jamanetworkopen.2020.19686.

Folstein, M. F., Folstein, S. E., McHugh, P. R., & Se, F. (1975). Mini-mental state. A practical method for grading the cognitive state of patients for the clinician. *Journal of Psychiatric Research, 12*(3), 189–198.

Frost, R., Beattie, A., Bhanu, C., Walters, K., & Ben-Shlomo, Y. (2019). Management of depression and referral of older people to psychological therapies: a systematic review of qualitative studies. *British Journal of General Practice, 69*, 171–181.

Gotlib, I. H., & Hammen, C. (2009). *Handbook of depression* (2nd ed). Guilford Press.

Greenberg, S. A. (2007). How to try this: The Geriatric Depression Scale Short form. *American Journal of Nursing, 107*(10), 60–69.

Greenberg, S. A. (2012). The Geriatric Depression Scale. The Hartford Institute for Geriatric Nursing: New York University; College of Nursing. Retrieved from: chrome-extension://efaidnbmnnnibpcajpcglclefindmkaj/https://wwwoundcare.ca/Uploads/ContentDocuments/Geriatric%20Depression%20Scale.pdf.

Gureje, O., Kola, L., & Afolabi, E. (2007). Epidemiology of major depressive disorder in elderly Nigerians in the Ibadan study of ageing: A community-based survey. *Lancet, 370*(9591), 957–964.

Hodges, J. R., & Larner, A. J (2017). Addenbrooke's cognitive examinations: ACE, ACE-R, ACE-III, ACEapp, and M-ACE. In *Cognitive screening instruments: A practical approach* (2nd edition, pp. 109–137). Springer.

Horackova, K., Kopecek, M., Machů, V., Kagstrom, A., Aarsland, D., Motlova, L. B., & Cermakova, P. (2019). Prevalence of late-life depression and gap in mental health service use across European regions. *European Psychiatry, 57*, 19–25.

Hyer, L., & Kramer, D. (2004). CBT with older people: Alterations and the value of the therapeutic alliance. Psychotherapy: Theory Research Practice. *Training, 41*(3), 246–291.

Hughes, C., Herron, S., & Younge, J. (2014). *CBT for mild to moderate depression and anxiety: A guide to low intensity interventions*. McGraw Hill.

Independent Age (accessed 2023): Older people and depression. https://www.independentage.org/sites/default/files/2020-02/Independent%20Age_older%20people%20%26%20depression_.pdf.

Jackson, R., & Baldwin, B. (1993). Detecting depression in elderly mentally ill patients: The use of the geriatric depression scale compared with medical and nursing observations. *Age and Aging, 22*, 349–353.

Jacobson, N. S., Dobson, K. S., Traux, P. A., Addis, M. E., Koerner, K., Gollan, J. K., Gortner, E., & Prince (1996). A component analysis of cognitive-behavioral treatment for depression. *Journal of Consulting and Clinical Psychology, 64*(2), 295–304.

Janssen, N., Huibers, M. J., Lucassen, P., Voshaar, R. O., van Marwijk, H., Bosmans, J., Pijnappels, M., Spijker, J., & Hendriks, G. J. (2017). Behavioural activation by mental health nurses for late-life depression in primary care: A randomized controlled trail. *BMC Psychiatry, 17*, 230.

Jonsson, U., Bertilsson, G., Allard, P., Gyllensvard, H., Soderlund, A., Tham, A., & Andersson, G. (2016). Psychological treatment of depression in people aged 65 years and over: A systematic review of efficacy, safety, and cost effectiveness. *PLoS One, 11*, Article e0160859. https://doi.org/10.1371/journal.pone.0160859.

Kavan, M. G., & Barone, E. J. (2014). grief and Major Depression-Controversy over changes in DSM-5 Diagnostic Criteria. *American Family Physician, 90*(10), 693–694.

Kraus, C., Kadriu, B., Lanzenberger, R., Zarate Jr, C.A. and Kasper, S. (2019). Prognosis and improved outcomes in major depression: a review. *Translational Psychiatry, 9*(127). https://doi.org/10.1038/s41398-019-0460-3.

Kroenke, K., Spitzer, R. L., & Williams, J. B. (2001). The PHQ-9 validity of a brief depression severity measure. *Journal of General Internal Medicine, 16*(9), 606–613.

Layard, R., & Clark, D. M. (2015). Why more psychological therapy would cost nothing. *Frontiers in Psychology, 6*, 1713.

Levis, B., Benedetti, A., & Thombs, B. D. (2019). Accuracy of Patient Health Questionnaire-9 (PHQ-9) for screening to detect major depression: Individual participant data meta-analysis. *British Medical Journal, 9*, 365.

Lewinsohn, P. M., & Graf, M. (1973). Pleasant activities and depression. *Journal of Consulting and Clinical Psychology, 41*(2), 261–268, doi: 10.1037/h0035142.

Linden, M., & Kurtz, G. (2009). A randomised controlled experimental study on the influence ofpatient age on medical decisions in respect to the diagnosis and treatment of depression in the elderly. *Current Gerontology and Geriatrics Research, 475958.* https://doi.org/10.1155/2009/475958.

Luck-Sikorski, C., Stein, J., Heilmann, K., Maier, W., Kaduszkie-wicz, H., Scherer, M., Weyerer, S., Werle, J., Wiese, B., Moor, L., Bock, J. O., König, H. H., & Riedel-Heller, S. G. (2017). Treatment Preferences for depression in the elderly. *International Psychogeriatrics, 29*, 389–398.

MacKenzie, C. S., Lippens, T., Mather, A., & Sareen, J. (2009). Older adults help-seeking attitudes and treatment beliefs concerning Mental Health Problems. *The American Journal of Geriatric Medicine, 16*(12), 1010–1019.

Marek, K. D., Stetzer, F., Ryan, P. A., Bub, L. D., Adams, S. J., Schildt, A., Lancaster, R., & O'Brien, A. M (2013). Nurse Care coordination and technology effects on health status of frail elderly via enhanced self-management of medication: Randomised clinical trail to test efficacy. *Nursing Research, 62*(4), 269–278.

Markowitz, J. C., & Weissman, M. M. (2004). Interpersonal psychotherapy: Principles and applications. *World Psychiatry, 3*(3), 136–139.

Maslow, A. H. (1954). *Motivation and personality*. Harper and Row.

Mitchell, A. J., Bird, V., Rizzo, M., & Meader, N. (2010). Diagnostic validity and added value of the geriatric depression scale for depression in primary care: a meta-analysis of GDS$_{30}$ and GDS$_{15}$. *J Affect Disorders 125*(1-3), 10–17.

Murray, J., Banerjee, S. B., yng, R., Tylee, A., Bhugra, D., & Macdonald, A. (2006). Primary care professionals' perceptions of depression in older people: A qualitative study. *Social Sciences and Medicine, 63*, 1363–1373.

Mulsant, B. H., Rosen, J., Thornton, J., & Zubenko, G. A. (1991). Prospective naturalistic study of ECT in late life Depression. *Journal of Geriatric Psychiatry and Neurology Neurology, 4*, 3–13.

National Insitute for Health and Care Excellence (NICE). (2022). Depression in adults: treatment and management. www.nice.org.uk/guidance/ng222

NICE. (2009b). Depression in adults with a chronic physical health problem: recognition and management. www.nice.org.uk/guidance/cg91

NICE. (2009a). *Depression in adults: Recognition and management.* https://www.nice.org.uk/guidance/cg90.

NICE. (2018a). Depression: The NICE guideline on the treatment and management of depression in adults. https://www.nice.org.uk/guidance/cg90/evidence/full-guideline-pdf-4840934509

NICE. (2018b). *Dementia: Assessment, management and support for people living with dementia and their carers.* https://www.nice.org.uk/guidance/ng97.

Nursing & Midwifery Council. (2018). The code: Professional standards of practice and behaviour for nurses, midwives and nursing associates. http://www.nmc.org.uk/globalassets/sitedocuments/nmc-publications/revised-new-nmc-code.pdf

Nursing and Midwifery Council (NMC, 2018). The code: professional standards of practice and behaviour for nurses, midwives and nursing associates.

Nursing & Midwifery Council. (2019). Standards framework for Nursing and Midwifery Education.

Nobler, M. S., Oquendo, M. A., Kegeles, L. S., Malone, K. M., Campbell, C., Sackeim, H. A., & Mann, J. J. (2001). Decreased regional brain metabolism after ECT. *American Journal of Psychiatry, 158*, 305–308.

Ostlin, P., Eckermann, E., Mishra, U. S., Nkowane, M., & Wallstam, E. (2007). Gender and health promotion: A multi-sectoral policy approach. *Health Promotion International, 21*(S1), 25–35.

Overend, K., Bosanquet, K., VBailey, D, Foster, D, Gascoyne, S, Lewis, H, Nutbrown, S, Woodhouse, R, Gilbody, S., & Chew-Graham, C. (2015). Revealing hidden depression in older people: A qualitative study within a randomised controlled trial. *BMC Family Practice*, 142.

Phelan, E., Williams, B., Meeker, K., Bonn, K., Frederick, J., LoGerfo, J., & Snowden, M. (2010). A study of the diagnostic accuracy of the PHQ-9 in primary elderly care. *BMC Family Practice, 11*, 63.

Pies, R. (2014). The Bereavement exclusion and DSM_5: An update and commentary. *Innovations in Clinical Neuroscience, 11*(7-8), 19–22.

Pocklington, C. (2017). Depression in Older Adults. *British Journal of Medical Practitioners, 10*(1), a1007.

Polenick, C. A., & Flora, S. R. (2013). Behavioral activation for depression in older adults: Theoretical and practical considerations. *The Behavior Analyst, 36*, 35–55.

Pomeroy, I. M., Clark, C. R., & Philip, C. I. (2001). The effectiveness of very short scales for depression screening in elderly patients. *International Journal of Geriatric Psychiatry, 16*(3), 321–326.

Rai, D., Garg, R. K., Malhotra, H. S., Verma, R., Jain, A., Tiwari, S. C., & Singh, M. H. (2014). Acute confusional state/delirium: An etiological and prognostic evaluation. *Annals of Indian Academy of Neurology, 17*, 30–34.

RcPsych (2014). Depression in older adults. https://www.rcpsych.ac.uk/mental-health/problems-disorders/depression-in-older-adults

Richards, D. A., & Whyte, M. (2011). *Reach out: national programme student materials to support the delivery of training for psychological wellbeing practitioners delivering low intensity interventions (3rd edition).* Rethink Mental Illness. http://cedar.exeter.ac.uk/media/universityofexeter/schoolofpsychology/cedar/documents/Reach_Out_3rd_edition.pdf

Reed, G. M., First, M. B., Kogan, C. S., Hyman, S. E., Gureje, O., Gaebel, W., Maj, M., Stein, D. J., Maercker, A., Tyrer, P., Claudino, A., Garralda, E., Salvador-Carulla, L., Ray, R., Saunders, J. B., Dua, T., Poznyak, V., Medina-Mora, M. E., Pike, K. M., & Saxena, S. (2019). Innovations and changes in the ICD-11 classification of mental, behavioural and neurodevelopmental disorders. *World Psychiatry, 18*, 3–19.

Reynolds, W. J., & Scott, B. (1999). Empathy: A crucial component of the helping relationship. *Journal of Psychiatric and Mental Health Nursing, 3*, 363–370.

Reyes, D. V., Patel, H., Lautenschlager, N., Ford, A. H., Curran, E., Kelly, R., Lai., R., Chong, T., Flicker, L., Ekers, D., Gilbody, S., Etherton-Beer, C., Giudice, Lo, D., Ellis, K. A., Martini, A., & Almeida, O. P. (2019). Behavioural activation in nursing homes to treat depression (BAN-Dep): Study protocol for a pragmatic randomised controlled trail. *BMJ Open, 9*, Article e032421.

Rogers, C. R. (1956). Client centred theory. *Journal of Counselling Psychology, 3*(2), 115–120.

Royal Society for Public Health (2018). That age old question. https://www.rsph.org.uk/static/uploaded/a01e3aa7-9356-40bc-99c81b14dd904a41.pdf

Saito, M., Iwata, N., Kawakami, N., & Matsuyama, Y. (2010). Evaluation of the DSM-IV and ICD-10 criteria for depressive disorders in a community population in Japan using an item response theory. *International Journal of Methods in Psychiatric Research, 19*(4), 211–222.

Seitz, D., Purandare, N., & Conn, D. (2010). Prevalence of psychiatric disorders among older adults in long-term care homes: a systematic review. *International Psychogeriatrics*, 1025–1039. DOI: https://doi.org/10.1017/S1041610210000608.

Shadtri, A., Aimola, L., Tooke, B., Quirk, A., Corrado, O., Hood, C., & Crawford, M. J. (2019). Recognition and treatment of depression in older adults admitted to acute hospitals in England. *Clinical Medicine Journal, 19*, 114–118. https://doi.org/10.7861/clinmedicine.19-2-114.

Sheikh, J. I., & Yesavage, J. A. (1986). Geriatric Depression Scale (GDS): Recent evidence and development of a shorter version. *Clinical Gerontologist, 5*, 165–173.

Short, J. (2017). Options in the care of people with depression. NIHR accessible at: https://evidence.nihr.ac.uk/collection/options-in-the-care-of-people-with-depression/

Social Care Institute for Excellence. (2006). *Guide 3 Assessing the mental health needs of older people.* https://www.scie.org.uk/publications/guides/guide03/.

Spitzer, R. L., Kroenke, K., Williams, J. B. W., & Lowe, B. (2006). A brief measure for assessing generalized anxiety disorder: The GAD-7. *Archives of Internal Medicine, 166*(10), 1092–1097.

Stark, A., Kaduszkiewicz, H., Stein, J., Maier, W., Heser, K., Weyerer, S., Werle, J., Wiese, B., Mamone, S., Konig, H. H., Block, J. O., Riedel-Heller, S. G., & Scherer, M. (2018). A qualitative study on older primary care patients' perspectives on depression and its treatments-potential barriers to

and opportunities for managing depression. *BMC Family Practice, 19*, 2.

Stiles, P. G., & McGarrahan, J. F. (1998). The Geriatric Depression Scale: A comprehensive review. *Journal of Clinical Geropsychology, 4*(2), 89–110.

Swift, H. J., Abrams, D., Lamont, R. A., & Drury, L. (2017). The risks of ageism model: How ageism and negative attitudes toward age can be a barrier to active aging. *Social Issues and Policy Review, 11*(1), 195–231.

The Royal College of Psychiatrists. (2018). Suffering in silence: Age inequality in older people's mental health care. https://www.rcpsych.ac.uk/docs/default-source/improving-care/better-mh-policy/college-reports/college-report-cr221.pdf?sfvrsn=bef8f65d_2#:~:text=The%20increase%20is%20still%20more,reach%20the%20age%20of%2085

Thomas, H. (2013). Assessing and Managing depression in older people. *Nursing Times, 109*(43), 16–18.

Van Orden K. A., O'Riley, A. A., Simning, A., & Podgorski, C. (2014). Passive suicide ideation: an indicator of risk among older adults seeking aging services? *The Gerontologist, 55*(6). DOI:10.1093/geront/gnu026.

Vieira, E. R., Brown, E., & Rue, P. (2014). Depression in older adults: Screening and referral. *Journal of Geriatric Physical Therapy, 37*(1), 24–30.

Wade, D. T., & Halligan, P. W. (2017). The biopsychosocial model of illness: A model whose time has come. *Clinical Rehabilitation, 31*(8), 995–1004.

WHO. (1992). *International classification of disease-10.* World Health Organization.

WHO. (2017). Mental health of older people: Key facts. https://www.who.int/news-room/fact-sheets/detail/mental-health-of-older-adults

WHO. (2018) https://www.who.int/news/item/18-06-2018-who-releases-newinternational-classification-of-diseases-(icd-11)

WHO. (2019). *ICD-11: International classification of diseases, eleventh revision (ICD-11).* https://icd.who.int/browse11

WHO. (2021). Depression: Key facts. https://www.who.int/news-room/fact-sheets/detail/depression

WHO. (2021). Suicide: Key facts. https://www.who.int/news-room/fact-sheets/detail/suicide

Wilkinson, P. (2013). Cognitive behavioural therapy with older people. *Maturitas, 76*, 5–9.

Williams, S. Z., Chung, G. S., & Muennig, P. A. (2017). Undiagnoised depression: A community diagnosis. *Population Health, 3*, 633–638.

Wiese, B. (2011). Geriatric depression: The use of antidepressants in the elderly. *BC Medical Journal, 53*(47), 341–347.

Wuthrich, V. M., & Frei, J. (2015). Barriers to treatment for older adults seeking psychological therapy. *International Psychogeriatrics, 27*(7), 1227–1236.

Yesavage, J. A., Brink, T. L., Rose, T. L., Lim, O., Huang, V., Adey, M., & Leirer, V. O. (1982). Development and validation of a geriatric depression screening scale: A preliminary report. *Journal of Psychiatric Research, 17*(1), 37–49.

Medicine Management

Sue Latter, Rebecca Henry

With advancing age, the likelihood of developing a long-term illness increases, or an existing complaint may be exacerbated. An individual in the prime of life is able to respond to environmental fluctuations through homeostatic control, but with advancing years this ability declines. Older adults are less able to adjust to changes of temperature and posture. Accidents are more common, risk of infection is greater and tissues heal more slowly than in the younger person. Many of these conditions can be treated with drugs, allowing the older person years of comfortable, independent living. In other cases medication is unnecessary if changes are made to lifestyle. For example, including fibre in the diet on a regular basis may reduce the need for aperients as gut motility decreases. Similarly, alterations to carbohydrate and fat consumption may obviate the need for drugs for a patient who has developed non–insulin-dependent diabetes mellitus.

At one time the symptoms of age-related disorders were regarded by patients and health professionals as an inevitable part of life. Today they are treated routinely. At the present time people over age 65 make up a high and growing proportion of the population and consume the highest proportion of the United Kingdom NHS's drug budget. The number of older people in the United Kingdom population is increasing, so nurses can expect to care for increasing numbers in the future, and more of them will be taking medication. In the past most of this care took place in hospital, but with the trend toward care in the community now firmly established, nurses are required to look after increasing numbers of older people in community settings. Working as part of a multidisciplinary team, including GPs, geriatricians and pharmacists, nurses are involved in assessing and monitoring the care of these patients. Often the hands-on, day-to-day care is delivered through a combination of nurses, health care assistants and lay carers whose activities are supervised and supported by the nurse. As part of their extended role, many nurses are now responsible for prescribing. Every nurse therefore needs to develop and maintain a sound knowledge of the pharmacology of the medicines in their scope of practice.

This chapter provides an overview of the physiological challenges posed by older age and how they relate to medicines' effectiveness. It draws on research to outline other key issues that influence good medicine management in older people and highlights the role of nurses in this important area, using evidence to identify possible actions for practice.

PROBLEMS ASSOCIATED WITH MEDICATION USE BY OLDER PEOPLE

As people get older, there are changes in the way the body handles medication (i.e., pharmacokinetic), most importantly age-related decline in renal function, which can necessitate medication dose reduction. There are also changes that alter the way the body responds to medication (i.e., pharmacodynamic)—for example, receptors become more sensitive to the effects of benzodiazepines, so lower doses are recommended. Any adverse reactions are also often vague and non-specific—for example, postural hypotension and falls with psychotropic medications and confusion or constipation with many medications.

In addition to the pharmacological differences, the ageing body causes symptoms of the disease to differ from those present in the younger age group. Signs and symptoms of illness frequently become vague and non-specific. This may be compounded by communication difficulties and the coexistence of more than one medical condition. For example, a urinary tract infection in a young woman typically manifests as urinary frequency, pyrexia and dysuria. In an older person, it may manifest as loss of continence, becoming less cooperative or less lucid, or just vague signs of deterioration. However, infection should always be suspected if urine appears cloudy and has an offensive odour. Because of the often vague nature of symptoms and adverse reactions, it is important not confuse them. It is also important not to confuse the natural ageing process with symptoms of an illness and vice versa.

As we age, the balance between benefits and risks of medications shifts more toward risks. However, suggesting stopping medications due to age can be perceived as ageist (O'Mahony et al., 2015).

To further confuse matters, most clinical trials are carried out in healthy adult populations of people aged 18–64 without comorbidities and age-related changes. Data are often extrapolated from these healthy adults to older people. There are often variations in the way healthy adults handle medications that are exacerbated in older people. It is not until real life post-marketing use of a medication that we discover additional or increased issues such as adverse drug effects or drug/disease interactions.

PHARMACOKINETIC CHANGES

Absorption

The most common route of administration of medications is oral. To get into the bloodstream and to the site of action, they must first pass through the gut wall and liver. Drugs are either in an ionised (i.e., the molecule has a negative or positive charge) or non-ionised (i.e., a neutral molecule) form. The degree of ionisation of a drug depends on its chemical properties, which changes depending on the pH of the environment. The more lipid-soluble the drug is, the easier this process is. Non-ionised drugs are more lipid-soluble. Acidic drugs are better absorbed from the acidic stomach and alkaline drugs from the higher-pH intestine. As our bodies age, we produce less gastric acid and the pH rises, causing a reduction of solubility/absorption of acidic drugs such as aspirin.

Gut motility (i.e., peristalsis) and the rate of gastric emptying are also reduced, increasing the overall transit time of drugs to the site of absorption, which can produce a slower peak and prolonged and increased absorption of medications. This is a problem if you need a rapid-peak concentration, such as analgesics for sudden acute pain. It also means gastric irritants such as non-steroidal anti-inflammatory drugs and levodopa stay in the stomach longer and are more likely to cause increased gastric discomfort. Dose reduction may be necessary. Reduced peristalsis increases the possibility of the person having constipation and the need for extra care when prescribing medications that cause constipation.

As we age there is a reduction in the number of actively absorbing cells in the gastrointestinal mucosa. Most drugs are absorbed passively through the gut wall. Drugs such as methyldopa and levodopa are absorbed through active diffusion and may have reduced absorption.

As ageing is associated with some reduction in first-pass metabolism, bioavailability (i.e., the amount of medication that reaches the circulation unchanged) of a few drugs is increased (Shi & Klotz, 2011).

Many of the factors that influence absorption are contradictory. This unpredictability may mean plasma levels and/or efficacy need to be assessed before dosage changes.

In addition, older people with frailty may have difficulty swallowing tablets, and if oral medications are left in the mouth, ulceration may develop. People should always be encouraged to take their tablets or capsules with enough fluid and while in an upright position to avoid the possibility of oesophageal ulceration. It can be helpful to discuss with the older person the possibility of taking the drug as a liquid if available.

When drugs are administered topically, we must take into account the fact that with age the elasticity, moisture and turnover of epithelial cells of the skin is reduced, and repeated application may result in irritation, soreness or breakdown of the epithelial layer. The area should be carefully inspected before each application, and the person's report of discomfort should be taken seriously.

When delivering drugs by injection, we must take into account that with increasing age comes a reduction in muscle tone through inactivity, which can cause the fluid to pool at the site of entry and delay in its action. Older people have delicate skin, especially if taking steroids, and bruise easily. It is vital to rotate the site when injections are administered frequently.

Distribution

After drugs have been absorbed in the body, they need to be distributed to the site of action. Distribution depends on the properties of the drug and specific physiological factors for the older person. It is these factors that are affected by the ageing process.

Older people have increased total body fat—18%–36% for men and 36%–48% for woman—but decreased lean body mass. There is more fat for lipid soluble drugs such as benzodiazepines to accumulate in. This accumulation results in a slower release of drugs from the adipose tissue for metabolism and excretion. Increased volume of distribution and prolonged half-life means older people take longer to recover from the effects (Shi & Klotz, 2011). General anaesthetic agents are generally lipid soluble; older patients can take several days to recover from the confusion and disorientation.

The total body water declines by up to 15% between the ages of 20 and 80. The reduction in fluid causes some drugs, particularly water-soluble drugs such as digoxin, to be more concentrated, and signs of toxicity may be exhibited, particularly likely during long-term therapy when the concentration of drug has accumulated.

Older people have a lower serum albumin, the most abundant plasma protein. Only free drugs, not drugs bound to the plasma protein, are available to diffuse into the tissues. By reducing the plasma protein, the amount of free drug and therefore its affects are increased. This is particularly important for highly protein-bound drugs such as digoxin, theophylline, phenytoin and warfarin (Fig. 31.1).

Cardiac output is reduced by approximately 30% between the ages of 30 and 65. The biggest reductions are seen in the liver and kidneys. These changes reduce the speed at which drugs are etabolized and excreted.

The overall effects in changes in distribution may necessitate the use of lower doses, particularly for drugs that are lipophilic (i.e., attracted to and dissolve in lipids) or highly protein bound.

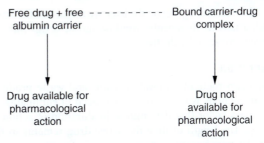

Fig. 31.1 Plasma carriage of pharmacologically active substances.

Metabolism

Drugs are treated by the body as foreign substances. In order to be rendered harmless and excreted, most drugs are converted into more water-soluble compounds. Most of the metabolism takes place in the liver by a process of oxidation or hydrolysis (phase 1) and conjugation (phase 2) using cytochrome P450 enzymes. In fact, drugs absorbed from the gastrointestinal tract pass through the liver before entering the systemic circulation, known as the first-pass effect (Fig. 31.2).

As we age, the liver reduces in size and has a decreased hepatic blood flow and impaired enzyme activity and hence metabolism. This is more important for drugs with a narrow therapeutic window (i.e., a small difference in dose between a therapeutic and toxic effect).

Drugs that are largely extracted by the liver display some age-related decrease in systemic clearance, but for most drugs with a mixed extraction profile (i.e., kidneys and liver), clearance is not reduced with advancing age. In general, activities of cytochrome P450 enzymes are preserved in normal ageing, and the genetic influence on drug metabolism is much more striking than age effects (Shi & Klotz, 2011).

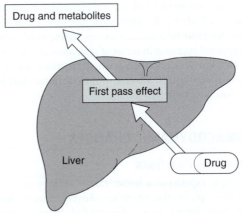

Fig. 31.2 First-pass effect in drug metabolism.

The effects of ageing on the liver are important for drugs with a narrow therapeutic window and/or drugs that are largely extracted by the liver.

Excretion

The main route of removal of toxins and waste products from the body is the kidneys. The speed of elimination is the main factor that determines the duration of action of drugs. The length of time the active drug remains in the circulation is known as the plasma half-life.

The most important effect of age is reduced renal clearance due to reduced renal function, blood flow and tubular function. Many older people excrete drugs slowly and are highly susceptible to nephrotoxic drugs. In addition to age-related reduction, acute illness can lead to rapid reduction in renal clearance, especially if accompanied by dehydration. A person stabilised on a drug with a narrow margin between the therapeutic and toxic doses (e.g., digoxin) can rapidly develop accumulation and adverse effects in the aftermath of a myocardial infarction or a respiratory-tract infection.

Shi and Klotz (2011) found one-third of older adults showed no decrease in renal function (GFR > 70 mL/min/1.73 m^2). In the other two-thirds, the age-related decline of renal function was associated with coexisting cardiovascular diseases and other risk factors.

Creatine is the consistent waste product from normal muscle tissue breakdown. It is almost completely filtered in the kidney and excreted in the urine. By knowing how much creatine is being cleared (i.e., creatine clearance), we know how well the kidneys are functioning. An alternative method of measuring renal function is by using estimated glomerular filtration rate (eGFR). However, eGFR is based on standard body surface area mean weight of 70 kg, but older people have a low body mass index. When measuring renal function in older people, it is therefore better to use creatine clearance.

Drugs can also be metabolised and excreted through bile, skin, lungs or body fluids. When renal function is impaired, these become more relevant, as does any decline in efficiency.

The general overview in terms of pharmacokinetics is to start with a low dose and then gradually increase the dose, balancing effects against adverse drugs reactions: start low and go slow (see Table 31.1).

PHARMACODYNAMIC CHANGES

Adverse Drug Reactions

Older people experience a higher rate of adverse effects to drugs than people in other age groups. Adverse drug reactions fall into three broad classes: dose-related, hypersensitivity and idiosyncratic. Dose-related adverse drug reactions may be due to exceeding the dose or pharmacokinetic changes.

Hypersensitivity adverse drug reactions are due to genetic or immunological abnormalities. These factors do not change with age, but as we get older we take more drugs, so we are more likely to come across a drug we are hypersensitive to. Idiosyncratic adverse drug reactions are due to a combination of generic, disease and age-related causes, and again the chance of being prescribed a particular drug increases with age.

Up to 11% of unplanned hospital admissions are attributed to harm from medicines, and more than 70% of these are due to older patients taking multiple medicines (NHS Scotland, 2018).

Drugs commonly associated with increased adverse drug reactions include antimicrobials, non-steroidal anti-inflammatory drugs (NSAIDs), diuretics, warfarin, angiotensin-converting-enzyme inhibitors/angiotensin receptor blockers, antidepressants, insulin and drugs with a narrow therapeutic drug range such as digoxin and lithium.

Organ Sensitivity

There is evidence some systems become increasingly sensitive to certain drugs as individuals age (Fixen, 2019). For example, the brain, and therefore older people, can experience excessive drowsiness, hangover effects and confusion with hypnotics.

In addition to the changes in organ sensitivity, older people have impairment in some of their homeostatic mechanisms, such as temperature regulation, static reflexes and postural instability, blood pressure regulation, bladder function, blood sugar levels and thirst sensation, leading to fluid and electrolyte balance. This impairment may lead to increased susceptibility to adverse drug reactions such as urinary incontinence, urine retention, confusional states, hypothermia and postural hypotension (for a summary see Table 31.1).

FALLS IN OLDER PEOPLE

Falls and fall-related injuries are a common and serious problem for older people. People above the age of 65 have the highest risk of falling, with 30% of people older than 65 and 50% of people older than 80 falling at least once a year. Falling has an impact on quality of life, health and health care costs (National Institute for Health and Care Excellence, 2013). See Chapter 18 for more information about falls.

The risk of falling is multifactorial; one of these risk factors is medications. Taking multiple medicines and the use of specific medicines can increase the risk of falls, such as drugs that can cause postural hypotension, such as antihypertensive drugs, and psychoactive drugs. Benzodiazepines are sedative, may cause reduced sensorium and impair balance; hypnotic Z-drugs such as zopiclone, zolpidem and zaleplon may cause protracted daytime sedation or ataxia. Antipsychotic drugs

TABLE 31.1	**Problem Drugs for Older People**		
Medications	**Pharmacodynamic**	**Pharmacokinetic**	**Recommendations**
NSAIDs	Increased risks from bleeding, more likely to be fatal; risk exacerbation of hypertension, heart failure, renal impairment	Increased risk of cardiac disease or renal impairment	Avoid if possible; use non-drug options such as weight reduction (if obese), warmth, exercise and use of a walking stick; paracetamol or low-dose NSAID plus proton pump inhibitor
Diuretics	Homeostatic upsets; particularly susceptible to side effects, including electrolyte disturbances	Slower elimination	Avoid long term for simple gravitational oedema; instead use increased movement, raising the legs and support stockings; titrate dose to effect
Warfarin	Increased sensitivity; bleeding more likely to be serious		May need a reduced dose
Benzodiazepines	Increased central nervous system sensitivity; impaired balance; increased risk of falls and confusion	Increased volume of distribution and half-life; increased sedation	Avoid or reduce dose (half)
Hypnotics		Slight decrease in hepatic metabolism; longer half-life; increased drowsiness; unsteady gait; slurred speech; confusion	Use non-pharmacological options; short courses of hypnotics with short half-lives; reduce doses
Beta1 and Beta2 receptor	Responsiveness decreased		Titrate salbutamol and terbutaline to response
Opioid analgesics	Increased central nervous system sensitivity and constipation		Reduce dose
Antipsychotics	Increased sensitivity to Parkinsonism, lethargy, hypotension, accidental hypothermia, falls; some have anticholinergic effects		Avoid or reduce dose
Tricyclic antidepressants	Increased risk of worsening cardiac conductive abnormalities and anticholinergic effects*		
Anti-Parkinsonian drugs	Increased sensitivity to anticholinergic effects*		Avoid or reduce dose
Digoxin	Narrow therapeutic index; increased risk of toxicity	Lower lean body mass	Reduce dose; check digoxin levels and monitor potassium levels
First-generation antihistamines	Risk of sedation and anticholinergic effects*		Avoid

*Anticholinergic effects include dry mouth, blurred vison, glaucoma, constipation, urinary retention, reduced cognition (confusion) and falls.

Note: See medicines.org.uk for full details.

may cause hypotension, gait dyspraxia or Parkinsonism, and sedative antidepressants causes sedation. When reviewing medications, consider that another risk factor for falls is having clinical depression (NHS Scotland, 2018).

COGNITION

Cognition includes the mental processes of memory, language, attention, executive functioning and visuospatial processing we use to help us acquire and understand knowledge.

Cognition declines naturally with age. When this decline is more than expected and interferes with normal functioning, it is known as dementia (see Chapter 29). Any cognitive decline could contribute to unintentional non-adherence with medication (see below). Several prognostic factors have been associated with dementia, including medical conditions such as diabetes and hypertension and medications with a high anticholinergic burden (NHS Scotland, 2018).

Some medications exert their effects through anticholinergic activity, such as oxybutynin, but for others, such as amitriptyline, the anticholinergic activity is an adverse effect. It is the total anticholinergic burden score that is important. This is made up of the sum of the individual medications.

Anticholinergic activity does not only cause confusion but can also lead to agitation, urinary retention, constipation, glaucoma and falls, which are all potential problems for older people (Quinn et al., 2020).

POLYPHARMACY

Polypharmacy is the use of many medications together, often more than four or five medications, or a medicine not matching a diagnosis (see Fig. 31.3). Hyperpolypharmacy is the use of 10 or more regular medications. The term is often used negatively, but it is important to note sometimes it is necessary for treatment of a single condition—for example, in the secondary prevention of myocardial infarction or if a patient has more than one condition.

Ageing is associated with a progressive decline in the functional reserve of multiple organs and systems. Older adults are therefore more likely to have multimorbidities and take more medications (Shi & Klotz, 2011). Common comorbidities include hypertension, diabetes, coronary artery disease and cardiovascular disease (Fillenbaum et al., 2000).

Polypharmacy increases an individual's risk of harm and contributes to hospital admissions and poor therapeutic outcomes (Kongkaew et al., 2013; Pirohamed et al., 2004). In fact, a person who takes 10 or more medications is 300% more likely to be admitted to hospital (Payne et al., 2014).

Common causes of problematic polypharmacy include therapeutic enthusiasm, the medication is not indicated or is no longer needed because the condition has subsided,

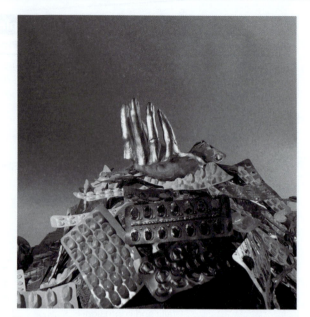

Fig. 31.3 Polypharmacy. (Picture courtesy of Rebecca Henry.)

the medication is being prescribed for adverse drugs reactions where there are alternative solutions, sub-therapeutic medications are prescribed, and/or there is poor communication on transfer of care (see below).

Polypharmacy is associated with increased risks of adverse drug reactions, drug–drug interactions and drug–disease interactions, leading to increased mortality and morbidity.

MEDICATION REVIEWS

With medication, less is sometimes better. All medication prescribing and deprescribing should be person-centred and will change over time. There are various tools to assist in this process.

The Medication Appropriateness Index (Hanlon & Schmader, 2013) includes 10 items to determine the appropriateness of a given medication: indication, effectiveness, correct dosage, practical direction, drug–drug interactions, drug–disease interactions, duplication, acceptable duration and expense. A higher total score indicates the medication is more inappropriate.

NHS Scotland (2018) suggest a seven-step approach.
1. Aim: What matters to the person?
2. Need: Identify essential drug therapy.
3. Need: Does the person take unnecessary drug therapy?
4. Effectiveness: Are therapeutic objectives being achieved?
5. Safety: Is the person at risk of or do they have adverse drug reactions?
6. Efficacy: Is drug therapy cost-effective?

7. Person-centred: Is the person willing and able to take drug therapy as intended?

Beers criteria (2019) lists drugs and drug classes to avoid, drugs and drug classes to avoid in certain diseases or syndromes, drugs to be used with caution, drug–drug interactions that should be avoided and dosage reduced in people with kidney disease (Fixen, 2019).

The Screening Tool of Older Persons' potentially inappropriate Prescriptions(STOPP)/Screening Tool to Alert to Right Treatment (START) criteria (2015) outline each of the body systems and which drugs or drug classes might be inappropriate and which medications should be considered in older people with specific conditions. It is considered to be more usable in clinical practice (O'Mahony et al., 2015).

Many acute hospitals and community services adapt the above criteria to produce more user-friendly tools. See Case Studies 31.1 and 31.2 for how these medication assessment tools can be used.

ADHERENCE TO MEDICATION

In addition to understanding the pharmacology of medicines, it's important to be aware of the issue of adherence and the evidence base nurses can draw on to promote it.

Adherence is the term used to describe a person's medicine-taking behaviour. How closely do people take

---

CASE STUDY 31.1

Doris is an 89-year-old who has been admitted to a medical ward with recent-onset increasing confusion. Her medications are as follows: amitriptyline 10 mg at night to help her sleep; oxybutynin 5 mg three times a day for urinary incontinence; codeine 60 mg three times a day, which she started last year when she broke her ankle and is still on her repeat prescription; and senna two tablets every night.

The doctor is ordering some tests to rule out physical causes. You have been asked to look into the medications.

Using NHS Scotland's polypharmacy tool (https://managemeds.scot.nhs.uk), table 3B page 37, what recommendations could you make about Doris's medications?

Answers
- Amitriptyline has a high cholinergic burden, which might be adding to her confusion. Consider non-pharmacological methods.
- Oxybutynin has a high cholinergic burden, which might be adding to her confusion. Consider changing to mirabegron.
- Codeine has a high cholinergic burden, which might be adding to her confusion. Review if any pain relief is needed. If so, try paracetamol.
- Senna may not be needed if she stops the codeine.

CASE STUDY 31.2

Derek is a 94-year-old man who fell at home and banged his head. On further discussion he confides he has been falling a lot recently but hasn't said anything as he did not want to be a burden to anyone. He knows how busy everyone is looking after sick people. He is taking the following medications: enalapril 20 mg once a day for hypertension, which he has been on for years; quetiapine 25 mg to help him sleep, which was started in the past couple of weeks; and warfarin as prophylaxis against a pulmonary embolism.

The doctor is ordering some tests to rule out physical causes. You have been asked to look into the medications.

Refer to the STOPP/START tool on the CGA Toolkit website (https://www.cgakit.com/m-2-stopp-start). What medication could be implicated?

Answers
- Enalapril can cause falls. Although he has been on it for years, as you get older, the dose needs to be monitored and adjusted.
- Quetiapine can cause falls. Suggest he tries non-pharmacological treatments.
- Warfarin should not be stopped because of falls, but the bleeding risks need to be considered. Give Derek instructions on what to do if he falls and cuts himself.

---

medicines according to how they were prescribed? The National Institute for Health and Care Excellence (NICE, 2009) defines medication adherence as the extent to which a person's action in medicine-taking matches agreed recommendations. These recommendations are usually outlined in the person's prescription and include details such as the dosage, number of times a day the medicine should be taken and any special administration instructions. The recommendations should also be based on an agreement between the patient and prescriber (see below). In the past, adherence was referred to as compliance with medicine-taking, but this term has connotations of professionals making unilateral decisions about what is in the best interest of an older person, with the person being in a passive role and only expected to obey instructions on medicine-taking. It is therefore no longer a preferred term to refer to patients' medicine-taking behaviours. Medicine management needs to actively involve the person mutually agreeing a treatment regime and to support the older person's self-monitoring of medication and symptoms; the latter is a key element of successful disease self-management (The Evidence Centre for National Voices, 2014).

Perhaps surprisingly, people often do not take their medicines according to agreed recommendations. The World

Health Organization (2003) estimated that up to 50% of people living with long-term conditions do not take their medicines as prescribed. As mentioned, people are increasingly living to an older age, often with one or more long-term conditions, and therefore the number of medicines they are taking is likely to increase. Although taking a number of different medicines may be helpful and clinically appropriate, problematic polypharmacy heightens the risks of non-adherence to agreed recommendations as the complexity of a regime, drug interactions and adverse effects are likely to increase (The King's Fund, 2013).

Unintentional Non-Adherence

Non-adherence can be divided into unintentional and intentional types. Unintentional non-adherence occurs when a person wants to follow the agreed treatment but is prevented from doing so by barriers beyond their control (National Institute for Health and Care Excellence, 2009). Unintentional non-adherence to medicine may be an issue for older people in particular; for example, cognitive decline may lead to memory problems with medicines being forgotten, or information about the importance of medicines may be less well understood. Or people may experience challenges balancing the complexity of instructions for taking several medicines—for example, carbamazepine bd with food for trigeminal neuralgia plus flucloxacillin qds 1 hour before food (for 7 days). In addition, physical problems such as arthritis or poor eyesight can make handling medicine containers and the information on them more difficult. Some interventions that address unintentional non-adherence are as follows.

Labelling

Since 1984 it has been a requirement of the British Pharmaceutical Society that all containers for medication are marked with large, typed labels so all members of the public, including older people, can read them. Instructions must be explicit. The label should contain clear details for administration and purpose of the medication. 'Two tablets to be taken four times a day if necessary for pain' is acceptable. Vague general instructions such as 'Take as directed' are not acceptable.

Memory Aids

Remembering when to take medicine can be difficult for everyone, old and young. The problem is increased in proportion to the number of medicines to be taken and the different regimens of administration. In a hospital environment, patients should be encouraged to be involved in medication management before discharge (Bucknall et al., 2019). Simple measures such as linking medicine-taking to events in a daily routine (e.g., getting up, mealtimes) may be

effective. Electronic means of reminding older people about taking medicines using smartphones, including texts and timed alarms, are also helpful. Voice-activated technology devices such as Alexa or Amazon echo can be programmed to remind people to take medications, attend important appointments, have a cup of tea or stand up every hour. Another memory aid is to give an older person a treatment card with an image or description of medicines and an easily comprehended outline of what each is intended for (e.g., 'water' tablet, pain tablet, breathing tablet). For individuals with greater difficulties, it may be necessary to make use of dose boxes such as the dosette box. Community pharmacies have check lists to assess who will benefit from a dosette box and who they will therefore fill one for. These are compartmentalised boxes or collections of tablet containers that are pre-filled with a supply of medicines, usually weekly. Each dose is placed in the appropriately timed compartment (e.g., 'morning'), and the person can check the medicine has been taken by seeing that the compartment is empty. This method may require the help of a relative, neighbour, friend or health professional to prime the box if the older person is unable to do so. Dosette boxes are not a universal solution for all medicine-taking; for example, some medicines should not be removed from foil packaging as it interferes with their pharmacological stability. The use of aids needs to be tailored and monitored for the individual.

Another resource for an older person who finds it difficult to remember medicine-taking is for someone else to help administer them. Relatives often begin to help when they observe signs of cognitive and physical impairment in an older adult. In people with dementia, family carers are an essential element of coping with medicines, performing tasks such as reminders and ordering, obtaining, storing and opening medicine (Lim & Sharmeen, 2018). Manias et al. (2019) pointed out activities often undertaken by relatives include assistance with administration, monitoring therapeutic and adverse effects, and clarifying information.

Aids for People With Physical Disabilities

Most medications are packaged in foil strips in boxes, but some are still supplied in bottles with child-proof lids. There are some instances where older people have difficulty opening child-proof drug containers or pushing medicine through the foil. Difficulties can be experienced by older adults with physical disabilities such as arthritis, which results in stiff, swollen finger joints and loss of manual dexterity. Pill popper gadgets are available, or tablets can be dispensed in conventional containers with non–child-proof lids or winged caps; these are very helpful for stiff hands. Small tablets may be difficult to handle; wide-necked bottles or tablet dispensers help with this problem. Pharmacists can be requested to provide a specific type of medication container.

Poor sight can be compensated for with large print or identifiable symbols to help an older person recognise the container. Different-coloured lids are available for easy identification. Braille labels are also available, although not all blind people read braille. Talking labels can be obtained, where a message is recorded and attached to the tablet boxes. Dose boxes can be helpful in this situation as an older person can feel which compartments are empty. For liquid medication, a measure marked clearly to the level of the exact dose or fixed-volume syringe is useful. These can be bought inexpensively from pharmacy stores. Special eyedrop dispensers and inhalers are also available. A range of aids are possible, and practical help can be provided by a community or hospital pharmacist. This is an indication of the need for multidisciplinary collaboration between different health professionals.

Whatever the method, it should be tried out with an older person to determine whether it is appropriate. Once an older person has started on a scheme of medication, their ability to cope should be monitored; as the person gets older, they may begin to need more help. For example, a nurse who can give an injection in a now-inaccessible site may be welcomed by an older person with diabetes. Assessment at repeated intervals is important.

Intentional Non-Adherence

Intentional non-adherence is a deliberate decision. It is not necessarily age-related—except perhaps because polypharmacy is more common with older age. This may increase the burden associated with medicine-taking or the unwanted effects of medicines on quality of life. For example, a person may omit their diuretic to avoid the risk of incontinence or the need to use a toilet urgently if they are going out for the day. In turn, this increases the likelihood of intentional non-adherence.

Over the past few decades there has been a considerable amount of research investigating the most effective ways of helping people take their medicines according to recommendations. Systematic reviews have brought together a body of research to answer this question. Nieuwlaat et al.'s (2014) Cochrane review of adherence interventions and Vermeire et al.'s (2005) Cochrane review of research into adherence in type 2 diabetes reached a similar conclusion: no single intervention has been shown to be effective in promoting adherence. They concluded current interventions for adherence in long-term conditions are complex or multifactorial and not very effective, according to the research available to date. Vermeire et al. (2005) found nurse-led interventions, home aids, diabetes education, pharmacy-led interventions, adaptation of dosage and frequency of medication-taking all showed a small effect on a variety of outcomes, including HbA1C, and therefore have

some limited evidence to support their use in practice. This highlights some of the methods nurses might consider using to help older people take medicines—for example, offering information (see Box 31.1) and education on medicine and prescribing appropriate dosages and formulations where required. It is also clear medicine management with older adults is undoubtedly a multidisciplinary team activity, where liaison with a person's prescriber and a community or hospital pharmacist is likely to be required to ensure prescriptions are tailored to their needs.

Many of the studies in these systematic reviews were conducted when compliance was the goal. More recently, there has been a shift in thinking to more actively acknowledge and discuss patients' views on medicines when making decisions about treatment regimes. In the early 2000s, the term *concordance* was introduced to capture the need to involve patients as partners in medicine discussions. As Bond et al. (2012) point out, this was at the forefront of a larger philosophical shift recognising the need for shared decision-making across a range of issues in health care. It was also linked to a body of evidence from psychology that patients' beliefs about medicine are an important predictor of whether they will take them as recommended. More specifically, the evidence suggests that what patients believe about the necessity of medicine in general and a particular medicine they are prescribed is weighed against their concerns about medicine in general and concerns about a specific medicine (Horne et al., 2013). The importance of exploring patients' beliefs and offering information about

---

BOX 31.1 Information Essential for Older People Receiving Prescribed Medication

- Name of the drug
- Strength
- Appearance (e.g., pink pills, red capsules, etc.)
- Purpose
- Dose
- Frequency with which it must be taken
- Storage (e.g., safety, how to dispose of unused medication if discontinued)
- Importance of expiry dates
- Common side effects that do not generally require further action
- Common adverse reactions and early signs they are occurring
- Common interactions and the need to mention existing medication when seeing a health professional
- Avoidance of OTC prescriptions when relevant
- Special instructions, perhaps maybe related to the route of administration or foods to avoid

medicine is reflected in the NICE guidance (National Institute for Health and Care Excellence, 2009) on adherence. The NICE, 2009 outlines that we should 'Be aware that patients' concerns about medicines, and whether they believe they need them, affect how and whether they take their prescribed medicines' (p. 7).

Communicating in partnership is important because nurses need to understand an older person's experience of taking medicines. For example, Campling et al. (2017) highlighted the work that is involved in self-managing medicine near the end of life, including ordering, obtaining, storing, scheduling and remembering to take it. Nurses need to understand the burdens that medicine-taking place on older people and consider ways of prescribing and medicine management that lighten the burden through, for example, altering dose frequencies or prescribing a liquid formula instead of tablets where swallowing is difficult.

Older people may adjust medicines, trading side effects with effectiveness, or alter their drug-taking to fit with their own priorities, such as fulfilling family and social obligations (Townsend et al., 2003). Nurses need to understand this from an older person's point of view, give information about alternative treatment options and consequences where possible or consider deprescribing, especially where polypharmacy is an issue. Deprescribing, especially for older frail people, may be important to reduce medicine burden, review whether any medicines are no longer necessary and/or deprescribe any that are causing potentially dangerous side effects or drug–drug interactions—for example, multiple analgesics, multiple anticoagulants or medicines that, when taken together, increase the risk of cumulative anticholinergic side effects (Polypharmacy Prescribing Comparators NHS England, 2021). The King's Fund (2013) suggested in the case of polypharmacy, best clinical practice might be to advise on the most effective interventions, then respect the person's preferences, realising a compromise might be required, as 'polypharmacy is likely to be futile if medicines are not taken as the prescriber intends' (p. 2).

There is evidence to suggest communicating in partnership works to improve adherence. Cox et al. (2003) concluded from their review of medicine-taking communication between patients and health care professionals that communication, such as encouraging patient participation and listening attentively to patients' views and concerns, may lead to improved outcomes, including enhanced adherence and satisfaction.

The Medicines Partnership (2003) outlines three essential components of concordance:

- *Patients have enough knowledge to participate as partners*: Offer patients information about medicines that is tailored to individual needs.

- *Prescribing consultations involve patients as partners*: Patients are invited to talk openly about their priorities, preferences and concerns about medicine-taking and treatment. They jointly agree on a course of treatment that reconciles as far as possible the professional's recommendations and the patient's preferences.
- *Patients are supported in taking their medicines*: All opportunities are taken to discuss medicine issues. Health professionals share medicine information effectively with one another, medications are reviewed regularly and practical difficulties in taking medicines are addressed.

MEDICINE MANAGEMENT AND SAFEGUARDING

Medicines have potential to harm as well as serve therapeutic purposes. The WHO (2017) recognises the global burden medicine-related harm can exert; in 2017 it launched its commitment to reducing the level of severe, avoidable harm related to medications by 50% globally over 5 years.

The NICE (2014) outlined that safeguarding issues in relation to managing medicines include

- Deliberate withholding of a medicine without a valid reason
- Incorrect use of medicine for reasons other than the benefit of a person
- Deliberate attempt to harm through use of a medicine
- Accidental harm caused by incorrect administration or a medication error

Although the NICE's guidelines refer to care homes, these potential hazards can also occur in other settings in which nurses regularly have responsibilities for safeguarding older people from medicine-related harms. In hospital it is the nurse's responsibility to ensure drugs are administered as prescribed and that the patient actually receives the drug. Omissions are possible if, for example, the drug was not available when required or because the patient was not present at a time when it was offered. In other cases, administration may be difficult because the older patient has difficulty swallowing tablets, or injections may be difficult to administer into loose folds of skin. Bruising frequently occurs with older patients. Such difficulties should be discussed with the pharmacist so that where possible, other routes of administration can be used on a temporary or permanent basis. It is not advisable to crush tablets without first checking with the pharmacist as it may interfere with the action of the drug. For example, the delayed action of slow-release preparations is lost if they are crushed, and enteric-coated medication might be destroyed in stomach acid.

The WHO (2017) also pointed out people are at increased risk during transitions of care; transitions increase the possibility of serious medication errors, which are often caused by communication errors. Older people may be transitioning between their own home and hospital and vice versa or between a care home and hospital; at these times prescribing responsibilities shift between, for example, a person's GP and a hospital specialist team, and furthermore new medicines may be added or others changed. Despite the risks associated with transition, there is evidence to suggest the older person's and carer's experience needs to be improved. Knight et al. (2013) found patients and families experienced inadequate explanations about medicine at discharge, leading to omission of medicine and incorrect dosages as well as anxiety and confusion. Manias et al.'s (2019) systematic review of family involvement in older people's medication at transitions of care found that although they were involved in information receiving and giving, and were provided support for medicine management at this time, health professionals did not acknowledge their role, and families had to persevere to have their voices heard. Communication about medication plans was haphazard and disorganised and not tailored to the person's needs. Nurses need to recognise care transitions are part of their safeguarding responsibilities. They need oversight of medication changes and omissions, to actively elicit and listen to the older person's and family's views, to provide information to them about medicine and to liaise with medical and pharmacy teams to reduce communication and medication errors.

ERRORS AND NEAR MISSES

The WHO (2017) acknowledges that medication errors are an inevitable part of health care, but efforts must be made to reduce them as far as possible. It is widely acknowledged that both human and system factors contribute to errors, which can occur at any stage of the medication process, including prescribing, dispensing, supply or administration, but they are particularly likely during the process of administration. The Care Quality Commission (2021) recommends a consideration of fatigue, staffing levels and environmental conditions. A recent systematic review (Manias et al., 2020) suggested increasing moves to IT-supported systems of medication management processes may reduce errors; more specifically, the review highlighted that medication administration errors were reduced by computerised (i.e., electronic) prescribing and the use of automated drug distribution systems as single interventions. Furthermore, combined interventions that included automated drug distribution and use of the electronic medical record, or prescriber education and pharmacist-led medication reconciliation, were found to be effective in reducing administration errors. Manias et al. (2020) recommended further research examining the effect of computerised medication reconciliation and electronic, computerised prescribing to confirm whether this combination is effective in reducing both prescribing and administration errors.

Near misses, or patient safety incidents, are defined by NHS England (2021) as any unintended or unexpected incident that could have or did lead to harm for patients. NHS England also pointed out that reporting incidents supports the NHS to learn from mistakes and to take action to keep patients safe. In England incidents can be reported on the National Learning and Reporting System, a central database set up to enable learning and analysis of incidents, including hazards, risks and opportunities.

OVER-THE-COUNTER MEDICATION

Selecting and purchasing medicines for your own use has an important role in self-care and maintaining independence. Traditionally the treatment of common ailments such as colds, coughs, headaches, constipation and mild aches and pains, together with first aid in the home, have rested with the individual, including the purchase of over-the-counter (OTC) medicines. Choice of drugs may be traditional, influenced by advertising or by advice from neighbours and friends. The range of products available is enormous. OTC medication can be obtained from community pharmacies where the advice of a pharmacist is readily available and from supermarkets where no information is forthcoming apart from the instructions included with the packaging. Controls placed by the Medicines Act 1968 relate to the number and strength of tablets on sale through different outlets. The sale of large quantities of most OTC drugs is permitted only when a pharmacist is present. This is important, as many OTC drugs, including the large number of 'cold cures' sold every day, contain aspirin, paracetamol, antihistamines and alcohol; it is not always obvious exactly what they contain, and all these may interact with prescribed drugs.

Problems Associated With OTC Medication

The potential for problems is enormous. The public may not consider patent medicines to be drugs or realise they can cause problems with prescribed medication. The chief dangers to accrue from frequent, uninformed use of OTC drugs include overdose, drug interactions, masking symptoms and abuse.

Overdose may result from patients doubling up on drugs already issued on prescription. For example, a patient might take a cold cure that contains aspirin in addition to soluble aspirin prescribed for rheumatic pain. This could result in frank overdose symptoms such as tinnitus or accentuated side effects such as gastrointestinal bleeding.

Interactions with prescribed medication can result if a person is not advised of the possibility they may occur. Cold cures may interact with drugs that belong to the monoamine oxidase inhibitor group. Aspirin and anticoagulants may interact.

Masking symptoms can be a problem; symptoms of illness in older adults often present in a vague, atypical manner. Pain that might be diagnostic of myocardial infarction in younger people is often mild or absent in older people. Thus the taking or giving of analgesia for mild pain or discomfort could rob the clinician of a useful diagnostic indicator.

The possibility of addiction to some OTC medicines, such as those that contain codeine, is also increasingly recognised.

DRUGS AND SOCIAL USES

Alcohol, tobacco, tea, coffee and herbs contain pharmacologically active ingredients with known actions on the body. Alcohol, caffeine and nicotine have addictive properties as well as social effects on behaviour and personality. In excess they can cause physical and mental damage. For example, caffeine is useful in treating apnoea of prematurity in neonates to reduce seizure thresholds in individuals receiving electroconvulsive therapy or for caffeine withdrawal migraines. However, in excessive doses, caffeine can cause anxiety, confusion, delirium, hallucinations, insomnia, palpitations and even arrythmias and seizures.

Some people think alcohol is a good sedative. In sufficient amounts, varying with the build, tolerance and other factors related to the make-up of an individual, it certainly induces sleep, but alcohol depresses rapid eye movement sleep, and many people wake up later in the night with rebound insomnia. The diuretic action of alcohol is also likely to disturb them. Many accidents among older people, especially those with frailty, are related to the use of alcohol or to sedatives, especially benzodiazepines, which should be prescribed with caution.

Herbalism has increased in popularity as an alternative to conventional medicine in recent years. For the most part it is considered safe, but the tests used on these preparations and the arrangements for quality control are less stringent than for conventional drugs, although many contain pharmacologically active ingredients. Herbs reputed to act on the heart (e.g., adonis, false hellebore, yellow foxglove) contain cardiac glycosides and therefore potentiate the effect of prescribed drugs such as digoxin. St. John's wort is another popular treatment that has numerous interactions, including with apixaban, antidepressants, combined hormonal contraceptives and warfarin. Glucosamine, an OTC supplement for joint pain, interacts with and potentiates the anticoagulant action of warfarin.

NURSE PRESCRIBING

In the United Kingdom over 35,000 nurses who have completed a post-registration prescribing training programme are able to independently prescribe, within their competence, any medicine from the formulary. Latter et al. (2012) established that nurse prescribers in the United Kingdom were prescribing clinically appropriately, and Tinelli et al. (2015) demonstrated nurse prescribing was acceptable to patients. Since then, systematic reviews (Gielen et al., 2014; Kroezen et al., 2011) have further established the effectiveness of nurse prescribing internationally, demonstrating that patient clinical outcomes are at least equivalent to prescribing by doctors.

Nurses may prescribe for older people living in their own homes, in GP settings or in hospital in-patient or outpatient contexts. Equipped with knowledge of pharmacology and the principles of discussing adherence described above, nurse prescribers have an important opportunity to discuss medicine with older adults and agree treatment regimes. In primary care they may work as part of a team, including GP practice–based pharmacist prescribers, to review older adults' medicines, including deprescribing some medicines when problematic polypharmacy and/or medicines burden is high. Naughton and Hayes (2017) pointed out that as deprescribing is part of the normal drug-prescribing pathway, nurse prescribers have a responsibility to see it as much a part of their role as prescribing, actively reviewing the risks and benefits of medicines using evidence-based tools.

As part of a community team, nurses who can prescribe for older people in their homes have an important role in offering rapid, direct access to medicine to prevent hospitalisation. As people approach end of life, research has found palliative care clinical nurse specialists play an important role in helping patients and carers access the medicine they need. Latter et al.'s (2020) survey of nurse specialists in England found two-thirds were prescribing two or three times a week, with the majority of health professionals reporting that nurse prescribers had a beneficial impact on patients' access to palliative care medicine.

TAKING DRUG HISTORIES

A drug history should be completed with older adults, taking time to record and discuss all that is relevant and providing time for questions and explanations. Tobiano et al.'s (2019) systematic review of patient engagement in admission and discharge medication communication in hospitals found patients view these activities as being concerned with two-way accurate information sharing. The review also found strategies to inform and empower patients include involving them in the assessment and encouraging them to communicate their understanding of medication. Tobiano et al. (2019) concluded person-centred communication is key to the success of patient engagement in medication communication.

Checklists are often used to ensure nothing is overlooked in taking a drug history. However, a checklist is of value only if its role as an aide-mémoire is kept in mind; it is of limited value if it is simply used to tick off items, then discarded in an effort to complete the task mechanically. A checklist is part of an assessment about a person's medications; that assessment then requires careful interpretation, planning and action. Frequently older adults tire or need time to recall all relevant details, so history-taking requires more than one session. It may be beneficial to defer some aspects until a family carer visits if they have been responsible for medication or need to be involved in future. As Manias et al. (2019) concluded from their systematic review of family involvement in older adults' medication at points of transition, greater efforts are needed to strengthen family involvement, including at admission and discharge consultations. Bearing these points in mind, the following checklists may be helpful for the nurse beginning to participate in assessment for older adults.

CHECKLIST TO RECORD A DRUG HISTORY ON ADMISSION TO HOSPITAL OR FOR A COMMUNITY CASELOAD

1. Information about prescribed drugs, including topical treatments, inhalers and injections: In hospital settings, medical staff may also obtain this information and record it in the medical case notes. When the nursing assessment is undertaken, the information should be obtained directly from the patient or a family carer and compared with the medical history. It should not be duplicated from one source to another because the purpose of the nursing history is to check and, when necessary, supplement information already given. Many patients are too ill when first admitted to hospital to tell the doctor everything, or they may feel overwhelmed.
2. Information about the drug-taking routine: This should include the times each drug is taken and the relationship between these times and other daily activities (e.g., sleep, meals). This may reveal unexpected problems that, with ingenuity, could be resolved. Thyroxine or diuretic drugs given too late in the day may lead to difficulty sleeping, and a small alteration in routine may obviate the need for night sedation. A change in the routine of taking drugs either before or after meals may alter the pattern of absorption and response. Discussion of the routine may additionally give an opportunity to assess and discuss adherence and highlight possible problems that may arise after discharge.
3. Information about OTC medication, including herbal and other substances: As pointed out earlier, mention of these drugs is frequently forgotten. Discussion should centre on medicine used routinely and occasionally and habits of use. This information may provide clues to symptoms such as diarrhoea when aperients are overused and may ensure abnormal readings are not obtained in tests. Some surprising incidents have been recorded; for example, throat lozenges that contain iodine have made the thyroid test of a hypothyroid patient appear to fall within the normal range.
4. Use of other substances, including, for example, dietary supplements or alcohol: Taking a drug history may be a good opportunity to discuss behaviour changes that will have a positive effect on health and well-being, as recommended in Making Every Contact Count (Health Education England, 2021).

MONITORING MEDICINE-TAKING

Here the nurse is in an ideal position to monitor the patient's progress, report response to treatment and discuss medicine-taking as many times as necessary, answering questions as they arise and negotiating an ongoing agreed regime if appropriate. Patients can be observed for problems that may arise on discharge (e.g., due to compromised vision or memory), and solutions can be sought and tested during a hospital stay or time on the community nursing caseload.

CHECKLIST TO RECORD A DRUG HISTORY ON DISCHARGE FROM HOSPITAL OR FOR A COMMUNITY CASELOAD

Preparation for a smooth transition to an ongoing home routine includes the following:
1. Ensuring the older person and family, if appropriate, has been given full verbal and written information about their medication and had an opportunity to discuss and agree a treatment regime
2. In hospital, ensuring appropriate medications are available to be given to the older person in good time before departure

3. Ensuring the older person or family knows where to obtain repeat prescriptions and the procedure this entails
4. Liaison with health professionals in the community such as the district nurse, GP and pharmacist as necessary

VALUE FOR MONEY AND SAFETY

Over the past 50 years, the development of modern medication has made a major contribution to reducing the burden of ill health in the population, especially among older people, who take more medicines per head than younger people. This has had major implications for organisations that provide health care, which have witnessed an enormous increase in the cost of medication. In England, the NICE stipulates criteria for establishing the value of new treatments and helping health service providers decide which products should be used routinely in clinical practice. As health care professionals, nurses should appreciate the role of organisations such as the NICE. Pressures on costs need to be viewed as part of the overall package of patient care. It has been suggested, for example, that for some conditions expenditure ought to be increasing because it is a cost-effective and therefore desirable way of increasing health gain for the population.

Biosimilars are a recent development in medicine manufacturing that have significant potential to reduce health care costs. Biosimilars are medicines that are highly similar to another biological medicine already licensed for use; they can be produced when the original exclusive patent for a biologic medicine expires. Biological medicines, prescribed for example for inflammatory bowel diseases, are among the most expensive drugs, so the expected growth in biosimilars over the coming years will offer significant potential for cost reduction. Nurses have a role in explaining the meaning and purpose of biosimilars to patients when and if they are asked to make a switch.

On the other hand, if people do not take their medicine as agreed, which may especially be the case where there is polypharmacy in older people, it can lead to medicine waste. Medicines are prescribed and dispensed, and represcribed, but not taken. This further highlights the value of discussing and agreeing a medication regime with an older person that is likely to lead to the best possible adherence. As mentioned, nurses may be involved in considerations of deprescribing as prescribers or members of the multidisciplinary team. Avery and Bell (2019), however, caution against deprescribing as primarily a cost-saving exercise: reviewing the evidence, they suggested given the complexity of the task, cost savings are likely to be modest. But from a shared decision-making and ethical point of view,

'deprescribing remains a worthwhile investment…and should be done in partnership with the patient and families who cope every day with burdensome polypharmacy' (p. 1570).

In addition, in any consideration of value for money, safety and medicines, nurses should be mindful of their role in antimicrobial stewardship. Inappropriate and overuse of antimicrobials is a major safety threat to health worldwide as well as being economically wasteful. Nurses can contribute to stewardship in a number of different ways. The Royal College of Nursing (2014) summarise them as
- Reducing demand for antimicrobial treatment—for example, through encouraging healthy living and public and patient expectations about antibiotic prescribing
- Enhancing the effectiveness of prescribed antimicrobials—for example, dispensing antibiotics at the right time in order to maintain therapeutic levels
- Providing specialist infection prevention advice—for example, to ensure guidance documents and standards are implemented
- Collaborating and acting internationally—for example, raising awareness and involvement by nurses and nursing bodies across Europe to support European Antibiotic Awareness Day and other affiliated promotions

According to the British Geriatrics Society (2018), infectious diseases account for a significant proportion of hospital admissions and deaths in older people. Infections include influenza and pneumonia, so we prioritise older people for vaccinations accordingly. However, older people have less of an immunological response to vaccines than younger people, and there is conflicting evidence on the outcomes. Randomised controlled trials show limited benefit, but cohort studies highlight that vaccinated older people have reduced hospital admissions and total mortality. Studies have shown age-related changes in the lungs and muscles have led to increased mortality rates with COVID-19, possibly due to reduction of lung reserves, airway clearance and defence barriers (Sanyaolu et al., 2020). Older people are therefore prioritised for COVID-19 vaccinations.

CONCLUSION AND LEARNING POINTS

Successfully managing medicine to treat symptoms is often a critical part of ageing well. This chapter outlines physical, psychological and social changes that occur with older age that may influence medicine management. These changes create needs that challenge nurses to respond as part of their role in nursing older people. Helping older adults manage medicine is enacted across a range of contexts, including community, primary care, secondary care and nursing homes.

KEY LEARNING POINTS

- Older people have more complex needs, with atypical presentations and coexisting functional, psychological and social needs.
- Start medications low, go slow and monitor.
- Simplify medication regimes whenever possible.
- It is important to review medication regularly for indications, interactions, adverse reactions and adherence and to consider dose reduction.

- Nurses can draw on an evidence base to promote adherence, including the importance of shared decision making and communicating in partnership.
- Medication patient safety issues include safeguarding, near misses and errors.
- Nurses have an important role in medicine management for older people, including taking drug histories, prescribing, monitoring medication-taking and promoting value for money.

REFERENCES

Avery, A. J., & Bell, B. G. (2019). Rationalising medications through deprescribing. *British Medical Journal, 364*, 1570.

Bond, C., Blenkinsopp, A., & Raynor, D. K. (2012). Prescribing and partnership with patients. *British Journal of Clinical Pharmacology, 74*, 581–588.

British Geriatric Society. (2018). Improving healthcare for older people. Vaccination programmes in older people. https://www.bgs.org.uk/resources/vaccination-programmes-in-older-people.

Bucknall, T., Digby, R., Fossum, M., Hutchinson, A. M., Considine, J., Dunning, T., Hughes, L., Weir-Phyland, J., & Manias, E. (2019). Exploring patient preferences for involvement in medication management in hospitals. *Journal of Advanced Nursing, 75*(10), 2189–2199.

Campling, N., Richardson, A., Mulvey, M., Bennett, M. I., Johnston, B., & Latter, S. (2017). Self-management support at the end of life: Patients', carers' and professionals' perspectives on managing medicines. *International Journal of Nursing Studies, 76*, 45–54. https://doi.org/10.1016/j.ijnurstu.2017.08.019.

Care Quality Commission. (2021). https://www.cqc.org.uk/guidance-providers/adult-social-care/reporting-medicine-related-incidents.

Cox, K., Stevenson, F., Britten, N., & Dundar, Y. (2003). *A systematic review of communication between patients and healthcare professionals about medicine-taking and prescribing.* Guy's. King's and St Thomas' Concordance Unit London.

Fillenbaum, G. G., Pieper, C. F., Cohen, H. J., Cornoni-Huntley, J. C., & Guralnik, J. M. (2000). Comorbidity of five chronic health conditions in elderly community residents: Determinants and impact on mortality. *Journal of Gerontology A: Biological Sciences and Medical Sciences, 55A*(2), 84–89.

Fixen, D. R. (2019). 2019 AGS Beers criteria for older adults. *Pharmacy Today, 25*(11), 42–54.

Gielen, S. C., Dekker, J., Francke, A. L., Mistiaen, P., & Kroezen, M. (2014). The effects of nurse prescribing: A systematic review. *International Journal of Nursing Studies, 51*, 1048–1061.

Hanlon, J. T, & Schmader, K. E. (2013). The Medication Appropriateness Index at 20: Where it started, where it has been, and where it may be going. *Drugs Aging, 30*(11), 893–900.

Health Education England. (2021). https://www.makingeverycontactcount.co.uk.

Horne, R., Chapman, S. C. E., Parham, R., Freemantle, N., Forbes, A., & Cooper, V. (2013). Understanding patients' adherence-related beliefs about medicines prescribed for long-term conditions: A meta-analytic review of the necessity-concerns framework. *PLoS One, 8*(12), e86033. https://doi.org/10.1371/journal.pone.0080633.

Knight, D., Thompson, D., Mathie, E., & Dickinson, A. (2013). 'Seamless care? Just a list would have helped!' Older people and their carer's experiences of support with medication on discharge home from hospital. *Health Expectations, 16*(3), 277–291. https://doi.org/10.1111/j.1369-7625.2011.00714.

Kongkaew, C., Hann, M., Mandal, J., Williams, S. D., Metcalf, D., Noyce, P. R., & Ashcroft, D. M. (2013). Risk factors for hospital admissions associated with adverse drug events. *Pharmacotherapy, 33*(8), 827–837.

Kroezen, M., van Dijk, L., Groenewegen, P. P., & Francke, A. (2011). Nurse prescribing of medicines in Western European and Anglo-Saxon countries: A systematic review of the literature. *BMC Health Services Research, 11*, 127. https://doi.org/10.1186/1472-6963-11-127.

Latter, S., Campling, N., Birtwistle, J., Richardson, A., Bennett, M. I., Ewings, S., & Santer, M. (2020). Supporting patient access to medicines in community palliative care: On-line survey of health professionals' practice, perceived effectiveness and influencing factors. *BMC Palliative Care, 19*, 148. https://doi.org/10.1186/s12904-020-00649-3.

Latter, S., Smith, A., Blenkinsopp, A., Nicholls, P., Little, P., & Chapman, S. (2012). Are nurse and pharmacist independent prescribers making clinically appropriate prescribing decisions? An analysis of consultations using the Medication Appropriateness Index. *Journal of Health Services Research and Policy, 17*, 149–156.

Lim, R. H., & Sharmeen, T. (2018). Medicines management issues in dementia and coping strategies used by people with living with dementia and family carers: A systematic review. *International Journal of Geriatric Psychiatry, 33*(12), 1562–1581.

Manias, E., Bucknall, T., Hughes, C., Jorm, C., & Woodward-Kron, R. (2019). Family involvement in managing medications of older patients across transitions of care: A systematic review. *BMC Geriatrics, 19*, 95. https://doi.org/10.1186/s12877-019-1102-6.

Manias, E., Kusljic, S., & Wu, A. (2020). Interventions to reduce medication errors in adult medical and surgical settings: A systematic review Therapeutic Advances in *Drug Safety, 11*, 1–29. https://doi.org/10.1177/2042098620968309.

Medicines Partnership. (2003). *Project Evaluation Toolkit*. Medicines Partnership.

National Institute for Health and Care Excellence. (2009). *Medicines adherence: Involving patients in decisions about prescribed medicines and supporting adherence Clinical Guideline (CG76)*. NICE.

National Institute for Health and Care Excellence. (2013). *Falls in older people: Assessing risk and prevention. Clinical guideline (CG161)*. NICE.

National Institute for Health and Care Excellence. (2014). Managing Medicines in Care Homes. Social Care Guideline (SC1). NICE.

Naughton, C., & Hayes, N. (2017). Deprescribing in older adults: A new concept for nurses in administering medicines and as prescribers of medicine. *European Journal of Hospital Pharmacy, 24*, 47–50.

NHS BSA Polypharmacy Prescribing Comparators NHS England. (2021). https://www.england.nhs.uk/patient-safety/report-patient-safety-incident/.

NHS England. (2021). https://www.england.nhs.uk/patient-safety/report-patient-safety-incident/.

NHS Scotland. (2018). *Scottish Government Polypharmacy Model of Care Group. Polypharmacy Guidance, Realistic Prescribing* (3rd Edition). Scottish Government. https://managemeds.scot.nhs.uk/.

Nieuwlaat, R., Wilczynski, N., Navarro, T., Hobson, N., Jeffery, R., Keepanasseril, A., Agoritsas, T., Mistry, N., Iorio, A., Jack, S., Sivaramalingam, B., Iserman, E., Mustafa, R. A., Jedraszewski, D., Cotoi, C., & Haynes, R. B. (2014). Interventions for enhancing medication adherence. *Cochrane Database of Systematic Reviews, 2014*(11), CD000011.

O'Mahony, D., Sullivan, D. O., Byrne, S., Connor, M. N. O., Ryan, C., & Gallagher, P. (2015). STOPP/START criteria for potentially inappropriate prescribing in older people: Version 2. *Age Ageing, 44*(2), 213–218.

Payne, R. A., Abel, G. A., Avery, A. J., Mercer, S. W., & Roland, M. O. (2014). Is polypharmacy always hazardous? A retrospective cohort analysis using linked electronic health records from primary and secondary care. *British Journal of Clinical Pharmacology, 77*, 1072–1082.

Pirohamed, M, James, S, Meakin, S, Green, C, Scott, AK, Walley, TJ, Farrar, K, Park, K, & Breckenridge, AM (2004). Adverse drug reactions as a cause of admissions to hospital: prospective analysis of 18,820 patients. *British Medical Journal, 329*, 15–19.

Quinn, T. J., Myint, P. K., McCleery, J., Taylor-Rowan, M., & Stewart, C. (2020). Anticholinergic burden (prognostic factor) for prediction of dementia or cognitive decline in older adults with no known cognitive syndrome. *Cochrane Database of Systematic Reviews, 2020*(2), CD013540.

Royal College of Nursing. (2014). Antimicrobial resistance: RCN position on the nursing contribution. Royal College of Nursing.

Sanyaolu, A., Okorie, C., Marinkovic, A., Patidar, R., Younis, K., Desai, P., Hosein, Z., Padda, I., Mangat, J., & Altaf, M. (2020). Comorbidity and its impact on patients with COVID-19. *SN Comprehensive Clinical Medicine, 2*, 1069–1076.

Shi, S., & Klotz, U. (2011). Age-related changes in pharmacokinetics. *Current Drug Metabolism, 12*(7), 601–610. https://doi.org/10.2174/138920011796504527.

The Evidence Centre for National Voices. (2014). *Supporting self-management: Summarising evidence from systematic reviews*. The Evidence Centre for National Voices.

The King's Fund. (2013). *Polypharmacy and medicines optimisation*. The King's Fund.

Tinelli, M., Blenkinsopp, A., Latter, S., Smith, A., & Chapman, S. (2015). Survey of patients' experiences of care for long term conditions provided by nurse and pharmacist independent prescribers in primary care. *Health Expectations, 18*(5), 1241–1255.

Tobiano, G., Chaboyer, W., Teasdale, T., Raleigh, R., & Manias, E. (2019). Patient engagement in admission and discharge medication communication: A systematic mixed studies review. *International Journal of Nursing Studies, 95*, 87–102.

Townsend, A., Hunt, K., & Wyke, S. (2003). Managing multiple morbidity in midlife: A qualitative study of attitudes to drug use. *British Medical Journal, 327*, 837–840.

Vermeire, E., Wens, J., Van Royen, P., Biot, Y., Hearnshaw, H., & Lindenmeyer, A. (2005). Interventions for improving adherence to treatment recommendations in people with type 2 diabetes mellitus. *Cochrane Database of Systematic Reviews, 2005*(2), CD003638.

World Health Organisation. (2017). Medication without harm: Global patient safety challenge on medication. https://apps.who.int/iris/bitstream/handle/10665/255263/WHO-HIS-SDS-2017.6-eng.pdf?sequence=1.

World Health Organization. (2003). *Adherence to long term therapies: Evidence for action*. World Health Organization.

Alcohol Misuse and Ageing

Margaret Orange

This chapter starts with a general overview of the developing role of alcohol in society, focusing specifically on older people. Prevalence, harm and the role of the nurse in developing evidence-based strategies to identify, screen and offer appropriate, individualised advice are subsequently outlined. The latter includes seeking the support of specialist services where indicated.

There is a growing evidence base and number of clinical guidelines on alcohol use, misuse and appropriate interventions (National Institute for Health and Care Excellence [NICE], 2010; 2011; Royal College of Psychiatrists, 2018), and emerging trends shed light on the complications and harms of excessive alcohol use in older adults (Phillips et al., 2020; Royal College of Psychiatrists, 2011; Wilson et al., 2013). The evidence demonstrates why now more than ever, nurses who care for older people are likely to encounter alcohol misuse and its associated problems in their everyday practice.

Alcohol has a well-established role within British culture, where its use is associated with pleasurable events related to socialising and celebrating. However, it is also associated with stress management and escape from pressure (Ling et al., 2012). Over recent decades, the drinking culture in the United Kingdom has gradually moved from social and more visible drinking environments such as pubs and clubs to the home environment. Here, drinking alcohol is often more discreet; the person drinking may find it harder to keep track of the amount consumed, and daily drinking can become the norm.

HISTORY AND POLICY CONTEXT

There is a general belief that the post-war generation was brought up surrounded by alcohol advertising, with drinking being 'normal' and socially acceptable, and non-drinking being the exception (Rao & Roche, 2017). Beliefs developed at this time are still held by many older people, leading to a problem drinking culture in this age group (Drugscope, 2014). This is only now becoming apparent and is likely to persist for the next two decades as the current cohort of older people live through their old age. These attitudes to drinking were formed when advertising focused on the social benefits of alcohol and there was less understanding of alcohol-related harm. Consequently, changing attitudes toward drinking in this age group is difficult, possibly more so than in other age groups, and measures to reduce harm may rely significantly on policy and legislative changes.

It has been highlighted that alcohol is becoming an increasing problem for the over 50 age group, with pensionable age adults accounting for 20% of hospital admissions due to alcohol, a rise of 50% in just 5 years (Office for National Statistics [ONS], 2018; Royal College of Psychiatrists, 2018). Public health leads have placed an emphasis on prevention and treatment, but, because price has an impact on how much people, particularly heavy drinkers, consume, there has also been an ongoing campaign for the control of alcohol through legislative changes to sales. This led to the campaign for a minimum unit price (MUP), recognising the role of cheap alcohol in the rise in alcohol-related harm.

With the evidence that the price of the cheapest alcohol was affecting the health of the heaviest drinkers, laws came into force in Scotland in May 2018 to enforce an MUP of 50 pence per unit. There is good reason to believe this measure of controlling the price of the cheapest alcohol is having some impact on the heaviest drinkers. *Monitoring and Evaluating Scotland's Alcohol Strategy* (Giles & Richardson, 2020) provided the latest data on alcohol consumption and measures related to an MUP, which showed a small decrease in the amount of alcohol sold per adult in Scotland since the MUP was introduced. Although NHS Health Scotland highlights this is the lowest-ever recorded level of consumption and the smallest gap in consumption recorded between Scotland, England and Wales, the changes are small. The MUP may need time to fully embed before meaningful comparisons can be made and its impact known. With no United Kingdom–wide approach in place, Wales saw the introduction of a 50 pence MUP in March 2020, and attempts continue to introduce an MUP in Ireland. In England, an MUP has not been agreed and remains an area for governmental debate.

Older individuals are now the age group at highest risk of alcohol misuse (ONS, 2017). However, there is a clear opinion that older people with substance misuse issues are a marginalised group, whose needs are not well served from a policy perspective (Royal College of Psychiatrists, 2011). There is criticism of the trend in public policy to focus almost solely on younger drinkers, and the ability of government to reduce alcohol-related harm in older people is likely to be hampered by a limited acknowledgement of the problem. However, with alcohol and drugs more recently being seen among the top 10 risk factors for mortality and morbidity in Europe, substance misuse in older people is becoming more visible. The public health burden of alcohol is a growing public health concern that is attracting policy attention (Burton et al., 2016). Drugscope (2014) highlighted the paucity of references to or mentions of older people in national substance misuse policy but did acknowledge public-health–focused guidance and policy

was starting to recognise issues such as alcohol-related hospital admissions and mortality in the older age group. This recently became evident in public health policy discussion (Commission on Alcohol Harm, 2020).

Many older people formed their attitude about drinking when alcohol was less understood and more widely available and acceptable. At that time people in middle age drank more in quantity and more frequently than the current generation of people in middle age. Fat et al. (2020) suggested there can be a cumulative impact of drinking on physical health, with drinking habits adopted in earlier life having long-term effects and accelerating the onset of some long-term conditions in old age. In their study, individuals with a history of hazardous (i.e., increasing risk) drinking at any point in their lifespan were more likely to have a range of predetermined physical health biomarkers, particularly cardio metabolic risk factors. Thus, not only are older people drinking more now, but there is also evidence to suggest they have already increased their risk due to drinking habits adopted earlier in the life course.

PREVALENCE

An increase in harms caused by alcohol use globally is well documented. It is cited as a leading risk factor in all-cause mortality and morbidity and places significant burden on health services globally (Phillips et al., 2020; Wilson et al., 2013).

Royal College of Psychiatrists (2018) evidenced the changing trend in older people's drinking habits, highlighting that adults over 55 are the only age group where increasing numbers of people are exceeding recommended limits. There was a 22% increase in people over 65 who exceed the government's recommended drinking levels (ONS, 2017).

Alcohol use disorders in older people are common and associated with considerable morbidity. The ageing of populations worldwide means the absolute number of older people with alcohol-use disorders is on the increase (Rao & Roche, 2017). Wadd et al. (2011, p. 3) suggested the United Kingdom may be on the verge of an 'epidemic of alcohol-related harm amongst older people', with an estimated 1.4 million people in this cohort thought to be exceeding government recommended alcohol limits. Alcohol consumption, hospital-related admissions and deaths are increasing among the older population and have become a concern for public health (Wilson et al., 2013). Adults over 65 form a significant proportion of individuals admitted to hospital, a figure that has doubled in the past 10 years.

The prevalence of alcohol use disorders in older people is generally accepted to be lower than in younger people, but rates may be underestimated because of underdetection and misdiagnosis (Butt et al., 2020; O'Connell et al., 2003).

The reasons for this are many and varied and explored later in the chapter.

It is suggested older drinkers may not be aware of the risks associated with their level of alcohol consumption (Bareham et al., 2019). The older population and many professionals are unaware of the previously mentioned impact of lifetime hazardous drinking on the normal ageing process (Fat et al., 2020).

DEFINITIONS

Recommended Drinking Guidelines

The recommended drinking guidelines for alcohol consumption (United Kingdom) were updated from the guidelines issued in 1995, to new guidance released by the chief medical officer (Department of Health, 2016). Although there is no intention to judge individuals or prevent people from drinking alcohol, the underlying objective of the current guidance is to support people in understanding the risks that alcohol may pose to their health, so they can make informed choices about their own use.

The current guidance (see Figure 32.1) states that to ensure the health risks from alcohol are reduced, no more than 14 units of alcohol should be consumed in a week, and these units should be spread evenly over 3 or 4 days, advocating several alcohol-free days each week. In changing the terminology used in the guidance from 'safe' to 'low risk', the chief medical officer made it clear there are no safe limits, and alcohol always has the potential to cause harm.

Although the chief medical officer's guidance addresses all-age adults and some specific areas of concern such as pregnancy, it is really important to recognise it does not address the specific issue of the ageing process and any increased risk in relation to ageing and alcohol intake.

Figure 32.2 illustrates the terminology used in these reviewed guidelines; the previously used terminology of *sensible*, *hazardous* and *harmful* has been replaced by *low risk*, *increasing risk* and *high risk*.

The new terminology reflects the fact that alcohol use should always be viewed in relation to risk. Even at low levels, it may pose some risk for some people. This terminology scale does not include individuals who are drinking to dependent levels, which sit above high risk.

There has been clear concern raised over a long period of time that due to the physiological changes associated with the ageing process, adult guidelines for alcohol consumption may not be suitable for older people, with the suggestion that even with relatively modest amounts of alcohol, older people are at an increased risk of adverse outcomes (Lang et al., 2007; Wadd et al., 2011). There has been support for some time that the adult recommendations should be reduced to one and a half units per day over 3 or 4 days, ultimately halving the current suggested limits (Dunne & Schipperheijn, 1989). More recently, caution has also been advised when applying drinking guidelines to older people due to their potential sensitivity to alcohol-related harm because of the ageing process, comorbid presentations and interactions with medications (Royal College of Psychiatrists 2018; Wilson et al., 2013).

- To keep health risks from alcohol to a low level, it is safest not to drink more than 14 units a week on a regular basis.

- If you regularly drink as much as 14 units per week, it is best to spread your drinking evenly over 3 or more days. If you have one or two heavy drinking episodes a week, you increase your risks of death from long-term illness and from accidents and injuries.

- The risk of developing a range of health problems (including cancers of the mouth, throat and breast) increases the more you drink on a regular basis.

- If you wish to cut down the amount you drink, a good way to achieve this is to have several drink-free days each week.

Note: This applies to adults who drink regularly or frequently (i.e., most weeks).

Fig. 32.1 Chief medical officer's guidelines for men and women. Source: Department of Health (2016).

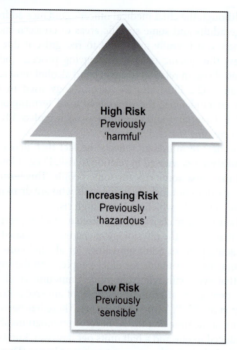

Fig. 32.2 Risk terminology. Source: Department of Health (2016).

However, the guidance acknowledges the low-risk drinking guidelines are based on average risks, and individuals can take account of other individual factors that could increase their personal risks from drinking. In consideration of this, the chief medical officer suggests (Department of Health, 2016) the following:

- Taking account of any previous negative effects experienced from alcohol
- Having an awareness of the possible interaction of alcohol and medications
- Understanding the relevant physical/mental health problems that alcohol may compound
- Considering other factors that could be relevant, such as low body weight or worries about falling

These factors should be considered by nurses when working with older people and are explored further throughout the chapter.

DRINKING HISTORY

Alcohol misuse, as described above, is often defined as drinking above the lower risk levels advised by the chief medical officer—in other words, adults who regularly exceed 14 units per week.

For the purpose of understanding care and treatment needs, distinctions can be drawn between when drinking began, which provides a useful starting point to define the problem and develop an understanding of need. Onset of drinking can be categorised in two ways:

- Early onset alcohol use: Alcohol that has persisted into older age from adulthood
- Late onset alcohol use: Alcohol use that began in older age

Drugscope (2014) discussed how estimations of use suggest that, of older people with alcohol problems, approximately two-thirds fall into the early onset category. This may imply alcohol use has been prevalent throughout adult life but has not previously been identified as an issue or addressed. Perhaps it has come to light more in old age due to the complications of coexisting physical or mental health problems.

The third of older people whose alcohol use is categorised as late onset may begin their relationship with alcohol because of changes in their physical or mental health or due to changes in their lifestyle associated with ageing. Social isolation, loneliness and loss in general have been cited as significant factors in the development of alcohol-related problems, but alcohol can also exacerbate and maintain these issues so they become a consequence of the alcohol use (Khan et al., 2006). However, late onset alcohol use does not always start due to negative reasons. Many older people are retiring younger and are more affluent than previous generations, with wide and varied social lives, where alcohol becomes a central focus or a social lubricant and has an important role in enhancing social engagement (Dare et al., 2014; Kelly et al., 2018).

Heavy or binge drinking among older people, whether early or late onset, is likely to be more widespread than dependant drinking. Coupled with a rise in life expectancy within this population, attention to older people and alcohol misuse is warranted in all health care environments (Johnson, 2000; O'Connell et al., 2003; Wilson et al., 2013).

EFFECTS OF ALCOHOL USE ON THE OLDER PERSON

It is well established, even before alcohol is considered, that due to the ageing process, older people are more likely than younger people to experience a range of chronic health problems alongside significant psychological and social changes. Moos et al. (2004) found that older people are more likely to receive medical management for the health problems caused by alcohol than for the alcohol-related health need itself. This could be due to the normalisation of drinking behaviour and the perception that any ill effects from alcohol are due to general health problems or deterioration (Wilson et al., 2013).

For this reason, it is crucial that health care practitioners understand that alcohol may play a part in every presentation.

A detailed account of the physical, mental and social or lifestyle factors associated with alcohol use is beyond the scope of this chapter, with excellent detailed texts already available, such as Royal College of Psychiatrists (2018). Wadd et al. (2011) also offers a comprehensive range of references on alcohol-related problems.

As the body's response to drugs changes with age, so too does its response to alcohol. Even with lower levels of alcohol, older people have an increased risk of its effects, which can be physical, psychological or social. Alongside this, the ageing process presents in a similar manner, and when both drinking and ageing occur simultaneously, these risks are exacerbated.

Table 32.1, adapted from Wadd et al. (2011), outlines some of the impacts of ageing and alcohol. There is a significant overlap, which makes the assessment and management of presentations particularly complex.

Alcohol is a central nervous system depressant. Its sedative effect impacts sleep pattern and tiredness, which in turn affects function and exacerbates problems already associated with the ageing process. As with other sedatives, gradual withdrawal of alcohol slowly improves functioning and physical symptoms such as sleep disturbance, leading to an observable improvement in symptoms. However, with sustained use, central nervous system depressants become less effective in achieving their desired result, leading to a need to increase the amount consumed in order to achieve the same effect. This can lead to alcohol dependence.

Understanding the effects of alcohol and its role in exacerbating changes in the ageing process, although well

TABLE 32.1 Impact of Ageing Process and Impact of Alcohol

	Impact of the Ageing Process	Impact of Alcohol
Physical	Reduced metabolism Chronic conditions Chronic pain Sleep problems High blood pressure, heart disease, stroke Incontinence Increased need for prescription hypnotics, anxiolytics and analgesics for a range of needs, including sleep, anxiety and pain	Prolonged effects of substances (e.g., alcohol) Alcohol dependency Liver problems Cancer, including liver, oesophagus High blood pressure, heart disease, stroke Stomach ulcers Gastrointestinal complaints Malnutrition, including poor absorption of nutrients and perceived decreased 'need' for food Pancreas problems Sleep problems Incontinence Interactions with medications
Psychological	Memory problems/cognitive impairment Dementia Depression Anxiety Loneliness Suicidality	Wernicke disease Korsakoff syndrome Central nervous system depressant, lowered mood Shame Embarrassment Suicidality
Social (life)	Life changes resulting in loss (e.g., bereavement, family changes, role changes, employment changes or retirement) Reduced social activities/social isolation Boredom, lack of purpose, lack of routine Financial strain Vulnerability to abuse Falls and accidents due to frailty or physical condition; requiring more assistance Homelessness	More likely to drink at home and exacerbate loneliness Loss of usual social networks and contacts More likely drinking will go unnoticed Falls and accidents when intoxicated Requires more assistance due to drinking More likely to rely on other people to support their needs Vulnerability to abuse

Source: Adapted from Wadd et al. (2011).

documented, is not necessarily well understood by non-specialists. Alongside this, as individuals age, the ability to treat alcohol-related problems becomes more difficult. This is reflected in the higher number of admissions to hospital in the older age group as treatment becomes more complex.

Increased risk drinking is common among older adults and may increase cardio metabolic risk factors. Population reductions in hazardous drinking are likely to result in improvements in liver function and blood pressure in older people and a reduced risk of stroke (Fat et al., 2020). Longer-lasting gains in health and well-being may accrue with earlier intervention in the life course, particularly in relation to weight gain. This supports a more preventative approach to alcohol by all services throughout the life course.

Wadd et al. (2013), having identified that between 50% and 80% of individuals with chronic alcohol problems experience cognitive impairment, discussed the significant degree of undiagnosed cognitive impairment in this group. In recognising that unlike many types of cognitive impairment that get worse with time, alcohol-related cognitive impairment can improve with a reduction in alcohol. The researchers called for better screening for cognitive impairment in alcohol services and equally for better screening for alcohol misuse in memory clinics. "Cognitive impairment can complicate the identification of alcohol problems and vice versa" (Wadd et al., 2013. p. 9).

It has been suggested that social isolation and loneliness contribute to all-cause mortality in older people (Perissinotto et al., 2012; Steptoe et al., 2013), and routine has been cited as an important factor in the well-being of individuals, particularly in relation to retirement, with a lack of routine being linked to mental health difficulties (Sewdas et al., 2017). Royal College of Psychiatrists (2018) recognised that social interaction is a key part of daily life, and not benefitting from such contact has been cited as putting individuals at higher risk of alcohol misuse. Therefore, social isolation may not only be an antecedent to alcohol problems but also one of the unintended consequences of problematic alcohol use. The increase in older people experiencing social isolation and loneliness during the COVID-19 pandemic is clearly documented (Hwang et al., 2020) and is of concern given the relationship highlighted with alcohol.

Older people are susceptible to frailty and falls, which can be intensified by alcohol use, as can incontinence, which may also then become an increasing risk for slips and falls. The relationship between the ageing process and alcohol use needs close attention.

Homelessness is rarely discussed as a risk in the older population, but there is emerging and concerning evidence that if undetected, alcohol misuse and subsequent social and behavioural issues can put an older person at risk of losing their accommodation (Giles, 2016).

TOWARD MORE EFFECTIVE MANAGEMENT OF ALCOHOL MISUSE IN OLDER PEOPLE

There is a need for better awareness and therefore education on alcohol misuse in the older population, not only in the general public but also among health professionals who deal with older people. Nurses in particular are in a prime position to recognise and intervene opportunistically when alcohol-related problems are developing in an older person.

Nurses have an important role in emphasising that, although alcohol may serve different purposes and have some perceived and actual benefits, the harms caused often compound the changes associated with the ageing process. The perceived benefits of alcohol can become more difficult to address if the older person does not understand the implications of alcohol for their current state. The older person also needs to have reassurance that support is available to overcome any perceived barriers to cutting down or stopping drinking in order to achieve a safer limit.

Role of the Nurse

The general or non-specialist nurse is unlikely to carry out a comprehensive addiction assessment of an older person and more likely to complete a general health questionnaire related to the purpose of the contact. However, alcohol questions should be included in the general assessment to ensure the potential role of alcohol in a person's presentation is always considered.

As the normal ageing process brings with it the significant and varying changes already highlighted (Table 32.1), alcohol use/misuse may be difficult to distinguish from problems associated with ageing. There is a need for professional curiosity and, given the prevalence, a degree of suspicion regarding alcohol in any general assessment. Crome et al. (2011) suggested that a high degree of clinical suspicion of addiction should be central to the assessment of non-specific or inconsistent clinical presentations, and this should trigger the implementation of formal screening for alcohol.

Identification and Brief Advice

It could be perceived, based on media coverage and focus of public health campaigns, that alcohol use is generally less prevalent in the older population as opposed to younger age groups, but significant factors may influence this, including poor detection rates and even a reluctance from professionals to screen older people (Johnson, 2000). Some reluctance may be attitudinal on the part of the practitioner and can lead to alcohol problems in this age group being undetected (O'Connell et al., 2003). Wilson et al. (2013) highlighted the need for non-specialist preventative approaches to avoid the continued harmful consequences of excessive alcohol use in older people and suggested brief interventions as being an effective means. Acute services such as emergency

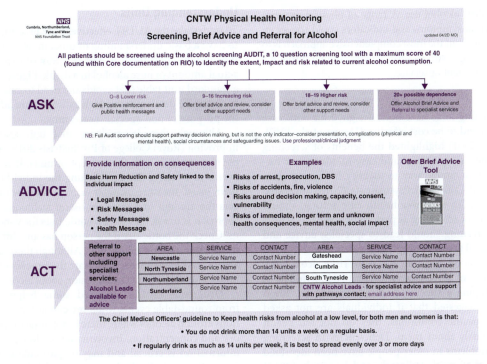

Fig. 32.3 Example screening, brief advice and referral for alcohol. Source: Cumbria, Northumberland, Tyne and Wear NHS Foundation Trust.

departments are well placed to pick up alcohol problems earlier in their development, when we know interventions are more likely to succeed (Hadida et al., 2001). This represents a significant opportunity to impact the prevalence discussed earlier in the chapter and reduce alcohol-related harm both in the older population now and for future generations.

Once there is established evidence of substance misuse in an individual, there is immense scope for the success of brief interventions across a variety of settings, including health settings such as accident and emergency departments, medical wards and outpatient departments. Such interventions include brief advice and providing information as well as an appraisal of motivation to alter substance misuse, all of which the non-specialist can deliver with some brief training or awareness raising.

Although the number of older people who are drinking at risky levels is concerning, individuals are not necessarily drinking to dependant levels, and most are not alcohol dependent. Therefore, the majority of people are not suitable for specialist addiction services but should be managed in universal settings. This means universal health care settings are an obvious place for the development of skills and competence in working with older people around alcohol use. It is of extreme importance that alcohol is considered on a patient group basis. Unless processes and protocols

are in place to ask everyone the same questions, the problem of identifying only individuals with significant issues is perpetuated, and the older person who is using alcohol in a risky way but not yet exhibiting visible signs or experiencing observable harms will continue to be missed.

For the purpose of illustration, the three-stage identification and brief advice approach of ask, advise, act is explained more fully. Figure 32.3 shows an example of this model in an NHS Trust—the Cumbria, Northumberland, Tyne and Wear NHS Foundation Trust. This approach is based on the fuller 5As model developed by Raw et al. (1998) in their work around smoking cessation. If this modified approach, estimated to take between 5 and 15 minutes, is adopted as a routine protocol with all service users in non-specialist settings, it offers comprehensive screening, brief advice and appropriate referral to specialist services.

STAGE 1: ASK (IDENTIFICATION AND SCREENING)

Identification

At the first stage of the process, there is an opportunity to identify service users who may be at risk and offer evidence-based screening of their alcohol use. A range of physical, psychological and social symptoms and indicators could trigger an alcohol screening, but the most comprehensive approach is to undertake this stage with all service users coming through a particular department or service.

Screening

Alcohol screening tools have been designed for both ease of application and to be cost effective (Derges et al., 2017). Hadida et al. (2001) highlighted the benefits of screening tools to be their simple, brief and easy-to-administer format, leading to a simple way to identify increasing alcohol risks. Royal College of Psychiatrists (2018) suggested all older people, in whatever health care setting, should receive an alcohol screening as part of their general assessment. This screening should lead to specialist advice and specialist referral where appropriate—essentially the provision of identification and brief advice for risky alcohol use.

The purpose of screening is to identify individuals at risk of developing a specific disease or condition. Blum et al. (1996) suggested that if individuals are not asked about these specific conditions, they do not tell health care professionals about them. Deficiencies in screening for alcohol problems in older people have been identified (Butt et al., 2020), with DiBartolo and Jarosinski (2017) suggesting that alcohol use disorder, although common, is underrecognised and undertreated in older adults. Within the addictions field, screening is the first stage in identification of individuals who exhibit increasing or high-risk alcohol use, with the offer of advice and education and also onward referral to specialist services where indicated (WHO, 2001).

There are many effective screening tools. For the purpose of illustration, the one recommended and endorsed by the NICE is shown in Figure 32.4, the Alcohol Use Disorders Identification Test (AUDIT) (NICE Clinical Guidance 115, 2011).

Screening tools such as the AUDIT, developed by the WHO, provide a simple method to identify risky drinking and a framework for intervention to help increasing risk (i.e., hazardous) and higher risk (i.e., harmful) drinkers reduce or cease their alcohol consumption. The AUDIT is now commonly used in a range of non-specialist settings.

The AUDIT is a single set of 10 questions, each with a score of 0–4, allowing a possible maximum score of 40. The AUDIT score gives an indication of the extent and impact of the alcohol problem, but health care staff can also develop the skills and competency to ask a range of individualised supplementary questions based on the personal information and context they are presented with. Possible supplementary questions are discussed later in the chapter.

Understanding Units

To undertake the AUDIT effectively, the practitioner needs to have a basic understanding of units in order to quantify the amount consumed. A unit is a way of expressing the actual amount of pure alcohol in a drink. Figure 32.5 shows a standard unit table that avoids the need to calculate units in any more detail. These rough estimates are adequate for the purpose of non-specialist screening.

Although there is evidence that unit knowledge is improving (Royal College of Psychiatrists 2018), older people may struggle with the concept of units. If so, there are means of working this out. Getting the individual to pour their 'usual' measure in water or to indicate with their fingers the amount in a glass are useful techniques. Another approach is to ask how long a bottle lasts for wine and spirits. Check the bottle size if the person has any difficulty with memory or understanding units. Although these approaches always lead to estimates, they start the process of assessing intake and begin an open discussion about alcohol.

Drugscope (2014) discussed some helpful feedback from round-table events when reviewing how to ask questions around alcohol where there is potential for poor memory and concentration. Involving family to obtain relevant information is crucial and may be particularly helpful in supporting an individual to complete drink diaries, which aid the development of a more comprehensive assessment. Alongside this, ensure questions are kept short and simple and recognise that the individual may find it difficult to engage in a lengthy discussion. Any support offered may need to be adapted to account for cognitive impairment, for example by using memory aids. It is important to remember cognitive impairment may complicate the diagnosis of alcohol problems, but alcohol use can also make the identification of age-related cognitive issues very difficult to detect. Both the long-term effect of alcohol misuse and advancing age can have a negative effect on cognitive functioning (Wadd et al., 2013), and nurses should be alert to possible underlying causes.

Scoring and Interpreting the AUDIT

The scores for each of the 10 questions should be totalled, with a final score out of 40. The score itself not only gives an indication of how to progress but also shows where the individual is in relation to their level of risk within the recommended drinking guidance (see Figure 32.6). This is often a good starting point to reflect on with the service user.

Once you have identified the level of risk, the score can be further interpreted to understand what level of intervention is required (see Figure 32.7).

Full AUDIT scoring can support pathway decision making in all settings but is not the only indicator. The nurse should consider presentation, complications (e.g., physical and mental

Alcohol unit reference

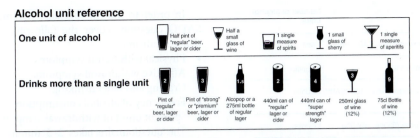

Questions	Scoring system					Your score
	0	1	2	3	4	
How often do you have a drink containing alcohol?	Never	Monthly or less	2 to 4 times per month	2 to 3 times per month	4 times or more per week	
How many units of alcohol do you drink on a typical day when you are drinking?	0 to 2	3 to 4	5 to 6	7 to 9	10 or more	
How often have you had 6 or more units if female, or 8 or more if male, on a single occasion in the last year?	Never	Less than monthly	Monthly	Weekly	Daily or almost daily	
How often during the last year have you found that you were not able to stop drinking once you had started?	Never	Less than monthly	Monthly	Weekly	Daily or almost daily	
How often during the last year have you failed to do what was normally expected from you because of your drinking?	Never	Less than monthly	Monthly	Weekly	Daily or almost daily	
How often during the last year have you needed an alcoholic drink in the morning to get yourself going after a heavy drinking session?	Never	Less than monthly	Monthly	Weekly	Daily or almost daily	
How often during the last year have you had a feeling of guilt or remorse after drinking?	Never	Less than monthly	Monthly	Weekly	Daily or almost daily	
How often during the last year have you been unable to remember what happened the night before because you had been drinking?	Never	Less than monthly	Monthly	Weekly	Daily or almost daily	
Have you or somebody else been injured as a result of your drinking?	No		Yes, but not in the last Year		Yes, during the last year	
Has a relative or friend, doctor or other health worker been concerned about your drinking or suggested that you cut down?	No		Yes, but not in the last year		Yes, during the last year	

Total AUDIT score

Scoring:
- 0 to 7 indicates low risk
- 8 to 15 indicates increasing risk
- 16 to 19 indicates higher risk,
- 20 or more indicates possible dependence

Fig. 32.4 AUDIT. Source: Aadapted from WHO 2001.

health), social circumstances and safeguarding issues. Ultimately, it is important that all professionals exercise their professional and clinical judgement on an individual basis.

Severity of Alcohol Dependence Questionnaire

The AUDIT tool is used to assess whether there is a problem with alcohol dependence, but it does not measure the severity of the alcohol problem if dependence is identified.

The severity of alcohol dependence questionnaire (SADQ) is a quick, reliable and valid instrument used to clarify the severity of dependence, most frequently in individuals who score 20 or more on the AUDIT. The SADQ was one of the first measures of alcohol dependence to be developed (Stockwell et al., 1979), based on the elements of alcohol dependence syndrome described by Edwards and Gross (1976). SADQ is a short, 20-item questionnaire,

Type of drink	Number of alcohol units
Single small shot of spirits* (25ml, ABV 40%)	1 unit
Alcopop (275ml, ABV 5.5%)	1.5 units
Small glass of red/white/rosé wine (125ml, ABV 12%)	1.5 units
Bottle of lager/beer/cider (330ml, ABV 5%)	1.7 units
Can of lager/beer/cider (440ml, ABV 5.5%)	2.4 units
Pint of lower-strength lager/beer/cider (ABV 3.6%)	2 units
Standard glass of red/white/rosé wine (175 ml, ABV 12%)	2.1 units
Pint of higher-strength lager/beer/cider (ABV 5.2%)	3 units
Large glass of red/white/rosé wine (250ml, 12%)	3 units

Fig. 32.5 Calculating units. Source: NHS (n.d.).

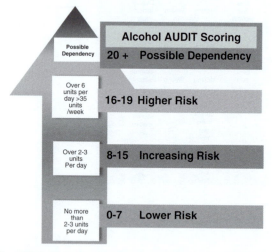

Fig. 32.6 Risk levels related to AUDIT scores. Source: Adapted from WHO (2001).

useful in informing the referral to specialist alcohol services and a treatment plan. Specialist alcohol treatment services generally repeat the AUDIT and SADQ, but availability of an initial score assists with prioritisation of the referral and therefore timely intervention for individuals in most need.

In order to inform specialist treatment decisions, the SADQ questions cover the following aspects of dependence syndrome:

- Physical withdrawal symptoms
- Affective withdrawal symptoms
- Craving and relief drinking
- Frequency of alcohol consumption
- Speed of onset of withdrawal symptoms

The questionnaire takes 2–5 minutes and can be self-administered. Scoring for each question is rated on a four-point scale ranging from zero for 'almost never' to three for 'nearly always', with a maximum score of 60 and a minimum of zero. A score of 31 or higher indicates severe alcohol dependence; 16–30 indicates moderate dependence, and below 16 indicates mild physical dependence. A medical detoxification regime is usually indicated for someone who scores 16 or higher on SADQ, and a score of 30 or higher often needs consideration of residential or in-patient detoxification.

It should be remembered that although universal services should develop the skills and competence to screen for risky alcohol use using a screening tool such as the AUDIT, at the point of identifying possible dependence, a referral should always be considered to specialist services, and specialist advice should be sought. Undertaking the SADQ is certainly not essential in non-specialist services, but developing skills in using these simple-to-administer tools significantly informs the assessment and subsequent referral.

STAGE 2: ADVISE (PREVENTION, EDUCATION AND HARM REDUCTION)

Although no further intervention is indicated for individuals who score less than 8 on the AUDIT, it is important the person is given positive feedback, which is a positive public health message in itself. It should be clarified that the score indicates current use is low risk, and positive reinforcement for maintaining recommended drinking limits should be given.

Brief interventions work by raising the issue, supporting people to recognise the problem and break a problem habit based on behavioural change. A number of approaches to behaviour change are possible, including the stages of change model (Prochaska & DiClemente, 1983), which described five phases, usually depicted in a cycle, that people go through in effecting habit-changing behaviour:

1. Pre-contemplation: Not considering change; may not have recognised the problem
2. Contemplation: Considering change but may not be fully committed or be ambivalent
3. Preparation: May be considering change and reflecting on what it means for them
4. Action: Starting to put some new behaviours into action

AUDIT score	Risk level	Non-specialist intervention
0–7	Lower risk	Clarification that current use is low risk Offer positive feedback for maintaining low-risk drinking levels
8–15	Increasing risk	Offer brief advice focusing on individual's presentation and risk and how to reduce it. Consider other support depending on individual presentation and needs.
16–19	Higher risk	Offer brief advice focusing on reducing risk (must be personalised) and consider other support depending on individual presentation. Consider referral to specialist services if there are complicating factors or comorbidity.
20 +	Possible dependence	Offer brief advice and referral to specialist services for assessment and diagnosis. If available, undertake SADQ to inform assessment for specialist services.

Fig. 32.7 Interpreting AUDIT scores. Source: Aadapted from WHO 2001.

5. Maintenance: Maintaining new behaviours and can self-manage; problem may not totally disappear

The model clearly recognises there can be a lapse at any point.

For individuals with drinking of increasing risk (i.e., AUDIT score of 8+), a brief intervention serves as a teachable moment to raise the issue around their drinking, offering the opportunity for recognition if pre-contemplative or reflection if there is already some awareness in the contemplation or preparation stages. Ultimately, brief interventions support the journey to the next stage of change for any individual and can be used in relation to any behaviour or habit. In this context, the teachable moment is a naturally occurring life transition or health event that motivates or activates individuals to spontaneously adopt risk-reducing health behaviours.

For individuals with higher risk and dependent drinking (i.e., AUDIT of 16+), a brief intervention provides an opportunity to clarify more specific harm reduction and provide advice with clear risk messages as well as discuss potential further intervention in relation to a specialist referral where indicated.

For individuals who score 20 or more, referral to specialist services is indicated due to possible alcohol dependence. Brief advice should still be offered as the therapeutic conversation about risks may be motivating and support the referral. If available and appropriate, a SADQ should also be completed.

Signposting individuals to specialist services is not recommended, as this is less successful in securing attendance and relies on further motivation to make contact independently at a later date. During an opportunistic brief intervention, if the individual understands the need to be seen by specialist services and agrees, it is a positive demonstration of motivation and should lead to a direct referral from the professional.

Within any brief advice, the practitioner should:

- Offer feedback on the assessment/screening undertaken in Stage 1
  - Discuss individualised score and what it means
- Raise concerns around the individual's drinking and its impact
  - Compare the individual's type of drinking and norms for this age group
- Identify some of the consequences of continued drinking specific to the individual
  - Physical, psychological, social (specific to ageing is also useful)
- Explore the benefits of cutting down or stopping drinking specific to the individual
  - Examples could include maintaining independence, feeling physically healthier, financial gains, cognitive improvements and improved family relationships
  - Explore the benefits vs. the risks (i.e., consequences) in order to make informed choices
- Advise how best to reach low-risk levels and strategies for cutting down
  - Opportunities that do not involve alcohol, such as social and recreational, and advice on lowering units can also be helpful

- Identify high-risk situations and coping strategies
  - Including boredom, loneliness, specific social contexts
- Provide written information (NHS has useful brief advice tools)
  - Include information for family and carers where appropriate for their own awareness and to reinforce messages

Some evidence suggests advice on the risks of alcohol use may be less meaningful and compete for an older person's attention more than in the younger population (Wilson et al., 2013), especially if the person already feels the benefits of using alcohol outweigh the risks. The long-term medical risks may seem distant or relatively unimportant given their age compared to the risk of losing the perceived benefits of socialisation and relaxation.

Messages delivered in the advice stage of the model must be personalised so they resonate and create cognitive dissonance, a situation where a disparity is highlighted between attitudes and behaviour. Examples include emphasising the impact of increasing alcohol intake on fall risk, quality of sleep and specific health conditions. Until individuals receive these personalised messages, they may remain in the pre-contemplative state of change, not recognising the impact of alcohol on other presenting situations. These personalised messages help the person move on. Brief advice is built on the premise of sowing seeds of doubt in an individual to prompt consideration of more informed choices and ultimately change. Customised information about safer or healthier ways of drinking is crucial. Advice may include how to reduce units. Evidence suggests older people are often poorly informed about the measurement of units.

For an individual who likes to have a couple of glasses of wine three or four times a week (which puts them in the increasing risk category), advice may be to have two single gin and tonics (or another spirit) as long drinks, which is an automatic reduction from six units in the wine to two units in the single measures and a reduction in risk level. Accurate measurement of units is important. Alcohol unit measures and marked glasses for measurement are widely available to support this approach.

Other advice includes the following:

- Switch to low-alcohol lagers.
- Drink soda with white wine to reduce the volume of wine (i.e., spritzer).
- Have a soft drink between alcoholic drinks.
- Make single units of spirits into long drinks that last longer.
- Always eat before drinking.
- Delay the time you start drinking.
- Tell people you are cutting down, so they don't tempt you to drink.
- Be prepared to say no to alcohol if it is offered to you (Case Study 32.1).

A WORD OF CAUTION

Although this middle phase of the model is termed the *advise* phase, the model is founded on the principles of motivational counselling techniques, which are clear that service users should be encouraged to make their own decisions. A practitioner who is advising rather than guiding is in danger of stimulating defensiveness, which can be counterproductive. An effective identification and brief advice is about not advising too much but encouraging individuals to identify the problems and any changes they

---

CASE STUDY 32.1

Ken, 74, recently presented to his GP, prompted by his family, with increasing forgetfulness. Ken talks with accuracy about his past, his time in the military and his wife, Liz, who passed away 2 years earlier following a short illness with cancer.

On taking a medical history, Ken was identified as having

- Two falls at home in the past 2 years, both needing hospital review
- Hypertension
- A myocardial infarction 5 years ago (stent in place)
- Treatment 10 years ago with low-dose mirtazapine for low mood and insomnia (stopped after 3 years; no further reports of low mood or insomnia on record)

It is of note that Ken rarely attends his primary care service except for medication review or organised follow-up such as flu vaccination.

Blood was taken to support any ongoing diagnosis and management. Ken says he is forgetful but puts it down to 'My wife used to do everything in the house'. He is dismissive of it being anything more than this. He says his mood is low, and it has been gradually deteriorating since the loss of his wife. Ken reports sleep disturbance, falling asleep easily but waking in the night. He puts this down to needing to use the toilet but wakes on several occasions.

He also reports an ongoing poor appetite and diet and again puts this down to the loss of his wife, as Liz did all

CASE STUDY 32.1—cont'd

the cooking. Getting used to doing this for himself has been difficult. He is not sure about weight loss but on asking reports his clothes are now loose.

On taking an alcohol history, Ken reports drinking two or three cans per night plus an 'occasional whisky' to help with sleep. He states he never gets any withdrawal symptoms. Ken reports going to the club with friends once weekly. He reports drinking more at these events and has occasionally tripped on the way home so is now getting a taxi home. Ken doesn't feel alcohol is a problem and says, 'I've been drinking all my life, but I am sensible'.

Although there were a number of other screening interventions related to the presenting problems of forgetfulness, potential low mood and physical health (including appetite/weight loss), a routine alcohol AUDIT was undertaken by the practice nurse, with a score of 13, suggesting increasing risk of alcohol-related harm. While continuing to investigate all other factors to support a clear formulation, the practice nurse was able to start a therapeutic conversation around alcohol following the ask, advise, act model.

ASK

The AUDIT score of 13 clearly identified increasing risk. The practice nurse was able to identify additional information by asking supplementary questions and discovered Ken has regularly drunk over the recommended limits on social occasions for many years, but this has significantly increased in the past 2 years since Liz died. He didn't drink every night before and is using alcohol to get to sleep but hasn't considered that his broken sleep is linked to the alcohol. He also rarely became intoxicated before, but in the last 2 years, he often feels intoxicated, particularly after a night at the club.

The practice nurse also identified the 'cans' are higher-strength alcohol by volume, with more units, and the 'occasional' whisky is actually most nights. Although it's one glass, it is a very large measure.

The practice nurse was able to ask Ken how he feels about it and to identify whether there was any motivation to change upon realising the risk.

ADVISE

When reflecting on the AUDIT score and supplementary questions, Ken became tearful, saying he knew he was

drinking more than usual but didn't think it was doing any harm.

The practice nurse asked if it was okay to talk to Ken about alcohol—how it might be affecting him currently and some ways of starting to deal with it. Ken was happy to have the discussion, which was specifically tailored to his current problems:

- Relationship between alcohol and accidents/falls
- Potential impact of alcohol on short-term memory and risks to cognitive functioning in the future
- Impact of alcohol on mood
- Impact of alcohol on nutrition and weight loss

While recognising the need to continue to fully investigate all presenting symptoms, the role of alcohol in the current presentation was highlighted, and possible solutions were discussed, including:

- The benefits of cutting down (and the risks of continuing to drink at these levels), essentially weighing up the pros and cons of current alcohol use
- Advice on how to reduce alcohol, ensuring Ken identified potential solutions while recognising any risk, and that Ken should not stop suddenly if there are any signs of dependence
- Identifying when he drinks most (i.e., high-risk situations) and exploring coping strategies

ACT

Because there was the facility to do so, the practice nurse agreed to see Ken again to review his progress. This allowed the opportunity to ensure there is clear action and no further deterioration.

The practice nurse also ensured the GP prescribed ongoing thiamine.

Ken was asked if he would like to take some reading materials so he could read about what was discussed, an alcohol brief intervention leaflet was provided.

Ken was also offered the opportunity to look at a range of support options, including local alcohol support groups and online support if preferable. Ken felt that a local support group might be helpful in getting him out of the house in an environment where there was no alcohol.

On reviewing him in the future, the practice nurse planned to review any changes and further action needed, including specialist referral for assessment from the clinical alcohol service if there were continued concerns.

wish to make themselves in order to move them through their own cycle of change. The question-and-response style used is important, and where possible, the individual should always be encouraged to identify the issues and suggest the solutions themselves. Some possible questions associated with different questioning styles are presented in Figure 32.8.

Style 1 is completely advisory and not encouraged with identification and brief advice; it should be avoided wherever possible. Style 2 is far more in line with the motivational interviewing style envisaged with identification and brief advice, where the individual is supported to find their own solutions and own their own change, and the professional can subsequently offer suggestions or information if needed as a conversation progresses.

Listening skills are very important. Allowing the individual to reflect on and explore their own ideas ensures their commitment and motivation to change. Questions such as "What else?" and "Anything else?" engage the individual in finding their own solutions, not only making them responsible for change but also ensuring they are fully engaged in the process.

The more the non-specialist practitioner engages in identification and brief advice and has these conversations, the more skilled they become, especially if they reflect on their own part in motivating behaviour change.

STAGE 3: ACT (NEXT STEPS AND ONWARD REFERRAL)

Non-specialists should know the process and pathway for referral to alcohol treatment in their locality and ensure it is offered where indicated.

There is clear evidence older people do well in treatment (Royal College of Psychiatrists 2018), so where there is a need for specialist support, this pathway should always be utilised fully.

Alcohol withdrawal in someone who is drinking to a dependent level needs to be managed carefully. Abrupt withdrawal can be life threatening, and specialist medical attention is always necessary where there are signs of acute withdrawal.

Where dependence or possible dependence (AUDIT score of 20+) is recognised by a non-specialist service, appropriate advice should always be given about continued alcohol use alongside the specialist referral. If a person has physical withdrawal symptoms like shaking, sweating or feeling anxious until they have had their first drink of the day, they should not stop drinking suddenly and should seek specialist advice and support. Likewise, where family are involved and have some responsibility for supplying alcohol, they should be advised not to stop the supply of alcohol abruptly and to seek specialist advice in order to deal with the situation.

Feedback question	Style 1 (Advisory)	Style 2 (Motivational)
Feedback on scoring	"From your AUDIT score, you are drinking at a really risky level and need to cut down."	Your score on the AUDIT questionnaire is (specific *score*), which suggests you are drinking at a level that might put you at risk from (specific personalised information—current presentation). How do you feel about that?"
Introducing brief advice	"Because of your score I need to give you some advice on how to cut down."	"Your AUDIT score has told us you are drinking above the recommended guidelines, and you know this might be having an impact on (specific current presentation). Are you okay if we have a brief chat about ways of dealing with this and possibly reducing the risk?"
Health/risk concerns	"Cutting down will be good for your health and might stop (current problems)."	"Can you think of any benefits you might get from cutting down?"
Finding solutions	"You should…"	"What else can you think of that you could do?" "Anything else?"

Fig. 32.8 Questioning styles.

SUPPLEMENTARY ASSESSMENT QUESTIONS

Brief intervention as a model is not the sole domain of alcohol interventions and is now used in a range of public health approaches to support behaviour change. However, screening and brief interventions specific to alcohol need to be routine and less sporadic in all services in order to have an impact on alcohol misuse in the ageing population.

As well as using a screening tool, non-specialist practitioners can ask further supplementary questions or simply probe further where it will add to the overall assessment and support the treatment pathway. Exploration of the context in which the older person is using alcohol is of crucial importance.

A more extensive alcohol assessment could include the following:
- More specific quantity and frequency questions, including current and past alcohol use and any changes
- Precipitants to the change/increase in drinking
- Any other drug use, including over-the-counter medication
- Triggers for alcohol use, including specific times, events or emotions
- Physical, psychological and social impact of alcohol use—what has changed for the individual as a result of drinking?
- Does having a drink help with... (presenting problem such as sleeping or loneliness)?
- Have you ever increased your drinking to cope with... (presenting problem such as sleeping or loneliness)?
- Any reported or objective evidence of alcohol dependence

Where possible, this information could be supplemented by mental state and physical examinations and appropriate investigations depending on the information elicited. However, if a referral to specialist services is made, these will also be undertaken in the specialist setting.

These supplementary questions focus on the issues and problems specific to the individual and make the assessment more natural and personalised alongside having the AUDIT score as a baseline. With the older population, supplementary questions may mitigate against any failings in the established screening tool to pick up on age-specific issues.

Another important consideration is an individual's readiness to change and their belief in their ability to change. This can be determined by asking a simple scaling question based on the action they are considering, such as cutting down or stopping their drinking.

"On a scale of 0–10, with 0 being not at all confident and 10 being totally confident, how confident are you that you can (change/reduce/stop) your current drinking?"

This scaling question can become an intervention in itself, as hearing the score can prompt a further brief conversation:

"So your confidence is at a 4. What makes it 4 and not lower?"

This ensures the individual recognises and names positive factors, which give them some confidence in their success, such as family support, etc. It can then be followed up with a further question:

"So your confidence is at a 4. What needs to happen to make it higher—say, a 7?"

This ensures the individual recognises and names the things that have to happen to give them more self-belief and confidence. It can be the start of identifying some personal goals.

All these brief advice techniques enable the non-specialist to have an informed and productive discussion with the individual once there is a recognition of risky alcohol use. The more they are used and practised, the more natural and effective they become.

DEPENDENCE

The International Classification of Diseases and Health Problems (ICD-10) (WHO, 1993) defines dependence syndrome as a cluster of physiological, behavioural and cognitive phenomena in which the use of the substance takes on a much higher priority for the individual than other behaviours that once had greater value (WHO,1993).

Essentially, the diagnosis of dependence seeks to identify when three or more of the identified criteria (Table 32.2) have been present together at some time during the previous year.

TABLE 32.2   ICD-10 Criteria for Alcohol Dependence Syndrome

- A strong desire or compulsion to drink alcohol
- Difficulties in controlling alcohol-using behaviour in terms of its onset, termination or levels of use
- A physiological withdrawal state when alcohol has ceased or been reduced
- Evidence of tolerance where increased amounts of alcohol are required in order to achieve effects originally produced by lower quantities
- Progressive neglect of previous activities or interests because of alcohol
- Increased amount of time taken to use alcohol and/or recover from the effects
- Persisting with substance use despite clear evidence of overtly harmful consequences, including physical and mental health issues

Source: WHO (1993).

However, specialist services also look at diagnosis of dependence on a spectrum of mild, moderate and severe, based on SADQ scoring and further comprehensive assessment that incorporates examining symptoms and consequences of alcohol use.

Diagnosis by specialist services is fundamental to ensuring the most appropriate, evidenced-based treatment pathway (NICE, 2011), hence the importance of ensuring practitioners understand the evidence around alcohol misuse in older adults and its implications for nursing. This includes the need to offer appropriate and timely referral to specialist services, as specified in the final stage of the 3As model—act.

IMPORTANCE OF THIAMINE

Wernicke encephalopathy is an acute neurological condition caused by thiamine deficiency and in developed countries is often related to chronic alcohol use disorder. The classic triad of symptoms are ophthalmoplegia with nystagmus, ataxia and confusion, but this triad presents together in only about 10% of people. Although often referred to as Wernicke/Korsakoff syndrome, the two conditions are distinct in their clinical presentation.

Wernicke encephalopathy is an emergency situation that presents with a mild confusional state and requires immediate parenteral thiamine supplementation.

Korsakoff syndrome is characterised by irreversible amnesia, usually with short-term memory loss, retrograde amnesia and confabulation, and personality changes related to frontal lobe damage.

The prognosis for Wernicke encephalopathy, if recognised and treated appropriately with a reduction or cessation of alcohol use, is generally good. However, for Korsakoff syndrome it is generally poor, as damage to components of the limbic system, such as mammillary bodies, is often permanent. Treatment comprises continued abstinence from alcohol, long-term thiamine and improved diet and support.

The NICE (2010) clarified the need to offer thiamine to people at high risk of developing Wernicke encephalopathy. Depending on the level of risk, guidance is available in relation to offering oral or parenteral thiamine, but thiamine itself is indicated where:

- There is malnourishment or a risk of it
- There is decompensated liver disease
- There is evidence of acute withdrawal from alcohol
- A medically assisted detoxification is planned

Although it is not expected that the non-specialist setting treats these complex presentations, understanding and recognition are vital to early intervention. Where there is any concern about Wernicke encephalopathy, early intervention with the use of thiamine is recommended.

BARRIERS TO SEEKING AND PROVIDING SUPPORT

The barriers to older people seeking help for alcohol-related problems have been discussed extensively but persist (Wadd et al., 2011). There is still a perceived stigma related to addiction, with people feeling embarrassment, guilt and shame—all common responses to the realisation there is a loss of control over alcohol and a fear it will be judged in some way.

Following a number of practitioner focus groups, Wadd et al. (2011) discussed the professional response to older people drinking, with practitioners reporting several reasons why they did not detect alcohol misuse in older adults. Some were simply not aware alcohol was a potential issue in this age group. Others were reluctant to ask potentially embarrassing questions and reported low confidence in their own knowledge and skills to address the problem. Crucially, personal judgements were discussed, with some practitioners reporting they felt it was wrong to deprive older people of their pleasures in life, and people were too old to change their behaviour. Practitioners have also reported they perceive alcohol-using behaviours to be a personal choice, and they may underestimate the extent of alcohol consumption, possibly due to limited knowledge about units and screening. All these practitioner responses and perceptions contribute to a failure to grasp the role alcohol plays in the presenting problem.

Given the sensitivities older people have around seeking help, there is a concern that asking individuals about alcohol may perpetuate these feelings, resulting from staff who are uninformed, lacking in confidence or don't believe in the appropriateness of asking the questions due to an ageist attitude.

For this reason, non-specialist practitioners, especially nurses, should have awareness and training and understand the importance of providing a comprehensive approach to managing alcohol in older adults.

The approach to any assessment of an older person should be informed by a person centred, non-confrontational and non-judgemental style that is above all non-ageist and underpinned with respect for privacy and dignity.

SUPPORT AND SAFEGUARDING

Although alcohol misuse can have a significant effect on a individual's family and carers, family and carers can also have a significant impact on an individual's recovery. Wadd et al. (2011) suggested that older drinkers are often motivated to seek treatment for their alcohol use because of family, and there is substantial evidence of the protective nature of support from family and carers within the field of substance misuse. That said, family-oriented approaches, while being recognised as a crucial element of effective treatment and recovery, can be undertaken only with consent and assurances around safeguarding.

It should be remembered that family are a useful resource for corroboration and collateral information when trying to understand alcohol use in an older person.

Older people, by the very nature of the ageing process, have increased physical, mental health and social care needs and subsequently may be more vulnerable to abuse. Alcohol can increase this risk and may be used as a means to control or to exploit the older person or to make them more compliant by controlling their supply of alcohol. Nurses should remain vigilant not only to the individual's alcohol use but also to its impact on the people around them and on the risk of abuse and/or exploitation. They should question the role alcohol plays in extended relationships and assess any reliance on others to provide alcohol.

Safeguarding should be considered throughout any presentation and care pathway and may include the use of alcohol by the carer, which can impact the care of the older person. There is evidence to suggest the impact of caring responsibilities can precipitate substance misuse in carers as a coping mechanism. Alcohol Change UK (2019), in its analysis of safeguarding adult reviews, highlighted that vulnerable adults are particularly at risk from alcohol and can be either deeply affected by their own excessive use or negatively affected by someone else's drinking. In relation to alcohol, Alcohol Change UK said, 'Misperceptions of these vulnerable adults by local services and practitioners may have contributed to a failure to fully grasp the role alcohol was playing' (p. 14). The analysis goes on to discuss how self-neglect in relation to alcohol was perceived to be a lifestyle choice, and this prevented further analysis and professional curiosity.

Complications of the ageing process and alcohol misuse can both cause vulnerability in an older person, and as pointed out by Alcohol Change UK (2019, p. 21), there should be 'better legal literacy' among practitioners in relation to the statutory powers available to them. Nurses should have a good awareness of the Care Act (2014) and the Mental Capacity Act (2005) (England) alongside any other relevant safeguarding legislation, including where alcohol fits within it, particularly in relation to self-neglect and fluctuating capacity. Adults with alcohol problems may be entitled to an assessment of care and support needs, but there can be limited understanding of how to apply the legislation in practice. Nurses should remember adults with chronic alcohol problems may be within the remit of safeguarding adults' processes, and advancing age may add to the complexity and subsequent need (see Chapter 14).

CONCLUSION AND LEARNING POINTS

Far from life becoming simpler, slower or easier as we move into retirement and older age, the ageing process, both from physical and mental health perspectives and together with social and lifestyle changes, can exacerbate and sometimes mirror the effects of excess alcohol use. It can leave older people particularly vulnerable to a range of harms, some of which are hidden.

Crucial to all nursing contacts with older people is the recognition that a person's relationship with alcohol is individual to them and so are their associated needs. Although choices about alcohol use should be made by the individual, nurses should endeavour to provide information and support in a clear, structured and motivational way, ensuring choices are fully informed. Older people are not a homogenous group, and therefore nurses need to have a range of tools available in order to offer the most appropriate support. They must also be prepared for the reality that abstinence is not everyone's goal. Some people may not wish to be alcohol free. Individual, informed choices should be made where possible with all the information and support available. Where choices are made to continue drinking, appropriate harm reduction advice can support a safer approach and ultimately reduce the risks.

The evidence is clear in relation to alcohol; the older population is drinking more, presenting to services more often and experiencing more harms. This chapter shows that nurses, when aware of emerging trends and risks around older people's drinking, can implement clear and simple processes to screen, identify and intervene in cases of risky alcohol use. Nurses see older people in a variety of settings for a range of different reasons. They are in a unique and privileged position of being able not only to intervene at the earliest stage to support individuals but also to adopt a public health approach to managing the current rise in, and harms related to, alcohol misuse in this age group.

The introduction of Commissioning for Quality and Innovation in 2009, a national framework for locally agreed quality improvement schemes, established the opportunity to create local quality improvement goals on an incentivised basis. It incentivised hospitals and other settings to deliver alcohol identification and brief advice, and programmes have been put in place to deliver identification and brief advice more routinely across a range of health care services. However, it does not appear to be translating into referrals to specialist services for older adults, and it is possibly too early to see its impact on morbidity and mortality. A concern is the extent to which the model is genuinely embedded and used in non-specialist practice. A future consideration may be the comprehensive rollout of identification and brief advice training for all non-specialist health workers as part of their core training and through mandatory updates. Escalating concern about alcohol use in older people supports the notion that alcohol use in the ageing population should be everybody's business and not dealt with solely by specialist mental health/drug and alcohol services, as was the case in the past.

RECOMMENDED READING

For a clear summary of the issues and concerns:
Royal College of Psychiatrists. (2018). *Our invisible addicts* (No. CR211). Royal College of Psychiatrists.

For a literature review and excellent case examples:
Wadd, S., Lapworth, K., Sullivan, M. P., Forrester, D., & Galvani, S. (2011). *Working with older drinkers*. University of Bedfordshire.

For a practitioner perspective, with honest and touching narratives from years of experience:
Rao, T. (2019). *Catch me when I fall*. Amazon.

REFERENCES

Alcohol Change UK. (2019). *Learning from Tragedies. An analysis of alcohol-related safeguarding adults reviews*. Alcohol Change UK.

Bareham, B. K., Kaner, E., Spencer, L. P., & Hanratty, B. (2019). Drinking in later life: A systematic review and thematic synthesis of qualitative studies exploring older people's perceptions and experiences. *Age and ageing, 48*(1), 134–146.

Blum, R. W., Beuhring, T., Wunderlich, M., & Resnick, M. D. (1996). Don't ask, they won't tell: The quality of adolescent health screening in five practice settings. *American Journal of Public Health, 86*(12), 1767–1772.

Burton, R., Henn, C., Lavoie, D., O'Connor, R., Perkins, C., Sweeney, K., Greaves, F., Ferguson, B., Beynon, C., Belloni, A., & Musto, V. (2016). *The public health burden of alcohol and the effectiveness and cost-effectiveness of alcohol control policies: An evidence review*. Public Health England.

Butt, P. R., White-Campbell, M., Canham, S., Johnston, A. D., Indome, E. O., Purcell, B., Tung, J., & Van Bussel, L. (2020). Canadian guidelines on alcohol use disorder among older adults. *Canadian Geriatrics Journal, 23*(1), 143.

Commission on Alcohol Harm. (2020). *'It's everywhere'— Alcohol's public face and private harm: Our response*. Alcohol Health Alliance.

Crome, I. B., Crome, P., & Rao, R. (2011). Addiction and ageing– Awareness, assessment and action. *Age and Ageing, 40,* 657–658.

Dare, J., Wilkinson, C., Allsop, S., Waters, S., & McHale, S. (2014). Social engagement, setting and alcohol use among a sample of older Australians. *Health & Social Care in the Community, 22*(5), 524–532.

Department of Health (DoH). (2016). *UK chief medical officers' low risk drinking guidelines*. Scottish Government.

Derges, J., Kidger, J., Fox, F., Campbell, R., Kaner, E., & Hickman, M. (2017). Alcohol screening and brief interventions for adults and young people in health and community-based settings: A qualitative systematic literature review. *BMC Public Health, 17*(1), 562.

DiBartolo, M. C., & Jarosinski, J. M. (2017). Alcohol use disorder in older adults: challenges in assessment and treatment. *Issues in Mental Health Nursing, 38*(1), 25–32.

Drugscope. (2014). *It's about time. Tackling substance misuse in older people. A briefing by Drugscope on behalf of the Recovery Partnership*. Drugscope.

Dunne, F. J., & Schipperheijn, J. A. (1989). Alcohol and the elderly. *BMJ: British Medical Journal, 298*(6689), 1660.

Edwards, G., & Gross, M. (1976). Alcohol dependence: Provisional description of a clinical syndrome. *British Medical Journal, 281,* 1058–1061.

Fat, L. N., Bell, S., & Britton, A. (2020). A life-time of hazardous drinking and harm to health among older adults: findings from the Whitehall II prospective cohort study. *Addiction, 115,* 1855–1866.

Giles, A. (2016). *Older people and alcohol misuse: Helping people stay in their homes*. Housing Learning & Improvement Network. Public Health England.

Giles, L., & Richardson, E. (2020). *Monitoring and evaluating Scotland's alcohol strategy: Monitoring report 2020*. Public Health Scotland.

Hadida, A., Kapur, N., Mackway-Jones, K., Guthrie, E., & Creed, F. (2001). Comparing two different methods of identifying alcohol related problems in the emergency department: A real chance to intervene? *Emergency Medicine Journal, 18*(2), 112–115.

Hwang, T. J., Rabheru, K., Peisah, C., Reichman, W., & Ikeda, M. (2020). Loneliness and social isolation during the COVID-19 pandemic. *International Psychogeriatrics, 32*(10), 1217–1220.

Johnson, I. (2000). Alcohol problems in old age: a review of recent epidemiological research. *International Journal of Geriatric Psychiatry, 15*(7), 575–581.

Kelly, S., Olanrewaju, O., Cowan, A., Brayne, C., & Lafortune, L. (2018). Alcohol and older people: A systematic review of barriers, facilitators and context of drinking in older people and implications for intervention design. *PLoS One, 13*(1), e0191189.

Khan, N., Wilkinson, T. J., & Keeling, S. (2006). Reasons for changing alcohol use among older people in New Zealand. *Australasian Journal on Ageing, 25*(2), 97–100.

Lang, I., Guralnik, J., Wallace, R. B., & Melzer, D. (2007). What level of alcohol consumption is hazardous for older people? Functioning and mortality in US and English national cohorts. *Journal of the American Geriatrics Society, 55*(1), 49–57.

Ling, J., Smith, K. E., Wilson, G. B., Brierley-Jones, L., Crosland, A., Kaner, E. F., & Haighton, C. A. (2012). The 'other' in patterns of drinking: A qualitative study of attitudes towards alcohol use among professional, managerial and clerical workers. *BMC Public Health, 12*(1), 1–7.

Moos, R. H., Schutte, K., Brennan, P., & Moos, B. S. (2004). Ten-year patterns of alcohol consumption and drinking problems among older women and men. *Addiction, 99*(7), 829–838.

National Institute for Clinical Excellence (NICE). (2011). *Alcohol-use disorders: Diagnosis, assessment and management of harmful drinking and alcohol dependence. Clinical Guidance 115.* NICE.

National Institute for Clinical Excellence (NICE). (2010). *Alcohol use disorders: Diagnosis and clinical management of alcohol-related physical complications.* NICE.

NHS. (n.d.). https://www.nhs.uk/live-well/alcohol-advice/calculating-alcohol-units/.

O'Connell, H., Chin, A. V., Cunningham, C., & Lawlor, B. (2003). Alcohol use disorders in elderly people—Redefining an age old problem in old age. *British Medical Journal, 327*(7416), 664–667.

Office for National Statistics (ONS). (2018). *Statistics on alcohol.* UK Government.

Office for National Statistics (ONS). (2017). *Adult drinking habits in Great Britain.* ONS.

Perissinotto, C. M., Cenzer, I. S., & Covinsky, K. E. (2012). Loneliness in older persons: A predictor of functional decline and death. *Archives of Internal Medicine, 172*(14), 1078–1084.

Phillips, T., Porter, A., & Sinclair, J. (2020). Clinical competencies for the care of hospitalized patients with alcohol use disorders. *Alcohol and Alcoholism, 55,* 395–400.

Prochaska, J. O., & DiClemente, C. C. (1983). Stages and processes of self-change of smoking: Toward an integrative model of change. *Journal of Consulting and Clinical Psychology, 51*(3), 390.

Rao, R., & Roche, A. (2017). Substance misuse in older people. *BMJ,* 358.

Raw, M., McNeil, A. N. N., & West, R. (1998). Smoking Cessation Guidelines for Health Professionals—A guide to effective smoking cessation interventions for the health care system. *Thorax, 53*(sup 5), S1–S18.

Royal College of Psychiatrists. (2011). *Our invisible addicts* (CR165). Royal College of Psychiatrists.

Royal College of Psychiatrists. (2018). *Our invisible addicts* (No. CR211). Royal College of Psychiatrists.

Psychiatrists, Royal College of (2018). Alcohol court victory. *Royal College of Psychiatrists,* (3), P12–P13.

Sewdas, R., De Wind, A., Van Der Zwaan, L. G., Van Der Borg, W. E., Steenbeek, R., Van Der Beek, A. J., & Boot, C. R (2017). Why older workers work beyond the retirement age: a qualitative study. *BMC Public Health, 17*(1) 672.

Steptoe, A., Shankar, A., Demakakos, P., & Wardle, J. (2013). Social isolation, loneliness, and all-cause mortality in older men and women. *Proceedings of the National Academy of Sciences, 110*(15), 5797–5801.

Stockwell, T. R., Hodgson, R. J., Edwards, G., Taylor, C., & Rankin, H. (1979). The development of a questionnaire to measure severity of alcohol dependence. *British Journal of Addiction, 74,* 79–87.

Wadd, S., Lapworth, K., Sullivan, M. P., Forrester, D., & Galvani, S. (2011). *Working with older drinkers.* University of Bedfordshire.

Wadd, S., Randall, J., Thake, A., Edwards, K., Galvani, S., McCabe, L., & Coleman, A. (2013). *Alcohol misuse and cognitive impairment in older people* (pp. 1–62). Tilda Goldberg Centre for Social Work and Social Care.

Wilson, G. B., Kaner, E. F., Crosland, A., Ling, J., McCabe, K., & Haighton, C. A. (2013). A qualitative study of alcohol, health and identities among UK adults in later life. *PLoS One, 8*(8), e71792.

World Health Organization (1993). *The ICD-10 classification of mental and behavioural disorders: diagnostic criteria for research* (Vol. 2). World Health Organization.

World Health Organization. (2001). *AUDIT: The alcohol use disorders identification test: Guidelines for use in primary health care* (No. WHO/MSD/MSB/01.6 a). World Health Organization.

33

Nursing Older People With Intellectual Disabilities

Daniel Marsden

People with intellectual disabilities are among the most disadvantaged in our societies and communities. This population experiences greater levels of ill health and significant difficulties accessing health care. Although some countries still segregate people into institutional care settings, most now are working toward community inclusion. However, in either circumstance it can be expected that this group will experience social exclusion and sometimes abuse, which incurs a further set of associated health and well-being issues. These disadvantages, inequalities and disparities can be measured in health outcomes, with people with intellectual disabilities having a significantly reduced life expectancy and more likelihood of avoidable deaths.

The life expectancy of people with intellectual disabilities is 20 years less than the general population, so it could be assumed the health conditions and issues associated with older age start appearing at a significantly younger age than the general population. Although this chapter considers both age-related and disability-associated health needs, it also reflects on determinants of health across the lifespan, as they allow us a perspective on the causes and resolutions to some of these challenges.

The care and support people experience is influenced by how their strengths and needs are defined and viewed. The chapter starts by outlining how intellectual disability is defined across the world and the prevailing perspectives on this population and society. These perspectives impact how this population is cared for and supported as well as where and by whom in different countries across the world, which are considered as wider influences on health status.

The chapter provides a contemporary outline of the increased physical and mental health conditions people with intellectual disabilities experience. The greater likelihood of multimorbidity presents unique challenges to specialist health care systems.

Disparities in health care can also be seen in end-of-life care and how people with intellectual disabilities experience death of family and friends. To help resolve some of these issues, we present a simple framework. This tool is intended to enable nurses who work with older adults with intellectual disabilities to make accommodations and deliver good quality care.

Throughout the chapter, case studies and learning activities are presented to provide the reader with an opportunity to reflect on their personal and professional experiences of people with intellectual disabilities and consider how this care and support could be improved. Finally, some additional resources are shared for further consideration.

DEFINITIONS

The World Health Organization (WHO, 2016) defines intellectual disabilities as a 'significantly reduced ability to understand new or complex information and to learn and apply new skills (impaired intelligence). This results in a reduced ability to cope independently (impaired social functioning) and begins before adulthood with lasting effects on development'.

In the United Kingdom, the term *learning disability* is used interchangeably with *intellectual disability*, but this can cause confusion in other countries. In North America, for example, learning disability describes cognitive disorders that affect the understanding, organisation and comprehension of information, including dyspraxia, dyscalculia and dyslexia, while in the United Kingdom this is termed *learning difficulty*. For the purposes of this chapter, the internationally recognised term *intellectual disability* is used.

It is estimated that people with intellectual disabilities make up between 1% and 2% of the population, but significant variability can be assumed across the world, based on context and the culturally influenced definition. Although global and European data appear to identify closer to 1%, North America identifies 1.3%, estimates in the United Kingdom are 2%, and estimates in Australia are 3%. Some states identify and track this population through their systems, but many people with intellectual disabilities are hidden from statistics and likely present in mainstream health services as vulnerable.

A range of diagnostic manuals provide further perspectives and add to the lexicon. In the last decade, the WHO has explored whether intellectual disability should be conceptualised as a health condition or a disability. Through this review, *intellectual developmental disorders* has replaced *mental retardation* (Bertelli et al., 2016; Salvador-Carulla et al., 2011). Similarly, the Diagnostic and Statistical Manual

of Mental Disorders 5th Edition (American Psychiatric Association, 2013) replaced *mental retardation* with *intellectual disability* and categorised it as a neurodevelopmental disorder. This process has redefined the levels of intellectual disability based on support required to live an independent life rather than that of IQ range:

- Mild intellectual disability: Better able to live independently with minimal support
- Moderate intellectual disability: Moderate levels of support required such as those available in group homes
- Severe intellectual disability: Daily assistance required with self-care and safety
- Profound: Around the clock care required

The more significant the intellectual disability, the greater the likelihood of other concurrent health conditions, with individuals with the most significant disabilities are identified as having profound and multiple disabilities. These include sensory impairments, physical disabilities and epilepsy. For more information, see 'Supporting Resources' at the end of the chapter.

While superficially these discussions appear to respond to the prevailing mood associated with the update in nomenclature, the depth of the consideration and debate indicates the complexity of our understanding and perspectives on disability. This has implications for national policy, resource allocation and legal implications for individuals' status and rights in nation states.

LEARNING ACTIVITY 1

Write a time line of the people with intellectual disabilities you have encountered during your life. Were these interactions through education or through work as colleagues or patients?

Models and Perspectives on Disability

As people with intellectual disabilities and their families and carers are required to negotiate systems, processes and services based on assumptions made about their perspectives and needs, it is important to consider these influencing perspectives. According to Haegele and Hodge (2016), the medical model of disability emerged when doctors and scientists replaced religious leaders as the cognitive authority in society. This authority was based on the ability to both define illness and heal the sick. This prevailing paradigm encouraged a biological perspective in which disability is comprehended as a medical issue that limits individual functioning and as such is viewed as deficient and disordered. From this perspective, disability is seen to reside with the individual, and disability is seen as a problem that requires medical intervention to 'heal' so individuals might live in society.

This perspective can be clearly observed in the early 20th century in the first medical textbook on the topic, *Mental Defectives: Their History, Treatment and Training* (Barr, 1904). It sought to differentiate between categories of intellectual disability to enable the development and selection of treatments and prognoses. Galton (1904) sought to align his theory of eugenics as a science for improving society; this quickly became prescient, leading to practical solutions for ensuring the 'feeble minded' were unable to reproduce. The development of large hospital institutions enabled society to be segregated, and in some places involuntary sterilisation laws were implemented (Sofair & Kaldjian, 2000).

Challenges to this mode of thinking arose initially in 1950s with policymakers in Denmark. Bank-Mikkelson (1980) coined the phrase *normalisation*; Nirje (1980) and Wolfensberger (1980) applied and adapted the concepts in Sweden and United States, respectively. Based on the values of equality and human rights, normalisation sought for people to live as normal a life as possible, particularly in areas such as housing, education and work. Critics of normalisation observed it was overly concerned with practicalities and service systems rather than the underpinning theory.

The social model of disability emerged to address some of these concerns. The social model posits that disability is imposed by society on individuals with impairments. In this context the impairment and disability are separate; the impairment resides with the individual, but the disability is caused by a society that has not taken into account the individual's impairments, which in turn has the effect of exclusion.

Allied to these ideas and perspectives, public reports of abuse in long-stay institutions changed public perceptions. This led to the closure of large long-stay hospitals, greater support for people living in the community and greater acknowledgement of this equality in legal frameworks and policy guided by the United Nations Convention on the Rights of Persons with Disabilities (CRPD) (United Nations, 2006).

However, the social model is not without its critics; commentators have acknowledged that not adequately recognising the implications of the significant impairments individuals might experience may also have a negative impact on the health and well-being of the individual. Along with this, swift resolution to these issues is not as easy to explicate. See Table 33.1 for more details Case Study 33.1 shares a vignette of Michael and his experiences through the health and care systems.

CASE STUDY 33.1

Michael is 63 years old and grew up in the south of England. He has autism and a mild intellectual disability. He has struggled with anxiety and mental health throughout his life and has been admitted to hospital three times. The first time was at the local long-stay institution, where his mental health improved, and he was discharged. In the 1980s he went to the social training centre, where he was friends with staff and other clients. Michael was an independent man; he was well known in his town and attended his local football team's home games. Although Michael had a high degree of independence, he wanted to work and live on his own.

Michael experienced services that were based on the medical model and social model, and although he developed his own independence and relationship with his support systems, these services were not able to support him to work, live independently or have a family of his own. Michael's story is based on an anonymised clinical experience.

COMMUNITY CARE CONTEXT

Given the heterogeneous population of people intellectual disabilities, it is likely that some, if not all, are reliant or interdependent on support systems and services for their activities of daily living. It is crucial for individuals who have a part to play in a person's health and care to know and understand the knowledge, skills and experience of individuals who offer care and support at home.

TABLE 33.1	Comparison of Medical and Social Models of Disabilities	
Measure	**Medical**	**Social**
Disability definition	Disorder of body or physiological system	Social construct; the environment that disables a person with an impairment
Intervention	Cure or treatment to give relief from the disability	Increased access and inclusion through activism
Environment	A health care service with health care professionals	At home, in the community with family, friends and social support
Advantages	Scientific and empirically designed advances in care and support	Distributes responsibility for accessibility among the community
Disadvantages	Paternalistic; inability to cure or repair disability	Inability to resolve issues without broad social change

Source: Adapted from Olkin (2002).

Although the CRPD (2006, article 19) demands signatory states provide for a range of residential and community support services to enable community living and inclusion, both the relative nature of intellectual disability to the society and the dynamic nature of these social structures contribute to a wide variation of services available. Mansell et al. (2010) observed three cohorts of countries in their analysis of readiness for implementation of the CRPD. The first cohort included countries well advanced in reducing dependence on large institutional care facilities, such as North American, Western Europe and Australasia. In the second cohort including some central and eastern European countries, there was a continued reliance on large-scale hospital services. The third group included states that had no policy position, leading to an assumed reliance on family and underdeveloped community support.

Woittiez et al. (2018) identified further distinctions between countries in the initial group, indicating smaller care services and reduced influence of the state can provide for a more individualised and personalised service. These countries also acknowledged the vital part played by families and friends, either through legislation or less formally through care provision.

These circumstances resulted in a proliferation of services provided by health services, social care and third-sector organisations (Cumella & Lyons, 2018), including residential care, nursing care settings, specialist mental health and behavioural units, smaller staffed homes, adult placements and shared life communities.

In the United Kingdom, smaller staffed homes are the type of support most funded by authorities. They tend to be small suburban houses with approximately four people resident, supported by a rota of staff who maintain and develop daily living skills. Socioeconomic issues have an impact on staff renumeration, which has a subsequent negative effect on recruitment and retention (Care Quality Commission, 2017). Although the aims and objectives of residential care services vary, the majority are concerned with maintaining and developing independent living skills. Staff knowledge and understanding of physical health treatments and programmes cannot be presumed. Evidence also indicates people with intellectual disabilities in residential care or supported living services are more likely to be the subject of adult protection investigations, indicating a greater likelihood of abuse (Beadle-Brown, 2010).

Although there is much focus on care and support services, a significant proportion of people with intellectual disabilities live either independently or are cared for at home by their families. For instance, in the United Kingdom, this accounts for an estimated 77% of the population with intellectual disabilities (NHS Digital, 2019), while in Ireland, it is estimated that around 65% are cared for in their family home (Linehan, 2014).

LEARNING ACTIVITY 2

In your country or culture, how are people with intellectual disabilities supported and cared for? What are the advantages and disadvantages of these systems? What impact do these systems have on the health of this population?

DEMOGRAPHICS

Life Expectancy and Premature Death

Medicine, nursing care and technology have led to an increase in global life expectancy. In 1930 life expectancy for people with intellectual disabilities was 20 years (Foundation for People with Learning Disabilities, 2003). Studies since the 1970s have consistently noted premature deaths of people with intellectual disabilities. Heslop et al. (2013) found over a quarter of this population were likely to die before the age of 50; the median age of death was 64. Heslop et al.'s (2013) study also showed a gender imbalance in this population, where men's life expectancy was 13 years less than in the general population, while women's was 20 years less.

The same themes have been echoed across other countries in North America, Europe and Australia (Heslop, 2015). In the United Kingdom, they have led to the commissioning of a national mortality review (University of Bristol, 2020). The continued evidence of disparities in life span were referenced in the most recent National Health Service (2019) strategy document, with specific objectives to resolve causes of preventable death in this population.

The more severe the intellectual disability, the shorter the life expectancy. Contextual factors that influence premature death include mobility, feeding ability, continence, sensory impairments and the care setting in which individuals reside. Secondary to these factors are the long-term health conditions associated with intellectual disabilities, such as epilepsy; specific conditions associated with particular disabilities—people with Down syndrome are at greater risk of hypothyroidism; and the various medications prescribed as treatment for these conditions that can be implicated in early death.

However, Heslop et al. (2014) advised of wider influences on premature deaths of people with intellectual disabilities, including inappropriate housing, care and support and difficulties accessing health services. Once in receipt of health care, contributory factors in premature deaths included health care professionals' inabilities to apply care and support, resolve issues of decision making and ability to work with family and carers (Heslop et al., 2014).

The causes of death are therefore somewhat distinct from those of the general population. The leading causes of death in the general population are cancers and coronary heart disease, but data from 2019 showed 41% of people with intellectual disabilities died from respiratory disorders such as pneumonia. People with intellectual disabilities were proportionally more likely to die from central nervous system disorders associated with epilepsy and cerebral palsy (University of Bristol, 2020).

HEALTH INEQUALITIES

Dahlgren and Whitehead's (1991) influential model presenting determinants of health is recognised throughout the world. It provides a visual representation of the external interconnected factors that shape our health and well-being and has application to people with intellectual disabilities.

Families with children with intellectual disabilities are less likely to work full-time and create a career path due to extra caring duties. Similarly, people with intellectual disabilities are less likely to have paid work, and when they do, they are unlikely to command a significant wage (Rickard & Donkin, 2018). These socioeconomic circumstances can impact living conditions, dietary intake and the communities and networks available. People with intellectual disabilities are more likely to be exposed to several risk factors that impinge directly on their health and lifestyle choices (Heslop et al., 2014). As they are highly unlikely to access to higher quality education activities, a cycle of deprivation can be drawn that provides some account for health outcomes evidenced in this chapter.

Diagnostic Overshadowing

One type of disparity that has gained some attention in recent years is diagnostic overshadowing. This refers to the process by which an individual receives a poorer or delayed treatment due to the misattribution of physical symptoms to the persons intellectual disability. Sheffer et al. (2014) suggest that this often occurs due to issues relating to poor communication and behaviours that might challenge health care staff, in crowded and busy environments, with some staff holding a stigmatising attitude.

Ethnicity

Evidence indicates different ethnic groups experience distinct health status across the world. These variations are believed not to be the result of biological differences but cultural and socioeconomic and influenced by the wider determinants of health. Robertson et al. (2019) suggests people with intellectual disabilities experience similar differences. In the United Kingdom, experience reflects the inequalities relating to mental health and behaviour deemed challenging rather than physical health conditions. They can be grouped into health status and health access, acknowledging that certain communities are less well represented in evidence.

Possible causes for this include language barriers and cultural attitudes.

In the United States, Magaña et al. (2016) indicate poorer physical and mental health of Black and Latino adults with intellectual disability than both their White counterparts and adults without an intellectual disability in similar ethnic groups.

In both cases, the intersection of race and disability present increased risks to health and mental health, and greater consideration is required in patient-facing nursing practice, public health programmes that promote health and research to better ascertain the nursing requirements of these cohorts.

Specific Health Needs

Ambulatory Care Sensitive Conditions

Ambulatory care sensitive conditions are defined as conditions that if managed effectively in the community should not result in a hospital admission, such as diabetes and asthma. Hoskin et al. (2017) identified in the general population that hospital admissions for these types of conditions can usually be correlated to poor access to primary care services, this provided a driver to develop the 10 ambulatory care sensitive conditions for people with intellectual disabilities:

- Convulsions and epilepsy
- Pneumonia
- Urinary tract infection
- Aspiration
- Cellulitis
- Dehydration and gastroenteritis
- Constipation
- Chronic obstructive pulmonary disease
- Asthma
- Diabetes complications

People with intellectual disabilities are more likely to experience hospital admission due to health conditions not being recognised or managed effectively in primary care. According to Hosking et al. (2017), people with intellectual disabilities in England were twice as likely to be admitted to hospital due to an ambulatory care sensitive condition compared to the general population and almost four times as likely to be admitted with lower respiratory tract infections and urinary tract infections.

Sepsis

There is growing evidence that disproportionate numbers of people with intellectual disabilities in the United Kingdom experience premature and avoidable deaths due to sepsis (Heslop et al., 2013; Simoes, 2016). The primary causes of infection leading to sepsis are reported to be pneumonias, constipation and urological infections (University of Bristol, 2020).

The Learning Disability National Mortality Review (University of Bristol, 2020) identified sepsis as the fifth most frequently recorded cause of death for adults and children with intellectual disabilities; but the top two causes—bacterial pneumonia and aspiration pneumonia—could be assumed to have caused sepsis, which means sepsis accounts for close to 50% of all deaths.

RESPIRATORY DISEASES

Dysphagia

Dysphagia is a feeding and swallowing disorder linked to many other conditions, including choking and airway blockages and reduced fluid and nutritional intake. It can cause secondary conditions like headaches, urinary tract infections and constipation. Of most significance is pneumonia, which is identified as the third-highest cause of death in this population and is a particular risk for individuals with profound and additional disabilities. Additional disabilities include physical disabilities, cerebral palsy and motor impairments (Robertson et al., 2018).

Gastro-Oesophageal Reflux Disease

Gastro-oesophageal reflux disease is a particularly common condition in people with intellectual disabilities, with recent Dutch evidence indicating half the population of individuals profound and multiple disabilities experience it (van Timmeren, 2016). Although heartburn and an unpleasant taste at the back of the mouth might seem like a nuisance, for some less mobile people with intellectual disabilities, it can increase the risk of chest infections such as aspiration pneumonia as well as oesophageal ulcers, Barrett's oesophagus and oesophageal cancer.

Pneumonia

Pneumonia is the leading cause of death of people with intellectual disabilities. In the United Kingdom, several practice-based programmes were established to minimise the risk of aspiration pneumonia (University of Bristol, 2018). They indicated several contributory factors, including poor oral health characterised by decaying teeth, excess or absence of secretions, tube feeding, dependence on others for oral care and feeding, and the knowledge and skills of carers who support the individual. Also implicated is the person's posture and mobility, which in many cases require individualised support systems and a consideration of other physical health issues, including diagnosis of particular cardio and respiratory health conditions and the medications used to treat them.

Gastrointestinal

Constipation is a common issue for older adults, but its prevalence is reported to be double in the intellectual disability population over the age of 50 (Peklar et al., 2017). This can be due to prolonged transit in the gut caused by neurological conditions and a series of risk factors such as poor diet, reduced mobility and lack of exercise, and increased use of polypharmacy. A recent study in Ireland indicated that 40% of the intellectual disability population of the over 40-year old had chronic constipation, a significant proportion of whom were taking more than one medication to manage the symptoms (AlMutairi, 2020).

People with intellectual disabilities have been found to be at greater risk of helicobacter pylori in institutional surroundings due to its infectious nature (Harper et al., 2020). While effective treatments are available, regular screening is required to ensure serious conditions such as a peptic ulcers and gastric cancer do not develop.

Genitourinary Systems

While urinary tract infections are linked to signs of aging in this population (Wark, 2016) and could be assumed to be normally identified and managed in primary care, people with intellectual disabilities are five times as likely to be admitted as an emergency to the hospital with this condition (Hosking et al., 2017). Unrecognised and untreated urinary tract infections can cause urosepsis, which accounts for 20%–30% of all cases of sepsis and is associated with high morbidity and mortality (Rhodes et al., 2017).

Evidence suggests that women with intellectual disabilities are more likely to experience precocious menopause (Robertson et al., 2020). This has been associated with increased risk of coronary heart disease, stroke, osteoporosis, dementia and premature death.

Androgen deficiency and hypogonadism are more common in men with intellectual disabilities (Winters, 2022).

Cancers

Global evidence indicates the rate of cancers in people with intellectual disabilities is comparable with that of the general population (McCarron et al., 2017). However, the incidence rises dramatically with age, and it could be assumed that as life expectancy increases, incidences of cancers are elevated. United Kingdom–based studies indicate people with intellectual disabilities are more likely to experience digestive and bowel cancers compared to the general population, where breast, lung and prostate cancer predominate (O'Leary et al., 2018). Men with intellectual disabilities may be more likely to develop testicular cancer than those in the general population, while women are less likely to experience cervical cancers. While people with fragile X syndrome may be at lower risk of some cancers, the incidence of leukaemia is higher in individuals with Down syndrome (Public Health England, n.d.).

Lifestyle and behaviour are significant to cancer risk, including tobacco and alcohol use, physical exercise, physical activity and body mass. Although people with intellectual disabilities are less likely to smoke or drink, as a population they are more likely to experience extremes of body mass, being ether obese or underweight (Public Health England, n.d.).

Endocrine

Several conditions have been found to be associated with a higher prevalence of type 1 diabetes, including Down, Turner, Klinefelter, Prader-Willi, Noonan and Williams syndromes and autistic spectrum condition (Taggart et al., 2013). The higher prevalence is further elevated by family history of the disease.

As previously identified, people with intellectual disabilities are more likely to experience many of the risk factors associated with type 2 diabetes, such as poor dietary intake, greater sedentary lifestyle and greater exposure to medications that increase body mass index. Some studies have indicated a higher prevalence of type 2 diabetes particularly in North America (Lunsky, 2011). Of particular concern in this group is the signs and symptoms may go unrecognised for a significant period, leading to urgent interventions for hyperglycaemia. Therefore, regular screening for individuals at risk is recommended.

Data from the United Kingdom (Public Health England, 2019) indicates that people with intellectual disabilities are almost twice as likely to have hypothyroidism as those from the general population; whilst Dutch study (Hermans & Evenhuis, 2014) states almost one in five people over 50 year old will have the condition. Screening for the condition is necessary among people with Down syndrome due to increased prevalence in this population; it is also recommended for other people with intellectual disabilities as the signs and symptoms can be challenging to elicit and interpret. Once diagnosed, the treatment and monitoring are relatively simple.

Neurological

Epilepsy has a high prevalence in people with intellectual disabilities, the proportion of which increases with the level of intellectual disability, with age, and is particularly linked with those with dementia (Robertson et al., 2015). Some studies have also linked psychiatric, behavioural issues and other physical impairments with the incidence of epilepsy. Other studies have confirmed people with intellectual disabilities have an increased risk of death compared to the general population, particularly for individuals who have recently experienced seizures (Young et al., 2015). Although sudden unexpected death through epilepsy is one cause, death through accident such as drowning is increased in this population, and greater risk of aspiration in this cohort has also been implicated (Bain et al., 2018).

Muscular Skeletal

Osteoporosis is characterised by low bone density, which can lead to fractures, pain, loss of mobility and independence. A recent study indicated low bone quality was of a high prevalence in both men and women with intellectual disabilities, although it is higher in women because of menopause (Burke et al., 2017). Authors have also speculated the rates increase based on level of intellectual disability due to increased exposure to risk factors such as use of anticonvulsant medications and reduced mobility (Bastiaanse et al., 2014). Older people with intellectual disabilities and those with a lower body mass index are at greater risk.

Adults with intellectual impairments are at greater risk of falls due to a higher prevalence of balance alterations and reduced mobility. Falls have a negative impact on quality of life, reducing participation in activities of daily living and leading to greater social isolation and dependence, although targeted exercise programmes for adults with intellectual disabilities can reduce these risks (Cortés-Amador, 2019).

Mental Health

People with intellectual disabilities are far more likely to have a mental health problem across all age ranges than people from the general population (Hughes-McCormack, 2017). Depression is common for adults with intellectual disabilities, and it appears episodes are more enduring than in the general population; one study found adults with intellectual disabilities were four times more likely to meet the criteria for chronic depression (Collishaw et al., 2004). A Swedish study concurred, indicating almost twice as many older adults with intellectual disabilities have a diagnosed mental illness compared to the general population (Axmon et al., 2018). However, accurate assessment, diagnosis and treatments can be challenging due to issues related to communication, physical health issues, misdiagnosis due to diagnostic overshadowing and a dearth of adapted and sensitive assessment tools for use with this population.

Sensory

Individuals with intellectual disabilities have a higher prevalence of sight impairment, sight-threatening disease and ocular pathology compared to the general population. Some evidence suggests up to 60% of older adults experience a sight impairment (Dunn et al., 2020) beyond what might be expected of age-related impairments. According to Li et al. (2015), significant adjustments to the regular assessment process are required to ensure an accurate diagnosis and lens prescription.

Similarly, it is estimated that 40% of adults with intellectual disabilities have a hearing impairment, which is significantly higher for those in older age (McShea et al., 2016). This figure is also increased for individuals with associated health needs such as Down syndrome.

Cardiology

As life expectancy rises, so do the risks of age-related health conditions. Excluding disability-associated congenital cardiac conditions, people with intellectual disabilities are as vulnerable to lifestyle-related risk factors, if not more so. For individuals with a mild intellectual disability, greater independence and reduced likelihood of employment can lead to increased levels of obesity, hypertension, diabetes and metabolic syndrome. For individuals with moderate and severe intellectual disabilities, there is greater likelihood of physical disabilities, reduced mobility and a more sedentary lifestyle, with an increased prescription of antipsychotic medications that increase risk of metabolic syndrome (De Winter, 2016).

Oral Health

Poor oral health has been linked to other quality-of-life measures such as pain, sleep disturbance, eating difficulties and reduced self-confidence (Marks et al., 2018). Evidence indicates people with intellectual disabilities have poorer oral hygiene, a greater prevalence and severity of gum disease, and a greater proportion of untreated tooth decay compared to the general population. This is particularly true for individuals over 40 with intellectual disabilities and those who rely on others to support them with mouth hygiene (Anders et al., 2010).

Dementia

Prevalence of early onset dementias of an Alzheimer's type have long been recognised and associated with people with Down syndrome, with almost all those over the age of 35 showing the neuropathological changes characteristic of the disease (Lott & Head, 2019). Although this does not reflect the requirements of clinical diagnosis, there is much evidence of this cohort having a significantly higher risk of its development in their 40s and 50s than that of the general population, and the majority will die as a result of complications of this functional decline in their 50s and 60s (Lott & Head, 2019).

There is some conjecture as to the relative incidence among individuals with intellectual disabilities who do not have Down syndrome. Strydom et al. (2013) found older adults in this cohort were five times or more likely than the general population to have dementia, while unlike in the general population, there are not higher rates of the disease in women.

Diagnosis for the condition can be challenging in this population due to the differences in presentation, the availability of sensitive assessment tools, reliance on third-party reporting and accessibility of physical screening associated with differential diagnosis. In many countries screening programmes are established to identify signifiers of functional decline.

The preceding sections give an outline of the evidence about the health of people with intellectual disabilities, including some comparisons with the general population. These health needs often go unobserved and unrecognised until they become acute, leading to distressing and costly admissions to hospital and ultimately premature and sometimes avoidable death.

LEARNING ACTIVITY 3

Plot the pathways through which people enter and exit your part of the service.

What assumptions are made about the people who access the service? Do you see people with intellectual disabilities regularly, on occasion, or not at all? Why?

MULTIMORBIDITY

Multimorbidity is the experience of having multiple diseases or conditions. It considers the various physical, psychological and social domains of the person. As life expectancy and the prevalence of long-term conditions increase, multimorbidity is fast becoming a challenge to health care professionals, systems and policy designers. The impact of multimorbidity for the individual can be reduced quality of life, increased use of health and social care services, and reductions in life expectancy.

The United Kingdom–based intellectual disability mortality review (University of Bristol, 2020) identified that over 70% of the cases reviewed experienced multimorbidity, with a significant proportion having three or more long-term conditions.

Although primary health care is considered a society-wide, generalist approach to health and well-being distributed based on people's needs, secondary care is more specialised and single-disease focused (World Health Organization, 2018). Benner (2001) observed the system design was not attending to the growing have observed this system design does not attend to the needs of a growing population of people with multimorbidity as they are not assessed and treated as whole people, more as lists of symptoms associated with a single condition.

Adults with intellectual disabilities are particularly likely to present with multimorbidity at a younger age than the general population (Hermans & Evenhuis, 2014). However, unlike population-based public health programmes, there is no correlation between geography, deprivation and the type of long-term conditions the person might experience. This is further complicated by health care systems that are primarily reactive and focused on a single condition rather than proactively screening and treating people holistically with a focus on ill health prevention, recognition and treatment in the community.

COVID-19

From the outset of the global pandemic, there were concerns about how people with intellectual disabilities would be affected, awareness of health inequalities and access to an increasingly rationed health care system (Lodge, 2020), increased likelihood of multimorbidity and significant alterations to lifestyle.

While initial findings (Turk et al., 2020) reassuringly indicated mortality rates were similar between people with intellectual disabilities and the wider population, the age ranges differed significantly, with most of the former group being in the younger adult range.

This was reinforced in the United Kingdom (Public Health England, 2020), where younger adults with intellectual disabilities featured more prominently in mortality figures, with the death rate being as much as six times higher. This data also provided evidence people who resided in residential care were also at a higher risk of death from the virus, although it is unclear how pre-existing multimorbidity and transmission played a part in these findings.

In the face of this data, debates across the world ensued pertaining to the prioritisation of populations for the COVID-19 vaccine. In the United Kingdom, only certain sections of the intellectual disability population were identified for early administration of the vaccine (Hatton, 2021; Lodge et al., 2021; Palliative Care for People with Learning Disabilities Network, 2021).

Allied to this, as community-based support services closed during lockdown, increased responsibilities and pressures were placed on families (Willner et al., 2020), causing increased rates of anxiety and mental health issues.

Evidence related to the pandemic continues to become available, but it would appear the well-observed and multiple vulnerabilities of this population were not being sufficiently offset by adjustments to health and care services.

Meeting the Health Needs of Older People With Intellectual Disabilities
Advanced Planning and End of Life

Although palliative care is increasingly recognised as a human right (Centeno et al., 2013), there are increasing concerns people with intellectual disabilities do not have equitable access to these services. This population has the same or similar needs as the general population toward end of life, but there are often additional and associated issues that make care more complex, including communication issues; expression of pain; understanding of their health, condition and treatment options; multimorbidity and polypharmacy; and social circumstances, which may mean reliance on care staff or older family members.

International consensus indicates getting end-of-life care right for people with intellectual disabilities requires adjustments to communication, how to support decision making, developing collaborative relationships and coordinating and managing care (Tuffrey-Wijne et al., 2015). See Table 33.2 for further information.

TABLE 33.2 Consensus for Palliative Care for People With Intellectual Disabilities in Europe
Equity of access
Communication
Recognising the need for palliative care
Assessment of total need
Symptom management
End-of-life decision making
Involving those who matter: family, friends and carers
Collaboration
Support for families and carers
Preparing for death
Bereavement support
Education and training
Developing and managing services

Source: Tuffrey-Wijne et al. (2015).

Making Accommodation for People With Intellectual Disabilities

The CRPD (2006) states signatories ought to mandate law where 'reasonable accommodations' can be made for people with disabilities. These relate to physical or mental health, religion, education and employment issues. A reasonable accommodation is defined as an adjustment that does not impose an undue burden to ensure individuals with disabilities can experience the service or activity on an equal basis with others.

While commentators and service providers have attempted to define reasonable accommodations, individualised needs are challenging to anticipate. However, frameworks are available to support individual nurses and health organisations to review their accessibility in the areas that are particularly significant for people with intellectual disabilities.

LEARNING ACTIVITY 4

Review and reflect on the pathway mapped out in Learning Activity 3. What actions could you take to improve access for people with intellectual disabilities?

Which of these are reasonable? Can you speak to your manager about these actions?

4C Framework for Making Reasonable Accommodation

Table 33.3 describes a tool created with nurses for making reasonable accommodation for people with intellectual disabilities (Marsden & Giles, 2017).

TABLE 33.3	**4C Framework for Making Reasonable Accommodations**

Communication	Choice Making
Collaboration	Coordination

Source: Marsden & Giles (2017).

Communication

Evidence indicates that close to 60% of people with intellectual disabilities over the age of 40 experience communication difficulties (Smith et al., 2020). Both health care professionals and people with intellectual disabilities indicate some concerns and worries about interacting with each other related to understanding and being understood (Chew et al., 2009). As such there are some useful guidelines to frame interactions.

First, consider the environment; it is advisable to select a quiet place to aid concentration. Facing the person supports the development of a rapport, and identifying the ground rules for the discussion can be helpful. This could entail identifying who needs to be part of the discussion: the individual and carer and acknowledging whether the person wants to speak to you on their own. If further information is required, you can ask whether it could be gained from the carer. It is also recommended to establish whether there are any communication adjustments the person might like you to make.

Gaining eye contact and speaking directly to the person and not the carer is crucial. Finding the rhythm of the conversation is important. You will want to leave extra time for a response before moving on.

Rephrasing and reflecting what you have heard from the person will offer useful feedback about the person's comprehension. Wherever possible, remain focused on one topic, and when it is time to move on to the next, clarify with the person if that topic is complete.

Some people with intellectual disabilities rely on augmentative and alternative communication tools (see Table 33.4). If they do, they may find it more difficult to interject or interrupt, so it is be advisable to invite them to ask questions.

Use of open questions is recommended to help you to establish and continue to adapt your communication and care to the individual. Closed questions have their place, but be mindful that you are able to establish the person's understanding.

As in all conversations, misunderstandings will occur, and it is recommended they are acknowledged with a question about what topic of conversation was or asking the person to say it in a different way James' case study outlines the use of clarifying questions to establish an agreeable form of terminology (Case Study 33.2). It always useful to be mindful of the broad interaction. Tiredness or boredom are not often referred to directly but can come from nonverbal communication such as fidgeting or yawning.

Resource to Support Communication

Beyond Words (see 'Supporting Resources') has a set of books on a range of topics that tell a story without words and allow the reader to interpret what might be happening.

TABLE 33.4	**Augmentative and Alternative Communication Tools**	
No Tools Required	**Low Tech**	**Aided Communication (High Tech)**
Body language, gesture, facial expressions, including pointing	Pen and paper to draw	Electronic devices (battery or main powered); most often speak or produce text
Verbal expression • Keep sentences short and simply • No jargon • Only one idea per sentence • Wait for a response; take time • Explain things in a concrete way, not abstract (e.g., "Take a tablet with your breakfast and one with your dinner" instead of "twice a day")	Communication charts; picture exchange systems	Device applications; software that can be downloaded to preferred device
Sign language; Makaton has a global reach; country-based sign language systems	Books with pictures such as available from Beyond Words Photo and symbol packages such as Photosymbols	

Source: Adapted from Curruthers et al. (2017), including guidance from Tuffrey-Wijne & McEnhill (2008).

CASE STUDY 33.2

James had an autistic spectrum condition and diabetes. On meeting him for the first time, the health professional asked about his health, but he appeared non-committal to having diabetes. Knowing this was the reason for the referral, the nurse asked about his blood sugar and finger-prick tests, which elicited a positive response from James. James said he did not always remember all the words, but he did test his blood sugar twice a day by pricking his finger.

Beyond Words has a number of books focused on health and healthy living, including *Going to the Doctors* and *Getting On with Cancer*.

Makaton (see 'Supporting Resources') is a sign language developed in the United Kingdom for people with intellectual disabilities that now has a global reach. It supports the development of vital communication skills such as listening, comprehension and expression, and it has an associated vocabulary and set of symbols.

Choice Making

Article 12 of the CRPD (United Nations, 2006) states people with disabilities have equal recognition before the law of all signatory countries. Of most significance to individuals with intellectual disabilities is autonomy and choice-making ability, referred to as capacity in some jurisdictions. There are two main responses to this requirement: a third party is permitted to make decisions on behalf of an individual (i.e., supported decision making), or a third party assists with the choice to be made (Devi, 2013). Many countries' statutes on supportive decision making also contain caveats for third-party decision making. A good example is therapeutic exception in the United Kingdom (Adams et al., 2018.)

Across the globe there have been several interpretations of the CRPD (United Nations, 2006) and the distinctions between third-party and supported decision making. One commonality are the elements of legal choice making, in which the individual

- Understands the information being presented
- Can recall the information
- Has an appreciation of the consequences
- Can express a choice to a third party

These are important questions to be mindful of, particularly for significant health-related procedures, including assessment and administration of treatment. The nurse or health care professional should be ready to account for themselves relating to this test and how they have adjusted the way in which the information has been presented.

If an individual has legally independent choice-making ability, the process can move forward. In the event an individual is unable to attend to one or more of the four

elements, a supported decision-making process is triggered, where a third party is consulted to determine what the individual would want if were they able to consent. In these cases, the professional who proposes the course of action, having established the individual requires additional support, engages a third party for this consultative support; this could be a family member or friend.

In circumstances where someone with severe and profound disabilities is without friends or family, a facilitator is engaged to proactively build a relationship to maximise their legal capacity.

In England and Wales, the Mental Capacity Act has five principles:

- Assume a person has the capacity to make a decision themselves unless it's proved otherwise.
- Wherever possible, help people make their own decisions.
- Don't treat a person as lacking the capacity to make a decision just because they make an unwise decision.
- If you make a decision for someone who doesn't have capacity, it must be in their best interests.
- Treatment and care provided to someone who lacks capacity should be the least restrictive of their basic rights and freedoms.

See Richard's case study for a practice example where capacity legislation has provided an explicit guide for safeguarding Richard's right to make a a an informed choice about the procedure and the health professional's responsibilities to make reasonable accommodations (Case Study 33.3).

CASE STUDY 33.3

Richard is a 48-year-old man with Down syndrome and a moderate intellectual disability who needs to attend the local phlebotomy clinic to have blood taken for thyroid-stimulating hormone and thyroxine levels. The nurse uses clear and simple language and some easy-to-read information about having a blood test to enable Richard and his mother to make a choice about the test.

These adaptations enabled Richard to understand the process and reasons for it, and on discussing it with his mother, he identified some ways the nurse could make the process easier for him.

The nurse adapted the environment to make it as relaxed as possible before Richard arrived. Richard was able to lie down on the bed and preferred not seeing the nurse and what they were doing preparing for the test.

This case study provides an indication of the main elements of England's and Wales's interpretations of the CRPD. The scenario indicates the accommodation the nurse made to effectively communicate with Richard, enabling an assisted decision to be made and a set of further adjustments to the process to enable a successful and timely outcome.

Collaboration

Facilitated choice making requires a good understanding of the individual and their health and social care circumstances. This is best achieved through collaboration with the individual and their family and support staff.

Older adults who live in the family home often have a more significant disability. By consequence their parent carers are usually significantly older, and women are the main carers in this context (Ryan et al., 2014). Family carers are similarly disadvantaged socially and economically to their children, with increased vulnerabilities to physical and mental health problems as a result. The functional relationship between parents and child also appears to shift into a mutual caring role, with the individual undertaking some practical tasks around the house where possible and providing a level of emotional support to the wider family.

Ryan et al. (2014) go on to observe that support for families who have retained this level of involvement ought to be supported and is implemented in some countries as part of statute and this can include welfare benefits, access to respite services and Carers assessments. It is also identified that families that care for family members are often not in receipt of the full support that authorities can offer and facilitating their access to these resources can enable the family to maintain their care and support.

Planning for significant life events is often lacking for individuals who live in co-dependent settings, and therefore the person may need to move home for safety purposes, unprepared. This can exacerbate both bereavement and feelings of loss. In some jurisdictions, primary care services keep records to enable their staff to monitor the situation holistically.

Having an awareness of a person's social circumstances is significant to ensure the right people are involved in decision-making processes, as they have insight into what further accommodations are required to enable the procedure to occur and the aftercare to be managed Sally's case study outlines how healthcare professionals can share more personalised information that will not cause further delay's and distress in the decision making processes (Case Study 33.4).

In certain circumstances families arrange a circle of support for the individual. This group can be made up of family friends

and staff who come together to support the person to achieve goals and make plans for the future. This person-centred planning approach can be proactive in planning for decision making with the individual, and where circumstances require it, could offer support where a significant medical decision or one where a change in home and community are required.

Coordination

As life expectancy increases, the incidence of multimorbidity increases and consequently the risks of premature and avoidable deaths. A number of actions and activities can be employed to resolve or mitigate this train of events. In an increasingly complex health and care environment, coordination of care is regularly identified as an important activity in confronting premature mortality. Care coordination is the deliberate organisation of care activities between two or more participants to enable the delivery of health services.

For nurses in the United States (Chappell & Mineo, 2015), care coordination is considered a leadership role involving six key principles:

- Know how care is coordinated in your setting
- Know who is providing care
- Establish relationships with multiple entities who can work together to improve transition management
- Know the value of technology
- Engaging patient and family
- Engaging all team member in coordination

Ruiz et al. (2020) presented two North American models led by nurse practitioners that provide clinic-, home- and community-based access to primary care services with a view to reduce and minimise the use of emergency care services. These are interdisciplinary teams made up of primary, specialist and consulting professionals, and the services provided include cognitive and physical assessment, needs assessment and resources dedicated to coordination with other providers to address health and social needs. It was found these teams were able to supplement the support group home managers could offer, and it allowed for proactive age-related health screening.

In the United Kingdom, the increased focus on choice within health care systems overlaid with the increase in multimorbidity and public health programmes to encourage healthy lifestyles prompted the role of health navigators to be evaluated. In some parts of the NHS, nurses' primary role is to support the individuals to access and make the best use of health services, ensuring information is exchanged effectively. A coaching role enables the person to make choices about their health and care (Academy of Medical Royal Colleges, 2015).

In several countries, nurses with a specialist nursing qualification in intellectual disabilities enable accommodations to be made across health services, enabling care that is coordinated and frameworks and tools to support coordinated care (Tuffrey-Wijne, 2014). Nicola's case study provides an

---

CASE STUDY 33.4

Sally is a 45-year-old woman with profound and multiple disabilities who was referred to a local hospital for an exploratory surgical procedure in day surgery. The referral included that the GP believed Sally would require assistance with making a decision about the operation, along with details of the important people in Sally's life. This enabled the admitting surgeon to ensure Sally's surgery was not delayed due to the facilitated choice-making process.

exemplar as to how specialist nurses in the field of intellectual disabilities can facilitate reasonable accommodations to be made in accessing health services (Case Study 33.5).

Health screening is also increasingly evident across health systems to help identify unrecognised health needs and ensure plans of care can be developed proactively to coordinate across health care systems. This is supplemented by dementia screening for older people with intellectual disabilities.

LEARNING ACTIVITY 5

Using the 4C framework, what adjustments could you be prepared to make the next time you are required to do so?

Do you need tools to do this? If so, where will you keep them?

CASE STUDY 33.5

Nicola is a 58-year-old woman with central palsy and a severe intellectual disability. The intellectual disability specialist nurse was alerted to Nicola's admission to hospital through the real-time tracking on their organisation's IT system. Nicola had had recurrent chest infections prior to the admission with aspiration pneumonia.

Nicola, her mother, the nurse and ward staff met on the ward to review the situation. The nurse used a hospital communication book to augment communication about her health. A percutaneous endoscopic gastrostomy (PEG) tube was proposed by the admitting doctor, which Nicola's mother was initially uncomfortable with.

Although intravenous antibiotics treated the pneumonia, and the nurses used the communication book to help communicate about simple issues, the intellectual disability nurse, family and carers discussed the implications and consequences of the PEG tube. Some information was prepared with pictures and simple sentences outlining Nicola's choice, including the risks and benefits of the procedure. A consensus between the surgeon, Nicola and her family and friends was found, and the procedure was undertaken. This enabled Nicola to return to the activities of daily living that she enjoyed like swimming and going out with friends to the cinema.

CONCLUSION

People with intellectual disabilities make up between 1∞ and 3% of every population around the world and may live in segregated communities either in institutions or isolated in the local community. Although this population has an increasing life expectancy that brings associated age-related health conditions, as a group they are more likely to die prematurely from avoidable deaths. Allied to this, older people with intellectual disabilities are more likely to have health conditions associated with their disability, which increases the risk of multimorbidity.

These individual factors are exacerbated by health care systems that are not always designed to make the anticipatory accommodations required through law. Nurses have a significant and crucial role to play in providing holistic care to this population through being aware of the legal duties required to make accommodations and being creative in how they augment their communication. Through these adjustments, nurses can support facilitated choice making, enabling patients' autonomy and ensuring they work holistically with individuals' families and care support to enable successful health interventions and healthy lifestyle choices.

This chapter provides tools and resources to support the nurse and includes a series of reflective activities to enable the nurse to reflect on their experiences, knowledge and work context.

KEY LEARNING POINTS

- Intellectual disability relates to impaired intelligence and social impairment.
- The prevailing social model of disability challenges us to consider how our knowledge, attitudes and services might further disable people with impairments.
- The health status is significantly poorer in this population and results in a life expectancy of approximately 20 years less than the general population.
- Equality legislation encourages and enforces countries to make reasonable accommodations for people with intellectual disabilities.
- Reasonable accommodations and adjustments for this group could be best organised by considering adjustments to communication, choice making, collaboration and coordination.

SUPPORTING RESOURCES

United Nations list of disability laws and acts by country/area: https://www.un.org/development/desa/disabilities/disability-laws-and-acts-by-country-area.html#menu-header-menu.

Hello, My Name is Ruth May: https://twitter.com/CNOEngland/status/1159423945147342849?s=20.

Getting Started with Makaton Signs and Symbols: https://www.youtube.com/watch?v=je16d8dmnWo.

Photosymbols: https://www.photosymbols.com.

Beyond Words: https://booksbeyondwords.co.uk/resources-dl/#health.

My Healthcare Passport: https://www.ekhuft.nhs.uk/EasySiteWeb/GatewayLink.aspx?alId=420924.

My Feral Heart: https://www.imdb.com/title/tt3184666/.

Future Learn: "Improving Health Assessments for People with an Intellectual Disability": https://www.futurelearn.com/courses/health-assessment.

REFERENCES

Academy of Medical Royal Colleges. (2015). *Coordinating care: In primary, community and outpatients settings.* Academy of Medical Royal Colleges. https://www.aomrc.org.uk/wp-content/uploads/2016/05/Coordinating_care_pcos_1015.pdf.

Adams, D., Carr, C., Marsden, D., & Senior, K. (2018). An update on informed consent and the effect on the clinical practice of those working with people with a learning disability. *Learning Disability Practice.* https://doi.org/10.7748/ldp.2018.e1855.

AlMutairi, H., O'Dwyer, M., Burke, E., McCarron, M, McCallion, P., & Henman, C. (2020). Laxative use among older adults with intellectual disability: A cross-sectional observational study. *International Journal of Clinical Pharmacy, 42*, 89–99. https://doi.org/10.1007/s11096-019-00942-z.

American Psychiatric Association. (2013). *Diagnostic and statistical manual of mental disorders* (5th edition). APA.

Anders, P. L., & Davis, E. L. (2010). Oral health of patients with intellectual disabilities: A systematic review. *Special Care in Dentistry, 30*(3), 110–117. https://doi.org/10.1111/j.1754-4505.2010.00136.x.

Axmon, A., Björne, P., Nylander, L., & Ahlström, G. (2018). Psychiatric diagnoses in older people with intellectual disability in comparison with the general population: a register study. *Epidemiology and Psychiatric Sciences, 27*(5), 479–491. https://doi.org/10.1017/S2045796017000051.

Bain, E., Keller, A. E., Jordan, H., Robyn, W., Pollanen, M. S., Williams, A. S., & Donner, E. J. (2018). Drowning in epilepsy: A population-based case series. *Epilepsy Research, 145*, 123–126.

Bank-Mikkelson, N (1980). Denmark. In R. J Flynn, & K. E Nitsch (Eds.), *Normalisation, social integration and community services* (pp. 51–70). University Park Press.

Barr, M. W. (1904). *Sketch of the history of the treatment of mental defect* (pp. 879–883). Charities.

Bastiaanse, L. P., Mergler, S., Evenhuis, H. M., & Echteld, M. A. (2014). Bone quality in older adults with intellectual disabilities. *Research in Developmental Disabilities, 35*(9), 1927–1933.

Beadle-Brown, J., Mansell, J., Cambridge, P., Milne, A., & Whelton, B. (2010). Adult protection of people with intellectual disabilities: incidence, Nature and Responses. *Journal of Applied Research in Intellectual Disabilities, 23*, 573–584. https://doi.org/10.1111/j.1468-3148.2010.00561.x.

Benner, P. (2001). From novice to expert. Excellence and power in clinical nursing practice. Prentice Hall.

Bertelli, M. O., Munir, K., Harris, J., & Salvador-Carulla, L. (2016). Intellectual developmental disorders": Reflections on the international consensus document for redefining "mental retardation-intellectual disability" in ICD-11. *Advances in Mental Health and Intellectual Disabilities, 10*(1), 36–58. https://doi.org/10.1108/AMHID-10-2015-0050.

Burke, E. A., McCallion, P., Carroll, R., Walsh, J. B., & McCarron, M. (2017). An exploration of the bone health of older adults with an intellectual disability in Ireland. *Journal of Intellectual Disability Research, 61*, 99–114.

Care Quality Commission. (2017). The state of health care and adult social care in England 2016/17. HC377. HMSO.

Centeno, C, Lynch, T, Doneo, O, Rocafort, J., & Clark, D. (2013). *Atlas of palliative care in Europe 2013* (full edition). EAPC.

Chappell, S., & Mineo, R. (2015). Joint statement: The role of the nurse leader in care coordination and transition management across the health care continuum. https://www.aonl.org/system/files/media/file/2019/04/care-coordination-nurse-leader.pdf.

Chew, K. L., Iacono, T., & Tracy, J. (2009). Overcoming communication barriers - working with patients with intellectual disabilities. *Australian Family Physician, 38*(1–2), 10–14.

Collishaw, S., Maughan, B., & Pickles, A. (2004). Affective problems in adults with mild learning disability: the roles of social disadvantage and ill health. *British Journal of Psychiatry, 185*, 350–351.

Cortés-Amador, S., Carrasco, J. J., Sempere-Rubio, N., Igual-Camacho, C., Villaplana-Torres, L. A., & Pérez-Alenda, S. (2019). Effects of a vestibular physiotherapy protocol on adults with intellectual disability in the prevention of falls: A multi-centre clinical trial. *Journal of Applied Research in Intellectual Disabilities, 32*, 359–367. https://doi.org/10.1111/jar.12531.

Cumella, S., & Lyons, M. (2018). Shared-life communities for people with a learning disability: A review of the evidence. *British Journal of Learning Disabilities, 46*, 163–171. https://doi.org/10.1111/bld.12224.

Dahlgren, G., & Whitehead, M. (1991). Policies and strategies to promote social equity in health. Background document to World Health Organisation—Strategy paper for Europe. Institute for Future Studies, Stockholm. Accessible in: Dahlgren, G., & Whitehead, M. (2007). *European strategies for tackling social inequities in health: Levelling up Part 2.* Copenhagen: WHO Regional office Office for Europe.

Department of Health. (2001). *Valuing people: A new strategy for learning disability for the 21st century.* The Stationery Office.

Devi, N. (2013). Supported decision-making and personal autonomy for persons with intellectual disabilities: article 12 of the UN convention on the rights of persons with disabilities. *The Journal of Law, Medicine & Ethics, 41*(4), 792–806. https://doi.org/10.1111/jlme.12090.

Dunn, K., Rydzewska, E., Fleming, M, et al. (2020). Prevalence of mental health conditions, sensory impairments and physical disability in people with co-occurring intellectual disabilities and autism compared with other people: A cross-sectional total population study in Scotland. *BMJ Open, 10,* e035280.

Foundation for People with Learning Disabilities (2003). Planning for tomorrow. Foundation for People with Learning Disabilities.

ICD-11 Beta Draft. http://www.apps.who.int/classifications/icd11/.

Haegele, J., & Hodge, S. (2016). Disability discourse: Overview and critiques of the medical and social models. *Quest, 68*(2), 193–206. https://doi.org/10.1080/00336297.2016.1143849.

Harper, L., Boulter, P., Ambridge, A., Griffin, P., & Ooms, A.(2020). Helicobacter pylori: Nurses' perceptions of diagnosis and treatment in adults. *Learning Disability Practice, 23*(2), 38–45.

Hatton, C. (2021). Beyond urgent: COVID-19 vaccination and people with learning disabilities. *Chris Hatton's blog* 11th January 2021. https://chrishatton.blogspot.com/2021/01/beyond-urgent-covid-19-vaccination-and.html.

Hermans, H., & Evenhuis, H. M. (2014). Multimorbidity in older adults with intellectual disabilities. *Research in Developmental Disabilities, 35,* 776–783.

Heslop, P., Blair, P., Fleming, P., Hoghton, M., Marriott, A., & Russ, L. (2013). *Confidential inquiry into premature deaths of people with learning disabilities.* Norah Fry Research Centre.

Heslop, P., Blair, P. S., Fleming, P., Hoghton, M., Marriott, A., & Russ, L. (2014). The confidential inquiry into premature deaths of people with intellectual disabilities in the UK: A population-based study. *Lancet, 383,* 889–895.

Heslop, P., Lauer, E., & Hoghton, M. (2015). Mortality in People with Intellectual Disabilities. *Journal of Applied Research in Intellectual Disabilities, 28,* 367–372. https://doi.org/10.1111/jar.12196.

Hosking, F., Carey, I., DeWilde, S., Harris, T., Beighton, C., & Cook, D. (2017). Preventable emergency hospital admissions among adults with intellectual disability in England. *The Annals of Family Medicine, 15*(5), 462–470. https://doi.org/10.1370/afm.2104.

Hughes-McCormack, L., Rydzewska, E., Henderson, A., MacIntyre, C., Rintoul, J., & Cooper, S. (2017). Prevalence of mental health conditions and relationship with general health in a whole-country population of people with intellectual disabilities compared with the general population. *BJPsych Open, 3*(5), 243–248. https://doi.org/10.1192/bjpo.bp.117.005462.

Li, J. CH., Wong, K., Park, A. SY., Fricke, T. R., & Jackson, A. J (2015). The challenges of providing eye care for adults with intellectual disabilities. *Clinical and Experimental Optometry, 98,* 420–429. https://doi.org/10.1111/cxo.12304.

Linehan, C., O'Doherty, S., Tatlow-Golden, M., Craig, S., Kerr, M., Lynch, C., McConkey, R., & Staines, A. (2014). *Mapping the National Disability Policy Landscape.* School of Social Work and Social Policy, Trinity College.

Lodge, K. (2020). Covid-19 shows that the lives of people with a learning disability are still not treated as equal. *BMJ Blog.* https://blogs.bmj.com/bmj/2020/09/01/covid-19-shows-that-the-lives-of-people-with-a-learning-disability-are-still-not-treated-as-equal/.

Lodge, K., Brown, C., & Hollins, S. (2021). People with an intellectual disability should be prioritised for vaccination. *BMJ Blog.* https://blogs.bmj.com/bmj/2021/01/14/people-with-an-intellectual-disability-should-be-prioritised-for-vaccination/.

Lott, I. T., & Head, E. (2019). Dementia in Down syndrome: unique insights for Alzheimer disease research. Nature reviews. *Neurology, 15*(3), 135–147.

Lunsky, Y., Timt, A., Robinson, S., Khodaverdian, A., & Jaskulski, C. (2011). Emergency psychiatric service use by individuals with intellectual disabilities living with family. *Journal of Mental Health Research in Intellectual Disabilities, 4,* 172–185.

Magaña, S., Parish, S., Morales, M. A., Li, H., & Fujiura, G. (2016). Racial and ethnic health disparities among people with intellectual and developmental disabilities. *Intellectual and Developmental Disabilities, 54*(3), 161–172. https://doi.org/10.1352/1934-9556-54.3.161.

Mansell, J., & Beadle-Brown, J. (2010). Deinstitutionalisation and community living: position statement of the Comparative Policy and Practice Special Interest Research Group of the International Association for the Scientific Study of Intellectual Disabilities. *Journal of Intellectual Disability Research, 54,* 104–112. https://doi.org/10.1111/j.1365-2788.2009.01239.x.

Marks, L., Wong, A., Perlman, S., Shellard, A., & Fernandez, C. (2018). Global oral health status of athletes with intellectual disabilities. *Clinical Oral Investigations, 22,* 1681–1688. https://doi.org/10.1007/s00784-017-2258-0.

Marsden, D., & Giles, R. (2017). The 4C framework for making reasonable adjustments for people with learning disabilities. *Nursing Standard, 31*(21), 45–53.

McCarron, M., Cleary, E., & McCallion, P. (2017). Health and health-care utilization of the older population of Ireland: Comparing the intellectual disability population and the general population. *Research on Aging, 39*(6), 693–718.

McShea, L., Fulton, J., & Hayes, C. (2016). Paid support workers for adults with intellectual disabilities; Their current knowledge of hearing loss and future training needs. *Journal of Applied Research in Intellectual Disabilities, 29,* 422–432. https://doi.org/10.1111/jar.12201.

National Health Service (2019) *The NHS long term plan.* https://www.longtermplan.nhs.uk/.

NHS Digital (2019) *Measures from the Adult Social Care Outcomes Framework* (ASCOF), England 2018-19. https://digital.nhs.uk/data-and-information/publications/statistical/adult-social-care-outcomes-framework-ascof/upcoming/indicator-files/1g-proportion-of-adults-with-a-learning-disability-who-live-in-their-own-home-or-with-their-family.

Nirje, B. (1980). The normalization principle. In R. J Flynn, & K. E Nitsch (Eds.), *Normalization, social integration and community services* (pp. 3149). University Park Press.

O'Leary, L., Cooper, S.-A., & Hughes-McCormack, L. (2018). Early death and causes of death of people with intellectual disabilities: A systematic review. *Journal of Applied Research in Intellectual Disabilities, 31,* 325–342. https://doi.org/10.1111/jar.12417.

Olkin, R. (2002). Could you hold the door for me? Including disability in diversity. *Cultural Diversity and Ethnic Minority Psychology, 8*(2), 130–137.

Palliative Care for People with Learning Disabilities Network. (2021). People with learning disabilities and COVID vaccinations. https://www.youtube.com/watch?v=w3mQYfHJ93M.

Peklar, J., Kos, M., O'Dwyer, M., et al. (2017). Medication and supplement use in older people with and without intellectual disability: An observational, cross-sectional study. *PLoS ONE, 12*(9), e0184390.

Rhodes, A., Evans, L. E., Alhazzani, W. et al. (2017). Surviving sepsis campaign: International guidelines for management of sepsis and septic shock: 2016. *Intensive Care Med, 43,* 304–377.

Rickard, W., & Donkin, A. (2018). A fair, supportive society. https://www.instituteofhealthequity.org/resources-reports/a-fair-supportive-society-summary-report/a-fair-supportive-society-summary-report.pdf.

Robertson, J., Chadwick, D., Baines, S., Emerson, E., & Hatton, C. (2018). People with intellectual disabilities and dysphagia. *Disability and Rehabilitation, 40*(11), 1345–1360. https://doi.org/10.1080/09638288.2017.1297497.

Robertson, J., Hatton, C., Emerson, E., & Baines, S. (2015). Prevalence of epilepsy among people with intellectual disabilities: A systematic review. *Seizure, 29,* 46–62. https://doi.org/10.1016/j.seizure.2015.03.016.

Robertson, J., Heslop, P., Lauer, E., Taggart, L., & Hatton, C. (2020). Gender and the premature deaths of people with intellectual disabilities: An international expert consultation. *Journal of Policy and Practice in Intellectual Disabilities, 18,* 80–103. https://doi.org/10.1111/jppi.12360.

Public Health England. (n.d.). Health inequalities: Cancer. https://fingertips.phe.org.uk/documents/Health_inequalities_cancer.pdf.

Public Health England. (2019). Health inequalities: Thyroid disorders. https://fingertips.phe.org.uk/documents/Health_inequalities_Thyroid_disorder.pdf.

Public Health England. (2020). Deaths of people identified as having learning disabilities with COVID-19 in England in the spring of 2020. https://assets.publishing.service.gov.uk/government/uploads/system/uploads/attachment_data/file/933612/COVID-19__learning_disabilities_mortality_report.pdf.

Ruiz, S., Giuriceo, K., Caldwell, J., Snyder, L. P., & Putnam, M. (2020). Care coordination models improve quality of care for adults aging with intellectual and developmental disabilities. *Journal of Disability Policy Studies, 30*(4), 191–201. https://doi.org/10.1177/1044207319835195.

Ryan, A., Taggart, L., Truesdale-Kennedy, M., & Slevin, E. (2014). Issues in caregiving for older people with intellectual disabilities and their ageing family carers: A review and commentary. *International Journal of Older People Nursing, 9,* 217–226. doi:10.1111/opn.12021.

Salvador-Carulla, L., Reed, G. M., Vaez-Azizi, L. M., Cooper, S. A., Martinez-Leal, R., Bertelli, M., Adnams, C., Cooray, S., Deb, S., Akoury-Dirani, L., Girimaji, S. C., Katz, G., Kwok, H., Luckasson, R., Simeonsson, R., Walsh, C., Munir, K., & Saxena, S. (2011). Intellectual developmental disorders: towards a new name, definition and framework for "mental retardation/intellectual disability" in ICD-11. *World Psychiatry, 10*(3), 175–180. https://doi.org/10.1002/j.2051-5545.2011.tb00045.x.

Shefer, G., Henderson, C., Howard, L. M., Murray, J., & Thornicroft, G. (2014). Diagnostic overshadowing and other challenges involved in the diagnostic process of patients with mental illness who present in emergency departments with physical symptoms—A qualitative study. *PLoS One, 9*(11), e111682. https://doi.org/10.1371/journal.pone.0111682.

Simoes, A. (2016). Hospital Mortality Review of Patients with Learning Disability. http://ldcop.org.uk/wp-content/uploads/2016/07/MorReview.pdf.

Smith, M., Manduchi, B., Burke, É., Carroll, R., McCallion, P., & McCarron, M. (2020). Communication difficulties in adults with intellectual disability: Results from a national cross-sectional study. *Research in Developmental Disabilities, 97,* 103557. https://doi.org/10.1016/j.ridd.2019.103557.

Sofair, A. N., & Kaldjian, L. C. (2000). Eugenic sterilization and a qualified Nazi analogy: The United States and Germany, 1930-1945. *Annals of Internal Medicine, 132*(4), 312–319.

Strydom, A., Chan, T., King, M., Hassiotis, A., & Livingston, G. (2013). Incidence of dementia in older adults with intellectual disabilities. *Research in Developmental Disabilities, 34*(6), 1881–1885. https://doi.org/10.1016/j.ridd.2013.02.021.

Taggart, L., Coates, V., & Truesdale-Kennedy, M. (2013). Management and quality indicators of diabetes mellitus. *Journal of Intellectual Disability Research, 57,* 1152–1163. https://doi.org/10.1111/j.1365-2788.2012.01633.x.

Tuffrey-Wijne, I., Goulding, L., Giatras, N., Abraham, E., Gillard, S., White, S., Edwards, C., & Hollins, S. (2014). The barriers to and enablers of providing reasonably adjusted health services to people with intellectual disabilities in acute hospitals: Evidence from a mixed-methods study. *BMJ Open, 4,* e004606. https://doi.org/10.1136/bmjopen-2013-004606.

Tuffrey-Wijne, I., & McEnhill, L. (2008). Communication difficulties and intellectual disability in end-of-life care. *International Journal of Palliative Nursing, 14*(4), 189–194.

Tuffrey-Wijne, I., McLaughlin, D., Curfs, L., Dusart, A., Hoenger, C., McEnhill, L., Read, S., Ryan, K., Satgé, D., Straßer, B., Westergård, B.-E., & Oliver, D. (2016). Defining consensus norms for palliative care of people with intellectual disabilities in Europe, using Delphi methods: A White Paper from the European Association of Palliative Care. *Palliative Medicine, 30*(5), 446–455. https://doi.org/10.1177/0269216315600993.

Turk, M. A., Landes, D. S., Formica, M. K., & Goss, K. D. (2020). Intellectual and developmental disability and COVID-19 case-fatality trends: TriNetX analysis. *Disability and Health Journal, 13,* 100942. https://doi.org/10.1016/j.dhjo.2020.100942.

United Nations. (2006). Convention on the rights of persons with disabilities (CRPD).https://www.un.org/development/desa/disabilities/convention-on-the-rights-of-persons-with-disabilities.html#menu-header-menu.

University of Bristol. (2018). Learning disability mortality review (LeDeR) programme: Learning into action bulletin. https://www.bristol.ac.uk/media-library/sites/sps/leder/WORKINGAspirpneumJulynewsletterfinal2.pdf.

University of Bristol. (2020). Annual report 2019. http://www.bristol.ac.uk/media-library/sites/sps/leder/LeDeR_2019_annual_report_FINAL2.pdf.

van Timmeren, E. A., van der Putten, A. A. J., van Schrojenstein Lantman-de Valk, H. M. J., van der Schans, C. P., & Waninge, A. (2016). Prevalence of reported physical health problems in people with severe or profound intellectual and motor disabilities: A cross-sectional study of medical records and care plans. *Journal of Intellectual Disability Research, 60,* 1109–1118. https://10.1111/jir.12298.

Wark, S., Hussain, R., & Edwards, H. (2016). The main signs of ageing in people with intellectual disability. *Australian Journal of Rural Health, 24,* 357–362. https://doi.org/10.1111/ajr.12282.

Willner, P., Rose, J., Stenfert Kroese, B., et al. (2020). Effect of the COVID-19 pandemic on the mental health of carers of people with intellectual disabilities. *Journal of Applied Research in Intellectual Disabilities, 33,* 1523–1533. https://doi.org/10.1111/jar.12811.

Winters, S. (2022). Hypogonadism in males with genetic neurodevelopmental syndromes. The Journal of Clinical *Endocrinology & Metabolism*, 107(10), e3974–e3989.

World Health Organisation. (2016). *Definition: Intellectual disability.* http://www.euro.who.int/en/health-topics/noncommunicable-diseases/mental-health/news/news/2010/15/childrens-right-to-family-life/definition-intellectual-disability.

World Health Organisation. (2018). *A vision for primary health care in the 21stcentury.* https://www.who.int/docs/default-source/primary-health/vision.pdf?sfvrsn=c3119034_2.

Wolfensberger, W. (1980). A brief overview of the principle of normalisation. In R. J. Flynn, & K. E. Nitsch (Eds.), *Normalisation, social integration and community services* (pp. 7–30): University Park Press.

Woittiez, I., Eggink, E., Putman, L. & Ras, M. (2018). An international comparison of care for people with intellectual disabilities: An exploration. https://english.scp.nl/publications/publications/2018/07/06/an-international-comparison-of-care-for-people-with-intellectual-disabilities.

Young, C., Shankar, R., Palmer, J., Craig, J., Hargreaves, C., McLean, B., Cox, D., & Hillier, R. (2015). Does intellectual disability increase sudden unexpected death in epilepsy (SUDEP) risk? *Seizure, 25,* 112–116.

34

End-of-Life Care: Dying, Bereavement and Loss

Jane Berg

CHAPTER OUTLINE

'Where there's life, death is inevitable. Dying's easy; it's living that's hard. The harder it gets, the stronger the will to live. And the greater the fear of death, the greater the struggle to keep on living.'

—*Mo Yan (Chinese author)*

Very few people expect to die soon, with the possible exception of those who have been exposed to significant poor health or experienced living with violence. This is the case for some older people. With the average age of death in the United Kingdom being almost 80 for men and 83 for women (Office for National Statistics [ONS], 2019), one may be deceived into assuming people who have achieved the age of 80+, 90+ or even 100+ are prepared for the end of their life. This is not necessarily so.

If one looks at the media, it is common to see older people living active lives, taking part in sports, remaining active in business and politics, and continuing to be vibrant and living life to the full. Most of us wish to be in this situation as we age (Fig. 34.1).

The reality is that the average number of years of healthy life has increased over time to approximately 63 (ONS, 2019).

This is variable according to a number of factors, which means in the final decades of life, many people experience poor health.

Many things influence when and how we die and our health status, including socioeconomic inequalities, ethnicity, geographical location, access to health and care services and prevalence of infectious diseases.

Palliative care is a branch of health care that spans the ages and is available from childhood onward. Palliative care is sometimes known as supportive care. The aim is to help preserve and improve the quality of life for people who have a progressive, advanced illness that cannot be cured and they are likely to die from. The illnesses considered progressive and advanced are wide-ranging.

Traditionally, palliative care services were designed primarily to support people with advanced cancer or children born with life-limiting conditions, but over the past few decades, people with other illnesses such as organ failure and neurological diseases have been recognised as benefitting from palliative care. More recently, dementia has been recognised as a life-threatening disease that requires palliative care.

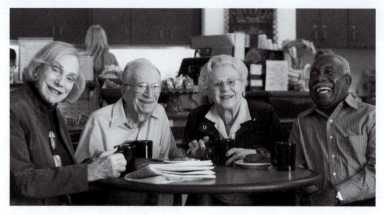

Fig. 34.1 Enjoying an active healthy old age. (monkeybusiness. Depositphotos.com)

There is also recognition that for some people, multiple comorbidities contribute to increasing frailty, which is known to increase risk of death and may be helped by taking a palliative approach.

WHAT IS PALLIATIVE CARE?

It is helpful to consider palliative care in two categories:

- **Palliative care approach:** Provided by many non-specialist health and social care providers, such as community nurses, hospital nurses, general practitioners, social workers and carers, to name a few. This approach focuses on support for a person's health and social care needs with the intention of improving quality of life.
- **Specialist palliative care:** Offered to people who experience complex symptoms that are not easily controlled. In the United Kingdom, it is provided by hospices, acute hospital palliative care teams and community-based palliative care teams.

The term *palliate* means to cover or ease without curing the underlying problem. Palliative care is directed at improving the quality of life for someone whose underlying condition has either progressed beyond the stage where it is possible to aim for cure, or whose illness is one for which no known cure is available.

Palliative care support is not just for people affected by the illness but also for their families through the illness and beyond into bereavement (Box 34.1).

Impeccable assessment is a key component of care and includes understanding what is happening to the person, what contributes to the cause and what the effect is on the individual and people close to them. It also allows for identification of signs and symptoms that may, with the right treatment, be reversed. The prevention of suffering is an integral component, so the palliative care approach tries to anticipate problems associated with the deterioration of a person's disease and avoid or alleviate the suffering. Palliative care isn't just about physical care. Living with a life-threatening disease affects every aspect of life, encompassing the social, psychological and spiritual. At the end of life there may be suffering in any or all these aspects. In order to assess and support someone experiencing distress, palliative care requires a holistic approach and a range of different and complementary skills. Therefore, palliative care teams are multiprofessional, drawing on the skills of doctors, nurses, physiotherapists, occupational therapists, chaplains, social workers and many others.

The development of the hospice movement in the United Kingdom is attributed to Dame Cecily Saunders, who founded

---

BOX 34.1   WHO Definition of Palliative Care

Palliative care is an approach that improves the quality of life of patients (adults and children) and their families who are facing problems associated with life-threatening illness. It prevents and relieves suffering through the early identification, correct assessment and treatment of pain and other problems, whether physical, psychosocial or spiritual.

Addressing suffering involves taking care of issues beyond physical symptoms. Palliative care uses a team approach to support patients and their caregivers. This includes addressing practical needs and providing bereavement counselling. It offers a support system to help patients live as actively as possible until death.

Source: WHO, 2020.

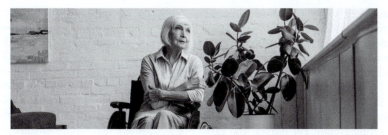

Fig. 34.2 Older people are more likely than others to die in a care home. (VitalikRadko. Depositphotos.com)

St Christopher's hospice in 1967. The hospice movement has developed over subsequent years and influenced the development of services worldwide (Clark, 2005).

Throughout her varied career, Cecily Saunders practised as a nurse, social worker, doctor, academic, researcher and writer. Her focus was on developing expertise to improve the care of dying people. She had a passion for and strong understanding of the way in which patients could benefit from different but combined professional approaches, specifically using expertise to address physical, psychological, social and spiritual needs. Working together, professional groups are able to deliver care using a holistic approach, with the patient and family at its centre.

PLACE AND CAUSE OF DEATH

Where someone dies varies according to their age. Across all ages most people die in hospital, but those aged 75 to 84 are more likely than other age groups to die there. People over 85 are more likely than others to die in a care home. Although increasing age reduces the probability of dying at home (Public Health England, 2018), most people would prefer to die where they normally live, either in their own home or a care home. It is important to know this because nurses are likely to encounter older adults in the last days of life, requiring a palliative care approach whatever setting they work in.

Homes and care homes are predicted to be increasingly common as a place of death over the next few decades, and the ability of nurses in these settings to manage end of life is vital to ensure rates of death in hospital do not increase (Bone, et al., 2018) (Fig. 34.2).

Over the past decade, the leading cause of death for older people changed from ischaemic heart disease to dementia (Office of National Statistics, 2020). A quarter of people over 75 have dementia as the cause or an underlying factor, and deaths from cancer and liver disease have increased. Chronic heart disease and stroke have fallen in the proportion of causes of death. Cause of death is an important factor that influences where someone dies (National End of Life Care Intelligence Network, 2019). Understanding cause of death is important, but as people age, there is a greater possibility they have more than one significant illness. This is known as comorbidity or multimorbidity. It is predicted that the number of older people living with four or more chronic diseases will double from 9.8% in 2015 to 17% in 2035 (Kingston et al., 2018). This has implications for the health and care system, including hospital and care home admissions, costs, quality of life and dependency on a range of services (Age UK, 2019). Multiple morbidity may be experienced alongside frailty, which is when the ageing process leads to multiple body systems gradually losing their in-built reserves (Turner, 2014). Frailty contributes to vulnerability of people to the challenges of long-term illness and slower, less complete recovery from acute episodes. A more in-depth discussion of frailty is given in Chapter 6.

Older people access specialist palliative care services less than younger people (Dixon et al., 2015). Although people 85 and above account for 39% of all deaths, only 16.4% of people in this age group access specialist palliative care services. Dixon et al. (2015) suggested a number of reasons. First, the proportion of older people dying from cancer is lower than that of younger people, and cancer is a trigger for referral to specialist palliative care. Second, older people may have less clinical need, or their needs are not recognised effectively, or perhaps they are under the care of geriatricians who are already providing palliative care. In another study, Lloyd et al. (2015) found the reasons were complex, but it was clear that older people have more unmet needs for symptom relief, less access to general or specialist palliative care and greater information needs than younger people. The triggers that would prompt a referral to specialist palliative care are less clear when someone has multiple morbidities, and therefore the dying phase is more difficult to recognise.

PALLIATIVE CARE AND END-OF-LIFE CARE

These terms are often confused, leading to the assumption that anyone who requires palliative care is approaching death, but palliative care, as illustrated in the World Health Organization's definition, Box 34.1 can be required at any stage of a person's illness. An example is someone who diagnosed with motor neurone disease, a progressive, life-threatening disease with varying survival rates. In this case the symptoms, which develop over time, require attention from specialists in palliative care who can help alleviate some of the distress associated with symptoms and enable the individual to 'live with' and cope with the symptoms.

End-of-life care is the care focused on the last months, weeks or days of a person's life when there may be clear signs they are deteriorating rapidly. For nurses who care for patients with progressive, life-threatening disease, recognising when the end of life is approaching is important but challenging. Clinicians have been shown to be inaccurate and unreliable in their predictions of life expectancy regardless of their professional background. The level of experience of the clinician improves accuracy, as does combining perspectives, where the prognosis is estimated using a team approach (White et al., 2016).

People who work in long-term settings such as care homes are often in a position to identify residents who are changing rapidly, and therefore they can provide background and insight to support decision-making in relation to end-of-life care. This issue is discussed later in the chapter in the section on recognising dying. Noticing changes and acting accordingly can be more difficult for nurses who work in an acute setting if they have been unable to establish an accurate picture of the patient's normal function, mood and behaviour.

Being aware of someone's likely prognosis is helpful, as it informs decisions about their support needs, what interventions are appropriate and how to guide conversations with the patient and their family. (see Case Study 34.1)

SOCIAL CIRCUMSTANCES

A significant proportion of older people (16%) live in poverty (Age UK, 2020). This has implications for choice in where they live and how they obtain care.

About a third of people over 65 live alone (ONS, 2019), and people reaching old age tend to experience a reduction in their social networks. As people become older, they commonly experience the loss of partners, friends and family, leading to a reduction in the social support systems available to them. Loneliness has a detrimental effect on wellbeing. Although age itself isn't thought to cause loneliness, old and very old people are more likely to experience circumstances that contribute to loneliness, such as living alone and reduced ability to participate in social activities.

BELIEFS

People's belief systems influence the way they approach the end of their life. These may be made up of a complex matrix of values, attitudes and a worldview that starts in childhood but is shaped by experience. This complex set of influences

---

CASE STUDY 34.1

Annie Brown was 87 and lived at Orchard Lodge care home. She moved there 5 years ago when her arthritis meant she was unable to manage by herself in the bungalow she had shared with her husband before he died 2 years earlier.

She had slight memory deficit but previously enjoyed joining in care home activities, particularly the Thursday quiz, where her vast knowledge of geography and music made her a popular teammate.

Caroline, Annie's daughter, lived two hours away and visited twice a month.

Care staff had noted over the past few months that Annie had become less mobile to the point where she needed two carers to help her stand and walk short distances. She frequently declined meals, telling staff she wasn't hungry. She lost 12 kg and now weighed 47 kg. Annie had become breathless and reported feeling a tightness in her chest. The GP visited, and she was referred to the hospital, where she had an extensive examination, blood tests, X-rays and a CT scan. She later attended the hospital again for a lung aspiration. The journey to the hospital was tiring for Annie, and each time she seemed to take a day or two to recover.

Annie was diagnosed as having stage 3 mesothelioma in her left lung. She was able to tell the consultant that as a teenager she had worked in a laundry washing workers' overalls from the local ship building yard. She recalled how asbestos dust flew off the laundry as she loaded it into the machines.

The consultant suggested chemotherapy would relieve the breathlessness, but it wasn't possible to cure the disease.

Annie felt strongly she didn't want to have to go back to the hospital for treatment. She asked to go back to the care home, where she knew the staff and felt they understood her. With the support of her GP and community palliative care team whe felt confident she would receive the care she needed.

---

shapes how we see ourselves in the world or universe and can be termed spirituality. Spirituality is a broad term but is often misinterpreted as religion. For some people, their faith is an important part of who they are, but people without a faith can equally have a strong spiritual belief.

We live in a multicultural society where individuals come from different cultures but interact throughout their lives with people who have a different view of the world, shaping and possibly incorporating other views into their own (Fig. 34.3).

It's important not to assume people can be categorised by specific aspects of their spirituality, so asking 'What is

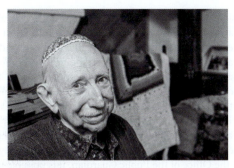

Fig. 34.3 Understanding and respecting the culture and religions of others is vital in end-of-life care. (creatista. Depositphotos.com)

important to you?' can be a very powerful question that helps a care team to understand a person's priorities and care for them in a way that respects their individuality.

TALKING ABOUT DYING

Older people are not a homogenous group. Many things influence their willingness to think and talk about death and dying, including culture, beliefs, experiences of death and who they are able to talk to.

Talking about dying is not easy for many people, including health and social care practitioners. Health care professionals have their own reasons why they may not be able to have these conversations, but in providing care for people toward the end of their lives, it is important to do so.

Planning ahead for someone's care involves knowing what is important to them in advance of the time information is needed. As a person deteiorates, they may lose the ability to communicate or think about what they want (Case Study 34.2). This is a particular feature of changed cognitive ability such as for people with dementia. Planning ahead, or advance care planning, is helpful in guiding care providers and allowing them to provide the care the person wants.

Advance care planning should be voluntary (NHS England, 2022). If a person has said that they do not want to discuss their future plans, it is important this is documented so the wider care team is aware, but as circumstances change, they may feel able to do so at a later stage.

Trigger points offer the opportunity for people to be able to think about their care, and nurses need to be able to recognise the cues and respond by supporting the person to make and record their plans.

Trigger points for planning ahead and discussing advance care include
- The death of a partner or friend
- A change in circumstances (e.g., moving to a care home)
- An acute episode of illness
- A hospital admission

CASE STUDY 34.2

Ada is 86 and lives alone in a bungalow. She has two daughters, who live a long distance away from her. Six months ago her husband died in a local care home where he had lived for a short time when his dementia meant he was no longer safe to live at home.

Following her husband's death, Ada has talked regularly about what she wants for when she dies. She has revisited her will to update it and made it clear to her daughters she wants to go to White Rose Care Home just down the road if she needs more care. She is familiar with the home, having helped out at their annual fete for some years. It is a cheerful, slightly untidy home her daughters would not have thought her first choice.

She has also told her daughers what she wants for her funeral. She wants a cremation and her ashes and her husbands' scattered on the local beach (Fig. 34.4) where they went for their Christmas Day walk for 10 years before he became too ill. She has planned a menu of smoked salmon sandwiches and champagne for the picnic they should take when they scatter the ashes—their traditional Christmas brunch.

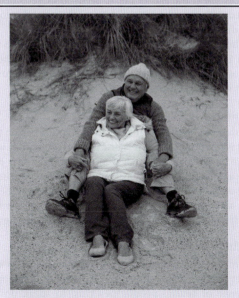

Fig. 34.4 Happy memories shape preferences for future decisions about the scattering of ashes. (Wavebreakmedia. Depositphotos.com)

The plan may include anything important to the person, such as ongoing contact with pets or continuing to observe relgious ceremonies. It may be focused on physical circumstances such as what treatments are acceptable or what they refuse. It can also include their preferences for after-death care such as what form of funeral they want. Kathryn Mannix is a strong avocate of talking openly about death and dying and emphasises the importance of learning what is important to the the individual and giving them the opportunity to plan ahead.

We are all individuals, and one persons plan may not be a good fit for another who, outwardly at least, appears to be in a similar situation. Enabling people to be architects of their own solution is key to respecting their dignity. They are only in a new phase of life: they have not abdicated personhood. (Mannix, 2017)

The people close to the person, their family and friends, may be a barrier to these discussions as they equally find it difficult to confront their own feelings about a loved one dying or contemplate a time in the future when more care is needed or the person dies. In some cases a professional caregiver asking about someone's end-of-life preferences can be a relief if they have not been able to talk this through with their family. (see Case Study 34.2)

TYPES OF ADVANCE CARE PLANNING DOCUMENTATION

Once someone has expressed a view about what their preferences are at the end of life, it needs to be recorded and shared with the relevant care teams. The type of information dictates where and how it is recorded.

The documentation below relates specifically to England. For other countries it is important to check the law, process and requirements that apply. The relevant government website is the best place to start.

Advance Statement

An advance statement is an opportunity for the person to say what is important to them—for example, where they would like to be cared for, who they want with them, if they prefer to be alone, and what personal habits or routines are important, such as wearing makeup, having a whisky in the evening and listening to music. These elements are important to helping the person retain their individuality and dignity.

Lasting Power of Attorney

If someone anticipates they may become unable to speak or act for themselves, it is possible in advance to appoint someone or several people they trust to speak on their behalf. Two aspects of life that may need an attorney are health and welfare and property and financial affairs. It is possible to appoint attorneys for one or both. A health and welfare lasting power of attorney comes into effect only if someone becomes incapacitated, but a property and financial affairs power of attorney may be used as soon as it is registered if the individual prefers someone else to take responsibility for their finances , or becomes unable to do this themselves (see Case Study 34.3).

The documentation for both lasting powers of attorney is available on the government website https://www.gov.uk/power-of-attorney. Once completed, it needs to be registered with the Office of the Public Guardian. It is possible to complete the process without legal advice, but if there is any doubt about a person's capacity, a solicitor should be involved.

CASE STUDY 34.3

Alice was fiercely independent and had lived alone since the death of her husband 15 years earlier. She was generally well and enjoyed going out and meeting friends from her church, and she took regular trips to the local supermarket, using a taxi when she felt unable to walk up the hill home. Her son and his family lived on the same street and saw Alice regularly.

She had always been very astute with money, and although she had known times of poverty, she took pride in always paying her bills on time.

Alice became ill very suddenly one evening, and an ambulance was called. She was diagnosed as having had a left-sided cerebrovascular accident. Over the next 3 weeks it became clear it had affected her speech, understanding and ability to walk.

Her son, Bill, and his wife visited regularly, and when it became clear she was not going to be able to return home soon, they collected her post, emptied her fridge and made the house secure.

Among the post were two bills Bill knew his mum would want paid as soon as possible. He considered himself fortunate to be able to pay for them knowing how important it was to her that she wasn't in debt.

He was able to reassure her all was well. She died a week later after a further cerebrovascular accident.

Bill felt some comfort in knowing that without having access to her money, he had been able to make sure she did not owe anything when she died , something he felt would have caused her great distress. He realised at other times in his life he would not have been in a position to pay the bills on her behalf and how distressing he and Alice would have found it.

Several months after her funeral, Bill appointed a lasting power of attorney for himself for property and financial affairs.

Someone who has been appointed as an attorney can make decisions about treatment, where the person lives and what care they receive. They can also sign medical consent forms on behalf of the person. It is possible to check if someone has appointed an attorney by consulting the Office of the Public Guardian at https://www.gov.uk/find-someones-attorney-deputy-or-guardian.

Advance Decision to Refuse Treatment

An advance decision to refuse treatment is a legally binding document also known as a living will that is used only when someone feels strongly that they don't want a particular treatment. It could be for a number of reasons, such as religious belief or because someone doesn't want life-sustaining treatment such as artificial ventilation or cardio-pulmonary resuscitation. It is possible to make an advance decision to refuse treatment independently. Documentation is available on a number of websites (e.g., https://compassionindying.org.uk/choose-a-way-to-make-an-advance-decision-living-will).

The document needs to be valid, signed and witnessed, and applicable to the situation. It needs to be worded in such a way that expressly says the treatment is refused 'even if my life is at risk or may be shortened as a result'. It is also necessary to specify the circumstances in which the treatment is refused. It is important that the person making the advance decision to refuse treatment understands its implications and when and how it will apply, so seeking legal advice may be helpful.

Do Not Attempt Cardio-Pulmonary Resuscitation

Many nurses have witnessed an attempted cardio-pulmonary resuscitation (CPR) and therefore have an appreciation they can be traumatic events that subject the patient to an aggressive form of treatment that, by its nature, is undignified. Nurses may also have cared for patients after a cardiac arrest and know about the potential for reduced quality of life, including musculoskeletal injury, neurological damage, further cardiac damage and psychological consequences such as depression (Resuscitation Council UK, 2015).

For someone in previous good health, a resuscitation may be able to return them to a good quality of life. For someone who is living with a life-threatening illness or becoming increasingly frail, there is a strong possibility the resuscitation will not be successful or that the added physical burden will reduce their quality of life.

When someone is in a situation where their heart stopping may be anticipated, it is best practice for the patient, significant family members and the doctor to agree what action will be taken when this happens. Unfortunately there is not a high level of awareness among the general public about the poor success rate of CPR and the consequences of the intervention. The conversation should include a discussion about the predicted success and consequences of a resuscitation attempt so the patient and family are fully informed and able to contribute meaningfuly to the discussion.

Some people believe the preservation of life is so important they will want an attempt to be made even if this results in reduction in quality of life. Others believe their heart will stop when it is their time to die so do not want an attempt to resuscitate. This is a personal decision.

People in the United Kingdom have the right to refuse a treatment by making an advance decision to refuse treatment order but do not have the right to insist on having a treatment, including CPR, if the doctor feels it would be futile. Ideally the decision should be a shared one. However, if the doctor or senior clinician completes a do not attempt CPR order without patient or family agreement, they must make the family aware it has been done.

The record of the decision not to attempt resuscitation is not legally binding and can be amended at any time. It should be reviewed regularly. In some settings the form can be signed by a senior nurse with appropriate training and experience if local policy allows (BMA;RCUK: RCN, 2016).

In some areas of the United Kingdom, the decision about resuscitation is incorporated into a recommended summary plan for emergency care and treatment, which allows for recording decisions about other potentially life-threatening situations as well as cardiac arrest.

Whatever method is used to record decisions, it is very important that all the care team are aware of them so the appropriate treatment can be given when a situation occurs.

Recognising Dying

Sometimes it is only in hindsight we can identify the deterioration in someone's condition as they move toward the end of life.

It is common to see subtle changes such as declining mobility, reduced appetite, increased susceptibility to infections and perhaps social and emotional withdrawal from previous interests and activities. These changes can happen over a period of months or quite suddenly.

In many cases it is possible to recognise when people are actively dying as opposed to gradually deteriorating. This is sometimes referred to as the terminal phase or the last few days/hours. The signs of active dying include
- Reduced engagement and lack of energy
- Long periods of sleep or semi-unconsciousness
- Reduced desire to eat or drink
- Reduced need to pass urine or stools
- Changes to breathing (e.g., becoming shallow or laboured)
- Changes to skin colour and cooling as circulation slows
- Changes to the colour of the lips or nail beds as breathing becomes less efficient
- Restlessness or confusion

It is important that the multidisciplinary and wider care team understand a person is approaching the end of their life. The emphasis of care then becomes comfort to support the person and their family to reduce distress as far as possible.

Communication

'How people die lives on in the memories of those who live on' (Saunders, 2006).

Communicating with dying people and their families can be challenging, but compassionate, open and clear communication is key to good care. Older people may have specific sensory deficits that mean there are barriers to communication that require communication skills. In-depth discussion of communication with older people is covered in Chapter 25.

Ideally, communication should be face to face, where the use of body language and touch can support what is communicated verbally, but sometimes circumstances mean communication needs to be done at a distance. This may be in cases where the family member is geographically distant and discussion or breaking bad news needs to be done by telephone or video link. If possible, the same principles and stages should be used to direct the conversation. Additionally, it is helpful to establish that there is immediate support available.

When people are unable to be present with the person who is dying, videoconferencing is increasingly used to help patients connect with their family and friends. Supporting an older person in a video call may involve instructing them on how to use the equipment or physically holding the device and connecting if they are unable to do it themselves. The value is that loved ones can say their goodbyes and have a sense of being involved. For the nurse, it may mean more awareness and closer involvement in final conversations that in other circumstances they might withdraw from to respect the privacy of the patient and family.

The need to communicate at a distance is often because of geographical distance or lack of access to transportation, but in 2020 distancing was caused by the risk of infection from COVID-19. The additional challenges of the need for face masks and visors meant voices were muffled and non-verbal communication such as facial expressions hidden. Importantly reassuring touch was limited for safety reasons. The effects were exacerbated if someone had dementia or hearing or vision impairment. To mitigate the effects of wearing personal protective equipment, conversations should be deliberately slower and clearer with introductions made even to people who have met before, as personal protective equipment may make people less recognisable or distinguishable from colleagues. Facial expressions may need to be exaggerated and the volume of voice raised.

There are two distinct forms of communication. The first is where time is set aside specifically for sharing some news. It is possible for the health care professional to set the scene and think in advance about how to apply a specific approach. Models of communication models are available, such as SPIKES (Buckman, 2005):

S Get the **s**etting right, and ensure privacy.
P **P**erception: find out what they know and understand.
I Ask the patient for an **i**nvitation to talk.
K Share your **k**nowledge.
E Address **e**motions using empathy.
S Agree on a **s**trategy and summarise.

Although it is often the role of medical colleagues to break bad news such as a diagnosis or prognosis, nurses also need to be prepared. Bad news is anything that negatively changes a person's view of their situation. Significant bad news in the context of end-of-life care may be having to tell a relative someone has died or deteriorated. Less significant but potentially distressing bad news may be that a visitor they were looking forward to having isn't able to come.

The second form of communication is more informal and can be initiated by the patient, family or health care professional.

It is important the whole care team be open to being asked questions and alert to cues about when someone might want to talk. Invitations to ask questions or share concerns should be part of every interaction with the patient and family. People choose who they feel comfortable sharing their feelings with. It could equally be the health care assistant who is helping them in the bathroom or the nurse responsible for their care plan. This is another example of where a coordinated team approach is important so the team can share and support each other where appropriate.

When someone feels able to talk, active listening and focusing on them can help alleviate distress. Conversations can be encouraged by questions such as 'You seem distressed today. May I ask what you are concerned about?' Using reflecting, summarising and paraphrasing can help to demonstrate active listening and attempt to understand and support.

Not only does the person choose who they talk to, but they also choose the setting (Fig. 34.5). The family member may need to have a separate conversation with the nurse away from the patient to be comfortable asking questions they don't want to ask in front of the patient. Nurses should be sensitive to cues that a family member is indicating they wish to continue the conversation as the nurse moves away from the patient to leave the room or patient's home. This may result in conversations being conducted in corridors or on front doorsteps, where the setting might not be ideal for privacy or comfort. In this case it is important to be certain that any information shared is done so while respecting the confidentiality of the patient (Fig. 34.6).

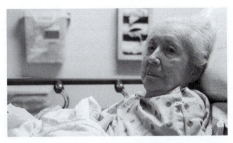

Fig. 34.5 Some settings are challenging when trying to have conversations about difficult issues. (fotoluminate. Depositphotos.com)

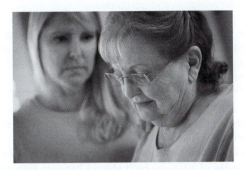

Fig. 34.6 Active listening skills are helpful in understanding the patient and family. (Feverpitch. Depositphotos.com)

MANAGING SYMPTOMS

Managing symptoms well is important to ensure the best quality of life as someone deteriorates and approaches the end of their life.

Common symptoms experienced toward the end of life are
- Pain
- Nausea and vomiting
- Dyspnoea
- Sore mouth
- Constipation
- Poor appetite
- Distress and anxiety

For all these symptoms, assessment is key to understanding and treating. A cycle of assessment, treatment, evaluation and reassessment is needed as the situation changes.

A variety of tools can be used to record assessment accurately; some are discussed below. Assessment can be done in a number of ways, including observation, clinical measurement and asking the person when possible.

It is important to find out from the patient what symptom they find most distressing and not to assume their priorities. For example, if someone has lived with a chronic lung condition, they may not be as distressed by breathlessness as observation might suggest. An individual's belief systems impact how they feel about the symptoms and what they would want the care team to focus on. To have an accurate assessment, a combination of observation, talking with the person and clinical measurements gives the most accurate picture. Recording of symptoms is important, as a person's condition may change hour by hour toward the end of their life, and the reassessment may be completed by a different member of the team. Recording 'pain improved' does not in itself help colleagues know if the treatment is the right one. The same statement reinforced with a numerical value, what treatment was given and any other contributing factors is far more helpful.

As a person approaches the end of their life, the treatment for each symptom needs to be balanced with the possible discomfort or side effects and the possible benefit. If the person has expressed views about their preferences at the end of life, they will be enormously helpful in deciding on the course of action. An example is someone who has an acute infection toward the end of their life and has stated they definitely don't want to die in hospital. The decision could be that oral antibiotics are given in their home. Another individual in the same situation who wants to live for as long as possible might be taken to hospital for administration of stronger intravenous antibiotics, even though there is a high risk it will mean they die in hospital.

The goal of treatment and care needs to be adjusted for someone who has a life-limiting condition. After any reversible cause of symptoms should be addressed. The overall goal is maintaining comfort, dignity and preserving independence for as long as possible.

Pain

Pain is an experience we all have, and a person's perspective on pain can change with many different factors. Cecily Saunders coined the phrase *total pain*, which acknowledges our experience of pain can be influenced by many factors: physical, psychological, social and spiritual (Saunders, 2001).

Many older people live with chronic conditions, some of which cause pain. It is important to maintain any treatments that have been found to help when possible. However, as the end of life approaches, modifications may need to be made. For example, someone living with chronic arthritis pain may have managed it with mild analgesics and exercise. As the end of life approaches, the medication needs to be reviewed, and as exercise becomes difficult, it may need to be replaced by passive limb movements and the use of warm/cool packs to control pain.

It is possible a person will experience more acute pain, which needs to be investigated and treated.

Assessing pain is vital to being able to treat it successfully, and the assessment needs to be ongoing. When

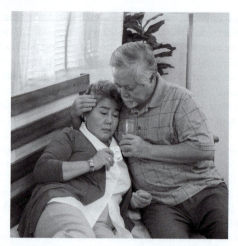

Fig. 34.7 Observing posture and facial expression can be important in assessing pain. (mkitina4. Depositphotos.com)

CASE STUDY 34.4

Sarah has lived at Downing Place Care Home for 9 months. She worked in the theatre as a director for many years until she retired 27 years ago. For many years after retirement, she ran the local branch of the Women's Royal Voluntary Service. She still has a large social circle with friends who visit most days.

Sarah was diagnosed with colon cancer 3 years ago and had surgery. She is known to have secondary abdominal deposits.

The abdominal pain Sarah experiences is treated with regular analgesia and top-up doses.

The staff regularly reassess her pain and note that her requests for top-up analgesia are much lower on some days than others. By careful observation and recording, they notice a pattern of higher analgesic use when Sarah does not have any visitors.

---

assessing pain, observation is an important element (Fig. 34.7). The things to note are as follows:

- Is the person holding themselves differently from usual?
- Do they appear agitated?
- What are their facial expressions?
- Are they moving in a way to guard a part of their body?
- Is there anything about where they are and what they are doing that seems to change the pain?
- Do they look pale or flushed?
- Are they groaning or calling out?

Observational assessment is always important (see Case Study 34.4) but becomes more so when people are unable to articulate details of their pain. This is often the case with people with cognitive or communication difficulties.

A number of tools exist assess pain using observation and recording the observations. Pain assessment in advanced dementia (PAINAD), the Abbey pain scale and Doloplus-2 are commonly used (Scofield, 2018), but the accuracy of tools is variable, and training on their use is important (Schofield & Abdulla, 2018).

If someone is able to answer questions about their pain, a simple question of level of pain can be a helpful guide.

Pain is complex, so using more in-depth questions provides more accurate assessment. The SOCRATES mnemonic is helpful to remember what questions to ask:

Site: Where is the pain?
Onset: When did it start? Does it change over time?
Character: How would you describe the pain (e.g., shooting, stabbing, aching)?
Radiation: Does the pain go anywhere else?
Associations: Are there any other signs such as redness or swelling?
Time: Is it worse at any particular time of day?

Exacerbation: Does anything make it worse or better?
Severity: What level is it?

It is possible an older person has a number of sources and types of pain, so each should have its own assessment. For example, if someone has a malignant tumour, there may be pain from the tumour itself, but a distinctly different pain could simultaneously be experienced from metastases or constipation. It is sometimes useful to have a drawing of a figure in the patient's notes so different pains can be drawn, described and identified separately.

Pain can be classified into two major types. The most common is nociceptive pain, which is the body's response to stimulation of the nociceptors. It can be either visceral (i.e., associated with internal organs) or somatic (i.e., associated with tissues such as bones and skin). The second type is neuropathic, which refers to damage to the nervous system (Watson et al., 2016).

Each type of pain presents with different patterns, and an accurate assessment helps identify the type of pain and therefore what treatments might help.

In 1986 the World Health Organization (WHO) devised a step approach to medications for cancer pain (https://www.who.int/cancer/palliative/painladder/en). Although it is helpful in guiding treatment for pain in palliative care, it has also been used in the management of chronic pain.

The WHO step approach guides prescribers through the use of non-opiates to mild opiates to strong opiate analgesics. At each stage an adjuvant could be prescribed alongside the analgesic. An adjuvant drug is one that is not an analgesic itself but is known to enhance analgesic action. An example is antidepressants, which can be very helpful with neuropathic pain.

In many situations pain is a useful protective mechanism the body uses to indicate potential or actual injury and warn us to change our behaviour or investigate the cause. However, in palliative care often the cause is known and cannot be treated. The use of PRN (i.e., as necessary) analgesia is not helpful, as the underlying cause may not be reversible. Palliative analgesia should be given regularly in order to keep the pain from returning.

The oral route is familiar for people and the preferred route when possible, but if it becomes difficult, injectable medication is required. Suppositories are also available, but the range of medications is limited, and administration can be less acceptable.

Drugs by intramuscular or subcutaneous injection can be fast and effective. In palliative care, medication may be needed regularly, so to avoid the discomfort of regular injections, a continuous subcutaneous infusion device such as a McKinley syringe pump is often used.

A syringe pump is a safe and comfortable way to control symptoms by administration of subcutaneous drugs if the oral route is inappropriate because the patient has become unable to swallow or has nausea and vomiting. It allows for the administration of several drugs at the same time. This can be extremely helpful when the patient is experiencing multiple symptoms, but care needs to be taken that the drugs mixed in a continuous subcutaneous infusion are compatible. Dickman and Schneider (2016) provided comprehensive information about how to use a syringe driver and drug compatibilities, but nurses also need to follow local policy about the training and competency required before using a syringe pump. Once pain is controlled, there needs to be regular reassessment, as it is likely to change over time. Depending on local policy and the care setting, regular analgesia may be prescribed over a dose range that can be varied according to the assessment or supplemented with PRN doses. Flexibility is particularly helpful if the pain is exacerbated by something like movement.

The care team needs to know what side effects to observe for when administering any drug and what action to take if they are observed. For example, morphine, the opiate of choice for severe pain (NICE, 2012 [reviewed 2016]), commonly causes constipation, nausea and drowsiness. A regular laxative should be prescribed prophylactically, and an antiemetic should be available if needed.

There is a proven close association between mind and body that is often seen in pain levels. Pain tends to be exacerbated by emotions such as fear, anxiety or boredom and can be less distressing when someone feels safe, secure or engaged in activity.

This is just one illustration of how important a team approach to palliative care is. Involvement of the wider team, such as activity coordinators, occupational therapists and faith leaders, may significantly contribute to the management of pain for some people in conjunction with the pharmacological methods.

Nausea and Vomiting

Although nausea and vomiting are often thought of together, they are two distinctly different things that can occur together or separately.

Assessment is the key to appropriate treatment. There may be a number of causes, including the following:

- Pain
- Constipation
- Raised intercranial pressure
- Anxiety
- Metabolic disturbance
- Post radiotherapy
- Gastrointestinal obstruction
- Infection
- Drug/substance induced (e.g., analgesics, antibiotics, alcohol)
- Poor oral condition
- Unpleasant smells

Understanding the cause helps identify what can be done to address the nausea or vomiting. Pharmacological treatments are one method, but there are many other things that may help, such as addressing constipation, removing or masking an unpleasant smell, ensuring the mouth is clean and comfortable, upright positioning and providing a breeze to the face through a fan or opening a window. Acupuncture and hypnotherapy may also help.

Dyspnoea

Shortness of breath is an unpleasant symptom of many diseases that can be particularly frightening. Assessment is the first stage of support. Understanding the cause informs treatment decisions.

The individual's history should indicate the possible causes. If the onset of breathlessness is sudden, it may be infection, cardiac arrhythmias, anaemia, pleural effusion, superior vena cava obstruction, pneumothorax, pulmonary emboli or infection, or psychological. These causes should be treated when possible.

Commonly used medications include bronchodilators, steroids and antibiotics. Low-dose opioids are sometimes helpful in reducing the sensation of breathlessness, and oxygen is used if the person is hypoxic.

A number of non-pharmacological interventions may help, including positioning upright to allow expansion of the chest or leaning forward to allow expansion of the back of the lungs. The patient should indicate which is most comfortable. The use of fans to the face or a breeze from an open window may also help, but fans are not advisable if there is the possibility of airborne or droplet infection such as COVID-19 due to the risk of spreading infection (Marshall, 2020)

Whatever position is comfortable is often maintained for some time, so the person needs to be supported in an appropriate bed or chair with pillows. The maintenance of one position clearly puts the person at risk of skin ulceration caused by pressure, so careful attention to skin care and the use of pressure-relieving devices needs to be a priority.

Physiotherapy and occupational therapy can be very important in managing breathlessness; however, the goal of any treatment is to maintain comfort and independence rather than seeking to rehabilitate in the conventional sense.

Whatever the cause of breathlessness, most people benefit from a calm, reassuring approach from those around them. Activity may exacerbate difficulty breathing, so it is helpful to think about activity levels and how they might be reduced. If a person is at home, it could mean suggesting rearranging the home to enable easier access to the toilet.

It may be helpful to have a conversation with the patient to find out what activities they want to prioritise so their efforts can be directed and help can be provided.

Fatigue

Fatigue is a common feature of end-of-life care. Energy levels drop, and daily activity becomes difficult and exhausting. Managing fatigue starts with assessment as fatigue can be caused by a number of things, including anaemia, sleep disturbance and poor diet.

Often the disease process is responsible, and managing fatigue is something to be approached by the multiprofessional team. Anaemia may be possible to reverse, and steroids are sometimes helpful in increasing energy levels and appetite.

People sometimes feel they need to carry on with activity during the day, but reassessing what their priorities are and discussing with them how energy can be managed can give them strategies to maintain the activities they most value (Case Study 34.5) (Fig. 34.8).

Possible strategies include
- Sitting down to complete activities such as washing, showering and food preparation
- Building rests into the daily routine
- Using convenience foods more
- Spreading out activity through the day
- Gentle exercise
- Accepting help with tasks
- Not sleeping for too long
- Good sleep hygiene

CASE STUDY 34.5

Harry lived alone. As a former soldier, he liked to keep his home neat and tidy. Routine was important to him. He became increasingly breathless with end-stage chronic obstructive pulmonary disease.

Harry received support from the community nursing team and was clearly struggling to continue to do all the household chores and maintain his hygiene. By the time his daughter Judith finished work and came to visit, he was exhausted and could tolerate only a short visit, frequently falling asleep as they watched the news together.

The community nurse suggested Harry would benefit from help in the home, but he frequently dismissed it as not necessary. He felt it was important not to 'give in' and to keep to his usual routine.

It was clear the fatigue was making everyday tasks extremely difficult.

The nurse talked to Harry and suggested it would be helpful to develop a strategy for managing his fatigue. The things identified as being most fatiguing were washing and dressing, making his meals, cleaning the flat and talking to Judith. The nurse suggested Harry consider which of these he felt he should 'spend' his energy for the day on. He identified being with Judith as his main priority and his second to be washing and dressing. He realised that to be able to continue to do those things, he needed help with cleaning and food preparation. He was still not happy but accepted the help as part of his fatigue management plan.

Anorexia

Culturally, food and drink are vitally important (Fig. 34.9). Family celebrations, religious festivals and ceremonies have food and drink as an integral component. In addition, most people see food as a way of nurturing loved ones—of showing love and affection and helping ill people recuperate.

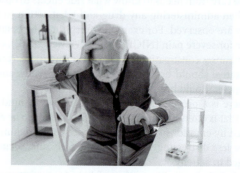

Fig. 34.8 Fatigue is a common symptom and affects all aspects of daily activity. (HayDmitriy. Depositphotos.com)

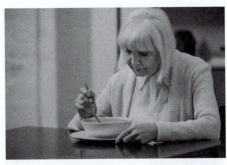

Fig. 34.9 Food and drink are an important part of life, both for physical well-being and for social and cultural reasons. (AllaSerebrina. Depositphotos.com)

It is no surprise that when someone approaches the end of their life, and their appetite wanes, it causes distress for their carers for them. As activity slows and the body becomes less able to process or utilise food, the amount required drops. Taste can change, as can the ability to manage different consistencies. Carers may become distressed at the reduced amount the person is eating. It is a common misconception that feeding someone at the end of life helps them stay stronger for longer. In fact, eating more than necessary is likely to make them tired and uncomfortable.

Conversations with concerned families about eating can be difficult, but it is helpful to acknowledge how important it is. Food at the end of life is not just for fuel for the body but for enjoyment and comfort.

Helpful strategies include the following:
- Small amounts more frequently
- Well-presented food (e.g., the use of smaller plates is less off putting)
- Experimenting with different tastes
- Using alcohol as an appetite stimulant if the person enjoys it
- Using finger foods if using cutlery is difficult
- Avoiding 'healthy' versions of food (e.g., low-fat yogurt if only a small amount is possible)
- Focusing on preferred foods

Supplement drinks can be helpful, but most people do not choose them over a favourite food, and they should be avoided as meal replacements.

Oral Discomfort

Oral health is important, as lack of attention can lead to unnecessary suffering and distressing physical and psychological symptoms. Someone who is breathless—particularly someone on oxygen therapy, has lost weight, is on certain medications or is drinking little can be particularly at risk. Issues encountered at the end of life include a dry mouth, ulceration, drooling and infection. Caring for the mouth is sometimes overlooked but can be of huge importance to the patient at the end of their life.

Assessment of the mouth should start with asking the person if they have any discomfort and what they normally do to look after their mouth. An examination of the mouth should be done using a torch. Oral assessment tools are available and guide a detailed assessment and record of findings.

As someone becomes dependent on others to perform oral care, ideally the tools they are accustomed to should be maintained and adapted if necessary. A small-headed toothbrush with toothpaste may be the most familiar and comfortable. Dentures should be cared for as usual.

Candidiasis or oral thrush is a common fungal infection in which white plaques are seen on the inside of the mouth or tongue. Antifungal treatments can help, but the form given needs to take account of the ability of the person to take medication or retain local treatments in their mouth. A dry mouth is very common. Small sips of fluid, ice chunks, sucking sweets and regular cleaning of the mouth can help (Health Education England, 2019).

Hygiene and Skin Care

Enabling a person to continue to care for their own hygiene needs may be important to them. Even when someone is very weak, it may be possible for them to do some of hygiene for themselves. Gradually there is a shift to a member of the care team taking over and helping maintain skin integrity and comfort. Poor dietary and fluid intake, lack of movement, poor circulation, lack of oxygen in the blood and incontinence are contributory factors to skin being at risk of damage. Skin care should be considered in the context of the patient's overall condition and aim to prevent damage when possible and use comfort measures when not. Assessment of the skin is covered in Chapter 24. In palliative care, it is important to note the colour, any areas of potential risk such as bony prominences, external moisture levels from sweating or incontinence, presence of breaks in the skin and changes such as swelling. The surface the person is lying on needs to be specifically designed for avoidance of pressure ulcers and extreme care taken with moving and washing. The frequency of moving the patient should be planned on an individual basis with the need to keep the patient comfortable as the primary goal. In addition to preserving skin integrity, the need to move joints to limit stiffness and the amount of distress caused by movement are factors to consider.

Individual hygiene and grooming are a big part of who we are as individuals. The patient or family can offer a guide about what is normal for the patient. Getting it wrong in terms of how they like to appear can be upsetting for the patient and family, so a care plan should include how they wear their hair, how often they shave, what makeup they

CASE STUDY 34.6

Jackie was 12 when her granny died. Granny had been admitted to hospital after a cerebrovascular accident and was unconscious before she got to the ward.

Jackie's parents debated if she should be taken to see her granny when it became clear she was going to die soon. They decided Jackie should be allowed to say goodbye as they were very close, and they felt she was able to cope with the reality of the situation. Jackie really wanted to do it.

When she visited, she was very quiet at first, then she cried and held her granny's hand as she said goodbye.

Many years later Jackie and her mum were talking about Granny and her last few days. What Jackie recalled as the most upsetting part of the visit was seeing Granny's facial hair. She had no idea women could grow hair like that. She was embarrassed to mention it as she knew Granny would be mortified at anyone seeing it. For her this was the ultimate indignity.

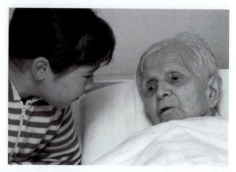

Fig. 34.10 Getting care right at the very end of life is important for everyone involved. (Anetta.Depositphotos.com)

like to wear, whether they use deodorant or perfume, and any other personal details (Case Study 34.6).

The Last Few Hours

Getting care right in the last few hours is extremely important not only for the patient but also their families and care team (Fig. 34.10).

Recognising when that stage is reached is challenging, particularly for staff who have not spent time with the patient. Often it is individuals in close proximity such as health care assistants who recognise subtle changes.

The changes that may be seen are the patient withdrawing from interaction with others, becoming semiconscious or unconscious, eating and drinking less, skin discolouration, changes to breathing, confusion and having visions.

Communicating that the end of life is close to family members can be very difficult, but the benefits are that it allows them time to prepare mentally and say goodbye.

The communication needs to be sensitive but clear and may need to be repeated to help people absorb the news. Usually, family want honest, clear communication, but predicting the amount of time left is extremely difficult. Admitting uncertainty but using phrases such as *soon* or *very soon* or saying someone is sick enough to die (Mannix, 2017) can help the family adjust their thinking and on a practical note decide who should be there and if any other family members need to be informed.

The understanding of what constitutes a good death has been explored many times in literature and is subject to much debate, but the important thing to remember is

the person dying and their family have their own set of circumstances that dictate if it is considered a 'good death'. Commonly in the literature, being free from distressing symptoms is a feature, as is the presence of family and accordance with the individual's belief system.

If the patient has a detailed advance care plan, it forms part of the blueprint for what the care team is trying to achieve.

Compassion, dignity and respect are key aspects of caring for someone at the end of their life. The patient and family should feel it in all interactions. Being with someone as they approach the very end of their lives is a privilege but a responsibility. Everything said and done by the health and care team involved may be remembered by the family as part of their reliving the experience.

When a death is expected, there is the opportunity to shape the experience to a certain extent. The way the dying person is approached, spoken to and touched while providing care and the willingness of the caregivers just to be there can influence the experience of death.

Supporting the psychological and spiritual well-being of the patient and family is equally important as managing their physical care.

Families need to be given time to be with the patient and talk to them, hug them and if appropriate perform rituals according to their beliefs. Being in such an intense situation is draining, and key family members may need time away from the bedside to eat, wash and change and just to reflect, cry or get angry. In situations where the family is unable to be at the bedside for a patient's final moments to say goodbye, kiss, hug and perform rituals, their experience of grief may be more complex. This was seen during the COVID-19 pandemic, when large numbers of people died and visitors were unable to be present, which is known to be a risk factor for complicated grief (Gesi et al., 2020).

The perceived wisdom is that people prefer not to die alone, but every death is unique, and anecdotally nurses have noted sometimes the moment when a key relative is away from the bedside for a few minutes is when the person dies. Although there is no way of gathering evidence on this, it may be some people prefer to take their last breath in private. Control over the moment of death cannot be proven, but many nurses have also noted sometimes the anticipated arrival of a significant person or date can delay death beyond the time predicted.

Knowing the wishes of an individual guides care in many ways, but there needs to be a balance between wishes and practicalities. For example, if someone expresses a wish to die at home, it needs to be balanced with understanding of the ability of the family to cope with their care needs with the services available to them. Older people living alone may not be able to achieve this, or if they are living with a spouse or partner, a lot depends on their ability to provide care when they themselves are likely to be older.

Once the place of death is certain and symptoms are controlled so the patient is comfortable, things can be done to support the patient and family through this time (Case Study 34.7).

Physical Changes in the Last Few Hours

Physical changes in the last hours of life can be alarming, but understanding them offers the opportunity to inform and support the patient and their families. Although the patient may appear unconscious, it is impossible to know if they can hear, so it is important everyone continues to address them as if they were conscious.

CASE STUDY 34.7

David had a history of cardiac problems starting when he was in his 50s when he experienced his first myocardial infarction. In his late 80s, he was dying in an acute hospital ward following another myocardial infarction and acute heart failure.

It was recognised that he was dying and would not survive discharge home. Reluctantly he agreed to stay on the ward. His friends and family visited him often. His son Tom told the nurses about how David loved music, mainly operatic and men's voice choirs.

Fortunately, a side room was available, and Tom was encouraged by the nurse to play David's favourite music as he drifted into unconsciousness and eventually died. The vicar from David's chapel visited him before he died, as did his friends from the Masonic lodge.

Recalling his father's death afterward, Tom reflected that although he was unable to be at home, David died as he lived—with friends, family and music around.

The ability to eat and drink may be lost, but maintaining the comfort of a moist mouth and lips can be done with small amounts of cool water or a favourite drink. Lips can be dry, so a salve may help. This is something the family can be encouraged to do if they are present.

Confusion and restlessness are common at the end of life, and some people appear to see visions of people who have already died. This can be either comforting or distressing. The restlessness may have a physical cause such as a full bladder or bowels. Elimination can be managed by providing urinals or bedpans as long as possible, but provision of pads that are changed regularly may be more comfortable than a urinary catheter. Adults usually have a strong aversion to urinating in bed, so they need to be reassured it is acceptable, and they will be cleaned and made comfortable afterward. These conversations can mark a loss of dignity so should be done as sparingly and sensitively as possible. In the last few hours, the kidney function slows as major organs shut down, so the amount of urine produced is likely to be very small. Bowel management can be problematic and should be guided by any discomfort. If the person hasn't had their bowels opened for some time but has no discomfort, it is better not to take any action.

If restlessness continues and is causing distress, sometimes anxiolytics or sedation are necessary. It is important to know what the person wants, and if possible it should be discussed with them and their family.

Hygiene and skin care need to be viewed in light of the current condition of the patient. There is no place for 'routine' washing in the last few hours, but a face or hand wash or a wash of the underarms and back might help if someone seems uncomfortable, particularly if they are sweating. Using the opportunity when changing a pad or bedsheet to check for pressure area damage is helpful, but turning someone for the sake of long-term skin protection is not appropriate. Gentle limb movements might prevent discomfort from stiffness. Junior or inexperienced staff may need support to understand why routine washing and moving are not always appropriate. Care should be individualised and based on knowledge of the patient and regular assessment.

Pain, nausea and vomiting or breathlessness may emerge as symptoms in the last few hours and should be assessed and managed as above.

Breathing patterns change in the last few hours, sometimes slowing and becoming shallower. Cheyne-Stokes is a pattern of breathing where periods of apnoea are followed by deep breaths. It can be alarming and tense as families wait for the person to take the last breath and die. In addition, sometimes the person's inability to clear their airway by sighing or coughing means a build-up of fluid in the airways results in a distinctive rattle, sometimes known as a death rattle. Once the rattle is heard, it is possible to prevent it from getting worse with medication such as hyoscine (e.g., butylbromide or hydrobromide) or glycopyrronium (Watson et al., 2016). The secretions already formed will not be helped, but a change of position for the patient may reduce the rattle. It is surprising that this rattle doesn't appear to distress the patient, but for relatives it can be very alarming, so reassurance that it doesn't cause the person to choke or feel uncomfortable may help.

As circulation slows, the person's extremities become cooler and tinged blue or grey.

Care After Death

The point of death is often very poignant. When a nurse is present, families often turn to them for confirmation. It's important the nurse is confident this is the case (Fig. 34.11). Depending on the setting, some nurses are able to officially verify death using a set procedure, but in others a doctor or senior nurse is called to confirm death has occurred. If the nurse is not able to confirm officially, saying, 'Yes, I believe so' and outlining the way it will be verified is helpful. Often the family knows, as the person appears to relax, there is a clear absence of breathing and pulse, and the extremities become colder.

Families may choose to spend time with the person who has died or begin rituals for the dead. The care given to the body depends on the situation and the beliefs of the person and their family. It is helpful to make sure before the family are left alone or leave the care setting that they have a clear idea of the next steps and where they can get help if needed.

Bereavement Loss and Grief

Loss is a profound human experience that refers to something or someone no longer being available. This can be an object or a relationship.

Bereavement is loss through death, and grief is the emotion felt following a death. Bereavement incorporates many different losses, such as the loss of companionship, security and lifestyle. Each bereavement is personal, and the grief people feel can be influenced by many things, such as their relationship with the deceased, their social and emotional support networks, the nature of the death and what the loss of that person means to their own life.

The way grief affects a person can be physical emotional, and cognitive (Fig. 34.12).

Physical reactions include
- Headaches
- Muscular aches

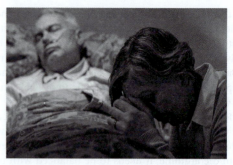

Fig. 34.11 During the last few hours of a patient's life, the family needs care and support. (CandyBoxImages. Depositphotos.com)

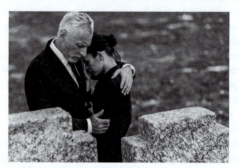

Fig. 34.12 Loss is a profound experience, and rituals are often comforting. (AndrewLozovyi. Depositphotos.com)

- Nausea
- Tiredness and exhaustion
- Menstrual irregularities
- Loss of appetite
- Pain
- Insomnia
- Tenseness
- Sensitivity to noise

Emotional reactions include
- Sadness
- Anger
- Guilt
- Jealousy
- Fear and anxiety
- Shame
- Relief
- Emancipation
- Powerless/hopelessness
- Pining
- Emotional pain
  Cognitive reactions include

- Obsessive thoughts
- Inability to concentrate
- Fantasising
- Apathy
- Dreams
- Disorientation and confusion
- Continued thoughts about the loss
- A sense of the deceased's presence (i.e., hallucinations)
- Attempts to understand or rationalise the loss (Gross, 2016)

Models of grief may aid in understanding the pathways people take on their journey. One often quoted is that developed by Kubler-Ross (Kubler-Ross, 1969), which identifies stages of grief through which people who are dying or bereaved may go: shock/denial, anger, bargaining, depression and acceptance. More recently a model proposed by Stroebe and Schut (1999) recognises people often oscillate between confronting the grief and returning to normality, or between loss and restoration.

There is no standard pattern, and each experience of grief is unique to the individual and the bereavement they have experienced. It is a natural reaction that varies in intensity over time. In most cases, particularly when death occurs after a long illness, grief eventually reduces to a level that allows the bereaved to return to their life, adjusted to incorporate the loss. For some people, the grief is complicated, and they may need specialist support to help them manage.

Nurses can help the bereaved by taking time to listen and remembering that bereaved people often need to tell their story many times as a way of transferring their experience into a memory instead of reliving it as a reality (Mannix, 2017). It is also important that bereaved people receive practical help in terms of their daily lives. In the acute stage of grief, the bereaved sometimes need reminding to eat, drink, sleep and look after themselves. Later there may be a need for help in learning new skills and tasks that help them to adjust to life without the deceased person. Volunteer services are available in some areas to provide listening and practical advice. Specialist services are available for people who are experiencing more complex or prolonged grief, and they may be delivered by volunteers or health care professionals.

Personal and Team Resilience

Caring for a dying person can be emotionally and professionally challenging for many reasons. It may be that staff working in a community setting or care home have known the patient/resident for some time, and the nurse or carer also experiences grief following the death.

It may also be that staff absorb some of the suffering associated with the situation. Sometimes it is difficult not to be reminded of personal loss. People have different levels of resilience, and it is important in working as a team that all members receive support to allow them to continue to deliver high-quality, compassionate care.

Team debriefs, clinical supervision and informal support mechanisms help. Nurses who manage a team should be aware of what is available and offer a variety of support.

CONCLUSION AND KEY LEARNING POINTS

Caring for people at the end of their lives is a privilege and a challenge.

KEY LEARNING POINTS

- Care should be individualised and recognise the uniqueness of the individual.
- To meet the variety of needs for an individual, a multiprofessional approach achieves the best outcome.
- Assessment is the starting point, and regular reassessment is needed as the situation changes.
- Older people and their families are not always prepared for the end of life.
- Many people live the last decades of their lives with diminished health and multiple morbidities.
- Nurses in all care settings need to be able to deliver end-of-life care and able to refer patients to specialist services when necessary.
- To ensure end-of-life care is person-centred, a thorough holistic assessment of physical, psychological, social and spiritual history and current status is needed.
- Giving people the opportunity to plan ahead for their future care needs ensures what is important to them is recognised.
- Recognising when someone is actively dying is especially difficult if they have been deteriorating over a longer period of time.
- Symptoms that cause distress should be actively managed until the moment of death and where possible anticipated.
- Grief is a normal reaction to bereavement; nurses are in a position to support people experiencing grief and refer to bereavement services if appropriate.

REFERENCES

Age UK. (2019). Later Life in the United Kingdom 2019, s.l.: Age UK.

Age UK. (2020). Reports and briefings. [Online] https://www.ageuk.org.uk/globalassets/age-uk/documents/reports-and-publications/reports-and-briefings/money-matters/poverty_in_later_life_briefing_2019.pdf#:~:text=The%20link%20between%20low%20income,relative%20poverty%20and%20material%20deprivation.

BMA, RCUK, & RCN. (2016). *Decisions relating to Cardopulmonary Resuscitation* (3rd ed., 1st revision). British Medical Association.

Bone, A., Gomes, B., Etkind, S. N., Verne, J., Murtagh, F. E. M., Evans, C. J., & Higginson, I. J. (2018). What is the impact of population ageing on the future provision of end-of-life care? Population-based projections of place of death. *Palliative Medicine, 32*(2), 329–336.

Buckman, R. (2005). Breaking bad news. The S-P-I-K-E-S strategy. *Psychosocial Oncology, 2*, 138–142.

Clark, D. (2005). *Cicely Saunders founder of the Hospice Movement Selected Letters 1959-1999.* Oxford University Press.

Dickman, A., & Schnieder, J. (2016). *The syringe driver* (4th edition). Oxford University Press.

Dixon, J., King, D., Matosevic, T., Clark, M., & Knapp, M. (2015). *Equity in the provision of palliative care in the UK: Review of evidence.* Personal Social Services Research Unit.

Gesi, C., Carmassi, C., Cerveri, G., & Carpita, B. (2020). Complicated grief: What to expect after the Coronavirus pandemic. *Frontiers in Psychiatry, 11*, 489.

Gross, R. (2016). *Understanding grief: An introduction.* Routledge.

Health Education England. (2019). Mouth Care Matters. [Online] http://mouthcarematters.hee.nhs.uk/wp-content/uploads/sites/6/2020/01/MCM-GUIDE-2019-Final.pdf.

Kingston, A., Robinson, L., Booth, H., Knapp, H., & Jagger, C. MODEM Project. (2018). Projections of multi-morbidity in the older population in England to 2035: Estimates from the Population Ageing and Care Simulation (PACSim) model. *Age and Aging, 3*(1), 374–380.

Kubler-Ross, E. (1969). On death and dying. Routlage.

Lloyd, A., Kendall, M., Carduff, E., Cavers, D., Kimbell, B., & Murray, S. A. (2015). Why do older people get less palliative care than younger people? *European Journal of Palliative Care, 23*, 132–137.

Mannix, K. (2017). *With the end in mind.* Harper Collins.

Marshall, K. (2020). Breathlessness: Causes, assessment and non-pharmacological management. *Nursing Times, 116*(9), 24–26.

National End of Life Care Intelligence Network. (2019). *Death in people aged 75 years and older in England in 2017.* Public Health England.

NICE. (2012, reviewed 2016). *Palliative care for adults: Strong opiates for pain relief.* NICE.

NHS England. (2022). *Universal Principles of Advance Care Planning.* NHS England.

Office for National Statistics. (2019). Health state life expectancies, UK: 2016 to 2018. [Online] https://www.ons.gov.uk/peoplepopulationandcommunity/healthandsocialcare/healthandlifeexpectancies/bulletins/healthstatelifeexpectanciesuk/2016to2018#healthy-and-disability-free-life-expectancy-in-the-uk.

Office for National Statistics. (2019). National life tables, UK: 2016 to 2018. [Online] https://www.ons.gov.uk/peoplepopulationandcommunity/birthsdeathsandmarriages/lifeexpectancies/bulletins/nationallifetablesunitedkingdom/2016to2018#:~:text=1.,for%20males%20and%20females%20respectively.

Office for National Statistics. (2019). Office For National Statistics. [Online] https://www.ons.gov.uk/peoplepopulationandcommunity/birthsdeathsandmarriages/families/datasets/livingaloneintheuk.

Office of National Statistics. (2020). Leading causes of death, UK: 2001 to 2018. [Online] https://www.ons.gov.uk/peoplepopulationandcommunity/healthandsocialcare/causesofdeath/articles/leadingcausesofdeathuk/2001to2018.

Public Health England. (2018). Statistical commentary: End of life care profiles, February 2018 update. [Online] https://www.gov.uk/government/publications/end-of-life-care-profiles-february-2018-update/statistical-commentary-end-of-life-care-profiles-february-2018-update#:~:text=Main%20findings,-This%20update%20shows&text=in%202016%2C%20almost%20half%20of,deaths%20.

Resuscitation Council UK. (2015). Guidelines Post—Resuscitation Care—Resuscitation Guidelines 2015. https://www.resus.org.uk/library/2015-resuscitation-guidelines/guidelines-post-resuscitation-care.

Saunders, C. (2001). The evolution of palliative care. *Journal of the Royal Society of Medicine, 94*, 430–432.

Saunders, C. (2006). *Selected writings 1958-2004.* Oxford University Press.

Schofield, P., & Abdulla, A. (2018). Pain assessment in the older population. What the literature says. *Age and Ageing, 47*, 324–327.

Scofield, P. (2018). The assessment of pain in older people. UK National Guidelines. *Age and Ageing, 47*, i1–i22.

Stroebe, M., & Schut, H. (1999). The dual process model of coping with bereavement: rationale and description. *Death Studies, 23*(3), 197–224.

Turner, G. (2014). *Introduction to frailty, fit for frailty.* British Geriatrics Society.

Watson, M., et al. (2016). Palliative Adult Network guidelines, 4th ed. Bedfordshire and Hertfordshire, London Cancer Alliance, Northern Ireland, PallE8, RM Partners, Surrey Sussex and Wales.

White, N., Reid, F., Harris, A., Harries, P., & Stone, P. (2016). A systematic review of predictions of survival in palliative care. How accurate are clinicians and who are the experts? *PLoS One, 11*(8), e0161407.

World Health Organisation. (2020). Palliative care, key facts. https://www.who.int/news-room/fact-sheets/detail/palliative-care.

35

The Role of Technology and Digital Tools in the Care and Support of Older People

Rebecca Jarvis, Jonathan Darley, Caroline Chill, Fay Sibley, Denis Duignan

CHAPTER OUTLINE

Our population is ageing, and there is a growing demand for care. This environment places increasing demands on the care system and care workers in terms of the location, quantity and type of care required. With the rapid emergence of digital technology, there is an opportunity to rethink the way services are delivered, reconfiguring the care system to better meet the challenges of caring for a population of older people that is larger and has more complex needs than ever before.

Digital technology is now part of everyday life for much of the population and is rapidly transforming the ways in which we both work and live. Communicating via email or videoconferencing is becoming the norm, and access to advanced digital technology in the form of smartphones and other internet-connected devices is widespread. It is crucial that health and care services keep pace with the constantly changing technological environment around us, and we are seeing how digitisation is requiring us to adopt new ways of working to benefit patients and improve efficiency and sustainability.

The adoption of digital tools and technology was accelerated by the COVID-19 pandemic, but other key factors driving it include

- Increased internet access and digital literacy among older people
- Increasing sophistication of technologies, enabling more effective monitoring
- A greater focus on data and use of artificial intelligence algorithms to improve clinical decision making

- Greater availability of devices that are easy to use and affordable
- Greater focus on interoperability between devices and electronic patient record systems
- More consistent assessment and evaluation criteria for approval of digital tools and apps for use within the NHS

The emerging technologies being introduced to support the delivery of care services can generally be broken down into the following categories, depending on their goals:

- Devices and technology used by individuals to promote and protect independence and well-being
- Tools to improve communication between people and health and care services
- Monitoring of long-term conditions and well-being
- Technology focused on assisting professionals in the delivery of care

Each of these categories is explored in this chapter, with examples to illustrate the rapidly evolving use of technology in care.

PROMOTING AND PROTECTING INDEPENDENCE

Living Independently

Most older people want to live independently and safely in their own homes. Technology can help them do that, even if they are living with frailty or have memory problems.

Telecare systems are designed to offer a safety net for people with care needs living independently. They operate by sending a warning to a call centre, carer, friend or family member if there is a problem detected in the home such as falling, inactivity, fire, flood or gas leak.

By remotely monitoring an older person's activity and other factors in their home, the technology helps keep them safe and independent. It also provides reassurance to family and friends who live far away. Telecare devices can prevent a problem before it occurs or send a timely alert if something goes wrong.

Many people are familiar with the concept of a personal alarm triggered by an individual if they need to call for help, but there is also a growing market in sophisticated activity-monitoring systems that raise an alert when sensors in the home detect potential problems.

There are two main types of telecare systems:
- Systems connected to a professional monitoring centre that is staffed at all hours
- Smart systems that send alerts and updates directly to family members via an app

Local authorities may fund the use of telecare systems as part of a care package for some people if they meet certain criteria, but many older people or their families are purchasing these systems privately to provide peace of mind.

Smart Technology

Smart technology is increasingly being used as a form of telecare. Smartphones can be used to monitor the movements or activity of individuals if they are equipped with specific apps. Alternatively, dedicated smart devices, such as movement sensors and smart plugs, can be connected to a base unit using a Wi-Fi signal.

Alerts from connected devices are then sent directly to family, friends or carers via a broadband or mobile phone connection. For example, alerts can be configured to be shared about what time the person gets out of bed, when they leave or return to the house, or when they put the kettle on.

One example is the Howz Home Care Kit. The Howz software learns patterns of behaviour and allows an older person and their friends, family or carers (with the right permissions) to monitor health indicators. It spots changes in routines, which are often an early indication of health deterioration. Case Study 35.1 depicts Howz in action.

Some people find it difficult to use a smartphone in a way that supplies enough information to be useful for monitoring purposes, especially if they have poor dexterity. For these people, voice-controlled smart hubs and smart speakers can be used instead.

Risks related to smart technology may not be immediately obvious, but they do need to be acknowledged and managed carefully. For example, voice-activated assistants rely on a Wi-Fi network and main power and thus are vulnerable to outages. In a scenario where a user is heavily reliant on their assistant, it could create unacceptable risks to a person's safety.

Data governance is also crucial. Participants in the Argenti Partnership Echo trial needed an Amazon account, meaning Amazon held some of their personal data, including any conversations held through the Echo device. Other smart hubs or digital assistant devices such as Google's Nest and Apple's Siri have similar information-sharing considerations to bear in mind. Robust data governance policies are a priority, and the person should be at the centre of making informed decisions about how their data is used wherever possible.

Although none of this technology replaces the need for human contact and physical care, it can provide an additional means to enable people to continue to live with the level of independence they want.

CASE STUDY 35.1

Ernest is 96 and enjoys getting out and about and meeting his friends for morning coffee. He stopped driving last year but catches a bus most mornings to the local supermarket, where he is the oldest of a little group who meet up in the café for a daily natter. He has lived in his three-bed semi for 54 years and plans to stay there for as long as possible. He has spent the last 14 years living on his own since his wife died.

Howz gives him the reassurance that his family will be alerted to any change in his routine.

Ernest said, 'I like to go out of a morning. If I do that, it helps with the rest of the day at home, and it is very good to stop loneliness. Apart from that, my son, Jim, comes up and collects me on a Saturday morning, and I go there for lunch.'

His independence and routine are very important to him. 'Having Howz is a comfort because I know if I didn't follow my routine and get up and about, someone would know. There was one occasion when I was sick and didn't get out of bed. Jim got an alert and called me. The system isn't intrusive at all; we are just all reassured it is there. I'm a lucky man. I have a caring family, and this lets them know everything is okay.'

Jim is glad he installed Howz in his dad's home, especially for the early warning he got when Ernest was

CASE STUDY 35.1— cont'd

poorly. He said, 'We tried one of the early Howz kits, and at first it was a great novelty. I kept joking with my dad about how many cups of tea I could see he was drinking. As time went on, I guess we both got more used to it, and I started to rely more on the alerts. Last year I was away on holiday in Malta, and I got an alert to say the usual movement hadn't been detected in dad's home. I called him straight away, and it turned out he had been really sick so was ill in bed. It wasn't life or death, but at his age, it could have become more serious. He is a very proud man and wouldn't have wanted to make a fuss, so I am not sure he would have called anyone. Although I was away, I was able to get hold of my brother, who popped in to check on him and see what he needed. It is a really practical example of Howz in action.'

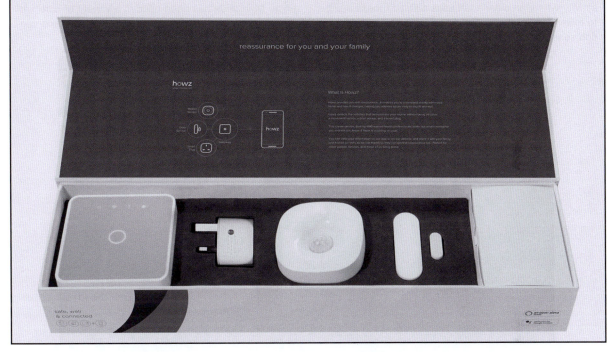

BOX 35.1   Argenti Partnership Echo Trial

The Hampshire Argenti Partnership—a partnership between Hampshire County Council, Argenti and the local government association—ran a trial in 2018 to use voice-controlled technology to help people live more independent lives (PA Consulting, 2020).

In the trial, Amazon Echo smart speakers were deployed in the homes of 50 people with care needs. The Echo's functionality was tailored to each person to provide personalised support for their daily routines. Functionality included setting reminders for medication and calendar appointments for people with memory problems, adding items to online shopping lists so carers could shop for housebound individuals, and turning on music, podcasts and the news to help people stay connected. The devices also helped people control their own environment by turning on appliances.

The results were very positive, with two-thirds of the people in the trial being able to regain some degree of independence for the first time in a significant period. Participants also reported feeling less isolated, and almost half the participants reported a reduced reliance on others. Additionally, the trial showed the technology could reduce the burden on informal carers.

Getting and Staying Active

Supporting older people to keep physically, cognitively and socially active is a key part of long-term care. Many studies have shown regular physical activity and meaningful interaction with wider society helps improve physical and mental functions as well as reverses some effects of chronic disease to keep older people mobile and independent (Cooney et al., 2014; McPhee et al., 2016).

Game-based interventions for older adults support these types of activities by keeping the brain and body stimulated and active (Kovisto & Malik, 2020) (see Box 35.2).

BOX 35.2   Memoride

Memoride is an example of physical, social and cognitive activity where an older adult uses a static fitness device to follow familiar cycle routes through a screen. The motion sensor allows the technology to work with the user as they cycle to create a unique and meaningful experience. Memoride has been used in a variety of care settings and proven to trigger positive memories and conversations.

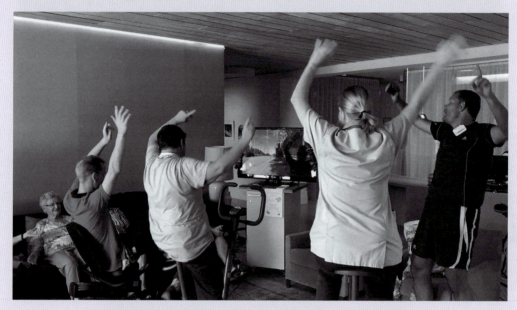

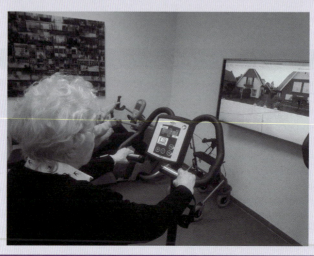

Virtual reality (VR) is also emerging as a technology solution to enhance the lives of older people and less physically able patients. VR games have been shown to have positive clinical effects for balance and mobility compared with no treatment or conventional interventions (Neri et al., 2017).

VR headsets are relatively easy to use and can allow older care home residents to explore immersive experiences to stimulate and entertain. A wide variety of virtual reality devices and programmes are available that aim to support the physical and mental well-being of older people, but the evidence supporting their effectiveness is only beginning to emerge.

IMPROVING COMMUNICATION

Patient Access and Digital Inclusion

In recent years, great progress has been made to help people communicate with health and care services, including giving patients access to important parts of their health care records.

BOX 35.3   Primary Care Digital Access Tools

- Patient Access by EMIS Health
- SystmOnline by TPP
- myGP by iPlato
- Evergreen Life by Evergreen Health Solutions
- NHS app

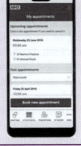

Note: Examples are not exhaustive.

In primary care, patients can generally make and view appointments, review prescriptions, see vaccination histories and interact with their GP via one or more digital tools. The precise functionality varies depending on the electronic record system used by the GP.

In secondary care, digital tools such as the NHS e-Referrals Service, Dr Doctor, Healthcare Communications and Zesty allow patients to view and manage upcoming appointments. These tools are evolving at pace, developing wide-ranging features designed to improve patient experiences.

Progress is also being made to enable patients to view records held by multiple organisations as a single unified record. For this to be achieved, significant technical infrastructure and cross-organisational working is required:

- Medical records must be digitised.
- Records from many different sources must be combined.
- Patients must have a secure platform to view their information.

Recently many portals, apps and websites have become available to patients, offering a variety of capabilities such as viewing clinical summary information, inputting patient reported outcome measures and managing appointments. These include the NHS App and products such as Zesty, patientsknowbest and mymedicalrecord.

GP practices have made rapid strides in digital communication, with many adopting options for consulting via secure email-based services such as eConsult and Doctorlink, which can direct patients to self-help information as well as enable a response from a clinician.

Increasing use of specialist digital communications platforms such as AccuRx can enable secure video consultations and act as a portal for patients to send information to their GP for inclusion in their health care record.

Shared Electronic Urgent Care Records

Shared electronic care plans enable patients' wishes and clinical recommendations about their future care to be viewed by the health and social care providers who care for them. Shared care records can also be accessed by urgent care providers 24/7 in a medical emergency, such as GP out of hours services, 111, ambulance services, urgent care centres and hospital emergency departments. See Box 35.4 illustrates

---

BOX 35.4   Coordinate My Care

Coordinate My Care (CMC) is a shared electronic urgent-care–planning system currently being used in London to provide more coordinated and personalised care to people in the event of an emergency or at the end of life. Most people want to die at home, and dying in the place of your choice is used as a marker of the quality for end-of-life care. But across most of the United Kingdom, only 45% of people actually do die at home or in a care home (Public Health England, 2018).

CMC (2020) data show a clear correlation between patients having a CMC plan and achieving urgent care and end-of-life wishes. Studies have shown that when people have a CMC plan, only 18% of them die in hospital compared with 54% nationally (CMC, 2020). There is also evidence that CMC plans enable more appropriate use of health care resources and reduce inappropriate hospital admissions (CMC, 2020). A study undertaken in 2013 demonstrated the average cost of treating patients in their last 6 months of life was over £2000 lower for individuals with a CMC plan than those without (Bakhai et al., 2014).

the power of digital communication across different parts of the health system that enables patients wishes be taken into account at the end of life.

Safe and effective sharing of patient care records supports provision of higher-quality person-centred care, giving a voice to the patient on how and where they wish to be cared for as well as supporting the patient in having to tell their story only once. Holding 'need to know' information, records include specific clinical information, the person's care preferences in anticipated deterioration as well as their end-of-life wishes.

Additional Considerations for Digital Communications Tools

There is a widespread expectation that using digital tools to change modes of communication and access to information can benefit patients and health systems. At this stage, the supporting evidence for this is mixed, as academic studies in this area often evaluate small sample sizes or very specific interventions. However, there is anecdotal and real-world experience to suggest these interventions can support individual-level or system-level improvements.

For example, considering an operational perspective, two studies at different NHS trusts suggested use of a digital, patient-facing appointment booking system reduced the appointment 'did-not-attend' rate by by 8.5% (Drdoctor. co.uk, 2020) and 17.2% (Bartlett et al., 2018).

Although more rigorous academic studies are required to validate these results, the data supports the simple hypothesis that making it easier for patients to see and change their appointment slot increases the likelihood they attend. This clearly benefits patients through providing access to the care they need. However, it can also significantly benefit health providers and systems, given the wasted time and cost of missed appointments (Bartlett et al., 2018; Drdoctor.co.uk, 2020).

As discussed earlier, digital tools are also being used to improve patient access to clinical information. It is suggested it may provide patients with a better understanding of their condition and give them a greater sense of control of their care. In turn, it may lead to improved clinical outcomes through better adherence to medicines and clinical advice. Many studies are assessing these approaches in different diseases and patient groups. One meta-analysis in diabetes supports the finding that sharing electronic health records with patients is effective in reducing HbA1c levels, a major predictor of mortality in type 2 diabetes (Neves et al., 2020). Although the results are promising, care should be taken in immediately assuming these trends would apply to other populations or disease areas.

An important implication of all digital health interventions is a potential to increase health inequalities through the concept of digital exclusion. People may be digitally excluded because they cannot access devices, cannot access the internet or do not possess the fundamental skills or confidence to use the devices or systems required. Although digital exclusion has been falling, in 2018, 10% of the United Kingdom adult population had never or not used the internet in the past three months (Ray et al., 2020).

Health care policy makers and providers therefore need to consider how to avoid increasing health inequalities as the use of digital communication tools becomes more widespread. This may involve more direct training and funding of digital skills in hard-to-reach patient populations and ensuring any new tools are designed with the needs of these users in mind.

The COVID-19 pandemic revealed and brought to prominence the vast disparities that have an impact on Black, Asian and minority ethnic communities within health and care. Improved access to digital support and services may provide new opportunities to reduce health inequalities.

Examples of work to improve digital access to older people; Black, Asian and minority ethnic communities; and other groups include the Good Things Foundation's Digital Health Lab (https://digital-health-lab.org/), which aims to widen NHS digital participation. The foundation works with the NHS and other partners to bring digital health inclusion to communities who are most excluded. One of the projects is the Tower Hamlets pathfinder, which assists Black, Asian and minority ethnic groups with the tools and information to access a GP or online services and to co-design ways to reduce exclusion. Other projects include work to support isolated older people, people who are homeless, people living with dementia, people with sensory impairments and people with long-term conditions.

There is also the question of maintaining adequate quality for digital tools used in health and care and ensuring common standards are adhered to in order to support interoperability. Digital tools endorsed by the NHS must go through robust acceptance and review processes to ensure they are technically sound, secure and fit for purpose, and they conform to modern accessibility standards. Currently, this process is managed by the government's digital transformation body for health and social care, NHSX.

Management of Long-Term Conditions

There is a growing use of digital tools and technologies in the management of long-term conditions, where there is a significant opportunity to improve patients' understanding of their disease and help them minimise the impact of the condition on their day-to-day life. Given older patients are more likely to be living with long-term conditions, digital solutions can play an important role in their care. In this section, we consider how digital technology is being used for the management of long-term conditions in older people.

Providing Information

Many organisations are developing apps and websites to provide condition-specific information to patients in their care. This is in addition to providing direct care, aiming to educate and reassure patients and improve experience and outcomes.

Care Providers

Example. Torbay and South Devon's Rheumatology Connect app includes

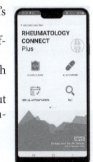

- High-quality information about different conditions and medications
- Specific information about the 6-month period post-diagnosis
- 'Meet the team' (i.e., information about the department's staff and direct contact details)
- Clinic locations
- Video instructions for exercises

There are numerous other examples, designed by NHS and non-NHS organisations, that patients will increasingly encounter. They are often offered through app stores where rankings are based on download statistics and user ratings, and previous work has shown there is little correlation between user ratings and whether an app adheres to established evidence-based practices (Wyatt, 2015).

It is increasingly difficult for clinicians to keep track of reliable digital sources of information and decide whether to endorse particular apps or websites. The current state of evidence for mobile health interventions, including apps, is relatively immature, as the clinical effectiveness of many health apps has not been established yet and cost-effectiveness information is only beginning to emerge (van Velthoven & Powell, 2017). The NHS has established a process to assess health apps. NHS staff should endorse only apps that have gone through this process and been added to the NHS Apps Library.

Remote Monitoring

Remote physiological monitoring uses devices to measure metrics such as blood pressure, temperature, weight, pulse rate and oxygen saturation. It can also refer to the measurement of disease specific measures (e.g., blood sugar for diabetic patients) outside of a hospital or care environment. It may involve the use of consumer technology or more specialised equipment. Examples include the Free-Style Libre blood glucose monitoring system for diabetes management and vital signs measurement technologies to

determine deterioration of patients in care homes using the National Early Warning Score (NEWS2) (NHS England, 2020).

Remote monitoring is a rapidly evolving area, with increasing attention being placed on the benefits and risks of these approaches for both patients and health and care systems. Some benefits include

- Reassurance of patients and empowerment to self-care
- Beneficial clinical outcomes from timely awareness of physiological changes
- Potential for earlier discharge of patients
- Reduced need for face-to-face follow up appointments
  However, there are also potential risks:
- Inducement of anxiety and worry from constant monitoring
- Difficulty managing increased clinical load from alerts, especially in cases of a false positive, where a clinical investigation or intervention is triggered where none is required

For remote monitoring to be effective, a number of challenges need to be overcome:

- Teaching and supporting patients and carers to use and maintain devices appropriately
- Appropriate and timely interpretation of the results, including an agreed understanding of how results are acted on and how they may alter management and care
- How information security risks are addressed if data is transferred between systems; although any devices in clinical use should have processes in place to minimize these risks, nurses and other caregivers should be mindful of security

As well as physiological measurements, digital tools allow patients to regularly self-report and share information on symptoms and well-being. Although patient-reported outcomes have been used in paper format in many medical facilities for some time, digital approaches significantly increase the frequency and ease of which they can be completed. Self-scoring may give clinicians greater insight into how the patient is feeling and help inform a more person-centred approach to care. See Box 35.5 of Safe Steps, a digital falls-risk assessment tool.

THE IMPORTANCE OF MANAGING EXPECTATIONS, PUBLIC CONFIDENCE AND TRUST IN DIGITAL HEALTH

The proliferation of health technologies issued to patients and those being adopted autonomously—such as smart weighing scales, blood pressure monitors and smart device

BOX 35.5   Safe Steps, A Digital Falls-Risk Assessment Tool

For the 11.6 million older people living in the United Kingdom, falls represent a major problem, with six people falling every minute. Forty percent of people who suffer from a fall are left with a moderate or extensive injury. Falls account for approximately 40% of hospital admissions from care homes across the United Kingdom and cost the NHS nearly £2.2 billion per year. The impact of falls often goes beyond the physical, with over one-fifth of people losing their confidence and being more at risk of falling again.

Safe Steps is a digital fall-risk assessment tool designed to reduce the number of falls in care homes. Based on the NICE guidelines, Safe Steps uses a set of assessment questions to create individual, personalised care plans that allow care homes to proactively implement a review process whereby vulnerable residents can be identified and receive appropriate care, thus reducing their risk of falling.

Accessed via a secure, cloud-based app, Safe Steps provides a digital audit trail for Care Quality Commission reporting requirements and reduces the amount of paperwork created in a care home. A study of 148 health and care organisations in the Wirral demonstrated the app reduced falls by 28% and ambulance calls by 20%.

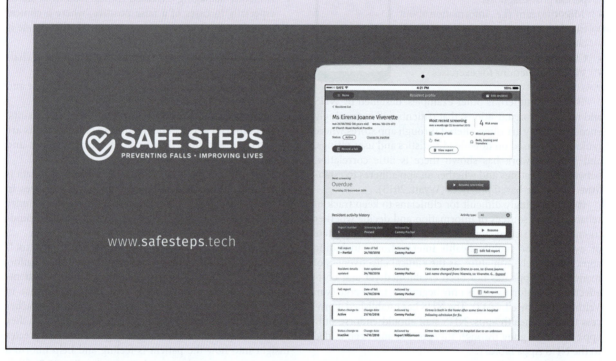

applications—presents challenges related to perceptions of risk, data transparency, privacy, ownership and agency. Recent high-profile cases such as the Facebook-Cambridge Analytica data scandal have raised awareness around data ownership and consent issues, negatively impacting the public's trust in digital and sharing data. In the United Kingdom, data from the Edelman (2019) Trust in Technology Study suggested a large majority of the informed public and general population do trust health technology businesses, but that trust is strongly related to the perceived benefit to the individual. A Doteveryone (2020) United Kingdom study on attitudes toward digital found 77% of respondents were concerned about their personal data being sold and nearly half felt they had no choice but to sign up to services despite concerns.

Many digital health approaches rely on the goodwill of individuals sharing their personal and sometimes sensitive data, and therefore establishing trust is vital to the uptake and subsequent delivery of the intended benefits (Nature Medicine, 2020). Establishing trust with digital health information and technology is complex, and a myriad of factors such as the recipient's perception of the authority of the publisher, quality of content, credibility and usefulness of the information contribute to trust judgements (Rowley et al., 2013).

The NHS has worked and continues to work to build public trust in its own data and digital services and those provided by industry. In recent years, approaches have included the application of open standards, attainment of cybersecurity accreditation for care providers and creation of procurement frameworks that vet products and suppliers to the highest standards to ensure the digital tools and technologies are safe, secure, transparent and fit for purpose for patients and staff (Department of Health and Social Care, 2018). In the context of nursing older people, it is important that clinicians are informed about any technology they endorse or prescribe (i.e., using only products that have been thoroughly vetted) and set out expectations with patients accordingly. It is vital that clinicians address the personal benefits and risks of specific innovations suggested for use in care settings and acknowledge and address concerns raised by patients and carers.

Assisting in the Delivery of Care
Robotics

Robots are not yet routinely used in the delivery of care. However, the potential of robotic devices is being explored in some countries.

Assistive care robots can provide essential support for individuals who need help carrying out everyday tasks and are starting to be used in countries like Japan, which has a super-ageing society and shortage of care workers.

Assistive robots carry out a range of everyday tasks such as helping people get in and out of bed and reminding people to take medication. There is also potential for assistive care robots to predict when patients might need to use the toilet, provide emotional support and assist nurses with routine tasks such as taking blood and monitoring temperature. This can free up nurses to focus on more complex tasks such as creating care and treatment plans.

Products like the Robear nursing robot, developed in partnership by the Riken research institute and manufacturing corporation Sumitomo Riko, are already assisting patients and nurses in Japan.

Robotic exoskeletons are wearable electromechanical devices intended to mimic, augment or enhance the body's own movements. Robotic exoskeletons can be used in rehabilitation to improve physical functioning (Fig. 35.1).

Therapeutic robots are starting to be used as companions for patients and residents of care and nursing homes and are being introduced into treatments for anxiety and depression. For example, PARO is a robotic baby harp seal covered in soft white fur and designed to elicit an emotional response from patients in hospitals and residents in care and nursing homes (Fig. 35.2). The intended effect is to calm the patient in a similar fashion to animal-assisted therapy. Researchers discovered that a robot companion

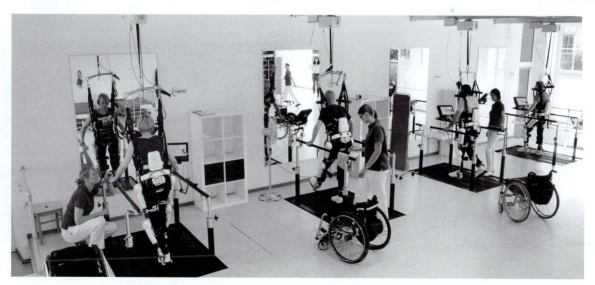

Fig. 35.1 Robotic exoskeletons used in rehabilitation to improve physical functioning.

such as the seal PARO offered benefits to older adults in a residential care facility in New Zealand that were similar to that of a living animal companion in terms of the effect on reducing loneliness (Robinson et al., 2013).

Similarly, early findings from the international Culture-Aware Robots and Environmental Senor Systems for Elderly Support (CARESSES) project found improved mental health and reduced loneliness in care home residents after they spent time with a friendly robot called Pepper (Booth, 2020). Pepper is a wheeled robot in a human form that moves independently and is designed to be culturally competent, meaning it learns about the interests and backgrounds of care home residents.

There is still a long way to go before robots are routinely used in care delivery. In addition to cost, one of the main barriers is mindset of the people working on the frontline of caregiving who are concerned that human care will be replaced by robots. A study by the United Kingdom recruitment specialist Randstad (2019) found more than 80% of people are opposed to using robots in care. However, there has been little research into attitudes of older people, and it is as yet unknown as to what extent older people would choose support from a robot rather than putting the burden on a family member or having care provided by a stranger.

Conclusion

In this chapter we discuss how technology and digital tools have the potential to transform how we manage, deliver and experience health and care services—for example, by

- Helping older people live independently for longer
- Improving the way patients interact with health and care services, providing them with a better experience
- Providing more joined-up care, as different parts of the system communicate better with each other
- Generating efficiencies in service delivery, giving health and care professionals more time to provide care
- Empowering patients by giving them the information they need to make decisions about the care and support they need

We also consider the potential risks of introducing technologies into our health and care system. To help mitigate these risks, some of the safeguards put in place must include

- Robust data governance so patient data is protected in line with the law, and patients are able to make informed decisions about how their information is used
- Designing health interventions that avoid creating health inequalities and ensuring the 'digitally excluded' are not overlooked.
- Appropriate assessment and evaluation of digital tools used by or endorsed by health and care professionals

Note: All the named products, digital tools and devices described in the chapter are examples of innovations being used to support older people. They are provided purely for educational purposes and not as promotion.

The authors would like to acknowledge the contribution of the Health Innovation Network and South London Academic Health Sciences Network in writing this chapter.

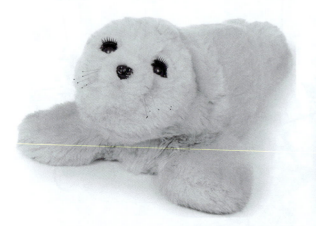
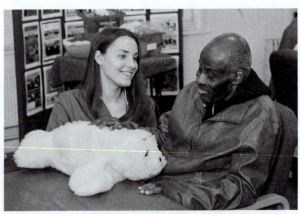

Fig. 35.2 PARO—the therapeutic robotic baby seal.

KEY LEARNING POINTS

- The increasing use of digital technologies puts new responsibilities on health and care professionals. It is important that care and nursing staff have the skills to set up and use these tools as well as be able to help their patients use digital platforms and services as required. Health and care professionals need to be able to explain the impact of digital tools to their patients and to make clear any balance of risks and benefits.

- With rising numbers of requests from patients seeking specific digital health tool recommendations, nursing professionals need to become familiar with validated tools within their specific clinical domains alongside more generic health apps such as those contained within the NHS app library.

- Nursing staff may also find it helpful to build knowledge around digital accessibility tools relevant for older people, such as magnifier applications for supporting patients with impaired vision, voice automation applications for motor difficulties and other technologies targeted at supporting people with cognitive impairments or deafness.

- Above all, health and care professionals must remember that digital tools and technologies offer value only if they support higher standards of patient and person-centered care, and decisions around how and when to use these tools must be taken with the person as the priority. While the specific platforms and devices being used will change rapidly in the coming years, the needs and desires of the person being cared for should always be front-of-mind when introducing or utilising digital technology for health and care purposes.

REFERENCES

Bakhai, K., Bell, M., Branford, R., Cilauro, F., Thick, M., Mansell, K., O'Sullivan, C., Woolley, N., & Riley, J. (2014). *Evaluation electronic palliative care coordination system-coordinate my care (CMC): A service evaluation.* [online]. https://www.coordinatemycare.co.uk/wp-content/uploads/2019/04/cmc-2014-darzi-fellow-service-evaluation.pdf.

Bartlett, M., Blazer, S., Hobson, G., & Abbs, I. (2018). The power of digital communications: Improving outpatient attendances in South London. *Future Healthcare Journal, 5*(1), 43.

Booth, R. (2020). *Robots to be used in UK care homes to help reduce loneliness.* [online]. *The Guardian.* https://www.theguardian.com/society/2020/sep/07/robots-used-uk-care-homes-help-reduce-loneliness.

Cooney, G., Dwan, K., & Mead, G. (2014). Exercise for depression. *JAMA, 311*(23), 2432–2433.

Department of Health and Social Care (2018). *The future of healthcare: Our vision for digital, data and technology in health and care.* https://www.gov.uk/government/publications/the-future-of-healthcare-our-vision-for-digital-data-and-technology-in-health-and-care/the-future-of-healthcare-our-vision-for-digital-data-and-technology-in-health-and-care.

Drdoctor.co.uk. (2020). *Improving outpatients attendances at Aintree University Hospital.* [online]. https://www.drdoctor.co.uk/customer-stories/improving-outpatients-attendances-at-aintree-university-hospital.

Edelman (2019). https://www.edelman.com/sites/g/files/aatuss191/files/2019-04/2019_Edelman_Trust_Barometer_Technology_Report.pdf.

Koivisto, J., & Malik, A. (2020). Gamification for older adults: A systematic literature review. *The Gerontologist, 61*(7), e360–e372.

McPhee, J. S., French, D. P., Jackson, D., Nazroo, J., Pendleton, N., & Degens, H. (2016). Physical activity in older age: Perspectives for healthy ageing and frailty. *Biogerontology, 17*(3), 567–580.

Nature Medicine. (2020). Build trust in digital health. *Nature Medicine, 26*(8), 1151.

Neri, S. G., Cardoso, J. R., Cruz, L., Lima, R. M., De Oliveira, R. J., Iversen, M. D., & Carregaro, R. L. (2017). Do virtual reality games improve mobility skills and balance measurements in community-dwelling older adults? Systematic review and meta-analysis. *Clinical Rehabilitation, 31*(10), 1292–1304.

Neves, A. L., Freise, L., Laranjo, L., Carter, A. W., Darzi, A., & Mayer, E. (2020). Impact of providing patients access to electronic health records on quality and safety of care: a systematic review and meta-analysis. *BMJ Quality & Safety, 29*(12), 1019–1032.

NHS England. (2020). *National Early Warning Score (NEWS).*: England.nhs.uk. [online]. https://www.england.nhs.uk/our-work/clinical-policy/sepsis/nationalearlywarningscore/.

PA Consulting. (2020). *"Alexa, Can You Support People With Care Needs?" Trialling Consumer Devices in Adult Social Care.* [online] http://www2.paconsulting.com/rs/526-HZE-833/images/Trialling%20Consumer%20Devices%20report%20-%20PA%20Consulting.pdf.

Public Health England. (2018). *Statistical commentary: End of life care profiles,February 2018update.* [online] https://www.gov.uk/government/publications/end-of-life-care-profiles-february-2018-update/statistical-commentary-end-of-life-care-profiles-february-2018-update.

Randstad. (2019). *Robots and carers, working together. | Randstad UK.* [online] www.randstad.co.uk. https://www.randstad.co.uk/about-us/industry-insight/robots-carers-working-together/.

Ray, A., Stevens, A., & Thirunavukarasu, A. (2020). Offline and left behind: How digital exclusion has impacted health during the Covid-19 pandemic - The BMJ. [online]. *The BMJ.* https://blogs.bmj.com/bmj/2020/07/03/offline-and-left-behind-how-digital-exclusion-has-impacted-health-during-the-covid-19-pandemic/.

Robinson, H., MacDonald, B., Kerse, N., & Broadbent, E. (2013). The psychosocial effects of a companion robot: A randomized controlled trial. *Journal of the American Medical Directors Association, 14*(9), 661–667.

Rowley, J., Johnson, F., & Sbaffi, L. (2013). *Insights into trust in digital health information* (pp. 4–6). Manchester, UK: CARPE. https://www.mmu.ac.uk/media/mmuacuk/content/documents/carpe/2013-conference/papers/future-of-health-care/Jennifer-Rowley-et-al.pdf.

van Velthoven, M., & Powell, J. (2017). Do health apps need endorsement? Challenges for giving advice about which health apps are safe and effective to use. *Digital Health, 3,* 2055207617701342.

Wyatt, J. (2015). *Avoiding 'apptimism' in digital healthcare.* [video] TEDxUniversity of Leeds. https://www.youtube.com/watch?v=HQxjDDeOELM.

Postscript: New Directions and Reflections on Caring for Older People

36

New Directions and Reflections on Caring for Older People

Fiona M. Ross, Ruth Harris, Joanne M. Fitzpatrick, Clare Abley

CHAPTER OUTLINE

In this chapter we return to and reflect on themes of the book that are not the subject of separate chapters because of their relevance to many. We draw on and integrate material from our contributors and the wider literature and listen to voices of older people. We highlight themes on images of ageing, valuing personal care and relationships, balancing rights and risks, rehabilitation and empowerment of older people, critical care, interprofessional issues and the contribution of nursing to improving quality in practice and education.

IMAGES OF AGEING

In this book we sought to convey a positive image of ageing by emphasising individual activity and social engagement as well as the nurse's role in contributing to maximising the potential for improvement and maintenance of function for people challenged by long-term conditions.

We write this chapter in the immediate aftermath of the death of Queen Elizabeth II, age 96, at Balmoral Castle in Scotland. She gave a long life of devoted public service and exemplified to us all a positive image of ageing well. Although the life of a monarch cannot be compared with individuals who have faced vicissitudes, poverty and stressful working lives, the image of her working to the very last (Fig. 36.1), despite visible frailty, is a powerful symbol. She was a role model to many.

This positive image of Queen Elizabeth II runs counter to stories common in many Western societies of an old

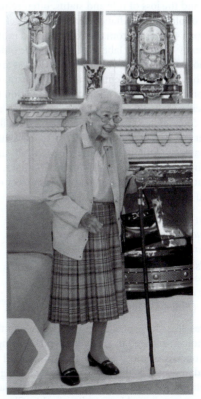

Fig. 36.1 Queen Elizabeth at the last public meeting of her long reign, 2 days before her death. (Photo by Jane Barlow—WPA Pool/Getty Images.)

person with failing faculties and diminished control of physical function.

> *An ageing man is but a paltry thing,*
> *A tattered coat upon a stick.*
> **(Yeats, 1973, pp. 82–83)**

In the context of negative images of ageing, some old people may resort to self mockery:

> *You know you're getting old when you stoop to tie your shoes and wonder what else you can do while you're down there.*
> **(George Burns, cited in Katz, 1988, p. 14)**

The factors that contribute to ageism are complex and are alluded to in a variety of contexts in this book. Christina Victor, in Chapter 2, discusses the various theoretical and empirical positions that influence our thinking, the questions we ask and the responses we make to older members of our families and people in our care. The biological model of ageing has been and continues to be pervasive and influential in policy and practice. It depicts ageing as a process of continual and inexorable decline with the onset of health changes and the loss of role and status, often reinforced by imagery of old, wrinkly hands. Even though definitions of old age span 40 years—from 60–100 years and more—there is a tendency to use lazy labels that stereotype older people as a homogeneous group with increasing illness and dependency. These ideas frequently underpin ageism, labelling, institutionalisation and an absence of innovation in care.

In their discussion of the biology of human ageing in Chapter 5, Brendan Garry and colleagues challenge the view that old age is often considered to be synonymous with disability. Although ageing impacts all the body's organs and systems, the authors emphasise that knowledge of the pathophysiological processes helps direct evidence-informed nursing care of older adults.

> *I'm an old woman now*
> *And nature is cruel,*
> *Tis her jest to make*
> *Old age look like a fool.*
> *The body it crumbles*
> *Grace and vigour depart.*
> **(Elder, 1977, p. 8)**

Figures 36.2–36.4 show older people making their own health choices, engaged in keeping fit and carrying on.

The concern of much sociological theoretical development and research is the social context of older people's lives, particularly housing, health, poverty and isolation. The social construction of old age is discussed in Chapter 2 and developed by Christina Victor through analysis of empirical findings from demographic and epidemiological studies in

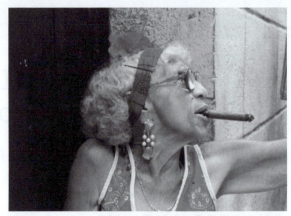

Fig. 36.2 In some cultures (this picture is taken in Havana) smoking is part of the identity.

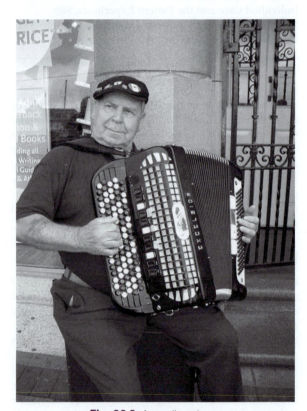

Fig. 36.3 Accordion player.

Chapter 3. The notion old age and dependence are social constructions, and society reinforces class, gender and income differentials in old age, is an important theme picked up throughout the book in relation to access to services, inequalities faced by individuals ageing in ethnic communities and underserved groups who are experiencing homelessness,

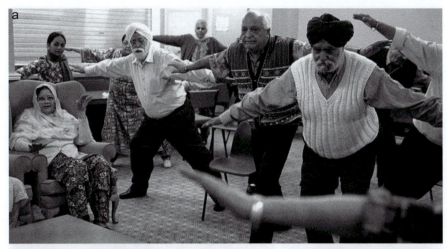

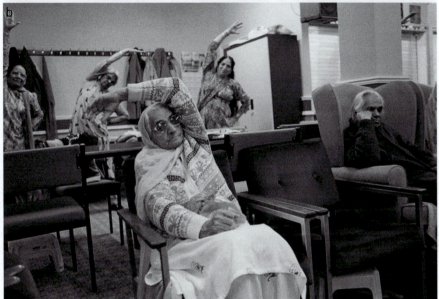

Fig. 36.4 (a, b) Keeping fit.

as discussed by Samantha Dorney-Smith and colleagues in Chapter 12. Maria Ponto, in Chapter 4, discusses the work on disengagement from the perspective of psychology and some of its unfortunate consequences for policy and practice that reinforce the biological model of ageing.

Countering ageism at system, professional and individual levels is vital to tackle concerns about poor, unresponsive, insensitive and discriminatory services. This issue is addressed in several chapters (e.g., Tommy Dickinson and colleagues, Chapter 26). The authors challenge ageist assumptions, such as that people become post-sexual or even asexual

as they reach advanced ages. Although the National Service Frameworks introduced in the first 10 years of this century have been rested, the challenges for health and social care and for nursing are clear in the way in which resources are allocated to services for older people, recruitment and retention of staff, the extent to which the age of service users influences clinical decision-making, and attitudes and behaviours expressed toward older people, which can be demeaning or, at the very least, thoughtless. This kind of thinking was exposed in the cynical and loose political language during the COVID-19 pandemic, such as 'bed blockers' and 'pile the

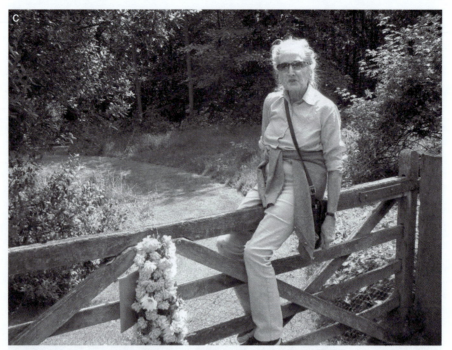

Fig. 36.4 (c) 90th birthday - keeping fit (cont'd).

bodies high'. This came when society and the health and care sectors were wrestling with unprecedented negative consequences for older people in terms of restrictions, social isolation and separation from loved ones and neighbours, especially at times of loss and grief.

The life history and biographical approach to ageing is introduced in Chapter 2, which has origins in both psychology and sociology. It takes account of how people see and value their own lives and the meaning of social events, thereby promoting self-esteem:

> I'll tell you who I am …
> I'm a small child of ten,
> with a father and mother
> brothers and sisters who
> love one another.
> **(Elder, 1977, p. 7)**

We hope this book, articulated by the different subject specialists, portrays the view that assumptions should not be made about older people as a homogeneous group with needs easily categorised into problems. We avoided age- and gender-biased language. We conveyed our views that older people have their own memories, experiences and outlook on the future and should be allowed choice. People now in their 80s and 90s have lived through immense social change, the aftermath of two world wars, massive technological innovation and now a digital revolution. The very old reared their children without the crutch of the welfare state, while the baby boomers, born after the Second World War, grew up with expectations the health service is there for them from cradle to grave. As this book emphasises, it is impossible to characterise people who have reached a century with the same label as those aged 60 who are socially engaged, in full-time work, and supporting growing and intergenerational families. For example, as an older mother, my youngest son was still at school when I reached pensionable age, and I was in a full-time and demanding job (Fiona Ross). Many older people don't feel old but are reminded of the fact when they look in the mirror. At Leonard Cohen's last concert in London, which he did in his eighties, he told his audience, 'Never look in a magnifying mirror of the kind you find in a hotel bathroom'. With a wealth of life experience, most people wish for a dignified older age characterised by stoicism, pride and forbearance that needs no condescending professional attitude. As Doris Lessing (1983, p. 174) said, 'They have already been felled several times, and picked themselves up, put themselves back together, each time with more and more difficulty, and their being on the pavement with their hands full of handbag, carrier bag, and walking stick is a miracle'.

No strangers to hard work, some old people have memories of leaving school on their 14th birthday to start work: 'In the cardboard factory, it was very tiring, standing all day from half past seven to six o'clock . . . I swore I would never let my children do the same'. As one of the authors' patients once said (Fiona Ross).

Some have memories of war:

When I had my son I went into the Nelson Hospital and that was tough when the bombing and doodle bugs started … one morning when I thought I've had enough of this, the sirens went and the nurse ran away. I'm in the ward with about twenty babies and I thought, well I can only save one and that is mine. I lay over the top of his cradle and held the other baby the nurse had left. When the bomb came down, there was flying glass, all in my hair, but at least we were safe.

Growing old while living in the home you know and love is something most of us want and is linked to ageing well, but it is not always possible (Fig. 36.6).

The book tries to take account of the indigenous population of White older adults who lived through major social change as well as groups of older people from Black and ethnic minorities who are diverse in terms of their reasons for settling in the United Kingdom, class, religion, culture and ethnicity. But we acknowledge there is always more to do here. Chronological age is determined by cultural systems, and in some communities, people are regarded as older adults from their mid-50s, which has implications for how individuals who were part of the Windrush generation and inward migration in the 1950s are treated. Figure 36.5 shows Emelda Antoine, 93, who lived in Grenada. Her children came to the United Kingdom as part of the Windrush generation.

The experience of ageing for Black and ethnic minorities is context-specific, with collective opportunities for enjoyment and prayer but also loneliness, as illustrated in the experience of a Hindu woman in her 80s:

Mrs A was brought up in a high-caste family in India and was active in the independence movement. She came to London in the swinging '60s and worked in a middle-ranking post in the civil service:

The men I realized do not want a woman as their equal … I became an alcoholic, because of the extreme loneliness of London, whereas in Delhi I was somebody, I had a group of friends and my own family, with a purpose in life … even though I got the job in the civil service, it meant nothing, because there was nobody to talk to, nobody to bother, suddenly this complete anonymity.

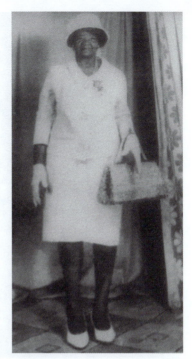

Fig. 36.5 Emelda Antoine. (Source: Annie Antoine and Fiona Ross.)

Ageism is not expressed only in social and professional attitudes but is often unfortunately an entrenched part of institutional policies and practice. The organisation of health services for older people and its development as a medical specialty are less well recognised and resourced than, for example, paediatric care. As Christina Victor discusses in Chapter 2, it was only in the 1950s that Marjorie Warren pioneered the work that made geriatrics a respectable specialty in medicine. Even so, in many medical schools, departments of ageing are small and often peripheral to the mainstream specialties. A career in the medicine of old age for a young graduate is perceived as a worthy but low-status choice. To some extent these attitudes prevail in nursing care of older people in that there are often difficulties in recruiting staff to work in care settings for older people, and the demand for post-registration training in gerontological nursing is always lower than for popular areas such as critical care. There are signs this is changing but perhaps too slowly, as described in the workforce section at the end of Chapter 7. Nursing development units and nurse-led units dedicated to the care of older people have sadly withered through lack of investment. But their legacy paved the way for nurse-led practice, expanding therapeutic benefits from relationship-based care and the development of more autonomous roles that maximise skills and leadership, such as the nurse consultant role (see

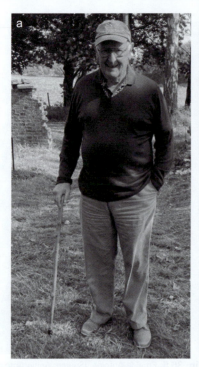
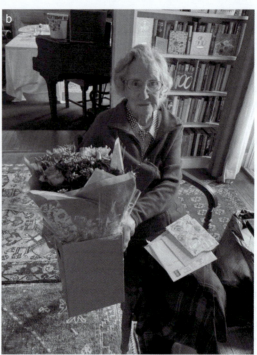

Fig. 36.6 a: Retired farmer, 96, living on the farm where he was born. (Source: Robert Tatam and Fiona Ross.) b: Centarian celebrating in her home. (Source: Desiree Roderick and Fiona Ross.)

Box 36.1). These issues are covered in various Chapters 6, 8, 9 and 10 and others.

Poor accessibility of services for older people is another example of the institutionalisation of ageism. Issues such as rationing, use of services and uptake are vital considerations in present social care policy for old people. The ageing population, with its increasing need for care, combined with reductions in length of stay in hospital and often inadequate community care provision available on discharge, has resulted in the pejorative but common term of 'bed blocker'. This term implies it is the individual who is responsible for being an obstacle and preventing others from receiving necessary care rather than the faulty system. Christina Victor, in Chapter 3, and later Fiona Ross, in Chapter 7, discuss issues of accessibility and use of services. The increasing shift toward a mixed economy of care, escalating costs of long-term care and political hesitancy in England to make social care free as it is in Scotland have serious implications for the choices and care alternatives available.

INDIVIDUAL CARE AND THE PATIENT EXPERIENCE

We hope the book conveys our beliefs about the importance of valuing individuals, their history and their concerns and needs within the caring relationship. Good communication is central, as Andrée Le May and Heather Elbourne describe in Chapter 15. Perhaps what is often overlooked is the emotional and challenging nature of nurses' work, who need to be supported by a cohesive team and positive organisational culture. There is increasing evidence from patients' surveys of perceived shortcomings in the delivery of essential nursing care, including nutritional support and basic personal care such as help with toileting. Case Study 36.1 is based on a true story that illustrates a failure in communication. Names have been changed to protect confidentiality.

What is striking about Janet's story is the apparent lack of effort to involve the patient on setting nursing-care goals. The tendency for society and professionals to display an alarming arrogance in asserting they know what is best for older people is illustrated, this time from literature:

Our campaign for Annie is everything that is humane and intelligent. There she is, a derelict old woman, without friends, some family somewhere but they find her condition a burden and a scandal and won't answer her pleas; her memory going, though not for the distant past, only for what she said five minutes ago; all the habits and supports of a lifetime fray-

BOX 36.1 A Consultant Nurse Role for Vulnerable Adults

One of the editors (Clare Abley) took up a post as nurse consultant for vulnerable older adults in 2000 (she is currently employed by the Newcastle upon Tyne Hospitals NHS Foundation Trust). This brand-new role provided an opportunity to combine expert practice with service and practice development, education and research, all focusing on the care of older people. The boundaries of the post were poorly defined at the start, including the patient group of vulnerable older adults. However, the experience provided the basis for a PhD (What is vulnerability in old age?) and the subsequent development of the post along the lines of a clinical academic with an honourary contract as a senior clinical lecturer at Newcastle University. The post focuses on dementia care and includes managing a small team of nurse specialists, leading the trust agenda for dementia care and undertaking post-doctoral research to improve hospital care for older patients with dementia (NIHR Clinical Lectureship 2014–2019). Twenty years later, and despite numerous organisational reconfigurations, the opportunity to lead developments and ultimately improve patient care for older people using all the key components of the role is sustained, providing an ongoing source of motivation and job satisfaction.

CASE STUDY 36.1 A Failure in Communication

Janet is 75 years old and married to a retired GP. She has ovarian carcinoma, for which she has had intensive treatment. Over a period of time she experienced increasingly frequent episodes of intermittent bowel obstruction, which, exacerbated by a fever and cellulitis, precipitated her admission to a local acute hospital unit. Her medical management was faultless, but the nursing care had serious shortcomings, some of which are summarised below:

- Although on admission a nutritional assessment was completed by the dietician, the recommendations were not implemented by the catering staff. Time went by before anyone did anything about it.
- The intravenous infusion was frequently interrupted, requiring recannulation, which on one occasion was delayed for 7 hours. A message was given but not followed up.
- She experienced constant disruption of her sleep due to late administration of intravenous medications. Task-centred drug rounds meant individual needs for sleep were overlooked.
- An attempt to test Janet's blood sugar was stopped as she had the foresight to ask the right question and establish they had the wrong patient. This error was averted by her alertness, but what else might have happened?

Janet's husband did not wish to complain formally, preferring to make a series of observations and concerns that were more difficult and painful to ignore. His view was that failure of communication was probably the root of all the problems, compounded by pressure of work and understaffing.

ing away around her, shifting as she sets a foot down where she expected firm ground to be . . . and she sitting in her chair suddenly surrounded by well wishing faces who know exactly how to put the world to rights.
(Lessing, 1983, p. 162)

Patronising attitudes conveyed by knowing how to put the world to rights are one thing, but even professionals who try their best to offer appropriate services and communicate sensitively in a humane and intelligent way may still miss the mark. It is frequently the case that 'off-the-shelf' services are not acceptable to an old person. When this happens, it is important other solutions are explored using approaches to assessment and care planning.

Situations where the balance between rights and risks are at their starkest are in the care of people living with dementia. Attempts to keep people living in the community for as long as possible mean many old people are deteriorating within their own homes. However, the family and neighbours are faced with an old lady going out in a nightgown to look for her dead daughter, forgetting to lock up, losing keys, forgetting to eat or leaving the gas on.

Introducing paid carers to support people living with the confusion of old age and dementia in their homes is not always the easy solution, because strangers and a series of different faces may further confuse or be the subject of suspicion. Innovative approaches to dementia care, discussed in Chapter 29 by Katie Davis and Rachel Price, must be disseminated widely to both lay and professional audiences. Frequently it is the community, neighbours and families who remonstrate for admission to care, because they can no longer cope with the anxiety and feeling of responsibility if something were to go wrong. On the other hand, for individuals who are looked after successfully, it is often the community network and families who make it work.

Older people are the best judge of their capabilities and limits. Why should it be any different than for the rest of us?

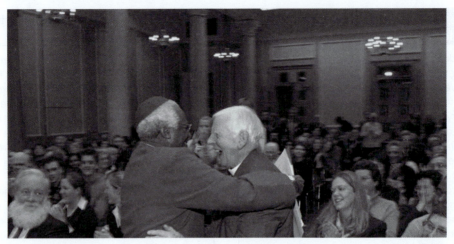

Fig. 36.7 Meeting of old friends—Archbishop Desmond Tutu and Reverend Professor Christopher Evans.

There are plenty of examples of older statespeople and figures from the world of the arts, both women and men, who in their 80s continue in public life with vigour and vision. We would not assume to give 'we know best' advice to Judi Dench, Joe Biden or Nelson Mandela, global icons for positive ageing (Fig. 36.7).

For the most part people know when and how to develop personal strategies to minimise risk and maintain as far as possible their normal activities. A 78-year-old woman, for example, who was travelling to Norfolk weekly to care for her dying brother, told us, 'There will be nobody to look after me. This doesn't worry me very much, because I want to look after myself, but I think that there is an insidious carefulness that has crept into my activities'. This woman was deciding to take fewer personal risks because of her knowledge of potential consequences.

REHABILITATION AND EMPOWERMENT OF OLDER PEOPLE

The concept of rehabilitation is a complex but continuous thread throughout this book. We take it to mean 'a set of interventions designed to optimise functioning and reduce disability in individuals with health conditions in interaction with their environment' (WHO, 2022). Some chapters are more explicit in their attention to rehabilitation than others—the chapters on safe mobility, eye health, hearing, nutrition, elimination, healthy skin, pain, depression and delirium, for example. In this section we bring together features of rehabilitation raised in earlier chapters to demonstrate its importance throughout the book. We identify aspects to which nurses could usefully give more attention, with the aim of enhancing feelings of empowerment and maximising people's independence.

Autonomy, choice and enabling people to create health on their own terms are important features of health promotion and are emphasised by Sarah Cowley and colleagues in Chapter 8. The principles of health promotion and public health they outline—enabling, mediating, advocacy, creating supportive environments, developing personal skills, valuing citizen participation—are fundamental to the provision of autonomy, choice and empowerment for older people and to their potential for rehabilitation. This means allowing people to make their own informed decisions. Family and social relationships are the core of well-being. Figures 36.8a and b show the importance of grandchildren and intergenerational relationships.

Maximising people's well-being and rehabilitation potential requires patience, listening, observation and skilled therapeutic nursing interventions. All are important to overcoming the many challenges to communication that occur for older people, particularly those with visual impairment, hearing loss, speech impairment, cognitive impairment and social isolation. Andrée le May, in Chapter 15, looks at these challenges and the process of therapeutic care skilled nurses provide. The aim of therapeutic nursing care is to define every person's potential for rehabilitation, maximising their independence. This applies to all potential and actual health deficits covered in this book and their consequences, be they pain, depression, immobility, breathing difficulties, malnutrition or incontinence. Separate chapters cover each of these areas. Promoting rehabilitation and self-determination and maximising independence are fundamental to nursing, whatever the focus. These principles apply equally to promotion and maintenance of health, care of people who are ill or have disabilities, and care of people who are dying.

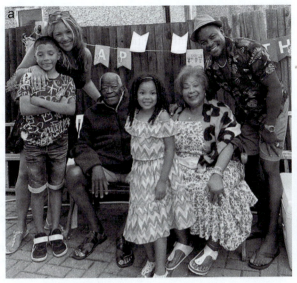

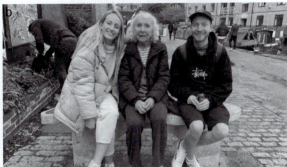

Fig. 36.8 a: Three generations celebrating together. (Source: Karlene Davis and Fiona Ross.) b: Grandmother in her late 90s enjoying the company of grandchildren. (Source: Kate Jackson and Fiona Ross.)

Empowerment is a concept we believe is important in every care setting for older people. Although this book does not deal specifically with critical care nursing, it is our view the principles of holistic nursing care apply equally to a seriously ill person. The challenges in critical care are different, the pace of decision-making is rapid, the emotions and anxiety of families and carers are raw and exposed, and the medical and nursing needs of older people are complex. Nurses who work in critical care need knowledge of the management of acutely ill people as well as an understanding of the different needs of the older person. Poet Michael Rosen's (2022) book *Many Different Kinds of Love* tells his COVID-19 story of 6 weeks in an induced coma in intensive care, slow recovery and return home (see Fig. 36.9):

I am learning to de-bed.
You have been good and kind to me
But I can't stay with you.
I will turn to mush
Bits of me will stop
I will fade
I will slip into your folds
And never wake up again.
I am de-bedding myself
(Rosen, 2021, p. 111)

Nurses who concentrate on prevention increase patients' independence. For example, nurses can play a part in the multidisciplinary team to detect depression, provide therapeutic support and prevent depression in older people—a problem that is easily missed and often goes unreported, as discussed by Colin Hughes in Chapter 30. Nurses see older people in a variety of settings and are in an unique position to improve quality of life. Assessment that takes a comprehensive, interprofessional approach and involves the patient and family detects problems that can be missed and expands the potential for rehabilitation and well-being. Focusing on delirium, in Chapter 28, Emma Vardy and colleagues discuss how nurses can play a central role in detection, treatment and prevention and in improving physical, psychological and social outcomes for older people.

Deafness, which is often linked to depression, causes feelings of powerlessness and rejection. Hearing loss is an invisible disability very different from blindness. The stigma is therefore far greater, especially when linked, as it often is, to the notion of senility and mental decay. Deaf people can be helped through rehabilitation, but they may refrain from seeking help because they fear being stigmatised or take the ageist view that to be deaf is part of being old and nothing can be done about it. Hearing aids have significantly improved and been more widely accepted in the past 10 years due to the introduction of digital technology. As we learn from Helen Pryce and Nisha Dhanda in Chapter 16, many environmental hearing aids are on the market now, such as alarm light systems and telephone, television and radio attachments that do not disturb other people. Public recreational halls are now often wired with a loop system for the benefit of people with hearing loss.

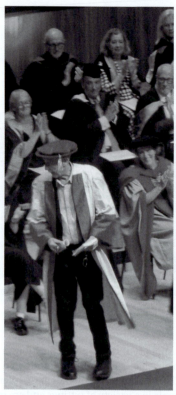

Fig. 36.9 Michael Rosen, 75, receiving an honorary fellowship at Westminster University in July 2022. (Source: Michael Rosen and Fiona Ross.)

Extending this requirement to locations frequented by older people, like hospital wards and nursing and residential care homes, would benefit many more people.

There is no doubt giving older people information about their treatments and medication increases the likelihood of adherence to a prescription even when faced with unpleasant side effects. People can cope with side effects if they know what they are and can balance them against the benefits of the treatment (see Chapter 31 by Sue Latter and Rebecca Henry). Encouraging self-medication for people who want to and can manage their own regimens reduces errors and increases concordance and the person's sense of control over the recovery process. Nurses have a major role in providing accurate information, giving evidence-based advice and promoting rehabilitation in this way.

Intermediate care schemes provide individual packages of care for people who want to stay at home even when their need for nursing care is substantial, as discussed by Caroline McGraw in Chapter 9. If more schemes were available, people could be offered a real choice, it would increase the potential for maintaining independence. On the other hand, some older people prefer to live in a residential or assisted living facility or nursing care home rather than struggling to cope with activities of daily living at home.

Residents of care homes may deteriorate and have diminished capacity for rehabilitation if they lose a sense of personal autonomy and control over their daily lives and are denied opportunities for self-help. Oversupportive environments in care homes exert too few demands on an older person and may encourage apathy, boredom and submissiveness. Care homes that offer residents genuine choice, freedom and privacy, and have a minimum of rules and regulations, are often rich in facilities and resources and have open access to the outside world. These environments promote rehabilitation, empower residents to take initiative themselves and maximise their independence. Care home managers who recognise the need for continuing education and training for their staff and invest in training provide a residential environment that optimises the balance between ensuring security and safety for residents and encouraging them to make choices, take control and be independent.

In Chapter 11 Richard Adams and Karen Spilsbury articulate the role of nursing to promote independence in long-term care settings. They discuss rehabilitation in the context of wider choice, which has implications for improved outcomes such as better resident morale, reduced morbidity of residents, better quality of life and the possibility of enabling some people to be discharged home. The hidden world of nursing and residential care homes was exposed during the COVID-19 pandemic, when the public and politicians became aware of staff shortages, lack of access to basic equipment and personal protective equipment and lower awareness of infection control policies that painfully put older vulnerable people at risk, as evidenced by the disproportionate mortality (Comas-Herrera et al., 2021).

Case Study 36.2 is intended to illustrate the support, advocacy and care found in nursing-home settings, even though increasing dependency unwittingly occurred.

Far-sighted health care professionals, who know their clients and their life histories well, encourage family carers, as well as the people they care for, to demand the kind of support they need—for information, training in skills and tasks, emotional support, social support, respite services and culturally sensitive services (see Chapter 13 by Nan Greenwood). If carers' demands for support are met, they are likely to want to continue caring, and the rewards of caring will increase. Raising the level of the service user's voice increases the rehabilitation potential of cared-for people and the range of choices open to carers. However, family carers can be forgiven if they feel they have little choice. Current policies on community care promote the notion it is better for social and health care agencies to

CASE STUDY 36.2   A Positive Experience

Peggy was admitted to a private nursing home about 15 miles from the small seaside village she had lived in for the last 30 years of her life. In her early 80s and without any close relatives, she had worked indefatigably as a volunteer for meals on wheels, nursed her mother and husband (both in their 90s) to the end of their lives and cared in numerous ways for friends and neighbours. She began to have difficulty living alone because of a rapidly failing memory. When admitted to a private nursing home, she deteriorated yet recognised friends with a sparkle in her eyes but without making connections they could understand. All her life she had given tremendous warmth to all around her, and it was remarkable to see her do this in an unfamiliar place when living at close quarters with strangers. The care staff did more than they should for her, feeding and helping her to the toilet when, given time and encouragement, she could do these things for herself. Essentially a gregarious person, she responded with smiles and giggles to the staff, and they loved her.

Over the last few months of her life she became increasingly frail and dependent. Although the general practitioner recommended admission to hospital, the matron of the home insisted Peggy could be cared for in the home. The nursing care was excellent with attention to detail, and there was someone with her when she died peacefully. For those looking on, the decision to admit her to a home seemed a compromise. However, the warmth and companionship she found, despite her mental confusion during her final frail months, was perhaps just what she needed and allowed her to continue to give in the only way she could—with her smiles, right to the end.

literature on the problems that exist with converting the policy rhetoric—that interprofessional work is a good thing—into reality. In the care of older people, there are some good models of multiprofessional care planning and discharge arrangements, but often these break down in practice when the system is under pressure. The reasons are speed of patient turnover, lack of organisational and professional commitment, inadequate resourcing or communication failure. In Chapter 10 on hospital care, Anthony Arthur emphasises the team-based nature of hospital care for older people, including the importance of multiprofessional discharge planning. A question that continues to arise from this debate is how far the patient or carer is involved in the decision-making with the professional team. A pervading theme in this book is, despite the professional rhetoric about empowerment and involving the patient and carer in the process of care, too often in reality this falls short.

As well as trying to ensure clients' and carers' needs are centre stage, more research is needed to establish how interprofessional teamwork can make a difference to the outcomes of care for older people and their families. In this book, various chapters cover interprofessional working for older people, for example Chapter 34 on end of life care. In Chapter 18 Julie Whitney discusses how rehabilitation works most effectively when it is person-centred, adheres to a biopsychosocial model and includes input from the multidisciplinary team. Bridget Penhale, in Chapter 14, discusses nurses and social workers working together to develop strategies to identify early signs of abuse and in system change represented by the development of integrated care, which brings together health, social care and local authority services, as described in Chapter 7.

SPECIALIST ROLES

There is much debate in the professional literature about specialist practice in nursing and nurse practitioner roles. A number of factors contribute to this debate, such as the changing boundaries between medicine and nursing that result from the reduction in working hours for junior doctors, the shift of services from acute to primary care, and professional aspirations. There has always been a central role for nursing and nurses in the care of older people. For reasons referred to earlier on the low status ascribed to the medical specialty of geriatrics, nursing has tended to play a reactive provider role rather than leading and innovating. There is tremendous scope both in acute hospital care and community settings for nurses to lead the way in giving patient- and family-centred care that does not lose sight of the people, their memories and the significance of their memories to their lives.

support people in their own homes, avoiding the negative effects of institutionalisation. This can mean very little choice for carers. They are expected to look after relatives at home whatever their preference. It also suggests care at home is never institutional. Yet the worst features of institutionalisation—unwanted routines, rules and regulations, depersonalisation, emotional distance from carers, segregation from the outside world and so on—can be just as much a feature of care at home.

INTERPROFESSIONAL WORKING

Care of older people frequently requires a collaborative approach between professionals. This should be at both interagency and interprofessional levels. There is growing

Examples of innovative roles in the United Kingdom include the consultant nurse and modern matron in addition to advanced clinical practitioners, as discussed in Chapters 8 and 9. It is not uncommon for community-based nurse practitioners, who may or may not have the job title of consultant nurse, to be nurse prescribers and to lead a multidisciplinary team with a specialist focus, for example frailty. Twenty years from the introduction of the first nurse consultant roles in the United Kingdom, posts have evolved and developed in response to service demands and sometimes according to the strengths of the postholder. An early but still relevant evaluation of the nurse consultant role demonstrated the impact consultant nurses had on making care more user-focused, developing new nurse-led services and improving current practice by developing procedures, processes and protocols in health care (Guest et al., 2004). In the first 2 to 3 years in their roles, consultant nurses demonstrated their impact more in terms of improving the processes of care than in showing a clearly defined effect on health outcomes for patients and clients. Case Study 36.3 provides an example of demonstrating impact. The extracts included are from a series of interviews conducted over time with a consultant nurse in care of older people (Guest et al., 2004). The case study conveys the job as demanding but exciting and extremely satisfying in the success with which the consultant was able to make a major impact on the quality of care. The researchers concluded the type of consultant role held by the individual was that of a designer-developer for services for older people (Guest et al., 2004).

Subsequent research focused on the leadership role of the consultant nurse for older people broke it down into the various processes involved—in other words, developing a vision for the service, acting as a mediator and champion and exerting control over complex change initiatives (McIntosh & Tolson, 2009). Consultant nurses were considered, and still are, ideally placed to provide leadership at strategic and clinical levels as well as influence operational development (Manley et al., 2008).

The need to demonstrate impact continues. In 2011 a systematic review found limited evidence that examined impact of the consultant nurse role (Kennedy et al., 2011). The same study led to the development of a framework to capture impact that comprised three domains: clinical significance, professional significance and organisational significance. This framework and the associated toolkit provides an excellent resource to measure impact. The toolkit can be used by consultant nurses or by managers to provide support for consultant nurses new in post (Gerrish et al., 2011).

CASE STUDY 36.3 Making an Impact as a Consultant Nurse

Service Development

On her first anniversary in the role, at the second interview, the consultant described herself as feeling good with respect to the service development activities she had initiated:

> It's starting to crystallize now, for me. Ummm. It still feels very positive … I really just hope that … you know it's one of these roles that gets the opportunity to grow and to blossom, and that people recognize that that does take time … .

At the third interview, she mentioned four service development projects she was working on. The first was an education project on incontinence of patients which was led by a community colleague and involved all medical staff (house officers, registrars and consultants) as well as herself and all nurses, with the result, she said, that 'we're getting consistent education right the way through, which is great'. She had been given responsibility for leading this project in the directorate together with the medical consultant. The project was designed initially to involve audit and education of all new medical staff although she was keen for other professionals to share the learning opportunity too, so as to promote multidisciplinary learning.

The second project was a re-evaluation of a nurse-led transient ischaemic attack service for which funds had been acquired from the trust. By the fourth interview, the consultant said the project had been set up and was progressing well. They had integrated medical and nursing documentation and sent out publicity material to the primary care trust and general practitioners with a view to starting data collection the following month.

The third project was a service development designed to ensure rapid access to health services for potential stroke patients. This would, the consultant told us, enable nursing practice to be more holistic, interdisciplinary and preventive. The trust had accepted the business plan and agreed to fund a 6-month pilot evaluation and audit facilitator. At the same time, the research group was bidding for a research grant to take the evaluation further jointly with medical and university colleagues; their bid had got through the first round. If successful, the university would provide research support in the trust, and nurses would be seconded to be involved in the research as data collectors.

CASE STUDY 36.3—cont'd

The fourth project was a multidisciplinary outreach team project due to start soon. The consultant, who was co-leader of the project with the consultant geriatrician and was coordinating it jointly with the superintendent physiotherapist, described the huge amount of work required to get the multidisciplinary team going. Following a successful bid for funds, they had to work very hard to set up the team of nurses, physiotherapists, geriatrician and primary care colleagues to meet the deadline for going live in a couple of weeks. Funds would cover appointment of an audit administrator to evaluate the outreach work using preset performance indicators. The consultant was looking forward to getting started:

> I think we've got a very forward-thinking team, they don't have a lot of problems with boundaries, they don't get very territorial.

At the fourth interview, the consultant described herself as having to troubleshoot in the outreach project, with a particular emphasis on advising how best multidisciplinary teams can learn to handle defensive staff in improving standards of care. Her approach was to encourage discussion of the difficulties among all staff, support the staff, engage in teamwork, act as a role model in providing good care and learn from each other. She was able to report a number of achievements: the clinical interprofessional pairs of staff were working well (e.g., nurses were paired for outreach work with physiotherapists, occupational therapists, speech and language therapists and social workers); they were well received and accepted by clients; they were overcoming challenges without difficulty; and improvement in patient care in the wards and in discharge arrangements was already apparent. The evaluation was continuing through audit and the consultant's doctorate work, both of which she said were going well. She hoped to demonstrate effectiveness of the project and get more funds from the trust for a further year.

By the fifth interview, the new outreach team had been set up, but the consultant was facing the problem of being unable to get adequate staffing cover:

> I think I told you—on the basis of ummm the senior nurses around the unit would be seconded on to the team, so of course that means that they still have their ward commitments as well … . And it's very, very difficult to get replacements for them when they're not able to do outreach work … . It needs to be somebody with expertise. So it's something we've struggled with a little bit over the last month … we've

been a bit of a victim of our own success, because it's been going very well … . Which is great, it's very positive … . At the same time it's quite frustrating because it's not about … it's not about money. It's actually about people with the right skills, the right expertise, and the authority to make decisions.

The problem was quickly resolved, however, when two part-time workers were employed to do outreach work.

Impact and Effectiveness

By the second interview, the project on implementing the multidisciplinary outreach team for older people was moving forward following the successful bid for funding. By the fifth interview, baseline data collection had been completed, and the consultant was pleased with progress:

> I've done all the baseline audits against [established performance indicator] standards, so in 3 months' time we'll be looking to see where we've been, who we've visited, what input we've been able to do. And I've been collecting sort of vignettes from each team, for sort of a newsletter to go out next week—we do a 3-monthly newsletter … . And to make people sort of aware that this is where we can help, this is the sort of thing that we've been able to do … . So that's been quite good.

Later on, the consultant reported success in acquiring funding from the trust to enable consolidation of the outreach work and to expand its influence:

> We were successful in bidding for another 2 years of funding for the outreach team [this came from the Department of Health's National Service Framework standard 4 implementation fund]—the team will now be full-time and focus on practice development as well as supporting inpatient management.

At the third interview, the consultant mentioned the progress achieved on a project evaluating nurse-led beds. The evaluation report had been particularly well received by the trust, which was to continue funding the project for another year. A positive outcome from the study was identified as a saving of some £134 000 by 24% of patients being discharged home rather than to a care home, as had been expected at the start. Also, the quality of care was better than before, she told us, with some patients destined for continuing care gaining sufficient improvement in their level of independence that an alternative discharge destination became a possibility:

Continued

CASE STUDY 36.3—cont'd

So we're all feeling sort of quite, you know that all of the work that we've been trying to do and push forward, is starting to come together now, with some support as well. So I think that's quite positive for people.

At the fifth interview, the consultant was jubilant about the progress made in developing the new transient ischemic attack service. The stroke unit had been trying for 4 years to get this new service going, and only now, since she had been in post, was it moving ahead:

Fantastic! Up and running. Started on the 2nd of June. Ummm. Got patients coming through. Everybody seems to be happy with that. We've had one or two minor glitches with radiography, trying to sort of book our CT scan sessions and things like that. So I've sort of again you know been wheeled in to try to iron those out, and am negotiating furiously. But things seem to be going all right at the moment. But the great thing is that the stroke unit actually feels as though it's achieving something that it's been trying to do for the last 4 years, and get this TIA service off the ground . . . they're getting the patients in through the doors and they're doing what they wanted to do—which is give people an easy-access, one-stop service.

After the final interview, she was delighted to be able to report continued good news: 'The TIA service is going really well, and the trust may well extend this next year.' It became clear that the consultant's work was being recognised as an important innovation by the trust when she was asked to advise on setting up more consultant posts in care of older people.

We have deliberately included detail from the evaluation here as it describes job content—the way nurse leaders in these roles shape and craft their contribution in an outcomes-focused way, enabling maximum impact for their service. This consultant's profile marks her as an achiever who thrives on challenge and has the skills to overcome problems, as occurred in turning a resistant ward sister into an enthusiastic and cooperative colleague. There are many more examples of achievements than problems in her story, and she was blessed with strong managerial and medical support. She seems to have developed a good balance between the different components of the job, including research and evaluation, which she integrated into service development initiatives and her professional doctorate. She seems to thrive on the continued opportunities for expanding the role rather than seeing them as an added burden to an already overstretched workload. Although she was active in clinical practice, this profile of the role suggests more of a designer-developer than a superspecialist. That is to say, rather than focusing the nurse consultant role on expert clinical practice working directly with patients, this consultant is more likely to act as a troubleshooter when complex clinical problems arise and leave the day-to-day clinical work in the hands of her nursing colleagues. Instead, her approach takes a broader, organisation-wide, more strategic focus that is facilitative and supervisory in working toward her main goal of developing and improving practice.

QUALITY IMPROVEMENT

Improving the quality of care is an underlying thread throughout the book. Assessment is the cornerstone of high-quality care and leads to successful care planning when all professionals—medical, nursing, therapy and social care practitioners—working collaboratively are involved in the assessment, planning and commissioning of care. The outcome of interprofessional collaborative work is duplication of effort is avoided and patients benefit.

Assessment of carers' needs is as important as those of patients, as discussed in Chapter 13. Where services are good, carers should participate in the assessment with special attention to the needs of ethnic-minority groups. The COVID-19 pandemic exposed stark inequalities in health provision and outcomes across minority ethnic groups, in part due to systemic problems in White ethnocentric services that fail to address cultural expectations and varying needs of different ethnic communities. This may mean a lack of advocacy services or translators to work with people whose first language is not English. Ensuring individual attention of this kind should be non-negotiable but may be challenging in today's climate of stretched resources, workforce shortages and demands for efficiency and cost-effectiveness.

There is also a need for development work with care homes to help them examine what they do and how their approach to care affects residents and direct care staff. This kind of scrutiny is important at all levels, from top leadership and management to direct care staff, and should include residents and their families and friends. Action research can ensure staff are involved in identifying their training and development needs and in taking decisions about making improvements. As discussed in Chapter 11, when nurses are valued and care workers are given recognition and respected for the job they do, their self-esteem rises, they value themselves as having status in health and care work, and the quality of care to residents improves. It is not good enough to do handclapping on a Thursday night, as we all did in the early phase of the COVID-19 pandemic. Pay and rewards that are both tangible and meaningful are paramount. One of the authors (Fiona Ross) managed a charity that ran end-of-life care in the community and a hospice. We were always strapped for cash as our services relied on charitable donations through fundraising, but as a board and senior managers, we were committed to rewards, which were sometimes monetary, sometimes celebratory with cake, but more importantly meant providing a menu of flexible working opportunities, progression pathways and always personal thank-yous from the chief executive.

More than ever, nurses have to demonstrate their worth. Older patients receive care in a wide range of surgical, medical and community settings and services, and all adult nurses need the diverse range of skills required to care for older people. Even where the need for skilled and qualified staff is acknowledged (Aiken et al., 2017), staff availability can be limited, most evident most recently in the United Kingdom in the wake of the pandemic.

Expert nursing is as important in the care of older people as it is for any age group and any condition. The definition of an expert nurse described by Benner et al. (1996, p. 145) holds true: someone who has '(1) clinical grasp and response-based practice; (2) embodied know-how; (3) [sees] the big picture; and (4) [sees] the unexpected'. The expert nurse intuitively understands a situation and its solution without having to rely on rules or guidelines and goes straight to the heart of the problem, uncluttered by having to consider other fruitless possibilities. Nurses with this level of expertise exist and work with older people and their families. They are specialists in their field. More research is needed not so much on whether nurses make a difference—it is known they do—but on what is different and how it is achieved. The knowledge gained and lessons learned would then be available for nurses and their colleagues to make improvements in areas of their practice they know to be weak.

Examples of bad practice such as exposed in the Francis (2013) public inquiry into the failures at Mid Staffordshire NHS Foundation Trust exist, but the media do not help with their sensationalist style of reporting cases of abuse. In contrast, examples of good practice are not often publicised. Nurses could do more to champion good care, using evidence not just in the nursing press but also in national and local newspapers, women's and men's magazines, social media and local radio and television. Safeguarding, codes of practice and regular auditing of hospitals and care

homes are important and are practised and welcomed by good centres. The National Audit of Dementia, commissioned by the Healthcare Quality Improvement Partnership on behalf of NHS England and the Welsh government, is a good example of a national programme aimed at driving up standards of care for older people (Royal College of Psychiatrists, 2019). Introduced in 2010, the audit has been undertaken every 3 to 4 years since and continues to have a high level of participation from general hospitals, although an audit has not been held since before the pandemic. Research is needed to identify the predictors of high quality and to use them as levers to promote good practice in all settings. It is much better to discover the correlates of high quality and apply them widely than to concentrate on rooting out the bad apples and going through the lengthy and often unsuccessful process of hospital closure, deregistering care homes and sacking staff.

Rotating students through long-stay settings can help raise standards of practice and is happening regularly. All settings need a budget for continuing education and training for staff; this is particularly important for staff of care homes given the increasing frailty and nursing needs of their residents.

A person who complains of unsatisfactory treatment or a member of staff who raises a concern should always be listened to and taken seriously even if it turns out to be different from what was first thought or that fears are unfounded. We are told the user's voice is being heard increasingly in this consumer age, but how much are individual needs really being met, given the relentless drive for efficiency and cost-effectiveness and the widening gap in health equality? The unglamorous areas of care are ones in which nurses can do much to improve practice—hearing loss, eye health, foot disorders, tissue viability, dentition, nutrition, elimination, sleep, dementia care and depression, for example. More research is needed into effectiveness of care of older people in these areas.

Nurses can do much to improve care by evaluating the effectiveness of different therapies, thereby enhancing patients' independence, comfort, dignity and well-being through rehabilitation and therapeutic programmes. The prevention and management of delirium is an area that requires considerable investment (i.e., nursing time and resources), as discussed in Chapter 28. The importance of informed, evidence-based and skilled care is emphasised throughout this book and notably in the clinical chapters, although there is always need for more and better evidence (Richards et al., 2018). Education at pre- and post-registration levels is also a key to good practice. Continuing education is crucial to ensuring the workforce maintains current and relevant knowledge and skills. The commissioning relationship between NHS trusts and education providers may mean priorities for purchasing education sideline courses on care of older people. Staff find it increasingly difficult to take time off when clinical areas are hard-pressed and understaffed. Recent initiatives in education are, however, taking account of the multiprofessional care team and offering work-based and interprofessional learning. There are increasing opportunities for students from different health professions to engage in joint clinical problem-solving and decision-making and together find solutions in the care of older people.

FUTURES

This book closes with a reflection on the United Kingdom health system. While nurses are a central part of care for older people, they cannot do their job without the individuals who 'change the bulb … and wheel the bin' or other members of the health care team (Rosen, 2022). No one expresses the importance of the whole health and social care system better than Michael Rosen. His poem is here printed in full with his permission.

> *These are the hands*
> *That touch us first*
> *Feel your head*
> *Find the pulse*
> *And make your bed.*
> *These are the hands*
> *That tap your back*
> *Test the skin*
> *Hold your arm*
> *Wheel the bin*
> *Change the bulb*
> *Fix the drip*
> *Pour the jug*
> *Replace your hip.*
> *These are the hands*
> *That fill the bath*
> *Mop the floor*
> *Flick the switch*
> *Soothe the sore*
> *Burn the swabs*
> *Give us a jab*
> *Throw out sharps*
> *Design the lab.*
> *And these are the hands*
> *That stop the leaks*
> *Empty the pan*
> *Wipe the pipes*
> *Carry the can*

> *Clamp the veins*
> *Make the cast*
> *Log the dose*
> *And touch us last.*
> **(Rosen, 2022)**

Rosen conveys the complexity of the health care system powerfully in this poem. We cover the breadth and depth of nursing practice in this book. We want to highlight the value of good communication and information-giving. Nurses need above all to respect, understand and address the needs of older people as diverse and individual. This is easier said than done, particularly in hard-pressed organisations with workforce shortages facing continuous demands to implement fast-moving policy and meet new service targets. For example, the challenge of providing high-quality care for people living with dementia in large, busy, acute hospitals cannot be underestimated. Even with the best intentions, person-centred care is difficult to deliver in these settings. Nurses need support and space to express their own feelings in order to be there with someone's distress and pain, or as Le May and Elbourne put it in Chapter 15, being alongside the 'ordeal'. We hope this book helps nurses work with others to gather and integrate the knowledge necessary to enable older people to be themselves and as Dylan Thomas says:

> *Do not go gentle into that good night,*
>
> *Old age should burn and rave at close of day; Rage, rage against the dying of the light.*
> **(Thomas, 1996, p. 63)**

REFERENCES

Aiken, L. H., Sloane, D., & Griffiths, P. (2017). Nursing skill mix in European hospitals: Cross-sectional study of the association with mortality, patient ratings, and quality of care. *BMJ Quality & Safety, 26*, 559–568.

Benner, P., Tanner, C. A., & Chesla, C. A. (1996). *Expertise in nursing practice: Caring, clinical judgment and ethics.* Springer.

Comas-Herrera, A., Zalakaín, J., Lemmon, E., Henderson, D., Litwin, C., Hsu, A., Schmidt, A. E., Arling, G., Kruse, F., & Fernández, J.-L. (2021). *Mortality associated with COVID-19 outbreaks in care homes: International evidence.* International Long-Term Care Policy Network. https://ltccovid.org/2020/04/12/mortality-associated-with-covid-19-outbreaks-in-care-homes-early-international-evidence.

Elder, G. (1977). *The alienated: Growing old today.* Writers' and Readers' Publishing Co-operative.

Francis, R. (2013). Report of the Mid Staffordshire NHS Foundation Trust Public Inquiry.

Gerrish, K., McDonnell, A., & Kennedy, F. (2011). *Capturing impact: A practical toolkit for nurse consultants.* Sheffield Hallam University.

Guest, D. E., Peccei, R., Rosenthal, P., Redfern, S., Wilson-Barnett, J., Dewe, P., Coster, S., Evans, A., & Sudbury, A. (2004). *An evaluation of the impact of nurse, midwife and health visitor consultants.* King's College London. http://www.nursingleadership.org.uk/publications/NurseConsReport.pdf.

Katz, E. (1988). *Old age comes at a bad time: Wit and wisdom for the young at heart.* Robson Books.

Kennedy, F., McDonnell, A., Gerrish, K., Howarth, A., Pollard, C., & Redman, J. (2011). Evaluation of the impact of nurse consultant roles in the UK: A mixed method systematic literature review. *Journal of Advanced Nursing, 68*(4), 721–742.

Lessing, D. (1983). *The diaries of Jane Somers.* Penguin.

Manley, K., Webster, J., Hale, N., & Minardi, H. (2008). Leadership role of consultant nurses working with older people: A co-operative inquiry. *Journal of Nursing Management, 16*(2), 147–158.

McIntosh, J., & Tolson, D. (2009). Leadership as part of the nurse consultant role: Banging the drum for patient care. *Journal of Clinical Nursing, 18*(2), 219–227.

Royal College of Psychiatrists. (2019). *National Audit of Dementia care in general hospitals 2018–2019: Round Four audit report.* Royal College of Psychiatrists.

Richards, D., Hilli, A., Pentecost, C., Goodwin, V., & Frost, J. (2018). Fundamentals of nursing care: A systematic review of the evidence on the effectiveness of nursing care interventions for nutrition, elimination, mobility and hygiene. *Journal of Clinical Nursing, 27*(11–12), 2179–2188.

Rosen, M. (2022). *Many different kinds of love.* Penguin Random House. Ebury Press.

Thomas, D. (1996). *Do not go gentle into that good night.* In *The nation's favourite poems.* BBC Books.

Yeats, W. B. (1973). Sailing to Byzantium. In P. Larkin (compiler) (Ed.), *Oxford book of twentieth century verse* (pp. 82–83). Oxford University Press.

World Health Organisation. (2022). Rehabilitation. https://www.who.int/health-topics/rehabilitation#tab=tab_1.

INDEX

Note: Page numbers followed by 'f' indicate figures, 't' indicate tables, and 'b' indicate boxes.

Infection transmission (Continued)
  physiological changes, 345
  portal of entry and exit, 340–341
Informal carers, 171–173
Information-processing model, 26
Integrated health and social care systems, 72–73, 75
Intellectual disability, 536
Intelligence, 26–27
Intentional non-adherence, 507
Intergenerational conflict, 10
Intergenerational relationships, 36f
Intermediate care, 116–117
International Classification of Functioning, Disability and Health (ICF), 252
International Classification of Sleep Disorders, 377
International Network for Prevention of Elder Abuse (INPEA), 190
International NPUAP-EPUAP Pressure Ulcer Classification System, 359t
Interpretative theories of ageing, 11
Intractable incontinence, management, 331–332
Ischaemic-reperfusion injury, 357
Ischaemic ulcers, 275

K

Korsakoff syndrome, 530

L

Learning disability, 536
Levinson's transitions in adult life, 31–32, 31t
Lewy body dementia, 460
Life expectancy, 8, 17, 64, 133, 135
  COVID-19 and, 8
Life review, 34
  stories, 90b
Listening, 224, 233f
Locus of control, 33–34
Loneliness, 93–94, 98, 103, 111, 226
Longevity, 93

M

Making every contact count (MECC), 54
Malnutrition, 43, 124
Maximum lifespan, 8
Medicine management, 5–6
Memory, 27–28
Mental Capacity Act, 464f
Mental capacity decisions, 164
Mental ill health, 18–19
Microcirculation, 356–357
Micturition, 324
  bladder dysfunction, 326
  incomplete voiding, 329
  lifestyle alteration and education, 326
  overactive bladder, 327

Micturition (Continued)
  stress urinary incontinence, 328
  urinary tract infection, 330
Mixed dementia, 460
Mobility, 444
  assessment, 256, 256f
  dementia, 255
  exercise and physical activity interventions, 264
  frailty, 255
  objective measurement, 257
  observing balance, 256
  observing gait, 257
  osteoarthritis, 255
  Parkinson's disease, 255
  rehabilitation, 263
  safe moving and handling regulations, 265
  self-management, 263
  stroke, 255
  walking aids, 265
Modernization theory, 9
Montreal cognitive assessment test (MOCA), 462
Morbidity, 17, 150
Mortality, 17, 150
  patterns in later life, 17
Multimorbidity, 18, 542
  implications for community nursing practice, 110
  prevalence of, 18
  risk of hospital admission, 110
Muscle fibres, types, 254
Muscle mass, 49–50
Musculoskeletal system, 49
  ageing effects, 252
Myocardial infarction, 446

N

National Assistance Act, 1948, 108, 113
National Health Service (NHS), 72, 108, 129, 134
  care payments, 76
  continuing health care, 77
  GP practices, 150
  long-term plan and integrated care, 72, 79–81, 138
National Homelessness Advisory Service, 161
National Service Frameworks, 587–588
Nausea, 563
Near-vision testing, 240
Negative life events and stresses, 35
Neglect, 189
Neuroischaemic ulcers, 276
Neuropathic ulcers, 275
NHS and Community Care Act, 1990, 115–116
Non-communicable diseases, 153

Norton scale, 362, 363t
Nutritional care, 5, 305
  ethical issues, 311
  evaluation, 311
  interventions, 308
  mouth care, 311
  nutritional assessment, 307, 368–369
  obesity management, 310
  oral nutritional supplements, 310
  planning care, 308
  risk screening and nutritional assessment, 306
  screening for malnutrition risk, 306
  third-sector interventions, 311

O

Observational learning, or modelling, 29
Ocular anatomy and physiology, 4–5
Onychauxis, 271
Onychogryphosis, 271
Onychomycosis, 271–272
Operant conditioning, 29–30
Opioids, 427
Organ sensitivity, 502
Orthostatic hypotension, 254
Osteoarthritis, 253, 255, 274, 420
Osteoporosis, 420, 541
Over-the-counter medication, 509

P

Pain, 384, 417, 420, 561
  acute, 418
  assessment, 422
  assessment scales, 425
  communication of, 418, 425
  experience of, 422
  intensity measures, 423
  management of, 443
  measurement of, 423
  musculoskeletal, 420
  physiology, 418
  sensory components of, 419
  syndromes, 420
Palliative care, 553–554
  end-of-life care, 554–555
Parasomnias, 385
Parkinson's disease, 47, 255, 409
  dementia, 461
Peripheral inflammation, 438
Personal health budgets, 109
Personal Independent Payment, 76
Personal protective equipment (PPE), 348
Person-centred care, 99, 100b, 138–139, 151, 402
Pharmacological solutions, 427
Place-based care, 72–73
Pneumonia, 540
Polypharmacy, 504